Handbook of EMERGENCY MEDICINE

EDITED BY

ANN HARWOOD-NUSS, M.D.
Professor
Division of Emergency Medicine
Department of Surgery
University of Florida
Health Science Center—Jacksonville
Jacksonville, Florida

ROBERT C. LUTEN, M.D.
Professor
Division of Emergency Medicine
Department of Surgery
University of Florida
Health Science Center—Jacksonville
Jacksonville, Florida

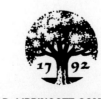

J. B. LIPPINCOTT COMPANY
PHILADELPHIA

Acquisitions Editor: Lisa McAllister
Developmental Editor: Paula Callaghan
Production Editor: Mary Kinsella
Manuscript Editor: Henry Bashwiner
Indexer: Barbara Littlewood
Cover Designer: Ilene Griff
Production Manager: Janet Greenwood
Production Service: Berliner, Inc.
Printer/Binder: R.R. Donnelley & Sons Company, Crawfordsville

Library of Congress Cataloging-in-Publication Data
Handbook of emergency medicine/edited by Ann Harwood-Nuss.

    p.   cm.
  Includes index.
  ISBN 0-397-51327-5
  1. Emergency medicine—handbooks, manuals, etc. I. Harwood-Nuss,
Ann.
  [DNLM: 1. Emergencies—handbooks. 2. Emergency Medicine—
handbooks. WB 39 H2358 1995]
  RC86.8.H353   1995
  616.02'5—dc20
  DNLM/DLC
  for Library of Congress   94-33278

3 5 6 4 2

The authors and publisher have exerted every effort to ensure that drug selection and dosage set forth in this text are in accord with current recommendations and practice at the time of publication. However, in view of ongoing research, changes in government regulations, and the constant flow of information relating to drug therapy and drug reactions, the reader is urged to check the package insert for each drug for any change in indications and dosage and for added warnings and precautions. This is particularly important when the recommended agent is a new or infrequently employed drug.

CONTRIBUTORS

Cynthia Aaron, M.D.
Stephanie B. Abbühl, M.D.
Khal Aboudan, M.D.
Thomas J. Abrunzo, M.D.
Mark C. Adams, M.D.
Stephen L. Adams, M.D.
Richard V. Aghababian, M.D.
Myrna E. Alexander, M.D.
Raymond H. Alexander, M.D.
E. Jackson Allison, Jr., M.D., M.P.H.
Jorge E. Alonso, M.D.
James T. Amsterdam, D.M.D., M.D.
Gail V. Anderson, Jr., M.D., M.B.A.
Charles Aprahamian, M.D.
Paul S. Auerbach, M.D.
Mark J. Ault, M.D.
William Banner, Jr., M.D., Ph.D.
Marvin Barnard, M.D.
Margaret Barron, M.D.
William J. Barson, M.D.
Edward J. Bayne, M.D.
Bonnie L. Beaver, M.D.
Julie L. Bellet, M.D.
Georges C. Benjamin, M.D.
Guy I. Benrubi, M.D.
Edward Bernstein, M.D.
Howard A. Bessen, M.D.
H. Stephen Beyer, M.D.
Philip B. Bhaskar, D.D.S.
Louis Binder, M.D.
Frank Birinyi, M.D.
Jorge Blanco
Mark Boehnert, M.D.
Michel A. Boileau, M.D.
G. Randall Bond, M.D.
J. Frank Bonfiglio, Ph.D.
G. Richard Braen, M.D.
Jeffrey Brent, M.D., Ph.D.
Michael Bresler, M.D.
Judith C. Brillman, M.D.
David C. Brittain, M.D.
Geoffrey Broocker, M.D.

Daniel Brookoff, M.D., Ph.D.
Jonathan Brooks, M.D.
Charles G. Brown, M.D.
Joseph A. Buckwalter, M.D.
Brent T. Burton, M.D.
Richard H. Cales, M.D.
William H. Campbell, M.D.
Donna A. Caniano, M.D.
Thomas R. Caraccio, Pharm.D.
Peggy Carlson, M.D.
Ross S. Carol, M.D.
C. Gene Cayten, M.D., M.P.H.
Donald R. Chabot, M.D.
Carey D. Chisholm, M.D.
Theodore Christopher, M.D.
Lowell Clark, M.D.
David M. Cline, M.D.
Joseph E. Clinton, M.D.
R. Kemp Crockett, M.D.
Marilyn K. Croghan, M.D.
Angel Cuadrado, M.D.
William Cuatico, M.D.
Steven C. Curry, M.D.
Rita Cydulka, M.D.
Philip S. Czekaj, M.D.
William Dalsey, M.D.
Daniel F. Danzl, M.D.
David Dansky, M.D.
Richard C. Dart, M.D.
K. Dauphinee
Steven J. Davidson, M.D., M.B.A.
Mohamud Daya, M.D.
Christopher J. Degnen, M.D.
Lucian K. DeNicola, M.D.
Heeten Desai, M.D.
Lynnette Doan–Wiggins, M.D.
J. Ward Donovan, M.D.
Craig E. Downs, M.S., D.O.
Steven C. Dronen, M.D.
Mitchell D. Drucker, M.D.
William R. Dubin, M.D.
Mary L. Dunne, M.D.

John J. Dymowski, M.D.
Philip A. Edelman, M.D.
Richard F. Edlich, M.D., Ph.D.
Joanne M. Edney, M.D.
Frank Ehrlich, M.D.
Teddi F. Eisen, M.D.
Michael Eliastam, M.E., M.D.
Fred Epstein, M.D.
Steven J. Eskin, M.D.
Roy G. Farrell, M.D.
Francis M. Fesmire, M.D.
Susan Fish, Pharm.D.
Arthur C. Fleischer, M.D.
Tim Flynn, M.D.
Alan T. Forstater, M.D.
Scott Freeman, M.D.
R. Scott French, M.D.
James C. Garlington, M.D., J.D.
Gregory G. Gaar, M.D.
Pierre Gaudreault, M.D.
Joel Geiderman, M.D.
Alan Gelb, M.D.
James E. George, M.D., J.D.
Richard D. Gerkin, Jr., M.D.
W. Brian Gibler, M.D.
Jonathan M. Glauser, M.D.
Jay M. Goldman, M.D.
Federico Gonzalez, M.D.
Marc J. Gorayeb, M.D.
Alana L. Grajewski, M.D.
Michael Greenberg, M.D.
Constance S. Greene, M.D.
Peter L. Gross, M.D.
Joanne Guay, M.D.
William Graham Guerriero, M.D.
Joseph L. Gugliotta, M.D.
Raymond Gyarmathy, M.D.
Alan H. Hall, M.D.
Matthew Hall, D.D.S., M.D.
C. William Hanson, M.D.
Cherie A. Hargis, M.D.
James L. Harper, M.D.
Ann Harwood–Nuss, M.D.
Elizabeth A. Hatfield, M.D.
Malcolm K. Hatfield, M.D.
Mark Hauswald, M.D.
Clifton A. Hawkes, M.D.
Christine E. Haycock, M.D.
Douglas J. Hayes, PA-C
Andrew J. W. Heath, M.D., Ph.D.
Mary A. Hegenbarth, M.D.

Irvin N. Heifetz, M.D.
Erica Heit, M.D.
Michael B. Heller, M.D.
Barry H. Hendler, D.D.S., M.D.
Fred M. Henretig, M.D.
Gregory L. Henry, M.D.
Charles A. Hergrueter, M.D.
James Hillman, M.D.
Robert S. Hockberger, M.D.
Dee Hodge, III, M.D.
Gwendolyn L. Hoffman, M.D.
Jerome R. Hoffman, M.D.
Robert P. Hoffman, M.D.
Lisa Horton, M.D.
John M. Howell, M.D.
David S. Howes, M.D.
Kathleen C. Hubbell, M.D.
Catherine Hudkins, M.D.
Michael Hunt, M.D.
Penny J. Hutchinson, M.D.
H. Range Hutson, M.D.
Ahamed Idris, M.D.
Richard Iseke, M.D.
Kenneth V. Iserson, M.D., M.B.A.
R. Scott Israel, M.D.
J. Edward Jackson, M.D.
Dag Jacobsen, M.D., Ph.D.
Sheldon Jacobson, M.D.
J. A. James, M.D.
Stanley Janasiewicz, M.D.
Michael S. Jastremski, M.D.
James Jenkins, D.O.
Robert Jorden, M.D.
Steven M. Joyce, M.D.
Andrew M. Kaunitz, M.D.
Thomas E. Kearney, Pharm.D.
Gabor Kelen, M.D.
J. William Kelly, M.D.
Kenneth W. Kizer, M.D., M.P.H.
Paul Klainer, M.D.
Bruce L. Klein, M.D.
Jane Knapp, M.D.
Katalin Koranyi, M.D.
David Kramer, M.D.
Edward P. Krenzelok, Pharm.D.
Ronald L. Krome, M.D.
Kenneth W. Kulig, M.D.
Donald B. Kunkel, M.D.
Peter G. Lacouture, Ph.D.
Michael D. Laufer, M.D.
Ann K. Leahy, M.D.

M. Andrew Levitt, D.O.

William J. Lewander

Neal A. Lewin, M.D.

Sergio Li, M.D.

Robert Linblad, M.D.

Christopher H. Linden, M.D.

Louis J. Ling, M.D.

James E. Lingeman, M.D.

M. Scott Linscott, Jr., M.D.

Toby L. Litovitz, M.D.

Neal Little, M.D.

Vivien Lloyd, R.N.

Ronald B. Low, M.D.

Robert A. Lowe, M.D.

Wayne Lucke, M.D.

Robert C. Luten, M.D.

Ronald B. Mack, M.D.

H. Trent MacKay, M.D., M.P.H.

Jon T. Mader, M.D.

Brian Franklyn Mandell, Ph.D., M.D.

Anthony S. Manoguerra, Pharm.D.

Steven M. Marcus, M.D.

Curtis E. Margo, M.D.

Vincent J. Markovchick, M.D.

Jose S. Martinez, M.D.

John A. Marx, M.D.

James Mathews, M.D.

James W. May Jr., M.D.

Suman Mayer, M.D.

Thom A. Mayer, M.D.

Kenneth McAllister, M.D.

Charles J. McCabe, M.D.

John B. McCabe, M.D.

Margaret M. McCarron, M.D.

Mark McCormick, M.D.

Mary A. McCormick, Pharm.D.

James H. McCrory, M.D.

Alison J. McDonald, M.D.

Newell E. McElwee, Pharm.D.

Mara McErlean, M.D.

Ted A. McMurry, M.D.

W. Kendall McNabney, M.D.

Robert M. McNamara, M.D.

Hubert S. Mickel, M.D.

Gary Miller, M.D.

Myron L. Mills, M.D.

Joyce M. Mitchell, M.D.

Howard C. Mofenson, M.D.

Ernest E. Moore, M.D.

Joseph Mueller, M.D.

Michael F. Murphy, M.D.

Daniel A. Muse, M.D.

Vinay M. Nadkarni, M.D.

Paul M. Nemiroff, PhD., M.D.

Kenneth Neuburger, M.D.

Constance G. Nichols, M.D.

James T. Niemann, M.D.

Eric Noji, M.D. M.P.H.

Robert C. Nuss, M.D.

Daniel J. O'Brien, M.D.

Michael L. Olinger, M.D.

Kent R. Olson, M.D.

David J. Orban, M.D.

Gary J. Ordog, M.D.

Joseph P. Ornato, M.D.

David T. Overton, M.D.

Gilbert Wolf Palley, D.O.

Paul Paris, M.D.

Richard K. Parrish, II, M.D.

Peter C. D. Pelikan, M.D.

Paul R. Pentel, M.D.

Paul E. Pepe, M.D.

Norman E. Peterson, M.D.

Yancy Y. Phillips, M.D.

Paul A. Pitel, M.D.

Stephen J. Playe, M.D.

George Podgorny, M.D.

Peter T. Pons, M.D.

D. W. Pope, M.D.

Franklin D. Pratt, M.D.

Madelyn Quattrone

Eugene Ragland, M.D.

Edward A. Ramoska, M.D.

Joel J. Reich, M.D.

Kevin M. Reilly, M.D.

Francis P. Renzi, M.D.

Troy M. Reyna, M.D.

Betty S. Riggs, M.D.

Gary R. Ripple, M.D.

Emanuel P. Rivers, M.D., M.P.H.

Raymond J. Roberge, M.D.

James R. Roberts, M.D.

Rebecca R. Roberts, M.D.

William A. Robinson, M.D.

George T. Rodeheaver, Ph.D.

Christopher C. Rose, M.D.

S. Rutherford Rose, II, Pharm.D.

Peter Rosen, M.D.

Robert E. Rosenthal, M.D.

David S. Ross, M.D.

John P. Rudzinski, M.D.

Barry H. Rumack, M.D.

Douglas A. Rund, M.D.
Marian C. Rutigliano, D.O.
Alfred Sacchetti, M.D.
Jorge A. Sallent, M.D.
Leonard Samuels, M.D.
Ricardo L. Sanchez, M.D.
Arthur B. Sanders, M.D.
Aysel K. Sanderson, M.D.
Diane Sauter, M.D.
Kusum Saxena, M.D.
Robert W. Schafermeyer, M.D.
Julie M. Schatz, Pharm.D.
Jay L. Schauben, Pharm.D.
Daniel T. Schelble, M.D.
David Schillinger, M.D.
Eric W. Schmidt, M.D.
David C. Seaberg, M.D.
Donna L. Seger, M.D.
Linda L. Settle, M.D.
Harry W. Severance, Jr., M.D.
Michael W. Shannon, M.D., M.P.H.
Robert Shesser, M.D., M.P.H.
Gerald A. Shiener, M.D.
Joseph Simon, M.D.
Jonathan I. Singer, M.D.
David C. Slagle, M.D.
Robert D. Slay, M.D.
Corey M. Slovis, M.D.
Martin J. Smilkstein, M.D.
Mark Smith, M.D.
R. Gregory Smith, D.D.S., M.D.
Peter L. Sosnow, M.D.
Gary G. Soud, M.D.
William H. Spivey, M.D.
David G. Spoerke, R., Ph.
James Sprague, M.D.
Cheryl L. Standing, M.D.
J. Stephan Stapczynski, M.D.
Christopher P. Steidle, M.D.
George Sternbach, M.D.
Charles Stewart, M.D.
Robert W. Strauss, M.D.
John B. Sullivan, Jr., M.D.
Ahimsa Porter Sumchai, M.D.
Douglas Swartz, M.D.
Ellen H. Taliferro, M.D.
Milton Tennenbein, M.D.
Thomas E. Terndrup, M.D.
John G. Thacker, Ph.D.
Harold Thomas, M.D.
Jessica L. Thomason, M.D.

Mark W. Todd, Pharm.D.
Theodore Tong, Pharm.D.
James Q. Touchy, M.D.
Paula L. Townsend, Pharm.D.
John F. Tucker, M.D.
Thomas W. Turbiak, M.D.
Timothy L. Turnbull, M.D.
Dennis T. Uehara, M.D.
Robert C. Urbanic, M.D.
Terence D. Valenzuela, M.D.
Phyllis A. Vallee, M.D.
Linda Van Le, M.D.
Michael V. Vance, M.D.
Brant L. Viner, M.D.
Gregory A. Volturo, M.D.
Scott R. Votey, M.D.
Barbara Insley Vuignier, Pharm.D.
David J. Vukich, M.D.
Alonzo Walker, M.D.
Ron M. Walls, M.D.
Frank G. Walter, M.D.
James J. Walter, M.D.
Robert L. Walton, M.D.
Jonathan Wasserberger, M.D.
Gary S. Wasserman, D.O.
W. Fred Watkins, M.D.
William A. Watson, Pharm.D.
Robert L. Wears, M.D.
Elizabeth A. Wedemeyer, M.D.
Larry D. Weiss, M.D.
Howard A. Werman, M.D.
Gerald P. Whelan, M.D.
Thomas A. Whitehill, M.D.
J. M. Whitworth, M.D.
David E. Wilcox, M.D.
Donald C. Willis, M.D.
Barry W. Wolcott, M.D.
R. Wayne Wolfram, M.D.
Allan B. Wolfson, M.D.
Joseph M. Woods, IV, M.D.
Alan D. Woolf, M.D., M.P.H.
John A. Worrell, M.D.
Martha S. Wright, M.D.
Collette Ditz Wyte, M.D.
Donald M. Yealy, M.D.
Gary Young, M.D.
Terry W. Zehr, M.D.
David N. Zull, M.D.
L. S. Zun, M.D.
Mark L. Zwanger, M.D.

PREFACE

The *Clinical Practice of Emergency Medicine* was developed with the intent that it serve as a comprehensive text focused on the diagnosis and management of medical emergencies. The text was written by academic and practicing emergency physicians—those most capable of directing discussion toward the undifferentiated, emergency patient. A new format was utilized to provide rapid access to information considered critical to the care of patients: basic disease, differential diagnosis, role of the consultant, patient disposition, indications for admission, guidelines for transfer, and perhaps the most popular section, the clinical pitfalls. We are gratified that the first edition has been enthusiastically embraced by both practicing emergency physicians and residency training programs.

We have designed the *Handbook of Emergency Medicine* to serve as a succinct guide for common emergencies. The handbook is not intended to replace the full-scale textbook; rather, it should serve as an extension of *The Clinical Practice of Emergency Medicine*. Each chapter in the handbook is derived from the corresponding chapter in the first edition of *The Clinical Practice of Emergency Medicine*. We have included sections on medical emergencies, surgical emergencies, environmental emergencies, pediatric emergencies, and trauma. In the interests of text size, we made certain editorial adjustments in content. For example, "Selected Toxicologic Emergencies" consists of the most commonly reported poisonings. Of course, the excellent and comprehensive toxicology section in the first edition supplements the handbook. The pediatric section of the handbook has also been limited, in the interest of text size, to true childhood emergencies and selected topics. We also excluded chapters on entities that were uncommon and better served in the full-size textbook. We retained the essential elements of design and organization that have made *The Clinical Practice of Emergency Medicine* so useful for clinicians. We have made extensive use of tables to facilitate the prioritization and understanding of importance clinical points. The 1992 Advanced Cardiac Life Support algorithms were reproduced to update the specific resuscitation sections. Finally, a new index was created that we believe will be more "user friendly."

We would like to thank the editors and contributors to the first edition of *The Clinical Practice of Emergency Medicine*. Although the handbook is the product of two editors, its chapters were developed from the expertise contained in the work of the original contributors. This work has been reorganized and rewritten in a style necessary for the handbook. We would like to thank our secretary, Ms. Dorothy Burgess, for her capable assistance. As always, a special word of thanks must go to Lisa McAllister, Senior Editor at J. B. Lippincott, who weathered the first edition and its companion handbook with great skill, persistence, humor, and equanimity.

Ann Harwood-Nuss, M.D.
Robert C. Luten, M.D.

CONTENTS

Section I—Surgical Emergencies

Section II—Trauma

Section III—Toxicologic Emergencies

Section IV—Environmental Emergencies

Section V—Medical Emergencies

Part I   Resuscitation

Part II   Cardiovascular Emergencies

Part III   Pulmonary Emergencies

Section VI—Pediatrics

Part IV   Pediatric Trauma

SECTION I

SURGICAL EMERGENCIES

Emergency Aspects of Ophthalmology

1 Acute Angle-Closure Glaucoma

Glaucoma is a group of disorders characterized by an elevated intraocular pressure to a degree sufficient to result in loss of vision. The clinical presentations and underlying pathologic mechanisms within this group of disorders are diverse. The two common classifications of primary glaucoma, open-angle glaucoma and angle-closure glaucoma, occur in approximately 1 out of 50 Americans over the age of 35, and represent, overall, the second leading cause of blindness in the United States.

There are three clinical types of primary angle-closure glaucoma. The chronic form is often subtle and difficult to diagnosis, with a gradual visual loss over a prolonged period. The subacute, or intermittent, form is characterized by periodic episodes of mild pain, blurred vision, and halos. In contrast, manifestations of the acute form of angle-closure glaucoma are dramatic, with the sudden onset of unilateral ocular pain and decreased visual acuity. Without appropriate therapy, acute angle-closure glaucoma is devastating and can result in blindness within a few days.

CLINICAL PRESENTATION

In acute angle-closure glaucoma, outflow of aqueous is suddenly and completely halted. This cessation is associated with a marked elevation of intraocular pressure, which can occur within 30 to 60 minutes. This acute pressure rise with distention of the ocular coats causes a sudden onset of severe pain that may be either localized to the eye, orbit, or brow, or generalized, as a severe headache. Vagal stimulation with the onset of sudden, severe pain often results in nausea and vomiting. On occasion the gastrointestinal distress dominates the presenting clinical picture, leading to an erroneous diagnosis of a gastrointestinal illness or an acute surgical abdomen. Blurring vision or the onset of rainbow-colored halos may occur simultaneously or shortly after the onset of pain (Table 1-1).

The patient with acute angle-closure glaucoma has a unilateral red eye with congested episcleral and conjunctival blood vessels, nonreactive mid-dilated pupil, corneal edema, shallow anterior chamber, and high intraocular pressure. The intraocular pressure is usually high, 60 mm Hg to 90 mm Hg (<21 mm Hg is normal). However, if the attack has been prolonged, the intraocular pressure may be low. The anterior chamber appearance is shallow. The cornea is usually hazy or steamy-appearing with epithelial edema. The untreated course of acute angle-closure glaucoma is varied. An attack damages the corneal endothelium, the lens, the retinal ganglion cell layer, and the optic nerve. The amount of damage is more dependent on the duration of an attack

---

TABLE 1-1. Diagnosis of Acute Angle-Closure Glaucoma

History
Acute onset of pain
Exposure to dim illumination (*i.e.*, movie theater)
Emotional upset or fatigue
Precipitating medications (anticholinergics, sympathomimetics)

Symptoms
Pain
Blurred vision/halos around lights
Loss of vision
Nausea
Vomiting

Signs
Conjunctival injection
Corneal edema (light reflex irregular or steamy appearance)
Mid-dilated, nonreactive pupil
Evidence of a narrow angle (fellow eye should also appear narrow)
Anterior chamber cells—no keratic precipitates

---

than on the degree of pressure elevation. Optic nerve damage is often generalized. In some patients the attack will continue and, if untreated, will result in pain and permanent blindness within 2 to 3 days. Visual prognosis improves with the initiation of prompt, effective treatment.

DIFFERENTIAL DIAGNOSIS

The differential diagnosis is shown in Table 1-2 and Figure 1-1. Causes not related to the corneal surface include acute iritis or anterior uveitis, acute angle-closure glaucoma, episcleritis, scleritis, orbital cellulitis, periorbital cellulitis, and septic cavernous sinus thrombosis.

EMERGENCY DEPARTMENT EVALUATION
HISTORY

Question the patient about the following factors:

Onset of symptoms (sudden, gradual, subsequent to accidental or surgical trauma)
Previous symptoms similar to those of the current complaint (brief episodes of pain, blurred vision, and halos around lights)
Visual acuity in the affected eye as well as in the fellow eye
Pain in or about the eye
Discharge or secretions from the eye (tearing is common with ocular pain; however, a purulent discharge may indicate an infectious cause)
Medical history of asthma or congestive heart failure and history of drug allergies (particularly sulfa drugs)

PHYSICAL EXAMINATION

VISUAL ACUITY
Visual acuity is one of the most important aspects of the ocular examination. If a distance or near visual acuity cannot be recorded due to inability to read the chart, the following should be recorded, including the distance at which each is tested: finger counting (FC), hand motions (HM), light perception (LP), or no light perception (NLP). Severe lacrimation or blepharospasm may pre-

TABLE 1-2. Differential Diagnosis

	Conjunctivitis	Keratitis	Iritis	Acute Angle-closure
Vision	Normal	Normal/blurred	Normal/blurred	Marked decrease in vision
Pain	None or minor; "irritated"	Moderate to severe; "sharp, irritated"	Moderate to severe; "ache, worse in light"	Severe/associated with nausea and vomiting
Discharge	Tearing	Tearing / Purulent if infected	None	None to tearing
Conjunctiva	Diffuse injection	Perilimbal to diffuse injection	Diffuse injection	Prominent perilimbal vessel dilation associated with diffuse injection
Pupil	Size: Normal / Reaction to light: Normal	Normal	Constricted	Mid-dilated
	Normal	Minimal reaction	Minimal or no reaction
Cornea	Clear or fine punctate erosions; slight haze	Minimal to moderate punctate erosions; hazy to opacification	Minimal to severe; hazy to steamy	Minimal to severe hazy to steamy
Intraocular Pressure	Normal	Normal	Low to elevated	Elevated / If prolonged attack, may be low
Anterior Chamber	Normal depth / No cells	Normal depth / Minimal cells	Normal depth (can be shallow) / Moderate to severe cell/KP present	Shallow (both eyes are shallow) / Minimal to moderate cell / No KP present

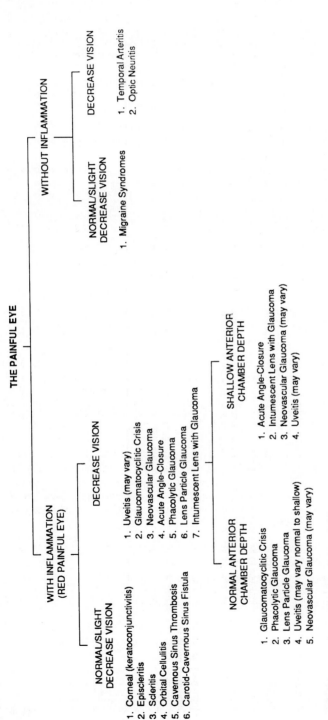

Fig. 1-1. Differential diagnosis of the painful eye.

THE PAINFUL EYE

WITH INFLAMMATION (RED PAINFUL EYE)

WITHOUT INFLAMMATION

NORMAL/SLIGHT DECREASE VISION
1. Corneal (keratoconjunctivitis)
2. Episcleritis
3. Scleritis
4. Orbital Cellulitis
5. Cavernous Sinus Thrombosis
6. Carotid-Cavernous Sinus Fistula

DECREASE VISION
1. Uveitis (may vary)
2. Glaucomatocyclitic Crisis
3. Neovascular Glaucoma
4. Acute Angle-Closure
5. Phacolytic Glaucoma
6. Lens Particle Glaucoma
7. Intumescent Lens with Glaucoma

NORMAL ANTERIOR CHAMBER DEPTH
1. Glaucomatocyclitic Crisis
2. Phacolytic Glaucoma
3. Lens Particle Glaucoma
4. Uveitis (may vary normal to shallow)
5. Neovascular Glaucoma (may vary)

SHALLOW ANTERIOR CHAMBER DEPTH
1. Acute Angle-Closure
2. Intumescent Lens with Glaucoma
3. Neovascular Glaucoma (may vary)
4. Uveitis (may vary)

NORMAL/SLIGHT DECREASE VISION
1. Migraine Syndromes

DECREASE VISION
1. Temporal Arteritis
2. Optic Neuritis

vent the examiner from testing visual acuity. These problems can be temporarily relieved in some cases with a topical anesthetic such as proparacaine hydrochloride or tetracaine hydrochloride.

LIDS AND ADNEXA

The lids and adnexa are first observed. Edema and erythema of the lids may be common to most of the conditions that present with a painful red eye. Some clues to diagnosis may include:

1. An enlarged preauricular node in the setting of viral conjunctivitis;
2. Localized swelling in the lid that is painful, as in a hordeolum (stye);
3. Lid edema and erythema in association with fever, indicating periorbital or orbital cellulitis (history of paranasal sinus infection or previous trauma);
4. Proptosis associated with lid edema and erythema, indicating orbital cellulitis (check for fever) or cavernous sinus thrombosis (check for cranial nerve involvement);
5. Decreased visual acuity associated with lid edema and erythema (consider acute angle-closure glaucoma, neovascular glaucoma, and lens-induced glaucomas)

CONJUNCTIVA

The conjunctiva is often nonspecifically injected; however, observation of the pattern of injection may be of some assistance. Perilimbal injection may indicate acute iritis or angle closure. Purulent discharge should alert the physician to a possible infectious cause.

CORNEA

A slit-lamp examination, using a small quantity of fluorescein, will help to identify corneal disease such as keratitis, ulcer, erosion, or foreign body as a possible cause to the painful red eye.

ANTERIOR CHAMBER

Assessment of the anterior chamber depth is essential in the evaluation of the painful red eye and the diagnosis of acute angle-closure glaucoma. Adequate estimation of the anterior chamber depth can be accomplished with an oblique flashlight and a slit-lamp examination.

SLIT-LAMP EXAMINATION   The central and peripheral anterior chamber depth can be estimated during the slit-lamp examination.

Pupils: The size and shape of the pupil and its reaction to light should be recorded for each eye. Unequal pupil size (anisocoria) should be noted, specifically with respect to the involved, red, painful eye. A mid-dilated nonreactive pupil is characteristic of acute angle-closure glaucoma. In contrast, the pupil in acute iritis is miotic (constricted) and poorly reactive.

Lens: Movement of the lens may indicate a dislocated or subluxed lens, secondary to trauma, or a systemic syndrome, most notably Marfan's syndrome. The dislocated lens may increase pupillary block and result in a secondary angle-closure glaucoma.

Intraocular Pressure: The range of intraocular pressure considered normal is from about 10 to 21 mm Hg. The applanation tonometer is usually mounted on a slit-lamp biomicroscope, but it can be hand-held. In applanation tonometry the cornea is flattened and the intraocular pressure determined by measuring the applanating force and the area flattened.

EMERGENCY DEPARTMENT MANAGEMENT

Patients with acute angle-closure glaucoma frequently present with nausea and vomiting due to vagal stimulation with the sudden increase in intraocular pressure. Acute angle-closure glaucoma is an ophthalmic emergency. Once the diagnosis has been established, the immediate goal is twofold: to consult with an ophthalmologist and to decrease the elevated intraocular pressure. If examination by a ophthalmologist is imminent, therapy should be delayed. However, if prompt consultation is not available, therapy to decrease intraocular pressure should be initiated with the goal to decrease aqueous production and increase aqueous outflow. The combination of topical medications, miotics and beta blockers, with systemic medications, carbonic anhydrase inhibitors and hyperosmotic agents, is often effective. The therapeutic options used in the medical management of acute angle-closure glaucoma are discussed below. The exact therapy depends on the patient's medical status.

TOPICAL THERAPY

TIMOLOL MALEATE (TIMOPTIC SOLUTION, 0.25% AND 0.5%)

Timolol is a nonselective beta blocker. Lowering of intraocular pressure occurs by decreasing aqueous humor formation. Timoptic solution should be used with caution in patients with known conditions that are contraindications for the use of systemic beta blockers, such as asthma, heart block, and heart failure. Side effects include decreased pulse rate, bronchial spasm, and altered mental state. *Recommended dosage for treating acute angle-closure glaucoma:* Timolol 0.5% solution 1 or 2 drops at 10- to 15-minute intervals initially for three doses and then 1 drop every 12 hours.

PILOCARPINE HYDROCHLORIDE 1% AND 2%

Pilocarpine is a direct-acting parasympathomimetic. The mechanism of action in acute angle-closure glaucoma is mechanical. With miosis the peripheral iris is pulled taut and away from the trabecular meshwork. Ocular side effects include a brow ache and diminished night vision. Systemic side effects, such as sweating, tremors, bradycardia, and hypotension, are uncommon in routine use of pilocarpine. *Recommended dosage for treating acute angle-closure glaucoma:* Pilocarpine 2% 1 drop every 30 minutes until the pupil constricts and then 1 drop every 6 hours. *Note:* Miotics cause congestion of the iris stroma and aggravate inflammation; for this reason concentrations higher than 2% are seldom used in an acute attack. Pilocarpine is not recommended if the diagnosis of acute angle-closure is unclear.

PREDNISOLONE ACETATE 1% (PRED-FORTE)

Topical corticosteroids reduce inflammation. *Recommended dosage for treating acute angle-closure glaucoma:* Prednisolone acetate 1% 1 drop every 30 minutes to 1 hour until surgical treatment is completed.

SYSTEMIC THERAPY

ACETAZOLAMIDE (DIAMOX)

Acetazolamide is a carbonic anhydrase inhibitor that inhibits aqueous humor formation. Give with caution in patients who have a history of allergy to sulfa drugs. *Recommended dosage for treating acute angle-closure glaucoma:* Acetazolamide 500 mg IV every 12 hours; or if a patient can tolerate oral administration, acetazolamide (250-mg tablets) 500 mg PO every 6 hours.

MANNITOL 20%

Mannitol is a hyperosmotic that can be administered parenterally. It can aggravate or precipitate congestive heart failure. Mannitol lowers intraocular pressure by increasing the blood osmolality. This creates a gradient between the blood and the vitreous and draws water from the vitreous cavity. Side effects include headache, mental confusion, congestive heart failure, and dehydration. *Recommended dosage for treating acute angle-closure glaucoma:* Mannitol 20% 1 g to 2 g/kg body weight IV over 30 to 60 minutes.

GLYCERIN 75% (GLYROL) AND ISOSORBIDE 45% (ISMOTIC)

These hyperosmotic agents can be administered by mouth. Glycerin should be avoided in diabetic patients, as it can produce hyperglycemia and ketosis. Isosorbide is not metabolized to sugar and is a useful oral hyperosmotic in diabetics. *Recommended dosage for treating acute angle-closure glaucoma:* Glycerin 75% 1.0 to 1.5 g/kg body weight PO (on ice with juice), or isosorbide 45% 1.5 g/kg body weight PO. *Note:* The hyperosmotic agents (mannitol, glycerin, and isosorbide) are not to be used simultaneously.

SURGICAL THERAPY

The definitive treatment of angle-closure glaucoma is release of pupillary block by an iridectomy. Laser iridectomies have recently replaced incisional iridectomies.

DISPOSITION

ROLE OF THE CONSULTANT   Acute angle-closure glaucoma is a ophthalmic emergency. Consultation with an ophthalmologist should occur immediately.

INDICATIONS FOR ADMISSION

INTRACTABLE PAIN, NAUSEA, AND VOMITING
Due to vagal stimulation as a consequence of the rapid and severe elevation of intraocular pressure, patients who present with acute angle-closure are systemically ill and usually require admission. Analgesic and antiemetic agents may be given if the patient is having severe pain, nausea, or vomiting.

INTENSIVE MEDICAL THERAPY AND MONITORING
Parenteral administration of medications should be given in the hospital to observe for possible untoward reactions.

COMMON PITFALLS

- The diagnosis of acute angle-closure glaucoma is often difficult and delayed.
- Complaints of pain, nausea, and vomiting are given primary attention. The overzealous treatment of these complaints (i.e., administration of analgesics and anticholinergics) may hinder a careful ophthalmologic examination and can exacerbate an angle-closure attack.
- Any patient with a painful red eye and decreased vision is considered an ophthalmic emergency and requires prompt consultation with an ophthalmologist.

2   Acute Visual Loss

Important historical questions: (1) Was the loss of vision unilateral or bilateral? (2) Painless or painful? (3) Was it preceded by other symptoms, either ocular or systemic? (4) Characterize the temporal course of the disorder—was it progressive, stationary, or transient? (5) If transient, how long did the loss of vision last? (6) Request the patient to be as specific as possible.

DIFFERENTIAL DIAGNOSIS

Table 2-1 lists common symptoms associated with visual loss and their clinical inference.

VISUAL FUNCTION TESTING

The visual experience consists of five basic functions: central vision, peripheral vision, color vision, night vision, and stereo acuity. To establish a cause of sudden visual loss, it is important to assess central acuity, peripheral vision, and color vision. *Central visual acuity* is measured with a Snellen eye chart. If the patient wears spectacles, they should be worn for the examination, and

TABLE 2-1. Symptoms Associated With Visual Loss

Symptoms	Clinical Inference
Colored halos around lights	Diffraction from corneal edema; angle-closure glaucoma
Photophobia, tender eye	Uveitis
Flashes of light in peripheral field of vision	Posterior vitreous detachment; predisposes to retinal detachment
Floaters	Vitreous hemorrhage; may precede retinal detachment
Peripheral monocular visual loss (veil), possibly progressing and affecting central vision	Retinal detachment
Distortion of straight lines	Macular dysfunction
"Spot" in center of visual field	Macular dysfunction, optic neuropathy
Decrease in peripheral visual field	Retinal detachment, chiasmal disease, advanced glaucoma, bilateral occipital lobe infarcts
Dramatic, sudden loss of vision	Vascular obstruction of retinal or optic nerve
Transient obscurations of vision (seconds), usually bilateral	Increased intracranial pressure
Transient visual loss lasting minutes (monocular)	Amaurosis fugax secondary to emboli or giant cell arteritis
Transient visual loss lasting minutes (binocular)	Transient ischemic attacks, migraine headache
Pain on eye movement	Can be associated with optic neuritis
Headache, temporal tenderness, jaw claudication, myalgias	Giant cell arteritis

each eye should be tested separately. The use of a pinhole may help to eliminate any residual refractive error. If pain prohibits examination, a topical anesthetic such as tetracaine can be administered. *Peripheral visual fields* can be mapped by the confrontation technique, and may be helpful in localizing lesions of the neuroretinal pathway. This test is a reliable means of detecting lesions of the optic nerve, optic chiasm, optic tract, optic radiations, and occipital cortex. Patients will often confuse a homonymous hemianopia with loss of vision in the eye on the involved side. *Central and paracentral visual fields,* which reflect macular function, can be assessed by use of an Amsler grid.

EMERGENCY DEPARTMENT EVALUATION AND MANAGEMENT

Vision can become impaired if there is (a) opacification of previously transparent parts of the eye (i.e., cornea, lens, or vitreous), (b) optic nerve dysfunction, (c) damage to the retina, or (d) injury to the intracranial optic nerve, optic tract, optic radiations, or occipital cortex. By systematically examining each anatomic component, the cause of visual loss can usually be determined. The cornea and conjunctiva are examined with a penlight or slit lamp for abnormalities of the surface epithelium and stroma. Corneal edema caused by a corneal abrasion or foreign body will often reduce vision and cause the patient to see colored halos around lights. Foreign bodies are most easily removed under the magnification of a slit lamp. Epithelial defects (i.e., abrasions) are easier to visualize when stained with fluorescein.

Measurement of intraocular pressure is necessary if acute glaucoma is suspected. Although chronic open-angle glaucoma causes slow, progressive visual loss, acute angle-closure glaucoma (about 5% of all cases of glaucoma) usually presents as a red, painful eye and visual loss. Blood in the anterior chamber (hyphema) can decrease vision by blocking the transmission of light. Hyphema most often occurs secondary to trauma but may also develop spontaneously due to systemic diseases. As senile cataracts opacify they cause slowly progressive visual loss. Uncontrolled diabetes mellitus, however, can lead to more rapid lenticular change.

The pupils are examined by the swinging flashlight test, which is the single most useful screening technique for optic nerve dysfunction. An abnormal result, referred to as a relative afferent pupillary defect (RAPD) or Marcus Gunn pupil, is a highly reliable sign of unilateral or asymmetrical optic nerve disease. Unilateral extensive retinal disease can also cause an RAPD. The patient's pupillary reactions should be observed in a dimly lit room with the patient fixating at a distant target. The pupillary responses are observed as bright light is directed into one eye and then briskly directed into the other eye. Normally a pupil does not constrict as the light is swung toward it because the direct and consensual light responses are equal. If there is unilateral optic nerve dysfunction or bilateral asymmetrical impairment, there is a relative difference in the consensual reflex and the direct response. An RAPD is detected as the swinging light produces apparent dilation in the affected eye.

The vitreous, optic nerve, and retina are assessed by direct observation using an ophthalmoscope. If the fundus cannot be visualized through an adequately dilated pupil, and the cornea and anterior chamber are clear, then there must be opacification of the lens or vitreous. If the fundus is seen, the examiner should study the color of the disk (is it pale or pink?) and determine whether the disk is flat or raised. The clarity of the disk margins should also be noted.

Vitreous hemorrhage is characterized by an acute painless loss of vision with absence of the normal red reflex of the fundus. Symptoms from vitreal blood will be described by patients as "floaters," as a "cobweb," or as profound visual loss. Visualization (ophthalmoscopically) of the fundus may be difficult. Vitreal hemorrhage occurs frequently secondary to vitreoretinal traction, diabetes, or trauma, but it may be related to retinal tears, tumor, or central retinal vein occlusion. Systemic diseases such as leukemia, anemia, macroglobulinemia, and thrombocytopenia may also predispose a patient to vitreous hemorrhage. Anticoagulants may also cause vitreal hemorrhage. Management revolves around treatment of the underlying conditions. If the hemorrhage does not clear, vitrectomy should be considered.

Retinal detachment can develop after trauma or spontaneously. Patients may notice flashing lights, floaters, or a visual field defect often described as a "shade being drawn." Often acuity will be normal when the macula, subserving central vision, is not affected. Inflammatory lesions of the retina may be caused by infectious disorders such as toxoplasmosis, syphilis, herpes zoster, and cytomegalovirus. Blunt trauma may cause retinal edema and account for transient visual impairment if the macula is involved. Resolution usually occurs within 1 week.

Central retinal artery occlusion causes acute, painless monocular visual loss, often to the level of bare light perception, associated with an RAPD. The entire posterior pole appears white secondary to nerve fiber layer edema. The fovea, which has no nerve fiber layer, appears red because of its choroidal blood supply. The pink fovea surrounded by a white retina in this setting has been termed a cherry-red spot. Narrowed arterioles may show sludging of erythrocytes. In a branch retinal artery occlusion, edema is limited to the area supplied by the affected arteriole. There are numerous causes that must be considered, including embolic disease from the carotids or cardiac valves damaged from rheumatic heart disease or mitral valve prolapse. Talc emboli from drug abuse are also visible. Giant cell arteritis, collagen vascular diseases, hypotension, homocystinuria, and sickle cell disease are other causes of retinal artery occlusion. In patients over age 50 without emboli, an erythrocyte sedimentation rate should be performed immediately to rule out giant cell arteritis. The goal of therapy for central retinal artery occlusion is to re-establish blood flow to the involved retina. This can be accomplished either by lowering intraocular pressure or by increasing arterial flow. The intraocular pressure can be decreased by performing an anterior chamber tap with a 25-gauge needle, or by digital massage. Digital massage can also mechanically dislodge an embolus. Instillation of topical medications such as beta blockers or systemic ingestion of a carbonic anhydrase inhibitor (e.g., acetazolamide [Diamox], 500 mg, PO or IV) will also effectively lower intraocular pressure. Inhalation of a mixture of 95% oxygen and 5% carbon dioxide will improve arterial blood flow by causing the retinal blood vessels to dilate. Treatment is usually not successful in regaining vision if more than 12 hours have elapsed since the initial event.

Central retinal vein occlusion presents as acute, painless visual loss. Depending on the type of venous obstruction, there may be an RAPD with large numbers of cotton-wool spots, optic disk edema, and flame-shaped retinal hemorrhages throughout the retina. Associated conditions include hypertension (60%), open-angle glaucoma (6%–20%), narrow-angle glaucoma, atherosclerosis (25%–50%), diabetes mellitus (15%–30%), and collagen vascular diseases. Polycythemia vera and dysproteinemia may be associated with bilateral central retinal vein occlusions. Neovascular glaucoma develops in 50% to 60% of patients within 3 months. Patients with central retinal vein occlusion need to be formally evaluated for possible panretinal laser photo coagulation to prevent the development of neovascular glaucoma.

The *optic chiasm* may be affected by pituitary adenomas, suprasellar meningiomas, craniopharyngiomas, or aneurysms. Involvement of the chiasm usually produces bitemporal hemianopia demonstrable on visual field examination.

Optic tract, optic radiation, or *occipital cortical impairment* produces homonymous hemianopia in the contralateral visual field. An RAPD may be present in optic tract lesions. Cerebrovascular accidents, neoplasms, and arteriovenous malformations are common conditions causing homonymous hemianopia that are localized by computed tomography and magnetic resonance imaging.

Bilateral occipital lobe infarcts may occur consecutively or synchronously. Central vision will not be impaired with occipital lobe infarction unless it occurs bilaterally. Cerebrovascular accidents that involve the occipital cortex may be caused by hypertension or hypotension. Arteriosclerosis is the most common predisposing condition; hypoperfusion during cardiac surgery is another situation that can lead to occipital lobe infarction. Visual loss from occipital lobe infarcts can occur in the pre-eclamptic woman. The diagnosis is confirmed with neuroimaging.

3   Acute Eye Infections

Conjunctivitis is the inflammation of the mucous membrane that covers the anterior sclera and inner eyelids. Infection of the conjunctiva is a common cause of the "red eye" treated in the ED. Most cases are self-limited, but severe cases may result in corneal scarring. Most commonly, infectious conjunctivitis is caused by viruses and bacteria. *Keratitis* is an inflammation of the cornea. The corneal epithelium may be involved in a superficial manner (with punctate erosions or ulceration), or there may be deeper involvement with infiltration. In either case keratitis is usually painful and often associated with viral or bacterial conjunctivitis.

Ocular conditions that cause a red eye create diagnostic dilemmas; infection is only one cause; the physician should make every effort to explore other causes. The urgency to treat conjunctival infection is not usually great unless corneal involvement is present. The anterior ocular surface is essentially a modified mucous membrane, and is easily "seeded" with pathogens through incidental contact or mild trauma. Corneal scarring is one of the leading causes of blindness worldwide. Treatment must, therefore, be accurate, and the patient carefully followed to avoid this complication.

VIRAL PATHOGENS

Viral pathogens include the adenoviruses, herpes simplex, and herpes zoster. A common agent is the adenovirus. Infection starts in one eye and becomes bilateral with a significant watery discharge and follicles. Preauricular adenopathy is common. Transmission occurs easily. Epidemic keratoconjunctivitis is caused by adenovirus types 8 and 19; there is marked discomfort, which may persist for weeks. Corneal infiltrates and pseudomembrane formation may be seen. Supportive care includes isolation, cool compresses, ocular decongestants, lubricants, and a broad-spectrum antibiotic to prevent secondary overinfection. Adenoviral keratoconjunctivitis does not respond to topical antibiotics. Progressive visual loss, increasing discomfort, and pseudomembrane formation are indications for urgent referral. Reduced discharge, swelling, and hyperemia are indicative of therapeutic success.

Herpes simplex conjunctivitis may present with unilateral conjunctival hyperemia associated with a clear discharge. Other findings may include malaise and lid vesicles or ulcerations in early or primary cases. Corneal spread can occur rapidly, resulting in a dendritic ulcer. Ophthalmologic consultation is indicated once the diagnosis is made. In simple, early epithelial herpes mechanical debridement is an important aspect of treatment and should be done by an ophthalmologist. Topical vidarabine 3%, trifluorothymidine 1%, or idoxuridine 0.5% may be used in consultation with the ophthalmologist.

Herpes zoster ophthalmicus, ocular involvement, should be suspected especially if the nasociliary branch of the fifth cranial nerve is involved. Punctate keratopathy, lid vesicles, or dendritic infiltrates may be present. Herpes zoster may mimic simplex. Immediate ophthalmologic consultation may be indicated. Topical cycloplegics and steroids are beneficial. There is evidence that systemically administered acyclovir may diminish the severity of the process and postherpetic neuralgia. Elevated intraocular pressure is quite commonly associated with the iritis of internal ocular involvement.

BACTERIAL PATHOGENS

Those pathogens of greatest clinical importance and frequency include *Staphylococcus,* *Haemophilus,* pneumococci (and other streptococci), *Neisseria gonorrhea,* diphtheroids, coliforms, *Pseudomonas, Proteus,* and *Moraxella.* Of lesser frequency are Parinaud's oculoglandular syndrome (cat-scratch fever) and luetic and tuberculous disease. Mucopurulent conjunctivitis is most commonly caused by *Staphylococcus aureus,* followed by *Streptococcus pneumoniae* and *Haemophilus influenzae.* The onset is often acute and unilateral but may rapidly become bilateral. Crusting of the lids is common. An epidemic form (pink eye) can be caused by pneumococci and *Haemophilus.* True pink eye is epidemic keratoconjunctivitis. Gram stain and culture are usually not necessary unless the case is quite severe, unresponsive to therapy, or in a compromised host. Treatment consists of warm compresses, lubricants, and broad-spectrum antibiotics (drops during the day and ointments at bedtime). Commonly used antibiotics include sulfacetamide 10%, gentamicin 0.3%, chloramphenicol 0.5%, and Neosporin. The sulfa drugs are less sensitizing than neomycin. Chloramphenicol is least sensitizing. Bacterial conjunctivitis should improve in 48 hours.

Gonococcal conjunctivitis usually causes unilateral conjunctival hyperemia, a severe purulent discharge with associated edema and erythema of the lids. The population at risk includes neonates, homosexuals, sexually active adults, and health care workers. The incubation period is from 1 to 3 days. Culture and Gram stain should be done and will reveal gram-negative intracellular diplococci. Urgent consultation is indicated as is admission for systemic therapy and frequent irrigation of the eye, since the gonococcus has the ability to penetrate the intact cornea. Topical antibiotics, irrigation, and parenteral penicillin or cephalosporins are used. Single-dose ceftriaxone may allow for selected outpatient therapy.

FUNGAL PATHOGENS

The common fungal pathogens include *Actinomyces, Aspergillus, Blastomyces, Candida, Coccidioides, Mucor* (in diabetics), and *Sporothrix*. Fungal infection is generally not fulminant. Patients taking corticosteroids and those with suppressed immune systems are at risk. A history of trauma involving vegetable matter is important. Beneath the corneal infiltrate an endothelial plaque may be seen. The hypopyon associated with this type of corneal infection may contain fungal elements. Gram and Giemsa stain and culture are essential. Fungal blepharoconjunctivitis can be controlled with lid hygiene and compresses. Due to the limited number of available topical antifungal agents, if the physician identifies fungal elements on corneal ulcer smears, natamycin 5% suspension (Natacyn) should be given every hour after appropriate consultation.

CHLAMYDIA

Mucopurulent inclusion conjunctivitis is extremely common, especially in sexually active young adults. The diagnosis is made by the lack of organisms on Gram stain and a positive immunofluorescent antibody screen. The presence or history of a urethral discharge may suggest concomitant gonococcal disease. Conjunctival scrapings may be helpful acutely. Systemic therapy is necessary and includes erythromycin or tetracycline, 1 g daily for 3 to 4 weeks. Ocular therapy (topical sulfa or erythromycin) is supportive only and not curative. Partners should be referred for treatment. Neonatal inclusion conjunctivitis occurs several days to 2 weeks after birth. The treatment is similar, but topical therapy with sulfacetamide 10%, four times daily for 3 weeks, is more effective. Systemic therapy is also indicated in the neonate. Trachoma continues to be a major cause of inflammatory blindness worldwide, although it is not prevalent in the United States.

CLINICAL PRESENTATION

Time of onset, contact with other infected persons or agents, use of medications, previous trauma, and associated illness are important; history of previous eye problems, eye surgery, contact lens wear, or trauma should be determined. The hallmark of anterior surface infection is the red eye. However, discomfort, visual loss, photophobia, discharge, and lids sticking shut in one or both eyes are common complaints. Uniocular disease demonstrates greater probability for certain conditions. Herpetic disease is usually unilateral. Adenovirus generally starts in one eye and "ping-pongs" to the other within a few days. Contact lens wearers are especially prone to all types of infectious disease, as well as to ischemic injury from overwear syndrome and toxic infiltrates from old and contaminated lenses. A history of trauma from vegetable matter (a tree branch) may cause a corneal infiltrate from a fungus. *Most* conjunctivitis is self-limiting. It is quite common in epidemic keratoconjunctivitis to see serious progression as immunologic responses increase. Pseudomembranes may indicate or aggravate severe corneal injury not present on the initial examination.

DIFFERENTIAL DIAGNOSIS

See Table 3-1.

EMERGENCY DEPARTMENT EVALUATION

Essential components include a careful history (use of contact lens), visual acuity in both eyes, and an external examination, including corneal inspection and slit-lamp examination.

TABLE 3-1. Differential Diagnosis of Red Eye

Factor	Infectious Keratitis/ Conjunctivitis	Iritis	Angle-Closure Glaucoma	Allergic/Toxic	Traumatic
Type of Injection	Diffuse	Diffuse, ciliary flush	Diffuse	Diffuse	Diffuse (hemorrhagic)
Discharge	Viral: watery; bacterial: purulent; fungal: mucopurulent, occasional pseudomembranes	Watery	Watery	Watery (± mucoid)	Watery
Itching	Minimal	None	None	Moderate to severe	None
Preauricular Node	Viral: fairly common; bacterial: occasional; fungal: occasional	None	None	None	None
Vision	Usually normal, may become markedly decreased if corneal involvement	Usually blurred	Usually markedly blurred (corneal edema)	Usually normal, unless corneal involvement	Usually markedly blurred (corneal, intraocular blood, retinal injury, etc.)
Pain	Usually mild but can be severe (especially adenovirus); more irritation than photophobia	Photophobia	Usually severe, but significant number have little discomfort	Usually very little, mostly irritation	Usually severe
Cornea	Usually clear unless epithelium involved; loses glassy appearance; infiltrates appear white	Usually clear	Generalized haze	Usually clear	If corneal injury, may be hazy
Intraocular Pressure (IOP)	Usually normal (elevated in zoster uveitis)	Usually down or normal; occasionally up	Elevated	Normal	May be normal, up or down (even with perforation)
Pupils	Usually normal	Usually smaller; poorly reactive	Mid-dilated (little or no reaction)	Normal	May be large, normal, small, or irregular
Scrapings/Stains	Viral: monocytic; bacterial: PMNs + stain inclusions; fungal: PMNs + stain			Eosinophils may be present (e.g., vernal)	

PMNs, polymorphonuclear leukocytes.
Modified from Vaughn D. Asbury T: General Ophthalmology, 11th ed. Los Altos, Calif, Lange Medical Publications, 1986.

15

LIDS   Crusting of the lids is common in bacterial overgrowth, infection, and dermatologic conditions (seborrhea). Ulcerations are common in herpetic and staphylococcal infections. Macro-organisms *(Phthirus)* and discoloration may also be seen. Lid eversion should be performed if indicated (foreign body, pseudomembranes).

CONJUNCTIVA   Note the presence of chemosis or discharge (serous, mucoid, or mucopurulent). Follicles represent lymphoid aggregates, which are a hallmark of acute adenoviral disease, but may, on occasion, be seen in other infectious, toxic, and allergic conjunctivitis. Membranes, or fibrinous pseudomembranes, are seen in severe conjunctivitis associated with adenovirus, occasionally in other conditions such as pneumococcus or streptococcus pneumoniae and diphtheria, and rarely in herpetic disease. Hemorrhage is usually petechial but may be more extensive, as seen in adenovirus, hemorrhagic conjunctivitis virus, *Haemophilus,* and pneumococcus or streptococcus pneumoniae. An acute, markedly purulent conjunctivitis should be thoroughly and rapidly evaluated before treatment. Corneal perforation is possible, especially in gonococcal disease.

CORNEA   The hallmark of epithelial injury, especially in viral disorders, is punctate areas of cell loss. These appear as stained specks with fluorescein and are diagnostic of adenovirus (superficial punctate keratopathy). However, many other conditions may mimic this, including herpetic disease. Ulceration implies a larger epithelial defect and is important to identify. Immediate referral is indicated because of the potential for permanent scarring or perforation. The description should include size, shape, and anterior stromal involvement. Herpetic ulcers are usually dendritic or geographic. Bacterial and fungal ulcers tend to be round with fluffy white borders and extend into the anterior stroma and are usually associated with a purulent discharge and lid-sticking. Infiltrates are epithelial, subepithelial, or stromal collections of inflammatory cellular debris that are nonspecific but common in viral (adenoviral, herpetic), chlamydial (inclusion), bacterial (in association with the ulcerative defect), and hypersensitivity reactions (small and near limbus).

ANTERIOR CHAMBER   The presence of white blood cells in the aqueous is the hallmark of iritis (uveitis), which occurs with severe anterior surface infections (herpetic disease, adenovirus). The grading of the reaction (1–4+) of these cells correlates with the severity of the iritis. Layering of the cells in the anterior chamber is called a *hypopyon,* a hallmark of severe ulceration of the cornea and endophthalmitis. Usually seen with bacterial and fungal infection, a hypopyon warrants immediate consultation and referral. In the presence of a small corneal ulcer without hypopyon, *consult first.* After stains and cultures have been performed, cover with "heavy" topicals (e.g., gentamicin drops every 30–60 minutes with bacitracin ointment every 2 hours). Fortified drops are most often used and are prepared by the pharmacy. If a hypopyon is present, or the ulcer is large or multiple, this is an ocular emergency, and the ophthalmologist should be called. Infectious ulcers of the cornea tend to be more central, whereas hypersensitivity immune ulcers (e.g., rheumatoid and staphylococcal) tend to be peripheral. Distant skin ulcerations or vesicles, including the lids, should suggest herpetic disease (simplex or zoster), as well as impetigo. *Moraxella* and *Staphylococcus* tend to cause ulceration and maceration in the lateral canthal regions.

DIAGNOSTIC AIDS

FLUORESCEIN

The eye is stained with a sterile fluroescein strip and viewed with a slit lamp. A small quantity is used. The examiner should look for areas of epithelial loss on both conjunctiva and cornea. The noninfected eye should be stained first.

LABORATORY STUDIES

With severe or unusual purulent conjunctivitis perform a Gram and Giemsa stain of the material. After cultures, conjunctival scrapings should be taken. Corneal scraping of ulcers must be performed at the slit lamp by an ophthalmologist. It is essential before initiation of antibiotics.

SPECIAL CONSIDERATIONS IN MANAGEMENT

It is important to avoid contagion. It is essential to maintain clean equipment and to avoid checking the intraocular pressure, unless necessary for the correct diagnosis, because of the risk of spreading contamination with the tonometer.

EMERGENCY DEPARTMENT MANAGEMENT

Table 3-2 lists topical antibiotics, while Table 3-3 indicates useful diagnostic and therapeutic drugs.

Therapeutic guides: It is important to recall that severe anterior surface disorders can result in iritis, with the potential to cause subsequent scarring of the pupil to the lens (posterior synechiae), as well as iris to cornea (peripheral anterior synechiae). Cycloplegics are essential and improve patient comfort. Longer-acting cycloplegics (scopolamine, homatropine, and atropine) may be necessary. Although corticosteroids play an important role in the management of iritis and may reduce corneal scarring, their use in the emergency setting is somewhat controversial. Sulfacetamide 10% or chloramphenicol 0.5% solutions given four to six times daily for several days will clear most simple surface infections. Gentamicin and tobramycin solutions are helpful, but they may be more beneficial when reserved for special situations. Drops are aesthetically superior and provide high levels quickly; however, they are cleared by tear drainage too quickly. Ointments reduce this clearing effect as well as the irritation but cause blurred vision. Use of ointments (chloramphenicol 1% or polymyxin–bacitracin combinations) may be helpful at bedtime.

DISPOSITION

ROLE OF THE CONSULTANT

Immediate consultation is indicated in the following circumstances:

> Conjunctivitis with a history or Gram stain suggesting gonococcal disease.
> Purulent conjunctivitis associated with a corneal infiltrate, especially if the infiltrate or ulcer is in or near the visual axis. Risk factors include trauma and contact lens history.
> Membranous conjunctivitis. Secondary injury to the cornea or severe corneal epithelial injury may occur.
> Consultation within 24 to 48 hours is indicated for relatively severe conjunctivitis or keratitis that suggests possible herpetic disease, especially if near the visual axis.

Consultation within 3 to 7 days is indicated in the following circumstances:

> Bacterial conjunctivitis that does not improve within 48 hours.
> Viral disease that is nonmembranous with intact vision (adenoviral disease [e.g., epidemic keratoconjunctivitis] may show persistent signs of involvement for weeks!).

INDICATIONS FOR ADMISSION

Emergency admissions are rare, but are indicated in corneal ulcers, endophthalmitis, and, occasionally, *Neisseria* conjunctivitis. It is uncommon to admit a patient with herpes simplex or zoster. The principal goal for admission is systemic therapy, frequent topical antibiotic administration, and subconjunctival or intravitreal injections. Topical therapy may need to be administered every 30 to 60 minutes.

SPECIAL CONSIDERATIONS

Most patients should be rechecked in 48 to 72 hours in moderately severe cases. Referral should be based on progression of the disease, lack of response, increased pain, and decreased vision.

TABLE 3-2. Antibiotics for Topical Use

General Principles of Administration

Topical antibiotics are given four times daily for simple infection, more frequently or fortified for serious infection (ulcers, gonorrhea). The most common infectious pathogens are *Staphylococcus aureus*, *Haemophilus* species, pneumococci, and staphylococcus *epidermidis*. Even though sensitivities show resistance to many of these antibiotics, they may still be bactericidal because of their high concentration (e.g., sulfa).

Antibacterial Agents

Bacitracin: Effective against most gram-positive organisms as well as diphtheroids, *Haemophilus*, and *Actinomyces*. Ointment form and in mixture with polymixin B (Polysporin). Fortified drops for ulcers prepared fresh only by pharmacy.

Chloramphenicol: Effective against many gram-positive and gram-negative organisms, especially *Haemophilus*, *Moraxella*, *S. aureus*, group B streptococci, and diphtheroids. Solution (0.5%) and ointment (1%) (Chloroptic, Econochlor, others). Low allergy index.

Erythromycin: Effective against gram-positive organisms, diphtheroids, *Haemophilus*, *Actinomyces*, and *Neisseria*. Only in ointment form (0.5%) (Ilotycin). Very effective for staph or rosacea blepharitis.

Gentamicin: Effective against most gram-negative organisms, especially *Pseudomonas*, as well as gram-positive organisms, including *Staphylococcus* species. Highly effective broad-spectrum agent, but has fairly high sensitizing as well as potential toxic effects. Available in solution and ointment form (Genoptic, Garamycin, Gentacidin).

Neomycin: Wide range of effectiveness (like gentamicin) but even more sensitizing and potentially toxic to corneal epithelium. Usually in mixtures in solution or ointment (Neosporin, Ocutricin).

Polymyxin B: Fairly effective against most gram-negative organisms (not effective against *Proteus* or *Neisseria*. Available in ointment form and only in mixtures (Neosporin, Polysporin, others).

Sulfacetamide: Effective against a wide range of gram-positive and gram-negative organisms; some *Staphylococcus* species, pneumococci, *Haemophilus*, *Moraxella*, and *Chlamydia*. Available in solution (10%, 15%, and 30%) and ointment form (10%) (Bleph-10, Sulamyd, others). Potential for allergy is fairly high.

Tetracycline: Effective against many *Staphylococcus*, *Streptococcus* species, also gonococci, *Actinomyces*, *Haemophilus*, a few gram-negative organisms, and *Chlamydia*. Available in solution and ointment (1%) (Achromycin). Allergy index is not bad, but irritating.

Antifungal Agents

Natamycin: Effective against many filamentary and yeast forms. Drug of choice for most mycotic corneal injuries (and only ocular formulation commercially available). Available as Natacyn, 5% suspension.

Antivirals

Idoxuridine: First antiherpetic drug available. Does not penetrate corneal epithelium well, but has been on market longest and fairly safe. Available as 0.1% solution and 0.5% ointment (Stoxil, Herplex). Resistance well known.

Vidarabine: Fairly effective by today's standards. Penetrates cornea only fairly well and is somewhat toxic to the epithelium (as is idoxuridine). Needs to be applied only five times daily (but ointment is annoying), rather than every 2 hours, as with most antiviral drops. Available as a 3% ointment (ARA-A, Vira-A).

Trifluorothymidine: Most popular antiviral for herpetic disease. Penetrates cornea fairly well. Toxic to epithelium. Available in 1% solution (Viroptic) and must be initiated at an every 2-hour dosage until ulcer is healing.

Acycloguarosine: Available for just about every other part of the body except the eye. In investigational studies it is highly effective in the treatment of ocular herpetic disease. It has a low toxicity. Acyclovir is available topically for genital use. It has a systemic preparation that has been helpful in reducing morbidity in herpes zoster (shingles), as well as for systemic zoster or simplex involvement.

TABLE 3-3 Common Ophthalmic Medications

Diagnostic Medications

These agents facilitate the ability to examine the eye.

Stains: Topical solutions that highlight epithelial abnormalities

  Fluorescein: Sterile paper strips are preferred to the 2% solutions owing to ease of contamination of the latter.
  Rose bengal: 1% solution stains devitalized epithelium, helpful in diagnosing herpetic ulcers, which may mimic abrasions

Anesthetics: Topical solutions that promote patient cooperation for the examination; also used in conjunction with stains; usually essential for determining intraocular pressure.
  Tetracaine hydrochloride (Pontocaine): 0.5% to 1.0% solution, lasts for 15 minutes; may sting.
  Proparacaine hydrochloride (Ophthetic, Ophthaine): 0.5% solution, less irritating
  Cocaine (0.25% to 0.5%): Effective but highly toxic to the epithelium

Mydriatics/Cycloplegics: Used diagnostically or therapeutically to dilate the pupil or paralyze the ciliary muscle. This permits evaluation of the internal ocular structures and gauges the baseline refractive error of the eye. In addition, these agents prevent synechiae formation (adhesions of the iris) by reducing intraocular inflammation through stabilization of the blood-aqueous barrier. These agents are usually capped in *red.*

Phenylephrine hydrochloride (Neosynephrine, Mydfrin): Dilates the pupil only, no cycloplegia; 2.5% solution is the only strength recommended because of the higher incidence of cardiovascular side effects with 10%. Dilation is fairly good and lasts for about 4 hours.

Tropicamide (Mydriacyl 0.5 & 1%): Provides an excellent short-term dilation of the pupil, plus cycloplegia (4 to 6 hours). Relatively easy to reverse; used most often by ophthalmologists.

Cyclopentolate hydrochloride (Cyclogyl 0.5%, 1.0%, and 2.0%): Best short-term cycloplegic for refraction but may last for 6 hours to 1 day!

Homatropine hydrobromide (1%, 2%, and 5%): Lasts for a few days and is useful for the treatment of short-term iritis cycloplegia caused by trauma or abrasions.

Scopolamine hydrobromide (Hyoscine 0.25%): Lasts for 3 to 5 days and is more effective for long-term inflammation seen postoperatively or in severe uveitis.

Atropine sulfate (0.25% to 2.0% solution, 0.5% and 1% ointment): Lasts for 10 to 14 days; most commonly used postoperatively and in severe uveitis. Epithelial and systemic toxicity are important features.

Therapeutic Agents

Lubricants: The most important layer of the eye for comfort and vision is the tear film. Abnormalities in this complex multilayered film are responsible for a significant percentage of complaints. Artificial lubricants can temporarily alleviate this problem.

Artificial tears (multiple brands): Usually contain methylcellulose and related compounds, as well as polyvinyl alcohols and others. The current trend is to use those that are minimally or not preserved. These agents are not only benign, but also relieve most anterior surface irritation from any cause. *Be liberal in dispensing these agents!*

Bland lubricating ointments (Hypotears Ointment, Duo-Lube, Ocu-Lube): Especially helpful for lubrication during sleep. Nonpreserved and non-lanolin types should be used.

(cont'd.)

TABLE 3-3 *(cont'd.)*

Therapeutic Agents *(cont'd.)*

Antibiotics: See Table 3-2

Anti-inflammatories: These agents are most often used to suppress allergic (*i.e.*, immunologic) reactions of the eye of all types, both externally and internally. It may be necessary to suppress severe external inflammation to avoid corneal scarring or permanent tear film abnormalities. Internally (eye), these agents help to prevent scarring (synechiae) and subsequent glaucoma. Topical application allows excellent penetration into the anterior chamber.

Medrysone 1% (HMS): Mild steroid, few side effects.

Fluorometholone 0.1% (FML): Slightly more potent, with fewer side effects than prednisolone and dexamethasone.

Prednisolone acetate and phosphate 0.125% and 1.0% (Pred Mild, Pred Forte, Inflamase Forte): Potent and highly effective for anterior segment inflammation. High risk for side effects (intraocular pressure and infection, especially herpes simplex activation).

Dexamethasone 0.1% (Decadron): Potent and highly effective. Very high risk for side effects.

Antiglaucoma Agents
These either suppress aqueous production, increase outflow facility, or both. Because the ciliary body and muscle are critical determinants of the intraocular pressure, autonomic neural agents and their blockers may affect the intraocular pressure. Carbonic anhydrase inhibitors block aqueous production because this enzyme is essential in the active production of aqueous humor.

  Miotics: *Pilocarpine 0.5% to 10%; carbachol 0.75%, 1.5%, and 3%; echothiophate iodide* (Phospholine Iodide) *0.06% to 0.25%:* Rarely cause systemic side effects. Miotics make the pupils small; usually capped in *green.*
  Adrenalin Agents: *Epinephrine cmpds 0.5% to 2.0%, dipivalyl epinephrine 0.1%* (Propine): Tachyphylaxis develops commonly, and eyes turn red!
  Beta Blockers: *Timolol 0.25% and 0.5%* (Timoptic), *betaxolol 0.5%* (Betoptic), and *levobunolol 0.5%* (Betagan): All have *yellow* tops and may cause systemic side effects, especially pulmonary. Betoptic is a slightly more selective beta-1.
  Oral Agents: Carbonic anhydrase inhibitors: *Acetazolamide* (Diamox 250-mg tablets, 500-mg capsules) and *methazolamide* (Neptazane 50 mg) are the principal agents used. These are mild diuretics and may cause potassium depletion when given chronically. If glaucoma therapy is given systemically, the incidence of side effects goes up dramatically. These agents are sulfa-related compounds; therefore, allergic reactions and rash are common. They may also precipitate renal stones in susceptible patients.
  Osmotic Agents: Oral *glycerin* 50% to 75% (1.0 to 1.5 g/kg) over ice frequently produces nausea and vomiting; *isosorbide* 45% (Ismotic), 1.5 g/kg, will lower pressure adequately over 1 to 2 hours. A rapid response is most often accomplished with a 20% solution of *mannitol*, 1 g to 2 g/kg IV over 30 to 45 minutes. These agents are used emergently to shrink the vitreous and rapidly lower the intraocular pressure. It is essential to know the patient's fluid, renal, and cardiovascular status when using these compounds.

COMMON PITFALLS

- Recognize high-risk situations, such as conjunctival pseudomembranes, post-traumatic reaction, and contact lens wear.
- Multiple antibiotics are often used when progression of the infection is really due to hypersensitivity (Neosporin) or toxicity to the drug. Prolonged therapy creates the risk resistant organisms or fungal growth.
- The red eye is not always infected!

- Initiating antibiotic therapy before diagnostic studies are performed generally forces the ophthalmologist into "shot-gun" therapy.
- Be cautious with the use of topical anesthetics and corticosteroids!

4   Orbital and Periorbital Infections

Orbital cellulitis and periorbital cellulitis are often used interchangeably, despite the fact that the single most important step in managing these diseases is to differentiate the two.

CLINICAL PRESENTATION

A more correct term than periorbital cellulitis is *preseptal cellulitis;* this includes any inflammation anterior to the orbital septum, a thin, broad, sheet-like layer of fascia that separates the orbit from the eyelids. Preseptal cellulitis presents with erythema, edema, warmth, and tenderness of one or both eyelids; chemosis and closure of the palpebral fissures. One or both eyes may be involved. Fever is more common than in orbital infection. A patient should *not*, by contrast, complain of ocular pain, pain with movement of the globe, ocular tenderness, or any limitation of globe mobility; these symptoms suggest postseptal (i.e., true orbital) infection. Orbital infection is inflammation of any of the tissues within the orbit posterior to the orbital septum. Preseptal cellulitis is invariably present, however, as are chemosis and proptosis. In addition to ocular pain, patients will (to varying degrees) exhibit internal and external ophthalmoplegia, pupillary paralysis, and decreased visual acuity, even to the point of blindness. They may also develop increased intraocular pressure and loss of sensation along the trigeminal nerve (V_1 and V_2).

DIFFERENTIAL DIAGNOSIS

The patient with apparent periorbital cellulitis should be presumed to have orbital cellulitis. Nearly 75% of all patients with an "acute orbit" will have periorbital cellulitis. The other 25% will have orbital cellulitis, subperiosteal abscess, orbital abscess, and cavernous sinus thrombosis. Subperiosteal abscess presents much like postseptal cellulitis, except there may be significant tenderness between the orbital margin and the globe itself. Orbital abscess is present in the postseptal tissues and resembles an orbital cellulitis, except that ophthalmologic findings of venous congestion and disk edema may be more prominent. Pus may be seen to spread into the lid and conjunctiva. Cavernous sinus thrombosis frequently presents as unilateral then bilateral axial proptosis with paralysis of cranial nerves III, IV, and VI. It is extremely difficult to distinguish from orbital cellulitis until infectious spread across the anterior and posterior intercavernous sinuses leads to bilateral involvement. Dilatation of the episcleral veins is a classic feature, and may be the first sign that the disease has worsened beyond orbital involvement. Both venous engorgement of the fundus and pupillary fixation and dilatation also suggest cavernous sinus thrombosis. There is no absolute continuum among these disorders. Cavernous sinus thrombosis, for example, may develop without evidence of abscess or cellulitis. Seventy-five percent of all patients with periorbital and orbital cellulitis will have an identifiable predisposing factor, with 50% due to sinusitis, upper respiratory tract infection, and otitis media with effusion. The orbit is a cone-shaped cavity, and the inferior, medial, and superior walls are immediately adjacent to the paranasal sinuses. It is easy to see why the likelihood of sinusitis rises to 75% in cases of orbital cellulitis.

In patients from whom bacterial pathogens are isolated, *Haemophilus influenzae* outnumbers all other pathogens. *Staphylococcus aureus, Staphylococcus epidermis, Streptococcus pneumoniae,* and other *Streptococcus* species constitute the remainder, with occasional reports of *Corynebacterium, Pseudomonas,* and mixed bacterial cultures. Even when there is strong evidence of hematogenous spread (most commonly due to *H. influenzae* type B or *S. pneumoniae*), blood cultures are positive only 11% to 34% of the time.

PEDIATRIC VERSUS ADULT PATIENTS

In general, patients with periorbital cellulitis tend to be younger than those with orbital cellulitis, although neonates with orbital cellulitis have been described. Both conditions are more common in childhood, both present acutely, and both may appear in a subacute form due to inadequate antibiotic therapy. The incidence of bacteremia falls strikingly with age. There is a 33% positive blood culture rate in patients under age 4, but only a 5% positive rate in adults. Streptococci, including *S. pneumoniae,* is noted in all age groups.

H. influenzae and *S. pneumoniae* represent 90% of positive blood cultures, with *H. influenzae* far more likely in patients under age five. *H. influenzae* should be strongly suspected, especially in the younger population, in the setting of sinusitis. Trauma and skin infections predispose to staphylococcal and streptococcal infections. The majority of periorbital and orbital cellulitides may be traced to these three causes (sinusitis, trauma, and skin infections).

EMERGENCY DEPARTMENT EVALUATION

Determining the cause and extent of inflammation is difficult. Preseptal (periorbital) cellulitis may present with sufficient swelling to inhibit visual acuity and ocular motility; fever is absent in 24% of all patients with preseptal and postseptal infections; and unilateral involvement is the rule rather than the exception for both. Blood cultures will be negative in 2/3 of children with orbital cellulitis. The negative culture rate rises to 90–95% in the adult. Cultures of eyelid aspirates and eye secretions correlate poorly with blood culture results. Cultures of cerebrospinal fluid are noncontributory unless meningeal signs are present. Sinus films do not differentiate between orbital cellulitis and orbital abscess and have been replaced by computed tomography (CT). CT of the orbit is advocated in all children with periorbital swelling in whom postseptal infection cannot be conclusively ruled out. Radiation exposure to the lenses can be considerable. There may be no advantage of contrast over nonenhanced CT. CT is inadequate in the differentiation of subperiosteal inflammation from mature orbital abscess. Ultrasound has been advocated because of its lack of ionizing radiation and its ability to discriminate between fluid and soft-tissue density.

EMERGENCY DEPARTMENT MANAGEMENT

If the infection appears to be localized to the preseptal tissues only and is not severe, antibiotics can be given orally on an outpatient basis to adults. In children, only the mildest cellulitis should be treated on an outpatient basis. This is controversial among pediatric experts; some recommend admission and parenteral antibiotics for all children with periorbital cellulitis. Either cefaclor or amoxicillin/clavulanate potassium (Augmentin) may be used with equal efficacy (40 mg/kg/day, q 8 hours). In cases of skin trauma or infection in which the suspicion of staphylococcal infection is high, dicloxacillin (25 to 40 mg/kg/day, q 6 hours) or, in the penicillin-allergic patient, erythromycin, (40 mg/kg/day, q 6 hours), may be given. The condition should be treated for at least 7 to 10 days. If the infection is secondary to sinusitis, treatment should last at least 2 to 3 weeks. If outpatient treatment has been selected, it is recommended that the patient be re-examined the next day, preferably by a specialist. If there is any question about the extent of the periorbital infection, intravenous antibiotics should be initiated. In the child under age 5 in whom either sinusitis is believed to be the source or in whom no clear cause can be found, coverage for both gram-positive cocci and *H. influenzae* should be begun until culture results are available. Cefuroxime, (75 mg to 100 mg/kg/day, q 8 hours) has been recommended as an alternative to the traditional regimen of ampicillin and chloramphenicol. The dose of cefuroxime should be increased to 240 mg/kg/day in cases of associated meningitis. Chloramphenicol may be used in the penicillin-allergic infant (50 mg to 100 mg/kg/day, q 6 hours); this dose is halved for neonates. In patients > age 5 or in patients whose infection is clearly related to a skin lesion, *H. influenzae* coverage may not be necessary. Nafcillin, (150 mg/kg/day, q 6 hours) or, for the penicillin-allergic patient, vancomycin, (40 mg/kg/day, q 6 hours) is recommended.

DISPOSITION

Any sign of true orbital (postseptal) involvement should prompt an urgent surgical consult. It may be necessary to perform decompression of the orbit to avoid damage to the optic nerve, and surgical drainage of the sinuses or any abscesses. Mild preseptal cellulitis in the adult may be treated on an outpatient basis, but only if the patient can be re-examined by an ophthalmologist the next day. If outpatient treatment is chosen, the first dose of the selected oral antibiotic should be given before discharge from the ED. If the periorbital swelling is considerable or involvement deep to the preseptal tissues is evident, intravenous antibiotics should be started in the ED. Children with periorbital cellulitis should be assessed with caution and an awareness that only the mildest of infections may be managed on an outpatient basis.

COMMON PITFALLS

- The most important task is to differentiate periorbital (preseptal) from orbital (postseptal) infections.
- All but the mildest cases of periorbital cellulitis warrant admission.
- Periorbital cellulitis may be easily confused with allergic periorbital swelling.
- Tests of little value in the differentiation of periorbital from orbital cellulitis include the WBC count, sinus films, cultures of eyelid aspirate or eye secretions, and routine cerebrospinal fluid cultures (in the absence of meningeal signs). Blood cultures in adults are of minimal value as well.
- Contrast-enhanced CT appears to be no more useful than an uninfused study in differentiating the type and extent of infection.
- Ultrasound may be significantly less useful in patients under age 4 because of the redundant mucosa.
- Patients under age 5 must be covered for *H. influenzae*.
- Periorbital and orbital cellulitis are seen infrequently. The key to treatment is rapid differentiation of the two conditions: proptosis, ophthalmoplegia, or loss of visual acuity suggests postseptal or true orbital cellulitis.

PART II

Emergency Aspects of Dental and Oral Surgery

5 Toothache and Common Periodontal Problems

Toothaches and "gum problems" are common presenting complaints. Attention should be paid to those patients who require prophylactic antibiotic coverage before any dental manipulations (e.g., history of rheumatic fever or orthopedic joint replacements). Recommendations for the prevention of bacterial endocarditis are outlined by the American Heart Association and should be reviewed before treatment. If signs of systemic toxicity are present, (major facial swelling, erythema, cellulitis, fever, and elevated white blood cell count) refer to the chapter on odontogenic facial infections.

ORAL EXAMINATION

The patient's face should be examined for external signs of dental disease, such as facial edema, erythema, and obvious lesions. The lymph nodes in the head and neck should then be palpated to document possible systemic involvement. The patient's maximum interincisal opening (usually 35–50 mm) should be checked by measuring between maxillary and mandibular incisors to rule out trismus. If the distance is diminished, this may indicate spread of dental infection outside the confines of the jaws. The soft tissues of the lips, buccal mucosa, vestibules, gingiva, tongue, palate, and floor of the mouth should be scanned for lesions. Ulcerations, parulis (gum boil) formation, erythema, swelling, purulence from the gingival crevice, and lesions of the edentulous ridge caused by irritation from a dental prosthesis should be noted. Next, the examiner should percuss each tooth on its occlusal surface with a tongue blade, checking for sensitivity. If sensitivity to percussion is found, the exact tooth location should be noted. If mobility is present, this is often indicative of advanced periodontal disease. With gloved fingers, the floor of the mouth should be bimanually palpated for masses.

CAUSES OF TOOTHACHE

DENTAL CARIES

Dental caries is characterized by the gradual demineralization and destruction of the hard dental tissues (enamel, dentin, and cementum). Treatment includes excavation and restoration of damaged dental structure by the general dentist.

PULPITIS

Pulpitis is defined as an inflammation of the confined structures within the dental pulp (connective, vascular, and nervous tissue), resulting in pain. The most common cause of pulpitis is infection secondary to deep dental caries. Acute pulpitis is characterized by intermittent attacks of sharp, throbbing pain and thermal sensitivity. Chronic pulpitis exhibits an intermittent dull pain and is less sensitive to thermal changes. A true pulpitis without periapical abscess formation will not be percussion sensitive. Treatment of acute and chronic pulpitis consists of removal of the cause (excavation of dental caries) and pulp capping or root canal therapy (endodontics). Emergency treatment is usually confined to prescribing analgesic medication and arranging for follow-up care. With severe pain, urgent dental consultation may be advisable.

PERIAPICAL (PERIRADICULAR) ABSCESS

When untreated, pulpitis due to dental caries can progress to pulpal necrosis and, eventually, periapical abscess. The involved tooth is usually nonvital and sensitive to both percussion and thermal testing. The toothache is characterized by an acute onset of constant, gnawing pain. The area adjacent to the tooth may be erythematous, tender, and distended. The treatment of choice of necrotic pulp with periapical abscess is either conventional root canal therapy or extraction of the involved tooth. The localized fluctuant buccal vestibular or palatal swelling secondary to periapical abscess should be incised and drained in the ED under local anesthesia. Gram's stain, culture, and sensitivity should be obtained. If the infection spreads and treatment is delayed, extension into the fascial planes of the head and neck may occur, resulting in a more serious odontogenic infection. Oral antibiotics (penicillin V potassium, 500 mg every 6 hours, or, if penicillin-allergic, erythromycin, 500 mg every 6 hours) are indicated as well as instructions for warm saline rinses (four times a day) and warm compresses. The patient should be given a follow-up appointment with the dental consultant as soon as possible.

A common pitfall is to delay incision and drainage of a localized abscess, which results in a more serious odontogenic infection.

PERIODONTAL DISEASE

The periodontium consists of the supportive dental structures, which are the gingiva, periodontal ligament, and alveolar bone. Periodontal disease is the inflammation and degeneration of these structures.

GINGIVITIS AND PERIODONTITIS

Gingivitis is the inflammation of the gingiva. It is most commonly caused by poor oral hygiene, but may be related to systemic disorders (AIDS, leukopenic disorders, allergic reactions, and diabetes mellitus), hormonal imbalances (puberty and pregnancy), and drug reactions (birth control pills, nifedipine, dilantin, and heavy metals). Treatment consists of control of local (plaque) and systemic factors. If gingivitis is left untreated, it can progress to periodontitis. Periodontitis is the extension of inflammation to the underlying bone with resultant bone loss. The cause and clinical presentation are similar to those of gingivitis, with the addition of tooth mobility. Neither gingivitis nor periodontitis is considered a dental emergency. However, either may be an indicator of systemic disease and should be referred to the general dentist.

PERIODONTAL ABSCESS (PARULIS)

With the progression of periodontitis and its associated bone loss, periodontal pockets form around the tooth. In these abnormally deep pockets both plaque and food debris accumulate. If a periodontal pocket becomes secondarily infected, a parulis, or gum boil, may form. Unlike the periapical abscess, the tooth associated with the periodontal abscess is vital and dental caries may not be present. Treatment consists of incision and drainage (under local anesthesia). The patient should be instructed in the use of warm saline rinses (four times a day) and referred to the dental consultant. Antibiotic therapy is not indicated unless the abscess is extensive. Follow-up care with a dental practitioner should be arranged as soon as possible.

PERICORONITIS

Pericoronitis is the inflammation and eventual infection of the gingival tissue (operculum) overlying the crown of an impacted tooth (usually a lower wisdom tooth). It is generally caused by normal oral bacterial flora (e.g., *Streptococcus* and *Bacteroides*). Occlusal trauma from the opposing maxillary third molar and a decrease in host defenses are contributing factors. Pericoronitis may present as a localized mild infection or as a severe infection with trismus, head and neck fascial space involvement, and systemic toxicity. Early pericoronitis presents as a reddened, tender swelling overlying the mandibular third molar or associated impacted tooth. A purulent exudate may be present. Emergency treatment may range from gentle gingival curettage, irrigation, or operculectomy to extraction of the opposing maxillary third molar tooth by the oral and maxillofacial surgeon. Appropriate antibiotics should be prescribed (penicillin v potassium, 500 mg every 6 hours, or erythromycin, 500 mg every 6 hours). If untreated, pericoronitis may progress and necessitate hospitalization for incision and drainage.

ACUTE NECROTIZING ULCERATIVE GINGIVITIS (VINCENT'S GINGIVITIS, TRENCH MOUTH)

Acute necrotizing ulcerative gingivitis is characterized by the development of painful, hyperemic gingivitis and punched-out erosion of the interdental papilla. It is noncontagious and thought to be caused by fusiforum bacteria and spirochetes. The disease generally occurs in the young adult and has a strong correlation with stress, nutritional deficiencies, smoking, and lack of adequate oral hygiene. The patient may present with fetid breath, fever, cervical lymphadenopathy, malaise, red and swollen gingiva, bleeding, pain, and necrosis of interdental papillae. The ulcerated area may be covered with a gray pseudomembrane. Definitive treatment consists of analgesic therapy, oral hydration, rest, and debridement of local factors (plaque and calculus) by the dental consultant. Palliative treatment with a mild anesthestic solution (equal parts by volume of kaolin-pectin suspension, viscous lidocaine, and diphenhydramine elixir) may be prescribed by the emergency physician. Oral antibiotics (penicillin or erythromycin) should be given, and follow-up care should be arranged.

RECURRENT APHTHOUS ULCERS (CANKER SORES)

Aphthous ulcers present as painful, recurring intraoral ulcerations of the mucous membrane. The lesions range in size from 2 mm to 20 mm and may be multiple. They appear initially as raised, red papules and progress to ulcerative lesions. The course may last for 7 to 14 days, with pain occurring during the ulcerative stage. Treatment is symptomatic. Both the anesthetic rinse described earlier and a tetracycline mouthwash (250 mg tetracycline in 5 mL H_2O four times a day) have been used with some success. One must be careful to avoid confusing recurrent aphthous ulcers with primary herpetic gingival stomatitis, variations of erythema multiforme, and other lesions of the mucous membrane. The patient should be referred to the dental consultant for evaluation, treatment, and follow-up care.

PRIMARY HERPETIC GINGIVOSTOMATITIS

Primary herpetic gingivostomatitis generally occurs in infants and young adults. It is caused by the herpes simplex virus type 1 and presents with pain, fever, headache, and regional lymphadenopathy. This is followed by oral vesicular ulcerative lesions that may become secondarily infected. The process is self-limited, and lesions heal in 7 to 14 days. Treatment includes supportive care, analgesic rinses, and prophylactic antibiotics.

DENTURE STOMATITIS

Ill-fitting dentures or chronic denture use may cause a localized or generalized inflammation of the underlying mucosa. The area may become red and painful. In addition, poor oral hygiene or contact allergy to the methyl methacrylate denture material may exacerbate the problem. Treatment consists of removal of the dentures at night or adjustment of the ill-fitting denture by the dental consultant. *Candida albicans* infections are often associated with denture stomatitis and can be treated with nystatin ointment or oral suspension.

ASPIRIN BURN

Aspirin (acetylsalicylic acid) as a home remedy applied topically on painful teeth or gums is common. The resultant burn causes a white irregular patch on the mucous membrane. As the necrotic tissue sloughs off, it leaves a painful, raw, red, bleeding surface. Normal mucosal healing occurs after discontinuance of topical aspirin use. Numerous cases of accidental acetaminophen or aspirin overdosage occur *in adults* as a result of toothaches.

6   Postoperative Complications from Oral and Maxillofacial Surgery

Oral surgery involves major facial surgery done in the hospital (e.g., osteotomies of facial bones) and minor procedures done in the office (e.g., removal of teeth). Patients who present to the ED may be referred directly from the surgeon's office after an intraoperative complication, or may have developed a problem several hours or days after hospital discharge or completion of office surgery. OMFS postoperative complications are unique for two reasons: (1) the airway may be compromised and (2) the patient may be in intermaxillary fixation (teeth wired together).

The evaluation must include: (1) assure adequate airway; (2) obtain history of surgical procedure (what, when, and by whom); and (3) after initial evaluation and stabilization, contact treating surgeon.

INTERMAXILLARY FIXATION

Intermaxillary fixation (IMF), wiring the upper and lower teeth together, is a common method of stabilizing the upper and lower jaws to allow for healing of jaw osteotomy procedures, jaw fractures, and jaw reconstruction procedures. Complications are rare, and the need to release the IMF on an emergency basis is infrequent. If release of IMF during the first 4 weeks postoperatively should be necessary, reoperation may need to be undertaken or a compromised surgical result will occur. The typical duration of fixation is 4 to 8 weeks, during which time the patient must consume only liquids. Speech is usually difficult to understand, and most patients lose 10% to 20% of their weight while the jaws are wired together. If an acrylic surgical bite splint is interposed between the teeth, the oral airway can be greatly restricted. Edema can further restrict the oral airway. If, in addition to a restricted oral airway, the patient has a restricted nasal airway, then adequate breathing becomes difficult. During the first 2 weeks postoperatively when IMF is used and some surgical edema remains, some patients become anxious about breathing and adequate nutrition, and may present to the ED. Reassurance and possibly a nasopharyngeal airway are all that are needed for treatment. Vomiting while in IMF is frightening to a patient but should not require release of IMF, since only liquids can be regurgitated.

Release of IMF can be done on an emergency basis when access to the airway is mandatory: (a) trauma in a patient previously in IMF; (b) significant airway restriction from acute infection or surgical edema; and (c) a severe medical emergency, such as status epilepticus, septic shock, or cardiac arrest. Release of IMF is accomplished by using small wire cutters to cut all the wires that cross from one dental arch to the other (all wires traversing from the upper teeth to the lower teeth). There may be from three to eight wire loops (6–16 wires) to cut. Occasionally rubber bands are used to hold the teeth together, and these can be cut with a scalpel or scissors. Release of IMF with wires may be time-consuming to those untrained in placing IMF. Consider emergency blind nasotracheal intubation or cricothyroidostomy in extreme situations. If wires are cut and not removed, small loose wires will remain in the mouth.

MANAGEMENT

1. Analyze blood gases;
2. Monitor the patient with a pulse oximeter;
3. Assess work of breathing and possibility of fatigue;
4. Consider nasopharyngeal airway;
5. Release IMF in extreme cases;
6. Consider cricothyroidostomy when immediate airway access is necessary and no experienced person is available to release wire IMF.

BLEEDING

Bleeding is one of the more common postoperative complications. The bleeding may be coming from the mouth or nose, or both. There is normally a small amount of bleeding that mixes with saliva during the first 12 hours after many intraoral procedures. Significant hemorrhage must be differentiated from this type of bleeding. Problematic hemorrhage is usually apparent during an office procedure or within the first 12 hours. Prolonged bleeding from a simple tooth extraction in the absence of a coagulopathy is usually minor, and controlled with oral gauze packs. For removal of lower wisdom teeth the occurrence of problem bleeding intraoperatively is 0.5% to 1.1% and postoperatively 0.5% to 0.8%. Possible sources of bleeding include the extraction socket, inferior alveolar artery, posterior superior alveolar artery, long buccal artery, facial artery, palatine artery, lingual artery, and maxillary artery.

MANAGEMENT

1. Suction the patient's mouth and determine the site of the bleeding;
2. Apply pressure using gauze packs and nasal packing;
3. Keep the patient's head elevated 45 degrees;
4. Decide whether the bleeding is caused by an anatomical problem or by coagulopathy, including excessive aspirin use;
5. Consider hematocrit and coagulation screen, type and cross match, and intravenous fluids;
6. Consider OMFS or ENT consultant for persistent or severe hemorrhage for possible suturing, electrocautery, or extraoral cutdown on facial, lingual, or external carotid arteries. Emergency ligation of the external carotid artery is seldom necessary, with local control preferred.

BLEEDING AFTER TOOTH EXTRACTION OR ALVEOLAR BONE SURGERY

The most significant hemorrhage related to alveolar bone surgery in the mandible is from damage to the inferior alveolar neurovascular bundle that runs in a bony canal below the roots of the posterior teeth. Damage to this structure can occur during surgical removal of teeth, odontogenic tumors, and cysts and the placement of endosseous dental implants.

MANAGEMENT

1. Place 4 × 4-in gauze packs directly over socket and have the patient bite down.
2. If, after two 30-minute sessions of biting on gauze, bleeding continues, then 1/4-in iodoform gauze, or Surgicel (oxidized cellulose) can be packed directly into bleeding sock-

ets or bone cavity, and 4 × 4-in gauze packs again placed over the area with the patient biting down. In order to place the packing into the socket, it may be necessary to administer a local anesthetic (e.g., 1% lidocaine with 1/200,000 epinephrine) into the mucosa circumferentially around the bleeding socket, and to perform an inferior alveolar nerve block in the mandible.

3. Electrocautery or sutures may be required. These should be done by the OMFS or ENT consultants.

SWELLING

Patients may present with acute swelling after OMFS procedures because of concern over the airway or swallowing, or for an explanation. The swelling may be from a hematoma, surgical edema, acute cellulitis, or abscess.

HEMATOMA AND SURGICAL EDEMA

Office procedures that may result in hematoma or surgical edema significant enough to warrant an ED visit are procedures in the floor of the mouth (e.g., excision of mandibular tori, excision of sublingual gland, and removal of stone from salivary gland duct).

MANAGEMENT

The airway is the primary concern.

1. Have the patient sit up and lean forward.
2. Perform appropriate monitoring (e.g., pulse oximeter), and consider admission for observation. With obvious airway compromise, consider the following interventions, in order of preference: insertion of a nasopharyngeal airway, oral or nasal endotracheal intubation, cricothyroidostomy, or tracheotomy.
3. Prophylactic antibiotics should be considered with both hematoma and surgical edema in the floor of the mouth to avoid development of a Ludwig's angina type of infection.

POSTEXTRACTION INFECTION

The most likely situation for a patient presenting to the ED is the rapid progression of an infection after removal of an impacted mandibular wisdom tooth, which can involve several tissue spaces, including parapharyngeal. Edema and infection in the masticator space causes trismus (limited mouth opening due to muscle spasm). This makes examination of the oropharynx difficult. The incidence of infection is 0.6% to 2.5%.

MANAGEMENT

1. Obtain the patient's history, including when and by whom the surgery was done, any immunocompromise, any preoperative infection and antibiotic use, current antibiotic.
2. Determine if significant limitation of mouth opening exists, and examine oropharynx for any parapharyngeal swelling.
3. Check temperature and extent of swelling (e.g., does it involve submandibular, submental spaces and extend across the midline?).
4. If the airway is compromised, consider insertion of a nasopharyngeal airway; cricothyroidostomy or tracheostomy is seldom necessary but must be considered for severe cases.
5. Consider hospital admission for intravenous antibiotics and surgical incision and drainage (I & D) in the operating room. Consult the OMF or ENT surgeon.
6. If the amount of trismus and swelling is minimal, oral antibiotics and daily outpatient follow-up for 3 to 4 days are essential.

SWELLING OF SALIVARY GLANDS DUE TO OBSTRUCTION OF DUCTS

Acute swelling of the submandibular gland(s) and, occasionally, the parotid can occur because of surgical edema or a suture obstructing the opening, as a result of intraoral surgery or placement of intraoral acrylic surgical stents. The swelling typically will be only mildly tender, without signs of infection. The patient may present hours to 3 days postoperatively.

EMERGENCY DEPARTMENT MANAGEMENT

1. The salivary ducts should be examined for any obstruction that can be eliminated (e.g., sutures or acrylic stents) and the OMF surgeon consulted. If edema is the only cause of the obstruction, the swelling will resolve in 3 to 4 days.
2 Prophylactic antibiotics may be important, especially if the surgery that has resulted in the swelling was for removal of a salivary duct stone that was causing chronic partial obstruction.

ASPIRATION OR SWALLOWING OF FOREIGN BODIES

Usually not a life-threatening condition, an evaluation can be done to determine the probable location of the object and whether arrangements need to be made to remove it. Teeth, dental restorations, bone, drill bit or dental instruments may all be swallowed or aspirated.

EMERGENCY DEPARTMENT MANAGEMENT

1. Obtain a description of the object and the events surrounding the aspiration or swallowing incident.
2. Order a chest x-ray or abdominal radiograph, to determine whether the object is in the lungs, stomach, or bowel.
3. Consider a pulmonary or gastrointestinal consult to remove the object by flexible fiberoptic endoscopy. Small, blunt objects may be allowed to pass through the gastrointestinal tract without intervention. Sharp or pointed objects in the gastrointestinal tract and all objects in the lungs should be removed as quickly as possible.

7   Temporomandibular Joint Disease

TEMPOROMANDIBULAR SYNDROME

Temporomandibular myofascial pain dysfunction syndrome, (TMJ syndrome) is a complex neuro-muscular disturbance, possibly resulting from and definitely aggravated by occlusal disturbances and the anatomy of the temporomandibular joint. Patients complain of nonspecific unilateral facial pain generalized to the region of the temporomandibular joint. The pain is dull, and increases throughout the day with continued jaw motion. Clinical examination frequently reveals spasm of the masseter muscle externally and the internal pterygoid intraorally. There is usually limitation of opening, with deviation toward the affected side. Temporomandibular joint x-rays are usually normal unless there is associated temporomandibular degenerative joint disease.

Routine radiographic evaluation of the temporomandibular joints should include a panoramic view, which is the easiest to read and requires the least sophisticated technique. The emergency physician can also order a temporomandibular joint series or tomograms of the joints, which should be taken in both open and closed positions. Tomograms avoid superimposition of other anatomical structures that make a regular temporomandibular joint series difficult to read. The panoramic survey and tomograms are necessary to distinguish arthritis, temporomandibular pain dysfunction syndrome, or internal derangement. Degenerative joint disease may involve one or both of the temporomandibular joints. Films may demonstrate flattening of the condylar head, erosions, or osteophyte formation. Rheumatoid arthritis should also be considered, but a good history should clarify the diagnosis. When any type of internal derangement is suspected, a computed tomographic scan of the joints should be ordered to assess bony architecture (i.e., arthritis). Magnetic resonance imaging is used to assess disk position, and arthrography can be used to assess disk position or perforation.

MANAGEMENT AND DISPOSITION

Temporomandibular joint pain or dysfunction, regardless of cause, is treated initially by a combination of physiotherapy (moist heat for 15 minutes four times a day) and a soft diet for approximately 2 weeks. Analgesics such as aspirin or aspirin-codeine combinations are effective in addition to muscle relaxants and tranquilizers such as diazepam. Bite plates (occlusal splints) are used to reposition the mandible to relieve spasm, correct oral habits, and "recapture" a displaced disk.

A documented internal derangement is usually referred to an oral and maxillofacial surgeon, who may perform arthroscopy or arthroplasty to permanently correct disk position or reconstruct arthritic joints.

COMMON PITFALLS

- Temporomandibular joint dysfunction is often called the "great imposter" because it mimics so many other facial pain syndromes.
- A failure to understand disk displacement and confuse it with muscle spasm. A history of joint noise is critical in this regard.

TEMPOROMANDIBULAR JOINT DISLOCATION

In acute dislocation of the mandible, the condyle moves too far anteriorly in relation to the eminence and becomes locked (the mouth is in open position as opposed to closed-lock). Subsequent muscular trismus prevents the condyles from moving back into the temporal fossa. The spasm and associated edema result in extreme discomfort and anxiety for the patient. Dislocation is likely to occur during maximum opening (yawning or laughing). Radiographs should be taken to rule out fracture. Relieve the patient's anxiety and intense muscle spasm with intravenous diazepam, 5 mg to 10 mg, titrated by slow injection. When the patient is sufficiently relaxed, the emergency physician should face the patient and grasp the mandible with both hands, one hand on each side with the thumbs (wrapped with gauze) placed on the occlusal surfaces of the posterior teeth. The fingertips are placed around the inferior border of the mandible in the region of the angle. Downward pressure is applied to free the condyles from their anterior position to the eminence. The chin is then pressed backward after the jaw has been forced downward. The mouth closes and the condyle returns into its position in the fossa. Postreduction instructions include a soft diet for 1 week, avoidance of wide opening of the mandible, and the use of analgesics and muscle relaxants. Severe cases may require intermaxillary wiring and fixation for added control. Patients should be referred to an oral surgeon for follow-up, since surgical alteration of the eminence may be necessary.

8   Dental, Oral, and Salivary Gland Infections

The presentation of dental, oral, and salivary gland infections can vary from a simple complaint of pain or gingival swelling to toxicity with massive facial swelling and a compromised airway. Variable factors include the origin and location of the infection and the degree to which the infection has been contained or spread to the deep spaces of the head and neck. The most common focus of infection is odontogenic, in addition trauma or surgery that may violate the natural anatomical barriers of the fascial planes of the head and neck, resulting in deep-space infection.

The key to diagnosis and management of dental infections and space infections of the head and neck is an understanding of the fascial planes of the head and neck. Cellulitis of odontogenic origin usually involves the middle and lower half of the face and neck. Although such infections are generally well contained, in a debilitated host or in the case of a virulent organism rapid spread of infection may have potentially lethal morbidity. The fascial spaces of the head and neck are potential spaces filled with loose areolar tissue that can rapidly break down when subjected to infection. In the case of oral infection the deep cervical fascia is the most important. The deep cervical fascia consists of several layers that surround the neck, including the superficial and investing layer that attaches to the inferior border of the mandible and splits to form the masticator space. Other spaces of importance include the lateral pharyngeal space (lateral to the pharynx and medial to the masticator space), the retropharyngeal space (between the deep cervical and prevertebral fascia), and the pharyngomaxillary space (from the base of the skull to the hyoid bone), which communicates with all deep spaces. The mylohyoid muscle of the mandible divides the sublingual (superior) and submaxillary (inferior) spaces. The submental space is anterior to the sublingual space. Infection involving the submaxillary, sublingual, and submental spaces with elevation of the tongue is called Ludwig's angina, a serious infection with a potential for airway obstruction. Infections that affect the midface involve the canine space, which is commonly infected by abscessed anterior maxillary teeth, and the buccal space, which is superficial to the buccinator and frequently infected by the molar teeth. Infections in these areas are especially important because of the possibility of cavernous sinus thrombosis due to the facial venous system.

EMERGENCY DEPARTMENT MANAGEMENT

Initial management begins with localization of the infection. Most infections will be of odontogenic origin and localized to a specific tooth. Patients with dental pain should be examined for the presence of infection. Pain to percussion with a tongue blade indicates involvement at the apex of the tooth (periapical abscess). Tender swelling over the gingiva adjacent to a tooth may indicate either a periodontal abscess or extension of a periapical abscess through the cortex of bone into the subperiosteal space. Differentiating these entities without a dental radiograph can be difficult. Management in either case would consist of incision, drainage, and antibiotic therapy (phenoxymethyl-penicillin or erythromycin, 250 mg four times a day). A fluctuant abscess requires drainage. In these localized infections, there is no need to open the abscess beyond a stab incision. The drain will allow for continued drainage and the source of the infection will be eliminated with extraction of the tooth, root canal (endodontic) therapy, or periodontal therapy.

The presence of cellulitis indicates that there has been spread of infection. Determine the following: (a) the extent of involvement of contiguous spaces, (b) potential for spread of infection to the fascial planes of the head and neck, and (c) potential for airway compromise. Once extensive involvement is recognized, the oral and maxillofacial surgeon should determine the site of the initial focus so that pus can be evacuated in the operating room.

The presence of more serious infections is indicated by fever, and involvement of the internal pterygoid or the masseter muscle will result in trismus (muscle spasm causing inability to open the mandible). The presence of trismus limits visibility of the oropharynx and makes the clinical diagnosis of retropharyngeal involvement difficult. If a toxic patient with trismus should vomit, the danger of aspiration is high, since the emesis cannot be quickly evacuated. Therefore, patients with severe trismus need an aggressive workup (including a computed tomographic scan of the retropharyngeal space) and admission for hydration and parenteral antibiotics. The oral cavity may be visualized under general anesthesia at the time of incision and drainage. The presence of Ludwig's angina requires aggressive attention to the airway. This may include nasoendotracheal intubation, tracheostomy, or observation in an intensive care environment in which such procedures can be rapidly undertaken.

Penicillin is the antibiotic of choice for the treatment of most orofacial infections, with the exception of some *Bacteroides* species. Second- or third-generation cephalosporins are useful in cases that involve *Bacteroides* or penicillin allergy, although crossover sensitivity must be considered. Clindamycin is a useful alternative, but potential side effects should be monitored, especially when oral therapy is initiated. Erythromycin is also a useful alternative, but it is more difficult to administer intravenously. Chloramphenicol is reserved for extreme situations in which there is no alternative therapy.

EMERGENCY DEPARTMENT DISPOSITION

THE ROLE OF THE CONSULTANT   Patients with a simple periapical abscess can be managed with intraoral saline rinses, analgesia, and oral antibiotics. A simple incision and drainage may be indicated. Follow-up should be arranged the next day with the oral and maxillofacial surgeon or the family dentist.

INDICATIONS FOR ADMISSION   All patients with suspicion of extension of infection to the fascial spaces of the head and neck should be admitted. Facial cellulitis with closure of the eye indicates potential spread of infection to the periorbital spaces and increased potential for cavernous sinus thrombosis. Patients with extensive trismus cannot be adequately evaluated by clinical examination. Patients with Ludwig's angina or impending Ludwig's angina (i.e., involvement of the three spaces without elevation of the tongue) are at risk for immediate airway obstruction and should be admitted. Such airway obstruction can occur precipitously and without warning, so anticipation is necessary. In most cases the patient will be admitted to the oral and maxillofacial surgeon. When the cause of the infection is not clear the patient may be managed by an otorhinolaryngologist.

COMMON PITFALLS

- All patients with complaints of orofacial pain or swelling must be carefully examined for the presence of infection and extension of infection from the initial focus.
- The emergency physician should aggressively manage infection that may be extending or has a high probability of extending, especially if the infection has the potential to spread to the mediastinum or involve the airway.
- Follow-up should always be recommended within 12 to 24 hours.
- The patient should always be encouraged to return to the ED in the case of high fever, increased swelling, inability to open the mouth, difficulty swallowing, or inability to open the eye.

PART III

Emergency Aspects of Otolaryngology

9   Adult Epiglottitis

Inflammatory disorders of the laryngeal region may primarily affect either supraglottic structures (supraglottitis, epiglottitis) or infraglottic structures (laryngotracheitis). *Supraglottitis* more appropriately defines the pathologic condition under discussion because the pathologic changes involve not only the epiglottis, but also the aryepiglottic folds and false cords. Epiglottitis does occur in adults, particularly in people aged 30 to 70 years. The causes of epiglottitis include infectious agents, physical agents, trauma, burns, and some medical disorders. The identification of a responsible infectious agent in adult epiglottitis has been difficult. Cultures are not only inadequate, but may also be frankly misleading. Blood cultures are not helpful, with the yield somewhere between 10% and 40%. The agent most commonly isolated in the blood is *Haemophilus influenzae* type B. Parainfluenza virus, adenoviruses, respiratory syncytial virus, and herpes virus have been suggested, but there is no evidence to confirm these as pathogens. *S. pneumoniae* epiglottitis has been associated with immunocompromise (malignancies and steroid dependency). Respiratory distress correlates with the degree of narrowing of the airway and indicates increased resistance to air flow.

CLINICAL PRESENTATION

The presentation of epiglottitis in an adult is often less dramatic than its presentation in a child. The typical presentation includes a sore throat out of proportion to physical findings, dysphagia, a muffled "hot potato" voice, and respiratory distress. The course of adult epiglottitis may vary from a fulminating course over hours to a subacute course over days or weeks. The clinical course of *H. influenzae* epiglottitis in an adult is usually severe, with rapidly developing airway obstruction. Any patient with a possible diagnosis of epiglottitis or airway obstruction should be evaluated for urgent and rapid nonsurgical and surgical airway control.

DIFFERENTIAL DIAGNOSIS

Possible associated conditions include peritonsillar or retro pharyngeal abscess, lingual tonsillitis, foreign body, angioedema, pharyngitis, drug allergy, inhalation or ingestion of toxic substances, acute thyroiditis, and epiglottic hematoma.

EMERGENCY DEPARTMENT EVALUATION

The potential exists for sudden airway obstruction and death despite a "benign" presentation. There is no typical time course for epiglottitis. The period from onset to presentation may be hours to days. Sore throat and dysphagia are consistent symptoms. There may be pain on protrusion of the tongue. Dyspnea, voice changes, and chills are less consistent. In the early stages fever may or may not be present; as the illness develops, however, temperature increases. Twenty percent to 30% of patients become moderately to severely ill with signs of airway compromise, such as drooling, stridor, use of accessory muscles, retraction, and cyanosis. Cervical lymphadenopathy and trismus may be noted. Adults should receive a limited physical examination, appropriate laboratory investigations, and intravenous therapy as indicated. Controversy exists about the instrumentation of the oral cavity to view the pharynx and larynx. Laboratory data are not useful. White blood cell counts are insensitive. Arterial blood gas analyses are predictable, redundant, and perhaps dangerous to the acutely distressed patient. Soft-tissue lateral neck x-rays are valuable in evaluating potential epiglottitis in adults. Several abnormalities may be evident, including enlargement of the epiglottis and aryepiglottic folds and ballooning of the hypopharynx with air. The "gold standard" in the definitive diagnosis of epiglottitis is direct and indirect laryngoscopy. The principal hazard of laryngoscopy is sudden, total airway obstruction; this procedure should not be performed by novices. For patients in moderate to severe respiratory distress, laryngoscopy should be performed with anesthetic and surgical staff and appropriate equipment to perform cricothyroidostomy, tracheostomy, and rigid bronchoscopy. Patients with no signs suggesting potential airway obstruction may undergo laryngoscopy in the ED if appropriate precautions are taken. Indirect laryngoscopy requires considerable technical facility. Direct laryngoscopy should be performed with a flexible fiberoptic instrument introduced nasally by an experienced operator. Diagnosis hinges on the ability of the operator to identify abnormal supraglottic structures.

EMERGENCY DEPARTMENT MANAGEMENT

The patient with possible epiglottitis should be evaluated in a resuscitation area and should not be left alone due to the risk of sudden airway obstruction. A vital piece of equipment is a bag for ventilation that does *not* have a positive-pressure relief valve ("pop off" valve). These bags are commercially available. Even a patient with a totally obstructed airway can usually be ventilated with such a device in experienced hands. Cooperative effort must involve the departments of emergency medicine, anesthesiology, and surgery (ear, nose, and throat). Airway management is controversial. Sudden upper airway obstruction is unpredictable in the patient with epiglottitis. Mortality is excessive when watchful waiting has been practiced. without active airway intervention. Opinion is divided on whether all patients with epiglottitis should be intubated prophylactically or should be observed until airway difficulty becomes apparent. Prophylactic airway intervention has reduced mortality in children. The benefits of intubation in adults outweigh the risks. Virtually all deaths caused by epiglottitis are preventable by this simple procedure. Orotracheal intubation under direct vision can be used. Once the airway has been established, a nasotracheal route may be preferred for patient comfort. The choice of antibiotics is based on the frequency and virulence of *H. influenzae* type B. The organism's resistance to ampicillin has led authorities to recommend that both ampicillin and chloramphenicol be administered until results of cultures and sensitivities are available. As an alternative, third-generation cephalosporins are effective and perhaps less toxic. Some authorities have advocated the use of corticosteroids, but scientific evidence of their efficacy is lacking. In the case of angioedema, however, steroids may be lifesaving. Aerosolized epinephrine and racemic epinephrine are not believed to be useful.

DISPOSITION

All patients should be admitted to an ICU. Recovery is monitored by laryngoscopy. Extubation commonly occurs in the operating room after 48 to 72 hours. Intravenous antibiotics are discontinued, but oral antibiotics should be continued for 14 days, pending culture results. If *H. influenzae* type B is isolated, case contacts should receive rifampin. If there are children younger than age 4 in the patient's household, all household contacts should be treated.

TRANSFER   No patient should be transferred unless airway control has been achieved. Appropriate airway equipment must also be available for intervention during transport.

┌─────────────────────────┐
│   **COMMON PITFALLS**   │
└─────────────────────────┘

- The most common pitfall is failure to consider the diagnosis of adult epiglottitis.
- Airway management for a patient with epiglottitis should be undertaken only by an experienced physician.
- Blind nasal or orotracheal intubation is contraindicated.
- Sudden airway obstruction should be anticipated.

---

10 Laryngitis, Pharyngotonsillitis, Peritonsillar Abscess, and Retropharyngeal Abscess

---

LARYNGITIS

Laryngitis is manifested by hoarseness, acute or chronic, inflammatory or traumatic. The voice change is due to edema of the vocal cords caused either by an inflammatory process or by trauma to the vocal cords. By far the most common cause of acute laryngitis is viral upper respiratory infection (URI). Typical viral agents include parainfluenza viruses 1 and 2, adenoviruses, rhinoviruses, and coronaviruses. Bacterial superinfection, especially in the immunocompromised host may cause a more virulent illness. Staphylococci and H. influenzae have been implicated.

CLINICAL PRESENTATION

Acute laryngitis of inflammatory origin is typical of viral URI and is easily recognized. Typical accompanying symptoms include cough, sore throat, low-grade fever and rhinitis. Hoarseness is due to inflammation of the vocal cords, edema from coughing, or tenacious secretions. The presence of hoarseness should draw immediate attention to the airway. A patient with impending airway obstruction of any etiology will present with complaints of shortness of breath, stridor, air hunger and possibly drooling in addition to a voice change. This is not simple laryngitis and constitutes a medical emergency. Voice change that presents with a more than 3- or 4-week history should be considered chronic, and possible etiologies include vocal cord nodules, vocal cord cysts and granulomas, malignant tumors of the larynx, neurological disorders, and gastroesophageal reflux.

EMERGENCY DEPARTMENT EVALUATION

(1) Is there an impending airway problem? (2) Is the voice change acute or chronic? Question patients regarding onset and duration of the illness, any associated symptoms, underlying medical problems, and any history of injuries to the throat. Most patients with routine URI-associated laryngitis present a few days into their illness. Patients with sudden onset or rapid progression of symptoms are most at risk for a potential airway problem and require a careful evaluation. Patients should be examined for signs of possible airway obstruction (i.e., shortness of breath or stridor). Laboratory investigation in viral laryngitis is not helpful. The only useful test is a soft tis-

sue lateral x-ray of the neck to rule out epiglottitis. Flexible fiberoptic laryngoscopy may be useful for patients in whom a possible airway obstruction is identified.

EMERGENCY DEPARTMENT MANAGEMENT

Acute viral laryngitis requires symptomatic management only. Mucolytic and expectorant agents, such as guafenisin and iodinated glycerol, are useful and well tolerated. These can be combined with decongestants and antitussives as necessary. Antihistamines have no role in this setting. Antibiotics are usually reserved for known immunocompromised states or in patients with a course prolonged more than a week, in which case bacterial superinfection is a possibility. Increased intake of fluids as well as humidification of room air at home are also useful. Voice rest is indicated in and recommended to patients who have overused their vocal cords. Any patient with signs of airway obstruction may require consultation with an otolaryngologist. A soft-tissue lateral x-ray of the neck must be obtained, and a complete blood count and IV fluids considered. Arterial blood gas in a patient with upper airway problems is not useful.

DISPOSITION

Patients with simple URI may be discharged and instructed to follow-up with their physicians if necessary. They are instructed that a 10- to 14-day duration of symptoms is likely. Any patient who presents with chronic laryngitis requires referral to an otolaryngologist for further evaluation of the larynx.

COMMON PITFALLS

- Failure to consider epiglottitis. The physician must remain alert to signs that suggest more than just laryngitis.
- All patients with chronic laryngitis should be referred to an otolaryngologist to rule out malignancy and neurologic disorders.

PHARYNGOTONSILLITIS

Sore throat is one of the most common presenting complaints in any outpatient facility. It affects patients of all ages, and is an integral part of upper respiratory tract infections. Transmission is by person-to-person contact by way of droplets of saliva. The causes of acute pharyngotonsillitis include bacteria, viruses, and fungi. Acute streptococcal pharyngitis caused by Group A beta hemolytic streptococci has received the most attention, since it was demonstrated in the 1950s that rheumatic fever could be prevented by treating the preceding pharyngitis. However, Group A beta hemolytic streptococci account for a minority of sore throats, usually limited to children, teenagers, and young adults. Other groupable streptococci (C and G), as well as *Neisseria gonorrhea, Staphylococcus aureus, Haemophilus influenza,* and *Corynebacterium diphtheriae,* are known causes of pharyngitis. Viral agents are probably the most common cause, including enteroviruses, adenoviruses, herpes simplex, parainfluenza virus, rhinoviruses, and cytomegalovirus. Special mention should be made of the Epstein-Barr virus, the causative pathogen of infectious mononucleosis (IM) and its accompanying pharyngitis, which is readily diagnosed. Candidiasis may be seen in the pharynx of the immunocompromised patient, or in the patient taking antibiotics for other reasons.

CLINICAL PRESENTATION

It is difficult to differentiate bacterial from nonbacterial infection of the pharynx on clinical grounds alone. All forms of pharyngitis may include fever, headache, dehydration, and dysphagia to varying degrees. Examination should include vital signs, palpation of the neck for associated adenopathy, particularly of the "tonsil nodes" at the angle of the jaw, and inspection of the throat. Typically, erythema of the soft palate, tonsils, and pharyngeal mucosa will be seen. It is useful to distinguish exudative from nonexudative pharyngitis. Exudates may appear as white or yellow spots on the tonsils or as patchy white-gray membranes, and are typical of group A beta hemolytic streptococci, IM, or, less commonly, gonorrhea or diphtheria. Nonexudative pharyngitis and ulcerated lesions of the tonsil surface are characteristic of viral pharyngitis other than that associated with IM. Petechiae may be present. The tonsils may be grossly enlarged, especially in young patients with IM. If this is the case, the voice will have a muffled quality. All lymph-node bearing areas as well as the liver and spleen should be palpated if IM is a consideration.

ƒPharyngitis and tonsillitis are somewhat difficult to separate. Arbitrarily, most physicians will call an acute process predominantly manifested by enlarged, erythematous tonsils, with or without exudate, and accompanied by fever and adenopathy an acute tonsillitis. A diffusely erythematous pharynx, without obvious enlargement of the tonsils or in a patient without tonsils is generally considered a pharyngitis. The etiologies and work-up are identical. The only significant difference is in their potential complications. Complications common to both are dehydration secondary to fever and poor oral intake due to difficulty in swallowing, as well as the nonsuppurative complications of strep (rheumatic fever, poststreptococcal glomerulonephritis). Tonsillitis may be additionally complicated by peritonsillar cellulitis and abscess, or partial airway obstruction from very enlarged tonsils.

EMERGENCY DEPARTMENT EVALUATION

Many institutions are using the rapid screens for group A beta hemolytic strep, which are specific, but less sensitive. If such a screen is used, it should be backed up with a standard throat culture if negative. A complete blood count and Monospot (heterophile agglutination) may be done in selected cases, as well as electrolyte levels if dehydration is a concern. A lateral neck film is essential for any patient with shortness of breath, noisy breathing, or stridor accompanying the sore throat. This radiograph is essential to exclude epiglottitis.

EMERGENCY DEPARTMENT MANAGEMENT

Admission should be considered any time a complication of pharyngotonsillitis is identified. The two most common reasons for admission are dehydration and the presence of peritonsillar cellulitis or abscess. Clearly, a patient who is unable to swallow will be unable to maintain adequate oral intake or take medication, and will probably fail to improve on outpatient management. An attempt to hydrate the patient and administer intravenous antibiotics over a period of several hours in the ED is a common alternative, provided suitable facilities are available and prompt family physician or otolaryngology referral is arranged after discharge. Peritonsillar cellulitis or abscess requires consultation with an otolaryngologist.

DISPOSITION

If the patient is not particularly toxic, and if no suppurative complication is suspected, many options for outpatient treatment are available. Some physicians reserve antibiotic therapy for positive throat cultures only. This approach requires a satisfactory method of patient contact in 2 days, when culture results are available, and may miss some patients. Many physicians treat patients strongly suspected of having group A strep infection before culture results are available. This would include patients with exudative tonsillitis, fever, or adenopathy; patients who have a history of rheumatic fever; patients with a history of close contact with someone with proven streptococcal pharyngitis; and any patient with a positive rapid test. Patients may be given two prescriptions—one for 2 days and one for the remaining 8 days, to be filled only if the throat culture is positive. Arrangements for phone contact or outpatient followup in 2 days if mandatory. Viral pharyngitis requires no specific treatment. Patients diagnosed with IM should be instructed to follow up with their family doctors within a week. Up to 25%–30% of patients with IM will have positive strep cultures.

Penicillin remains the drug of choice for streptococcal tonsillitis. It may be given as a single intramuscular dose of 1.2 million units of penicillin G benzathine, if compliance is questionable, or as a 10-day course of oral penicillin, 250 to 500 mg every 6 hours. In the penicillin-allergic patient, erythromycin, 250 to 500 mg every 6 hours is used.

COMMON PITFALLS

- The chronic sore throat, especially in a patient who smokes or drinks, may represent the earliest symptom of cancer, and prompt referral to an otolaryngologist should be arranged. Possible legal implications exist for a delayed diagnosis of cancer.
- Adult epiglottitis is uncommon and easily overlooked. Any patient who complains of a significant sore throat of sudden onset without pharyngeal findings to account for the degree of symptoms, respiratory symptoms accompanying the throat pain, or complains of feeling a "lump" in the throat should have a lateral neck film. Missing this diagnosis can have fatal consequences.

PERITONSILLAR ABSCESS

Peritonsillar abscess is a complication of tonsillitis. It usually occurs in teenagers and young adults, but can occur at any age, especially in people who are immunodeficient or have diabetes. It may occur following infectious mononucleosis. The abscess forms in the potential space that exists between the tonsil capsule and the superior constrictor muscle against which it lies. When tonsillitis spreads beyond the tonsil capsule, inflammation in this space results, leading to abscess if not treated. These are truly polymicrobial abscesses, and cultures will show a mixture of aerobes (usually group A beta hemolytic streptococci, but also pneumococcus, *Haemophilus influenzae*, and *Staphylococcus)* and anaerobes, especially *Bacteroides*.

CLINICAL PRESENTATION

The usual clinical setting is a young patient who has had a sore throat and fever for two or more days. The pain increases, becomes localized to one side, and is accompanied by dysphagia. As symptoms progress the voice becomes muffled, and progressive inability to swallow even saliva results in drooling and dehydration. Most patients notice earache. Some of these symptoms may occur with severe tonsillitis, but it is the lateralization of symptoms that is most suggestive of abscess. Inquiry into respiratory complaints and intercurrent medical problems should be made.

DIFFERENTIAL DIAGNOSIS

It is important to realize that there is a continuum of illness from simple tonsillitis to frank peritonsillar abscess. The patient may present at any point along this pathway, and symptoms and treatment vary accordingly. The first stage—inflammation without suppuration—is peritonsillar cellulitis. There is mild or absent trismus, fullness on the side of the affected tonsil, and unilateral erythema extending onto the soft palate. The palate is not bulging, nor is the uvula displaced. At the other extreme is the overt abscess with marked trismus, making examination of the oral cavity difficult. Once the mouth is opened, the soft palate on the involved side is seen to be markedly erythematous and obviously bulging forward and medially. The tonsil is pushed downward and the uvula pushed toward the opposite side by this expanding mass. It may be difficult to distinguish cellulitis from an early abscess.

All asymmetrical swellings of the oropharynx are not peritonsillar abscesses. Unilateral enlargement of a tonsil may occur from squamous cell carcinoma, lymphoma, leukemia, or vascular lesions and neoplasms of the lateral pharyngeal space. Such an enlargement can usually be distinguished from abscess by history and presentation. Lateral neck abscess of dental origin may be confused with peritonsillar abscess, but a history of a toothache should serve to differentiate the two.

Complications of peritonsillar abscess include extension into contiguous neck spaces, with risk of a deep neck abscess and possible subsequent catastrophic hemorrhage from erosion into the carotid artery or septic thrombosis of the internal jugular vein. Mediastinitis, airway obstruction, sepsis, and necrotizing fasciitis have all been described. Most of these complications occur in diabetics, immunocompromised patients, and neglected cases.

EMERGENCY DEPARTMENT EVALUATION AND MANAGEMENT

After examination a complete blood count, serum electrolytes, Monospot, and throat culture should be obtained. Intravenous fluids should be started to correct the dehydration that is almost invariably present, and intravenous antibiotics begun. Penicillin, 1 million to 2 million units IV every 4 hours, or clindamycin, 600 mg IV every 8 hours, should be given. Consultation with an otolaryngologist will be necessary for definitive management. Cellulitis may be adequately treated with antibiotics alone, although this condition frequently necessitates hospitalization for administration of intravenous fluids and antibiotics and observation for possible abscess formation. Early cellulitis may be treated with oral antibiotics and hydration, provided the patient has been evaluated by an otolaryngologist and follow-up within 24 hours arranged. Needle aspiration, incision and drainage, and acute tonsillectomy all have their advocates. The need for admission will be determined by the consultant and based on the selected form of treatment. Because of the great symptomatic relief that follows evacuation of a peritonsillar abscess, either by incision and drainage or by aspiration, many cases may be safely managed on an outpatient basis after drainage at the discretion of the responsible otolaryngologist. Patients who are toxic, who cannot swallow, who have complicating medical problems, or in whom cellulitis is diagnosed should be admitted.

COMMON PITFALLS

- The most common mistake is failure to recognize an impending abscess.
- Because of the risks and complications involved, needle aspiration and incision and drainage should be attempted only by trained personnel.
- Asymmetrical swelling of the pharynx is always abnormal even if asymptomatic, and necessitates further evaluation.

RETROPHARYNGEAL ABSCESS

The retropharyngeal space lies between the fascia that is densely adherent to the paraspinal muscles and the posterior pharyngeal mucosa that can be seen directly through the open mouth. There are actually three fascial layers with intervening potential spaces. These potential spaces extend to the mediastinum and offer a direct, unimpeded path for the spread of infection. Retropharyngeal abscess is primarily considered a disease of young children, due to suppuration of the lymph nodes into the space. These same nodes involute by puberty. Not surprisingly, the causes of retropharyngeal abscesses in adults are quite different. Trauma is the predominant cause, including iatrogenic injuries secondary to intubation or endoscopy, and ingested foreign bodies, any of which may penetrate the posterior pharyngeal mucosa. Blunt and penetrating neck injuries may cause an abscess, but this is usually a late complication and not likely to be the presenting problem in the ED. Cervical tuberculosis used to be a frequent cause of retropharyngeal abscess in adults. Finally, even in adults, an infection in the sinuses or ears may result in an abscess. The usual organisms are oral organisms. As with most neck abscesses, this process is polymicrobial, with Staphylococcus and anaerobes most commonly recovered.

CLINICAL PRESENTATION

The patient presents with fever, neck pain, and sore throat. Dysphagia and drooling are prominent features. If the abscess is high in the neck, nasal obstruction and a hyponasal voice result. The voice may sound muffled if the swelling is above the level of the larynx, and sounds normal if the abscess is lower in the neck. As the swelling enlarges, difficult or noisy breathing may be observed. Chest pain that may accompany this constellation of symptoms strongly suggests medi-astinal extension. On examination these patients are invariably toxic, dehydrated, and febrile. The head is held stiffly, and passive or active motion of the head is painful. Inspection of the neck does not reveal any redness or swelling, although anterior displacement of the larynx may be appreci-ated. Palpation of the neck reveals deep tenderness only. No fluctuance is felt because the abscess is deep; this negative finding should not mislead the clinician. There is no trismus with an uncomplicated retropharyngeal abscess, and direct visualization of the posterior pharyngeal wall should be possible. It appears erythematous, boggy, and displaced forward toward the uvula if the abscess is located at this level. A process lower in the neck may show no abnormalities on oral examination. Palpation of the posterior wall may confirm the diagnosis, but because of the risk of rupturing the abscess into an already compromised airway, this maneuver is not recommended.

Possible complications are many and serious. The airway is always at risk, either from obstruction of the upper airway by mass effect or from sudden rupture of the abscess with resul-tant aspiration or asphyxia. Direct extension inferiorly into the mediastinum is possible by way of the fascial planes. Extension into the lateral neck spaces may lead to hemorrhage from the great vessels or to jugular vein thrombosis. Overwhelming sepsis may occur, especially in the immuno-compromised patient.

DIFFERENTIAL DIAGNOSIS

The differential diagnosis of retropharyngeal abcess is not extensive. Other deep neck infections or even meningitis may be considered, but examination and radiographs should clarify this. All bulges on the posterior wall are not inflammatory. Hematomas (i.e., in the anticoagulated patient), osteophytes of the cervical spine, the rare neoplasm, or an occasional lymph node may present as a bulge on the posterior wall, but history should distinguish these from an abscess.

EMERGENCY DEPARTMENT EVALUATION

When retropharyngeal abscess is suspected, a complete blood count, blood cultures, and elec-trolytes should be obtained and intravenous fluids started. A soft-tissue lateral radiograph of the neck should be taken immediately, as well as a chest x-ray. The neck film remains the most impor-tant initial diagnostic test in evaluating pathologic processes in the retropharyngeal space. Positive findings include air in the retropharyngeal space, an air-fluid level behind the pharynx or esophagus, and widening of the retropharyngeal soft tissues. More than 7 mm from the anterior border of the body of C-2 and the posterior border of the air column, or more than 22 mm at C-6 is abnormal. Another rule of thumb is that the soft tissues should be no wider than one third the width of a vertebral body at C-2 and no more than the width of the body at C-6. A true abscess usually presents as a localized widening of the space, whereas cellulitis is more diffuse. A normal lateral neck film effectively eliminates this diagnosis. A chest radiograph should be taken to rule out possible mediastinitis. A CT scan of the neck and mediastinum should be obtained as soon as possible in all patients suspected of having a retropharyngeal abscess to confirm the diagno-sis, distinguish cellulitis from frank abscess, and to determine the extent of the abscess.

EMERGENCY DEPARTMENT MANAGEMENT

Intravenous fluids and intravenous antibiotics (penicillin plus penicillinase-resistant penicillin, clindamycin, or cephalosporins) should be started immediately, and consultation with an otolaryngologist sought. Equipment for management of the airway, including a tracheostomy set, must be available, and the patient carefully monitored for respiratory distress. These patients are always admitted to the hospital either to an ICU or directly to the operating room. Management includes incision and drainage in the operating room. Some cases of cellulitis may be adequately treated with intravenous antibiotics alone, but this decision rests with the otolaryngologist.

A retropharyngeal abscess is a true emergency. Mediastinal extension or airway obstruction can occur at any time, and expeditious diagnosis and aggressive treatment, as well as careful monitoring in the ED are necessary to avert a potentially disastrous outcome.

11   Sinusitis

Dysfunction of the sinuses ranges from mild congestion to severe, rapidly progressive infection that can result in lethal complications. The paranasal sinuses are part of the upper respiratory tract, and have direct communication with the nasopharynx. Normally the sinuses are sterile, but their direct proximity to the microflora of the nasopharynx can give rise to infection. Bacterial infection of the sinuses is usually preceded by antecedent dysfunction of the upper respiratory tract secondary to allergic-vasomotor changes, atmospheric pressure changes, chemical irritants, mechanical obstruction, systemic disease, or viral infection. Such processes can incite local tissue reactions, including vasodilation, increased viscosity of mucous secretions, and edema of the involved mucosa. Mechanical trauma to the nasopharynx secondary to nasotracheal intubation or nasogastric tube insertion has been associated with parasinus infection. These predisposing processes result in loss of patency of the relatively narrow channels that drain the sinuses. In adults with acute (<3 weeks) maxillary sinusitis the predominant infecting bacteria are *Haemophilus influenzae* and *Streptococcus pneumoniae*. Other aerobic and anaerobic bacteria have been implicated as the cause of acute maxillary sinusitis, and include beta hemolytic *Streptococcus pyogenes, Staphylococcus aureus,* and *Branhamella catarrhalis*. Chronic maxillary sinus infection (illness >3 months) often fails to grow organisms.

CLINICAL PRESENTATION

The signs and symptoms of acute sinusitis relate to the location of the involved sinuses. The classic description of acute maxillary sinusitis includes malar facial pain, referred ear pain, maxillary dental pain, purulent nasal discharge, and low-grade fever. There may be retro-ocular pain, conjunctivitis, and drainage of purulent material from the middle meatus of the nasal turbinate. Acute frontal sinusitis is associated with pain and tenderness over the lower forehead and purulent drainage from the middle meatus of the nasal turbinates. Bending forward or finger percussion over the forehead frequently exacerbates the pain; there may be associated fever. Acute ethmoidal sinusitis is predominantly a disease of children. It is frequently associated with retro-orbital pain and fever. Chronic sinusitis is characteristically associated with a paucity of signs and symptoms but has most often been associated with chronic purulent nasal discharge without facial pain or significant fever.

Special consideration should be given to any debilitated patient with acute sinus infection. Opportunistic rhinocerebral fungal infection with rapidly progressive extension is characteristic of the phycomycoses (mucormycosis) and is associated with a high mortality. Adults or children with uncontrolled acidosis associated with diabetes, leukemia, renal failure, or immunosuppression who present with signs of unremarkable sinus infection warrant emergency consultation and admission. Suspicion of phycomycetous sinus infection is heightened by the findings of nasopharyngeal necrosis, a dark nasal discharge, bony involvement on sinus films, ocular findings, cranial nerve involvement, or new onset diabetic ketoacidosis.

EMERGENCY DEPARTMENT EVALUATION

In acute maxillary sinusitis, the diagnosis can best be made by finding complete opacification of the sinus to transillumination. Partial opacification or dullness to transillumination is nonspecific and does not correlate with bacteriologic verification of infection. Sinus films are the most important diagnostic test available in the ED. In proven maxillary sinus infection, radiographs that show mucosal thickening greater than 8 mm correlates with infection. Radiographic findings of complete or partial opacification, an air–fluid level, and mucosal thickening are accepted as indirect evidence of infection. A "sinus series" should include Water's, Caldwell, lateral, and submental–vertex views. When indicated, skull tomograms and CT scans can further augment assessment.

EMERGENCY DEPARTMENT MANAGEMENT

In uncomplicated acute sinusitis the goal is to relieve obstruction to sinus drainage. Antibiotics are indicated in fever, sinus pain, purulent nasal discharge, and radiographic evidence of infection.

Ampicillin, 250 to 500 mg orally, four times a day for 10 days
Pseudoephedrine (Sudafed), 30 mg to 60 mg orally, four times a day for 10 days
Oxymetazoline (Afrin), two sprays in each nostril every 4 to 6 hours, for 3 days *only* or phenylephrine nose drops

Acceptable alternatives:

Trimethaprim-sulfamethoxazole
Cefaclor
Erythromycin, 250 to 500 mg orally, four times a day for 10 days
Cephalexin (Keflex), 250 to 500 mg orally, four times a day for 10 days

Other measures include a vaporizer, warm soaks to the face, and analgesia. Improvement usually occurs within 48 to 72 hours after the initiation of therapy. Most patients require a standard 10-day course of treatment. Follow-up in the ED is appropriate for patients who fail to improve after 72 hours of treatment.

DISPOSITION

Healthy patients with uncomplicated sinus infection can be treated as outpatients. If they complete a full course of treatment with total resolution of symptoms with no history of recurrent infection, they do not need further evaluation or referral. Those who fail to totally resolve their symptoms with a course of treatment should be re-evaluated, including repeat sinus radiographs. They should be referred to an otolaryngologist. Special consideration should be given to older patients, the debilitated, the immunocompromised, and diabetics. Such patients are at risk for rhinocerebral fungal infection and should be admitted with emergent specialty consultation. Likewise, patients with a history of chronic, recurrent sinus dysfunction should be referred to the specialist. Toxic patients with sinusitis, or those with any signs or symptoms that suggest CNS involvement, merit emergent consultation (otolaryngologist and neurosurgeon) and admission to ICU. Osteomyelitis, orbital cellulitis, or CNS extension should be suspected in all toxic-appearing patients. Obtain appropriate cultures, intravenous broad-spectrum antibiotics, and perform an emergent CT scan.

COMMON PITFALLS

- The most common error is inadequate treatment. Patients may become asymptomatic during treatment, do not complete a full course of antibiotics, and, harbor an indolent infection with subsequent chronic sinusitis. Stress the importance of completing the full 10 days of antibiotics.
- Failure to refer to a specialist when a history of recurrent or chronic sinus dysfunction is noted. This may be due to systemic disease, allergic rhinitis, nasal polyps, retention cysts, cocaine abuse, or chronic sinusitis. Multiple ED visits for a recurring sinus problem warrant specialty referral.
- Obtaining inadequate or inappropriate radiographic studies to properly document sinus infection is a common error. It is advisable to get a complete "sinus series" in adult patients with probable sinus infection, since multiple sinuses can be involved.
- Failure to consider rhinocerebral fungal infection in high-risk patients. Delay in diagnosis decreases survival. In a high-risk patient with a seemingly unremarkable sinus infection the diagnosis should be suspected and vigorously pursued.

12   Nasal Hemorrhage

Epistaxis occurs with an initial peak in early adolescence and a second, broader peak between the fifth and eighth decades. A seasonal variation exists between January and March.

CLASSIFICATION

Nasal hemorrhage is traditionally classified as either anterior or posterior. Anterior epistaxis can be directly visualized and most easily controlled. It is responsible for approximately 80%–90% of all cases. The most frequent bleeding source is Kiesselbach's plexus or Little's area. Posterior epistaxis is a functional rather than an anatomical term: it cannot be directly visualized, is difficult to access, tends to be more severe, and is not amenable to simple outpatient maneuvers.

EMERGENCY DEPARTMENT EVALUATION

A brief, thorough, directed history and physical examination will provide the information necessary to determine the cause of the bleeding, effect control, and make the appropriate disposition. Key points include the nature, onset, duration, and amount of bleeding, a personal or family history of epistaxis or bleeding disorder, a medication history (especially warfarin sodium [Coumadin]), a history of acute or chronic illness, and the possibility of trauma or foreign body insertion. Physical signs such as ecchymosis, purpura, spider angioma, hemarthrosis, and hepatomegaly may suggest an underlying bleeding disorder.

EMERGENCY DEPARTMENT MANAGEMENT

The ABCs of stabilization should be addressed. An adequate airway should be maintained. If there is hemodynamic compromise, parenteral crystalloid resuscitation should be initiated. Supplemental oxygen and cardiac monitoring may be required. Attention should be directed to the control of the epistaxis. After bleeding is controlled with direct external pressure or in conjunction with plain or vasoconstrictor-soaked pledgets inserted into the nose, the bleeding site must be identified. Removal of clots can be accomplished by having the patient gently blow his nose, by using point suction, or by using moistened cotton swabs to expose the nasal mucosa. Focal areas of anterior epistaxis can frequently be controlled with chemical cautery (silver nitrate application) or the use of small amounts of a topical hemostatic agent. If this fails, consideration can be given to the use of electrocautery. For persistent bleeding an anterior pack consisting of a petroleum jelly–impregnated gauze strip smeared with antibiotic ointment should be placed, using the nasal speculum and bayonet forceps. Patients who require anterior packs should be placed on either penicillin or a first-generation cephalosporin to prevent sinusitis or otitis media arising from obstruction of the sinus ostia or eustachian tubes. The patient should be observed for at least 15 minutes after the procedure to confirm adequate hemostasis.

Failure to control bleeding or the inability to visualize an anterior source denotes a posterior hemorrhage and mandates the application of a posterior pack. A more expedient, perhaps safer, and cost-effective method is to pass a #14 French Foley catheter (or similar commercial device) into the nose and inflate the balloon with air while it is in the nasopharynx. Frequently an anterior pack is required in conjunction with either of these two methods.

Placement of a posterior pack mandates hospital admission. The potential for morbidity is high. Complications include aspiration, hypoxia, and local or systemic infections, including toxic shock. Patients who are overanticoagulated and those with chronic, debilitating illness or recurrent epistaxis are also candidates for admission. For epistaxis unresponsive to the measures described above, otolaryngologic consult is required for consideration of alternative treatments, such as arterial ligation, embolization, or intranasal freezing.

COMMON PITFALLS

- Failure to adequately prepare for control of the epistaxis with necessary equipment causes unnecessary inconvenience and delays.
- Most patients do not require lab studies; reserve for the patient with excessive hemorrhage or suspected coagulopathy.
- Failure to adequately identify the source of anterior epistaxis and properly place the anterior pack results in return visits for hemorrhage control and repacking.

13   Acute Otitis Media in Adults

Acute otitis media is a well recognized disease. Figures 13-1 and 13-2 present the anatomy of the middle ear and tympanic membrane. Acute otitis media is defined as inflammation of the middle ear. An effusion is almost always present in the middle ear space. The effusion is usually assumed to be suppurative (generated by bacterial pathogens), hence the terms acute suppurative, purulent, and bacterial otitis media. Effusions that do not appear to be suppurative are often called

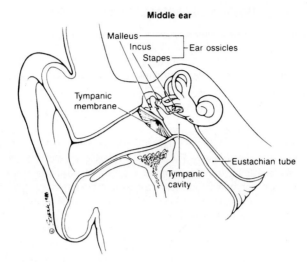

Figure 13-1. Anatomy of the middle ear.

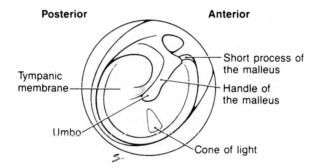

Figure 13-2. Anatomy of the tympanic membrane.

serous or secretory, and may present acutely. Classically, serous effusions are thought to be non-bacterial, although bacteria and other pathogens have been isolated from a serous effusion.

EPIDEMIOLOGY

Although acute otitis media is one of the most common and well-reported diseases of children, it is infrequently reported in adults. Twenty percent (2.4 million) of visits for otitis media occur in patients older than 15 years.

The etiology of acute otitis media has been studied in large pediatric populations over many years. Adult etiologies have been assumed to be similar. One recent prospective study in adults cultured purulent middle ear effusions. The predominant organism was *S. pneumoniae* (62.5%), followed by *S. aureus* (11.5%), H. influenzae (10.5%), *Streptococcus pyogenes* (7.3%), and other bacterial pathogens (8.8%).

CLINICAL PRESENTATION

In adults the usual presenting complaint is ear pain or discomfort. Often only one ear is affected, and the ear may have been the site of previous infection. There is usually a history of concurrent or recent upper respiratory tract infection. Other common presenting complaints are hearing difficulty, tinnitus, and vertigo. Fever may be variably present. Occasionally the adult patient will present with spontaneous rupture of the tympanic membrane and serosanguineous or purulent discharge from the affected ear.

EMERGENCY DEPARTMENT EVALUATION

The evaluation of ear pain should include a thorough examination of the head and neck to rule out other causes. Teeth and gums should be examined and percussed. The oropharynx and nasopharynx should be inspected for inflammation, sinusitis, and other disease entities. Parotid, submandibular, and submaxillary glands should be palpated and the temporomandibular joints examined. The soft tissue around the auricle should be inspected and palpated. The auricle and tragus should be manipulated. The neck should be inspected and palpated, and the carotids auscultated for bruits. The eyes should be briefly examined to rule out signs of glaucoma or other ocular pathology.

The hallmark of the middle ear examination is otoscopic visualization of the tympanic membrane. All wax, debris, and discharge that obstruct visualization must be removed. The tympanic membrane should be noted for appearance, landmarks, and light reflex. Signs suggestive of otitis media are loss of normal concavity of the membrane, bulging of the membrane, visual loss of the bony landmarks, and erythema or an opaque or bluish appearance of the membrane. A fluid level or bubbles behind the tympanic membrae may also be seen. Pneumatic otoscopy is the most sensitive and simple bedside test for effusion behind the tympanic membrane. Pneumatic otoscopy is available and noninvasive, and should be part of the routine examination. Tympanocentesis by the consultant may be considered in immunocompromised patients or treatment-failure patients when knowledge of the exact cause is important. Adults who present with symptoms of otitis media and high fever or signs of systemic toxicity should receive a thorough examination. A white blood cell count, blood cultures, chest radiograph, and studies of cerebrospinal fluid should be done as indicated.

EMERGENCY DEPARTMENT MANAGEMENT

Acute, uncomplicated otitis media with effusion in pediatric populations is usually assumed to be bacterial. *S. pneumoniae* and *H. influenzae* are the usual pathogens. Amoxicillin is the drug of choice. The treatment period is 10 days. Patients in whom signs and symptoms continue after initial antibiotic therapy or those who are allergic to penicillin should receive other antibiotics. Cefaclor, cefixime, trimethoprim-sulfamethoxazole, and amoxicillin–potassium clavulanate (Augmentin) are accepted alternative drugs. Supportive therapy includes fever control, local pain relief, and treatment of associated upper respiratory tract symptoms. Acetaminophen is adequate to treat pyrexia and local pain symptoms in most adults. Severe pain that requires narcotic analgesia should prompt a search for other causes of the pain. Decongestants and antihistamines are effective in reducing the symptoms of upper respiratory tract infection and should be considered in adults.

DISPOSITION

ROLE OF THE CONSULTANT   Adults with uncomplicated acute otitis media can be safely discharged on antibiotics and symptomatic therapy. Patients should be instructed to seek follow-up for worsening of symptoms or for symptoms of systemic illness. Follow-up examination of the ear after completion of therapy has not been evaluated in adults.

Patients who return with continued symptoms despite therapy should be re-evaluated for other causes. In their absence a trial of alternative antibiotics should be instituted. These patients should be cautioned to return immediately for worsening of symptoms. Follow-up at the completion of antibiotic therapy is mandatory. The patient who returns during or after therapy with worsening symptoms should be seen by an otolaryngologist and tympanocentesis considered. Patients with known immunocompromise or other disabling illness should have early referral. An otolaryngologist or primary physician must assess the results of therapy. The patient with signs of systemic toxicity deserves an immediate, thorough systemic examination. Immediate consultation is indicated. Hospital admission and parenteral antibiotics may be indicated.

INDICATIONS FOR ADMISSION   Most adults with otitis media are successfully treated as outpatients. The rare adult with systemic toxicity or severe localized spread should be admitted.

COMMON PITFALLS

- Failure to visualize the tympanic membrane
- Failure to test the mobility of the membrane
- Confusing a ruptured tympanic membrane with drainage with otitis externa

14   Acute Otitis Externa in Adults

Otitis externa is a general term that encompasses all of the irritative and infective processes that involve the skin of the external auditory canal. An accepted system is to subdivide otitis externa into three major groups: *inflammatory otitis externa,* which is caused by infectious pathogens; *eczematoid (allergic) otitis externa;* and *seborrheic otitis externa.* Inflammatory otitis externa can be further subdivided into acute forms, in which the predominant pathogens are bacterial, and chronic forms, in which fungal organisms predominate.

Acute inflammatory otitis is by far the most common type of otitis externa, defined as an inflammatory condition of the auricle, ear canal, or outer surface of the tympanic membrane. Acute inflammatory otitis externa can be further subdivided into diffuse and localized forms. Acute diffuse otitis externa is the most common form of all external ear infections and is often called "swimmer's ear." Acute localized otitis externa is commonly an infection involving a hair follicle in the area of the ear canal. Initial presentation of these two processes are similar.

ACUTE DIFFUSE OTITIS EXTERNA

Acute diffuse otitis externa is found in all age groups and in all climates and seasons. However, there is a greatly increased incidence during the summer months, especially among swimmers, hence the term "swimmer's ear." Acute otitis externa is the result of introduction of infectious agents into the ear canal. These agents are predominantly bacterial. Commonly cultured organisms are *Pseudomonas aeruginosa, Proteus vulgaris, Staphylococcus aureus,* and non-group A streptococci. Fungal organisms are less frequently responsible for acute disease, but are most often found in hot, moist environments or among people with compromised immune systems (*Aspergillus niger, Candida* species, *Actinomyces,* and yeasts).

The usual precipitating factor in acute otitis externa is the introduction of infectious organisms into a traumatized ear canal secondary to the insertion of cotton-tipped applicators, pencils, and other foreign bodies or to prolonged water exposure from water sports or bathing.

Predisposing factors include previous ear surgery or tympanic membrane rupture, narrow or abnor-mally angled canal, and excessive cerumen production. Symptoms develop over several hours or days; untreated, the infection can resolve, persist as a chronic infection, or, with some organisms (usually *Pseudomonas*), progress over weeks or months to malignant (necrotizing, invasive) otitis externa. This latter entity is seen almost exclusively in diabetics and other immunocompromised patients. Malignant otitis externa can result in a high incidence of neurologic sequelae or death.

CLINICAL PRESENTATION

Itching or pain in the affected ear is the usual presenting symptom, often heightened by manipu-lation of the auricle or tragus. Edema and erythema are present, and the canal may be closed. There is usually a discharge described as yellowish, greenish, or watery. Fungal infections pro-duce a dark or cheesy discharge. If the canal is visualized, it often appears pale, soggy, and ede-matous, occluded by cerumen and desquamated epithelium. Visualization of the tympanic membrane may be impossible, or it may appear erythematous. However, it should have normal mobility if tested. In more severe infections there can be periauricular inflammation, cellulitis, lym-phadenitis, and erythema. Fever is variably present, and pain can be intensified by any manipula-tion of the jaw or the affected side of the face.

EMERGENCY DEPARTMENT EVALUATION

This includes manipulation of the auricle and tragus, and periauricular area inspection for inflam-mation, cellulitis, folliculitis, and eczematous conditions. The canal should be inspected and its condition noted. The tympanic membrane should be visualized, if possible, and mobility tested to rule out otitis media. Fungal cultures should be included if the history is suggestive, the exudate is cheesy or black, or a candidal rash is present. In elderly patients with diabetes and other immunocompromised patients with otorrhea and intense ear pain the possibility of malignant oti-tis externa should be considered. Patients who have had symptoms for weeks or months and those who return with worsening or unresolved symptoms after previous evaluations and thera-pies should also be suspected. White blood cell (WBC) counts and erythrocyte sedimentation rate (ESR) should be obtained in these patients. Signs of systemic toxicity, local extension of infection to periauricular areas, nuchal rigidity, and facial nerve palsy should be sought.

Spread of infection to the mastoid or base of the ear may be detected with plain films and computed tomography (CT) (bony erosions of advanced disease), but radiographs are little help in early presentations. Bone scanning and gallium scanning are far superior in sensitivity in detecting early disease, and are preferred by many otolaryngologists. However, low specificity and decreased availability limit their usefulness. CT is the current modality of choice for defining the anatomical extent of disease. Significant destruction of trabecular bone is often necessary to define osteomyelitis by CT. CT has the benefit of being more available.

EMERGENCY DEPARTMENT MANAGEMENT

Management includes hygiene, elimination of microbes, and analgesics. Hygiene involves cleans-ing of the ear canal, and is considered by some to be the single most important part of therapy. For mild infections dry-mopping with a small tuft of cotton attached to a wire applicator may be sufficient and sometimes is even curative. In more severe infections, with an inflamed, edema-tous canal with cheesy secretions and debris, removal by suctioning is recommended. In severe cases, suctioning may be done with the operating microscope. After all major debris and exudate are removed, careful irrigation with warm, sterile saline solution or a 2% acetic acid solution is recommended. Forceful irrigation is contraindicated, as this could further traumatize the macer-ated epithelium of the canal and promote suprainfection. After irrigation, the canal may be dried with suction. Topical otic solutions are recommended. There is no consensus, on a solution of choice. There is a consensus that otic solutions are preferable to suspensions, except in cases of perforation of the tympanic membrane or presence of a ventilation tube. In canals that are severely inflamed and edematous an ear wick may be necessary for application of otic solutions. Expandable ear wicks of hydroxycellulose or similar materials are commercially available and are preferable to cotton. Ear wicks are usually used for 24 to 48 hours and then removed. Often they spontaneously fall out as inflammation subsides. Otic solutions are applied three to four times daily to the affected canal, two to four drops per application. There is no absolute consensus on length of treatment, but 10 days of therapy with resolution of symptoms is reasonable.

Pain from otitis externa can be intense, and some patients may require narcotic analgesia during the initial evaluation, cleaning, and wick insertion and during the first few days of therapy. Continued severe pain after therapy is begun should prompt re-evaluation. Mild, locally applied heat often seems to help in pain management. During the course of treatment swimming is prohibited, showers should be brief, and hairwashing infrequent and followed by installation of otic drops.

The role of oral antibiotics in acute diffuse otitis externa is unclear. There are no firm guidelines for empiric oral antibiotic therapy. In the vast majority of uncomplicated cases the measures above should bring about resolution of symptoms. Some authors suggest the addition of an oral antibiotic regimen for patients with intense pain or ear wick insertion. Penicillin V, trimethoprim-sulfamethoxazole, and erythromycin have all been advocated. The patient on an oral antibiotic who is improving should complete a 10-day course. Almost all cases resolve with institution of the measures above.

However, patients with progressive, unresponsive, or severe infections may require parenteral antibiotic therapy. Cultures of ear aspirate should be done on all such patients, and the possibility of malignant otitis should be considered, especially in predisposed patients. A combination of an aminoglycoside and an antipseudomonal penicillin should be begun. If *S. aureus* infection is suspected, a cephalosporin or penicillinase-resistant penicillin should be given. For patients with proven or suspected malignant otitis externa the infectious agent is almost invariably *P. aeruginosa;* parenteral treatment consists of an aminoglycoside and antipseudomonal penicillin.

DISPOSITION

Most patients with acute diffuse otitis externa may be discharged home with instructions for good otic hygiene, topical antibiotic drops, and symptomatic therapy, including analgesia. Discharge instructions should include avoidance of water sports during therapy and for up to 2 to 4 weeks after resolution of symptoms. A 10-day follow-up is encouraged. All patients with ear wicks and severe pain and those on oral antibiotics should be re-evaluated in 12 to 24 hours to ensure that symptoms are resolving. Patients with severe edema, exudative discharge, and pain may require aggressive hygiene with daily irrigation, suctioning, and drying of the ear canal until symptoms regress.

Otolaryngologic consultation should be considered in patients who require daily follow-up for hygiene irrigation. All patients with worsening of symptoms or failure to resolve with initial management should be evaluated by an otolaryngologist. In patients with worsening symptoms, consultation should be immediate to consider hospitalization and parenteral antibiotic therapy. Patients with systemic toxicity, meningeal signs, or facial palsy need immediate admission and parenteral antibiotic therapy. A workup to rule out malignant otitis externa is indicated, including lumbar puncture, CT, and bone scan.

15   The Neck Mass

The neck mass is a complaint or finding that may accompany a large number of disorders. It may be congenital or acquired, infectious or neoplastic, benign or malignant. In the pediatric population most neck masses are relatively common and minor, whereas the incidence of neoplastic lesions is high in the adult population. In neither group does the neck mass commonly present as an acutely emergent or life-threatening problem.

CLINICAL PRESENTATION

An accurate history and careful physical examination are critical in the evaluation of the neck mass. The primary goal is to determine the most likely site and cause. The history should address the seven cardinal symptoms of head and neck disease: dysphagia, odynophagia, referred pain with swallowing, hoarseness, stridor, speech disorder, and globus phenomenon. Dysphagia and odynophagia do not have to be present concomitantly but may allow the patient to localize the lesion to the upper aerodigestive tract. Referred pain is typically to the ear and has the same significance as odynophagia. A major concern suggested by neck pain is the presence of an infection or disease process extending to the deep spaces of the neck. Masses or space-occupying lesions can present as problems with speech or as airway obstruction, the latter the most likely emergency the physician may encounter with the neck mass. The globus phenomenon is the sensation of a lump in the throat that is present between meals and may be described as excessive postnasal drip, "worms" in the throat, trouble swallowing saliva, or excessive mucus. The globus phenomenon is *not* associated with difficulty swallowing food.

Other important features include the use of tobacco in any form, the excessive use of alcohol, previous radiation exposure of the neck, current or recent illnesses, current or recent injuries, infection of the head and neck, and other associated local or systemic symptoms. Specific questions about the mass should include duration, changes or fluctuations in size, associated pain or inflammation, and sites of any drainage.

The examination is critical and should include a thorough evaluation of the scalp, face, skin, nose, ears, oral cavity, dental structures, pharynx, nasopharynx, and the mass itself. Also included in this examination are indirect visualization of the nasopharynx and larynx with a mirror and head light, and manual digital palpation of the nasopharynx and base of the tongue. The neck mass is examined and palpated for size, shape, consistency, mobility, and tenderness. When attempting to determine whether a neck mass may be a lymph node, it is important to recognize the location of the normal chain of cervical lymph nodes.

DIFFERENTIAL DIAGNOSIS

The differential diagnosis of a neck mass is quite extensive and age dependent. The "80% rule" states that 80% of isolated neck masses in children are benign; in adults 80% of nonthyroid neck masses are neoplastic and 80% of neoplastic masses are malignant. Furthermore, 80% of these malignant masses are metastatic and 80% of the primary tumors are located above the clavicle.

INFECTIOUS NECK MASS

The most common cause of a benign neck mass in children is cervical adenopathy secondary to an upper respiratory tract infection. The most common viral cause of acute cervical lymphadenitis is mononucleosis.

Deep neck infection is a serious but uncommon problem that may lead to airway obstruction, septicemia, erosion into the carotid artery, and extension into the mediastinum. Ninety percent of deep neck space abscesses occur in either the retropharyngeal, the lateral pharyngeal, or the submandibular space. *S. aureus* and hemolytic streptococci are the pathogens most frequently found in children. Anaerobic streptococci and *Bacteroides* may occur in adults, especially when dental infection is the primary underlying problem. With increasing numbers of geriatric patients, especially those from nursing homes and those who are victims of self-neglect, infections of the salivary glands and submandibular space are seen. These infections are associated with poor oral hygiene, dental disease, dehydration, and general debilitation. Parotid gland infection, cellulitis, and abscess of the floor of the mouth or submandibular space (Ludwig's angina) are common examples.

CONGENITAL NECK MASS

About 6% of neck masses are congenital. The most common of these are thyroglossal duct cysts, dermoid cysts, branchial cleft cysts, and cystic hygromas (lymphangiomas). The first two present as midline neck masses; the latter two, typically as lateral neck masses. Thyroglossal duct cyst is the most common benign congenital neck mass. The vast majority occur between 1 and 9 years of age with a peak incidence between 3 and 5 years.

An epidermoid cyst is the most common of the dermoid cysts that occur in the head and neck. It is estimated that 27% of midline cervical masses are dermoid or epidermoid cysts.

Branchial anomalies may present as cysts, sinuses, or fistulas. The second branchial cleft is responsible for most anomalies, of which cysts are the most common.

NEOPLASMS IN CHILDREN

Benign neoplasms in children that present as neck masses include hemangiomas, lymphangiomas, fibromas, neurofibromas, and lipomas. Only 20% of neck masses in children are malignant. Of these, more than 50% are lymphomas in the Hodgkin's disease and histiocytic lymphoma (lymphosarcoma) groups.

Malignant neck neoplasms in children tend to be single, nontender, and fast-growing, and are located in the posterior triangle of the neck. Age is a key element in the occurrence of the various malignant neck neoplasms. From ages 1 to 5 neuroblastoma, rhabdomyosarcoma, histiocytic lymphoma, and Hodgkin's disease are more common. In the older child histiocytic lymphoma and Hodgkin's disease occur equally often. The adolescent most commonly acquires Hodgkin's disease. Even though histiocytic lymphomas occur twice as often as the Hodgkin's lymphomas in children, they present with nearly equal frequency in the head and neck. Eighty percent of Hodgkin's disease and only 40% of histiocytic lymphomas present with a neck mass. Histiocytic lymphomas occur at any age, whereas Hodgkin's disease is very uncommon before age 5, peaking in the 5-to-9 age group.

Rhabdomyosarcoma is the most common solid tumor of the head and neck in childhood and is one of the most common tumors in children under 6 years of age. It is seen less frequently in the nonwhite population. Rhabdomyosarcoma presents with rapid growth in the orbit, nasopharynx, ear, mastoid, face, or tongue. The neuroblastoma is the most common solid tumor in children overall, but presents as a neck mass only about 5% of the time. Five percent of malignant neck neoplasms are thyroid cancer (medullary, papillary, mixed papillary, or follicular). There is a 2:1 female predominance. Roughly three fourths of preadolescent children with a single thyroid nodule have a thyroid cancer. About 25% of neurofibromas and neurofibrosarcomas present in the neck and head, but represent only 5% of malignant head and neck neoplasms. Unlike in the adult, metastatic squamous cell cancer that presents as a neck mass occurs in less than 1% of the total neck masses in children.

ADULT NEOPLASMS

Benign neck neoplasms in the adult are of the same origin as those found in children but are significantly less common. Only 20% of adult neck masses are benign. Neck neoplasms account for 5% of all cancers. It is estimated that up to 90% of malignant neck masses in patients over 50 years of age are metastatic. Most often squamous cell carcinoma from a primary site in the upper aerodigestive tract metastasizes to the lymph nodes of the upper, middle, and lower aspects of the neck. When a neoplasm below the clavicle metastasizes to the neck it tends to involve the supraclavicular nodes. Figure 15-1 shows the lymph node groups and the anatomical areas from which metastasis occurs.

In most, the primary site for a metastatic node can be found with a history and physical examination. Of those with an occult primary lesion, 75% have a primary lesion in the head and neck; the remainder have a primary lesion below the clavicle. Sadly, lymph node spread is an ominous development, reducing the chance of control of most head and neck cancers by at least 50%.

Benign and malignant thyroid disease should always be in the differential diagnosis. This includes simple goiter, primary thyroid cancer, and metastatic thyroid cancer. Difficulty swallowing and voice change are especially suggestive of thyroid cancer in the presence of a thyroid mass or enlargement. Papillary and follicular carcinomas are the more common forms of thyroid cancer in the adult. Graves' disease and autoimmune thyroiditis should also be considered when there is an enlarged or painful thyroid with associated weight loss, tachycardia, and tremors.

Three fourths of salivary gland tumors are in the parotid gland, and one sixth of these parotid tumors are malignant. A painful mass in the parotid gland that is adherent to the skin or deep tissues is suggestive of a malignant neoplasm.

EMERGENCY DEPARTMENT MANAGEMENT

The nasopharynx, base of the tongue, and larynx should be examined both by digital palpation and indirect mirror visualization. Emergencies associated with neck masses are uncommon, but when they occur they are almost always caused by airway compromise from tracheal displacement and compression or from upper airway obstruction by a mass. Infectious complications such as sepsis, deep neck space infection, and extension into the mediastinum are other life-threatening problems that may occur. Labs include a CBC, monospot, and thyroid function studies. Radiographic studies may include the chest, sinus series, and lateral view of the neck. Needle aspiration of a neck mass in the ED is **not** recommended. Endoscopic examination, sialography, ultrasound, computed tomographic scan, magnetic resonance imaging, angiography, upper gastrointestinal series, barium enema, and biopsies are usually unnecessary in the ED but will be completed by the consultant(s).

EMERGENCY DEPARTMENT DISPOSITION

ROLE OF THE CONSULTANT   Consultation with a head and neck surgeon is required for any patient with signs or symptoms of airway compromise or if there is suspicion of a deep neck space infection. Any adult, especially one >40, with a history of tobacco or heavy alcohol use who presents with a neck mass of any size requires referral to a head and neck surgeon within a reasonably short period of time. Children should be treated according to the most likely cause of the mass and referred to their primary physician within a 2-week period if the mass has not resolved or is changing shape. Children with a lymph node greater than 3 cm in size should be referred for evaluation regardless of their age. Children with an asymptomatic mass of presumed congenital origin should be referred for follow-up with their primary physician or a surgeon skilled in head and neck surgery.

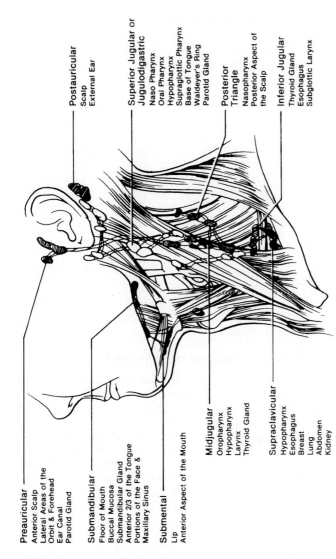

Preauricular
Anterior Scalp
Lateral Areas of the
Orbit & Forehead
Ear Canal
Parotid Gland

Submandibular
Floor of Mouth
Buccal Mucosa
Submandibular Gland
Anterior 2/3 of the Tongue
Portions of the Face &
Maxillary Sinus

Submental
Lip
Anterior Aspect of the Mouth

Midjugular
Oropharynx
Hypopharynx
Larynx
Thyroid Gland

Supraclavicular
Hypopharynx
Esophagus
Breast
Lung
Abdomen
Kidney

Postauricular
Scalp
External Ear

**Superior Jugular or
Jugulodigastric**
Naso Pharynx
Oral Pharynx
Hypopharynx
Supraglottic Pharynx
Base of Tongue
Waldeyer's Ring
Parotid Gland

**Posterior
Triangle**
Nasopharynx
Posterior Aspect of
the Scalp

Inferior Jugular
Thyroid Gland
Esophagus
Subglottic Larynx

Figure 15-1. Major cervical nodes and drainage patterns.

INDICATIONS FOR ADMISSION   The patient with a compromised airway or suspected deep neck space or mediastinal infection must be admitted. The toxic-appearing child or adult who is unable to swallow or tolerate oral fluids adequately should also be admitted for intravenous antibiotic therapy and hydration.

COMMON PITFALLS

- An incomplete or inadequate history and physical examination will result in the failure to find an apparent primary lesion in an adult. Ninety percent of the primary lesions can be determined from the history and physical examination.
- Failure to recognize the significant incidence of malignancy of neck masses in the adult results in unnecessary delays in evaluation and definitive treatment.
- Failure to provide and educate parents on the need for follow-up if their child has a suspicious cervical lymph node or mass will also result in unnecessary delays in definitive evaluation.

---

16 Emergency Aspects of Head and Neck Neoplasms

Neoplasms of the upper aerodigestive tract are common in 50- to 60-year-old men and women who smoke and drink. Oral cancer is not uncommon in men and women who have used smokeless tobacco for more than 15 years. Major salivary gland tumors affect both sexes, are not related to smoking or drinking, and usually occur in people aged 40 to 60. The emergency physician must never forget neoplasm as a cause of head and neck complaints in people aged 40 to 60. People who are afflicted with a neoplasm of the head and neck may be divided into two groups: (1) those whose tumors are symptomatic but who are unaware that they harbor a neoplasm and (2) those who know of their tumor. People in the first group are primarily diagnostic problems, whereas those in the second group are management problems.

NEOPLASMS OF WHICH THE PATIENT IS UNAWARE

A neoplasm of the head or neck is normally symptomatic early in its course. Symptoms are similar to or identical with symptoms of infection of the upper aerodigestive tract. Caveats include the following: (a) A sore throat of more than 2 weeks' duration in a person over 40 is cancer until proved otherwise. (b) Hoarseness or voice change that persists longer than 2 weeks in an adult over 40 is cancer until proved otherwise. (c) An otherwise unexplained unilateral serous effusion of the middle ear in an adult over 40 suggests cancer of the nasopharynx. (d) A nonhealing ulcer of the mucous membrane of the upper aerodigestive tract of more than 2 weeks' duration in an adult over 40 is suggestive of cancer.

Differentiating between infection and a tumor begins with a history and a physical examination with special attention to the upper aerodigestive tract. With the aid of the fiberoptic endoscope, emergency physicians should be able to visualize the entire upper aerodigestive tract. Head and neck squamous cell carcinomas are usually ulcerative, locally expansive, and invasive. Carcinoma of the base of the tongue is an exception to this generalization, as this tumor may initially be entirely submucosal. As squamous cell carcinomas grow they involve contiguous structures and later metastasize by way of the local lymphatics centripetally, ultimately reaching the lungs. Hematogenous spread of these tumors is not common early in the course.

CARCINOMA OF THE NASOPHARYNX

Carcinoma of the nasopharynx often makes its presence known by unilateral obstruction of the eustachian tube. This causes a sense of fullness or pressure and hearing loss in the affected ear. Other significant symptoms and signs are persistent sore throat, with pain not usually exacerbated by swallowing; blood-tinged nasal mucus; and expectoration of blood-tinged mucus. Otoscopic examination reveals fluid in the affected middle ear or a retracted eardrum. Visualization of the nasopharynx shows a tumor mass in the vicinity of the affected ear's eustachian cushion. The differential diagnosis includes nasopharyngitis (viral or bacterial) and lymphoma. Viral or bacterial nasopharyngitis is associated with diffuse inflammation of the entire nasopharynx and frequently a purulent exudate. Nasopharyngitis is often not accompanied by pharyngitis.

When a nasopharyngeal tumor is detected or strongly suspected, an extensive diagnostic workup is best done by the consultant. The emergency physician should not biopsy the tumor. The patient should not be discharged from the ED until a definite appointment has been made for follow-up care, usually within 3 to 5 days. ED treatment should be limited to measures directed toward pain relief and combating infection, if present.

COMMON PITFALLS

- Failure to associate an otherwise unexplained unilateral middle ear effusion in an older adult with carcinoma of the nasopharynx
- Failure to visualize the nasopharynx

CARCINOMA OF THE MOUTH
(INCLUDING LIPS AND ANTERIOR TWO THIRDS OF THE TONGUE)

The person with carcinoma of the mouth usually comes to the ED because of a sore, nonhealing ulcer. If the ulcer is on the anterior tongue, the person will also complain of exacerbation of the pain with tongue motion.

Physical examination reveals a discrete mucous membrane ulceration and varying amounts of local induration. The differential diagnosis includes herpetic ulcers, aphthous ulcers, lichen planus, pemphigus vulgaris, pemphigoid, and traumatic ulcerations secondary to dentures. It is usually impossible to differentiate between these various diseases by history and physical examination, except in a florid case of carcinoma. If the ulcer has not healed in 2 weeks with application of various topical or systemic agents, the person should be seen by a consultant within 3 to 5 days. The emergency physician should not biopsy the ulcer, but provide adequate analgesics, either systemic or topical, to relieve pain until the person can be seen by the consultant. A definitive diagnosis is usually made by biopsy of the lesion and the surrounding mucous membrane.

COMMON PITFALLS

- Failure to consider cancer as the cause of the ulcer

CARCINOMA OF THE POSTERIOR ONE THIRD OF THE TONGUE

A patient with carcinoma of the posterior one third of the tongue characteristically complains of a persistent sore throat of longer than 2 weeks' duration and some degree of dysphagia. The person often notes that the sore throat did not improve with antibiotics, but worsened. Direct visualization may show an ulcerating lesion, but frequently there is no mucosal aberration. The base of the tongue should be digitally palpated. This will reveal an area of induration. The differential diagnosis includes lingual thyroid, lingual tonsillitis, and lymphoma. A lingual thyroid gland is usually situated in the midline directly beneath the cecal foramen, whereas an early carcinoma of the posterior tongue is usually a unilateral lesion. Lingual tonsillitis ordinarily occurs in an adult who has previously undergone palatine tonsillectomy, and is recognized by the presence of diffuse inflammation, fever, and an elevated white blood cell count. When carcinoma of the base of the tongue is diagnosed, or strongly suspected, the emergency physician should evaluate the person's hydration and ability to swallow. If the person cannot maintain hydration or swallow sufficiently to obtain pain relief with oral medication, admission to the head and neck surgical oncologist is appropriate. If no specialist is available, arrangements should be made for transfer. If the person can swallow adequately to maintain hydration and obtain pain relief with oral medication, the person should be seen within 3 to 5 days by the oncologic surgeon.

COMMON PITFALLS

- Failure to visualize the base of the tongue
- Failure to digitally palpate the base of the tongue

CARCINOMA OF THE OROPHARYNX

Carcinomas that arise in the oropharynx usually involve either the palatine tonsil or the soft palate. Often the patient will complain of a persistent sore throat, some degree of dysphagia, and, not infrequently, fetid breath. Physical examination shows an ulcerative lesion that may contain impacted food debris. The differential diagnosis for tonsillar lesions includes lymphoma and granulomatous infections. When the soft palate is the tumor's primary site, neoplasms of minor salivary gland origin must also be considered. The definitive diagnosis is by biopsy of the lesion and the surrounding mucous membrane. This biopsy should not be performed by the emergency physician.

When carcinoma of the oropharynx is diagnosed or strongly suspected by the emergency physician, hydration and ability to swallow should be assessed. If the person can swallow enough to maintain hydration and to obtain pain relief from oral medication, follow-up care within 3 to 5 days with a head and neck oncologic surgeon should be arranged. If the patient's swallowing function is compromised, inpatient care for the patient on the service of a head and neck surgical oncologist is appropriate.

COMMON PITFALLS

- Failure to consider cancer as the cause of the ulcerative lesion

CARCINOMA OF THE LARYNX

A person who is afflicted with carcinoma of the larynx may present with a constellation of symptoms, ranging from persistent hoarseness to chronic sore throat, cough, and shortness of breath. Suspected epiglottitis is no contraindication to laryngoscopy. Laryngeal neoplasms are readily visible to direct and indirect laryngoscopy. When visualizing the larynx it is important for the examiner to note the location and size of the tumor, vocal cord function, and airway adequacy. The differential diagnosis includes vocal cord nodule (singer's nodes), vocal cord polyp, Reinke's edema of the vocal cord, hemorrhage into the cord, granulomas of the cords, leukoplakia of the cords, juvenile papillomatosis, tuberculosis, syphilis, acute epiglottitis, and acute laryngitis.

When carcinoma of the larynx is diagnosed or strongly suspected the emergency physician must evaluate the person's laryngeal competence. Laryngeal competence involves an adequate airway for respiration and the ability of the larynx to prevent tracheal aspiration. If laryngeal competence is lacking, supportive measures must be made (such as supplemental oxygen, endotracheal intubation, or emergency tracheostomy, depending on the severity of the problem). The greater the airway obstruction, the more cautious one should be in administering narcotics or relaxants, to avoid precipitating respiratory obstruction. An otolaryngologist should be contacted for emergency consultation. If the larynx is competent, follow-up care with an otolaryngologist should be arranged.

COMMON PITFALLS

- Failure to visualize the larynx
- Underestimation of the degree of laryngeal obstruction

MAJOR SALIVARY GLAND NEOPLASMS

Tumors of the parotid gland are roughly four times more common than tumors of the submandibular gland. These neoplasms grow slowly and are essentially symptom-free. Most are benign. Often it is another who discovers the growth and points it out to the affected person. Others discover their tumor, but relate it to a sore throat or some minor trauma. These people usually do not seek attention until the tumor size alarms them. The differential diagnosis includes acute parotitis, sialolithiasis with obstruction of the duct, and Sjögren's syndrome.

Physical examination may reveal a discrete tumor mass in a major salivary gland. The mass is usually firm, but a Warthin's tumor usually feels cystic. If "stripped," the gland will produce clear saliva. Acute parotitis is usually of abrupt onset. The gland is diffusely enlarged and very tender. "Stripping" the gland produces purulent saliva. Stones that obstruct the duct also become symptomatic abruptly. Eating greatly exacerbates the pain and swelling. "Stripping" produces no saliva. Frequently stones can be palpated along the course of the duct. The vast majority of stones are found in Warthin's duct. Sjögren's syndrome usually produces diffuse bilateral parotid enlargement. "Stripping" the gland produces thick mucoid saliva or none at all.

When a major salivary gland neoplasm is diagnosed follow-up care with an otolaryngologist should be done. Because these tumors are slow-growing and the majority are benign, there is no urgency for the referral. The emergency physician should not attempt to incise and drain cystic salivary gland masses or to perform excisional or incisional biopsies.

COMMON PITFALLS

- Misdiagnosis of intrinsic salivary gland tumors as inflamed lymph nodes

PREVIOUSLY DIAGNOSED NEOPLASMS

Patients with diagnosed head and neck neoplasms often seek emergency care because of complications associated with therapy or complications secondary to the neoplasm. Complications of therapy include dislodged feeding tubes, dehydration, nausea, vomiting, dislodged voice prosthesis, and obstructed tracheostomy tube. Complications secondary to the neoplasm are hemorrhage, wound infection, salivary fistula, esophageal obstruction, and airway obstruction.

COMPLICATIONS ASSOCIATED WITH THERAPY

TUBES   Feeding tubes (nasogastric [NG], gastrostomy, or feeding jejunostomy) are used to secure entry to the gastrointestinal tract for nutrition and hydration. Most often this follows extensive primary resection, salvage surgery, and radiation therapy. NG tubes are difficult to secure for long periods; therefore, accidental removal is not uncommon. Replacement of the NG tube is usually possible, but before the emergency physician attempts to do this, the head and neck surgeon should be contacted for specific instructions. The attending physician may prefer that no attempt be made to reintroduce the NG tube. Conversely, because of special circumstances, the surgeon may prefer to do this himself. Gastrostomy tubes are less prone to accidental removal because they are anchored by either a balloon-tipped catheter or a mushroom-tipped tube. However, balloons may rupture and deflate, resulting in accidental removal.

Current surgical technique favors suturing the stomach in the vicinity of the gastrostomy ostia to the anterior abdominal wall to minimize the possibility of a gastric "leak" even if the tube comes out. This maneuver also makes it easier to change the gastrostomy tube. When confronted with a dislodged gastrostomy tube, the emergency physician should contact the surgeon about which type and size tube to reinsert, if the patient has not brought the tube to the ED. A gastrostomy fistula will contract quickly if the tube is left out for more than a few hours. If this problem has occurred, the fistula can be dilated to its original size by *gently* passing a series of catheters of increasing diameter. Intragastric position should be checked by instilling and removing a small amount of sterile water or saline solution. Jejunostomy feeding tubes are not frequently dislodged because they are sutured to the abdominal wall. If one comes out, the emergency physician should not attempt to replace it. The attending surgeon should be contacted for further care.

VOICE PROSTHESIS   After total laryngectomy an increasing number of patients elect to have a small tracheoesophageal (TE) fistula established so they can use a voice prosthesis for speech. This prosthesis frequently dislodges. Although patients who use the prosthesis are taught how to insert the device, their attempts at insertion are not always successful. Occasionally the prosthesis is lost. A TE fistula will close rapidly if patency is not maintained. If an emergency physician has no training or experience in inserting a voice prosthesis, he or she should not attempt the procedure. Patency of the TE fistula can be ensured by passing a #16 French catheter through the trachea into the distal esophagus. The catheter can easily be secured to the chest wall. Once patency of the TE fistula is assured, the prosthesis can then be inserted by the surgeon at a later time. A voice prosthesis is small, and can be aspirated into the distal tracheobronchial tree. The irritation of the prosthesis usually causes a chronic cough, but when the prosthesis cannot be accounted for, a chest radiograph is indicated.

RADIATION AND CHEMOTHERAPY   Radiation therapy and chemotherapy are frequently associated with nausea, vomiting, and dysphagia. These problems lead to dehydration and an inability to obtain pain relief from oral medications. Emergency treatment for such patients depends on the severity of dehydration and the nature of the dysphagia, and should be approached in consultation with the surgeon. The decision whether or not to admit is generally made by the attending surgeon.

TRACHEOSTOMY PROBLEMS   A tracheostomy tube obstructs for one of three reasons: (1) the tube is occluded by secretions, (2) the tube is lying outside the tracheal lumen, or (3) the tube is blocked by an overinflated cuff. The quickest solution to the problem is the removal of the entire tracheostomy tube. This maneuver should result in immediate improvement in the airway. An obturator should always be used when reinstating the tracheostomy tube. Once the tube has been replaced, a sterile catheter should be passed into the trachea to confirm the intraluminal position of the tube. A tracheocutaneous (TC) fistula more than 72 hours old will not close immediately on removal of a tracheostomy tube. However, if the tracheostomy tube has been out for a number of hours, it may not be possible to reinsert the tube until the TC fistula has been gently dilated using the graduated tube technique. The same caveats for this technique are listed under the section for the gastrostomy tube.

COMMON PITFALLS

- Use of excessive force when replacing feeding tubes
- Failure to preserve the TE fistula after a voice prosthesis becomes dislodged
- Failure to rule out aspiration of a voice prosthesis
- Failure to check the intraluminal position of a tracheostomy tube by passing a sterile catheter into the distal trachea

COMPLICATIONS SECONDARY TO THE NEOPLASM

HEMORRHAGE   Hemorrhage from a ruptured major vessel is associated with an active, enlarging tumor, prior irradiation, wound infection, and a salivary fistula. Of head and neck vessels, rupture of the carotid artery is most frequent, but rupture of the lingual artery is not uncommon. Catastrophic hemorrhage is often heralded by a "sentinel" bleeding episode, which may be manifested by the coughing up of a moderate amount of blood or bleeding from the neck. Often the sentinel bleeding has ceased by the time the person arrives in the ED. A life-threatening situation exists. If examination reveals a blood clot over the carotid artery area or the surface of the tongue, **no** attempt should be made to remove the clot. An intravenous should be started, a CBC and type and crossmatch. Catastrophic hemorrhage from the carotid artery may be external through the neck or internal into the trachea. Internal hemorrhage is uniformly and rapidly fatal. External hemorrhage can be controlled by directly occluding the carotid artery. Definitive treatment of carotid artery rupture is usually ligation of the artery, although in selected cases angioplasty of the carotid artery is successful.

Massive bleeding from rupture of the lingual artery at the base of the tongue requires that the physician simultaneously maintain the airway while occluding the ruptured vessel. The patient should be in an upright position. Initially, the blood should be removed with suction and then pressure applied to the base of the tongue with a tonsil sponge or 4×4-in gauze pad on a curved hemostat. Measures to support the blood pressure should be taken. The patient must be admitted and taken to the operating room for definitive surgical treatment as rapidly as possible.

AIRWAY OBSTRUCTION   Airway obstruction secondary to an enlarging neoplasm is a frequent cause of ED visits. Obstruction can be mild or severe. Supplemental oxygen administered before and during laryngoscopy may enable the person to cooperate better during the examination. Visualization of the larynx is critical in planning immediate treatment and allows the emergency physician to quantitate the degree of obstruction and its location, and the feasibility of intubation directly or with the aid of a fiberoptic endoscope. Occasionally the airway obstruction is so severe that the person must either be intubated immediately or undergo a tracheostomy or cricothyrotomy. Rapid intubation with the guidance of a fiberoptic bronchoscope can often prevent the need for a tracheostomy. Tracheostomies are best performed in the operating suite but every emergency physician should be able to perform a cricothyrotomy.

FISTULAS   Salivary fistulas may develop weeks or months postoperatively. They are more common in patients who received preoperative radiation therapy. The appearance of a salivary fistula is often frightening to the patient and, if untreated, may lead to aspiration pneumonia. The emergency physician should suction and divert the salivary stream away from the trachea and call the attending physician. An NG tube may be indicated. Once the saliva has been diverted or absorbed and an NG tube has provided a feeding bypass, the patient can be discharged for follow-up care. The patient should be instructed not to eat or drink by mouth.

PAIN   Constant pain is a hallmark of the later stages of uncontrolled head and neck neoplasms. Although oral medication can successfully control such pain, often the cancer patient will report to an ED because of inability to obtain pain relief. A call to the attending surgeon is useful for the information necessary to calculate a dosage of narcotic adequate to control the person's pain.

COMMON PITFALLS

- Failure to recognize a sentinel hemorrhage
- Underestimation of the degree of airway obstruction
- Inability to establish an airway or perform a cricothyrotomy

PART IV

Emergency Aspects of General Surgery

17 Abdominal Pain in the Elderly

Elderly patients with acute abdominal pain present a special challenge. Older patients tend to have subtler presentations, but more serious and more urgent conditions. Of patients hospitalized with acute abdominal pain, surgical intervention occurs twice as often in the 65-and-older group, and the mortality is tenfold. Elderly differ from younger patients in several significant respects: higher pain threshold, tendancy to underreport complaints, delay seeking medical attention, lack of specific symptoms, diminished physiologic response, more insidiously atypical and nonspecific symptoms. Fever may be absent or below normal in the elderly person with abdominal infection. Renal, immune, cardiac, pulmonary, and homeostatic functions decline with age. The number of diagnostic possibilities increases with age. The elderly may have multiple simultaneous disease processes.

CLINICAL PRESENTATION
HISTORY

An accurate history may be difficult to obtain. Communication may be limited by impaired hearing (22% of the elderly), visual handicaps (15%), and dementia (22%). Increased physician skill, time, and patience may be required. All available sources of history should be used, including prior medical records and family. Pain may be perceived very differently, depending on the patient's social and cultural background and more immediate psychological stresses. Certain patterns of pain may help to narrow the focus: nature, course, and location. Abrupt onset is associated with perforation and some obstructions, an insidious onset occurs with inflammatory processes. Movement of pain suggests progression. A review of systems should include questions about swallowing, appetite, nausea, vomiting, change in bowel habits, diarrhea, blood in stool, and weight change.

PHYSICAL EXAMINATION

The *entire* patient should be examined. Vital signs should be evaluated. Low body temperature is common in elderly patients, especially in those who are seriously ill. Tachycardia and tachypnea may reflect pain, distress, volume depletion, sepsis, hypoxia, or acidosis. General appearance and mental status should be noted, as should abnormalities in the temperature, color, and moisture of the skin. A thorough examination of the cardiac and pulmonary systems may reveal an extra-abdominal source of the abdominal pain.

The abdomen should be inspected for scars, masses, peristalsis, and pulsations. The examiner should particularly note the contour of the abdomen, looking for the localized bulging of a hernia. A more generalized protuberance may suggest ascites or gaseous distention. The abdomen should be auscultated, noting the character and frequency of bowel sounds and bruits. Percussion of the abdomen helps to determine the size of the liver and spleen as well as the presence and distribution of tympany and dullness. The abdomen should be carefully and gently palpated, beginning in an area remote from the area of pain and slowly working toward the area of maximum tenderness. Rebound tenderness, suggesting peritoneal inflammation, should be sought. The back should be inspected for deformity and assessed for bony or flank tenderness. The rectum and genitalia must be examined. The rectal exam may reveal evidence of bleeding, a mass, or perirectal inflammation from abscess, appendicitis, or prostatitis. The stool should be examined for gross or occult blood. Evaluation of the genitalia may demonstrate a hernia or pelvic disease.

LABORATORY EVALUATION

The laboratory evaluation may be helpful but normal laboratory tests do not exclude a pathologic condition. A CBC may be useful. The WBC count is elevated (>10,000) much less often in the elderly with an inflammatory process than in younger counterparts. In those older than age 65 with a condition that requires immediate surgical intervention, only 39% have an elevated WBC count. Electrolytes, blood urea nitrogen, and creatinine should be selectively pursued, especially in patients who are taking cardiac glycosides or diuretics. Liver function tests are nonspecific but may be helpful when considering hepatobiliary disease. An elevated amylase level may suggest pancreatitis, obstruction of the pancreatic duct, or a perforated or penetrating ulcer. A urinalysis should be performed to exclude urinary tract pathology. An electrocardiogram will help to exclude myocardial infarction or arrhythmias. Radiographs of the chest and abdomen may also be helpful when ordered selectively. Literature encouraging cost-effective use of radiographs is not pertinent to the elderly.

DIFFERENTIAL DIAGNOSIS

Classic presentations in the elderly patient are less common due to less precise information, less definitive physical examination, mental confusion, or cardiovascular collapse. These factors, combined with multiple medications, chronic medical problems, and decreased physiologic reserve, result in delayed diagnosis and significantly increased morbidity and mortality. Causes of pain are:

1. Biliary colic or cholecystitis (12–33%)
2. Nonspecific abdominal pain (15%)
3. Intestinal obstruction (hernias, adhesions, malignancies) (12–25%)
4. Appendicitis (5–14%)
5. Perforated viscus (7–10%)
6. Gastrointestinal bleeding (9%)
7. Pancreatitis (7%)
8. Diverticular disease (6%), appendicitis (5–7%)
9. Cancer (4%)
10. Vascular (mesenteric ischemia, aortic aneurysm) (2%)

Other important causes of abdominal pain include peptic ulcer disease and nephrolithiasis. In addition, nonabdominal diseases can cause acute abdominal pain, including pneumonia, acute myocardial infarction, diabetic ketoacidosis, and drug toxicity. Remember that although 25% of elderly patients will have no discernable cause of their abdominal pain identified in the ED, up to 10% will be diagnosed with cancer within 6 months, the most common site being the colon.

BILIARY TRACT DISEASE

Biliary tract disease is the most common abdominal surgical emergency in the elderly, accounting for 25% to 30% of cases. The incidence of gallstones increases with age to about 30% in
those over age 70. Eighty percent present with complications of cholecystitis, cholangitis, or pancreatitis. Cholecystitis is associated with a higher risk of empyema, gangrene, and perforation of
the gallbladder. Cholangitis may present as septic shock. A rare form of cholecystitis seen exclusively in the elderly is emphysematous cholecystitis, caused by gas-producing organisms; the
diagnosis may be made on abdominal film with gas in the gallbladder or biliary tree.

Biliary tract disease may result in either acute or chronic symptoms, with classic symptoms blunted or absent in the elderly. Pain usually begins in the right upper quadrant (RUQ) or epigastrium and extends along the right costal margin to the infrascapular region. The pain is initially
crampy or colicky, but with time becomes continuous. Nausea is frequent and vomiting common.
Tenderness, guarding, and rigidity are noted in the right upper quadrant and epigastrium in 90%
of patients, while a palpable mass is present in less than 25%. Fever is not common; if present,
it suggests cholangitis or infection elsewhere (pyelonephritis, diverticulitis, or pneumonia).

Laboratory findings are nonspecific, with the WBC count usually mildly elevated. The most
common positive radiographic finding is an ileus pattern or "sentinel loop" in the RUQ. Isotopic
scans and sonographic studies are diagnostic. Acute cholecystitis with fever mandates hydration,
antibiotics, and urgent surgical consultation.

BOWEL OBSTRUCTION

Bowel obstruction is the second most common cause of abdominal pain that requires surgical
intervention. In a study of 300 consecutive elderly patients with bowel obstruction, the site of
obstruction was large bowel (33%), small bowel (33%), and obstruction caused by hernias (33%).
Large-bowel obstruction was caused by tumors, sigmoid volvulus, and fecal impaction in 98%.
Adhesions, gallstone ileus, and tumors accounted for 94% of small-bowel obstructions. Cardiac,
pulmonary, and sepsis were responsible for most of the 234 complications and 84 deaths. The
diagnosis of obstruction in the elderly is usually not difficult. A history of crampy abdominal pain
in the periumbilical or hypogastric area, nausea (95%), vomiting (85%), and constipation (85%)
frequently occur. A history of previous surgery is suggestive. Temperature elevation >1°F is
unusual and is associated with peritonitis. Examine for scars and hernias, particularly femoral and
inguinal. Tenderness is almost always present (90%); distention (63%), when present, is suggestive of obstruction. Auscultation may reveal increased frequency of high-pitched tinkling sounds
or absence of bowel sounds, depending on the stage of obstruction and the presence of complications. Rectal and external genitalia may reveal impaction or carcinoma.

WBC count is elevated in fewer than 50%, most often when severe dehydration is present.
Radiographs may confirm the obstruction, demonstrating dilated loops of bowel and air–fluid levels. In early obstruction, a nonspecific ileus pattern may be seen. Radiographs may also demonstrate the cause of the obstruction (e.g., volvulus, gallstone ileus, or bezoar).

APPENDICITIS

Appendicitis should be considered in any elderly patient with poorly defined abdominal pain. It is the
third most common cause of abdominal pain that requires surgical intervention, and presents with
the most confusing clinical picture. Classic symptoms (epigastric or periumbilical pain localizing to
the RLQ) are seen in <50%. In one study, only 15% presented within 24 hours of the onset of pain
at operation, <10% had simple appendicitis, 50% had gangrene or perforation, and 1/3 had
abscess formation. The only consistent finding was a history of abdominal pain and tenderness.
Temperature elevation was seen in about 75%. Fifteen percent of patients died of complications of
the disease or surgery. The most suggestive radiographic finding is an appendolith (an oval or round
calcification usually found in the RLQ). Abnormal, persistent gas collection suggests an abscess.

PANCREATITIS

Pancreatitis is the most common nonsurgical cause of acute abdominal pain in the elderly. Its incidence increases with age, often secondary to other gastrointestinal disorders, (biliary tract disease, peptic ulcer disease, and complications from therapeutic agents). It is characterized by severe and continuous epigastric pain associated with nausea and vomiting. Pain may be absent in 10% of elderly patients. The diagnosis may be found after investigation of unexplained hypotension or change in mental status. Fever is uncommon unless the illness is secondary to another process or complications. Although most patients complain of severe pain, severe tenderness on exam is not consistent. An elevated serum amylase level and WBC count are characteristic. The abdominal radiograph may reveal a localized ileus pattern (sentinel loop) early in the disease or a more generalized ileus pattern after prolonged inflammation.

DIVERTICULITIS

Sigmoid diverticula are common in the elderly and the incidence increases with age, present in 50% of patients over age 80. Diverticulitis represents an inflammatory response to a diverticulum that has ruptured into surrounding tissue. It is a common cause of abdominal pain in the elderly, accounting for 10% of ED visits. Diverticulitis usually presents with LLQ pain and change in bowel habits, usually constipation. However, symptoms may be nonspecific. The pain, usually crampy, may be continuous, and the lack of severity may lead to significant delay in seeking medical care. Bloody diarrhea occurs infrequently. Exam may reveal a mild to moderate elevation in temperature. The abdomen may show decreased bowel sounds and LLQ tenderness, but RLQ, suprapubic, or generalized tenderness may also be observed. The laboratory examination is seldom helpful; the diagnosis is clinical. The WBC count may or may not be elevated, and abdominal radiograph may reveal a nonspecific ileus pattern. Ultrasound may be useful.

PEPTIC ULCER DISEASE

Peptic ulcer disease is common with morbidity increasing with age. Complications such as perforation and bleeding are often seen and associated with high mortality. Signs and symptoms depend on the stage of the disease but are often nonspecific until late in the disease process. Less severe presentations may be characterized by intermittent gnawing or burning pain localized to the epigastric, substernal, or periumbilical region. Epigastric tenderness may be noted. Posterior penetration causes pancreatitis with associated symptoms; perforation causes excruciating pain. Associated peritonitis results in fever, generalized tenderness, guarding, and board-like rigidity. Others may present with upper gastrointestinal hemorrhage and shock. Anemia is often noted and depends on the severity and duration of the disease. Marked elevation of the WBC count and free intraperitoneal air are usually seen with perforation.

ISCHEMIC BOWEL

Mesenteric vascular occlusion should always be considered in the elderly patient who presents with an acute abdomen. There are several types of ischemic bowel disease; the presentation will vary depending on location, degree of collateral circulation, and underlying disease process. Thrombosis may result in an insidious onset of pain, anorexia, and diarrhea with or without blood loss. The physical examination may be nonspecific. The patient with an acute mesenteric vascular occlusion (whether thrombosis or arterial embolism) usually presents with catastrophic pain, poorly localized tenderness, bloody diarrhea, and, perhaps, vascular collapse. Radiographic studies may be helpful in establishing a diagnosis. An ileus may be present early. Abdominal studies with or without contrast may reveal diagnostic "thumbprinting" from edema or hemorrhage in the bowel wall.

CONSTIPATION

Slowing of gut motility and complaints of infrequent and insufficient defecation are common among the elderly. Constipation of recent onset requires investigation, as it is frequently a symptom of underlying pathology: carcinoma, volvulus, toxic etiologies, and drugs (especially laxatives, tricyclic antidepressants, and muscle relaxants). Paradoxical diarrhea, the passage of loose watery bowel movements past an incompletely obstructing fecal mass, may confuse the presentation. Rectal examination may demonstrate a fecal mass that requires digital disimpaction. Radiographs may reveal a colon full of stool, volvulus, or evidence of a proximal obstruction.

OTHER CAUSES

An exhaustive discussion of other causes of acute abdominal pain in the elderly is not possible. However, the clinician should be aware of the challenging spectrum of etiologies, including inflammatory bowel disease, intraperitoneal abscess, prostatitis, aortic aneurysm, and hernia; nephrolithiasis, pyelonephritis, and extra-abdominal etiologies such as myocardial infarction, congestive heart failure, pneumonia, thyroid disease, diabetic ketoacidosis, and drug toxicity.

EMERGENCY DEPARTMENT MANAGEMENT

Life-threatening problems take priority: airway, adequate ventilation, and circulation. Fluid challenges should be given cautiously and their effect closely observed, with frequent monitoring of vital signs, urine output and repeat physical exam. Central venous pressure is helpful if extensive fluid resuscitation is required; invasive hemodynamic monitoring may be necessary. A nasogastric tube (evacuate the contents of the stomach and maintain decompression) and Foley catheter are indicated.

DISPOSITION

The elderly patient who presents with abdominal pain must be evaluated with great caution. The physician must differentiate benign causes from the more serious, life-threatening diseases that present with vague or confusing symptoms. It is not always possible to determine the specific cause of abdominal pain in the ED. Many patients will be admitted for further evaluation and observation without a specific diagnosis. The emergency physician must be absolutely certain that a potentially life-threatening problem does not exist before discharging the patient. The patient's functional status and home environment are important. Appropriate instructions for follow-up should be given. Only the patient with an obviously benign condition should be discharged. Pain that has persisted for more than 6 hours should receive aggressive evaluation and surgical consultation for possible admission or observation.

COMMON PITFALLS

- Elderly patients with abdominal pain may under-report symptoms and delay seeking medical care.
- They may have atypical presentations, no fever or WBC count .
- The elderly are twice as likely to require surgery as younger patients with the same complaint, with more serious illness and more frequent complications.

18   Breast Masses and Breast Infection

Evaluation of a breast mass includes recognition of cancer and infection. A breast abscess usually occurs in lactating women, but it may also represent inflammatory carcinoma in the elderly. Cancer may present in a manner similar to fulminant mastitis. Experienced physicians are able to diagnose only 70% of breast cancers by examination alone. The initial evaluation of a breast mass may be difficult but relevant to patient outcome.

DIFFERENTIAL DIAGNOSIS

The differential diagnosis for breast mass includes cancer, mastitis, Paget's disease, benign neoplasms, lipoma, fat necrosis, Mondor's disease, and abscess.

CANCER

One out of ten women in the United States will develop breast cancer. Risk factors include a family history of breast cancer, obesity, nulliparity, initial pregnancy past age 30, and history of breast, ovarian, or endometrial cancer. Masses that are smooth, movable, and firm with distinct margins are usually benign. Seventy-five percent to 80% of cancerous lesions are hard and cartilaginous, with distinct edges that are serrated and irregular. Twenty percent to 25% of cancerous nodules are less hard and less fibrotic in consistency, making accurate clinical diagnosis more difficult. Cancerous nodules are usually located in the upper outer quadrant. Skin changes range from none to local edema or frank ulceration. Fibrosis may shorten Cooper's ligament and cause skin dimpling, a process also seen in fat necrosis. Bloody nipple discharge suggests ductal carcinoma or an intraductal papilloma.

Lymph nodes involved in the spread of breast cancer are initially rubbery and shotty, but eventually they become hard and matted with progressive infiltration. Axillary glands are most commonly involved, although spread to the parasternal and supraclavicular regions may also occur. Breast cancer cells disseminate through the lymphatics to lung, liver, and bony skeleton.

Patients suspected of metastatic breast cancer should have a complete blood count, calcium, electrolytes, liver enzymes, and chest radiography. Erythema, edema, tenderness, and induration are late skin changes, but they may also be seen in acute mastitis. Most breast infections occur 1 to 3 months postpartum, so mastitis or abscess in a nonlactating woman, as well as delayed resolution of a puerperal infection, is a warning sign of inflammatory cancer.

BENIGN NEOPLASMS

Fibroadenomas are the most common benign neoplasms of the breast. They usually present during the third to fourth decades of life and are spherical, firm, mobile, and well defined. Fibroadenomas should be removed to rule out cancer and preclude continued enlargement. Fibrocystic disease causes cyclical pain and swelling of one or both breasts just before menses. The nodules or cysts range from 2–3 mm to several centimeters in diameter. Treatment includes a well-fitting brassiere, heat, and analgesics. Danazol, an androgen derivative, may be effective if hormonal treatment is indicated.

FAT NECROSIS

Fat necrosis may present as a tender lump in the breast and follows trauma in 50% of cases. The mass usually does not enlarge, but nipple retraction may be seen. Excision for definitive diagnosis is indicated.

LIPOMAS

Lipomas are superficial in location and occur in any quadrant of the breast. These benign tumors vary greatly in size and transilluminate easily. Mammography is usually diagnostic.

MASTITIS AND ABSCESS

Most breast abscesses occur 1 to 3 months postpartum, but postmenopausal women may also develop mastitis. A postpartum breast abscess is caused by normal skin pathogens that invade through cracks in the nipple. Breast milk is an ideal culture medium. Unrecognized infection coalesces into abscesses, usually located away from the areola. Staphylococci are the most common causative agents; streptococci are cultured less often. Preventive measures include nipple hygiene, hand washing, cleansing the infant's skin, and early recognition. Mastitis in the lactating breast causes pain, fever, erythema, edema, tenderness, and induration. Fluctuance in a centrifugal location is the hallmark of a superficial abscess. Intramammary and retromammary loculations occur deep in breast tissue and near the pectoralis musculature, respectively. For this reason fluctuance may not be readily apparent. The breast appears indurated, and the patient withdraws to palpation. Paradoxically, decreasing induration and diminished pain may reflect the need for wide incision and drainage.

Postmenopausal breast abscesses are distinct from puerperal forms in cause and presentation. Causative bacteria include *Escherichia coli,* group D streptococci, staphylococci, and anaerobes, including *Bacteroides* sp. These are often found in the subareolar region in association with ductal ectasia, a chronic inflammation of major ducts below the nipple and areola. Recurrence rates after simple incision and drainage exceed 39%. Mamillary fistulas occasionally form between the areola and infected lactating glands. Although most breast abscesses occur postpartum, cancer may mimic mastitis. Mastitis or abscess in a nonlactating woman, as well as delayed resolution of a puerperal infection, are warning signs of inflammatory cancer. Tuberculosis remains the most common cause of persistent breast abscess. Chronic infection also occurs after inadequate drainage of partitioned areas within an abscess. Untreated chronic infection may result in substantial morbidity and cosmetic deformity.

Paget's disease of the nipple reflects carcinoma of the mammary ducts underlying the areola. The nipple initially appears dry, scaling, cracked, and eczematoid. The condition may progress to chronic skin inflammation and a surface crust. Subareolar fullness may or may not be palpable.

EMERGENCY DEPARTMENT MANAGEMENT

Simple mastitis in the lactating woman is treated with antimicrobials that are effective against staphylococci and streptococci. Dicloxacillin, 250 to 500 mg four times a day, or erythromycin, 250 to 500 mg four times a day in penicillin-allergic patients, is appropriate. Breast milk should be cultured for aerobes and anaerobes. Feedings may be discontinued for up to 48 hours if there is concern about infant diarrhea; however, drainage must be accomplished by either continued feeding or pump. Local heat should be applied. Superficial abscesses may be drained and treated in the ED if there is no fever or toxicity. Incision and drainage may also be performed by an emergency physician who is appropriately credentialed. Incision is performed in a curvilinear manner along skin lines or in a radial manner. A circumareolar approach may also be used. Care should be taken to ensure that there are no loculations that might result in a chronic abscess. Culture (anaerobic and aerobic) and Gram's stain of the drainage should be performed. The patient should be given an appropriate antimicrobial and instructed in the same local measures as for simple mastitis.

DISPOSITION

ROLE OF THE CONSULTANT   Patients with nontoxic mastitis or superficial abscess should be re-evaluated in 24 hours. Mamillary fistulas should be referred to a surgeon for excision and definitive closure. Postmenopausal inframammary abscesses necessitate surgical consultation because of the high recurrence rate after simple drainage. Incision and drainage of superficial abscesses may be referred to a surgeon for cosmetic reasons if the operator is not facile with the procedure.

INDICATIONS FOR ADMISSION   Women with marked temperature elevation or toxicity should be admitted and placed on intravenous antibiotics that are effective against staphylococci and streptococci. Women with simple infections that do not improve or that worsen after 24 hours should also be admitted. Patients with deep intramammary and retromammary abscesses are hospitalized for operative drainage.

COMMON PITFALLS

- Inflammatory cancer may present with erythema, edema, and tenderness. Infection in a non-lactating breast and failure of a postpartum infection to abate in a timely manner is suggestive of cancer.
- Inadequate drainage of a breast abscess may lead to chronic infection with morbidity and cosmetic deformity.
- Subareolar abscesses in postmenopausal women are usually associated with ductal ectasia (chronic subareolar inflammation) and may recur, necessitating removal of the involved duct system. These patients require surgical consultation.
- Subareolar abscesses may also present with mamillary fistula, demonstrated clinically by expressing pus from the nipple area. Surgical removal of the tract and definitive closure are indicated.

19   Acute Diseases of the Gallbladder

Acute cholecystitis is common disease, most often caused by cholelithiasis. It is estimated that 20 million Americans have gallstones. More than 500,000 cholecystectomies are done in the United States every year, making it one of the ten most frequently performed operations. Cholelithiasis is found among people of all ages, but it is most common in white women between the fourth and eighth decades of life. Cholelithiasis is the result of formation of stones in the gallbladder. The major elements in gallstones are cholesterol, bile pigment, and calcium. "Pure" bile pigment stones are usually associated with hemolytic anemia and sickle cell disease. Most stones are thought to originate in the gallbladder; acute biliary colic occurs when the stone(s) attempt to pass down the cystic duct or become lodged in the neck of the gallbladder. As the stones attempt to pass the cystic duct, biliary colic may be experienced, right upper quadrant crampy pain radiating to the back. The cystic duct may become occluded from the stone or obstructed secondary to edema with secondary infection, a condition called *cholecystitis*. If the stone is single and large, cholecystitis may be complicated by the stone eroding through the gallbladder into adjacent viscera. The stone passes through the gastrointestinal tract by way of the biliary-enteric fistula and usually lodges in the distal ileum. Small-bowel obstruction results from the *gallstone ileus*. If the stones are small and are passed into the common duct, they can occlude the distal common duct, resulting in *choledocholithiasis*. The obstructed common duct may result in cholangitis, infection of the biliary tree. Table 19-1 summarizes these diseases of the gallbladder.

ACALCULOUS CHOLECYSTITIS

Acalculous cholecystitis is acute and chronic inflammation of the gallbladder in the absence of gallstones. This condition most commonly affects patients with diabetes, chronic disease, sepsis, or multiple system failure. The incidence in the United States is 5%.

ASYMPTOMATIC CHOLELITHIASIS

Asymptomatic cholelithiasis is rare. Most stones ultimately cause symptoms. Dyspepsia or abdominal discomfort is often minimal and endured without treatment or diagnostic procedures.

ACUTE CHOLECYSTITIS

Acute cholecystitis accounts for 85% to 95% of cases, and involves gallstones that obstruct either the neck of the gallbladder or the cystic duct. Persistent obstruction of the cystic duct causes an increase in gallbladder pressure, with resultant ischemia and inflammation. The onset of constant pain in the right upper quadrant or epigastrium usually occurs after a heavy meal of fatty or fried foods. The patient may complain of previous, similar attacks. Nausea and vomiting are common. Fever, chills, and localized peritoneal signs in the right upper quadrant are strongly suggestive of acute cholecystitis. The gallbladder will dilate and become palpable in 30% of patients. Murphy's sign (increased right upper quadrant tenderness and arrest of inspiration during deep palpation) occurs when the inflamed gallbladder descends and contacts the examiner's fingers. Signs of systemic sepsis occur with progressive inflammation. Jaundice suggests common duct stones but may occur in acute cholecystitis. The differential diagnosis includes peptic ulcer disease with penetration or perforation, acute pancreatitis, retrocecal appendicitis, acute hepatitis, pneumonia, and hepatic abscess. Early cholangitis may mimic cholecystitis and should be considered, especially in the toxic-appearing patient.

Emergency management includes intravenous fluids and nasogastric tube suction. Laboratory studies may be supportive, but none are diagnostic of acute cholecystitis. Liver enzyme, alkaline phosphatase, and bilirubin levels may be slightly elevated. A mild leukocytosis may be present. A urinalysis should be done to rule out urinary tract disease. An elevated serum amylase level may indicate primary pancreatic inflammation or pancreatitis secondary to biliary tract disease (the most common cause of pancreatitis). Abdominal plain films may demonstrate gallstones. A sentinel loop in the right upper quadrant suggests the presence of inflammation, but this may also be caused by pancreatitis.

The choice of diagnostic studies depends on local institutional preferences. Ultrasonography can determine the presence of calculi, with an accuracy approaching 100%. However, the presence of stones is not specific for acute cholecystitis. In 5% to 10% of cases of acute cholecystitis no cystic duct stones are found at the time of surgery (acalculous cholecystitis). Ultrasonography has the advantage of discovering other sources of right upper quadrant pain, including diseases of the liver, pancreas, and kidneys. It is rapid, noninvasive, and less expensive than cholescintigraphy and is the initial study of choice for imaging the gallbladder. Cholescintigraphy utilizing various analogs of N-substituted iminodiacetic acid is the best test for detecting acute operable disease of the biliary tree. It is a study of function rather than of anatomy. HIDA scans are helpful in the setting of high suspicion and normal ultrasound, since the latter does not unequivocally exclude acute cholecystitis. In normal subjects, within 1 hour of injection, the isotope appears in the liver, intrahepatic bile ducts, gallbladder, common duct, and duodenum. In the presence of cystic duct obstruction by a stone, the gallbladder will not be visualized. A negative scan (the appearance of isotope in the gallbladder) virtually excludes acute cholecystitis.

Acute cholecystitis is a surgical disease, and surgical consultation in the ED is appropriate. Meperidine is the preferred analgesic, since morphine is thought to enhance sphincter spasm. Intravenous fluids and antibiotics should be administered. Elderly patients with medical problems

TABLE 19-1. Features That Differentiate Diseases of the Gallbladder

	Cholelithiasis	Acute Cholecystitis
Presentation	Usually asymptomatic, biliary colic—RUQ or epigastric pain (severe, persistent), nausea, vomiting	Pain—RUQ, severe usually associated with meal; nausea, vomiting
Physical Findings	Asymptomatic—normal exam, biliary colic—tenderness (RUQ, epigastrium)	Temperature elevation common, but slight; tachycardia, peritoneal irritation—RUQ (+ Murphy's sign); palpable mass in RUQ + 1/3 of patients; clinical jaundice unusual
Laboratory	WBC count normal, hepatic enzymes normal, bilirubin normal	Leukocytosis (mild); liver chemistries—slight elevation; bilirubin may reach up to 4.0 mg/dL
Radiographic Studies	Ultrasonography → stones	Abdominal films not diagnostic; help to rule out other conditions. Ultrasonography—low sensitivity; specificity and accuracy for cholecystitis only suggestive. Identify presence of gallstones. 99mTc-HIDA scans—high sensitivity, specificity, and accuracy; most reliable diagnostic test.
Differential Diagnosis	When biliary colic present—gastric/duodenal ulcer, pancreatitis, hepatitis, renal colic, gastroesophageal reflux, angina, hiatal hernia	Appendicitis, perforated ulcer, acute pancreatitis, hepatitis, RLL pneumonia

(cont'd.)

and diabetic patients require aggressive stabilization. Persistent pain, peritoneal signs, sepsis, and dehydration are indications for admission. Emergency cholecystectomy is seldom indicated unless the patient is severely ill with a palpable gallbladder. The timing of the cholecystectomy is controversial. Some prefer to admit the patient and administer intravenous hydration, nasogastric suction, and antibiotics. Others prefer to allow the acute episode to defervesce, to be followed by an elective cholecystectomy. The patient with resolving cholecystitis may be treated as an outpatient, but follow-up must occur within 3 to 4 days. Exacerbation of symptoms may result in a return visit.

CHOLEDOCHOLITHIASIS

Choledocholithiasis is the presence of gallstones in the common duct. Most common duct stones are believed to form within the gallbladder and then migrate down the cystic duct. The incidence of common duct stones in acute and chronic cholecystitis is 7% to 15%. The clinical manifestations may vary, depending on the acuity and degree of obstruction. Most often, colicky, severe epigastric pain is present. Jaundice may occasionally accompany the pain or, less often,

TABLE 19-1. *(cont'd.)*

Gallstone ileus	Choledocholithiasis	Cholangitis
Abdominal distention, pain, vomiting; usually elderly patient, 65–77 years; associated medical disorders frequent (diabetes, cardiovascular disease, h/o gallbladder disease)	May be asymptomatic; pain—RUQ	Usually elderly patient; H/O biliary tract disease; colicky RUQ pain, fever, chills
Appears acutely ill, dehydrated, abdominal distention, abdominal pain on palpation, clinical jaundice—unusual	Normal exam, or common duct obstruction → clinical jaundice → RUQ tenderness	RUQ tenderness, clinical jaundice (mild); temperature 104–105°F; Charcot's triad/Reynold's pentad not always present; hypothermia not uncommon
Leukocytosis (mild); electrolyte imbalance and dehydration—↓ Na, ↓ Cl-, ↓ K+, ↑ BUN; bilirubin not elevated	Asymptomatic—normal common bile duct obstruction; ↑ bilirubin, ↑ alkaline phosphatase, ↑ transaminase (minimal)	Leukocytosis >20,000 or <10,000 with left shift; bilirubin ↑ slight, alkaline phosphatase ↑
Abdominal films—pneumobilia—evidence of mechanical bowel obstruction; stone in GI tract	Abdominal films rule out other diseases; ultrasonography—stones in common bile duct, dilation of common bile duct, if obstruction	Abdominal film—pneumobilia may be present
Other causes of intestinal obstruction (hernia, adhesions, tumor)	Causes of obstructive jaundice—tumor in common bile duct, hepatic duct, head of pancreas, ampullar, duodenal	Nonsuppurative cholangitis; amoebic/pyogenic hepatic abscess

be present in the absence of pain. A patient with prior cholecystitis or cholecystectomy should be suspected of having common duct stones. The lab will reveal elevated liver enzymes, alkaline phosphatase, and bilirubin levels. Although hepatitis may also be associated with these laboratory abnormalities, the levels caused by choledocholithiasis with obstructive jaundice are seldom greater than two to three times normal. The prothrombin time may be prolonged. Abdominal plain films are usually negative but may provide information relative to the stomach, bowel, and kidney. Ultrasonography should be performed to establish the degree of extrahepatic biliary dilation and the presence of stones in the gallbladder or common duct. A dilated biliary tree in a jaundiced patient is indicative of extrahepatic obstruction. Treatment is surgical; early surgical consultation is appropriate.

CHOLANGITIS

Cholangitis, infection within the biliary duct system, is most often associated with choledocholithiasis. It is characterized by intermittent fever, upper abdominal pain, and jaundice. The triad of upper abdominal pain, fever and chills, and jaundice (Charcot's triad) suggests infection of the biliary tree. The addition of mental status alteration and hypotension is Reynold's pentad and is strongly suggestive of cholangitis, almost exclusively seen in the elderly. The patient appears septic; the white blood cell count is depressed in more than half the patients, transaminase levels are elevated, and amylase level is normal. Abdominal plain films may reveal air in the biliary tree. Ultrasonography may demonstrate the presence of stones in the gallbladder or common duct. Hepatic abscesses may develop secondary to suppurative cholangitis. Antibiotics should be effective against *Escherichia coli,* the most common pathogen. Antipseudomonal penicillin, ticarcillin clavulanate, and ampicillin/sulbactam are the antibiotics of choice. Surgical consultation should occur early, since intervention is indicated. The correct preoperative diagnosis is usually not made; mortality is high (30%–40%).

PERFORATION OF THE GALLBLADDER

Perforation of the gallbladder involves rapid necrosis of the gallbladder wall with subsequent bile peritonitis. Perforation of the gallbladder primarily affects the elderly and diabetics; it is a surgical emergency.

20   Acute Appendicitis

Appendicitis is an acute inflammation and obstruction of the appendix. It is the most common acute surgical condition of the abdomen. The classic presentation of appendicitis is that of periumbilical pain migrating to the right lower quadrant, associated with anorexia, nausea, vomiting, and a low-grade fever. The diagnosis can be difficult. No single diagnostic test exists. There has been no improvement in diagnostic accuracy in the past 20 years, with false-negative laparotomy rates at 20% in most institutions. The incidence of acute appendicitis is 1:1000 in the general population. It is the most common cause of emergency surgery and surgery during pregnancy in the United States. The highest incidence occurs in the second and third decades of life, but it is seen in all ages. The sex ratio is equal before and after puberty. During puberty the frequency of appendicitis is greater in boys. The single most important factor in morbidity and mortality is the presence of perforation at the time of surgery. Few complications occur in the absence of perforation.

At the extremes of age there is increased morbidity and mortality, the cause of which is multi-factorial. Less than 10% of patients operated on for acute appendicitis are greater than age 60, but more than 50% of all deaths from appendicitis are in this age group. In the older patient appendicitis may be a more fulminant disease, with a nearly 50% perforation rate at the time of surgery. The morbidity and mortality are due to delays in seeking treatment, delays in surgery, high incidence of perforation, and associated diseases. Nearly 50% of all patients with proven perforated appendicitis have sought medical attention previously. Perforation of the appendix is associated with a significant increase in morbidity and mortality. The mortality of simple unperforated appendicitis is 0.1%. It rises to 2%–6% in the general population with perforation, and to 15% in the elderly. The incidence of rupture varies not only with age, but also with locale. In charity hospitals the incidence of perforation is 25% to 30%; in a private hospital the incidence is 15%.

The anatomical position of the appendix significantly affects the clinical presentation of its pathologic state. Most commonly (65%) it lies adjacent to the cecum within the peritoneal cavity.

The second most common location is at the brim of the pelvis, where the tip of the appendix lies extraperitoneally behind the cecum. Malrotation, maldescent, and situs inversus all produce abnormal locations and atypical presentations.

CLINICAL PRESENTATION

The characteristic sequence of events includes malaise, anorexia, and vague periumbilical abdominal pain. Although anorexia may precede the onset of pain, most often pain is the initial complaint. Persistent pain for 6 to 8 hours' duration associated with anorexia, nausea, and, occasionally, vomiting is an important feature of the history. In greater than 50% the pain is initially diffuse, visceral, and central. Severe somatic pain follows, localizing to the right lower quadrant. Nearly half of all cases present *without* this classic picture, especially in the young, elderly, or pregnant woman. These three groups often present with confusing clinical pictures. In the child it is difficult to obtain a history. Early signs may include irritability and annoyance at being handled, refusing to eat, and assuming a fetal position. Patients over age 50 have a spontaneous perforation rate of 30% to 60%. The classic pattern of nausea, vomiting, anorexia, and generalized abdominal discomfort is seen in less than 50% of older patients. Anorexia is not common in the elderly; if present, perforation is more likely. Nausea is seen in 90% of older patients and occurs after the onset of pain. Many older patients perceive only diffuse abdominal pain, with no localization to the right lower quadrant.

The diagnosis of appendicitis is more difficult to make in pregnant patients than in any other subset. The problem of diagnosis is due to two main features of normal pregnancy: (1) the anatomical dislocation of the appendix and (2) changes in the abdominal wall. Acute appendicitis is the most common nonobstetric surgical condition in pregnancy, occurring with the same frequency during pregnancy as during the nonpregnant state. Cases are distributed evenly among the three trimesters. Anorexia is found in only 2/3 of pregnant patients with appendicitis. Classic right lower quadrant pain is felt by all patients with appendicitis in the first trimester, by 71% in the second trimester, and by only 27% in the third trimester. The right upper quadrant is the site of greatest pain in the third trimester. Pain that follows the classic periumbilical-to-right lower quadrant sequence occurs with variable frequency (10%–55%).

The abdominal examination is significantly altered by normal changes of pregnancy. The enlarged uterus causes displacement of the appendix from the right lower quadrant toward a more cephalad and lateral position. At 5 months' gestation the appendix is located in the right upper quadrant; at term the appendix is at the level of the right costal margin. Postpartum, the appendix does not return to its usual location until involution is complete (6–8 weeks). Tenderness in the right upper quadrant or the entire right abdomen is common in the presence of a 12-week or greater size uterus. The enlarged uterus lifts the abdominal wall away from the inflamed appendix. The laxity of the abdominal musculature and the abdominal wall changes minimize clinically apparent signs of peritoneal irritation. In the third trimester peritoneal signs are present in fewer than half of all patients with appendicitis. Leukocytosis does not differentiate appendicitis from other inflammatory causes of abdominal pain. The leukocytosis of pregnancy (12,000–15,000/μL) and puerperium (20,000–25,000/μL) may be present in the absence of disease. Graded-compression ultrasonography may be useful in identifying uterine, adnexal, and hepatobiliary abnormalities as well as in assessing fetal and placental status in the obstetric patient. Laparoscopy has also been used in unclear cases. Increased mortality is probably due to the delay in diagnosis and treatment; obvious delays in diagnosis approach 75% in the third trimester; in the first trimester there was insignificant delay before diagnosis. Appendiceal perforation appears to occur in pregnancy with an incidence of 25% to 60%, which exceeds that of the general population (29%).

The single most important factor that influences the physical examination, as well as morbidity and mortality, is the presence of perforation. The patient with acute appendicitis prefers to lie quietly in the supine position with his right leg drawn up. Vital signs are unremarkable in simple appendicitis. Low-grade fever and mildly increased heart rate may signify perforation or early appendicitis. Significant abnormalities of the vital signs indicate either complications of appendicitis or another diagnosis. The physical examination is primarily influenced by the location and presence of rupture. The hallmark is localized, deep abdominal tenderness over the right lower quadrant. This is the most significant physical finding in all age groups. McBurney's point, the usual point of maximal tenderness, is described as being 1 to 2 inches medial to the right anterior spinous process of the ilium on a line drawn to the umbilicus. Voluntary and involuntary abdominal guarding and rebound tenderness suggest significant peritoneal irritation.

Muscle resistance corresponds to the degree of inflammatory process. As peritoneal irritation progresses muscle spasms increase and become involuntary (i.e., true rigidity). Rovsing's sign is referred pain from the left to the right lower quadrant with palpation. The use of "cough" rebound may yield more consistent information. A positive obturator sign suggests peritoneal irritation, and is elicited by flexing the patient's knee and hip with external rotation of the hip. Increased stress on the obturator muscles results in pain. The rectal examination frequently elicits pain, especially in the right lower quadrant.

The physical findings in the presence of a ruptured appendix are more defined than in simple appendicitis. The patient usually appears toxic and has right lower quadrant pain. Often a mass effect is appreciated due to an abscess. Rebound tenderness and rigidity, abdominal distention, and ileus are often present, and relate to the severity and duration of inflammation.

DIFFERENTIAL DIAGNOSIS

The differential diagnosis of acute appendicitis is that of the acute abdomen. The diagnostic possibilities are influenced by (1) location of the appendix, (2) stage of process, (3) patient's sex, and (4) patient's age. The rate of incorrect diagnoses is highest in young women. The most common erroneous diagnoses, in descending order of frequency, are acute mesenteric lymphadenitis, no organic pathology, acute pelvic inflammatory disease, twisted ovarian cyst or ruptured graafian follicle, and acute gastroenteritis. A complete differential diagnosis can be found in Table 20-1.

EMERGENCY DEPARTMENT EVALUATION

A thorough history and physical examination (abdominal, rectal, and vaginal examinations) should be performed on all patients with abdominal pain. The patient's age and sex will influence the diagnostic considerations. Laboratory studies may rule out other conditions. A complete blood count, urinalysis, and rapid, sensitive pregnancy test should be done. The complete blood count in acute appendicitis may demonstrate a leukocytosis with a minimal left shift, although the sensitivity and specificity of this test remain controversial. The urinalysis may contain leukocytes and erythrocytes, which may be due to urinary tract disease or an inflamed appendix in proximity to the ureter. Abdominal plain films are seldom diagnostic unless an appendolith can be visualized. An appendolith over the right sacroiliac

---

TABLE 20-1. Differential Diagnosis of Acute Appendicitis

Gastroenteritis	Right kidney stone
Acute diverticulitis	Crohn's disease (often diagnosed
Mesenteric adenitis (common in	at the time of laparotomy)
children after a viral illness)	Pyelonephritis
Perforated duodenal ulcer	Endometriosis
Acute cholecystitis	Ovarian torsion
Ruptured graafian follicle	Bowel obstruction
Mittelschmerz	Mesenteric infarction
Ectopic pregnancy	Meckel's diverticulum
Pelvic inflammatory disease	

joint is a reliable, but not absolute sign. There are a number of nonspecific radiographic signs indicative of right lower quadrant inflammation: right lower quadrant ileus, loss of psoas margin, blunting of the flank stripe, dilated transverse colon, relatively airless intestine or reactive ileus, and lumbar scoliosis to the right. Ancillary studies, such as pelvic ultrasonography, laparoscopy, computed tomographic scanning, and barium enema, have been recommended by various authors.

EMERGENCY DEPARTMENT MANAGEMENT AND DISPOSITION

The patient should be made comfortable and given nothing by mouth. An intravenous line should be established to ensure adequate hydration and venous access. Pain medications should be deferred until the surgical consultation is complete. In the old, very young, or pregnant patient, evaluation and surgical consultation should be more aggressive because of the difficulty in diagnosis and the higher rate of perforation. ED or inpatient observation may be indicated according to local practice. If the diagnosis remains unclear and the patient is reliable, outpatient re-evaluation may be considered with close follow-up.

COMMON PITFALLS

- Pain usually occurs before the onset of other symptoms.
- The emergency physician should be particularly wary of abdominal pain in the young, elderly, or pregnant patient.
- Acute appendicitis is the most common cause of surgery during pregnancy. An understanding of the anatomical and physiologic changes of pregnancy should assist in the diagnosis.
- Delay in diagnosis increases the incidence of perforation with resultant increased morbidity and mortality.
- Surgery in the elderly is less dangerous in suspected appendicitis than awaiting perforation. Early surgical consultation should be obtained.
- The diagnosis of appendicitis should be questioned in the absence of anorexia.
- The emergency physician should watch for atypical presentations and not be reassured by subtle findings, especially in the young and old.
- Acute appendicitis remains one of the more commonly missed surgical diagnoses. Failure to diagnose appendicitis remains a significant risk management issue for emergency physicians.

21   Intestinal Obstruction

Intestinal obstruction is a major source of morbidity and mortality. The challenge is to quickly identify those patients with bowel obstruction, initiate proper therapeutic maneuvers and obtain appropriate surgical consultation. Interference with the normal passage of intestinal contents can occur from mechanical or neurogenic causes. Any portion of the large and small bowel may be affected. Mechanical obstruction is usually classified as simple, implying an intact blood supply, or strangulated, in which mesenteric vessel compromise occurs. Most series show a significant increase in patient morbidity and mortality when a simple obstruction is allowed to progress to strangulation. Early diagnosis and intervention are crucial for optimal patient outcome. Obstruction of the intestinal tract accounts for about 20% of all acute surgical admissions. The vast majority of small-bowel obstructions are caused by adhesions from prior abdominal procedures. Other causes in the adult include hernias, colon carcinoma, diverticulitis, and fecal impaction. Intussusception, seen in the pediatric age group, may also occur in the older patient. Strangulated inguinal hernia and complications from Meckel's diverticulum are other causes in infants. The overall mortality from intestinal obstruction is 5% to 10%.

CLINICAL PRESENTATION

The most frequent complaint of the obstructed patient is abdominal pain. It is often severe at the outset and may be referred to the epigastrium, the umbilical region, and, sometimes, the hypogastrium. Pain is usually colicky, with spasms lasting up to several minutes. Vomiting is a frequent symptom. If the vomitus is copious at the onset, a proximal small-bowel obstruction is likely. More often the early vomitus is not voluminous and consists of semidigested food. Later it becomes bilious and eventually dark brown and foul-smelling from the profuse bacterial growth in the stagnant lumen. Feculent vomiting usually signifies distal small-bowel obstruction and, in the absence of peritonitis, is diagnostic of intestinal obstruction. One must note that if the distal ileum or colon is obstructed, the patient may have no vomiting and may even progress to a near fatal condition without ever vomiting. Another common symptom is obstipation (no passage of feces or flatus). The patient may not present with this complaint, since the bowel distal to the obstruction can continue to empty as the condition progresses. Abdominal distention is a frequent complaint. The degree depends on the site and duration of the obstruction. In proximal jejunal obstruction the epigastrium is distended, whereas ileal blockage results in bloating of the central abdomen. Colonic obstruction is more likely to cause diffuse distention, particularly in the flanks.

Vital signs are usually within normal limits if the patient presents early in the clinical course and has no concomitant illness. However, the patient who ignores the early symptoms and presents later in the course may appear pale and anxious, with tachycardia, slight fever, and hypotension.

The abdomen should be inspected for scars indicating prior abdominal or pelvic surgery. Auscultation may reveal high-pitched, hyperactive, rushing bowel sounds associated with the patient's pain. Palpation, which usually reveals diffuse tenderness, must include careful attention to hernial orifices (inguinal, femoral, and previous abdominal incisions). Marked guarding and rebound tenderness are suggestive, but not confirmatory, of strangulation. Rectal examination may reveal impacted feces or a tumor. Gross or occult blood should be noted. Air can be introduced into the rectum by way of digital examination; therefore, the emergency physician may want to defer this evaluation until after the abdominal films are obtained.

DIFFERENTIAL DIAGNOSIS

If signs and symptoms of small-bowel obstruction are present but abdominal distention is absent, perforated ulcer, pancreatitis, appendicitis with peritonitis, and cholecystitis should be considered. These conditions are usually characterized by abdominal rigidity and the absence of feculent vomiting. The pain of renal and biliary colic is distinguished by its location and radiation. If distention is present, uremia, mesenteric thrombosis, and late peritonitis should be considered. Large-bowel obstruction can be confused with peritonitis, colitis with distention, and ileus (postoperative adynamic type is most common). Uremia can be accompanied by abdominal distention and vomiting.

EMERGENCY DEPARTMENT MANAGEMENT

Blood should be sent for complete blood count and electrolytes, creatinine, blood urea nitrogen, and amylase. Urinalysis should be performed. Leukocytosis should be noted. (In one study of 128 patients with small-bowel obstruction only leukocytosis and continuous pain were statistically significant for strangulation.) Abnormally high hemoglobin levels suggest hemoconcentration, whereas low values indicate possible bleeding into the bowel lumen. Electrolyte abnormalities from gastrointestinal fluid loss need to be monitored and corrected. The plain abdominal film (both supine and erect views) must be done. A left lateral decubitus view may be substituted for the erect view if there is difficulty in positioning the patient. Gas and fluid accumulation above the blockage gives rise to air–fluid levels when the patient is erect. The supine view shows the amount and distribution of air within the gut. Distended loops of small bowel can appear in a "stepladder" pattern across the central abdomen. In 5% of cases of intestinal obstruction abdominal films are normal. Small air pockets may appear as the "string of pearls" sign on the upright view. Dilated fluid-filled loops of small intestine and evidence of air in the colon indicate a partial small bowel obstruction. Colonic gas usually outlines the haustral folds that appear to extend into but do not completely traverse the width of the large intestine. Absence of air in the rectum is a sign of obstruction, but if the abdominal films are obtained after rectal examination, the presence of rectal air loses its significance.

Intravenous replacement of fluid and electrolyte loss is crucial. Normal saline solution or Ringer's lactate, dextrose in water, and appropriate potassium supplementation are recommended. Foley catheter and, if indicated by the patient's condition, a central venous line facilitates accurate monitoring of fluid replacement. A nasogastric tube should be inserted to decompress the stomach in anticipation of the need for surgical intervention. Antibiotics may be administered in consultation with the surgeon.

DISPOSITION

ROLE OF THE CONSULTANT   Early surgical consultation is of utmost importance. The challenge facing the surgical consultant is deciding whether strangulation is present. This often may only be determined at the operating table.

INDICATIONS FOR ADMISSION   All patients with mechanical intestinal obstruction should be admitted to the hospital for surgical management.

COMMON PITFALLS

- Delay in diagnosing intestinal obstruction and obtaining surgical consultation are factors that result in poor patient outcome.
- Patient procrastination in seeking medical attention compounds the problem.
- The goal is intervention before strangulation occurs.
- Failure to replenish lost fluid and electrolytes. Uncorrected losses result in a poor surgical candidate and contribute to increased morbidity and mortality.

22   Hernias

An inguinal hernia is not a major challenge to the emergency physician unless incarceration or strangulation exists. It is thought that up to 5% of the population have a hernia; 2% of the population have a demonstrable hernia. Inguinal hernias usually occur at the extremes of age. Hernias seen in children represent congenital defects and are indirect inguinal hernias. Hernias seen in older patients are direct hernias that result from relaxation of the abdominal musculature. Operations for various hernias are routine and the success rate is excellent. An inguinal hernia is much less common in females.

Seventy-five percent of all hernias occur in the groin. Two thirds are indirect and one third are direct hernias. Six percent of hernias are femoral and are much more common in women. Eighty-six percent of all groin hernias occur in men; 84% of all femoral hernias occur in women. However, the most common hernia in a female is not a femoral hernia, but an indirect inguinal hernia. Hernias in infants and children are almost always indirect. Ten percent of hernias are incisional, another 3% are umbilical, and the remaining 3% constitute unusual hernias.

Incarceration occurs when the protruding hernia is caught by the narrowness of the neck of the ring and cannot return into the abdominal cavity. In time the incarcerated hernia may become strangulated. The blood flow to and from the portion of the bowel caught in the hernia sac is compromised, eventually resulting in necrosis of the bowel. Early in the course of incarceration it is difficult to differentiate between incarceration and strangulation. Patients with strangulated hernias are usually more ill than those with incarcerated hernias. Because the loop of the bowel is outside of the general confines of the peritoneal cavity, strangulation often has a delayed onset of peritonitis, which makes the diagnosis more difficult. The hernias that are most prone to strangulate are those that protrude through a small ring. Typically, these include the femoral, indirect inguinal, and umbilical hernias.

Less common hernias include Richter's, Littre's, Velpeau's, Hesselbach's, pantaloon, and Cloquet's. Richter's hernia is a specific type of hernia in which only one side of the loop of the intestine is within the hernia sac. Littre's hernia is a rare hernia caused by an incarcerated or strangulated Meckel's diverticulum within the hernia. A pantaloon hernia is seen when indirect and direct hernias coexist on the same side of the groin. When there is a femoral and indirect hernia on the same side it is called Hesselbach's hernia. The umbilical hernia is common, particularly in black infants, in whom the incidence is as high as 65%; 10% of white infants have an umbilical hernia. Most umbilical hernias close spontaneously by age 2. Umbilical hernias are more common in females. Epigastric hernias are small herniations through defects in the linea alba. Such hernias are more commonly found above the umbilicus than below. A spigelian hernia appears at the semilunar line of Douglas, and is often confused with an inguinal hernia.

The differential diagnosis of an inguinal mass includes inguinal adenitis, ectopic testis, hydrocele, and varix.

CLINICAL PRESENTATION

The two most common presentations in adults are a bulge and pain or discomfort in the inguinal or scrotal area. The diagnosis of a hernia depends on the physical examination. The exception to this is in an infant or child. Commonly, parents will report a groin bulge that cannot be demonstrated at the time of examination. The patient should stand, with the examiner seated in front of the patient. The groin should be observed for a bulge during coughing and straining. If a bulge is not seen, then a finger should be inserted by invaginating the scrotum into the inguinal ring. The acts of coughing and straining should be repeated in order to allow the examiner's finger to feel the impulse of the bulging hernia. The examination should be repeated with the patient in the supine position.

EMERGENCY DEPARTMENT MANAGEMENT

After a brief history and appropriate physical examination a patient with a reducible hernia should be given instructions concerning avoidance of straining and exercise and the danger signs of incarceration and strangulation. Referral to a general surgeon for further evaluation and repair should be accomplished before discharge. The use of an inguinal truss remains common in Europe and elsewhere; occasionally it is used in the United States in cases that represent unacceptable surgical or anesthetic risks. A hernia that does not reduce spontaneously should be gently manipulated by pulling and pushing steadily until it returns to the abdominal cavity. A slight Trendelenburg position can facilitate this maneuver. Undue force should be avoided. Frequently an adult patient or the parent of an infant is more adept at reduction than the examiner. After reduction and lacking any signs suggestive of an intestinal obstruction the patient should be referred to a general or pediatric surgeon. An incarcerated or strangulated hernia needs urgent surgical attention. Intravenous fluids should be initiated, a nasogastric tube inserted, and appropriate laboratory studies ordered so that the patient can be promptly taken to the operating room. Flat and upright films of the abdomen may be useful.

DISPOSITION

INDICATIONS FOR ADMISSION   Indications for admission include incarceration, strangulation, signs of intestinal obstruction, peritonitis, significant vomiting, and unremitting pain.

COMMON PITFALLS

- Misdiagnosis of a high groin saphenous varix
- Confusing hernia with inguinal lymph node
- Being unaware of a small incarcerated hernia
- Failure to make an appropriate referral to a surgeon
- Failure to diagnose incarceration or strangulation

---

23   Colonic Diverticular Disease

The prevalence of diverticular disease has increased with our advancing age of the population. The incidence increases from 5% in the fifth decade to 50% in the ninth decade. It is estimated that in the population over age 60, the prevalence of diverticulosis is more than 30%. Diverticulosis in young adults has been diagnosed in association with Marfan's disease. The common causative agent appears to be a reduction in dietary fiber content. The pathophysiology is related to a pressure gradient between the colonic lumen and the serosa and areas of relative weakness in the bowel wall. The sigmoid colon is involved in more than 90% and in 50% it is the only segment of the bowel involved. The cecum is involved in 2%, the ascending colon and rectum in 4% each, and the transverse colon in 10%. Most people with diverticulosis remain asymptomatic throughout their lives, although 17% eventually showed signs of diverticulitis. The longer a patient has diverticulosis, the greater the probability of complications, primarily diverticulitis and bleeding. Diverticulitis results from inflammation of diverticula with either microperforation or macroperforation (abscess, fistula, peritonitis, or obstruction). Of patients > 60 with diverticulosis, about 1/3 will develop diverticulitis and about one third of these will have persistent symptoms and further complications. There is no relation between the number and size of diverticula and the incidence of complications or probability of recurrent disease. Bleeding from diverticulosis is massive in about 25%. The bleeding comes from an arterial lesion in the vasa recta. A disproportionately high tendency exists for right colon diverticula hemorrhage.

CLINICAL PRESENTATION

Patients with diverticulosis present with three common patterns: (1) mild left lower quadrant pain; (2) acute left lower quadrant pain, tenderness, and fever; and (3) massive lower gastrointestinal (GI) bleeding.

MILD LEFT LOWER QUADRANT PAIN (SYMPTOMATIC DIVERTICULOSIS)   Diverticulosis most frequently presents with left lower abdominal pain. The pain is usually dull, but sometimes it is crampy and intermittent.

ACUTE LEFT LOWER QUADRANT PAIN, TENDERNESS, AND FEVER (ACUTE DIVERTICULITIS)
Patients with acute diverticulitis present with acute left lower quadrant pain with or without a mass, tenderness, and rebound associated with fever and leukocytosis. Occasionally the pain and tenderness occur in the left upper quadrant. Patients may present with a picture of a ruptured viscus with diffuse tenderness, rebound, guarding, and diminished or absent bowel sounds. Diffuse abdominal pain is more commonly found in immunocompromised patients. Rarely, diverticulitis may present with signs of fistulization such as pneumaturia and draining infections of the lower abdomen or medial aspect of the upper thigh.

MASSIVE LOWER GASTROINTESTINAL BLEEDING (DIVERTICULOSIS)   Patients may present with painless, massive rectal bleeding. Such bleeding is characteristically sudden, often profuse from the onset, and more frequent in older people. The blood is usually bright or dark red, and although the patient may feel faint, initial hypotension is not common. Many patients with massive rectal bleeding have had a previous episode, suggesting diverticulitis.

DIFFERENTIAL DIAGNOSIS

DIVERTICULOSIS   When diverticulosis presents as mild, sometimes colicky left lower quadrant pain it must be differentiated from irritable bowel syndrome, Crohn's disease, and colon cancer.

ACUTE DIVERTICULITIS   Acute diverticulitis must be distinguished from more severe presentations of Crohn's disease, ulcerative colitis, and ischemic colitis, although diverticulitis and inflammatory bowel disease may coexist. It must also be distinguished from appendicitis. Although acute diverticulitis is usually left-sided and appendicitis usually right-sided, there are certainly cases of appendicitis that present with left lower abdominal pain as well as cases of solitary cecal diverticulitis and sigmoid diverticulitis adherent to the right lower quadrant. In women, diverticulitis that presents with a left lower quadrant mass has been misdiagnosed as a gynecologic mass. High fever, leukocytosis, and left lower quadrant mass should suggest a perforation and abscess. This may be due to inflammatory bowel disease, colon cancer, sigmoid volvulus, iatrogenic perforation of the rectosigmoid, or a tubovarian abscess.

DIVERTICULAR BLEEDING   Diverticular bleeding must be distinguished from other causes of profuse lower GI bleeding, such as angiodysplasia, ischemic colitis, and, occasionally, ulcerative colitis and colonic or rectal cancer. It is most difficult to distinguish between diverticular bleeding and angiodysplasia; however, the evaluation and the medical and surgical therapy are essentially identical.

EMERGENCY DEPARTMENT EVALUATION

LEFT LOWER QUADRANT PAIN   The history should focus on GI symptoms, previous similar attacks, prior diagnostic studies, change in bowel habits, duration of the attack, characteristics of the pain, and history of fever. With diverticulitis, the pain may be intermittent, crampy, and associated with nausea and vomiting. The attack may be associated with either constipation or diarrhea. The physical examination should note the temperature, pulse and blood pressure. Complete abdominal, pelvic, and rectal examinations are essential. In rare cases tenderness may be found only on rectal examination. Palpation may reveal the outline of the sigmoid colon as a rope-like mass. Minimal tenderness and mobility point to an irritable colon; a large, sausage-like, markedly tender fixed mass points to diverticulitis. Signs of peritonitis and the presence of a mass on pelvic and rectal examinations are important. Abdominal x-rays should be done to look for a mass in the left lower quadrant or free air. A complete blood count with a differential white blood cell count is indicated. Leukocytosis with a left shift is compatible with the diagnosis of diverticulitis.

LOWER GASTROINTESTINAL BLEEDING   The history should focus on the onset, color, amount, and frequency of bloody bowel movements. A history of previous attacks, bleeding tendencies, and bowel habits is important. Hemodynamic instability should be assessed (blood pressure, pulse, and ortho-static changes). Abdominal and rectal examinations are critical; focus on areas of tenderness and the presence or absence of a mass. The rectum should be palpated for masses and the color of the blood in the rectal vault noted. A sigmoidoscopic examination can be performed in the ED to rule out rectal causes of lower GI bleeding.

EMERGENCY DEPARTMENT MANAGEMENT

DIVERTICULOSIS   For the patient with left lower quadrant pain with no mass, fever, or leukocy-tosis, symptomatic therapy with a mild sedative-anticholinergic preparation can be recommended. A high-fiber diet and a follow-up flexible sigmoidoscopy should also be recommended.

DIVERTICULITIS   For the patient with severe diverticulitis, an intravenous line, nasogastric tube, blood and urine cultures and intravenous antibiotics should be begun. Sigmoidoscopy and bar-ium enema are generally contraindicated in acute diverticulitis. Sigmoidoscopy is very painful, and a barium enema could cause peritonitis if there is a perforation or if one develops as a result of the examination. The intravenous antibiotics used should either be an aminoglycoside (gentam-icin or tobramycin, 5 mg/kg/day) and clindamycin or cefoxitin (4 g to 6 g daily every 6 hours).

DIVERTICULAR BLEEDING   For the patient with massive lower GI bleeding, two large-bore intra-venous lines (16 gauge or larger) should be inserted, Type and crossmatch for 4 to 6 units of blood, Foley catheter, and lactated Ringer's infused at a rate depending on the patient's vital signs and cardiac status. If the patient is not stabilized after 2 liters of crystalloid infusion, a central venous line should be inserted and blood given. Hourly urine output should be monitored.

DISPOSITION

A surgical consultation should be requested for patients in whom the diagnosis of acute divertic-ulitis is suspected and in all patients with rapid lower GI bleeding. The patient with lower GI bleed-ing who is hemodynamically unstable should have an immediate surgical consultation.

INDICATIONS FOR ADMISSION   Patients suspected of having severe acute diverticulitis and those with gross lower GI bleeding must be admitted. Patients obviously septic, with severe concomitant diseases, or with massive lower GI bleeding should be admitted to an intensive care unit.

COMMON PITFALLS

- Although less frequently encountered in patients under age 40, diverticulosis is more likely to be complicated and require surgery in younger patients than in older patients.
- In women, diverticulitis presenting with a left lower quadrant mass is frequently misdiag-nosed as a gynecologic mass.
- Barium enema and sigmoidoscopic examinations using air insufflation may cause perfora-tion and peritonitis in patients who present with acute diverticulitis.
- Abdominal tenderness in less likely to be localized to the left lower quadrant in immuno-compromised patients; it is more likely to be generalized.

24   Perianal, Rectal, and Anal Diseases

The anorectal area is the site of few true emergencies, but many uncomfortable conditions.

ANORECTAL ABSCESSES

Anorectal abscesses are serious because they may spread rapidly, dissecting into deep tissue spaces. Perianal abscesses are located immediately adjacent to the anus; there is no induration noted on rectal examination. Ischiorectal abscesses are deeper, with diffuse and lateral perianal swelling; induration is present on rectal examination. Intersphincteric, intermuscular, and supralevator abscesses generally do not have external signs, but swelling and tenderness at various depths are noted during rectal examination.

CLINICAL PRESENTATION

Ischiorectal and perianal abscesses normally present with severe perianal pain and a "boil." Patients with deeper perirectal abscesses often present with fever, systemic toxicity, and a sensation of rectal fullness or heaviness. A perirectal abscess may extend intra-abdominally and cause systemic toxicity, peritonitis, and an abdominal or a pelvic mass. Although simple ischiorectal and perianal abscesses are the most common, an abscess may track into several tissue planes and have deep components in addition to superficial ones.

DIFFERENTIAL DIAGNOSIS

Swelling and pus can be present due to a local abscess or a sinus tract from a distant source. Pilonidal abscess, Bartholin gland abscess, deep perirectal abscess, and, rarely, intra-abdominal abscess fistula (Crohn's disease) can generate sinus tracts that may initially resemble a superficial buttocks abscess. Careful palpation is the most useful technique to differentiate a sinus tract from an abscess. Coexisting and predisposing illnesses should also be sought. They include inflammatory bowel disease, tuberculosis, various blood dyscrasias, sepsis, diabetes, and steroid therapy. Local trauma and local infectious processes (such as hidradenitis suppurativa, infected hair follicles, or a poorly healing episiotomy) also predispose toward abscess development. An aneurysm in the rectal region may simulate an abscess. Abscess aspiration results in accurate diagnosis and prevents catastrophe.

EMERGENCY DEPARTMENT EVALUATION AND MANAGEMENT

The extent of a perirectal abscess and its anatomical location are usually determined with a careful digital examination. The emergency physician should drain only relatively superficial abscesses that can be drained through perianal skin (ischiorectal and perianal abscesses). Adequate drainage is important. Some authors recommend culture of the abscess by needle aspiration before drainage. Although *Escherichia coli, Staphylococcus aureus,* and fecal anaerobes are the most common organisms in perirectal abscesses, other organisms also cause abscesses. Patients with rheumatic fever, mitral valve prolapse, endocarditis, or immunosuppressive conditions should receive intravenous antibiotics 30 minutes before incision. Cefoxitin is recommended, although penicillins and cephalosporins do not penetrate abscess cavities well. Incision and drainage should be performed with the patient prone or in the jackknife position with the buttocks taped apart. Local anesthesia with 1% lidocaine should be adequate, but some patients require meperidine or morphine. The incision should be radial; removal of an ellipse of skin may be helpful in facilitating drainage. Loculations should be broken up with a hemostat, and the wound should be copiously irrigated. Loose packing with a single piece of gauze should be removed in 48 hours. Sitz baths encourage drainage. Routine abscesses usually heal without the patient needing antibiotics. Indications for antibiotic therapy include systemic toxicity, a large area of cellulitis, lymphangitis, and immunocompromise. Patients with these symptoms should be considered for admission. Drainage of multiple abscesses may result in a residual fistula that will require further attention. The patient should be warned of this possibility and referred for follow-up surgery.

DISPOSITION

Deep abscesses with systemic symptoms necessitate urgent surgical consultation for drainage and admission to the hospital. Prompt therapy is important to prevent spread of the infection and septic shock. Poor outcomes have been associated with delay in therapy, inadequate treatment, and significant concomitant disease.

COMMON PITFALLS

- Failure to identify deep abscess
- Failure to identify an abscess as complex or of pilonidal origin
- Treatment in the ED of an abscess that requires extensive surgical management
- Failure to identify conditions that warrant preincisional antibiotics

ANORECTAL FISTULAS

An anorectal fistula is an abnormal communication between the anorectum (primary opening) and another site, usually after drainage of an anorectal abscess. The tract is usually single. A fistula or sinuses in the perianal area can also originate from nonanorectal sites, such as diverticulitis of the sigmoid colon, appendicitis, inflammatory bowel disease, periurethral infection, and presacral tumors.

Anorectal fistula is treated by uncapping the fistula and allowing it to heal outward from its base. The procedure should be performed by a surgeon. Treatment of fistulas that necessitates incision through the anorectal ring can result in incontinence.

HEMORRHOIDS

Hemorrhoids are varicose veins at the rectal outlet, and are the most frequent cause of rectal bleeding. Increased pressure in the hemorrhoidal veins is thought to be the major predisposing factor. Conditions believed to cause rectal venous outflow obstruction include pregnancy and bearing down when stooling (increased abdominal pressure), repeated storage of firm stool in the rectal ampulla (local obstruction of venous return), and hepatic fibrosis (shunting of venous return).

Internal hemorrhoids occur above the anorectal line. They are covered by mucosa and insensitive to painful stimuli. These features differentiate them from external hemorrhoids. When thrombosis is present hemorrhoids may be painful and a hard clot is palpable in the hemorrhoidal vessels. Hemorrhoids may itch but are usually not painful unless thrombosis is present. When pain is the chief complaint and hemorrhoidal disease is not extreme, another source for the pain should be carefully sought.

Acute exacerbations of hemorrhoidal disease characterized by prolapse of part of the anal canal and thrombophlebitis of the hemorrhoidal plexus require conservative treatment with stool softeners, sitz baths, pain-relieving ointment or suppository, and analgesics. Topical hydrocortisone is of value only if there is itching. With the exception of chronic or constantly prolapsed internal hemorrhoids, most episodes of hemorrhoidal disease are self-limited. A thrombosed external hemorrhoid can be treated conservatively or surgically. After local anesthesia the clot can be evacuated through a short incision made over the clot. Sitz baths and a pad to absorb the oozing are helpful after treatment. A thrombosed internal hemorrhoid should be managed by a surgeon.

RECTAL PROLAPSE

Rectal prolapse is a full-thickness protrusion of a portion of the distal rectum through the anal opening. The protrusion has a tubular appearance with concentric folds on the end. Mucosal prolapse occurs when the rectal mucosa loses its connection to the underlying muscle and protrudes out the anal opening; it differs from rectal prolapse in that there is no protrusion of muscle and the protruding tissue forms a circle with radial grooves. Internal rectal prolapse is also possible, in which the upper rectum and sigmoid have prolapsed into the rectal ampulla but not through the anal orifice. Women most often suffer from the latter condition. They may complain of incontinence of flatus or feces, tenesmus, rectal pressure, pelvic fullness or pain, lower back pain, or a sensation of incomplete evacuation.

A patulous anus is commonly found when repeated rectal prolapse is the presenting complaint. If the lesion has reduced at the time of examination, the most effective way to provoke prolapse is to have the patient strain. Rectal pain from rectal prolapse is uncommon and should suggest a secondary lesion or incarceration. Occasionally a polyp or rectal tumor may protrude through the anus and simulate prolapse. Examination after reduction helps to differentiate the conditions. Mental illness, multiple sclerosis, tabes dorsalis, and cauda equina syndrome are associated with rectal prolapse, although they are responsible for only a small percentage of cases.

Reduction of most prolapses can easily be accomplished in the ED but such reduction is usually short-lived. Incarceration of a rectal prolapse necessitates emergency operative therapy. Incarceration can progress to strangulation, bleeding secondary to ulceration, and rupture. Adults eventually require surgery for recurrent rectal prolapse. Most authorities recommend early surgery, since once incontinence develops from weakening of the sphincter, surgery to correct the prolapse may not restore continence.

VENEREAL DISEASE AND WARTS

Condylomata acuminata is caused by the human papillomavirus. The warts may be pedunculated or sessile. Patients with even modestly compromised cellular immunity are more vulnerable to wart infection, but the warts are also very contagious among nonimmunocompromised people. At least 25% of the sexual partners of patients with warts are also afflicted. Anogenital warts are associated with other sexually transmitted diseases. Data from sexually transmitted disease clinics suggest that 12% to 34% of patients with genital warts have gonorrhea, chlamydial infection, or syphilis. Condylomata lata are wart-like lesions caused by syphilis. They are smoother than anogenital warts and are nearly always moist. Syphilis should be recognized and treated by the emergency physician. Treatment includes penicillin G, 2.4 million units I.M., or a 10-day course of tetracycline or erythromycin. Venereal diseases such as herpes simplex, lymphogranuloma venereum, and gonorrhea can also manifest as rectal diseases.

CARCINOMA

The symptoms of anal cancer are often indistinguishable from those of benign lesions. The most common symptoms are pain and bleeding. A palpable mass is present in 25% of cases; pruritus is present in about 15% of cases. In about 25% of cases patients are asymptomatic, and cancer is detected by routine rectal examination. The predictive value in older people of a positive guaiac test result for colorectal carcinoma is about 5% to 10%. In addition, adenomas are found in approximately 30% to 40% of patients with positive guaiac test results. Squamous cell tumors account for 70% of tumors of the anus. Adenocarcinomas are common in the rectum. Risk factors for colorectal carcinoma include prior adenoma, family history of large-bowel cancer, history of breast or uterine carcinoma, exposure of pelvis to radiation, and presence of ureterosigmoidostomy. Familial polyposis, ulcerative colitis, and Crohn's disease of the colon are also risk factors. Leukemic infiltration into the anal area can result in severe anal pain, but in minimal physical findings except for superficial induration. The patient may appear quite ill. The white blood cell count is usually diagnostic. Persistent coccygeal pain suggests a tumor of neural origin in the coccyx and lower back. Spasmodic pain is more characteristic of benign conditions such as coccygodynia, a syndrome (secondary to trauma) of sharp pains precipitated by movement of the coccyx.

PILONIDAL DISEASE AND HIDRADENITIS SUPPURATIVA

Pilonidal disease is a syndrome of infection in the presacral midline that causes sinus tracts, abscesses, and pits. Hidradenitis suppurativa is a chronic inflammatory disease that originates in areas of apocrine sweat glands and results in superficial, often multiple, and interconnected abscesses. Treatment of both conditions involves incision and drainage of abscess cavities, moist heat or soaks, and antibiotics. Both conditions necessitate more extensive surgical procedures by a surgeon for definitive treatment; otherwise, recurrence is inevitable.

25   Abdominal Aortic Aneurysm

The timely recognition of an abdominal aortic aneurysm (AAA) can be a major challenge. The presentation may be confusing, accurate diagnosis difficult, and the price of delay or diagnostic error devastating. AAAs are present in nearly 2% of the elderly population, with 75% occurring in the over-60 age group. The incidence is increasing, although it is not clear whether this merely represents better diagnosis. Because the proportion of the population expected to survive to age 60 or more continues to increase, emergency physicians can expect their encounters with patients suffering from AAAs to increase as well. Virtually all AAAs are due to atherosclerosis, and thus the majority of patients are men. Similarly, many patients have evidence of other serious atherosclerotic lesions, such as coronary artery or cerebrovascular disease.

The natural history of the AAA is one of gradual expansion (although sudden changes in size do occur), followed by rupture, exsanguination, and death. Occasional cases of "closed, chronic rupture" have been reported. Most AAAs are symptomless until rapid expansion or leakage occurs. The onset of symptoms referable to the aneurysm is a serious prognostic sign. Eighty percent of patients with untreated symptomatic AAA will be dead within 1 year (33% in 1 month, 74% in 6 months). Ninety-five percent die within 5 years, and virtually none survive 10 years. The risk of rupture and death depends on the size of the aneurysm. A rough rule of thumb is that the risk of rupture within 5 years is equal to ten times the size of the aneurysm. For example, a 6-cm aneurysm carries a 60% risk of rupture, a 7-cm aneurysm 70%, and so on. However, even small AAAs can rupture. If AAA is discovered early and operated on electively, 80% of patients survive 1 year, 50% survive 5 years, and 25% are alive at 10 years. Operative mortality with elective surgery is roughly 2% to 5% in all age groups, compared with mortality from rupture (50% to 75% if in shock, 20% if ruptured but not in shock). Thus elective resection is generally recommended for aneurysms of 5 cm or more.

CLINICAL PRESENTATION

AAA can present in a wide variety of ways. However, presentations fall naturally into three major classes: asymptomatic, symptomatic, and ruptured.

ASYMPTOMATIC ANEURYSM

In the asymptomatic patient an AAA is discovered on routine examination for some other problem. Frequently the aneurysm is noted on abdominal plain films. The emergency physician's task in this setting is to ascertain that the aneurysm is truly asymptomatic, clearly and unequivocally unrelated to the patient's chief complaint. Appropriate referral for further evaluation and elective operations should be made.

SYMPTOMATIC ANEURYSM

Patients with symptoms referable to an AAA can be further subdivided into nonacute and acute presentations. In the nonacute patient abdominal, low back, or flank pain is the cardinal symptom. The pain may be associated with syncope at the time of onset. The discomfort occasionally radiates to the testis or leg, causing the symptoms to be attributed to renal colic, inguinal hernia, or lumbar spine disease. The pain is usually nonspecific, is not much affected by movement, and can vary considerably in location. Radicular findings or hematuria may occasionally be present, further misleading the physician. Other presentations of symptomatic, nonacute AAA include hydronephrosis or leg swelling (usually left) from compression, foot drop or sciatica, or new-onset (or worsening of previously controlled) hypertension secondary to renal artery compression. Less common presentations include testicular swelling or evidence of systemic embolization. Aortocaval fistulas are uncommon, and usually present as high-output failure with marked distention of the lower abdominal and leg veins. About 10% of symptomatic AAAs present with severe pain and marked abdominal tenderness. Patients in the symptomatic-acute category require immediate surgery without the usual preoperative evaluation and preparation, as rupture is either imminent or has already occurred but has been temporarily confined to the retroperitoneum. Because these patients typically have the appearance of an acute abdomen, identifying them as "emergent"cases is not as much of a problem as identifying the nonacute patients, even though the presumptive diagnosis may be erroneous (e.g., perforated viscus). An uncommon, acute presentation of an AAA is gastrointestinal bleeding secondary to an aortoenteric fistula. Such bleeding may be massive, and can distract the emergency physician from suspecting vascular disease. Aortoenteric fistula should be assumed whenever a patient who has had a resection of an AAA presents with gastrointestinal bleeding. Finally, AAA may present acutely as complete aortic occlusion with a clinical picture similar to that of a saddle embolus or acute Leriche syndrome. This complication requires prompt operation and still carries approximately a 50% mortality.

RUPTURED ANEURYSM

Most patients with ruptured AAA will have severe pain and a pulsatile mass. Seventy percent will be in frank shock. Some will have sustained cardiac arrest from which they have been resuscitated. There may be no history of AAA, since half the patients with ruptured AAA are asymptomatic immediately before rupture and death. Because this is an older population with a high prevalence of coronary artery disease, the emergency physician may be easily fooled into assuming a diagnosis of acute myocardial infarction with cardiogenic shock. Indeed, unless autopsy is routinely performed, death is frequently ascribed to acute myocardial infarction, pulmonary embolism, or cardiac arrest. However, one autopsy study has shown that 80% of patients lived 6 hours after the rupture, 50% survived more than 24 hours, 30% more than 6 days, and 10% more than 6 weeks. Thus most patients with ruptured AAA will survive long enough to reach the ED, where prompt diagnosis and operative intervention are possible. Rupture of an AAA is correctly diagnosed preoperatively about 60% to 70% of the time. If the diagnosis is delayed 10 hours, mortality increases; if the diagnosis is missed altogether, mortality may approach 100%.

DIFFERENTIAL DIAGNOSIS

The differential diagnosis of AAA includes the differentials of shock and the acute abdomen. If shock is present, the differential typically includes acute myocardial infarction, hemorrhagic pancreatitis, perforated ulcer (or other hollow organ), and mesenteric infarction. In patients whose presentation is less severe, renal or biliary colic, diverticulitis, and lumbosacral disk disease also need to be considered.

EMERGENCY DEPARTMENT EVALUATION AND MANAGEMENT

The evaluation of a patient with a suspected AAA must be tempered to the presentation. Patients in shock from an acute rupture need vigorous resuscitation, life support, and prompt operation. In less acute situations the following points should be addressed. The history should determine the character, location, and radiation of the patient's discomfort. Information about the nature of onset should be sought. The past history should document the presence or absence of risk factors for cardiovascular disease (e.g., diabetes, hypertension, and smoking) as well as any associated chronic illnesses, such as chronic obstructive lung disease and coronary artery disease.

Physical examination is the key to diagnosis, since more than 90% of AAAs are palpable. Size is difficult to estimate because of overlying tissue, and because AAAs frequently are larger in the anteroposterior diameter than in the transverse. Once an aneurysm is detected, the physical examination should attempt to determine the cephalad extent, size, and degree of tenderness and whether distal pulses are present. Any palpable abdominal pulsation in an obese patient should be suspected of being an AAA, even if a mass cannot be clearly discerned. Most aneurysms can be palpated in the epigastrium extending to the paraumbilical areas on both sides of the midline. A bruit is immaterial, since one is frequently present in patients over age 50 who do not have aortic disease. False-positive physical findings occasionally are caused by adhesions, thickened scars, tumors, or a palpable tortuous aorta.

Laboratory evaluation is pertinent only in nonruptured cases. Routine preoperative tests should be ordered if time permits. Because 60% to 75% of patients with AAA have severe, correctable coronary artery disease, preoperative cardiac screening is important, if the patient does not require an emergency procedure.

Radiologic evaluation is occasionally helpful, in that three fourths of AAA have calcified walls that are visible on plain abdominal or lateral lumbosacral spine films. Calcified walls indicate the presence of an aneurysm, but not whether it is enlarging or leaking. If they are absent, this finding is of no value in ruling out the diagnosis. Other radiologic evidence suggestive of a ruptured AAA includes loss of the psoas or renal shadows, the properitoneal fat line, or the presence of a soft-tissue mass. Two-dimensional ultrasound scanning is useful in quickly and accurately establishing the presence of an aneurysm. However, like plain film radiography, it is not as useful in determining whether rupture has occurred. Computed tomography takes somewhat more time than ultrasonography, but it is useful in selected cases to measure size. It is approximately 80% sensitive and close to 100% specific in identifying leakage or rupture. The usefulness of magnetic resonance imaging is still undetermined. Aortography is not routinely used and is usually not important for the emergency physician to consider. It may be useful to the surgeon if renal artery involvement is suspected, to demonstrate outflow in patients with significant peripheral disease, or to assess suspected visceral lesions (e.g., horseshoe kidney).

Initial management for patients in the symptomatic or ruptured categories should address the ABCs. This includes starting four large-bore intravenous lines followed by fluid resuscitation to a systolic blood pressure of 90 to 100, and crossmatching 10 to 12 units of blood. The pneumatic antishock garment has been helpful in stabilization in some cases.

DISPOSITION

Patients who are truly in the asymptomatic category should be referred to a vascular surgeon for further evaluation for elective resection. Even though these patients are older, it is generally felt that AAAs greater than 5 cm in diameter should be electively repaired. Smaller aneurysms should be evaluated by the surgeon and may be managed expectantly. Patients who present with symptomatic AAA should be admitted for close observation and further evaluation. The majority of these patients will require prompt surgery if it becomes clear that the aneurysm is the source of their symptoms. Patients who present with rupture of their AAA obviously should go straight to the operating room.

ROLE OF THE CONSULTANT   All patients who are suspected of suffering from a symptomatic or ruptured AAA should have a prompt surgical consultation, preferably with a vascular surgeon. Patients in whom the AAA is truly an incidental finding may be referred for later consultation if otherwise appropriate.

INDICATIONS FOR ADMISSION   All patients with symptomatic AAA should be admitted to the hospital for close observation and further investigation. One should assume that abdominal or back pain in the presence of AAA is due to sudden expansion or rupture.

TRANSFER CONSIDERATIONS   If the initial receiving hospital does not have sufficient surgical capability to treat an AAA, then transfer to a more appropriate institution may be indicated. The decision to transfer may be a difficult one for patients who present with cardiovascular instability. The current hospital's capabilities, the length of time in transit, and the likelihood of survival to the second hospital must be considered.

COMMON PITFALLS

- AAAs are frequently misdiagnosed, especially in the obese. Back pain is a common symptom, and because peritoneal signs may not be present unless free rupture into the abdominal cavity has occurred, the emergency physician may be misled to one of the common misdiagnoses of AAA, such as renal colic or lumbosacral disk disease. Because early recognition of AAA is most important to ensure maximum survival, it is a sound practice to perform a physical examination specifically aimed at ruling out an aneurysm in all patients over 50 who present with abdominal or back pain.
- A second major pitfall is assuming that an aneurysm discovered on physical examination is incidental and not the source of the patient's symptoms. Any back or abdominal pain in the presence of an AAA should be assumed to represent expansion or leakage in the absence of overwhelming evidence to the contrary.

26   Mesenteric Ischemia and Infarction

Mesenteric ischemia is the failure of normal oxygenation of the small or large intestine due to interruption of vascular flow. The consequences of this failure of oxygenation lie on a spectrum from intermittent, nonspecific intestinal symptoms to frank gut infarction with demise of the patient. Unfortunately, mortality remains well over 50%, primarily attributable to delay in diagnosis. The mechanism of the vascular interruption in mesenteric ischemia can be divided into three categories:

arterial occlusion, venous occlusion, and nonocclusive ischemia and infarction. Approximately one half to two thirds of all cases are due to superior mesenteric arterial occlusion; the remainder is split equally between mesenteric venous thrombosis and nonocclusive infarction. Of those cases that involve occlusion of the superior mesenteric artery, approximately one half are caused by embolus, one half by thrombus. Once ischemia is established, the pathologic sequence is identical, regardless of the mechanism of the ischemia. Initially, the mucosa and submucosa become edematous. Fluid, and then blood, is lost into the intestinal lumen, and finally, frank gangrene with bacterial invasion or perforation ensues. Hypotension occurs on the basis of blood and fluid losses and is exacerbated when sepsis supervenes. The hypotension leads to further compromise of vascular flow to the gut, and the process becomes self-propagating. All attempts to establish reliable diagnostic criteria for the condition have failed because the symptoms are nonspecific and the presentation unremarkable until the compromised gut (and often the patient) is not salvageable. There is a distinct epidemiological preference for the elderly, with mean ages reported at 60 to 78 years. Sporadic cases have occurred in otherwise normal young women who were taking oral contraceptive pills, but aside from these exceptions there is no sexual predilection. Most patients have evidence of significant pre-existing cardiovascular disease, especially congestive heart failure. Use of digoxin or diuretics is commonly reported. More unusual predispositions, such as radiation-induced arteritis and connective tissue diseases, have been implicated.

CLINICAL PRESENTATION
HISTORY

Presentation is highly variable. The only symptom that is universally present is abdominal pain, which may be localized or diffuse, and may have either a colicky or a constant character. Suddenness of onset is not a reliable symptom, as pain may develop over seconds, minutes, hours, or even days or weeks, depending on the underlying process. Vomiting, diarrhea, or both are reported or observed in 50% to 70% of patients. In 25% of cases vomitus or stool may be obviously bloody. Historically, the patient usually has a combination of the following: advanced age, a history of significant cardiovascular disease, a history of previous thromboembolic events, and concurrent medication with digitalis and a diuretic. The patient may report episodes of vague abdominal fullness or discomfort after meals, and unexplained weight loss is often present, if sought.

PHYSICAL EXAMINATION

Physical examination may be remarkably normal. The patient may appear completely well apart from the presenting pain. Approximately 20% to 40% of patients appear dehydrated, some to the point of frank circulatory shock. Fever and modest tachycardia are often, but not invariably, present. Hematemesis or melena may occur. Abdominal examination is fully normal in only a few cases, but often does not warn of the catastrophic nature of the disease. Signs of peritoneal irritation are present to some degree in 30% to 50% of cases. Less urgent abdominal findings, such as increased or decreased bowel sounds, localized or diffuse tenderness, distention, bruit, and mass, are present to some degree in virtually all cases. Most cases have occult blood in the stool, especially later in the course of the process. Approximately 10% present with catastrophic hemodynamic collapse, signs of severe systemic toxicity, altered mental status, and signs of frank peritonitis. The process is universally fatal.

DIFFERENTIAL DIAGNOSIS

The differential diagnosis of abdominal pain in the elderly is notoriously difficult. Symptoms are often vague or poorly represented. The patient may have other serious medical illness or dementia, which interferes with the history and examination. Physical examination is unreliable in the elderly, and may be falsely reassuring. Nevertheless, abdominal pain in a patient over age 50 must be considered representative of an ominous process. As the patient ages the likelihood of vascular disease increases. The principal diagnostic approach is the determination of whether a surgical condition is present, and whether the situation is urgent. In mesenteric ischemia, although both of these criteria are universally present, they are seldom appreciated.

EMERGENCY DEPARTMENT EVALUATION

It is of paramount importance that patients over 50 with abdominal pain undergo timely diagnostic workup to ensure that serious conditions, especially mesenteric ischemia, are not missed. More than 80% of patients who present to EDs with mesenteric ischemia are misdiagnosed or undergo extensive and time-consuming evaluations. ED evaluation is dictated by the patient's condition. When the patient presents in hemodynamic or septic crisis immediate therapeutic measures must precede definitive diagnosis. The upper airway must be assured, high-flow oxygen, and the need for immediate intubation assessed. Two intravenous lines should be established, and crystalloid solution administered. Although patients are elderly, crystalloid is rapidly administered, since hypovolemia aggravates the mesenteric hypoperfusion. Glucose, complete blood count, electrolytes, amylase, urea, creatinine, and glucose, coagulation parameters, and crossmatch, should be sent. Additional studies may be indicated. Continuous monitoring and a 12-lead electrocardiogram are obtained. The ultimate diagnosis may be obscured by the systemic nature of the presentation, and the prognosis is grim. Most patients present complaining of abdominal pain, usually with other symptoms, and undergo a less hurried evaluation. In all cases it is advisable to establish intravenous access, as the patient may deteriorate rapidly, especially if the presenting problem is vascular in nature.

LABORATORY AND ANCILLARY STUDIES

Laboratory studies are nonspecific. Although it has been said that the principal use of the laboratory in mesenteric ischemia is to exclude other entities, this is often not possible. The hemoglobin is almost universally elevated because of hemoconcentration late in the course of the disease, but it may be fully normal earlier on. Leukocytosis is present in almost all cases, and is often marked. Approximately 25% of patients have white blood cell (WBC) counts of 10,000 to 15,000, 50% have WBC counts of 15,000 to 30,000, and 25% exceed 30,000. Serum amylase levels show a modest elevation. Occasionally profound elevations are seen. Metabolic acidosis is widely thought to be a universal companion of gut ischemia, presumably on the basis of the anaerobic metabolism initiated by the ischemic process. This is, in fact, not reflected in the literature, and one recent large series noted normal serum bicarbonate levels in 60 of 60 patients. Other laboratory findings, such as azotemia, hyperbilirubinemia, elevated enzyme and inorganic phosphate levels, and other, more exotic determinations, are of no value.

Plain radiography is likewise nonspecific. Abdominal gas may be absent, sparse, or normal, or it may demonstrate an ileus pattern. In most cases the films are normal or not suggestive of any particular pathologic process. The finding of gas in the intestinal wall or in the portal venous system invariably occurs only late in the process, usually after the opportunity to salvage the patient has passed. Thumbprinting of the intestinal mucosa, shown in relief against air or barium, is strongly suggestive, but not specific. Contrast radiography, including computed tomography scanning, offers little advantage over plain films, except in the exclusion of other pathology. Endoscopy yields useful information only if the involved segment of gut is within reach of the endoscope, a distinctly unusual circumstance.

The definitive diagnostic maneuver in the evaluation of a patient with suspected mesenteric ischemia is aortic and mesenteric angiography. This establishes the diagnosis. Angiography also allows the selective infusion of vasodilating agents, such as papaverine, directly into the affected vessels. Elderly patients who present with abdominal pain, especially those with risk factors for mesenteric ischemia, must undergo a rapid diagnostic sequence leading to a solid provisional diagnosis. The additional features of *pain out of proportion to the physical examination,* significant leukocytosis, clinical signs of dehydration or hemoconcentration, and other clinical features of mesenteric ischemia mandate consideration of early angiography to confirm or exclude the diagnosis. Many patients have their diagnosis made only at autopsy, or at laparotomy when the disease has progressed to frank infarction. Early surgical consultation must be sought in cases of suspected mesenteric ischemia. Waiting for "confirmation" of the diagnosis by development of significant metabolic acidosis, circulatory collapse, frank peritoneal signs, definitive findings on plain radiography, or other unambiguous events will place the patient in profound jeopardy. If any reasonable doubt exists as to the diagnosis, and the patient is not in obvious need of immediate laparotomy, angiography should be obtained. Admission to hospital with a diagnosis of "Rule out mesenteric ischemia" is unacceptable.

DISPOSITION

ROLE OF THE CONSULTANT   Mesenteric ischemia is a surgical disease. Temporizing measures, such as selective papaverine infusion during angiography, do not obviate the need for revascularization. Surgical and radiographic consultation should be sought early. If facilities for vascular surgery or invasive radiography are not available in the institution of presentation, immediate general surgical consultation should be sought and early transfer arranged.

INDICATIONS FOR ADMISSION   The decision to admit an elderly patient with undiagnosed abdominal pain should not be difficult. The list of serious causes of abdominal pain in the undiagnosed elderly patient significantly outweighs the list of trivial or benign conditions. In addition, elderly patients with "benign"conditions, such as biliary colic, often fare poorly and deteriorate precipitously. In patients with a clear diagnosis that is not felt to require hospitalization, close consultation with the primary physician and early follow-up examination are mandatory. When the diagnosis is in doubt, or when the patient carries an established prior diagnosis such as "diverticulosis" but appears to be developing another acute process, admission and early surgical consultation are indicated.

COMMON PITFALLS

- The most common pitfall is failure to make the diagnosis while the patient is still living or salvageable.
- Admission of a patient to hospital with suspicion of mesenteric ischemia mandates immediate angiography. Without angiography the condition will only become apparent when it is too late to save the patient.
- Perhaps the greatest pitfall is the reluctance to obtain angiography. Angiography carries a low risk of morbidity, and is even more appealing when balanced against a universally fatal condition.
- Early radiographic consultation and refusal to "wait until morning" are essential to a good outcome.
- From the medicolegal standpoint it is of paramount importance to establish a sound diagnosis in all patients who present with abdominal pain. If the patient is elderly, consultation and admission should be considered in any uncertain circumstances.

27   Aortic Dissection

Aortic dissection is the most frequent catastrophic event involving the aorta but it remains a diagnostic challenge to the emergency physician. The term "dissecting aneurysm" is often used; this term is misleading. A true aneurysm seldom is present during dissection. Aortic dissection is the preferred nomenclature. Dissection of the aorta begins with an intimal tear, usually (70%) in the ascending portion of the thoracic aorta. The intimal tear allows blood to penetrate down to the media separating intima from adventitia. The length of time required to dissect the entire aorta can be seconds. The site of the initial intimal tear is usually at the aortic root or between the origin of the left subclavian artery and the ligamentum arteriosum. These two areas of the aorta are relatively fixed, and it is felt that maximum stress is applied to these areas during systole. Dissection then proceeds either distally or proximally. Atheromatous plaque throughout the length of the aorta is the main factor that limits dissection. For this reason patients <40 usually have diffuse dissections, whereas patients >65 tend to have localized dissections. The role of the underlying structural defect of the aortic wall remains unclear, but it is certain that hypertension plays a leading role in the development of aortic dissection. Dissection may be a multifactorial disease, with hypertension the principal risk factor. Approximately 90% of patients with Marfan's syndrome die of the cardiovascular complications of dissection or ruptured aneurysm.

CLASSIFICATION   The daily classification demonstrates involvement of the ascending aorta *(type A)*; if the dissection is limited to the descending aorta, it is classified as *type B*. This scheme reflects prognosis and aids in the decision of whether surgical or medical treatment should be instituted. Type A dissections are more common (60%–70%) and are considered surgical emergencies. The only contraindication to surgery is an evolving stroke. Heparinization is used in the operative repair, and restoration of flow often results in intracerebral hemorrhage. Mortality of medically treated type A approaches untreated type A (70%–80%), whereas mortality of surgically treated type A is 15% to 20%. Type B dissection is managed medically. The surgical mortality of type B dissections is the same or greater as the mortality associated with medical management (11%). Some surgeons prefer surgical repair for uncomplicated type B dissections. Indications for repair of type B dissections include hemorrhage, limb or organ ischemia, intractable pain, or progression of dissection despite medical management.

MORTALITY   The 10-year survival is 40%. The most common cause of death (86%) is rupture of the aortic wall into the pericardial sac. The site of rupture is most commonly into the pericardial sac (65%), the pleural space (35%), followed by the mediastinum (12%). Death from congestive heart failure occurs in about 3% of cases, and death secondary to myocardial infarction in 3%.

CLINICAL PRESENTATION

To make the diagnosis of dissection it must be in the differential diagnosis. The history should focus on risk factors for aortic dissection, especially hypertension. Marfan's syndrome is a major risk factor. Sudden onset of excruciating pain is the most common presenting symptom (80%–90%). The pain is described as "ripping or tearing"and reaches full intensity immediately. The location of the pain can vary from substernal (32%) to back (21%) to precordial (21%). Another classic feature of aortic dissection is the migratory nature of the pain. As the dissection proceeds, the pain shifts in location from the chest to the back, the neck, and, finally, the extremities. About 10% to 20% of cases present without pain.

A variety of signs and symptoms that result from vascular compromise as the dissection proceeds have been described. Neurologic findings are seen as the initial signs of a proximal dissection. Syncope is the initial presentation in 9% of cases. The aorta's proximity to other mediastinal structures can cause hoarseness (laryngeal nerve compression), dyspnea with wheezing or stridor (tracheal compression), and dysphagia (esophageal compression). Gastrointestinal symptoms include midepigastric pain, hemorrhage, or melena secondary to splanchnic vessel infarction. Renal artery involvement may lead to hematuria (9%), flank pain, oliguria, or uncontrollable hypertension from renin release.

On examination the patient may appear to be in shock, yet paradoxically have a normal or elevated blood pressure (75% to 85% are initially hypertensive). Jugular venous distention may be secondary to congestive heart failure, cardiac tamponade, or an expanding hematoma around the aorta causing outflow obstruction. Proximal dissection of the aorta may lead to aortic insufficiency (50% to 60%). An aortic stenosis murmur can often be heard if a sufficiently large hematoma forms at the base of the aorta.

Poor prognostic factors include pleural effusion, cardiac tamponade, and pericardial friction rub. The presence of these signs implies leakage of the dissection into the pericardial space. The abdominal examination may reveal tenderness to palpation, rigidity or a palpable pulsatile mass. Examination of the limbs may reveal unequal, decreased, or absent peripheral pulse with proximal dissection (50%) and distal dissection (60%). Differential blood flow to the extremities often manifests itself by a marked discrepancy in blood pressure between arms.

DIFFERENTIAL DIAGNOSIS

Myocardial infarction is the principle diagnosis of exclusion. It is also the most common misdiagnosis (16%). Other conditions (and the incidence of misdiagnosis) include nondissecting thoracic aneurysm (7%), mediastinal cyst or tumor (7%), pericarditis (5%), cholelithiasis or cholecystitis (4%), and pulmonary embolus (2%).

Four factors favor the diagnosis of aortic dissection:

1. History of hypertension
2. Duration of symptoms <24 hours
3. Migratory pain
4. Left ventricular hypertrophy on EKG

The following features should further suggest the diagnosis:

Aortic insufficiency with chest or back pain
Symptoms of acute regional ischemia, such as hemiparesis
Flank pain and hematuria without an obvious source of arterial embolism
Multiple areas of acute ischemia
Acute, unexplained left ventricular failure
Atypical chest or back pain
Disappearance and reappearance of proximal pulses
Presence of neurologic symptoms

EMERGENCY DEPARTMENT EVALUATION

The patient should be placed on a cardiac monitor and intravascular access established with two large-bore catheters. Type and crossmatch, complete blood count, electrolytes, amylase, cardiac enzymes, urinalysis, should be carried out, and a 12-lead EKG established. Twenty-three percent with aortic dissection have ECG changes compatible with myocardial infarction and 10% have ECG changes compatible with pericarditis.

Radiologic studies establish the diagnosis. The most available study is the chest radiograph. In 80% to 85%, the chest radiograph demonstrates some abnormality. A widened mediastinum is the most common finding, but a left-sided pleural effusion or an indistinct aortic knob may also be seen. A calcified aortic intima may be seen and if separated by >6 mm from the outer wall, this is considered to be pathognomonic for dissection. If the diagnosis of dissection is considered, radiologic confirmation with aortography or computed tomography (CT) is indicated. The aortogram is the "gold standard." It reveals the extent of dissection, the condition and patency of the distal vessels, and the pattern of blood flow in the true and false lumens. The main disadvantage of the aortogram is the large dye load that must be administered. A second disadvantage is that a dissection may not be detected if the false lumen is not perpendicular to the x-ray beam. The aortogram has a sensitivity and specificity of approximately 90%. CT permits superior visualization of fluid collections in the pericardium, pleura, and mediastinum, moderate demonstration of distal vessel patency, noninvasiveness, and sensitivity and specificity equal to aortography. The main disadvantage of CT is the large dye load.

Echocardiography is noninvasive and requires no contrast. Transesophageal ECHO appears promising.

EMERGENCY DEPARTMENT MANAGEMENT

It is critical to reduce arterial blood pressure and the forceful contractility of the left ventricle. These measures should be initiated before confirmatory tests are performed if clinical suspicion for dissection is high. Systolic blood pressure control is important because the rate of dissection is directly proportional to the blood pressure, especially to the rate of rise of arterial blood pressure. The drug of choice is intravenous nitroprusside at an initial rate of 0.5 µg to 1.0 µg/kg/min. The systolic blood pressure should be maintained at 100 mm Hg to 110 mm Hg. Oral agents should not be used. Once a systolic blood pressure of 100 mm Hg is achieved, beta adrenergic blockade must be achieved to reduce arterial wall shearing forces (propranolol, 1 mg IV every 5 minutes until the pulse rate reaches 60–80 beats per minute). Congestive heart failure, chronic obstructive pulmonary disease, heart block, and bradycardia are contraindications to the use of propranolol. In such cases the use of cardioselective agents (atenolol or metoprolol) may be indicated. The role of calcium channel antagonists is promising.

DISPOSITION

Management of the patient with aortic dissection requires urgent multispecialty involvement. The radiologist should be consulted for CT or aortography. The internist and thoracic surgeon should also be notified. All patients suspected of having acute aortic dissection should be admitted to an intensive care unit. Indications for transfer include inadequate facilities or personnel to make the diagnosis or treat the condition. If transfer is indicated, air transport should be used in order to minimize the time required. If ground transportation is used, an ALS unit should be used.

COMMON PITFALLS

- The most common mistake is failure to consider the diagnosis of aortic dissection.
- The internist, radiologist, and thoracic surgeon should be consulted early.
- The most important aspect of emergency department management is control of the blood pressure.

PART V

Emergency Aspects of Orthopedic Surgery

28   Low Back Pain

Between 50% and 80% of all adults have at some time had low back pain. In the United States the estimated cumulative lifetime prevalence of low back pain ranges between 13.8% and 18%. More than 18 million Americans have chronic low back pain, 5.4 million are disabled by it, and the cost is greater than $16 billion each year. The natural history of low back pain is good: 60% of those afflicted will return to work within 1 week, and 90% will do so within 6 weeks. Although there are many mechanical and nonmechanical causes of back pain, rarely will these be life-threatening or neurologic emergencies.

CLINICAL PRESENTATION AND EVALUATION
HISTORY

A general review of systems is indicated (constitutional symptoms as fever, chills, night sweats, weight loss, and sleep disorder). Chronic illnesses (hypertension, heart disease, angina pectoris, cancer, peptic ulcer disease, pancreatitis, and pyelonephritis) should be noted. Dysuria, alcohol or drug abuse, bladder or bowel dysfunction, and depression are key findings. The character, location, radiation, and duration of the back pain can be revealing. Pain of sudden onset and short duration is frequently associated with facet joint disorders, whereas pain that gradually increases over weeks more often involves the disks. Facet or disk pain tends to be more severe in the back, buttocks, and posterior thigh, whereas pain that arises in an inflamed nerve root radiates distally beyond the knee. Radicular pain, particularly if accompanied by paresthesia or loss of sensation, is an indication of mechanical nerve root compression.

    Factors that aggravate or relieve pain should be explored. As a rule, nonmechanical pain is usually continuous and not made worse by exercise; mechanical pain is usually worse with movement and relieved by rest. Pain that is caused by a bulging or herniated disk is usually made worse by forward bending, rotation, and coughing or sneezing. Pain that is made worse by back extension occurs in patients with disorders of the facets and ligaments. Spinal stenosis with cauda equina claudication is generally limited to patients over age 50. These patients commonly complain of intermittent bilateral leg pain, numbness, tingling, or weakness brought on by walking or standing, and that is relieved by rest, sitting, squatting, or lying down. Patients with degenerative joint disease that involves the spine may report back stiffness that is worse in the morning and improves with movement through the day.

DIFFERENTIAL DIAGNOSIS

See Table 28-1.

The cause of low back pain is unknown in as many as 85% of cases. Although serious disease is rare in patients who present with low back pain, it is mandatory to consider and to exclude those who require emergency treatment. Patients with low back pain from significant acute trauma should have spinal films taken. Significant axial loads result in compression fractures of the vertebral bodies. Shearing forces, such as those that occur with seat belt injuries during sudden, unimpeded flexion of the lumbosacral spine, may cause subluxation or dislocation of vertebrae. Spinal stenosis, a narrowing of the central spinal canal, can be congenital or result from herniated disk, surgery, spondylolisthesis, and, most often, hypertrophic degenerative joint disease of the disks and facet joints. Patients complain of muscle weakness, loss of strength, and paresthesia, commonly in both legs. These symptoms are brought on by walking or prolonged standing, but they may be absent on examination when the patient is at rest. The symptoms can often be revealed by having the patient exercise during observation.

TABLE 28-1. Causes of Low Back Pain

Neoplasms

Benign bone and neural tumors: Meningioma, neurofibroma, ependymoma (can have high grade of malignancy), osteoid osteoma, hemangioma, osteoblastoma, eosinophilic granuloma

Malignant bone and neural tumors:

Primary—multiple myeloma, osteosarcoma, chordoma

Secondary (metastasis)—breast, lung, prostate, kidney, uterus, ovary, thyroid, colon

Trauma

Compression fracture, fracture dislocation, transverse process fracture, facet subluxation, ligamentous tear, muscle strain

Congenital Disorders

Facet asymmetry, transitional vertebrae, spondylolysis, spondylolisthesis

Degenerative Disorders

Osteoarthritis of spine or hip, herniated disk, spinal stenosis, nerve root entrapment

Metabolic Disorders

Osteoporosis, alcoholic and diabetic neuropathy, Paget's disease, gout, acromegaly, hyperthyroidism

Inflammatory Disorders

Ankylosing spondylitis, arachnoiditis, rheumatoid arthritis

Infections

Tuberculosis, epidural and subdural abscess, disk space infection, osteomyelitis, syphilis, herpes zoster, meningitis, bacterial endocarditis, urinary tract infection, psoas and paraspinal muscle abscess

Vascular Disorders

Aortic aneurysm, arteriovenous malformation, aortoiliac arteriosclerosis

Psychosocial Disorders

Depression, conversion reaction, malingering, narcotic addiction

Miscellaneous

Visceral inflammation (*e.g.,* pancreatitis, pyelonephritis, cholecystitis, penetrating peptic ulcer), renal calculi, endometriosis, prostatic disease, scoliosis, lymphoma, hernia of the inferior lumbar space, leg length inequality, sickle cell anemia

Aortic aneurysm and aortic dissection can present as back pain. Most aortic aneurysms occur in the abdominal aorta immediately distal to the renal arteries; the vast majority are caused by arteriosclerosis, usually in men > age 60. The vertebral column is the most common site of bone metastasis, and the primary site may be asymptomatic. Pain is the first symptom in more than 90% of patients with epidural cord compression. Patients at risk are over age 50 with a history of weight and appetite loss. Back pain limited to the thoracic area is unusual and should raise suspicion of a structural mass lesion. Herniated disk usually causes a unilateral bulging that irritates or compresses one nerve root, thereby producing unilateral signs and symptoms of sciatica. The hallmark of sciatica is pain and paresthesia that radiate down the posterior or lateral leg in a radicular manner, along with weakness and neuropathy. Chronic prostatitis or cancer may cause lumbosacral pain, but with lesions of the bladder or testes back pain is unusual. Infection of the vertebrae commonly presents with only back pain early.

Osteomyelitis is an infection of bone that results from the seeding of bacteria by one of several routes: hematogenous, extension from a contiguous site of infection, or through direct introduction (e.g., open fractures or surgery). The lumbar vertebrae are the most frequent sites of hematogenously spread osteomyelitis in adults. Infection is most commonly caused by either *Staphylococcus aureus,* coliform bacilli, or tuberculosis. Urinary tract infection, pelvic surgery, and pelvic infection are associated with vertebral osteomyelitis. A primary hematogenous source of infection can be identified in more than 40% of cases. Genitourinary infection is the most frequent source, followed by skin and respiratory infection. Intravenous drug abusers are at increased risk for osteomyelitis. Patients at risk include those with endocarditis or diabetes, those who chronically use steroids, and those who are otherwise immunocompromised. Patients with sickle cell disease and SC hemoglobinopathy are also subject to osteomyelitis, usually of the long bones, but occasionally involving the vertebrae. *Salmonella* is the organism that causes osteomyelitis in sickle cell patients.

Low back pain that arises in the synovially lined facet joints is the consequence of degenerative changes that often develop simultaneously with disk changes at the same level. This syndrome is characterized by recurrent acute episodes of low back pain that lasts for a few days, without radicular symptoms. On physical examination the pain is exacerbated by back extension and relieved by rest in the recumbent position. There are no neurologic deficits unless degenerative changes are severe enough to cause stenosis of a nerve root foramen or narrowing of the spinal canal.

PHYSICAL EXAMINATION

Attention should be paid to fever, muscle wasting, heart murmurs, abdominal tenderness, abdominal bruit or pulsatile mass, leg pulses, pelvic or adnexal tenderness, needle tracks, or lymphadenopathy. The prostate should be examined for tenderness or masses. Women should have a pelvic exam, in general. The back examination involves the musculoskeletal and neurologic systems. Because more than 90% of disk herniations occur at the L4–5 or L5–S1 levels, the neurologic examination focuses on the L5 and S1 nerve roots.

ISOLATING NERVE ROOTS
L5: The patient should be sitting in a chair with the heel of the affected leg on the floor. The patient elevates the forefoot against strong downward pressure applied by the examiner. One must differentiate between true release seen in nerve root compression and voluntary release. The S1 nerve root is tested by observing the power of plantar flexion; the patient is asked to perform ten toe raises on both feet and ten more on each foot separately.

Knee reflexes test nerve roots L2, L3, and L4, and the ankle reflexes test S1 and S2. Asymmetrical reflexes on repeated testing are an important indicator of nerve root pathology and are more reliable than the absolute degree of response. With the patient sitting on the examination table with the legs dangling free, extension of the leg at the knee stretches the sciatic nerve and places traction on spinal nerve roots in the same manner that straight-leg raising does with the patient supine. In discogenic low back pain this maneuver should increase the pain radiating down the leg and induce the patient to lean back in an attempt to relieve the tension on the sciatic nerve. With the patient lying supine, the hip joint is tested by flexing the hip and then rotating the joint. Pain that originates in the hip tends to radiate into the groin and down the anteromedial thigh, whereas back pain usually radiates down the buttock and posterior thigh. The straight-leg raising test is also performed in the supine position and is a sign of sciatic nerve root irritation if pain radiates down the extended leg when it is raised 60 degrees or less. Crossover leg pain, a sign of central disk herniation, is noted when pain radiates down the usually asymptomatic leg when the opposite painful leg is raised. L5 can be tested by noting the power of hip abduction against resistance. Sensation in the saddle area of the buttocks is supplied by S3, S4, and S5 and should be tested with pinprick along with anal sphincter tone and reflex. If neurologic deficits are revealed through these maneuvers, together with the presence of crossover leg pain, then central disk herniation with spinal cord compression should be strongly entertained. This particular syndrome is a *surgical emergency*.

RADIOGRAPHY

Low back pain accounts for nearly 7 million lumbosacral spine series each year. Spine films are not essential for evaluating every patient with low back pain. The following criteria would be expected to increase the yield of lumbar films:

1. Over age 50
2. Fever, weight loss, adenopathy, elevated erythrocyte sedimentation rate, or other signs of systemic illness
3. Findings suggestive of ankylosing spondylitis
4. History of previous malignancy
5. Significant trauma
6. Motor neurologic deficits (including cauda equina syndrome)
7. Intended litigation or compensation
8. Chronic use of corticosteroids
9. Drug or alcohol abuse
10. Symptoms that continue after 2 to 4 weeks of conservative therapy

Other laboratory tests that might be useful include a complete blood count, a urinalysis, and an erythrocyte sedimentation rate.

EMERGENCY DEPARTMENT MANAGEMENT

If there are no signs of systemic illness or major neurologic disorder, initial therapy should be conservative and directed toward relieving symptoms. The duration of symptoms, presence of neurologic deficits, prior back surgery, symptoms of depression, involvement in litigation or disability determinations, and the presence of trauma should be elicited. Narcotic analgesics may be helpful for patients with severe acute low back pain or cancer pain, but may be inappropriate for patients with chronic low back pain. Bed rest reduces or eliminates the pain and symptoms of most mechanical back pain. Further investigation is warranted if the pain persists for longer than 2 weeks.

INDICATIONS FOR HOSPITAL ADMISSION OR SURGICAL INTERVENTION

Central disk herniation, cauda equina syndrome: incontinence of urine or stool, bilateral leg
     weakness or reflex loss, loss of rectal sphincter tone, saddle distribution anesthesia
Muscle weakness that is progressive or fails to improve with conservative therapy
Reflex loss
Persistent disabling sciatica

Unstable fractures, dislocations, or subluxations
Spinal infections or meningitis
Spinal cord tumors

SPINAL CORD NEOPLASMS

Spinal cord neoplasms associated with neurologic deficit demand immediate intervention: intravenous steroids, radiation therapy, and surgical intervention. Intravenous steroid therapy is usually recommended for all patients, 100 mg IV dexamethasone, followed by 24 mg dexamethasone every 6 hours. Controversy surrounds the decision to perform immediate decompressive laminectomy. There is no difference in outcome between two groups treated with radiation therapy alone versus primary surgical intervention followed by radiation therapy. Patients with back pain associated with new or progressive neurologic deficit require admission for further evaluation. Patients with back pain and newly diagnosed neoplasia, and especially those with associated neurologic deficits, must be emergently treated. Patients with previously diagnosed malignancy who present with back pain but lack both neurologic signs on careful examination as well as abnormality on diagnostic imaging, including CT scan, may be treated on an outpatient basis with appropriate analgesics and early follow-up. Consultation is advisable for all such patients. The remaining patients, having neither evidence of neoplasia (despite adjunctive testing) nor neurologic deficit, may be treated with appropriate analgesics and routine referral for outpatient follow-up.

COMMON PITFALLS

- The ease of diagnosis in the evaluation of patients with spinal cord tumors correlates inversely with the prognosis.
- The potential reward is prevention of irreversible loss of function, which can only follow accurate and timely diagnosis and treatment.
- The physician must suspect potentially serious pathology, despite the large numbers of patients who present with the common complaint of back pain.
- The importance of a methodical neurologic examination of all such patients cannot be overstated.
- Failure to diagnose metastatic disease of the spine in the patient with a previously diagnosed malignancy risks preventable but permanent disability and allegations of negligence. The devastating impact on the quality of remaining life in such patients is evident.

29   Carpal Tunnel Syndrome

Carpal tunnel syndrome is a syndrome caused by the compression of the median nerve at the wrist. It is the most common compression neuropathy in the upper extremity. Conditions that either decrease the size of the canal or increase the volume of contents in the canal can potentially produce carpal tunnel syndrome. Numerous conditions have been shown to cause the carpal tunnel syndrome, although the idiopathic variety is probably the most common.

CLINICAL PRESENTATION

Carpal tunnel syndrome occurs most frequently in women (2:1) and ages 40 to 60. It is frequently bilateral. The patient typically complains of numbness, tingling, burning, or paresthesias in the hand along the distribution of the median nerve (the thumb, index, middle, and radial aspect of the ring fingers). The symptoms characteristically awaken the patient and may be relieved by shaking the hand. As the syndrome progresses, the symptoms become more frequent, often exacerbated by activities that maintain the wrist flexed, such as driving and holding a book, and by use of the hand such as with knitting, sewing, and hammering. Patients may also complain of weakness or clumsiness in the hand. On examination there may be decreased sensation to light touch or decreased two-point discrimination in the median nerve distribution. Phalen's wrist-flexion test and Tinel's sign are frequently positive with carpal tunnel syndrome. Phalen's test is positive if holding the wrist in complete, but unforced flexion for 30 to 60 seconds reproduces or exaggerates the numbness and paresthesias in the median nerve distribution. Tinel's sign is positive if light tapping over the median nerve at the wrist causes a tingling sensation distally along the median nerve. In more advanced cases there may be weakness of the median-innervated thenar muscles, the abductor pollicis brevis and the opponens. Thenar atrophy is best seen as a guttering appearance along the radial aspect of the thenar eminence that exposes the first metacarpal. In cases of carpal tunnel syndrome caused by an inflammatory synovitis (rheumatoid arthritis) there may be swelling along the volar aspect of the wrist.

EMERGENCY DEPARTMENT EVALUATION

Radiographs of the wrist, including a carpal tunnel view, may show structural abnormalities such as callus, osteophytes, and calcific deposits. Cervical spine films are useful if the symptoms suggest a cervical radiculopathy. Thyroid function tests, fasting blood sugar, erythrocyte sedimentation rate, rheumatoid factor, antinuclear antibodies, serum calcium, uric acid and a white blood cell count may all be useful.

EMERGENCY DEPARTMENT MANAGEMENT

Most patients can be treated conservatively. Wrist splints in neutral or slight extension can be worn when symptoms arise, especially at night. The patient should be told to avoid any hand activities that obviously aggravate the symptoms. Underlying medical causes (e.g., hypothyroidism, rheumatoid arthritis, and gout) should be treated. Diuretics may be useful if carpal tunnel syndrome is associated with pregnancy but should be given with the approval of the patient's obstetrician.

DISPOSITION

Patients with symptoms of carpal tunnel syndrome should be referred for evaluation and treatment. Outpatient electromyographic and nerve conduction studies may help differentiate carpal tunnel syndrome from other causes. The injection of steroids into the carpal canal frequently results in significant improvement and often complete relief. However, the symptoms often recur. Indications for operative treatment include muscle weakness, thenar atrophy, and no response to or recurrence after conservative treatment. Surgery consists of the division of the transverse carpal ligament and affords excellent results.

PART VI

Emergency Aspects of Neurosurgery

30   Intracranial Neoplasms

Intracranial neoplasms (INs) are benign or malignant tumors located within the cranial cavity. They include masses that arise from or are metastatic to the pituitary or pineal glands, meninges, intracranial portion of the cranial nerves, intracranial blood vessels, or the brain tissue itself. About 75% of central nervous system (CNS) tumors in children are infratentorial, whereas 75% of such tumors in adults are supratentorial. The most common brain tumors in adults are metastatic tumors, malignant gliomas, meningiomas, and pituitary adenomas. Cerebellar astrocytomas, medulloblastomas, and fourth ventricle ependymomas predominate in children. Gliomas are neoplasms of glial lineage and constitute 50% of primary intracranial tumors. They include multiple types, from the highly malignant glioblastoma multiforme to the relatively benign astrocytoma. These tumors have a predilection for the cerebral hemispheres in adults. Increasing age of the patient correlates with poor prognosis. Meningiomas are the second most common adult brain tumor, constituting 20% of primary intracranial neoplasms. They are histologically benign slow-growing tumors of arachnoid tissue and are usually very vascular. Of all INs, meningiomas have the highest association with extraneural tumors. Meningiomas usually compress but do not invade brain tissue. Changes in the underlying skull are frequent and may be seen on plain radiograph. They also contain a high concentration of progesterone receptors, rendering them hormone sensitive.

Pituitary adenomas represent 15% of all primary intracranial tumors. Only one third of the patients reveal the characteristic sign of bitemporal hemianopia from compression of the optic chiasm by superior extension of the tumor. Some patients present with only endocrine symptomatology, such as secondary amenorrhea, galactorrhea, impotence, and Cushing's syndrome. Diagnosis is aided by an enlarged sella turcica on lateral skull films, a pituitary mass on computed tomography (CT), or an abnormal signal on magnetic resonance imaging (MRI). An elevated serum prolactin level is present in two thirds of these patients.

Acoustic neuroma is a benign schwannoma of the eighth cranial nerve that is usually located within the internal auditory meatus. It constitutes 7% of all primary intracranial tumors. More than 95% of patients with this tumor present with unilateral neurosensory hearing loss. Other symptoms include tinnitus, vertigo, dysequilibrium, facial paresthesias, dysphagia, and hoarseness.

Metastatic tumors are the most common intracranial tumor in late middle life and account for 20% to 30% of all adult INs. Lung and breast cancer are the number one primary tumors in men and women, respectively. Malignant melanoma, hypernephromas, and colon carcinomas complete the five most frequent primary lesions. Cerebral metastases, like emboli, tend to be found along the middle cerebral artery distribution in the parietal lobe. They are usually multiple. Thus a neurologic examination and enhanced CT or MRI findings of several lesions should suggest the possibility of metastatic disease. Meningeal carcinomatosis is a diffuse infiltration of the meninges by tumor cells that can occur with systemic cancer. Clinical suspicion is warranted in the presence of multifocal neurologic signs and symptoms, and suspicion is verified by an abnormal cerebrospinal fluid (CSF) analysis, typically revealing increased intracranial pressure (ICP), increased protein concentration, decreased glucose, pleocytosis, and, occasionally, malignant cells.

CLINICAL PRESENTATION

A slow onset and gradual worsening of symptoms are typical for INs.

HEADACHE
A recent onset or change in the character of a headache may signal the presence of an IN. Although most patients with headache do not have tumors, 60% to 90% of patients with brain tumors complain of headache at some point in their illness, and 20% have headache as the initial symptom. Headaches are described as steady, nonthrobbing, dull, aching pain relieved by analgesics. They may be mild and intermittent at first. With tumor growth the headaches become more severe, more frequent, and persistent. Other characteristics of tumor-induced headaches include early-morning occurrence, aggravation by Valsalva maneuvers, and association with vomiting, particularly in the absence of preceding nausea. Any headache—no matter the character—associated with seizure activity, abnormal mental status, focal neurologic signs, or papilledema is due to IN until proven otherwise.

SEIZURES
New onset of seizure activity is another common presentation of patients with IN. Thirty-five percent of cerebral tumors are associated with seizure activity, and seizures are the initial symptom in 15%. In patients under age 20 the incidence of cerebral tumors causing epilepsy is almost negligible at 0.02%. In patients with new onset of seizure activity and focal neurologic deficits the incidence of tumor increases to 50%. Half of the patients without history of prior seizure who present with status epilepticus also have IN. Besides initial status or focal neurologic findings, clinical suspicion of IN should also be aroused in any patient over age 20 with a first episode of seizure, particularly if the seizure is followed by a prolonged postictal period or Todd's paralysis. The risk of IN is also increased if the seizure has focal motor, sensory, or psychomotor features.

MENTAL STATUS
Mental status or behavioral changes are commonly seen with IN, particularly with frontal and temporal lobe lesions. Because of their often subtle nature, such changes may be overlooked until focal neurologic signs develop. Alterations of mental status may be disclosed by questioning families and friends. Symptoms can mimic a depressive disorder or Alzheimer's disease with a predominance of apathy, irritability, restlessness, depression, loss of spontaneity, or memory loss. Changes in mental status seem to occur most often with rapidly growing tumors, such as glioblastomas.

FOCAL NEUROLOGIC DEFICITS
Progressive focal neurologic defects may also be produced by intracranial masses. Common findings include aphasia, hemiparesis, sensory or visual deficits, and cranial nerve palsies. The sixth cranial nerve is involved most commonly because it has the longest intracranial course. The characteristic unique to IN-induced focal neurologic deficits is that these deficits tend to be slow in onset with only gradual increase in severity. Rarely the onset of symptoms is sudden, and intraneoplastic hemorrhage must then be a consideration.

MISCELLANEOUS
Vomiting occurs in 70% of patients with IN, but it is the presenting symptom in only 10%. It is characteristically projectile, unrelated to food, more frequent in the early waking hours (as is headache), and usually not preceded by nausea. Like headache and papilledema, it is one of the cardinal signs of chronically increased ICP.

PRESENTATION BY LOCATION

Clinical presentation depends on the presence or absence of elevated ICP and the location of the tumor. Mixed clinical pictures are often present, since tumors usually spread to involve more than one brain region. Frontal lobe tumors may produce personality change, particularly in respect to acquired social behavior. Uninhibited behavior may be prominent, and reflected in the use of inappropriate language or actions without regard for their effect on others. Apathy and poor hygiene are common. A severe decline in intellect and memory may also ensue. These changes develop slowly over months to years, until an obvious dementia occurs. Patients may also experience loss of bladder control. Generalized tonic-clonic seizures and jacksonian or partial motor seizures are also characteristic of frontal lobe tumors.

Parietal lobe neoplasms present with dysphasia if the dominant lobe is affected, and dyspraxia if the nondominant lobe is involved. Sensory loss, inattention, homonymous hemianopia, and loss of opticokinetic nystagmus also occur.

Temporal lobe masses can also present with personality changes, but these tend to be subtler than those associated with frontal lobe tumors. They are characterized by alterations in affect, imitating psychotic disorders rather than the demented picture of frontal lobe tumors. Other symptoms include complex partial seizures with prodromal gustatory, olfactory, auditory, or formed visual hallucinations and upper quadrantic homonymous hemianopia.

EMERGENT PROBLEMS

Although the *sine qua non* of IN is slow, progressive deterioration in clinical status, occasionally a rapid decline occurs. This is often caused by an acute increase in ICP that develops in minutes to hours, and is characterized by a sudden and marked increase in headache, with stiff neck, opisthotonus, facial flushing or pallor, and drowsiness that may progress to coma. Characteristically, the patient develops bradycardia with an elevation of blood pressure. This is termed the Cushing response and is the physiologic rise in systemic blood pressure as a consequence of increased ICP. Reflex bradycardia secondary to elevated mean arterial pressure (MAP) is another component of this response. The respiratory rate slows and deepens and may progress to a Cheyne–Stokes pattern. This acute alteration in ICP is usually caused by an intracranial bleed; however, it can be seen with hemorrhage into an IN. Such hemorrhages occur with glioblastoma multiforme and metastatic brain tumors.

DIFFERENTIAL DIAGNOSIS

Depending on which of the multiple presentations occurs, IN can be mimicked by a multitude of neurologic and psychiatric disorders.

HEADACHE
Migraine headaches share similar characteristics with IN-induced headaches. They are intermittent but not worse in the early waking hours, as are IN headaches. They are often associated with vomiting that is preceded by nausea. In tumors, neurologic deficits are progressive, in migraine headaches they are fleeting. Although the migraine headache is typically unilateral, it is a throbbing, severe pain, unlike the characteristic dull aching of a tumor. Also, the duration of a migraine headache is hours to days, which is usually longer than the duration of a tumor-induced headache.

CEREBROVASCULAR ACCIDENT
Tumors occasionally present in an apoplectic manner and mimic stroke, particularly if there is hemorrhage into the tumor. IN characteristically has an insidious onset with progressive worsening of symptoms over time. The distinction between tumor and CVA may be made with CT.

BRAIN ABSCESS

Brain abscesses are characterized by headache, papilledema, pyramidal signs, and seizures. Often the patient will present with tachycardia, fever, leukocytosis, and other signs of infectious etiology. The patient may give a history of head injury, previous meningeal symptoms, or rheumatic or cyanotic heart disease. However, in chronic brain abscess these latter signs and symptoms may not be present. It may be difficult to distinguish an abscess from a neoplasm even with the enhanced CT or cerebral angiography. A brain biopsy may then be necessary for definitive diagnosis.

Acute infection of the meninges may simulate symptoms of brain tumors. The diagnosis may be made on examination of the CSF after a negative CT scan.

PSEUDOTUMOR CEREBRI

Pseudotumor cerebri is a syndrome consisting of nonspecific intermittent headache, papilledema, constricted visual fields, and an enlarged blind spot. It is often seen in obese young women with menstrual irregularities.

EMERGENCY DEPARTMENT EVALUATION
HISTORY

ED evaluation of a suspected intracranial neoplasm should begin with a careful history. Direct questioning regarding change in behavior or affect, visual disturbances, weakness, changes in sensation or speech, history of headache or vomiting, and new onset of seizures should be elicited.

PHYSICAL EXAMINATION

The physical examination should include a detailed neurologic and mental status examination. The most frequent finding in IN is papilledema, seen in 50% to 90%. A fundoscopic examination is imperative. Visual field confrontation testing must also be performed. Papilledema is a nonspecific, nonlocalizing consequence of increased ICP. Venous pulsations, although not always visible, rule out increased ICP when seen. Focal neurologic deficits may be identified, including hemiparesis, positive Babinsky's sign, cranial nerve palsies, dysarthria, ataxia, dysphasia, and abnormalities in sensation. These signs may have localizing potential, but this is usually lost in the face of increased ICP. Patients who present with acutely elevated ICP may manifest headache, meningismus, bradycardia and hypertension, and altered levels of consciousness. The classic ipsilateral fixed and dilated pupil with contralateral hemiparesis or terminal findings of bilateral fixed and dilated pupils, decerebrate posturing, hypoventilation, tachycardia, and hypotension signify an impending herniation and demand immediate treatment. In patients suspected of having brain malignancies, a thorough breast, pulmonary, abdominal, and skin examination should be performed to identify possible primary malignancies.

LABORATORY STUDIES

Laboratory workup of patients with suspected IN or of patients who present with altered mental status, new-onset seizures, focal neurologic deficits, or evidence of elevated ICP include complete blood count and determination of serum levels of electrolytes, calcium, magnesium, glucose, and blood urea nitrogen. These are ordered to rule out metabolic or infectious abnormalities. Baseline serum osmolalities should be obtained if mannitol therapy is to be initiated. Liver function tests and measurement of serum ammonia levels may be helpful if hepatic encephalopathy is in the differential diagnosis. Coagulation studies and type and crossmatch should be ordered if urgent neurosurgical intervention is a consideration.

RADIOLOGIC STUDIES

Plain films of the skull demonstrate abnormalities in only a small percentage of cases. CT or MRI should be obtained regardless of the plain film findings if IN is clinically suspected. The major diagnostic tool available for the ED evaluation of IN is CT. CT may be used to rule out IN in suspected patients, since the accuracy of CT for diagnosing brain tumors is approximately 85% in nonenhanced studies and rises to 95% when intravenous contrast agents are used. Metastatic tumors that are 1 cm or greater in size are visualized with CT. For the ED patient, because of implanted or attached metal devices and ferromagnetic life-support systems, CT remains the imaging modality of choice. In addition, acute hemorrhage less than 48 hours old may not be seen on MRI. The long scanning time for MRI (5–15 minutes, compared with 3–4 seconds for CT) requires a cooperative, immobile patient.

MISCELLANEOUS STUDIES

Lumbar puncture is relatively contraindicated in the presence of an IN, but it may be warranted after a negative CT if meningeal carcinomatosis, meningitis, or subarachnoid hemorrhage is suspected.

EMERGENCY DEPARTMENT MANAGEMENT

Management of patients with IN is directed at associated symptoms and complications: airway control, ventilation, and stabilization of circulation. An intravenous line should be established. Once stabilized, acute intervention depends on the presentation of the patient. When a confused or comatose patient presents, stabilization should include administration of 50% dextrose in water, naloxone (Narcan), and thiamine (vitamin B_1) to rule out the more common and easily treatable causes of coma such as hypoglycemia and narcosis and to prevent or even treat Wernicke's encephalopathy. The patient should be placed on a cardiac monitor and vital signs should be closely followed.

SEIZURES
Prevention of further seizures or treatment of an actively seizing patient should be done without further depressing mental status when possible. Phenytoin loading (10–15 mg/kg IV piggyback over 20 minutes) is the therapy of choice. Diazepam should be given to actively seizing patients to control status, in addition to phenytoin. Phenobarbital is reserved as a last-line drug because of CNS depression, but when necessary it may be given 2 mg to 3 mg/kg initially to a total of 15 mg to 18 mg/kg.

INCREASED ICP
For patients suspected of elevated ICP the head of the bed should be raised 20 to 30 degrees to aid cerebral venous outflow and thus potentiate ICP lowering. Fluids should be given at KVO rate unless the patient is simultaneously hypotensive. In this situation shock management supercedes, and isotonic fluid resuscitation with possible Trendelenburg positioning is warranted. In the absence of hypotension, normal saline 0.45% or 0.9% administered at KVO rate is preferred over dextrose 5% in water or other hypotonic solutions, as the latter may precipitate or aggravate cerebral edema.

HYPERVENTILATION
Patients with IN seldom present with acute elevation of ICP, but when they do emergent treatment is necessary. Intubation with hyperventilation is the fastest method to decrease ICP. The goal is to keep PCO_2 between 25 and 30 torr. Excessive hyperventilation with a PCO_2 below 20 torr restricts cerebral perfusion and may result in ischemic sequela. Oxygen supplementation is used to ensure adequate tissue oxygenation and to prevent hypoxia. The use and route of lidocaine before intubation are somewhat controversial, but most investigators conclude that 100 mg lidocaine given intravenously 1 to 5 minutes before intubation lowers the risk of transient ICP elevation.

OSMOTIC AGENTS
Osmotic agents include urea, glycerol, and mannitol, of which mannitol is the agent of choice. These drugs are used in patients with ICP elevation to stabilize the patient until surgical decompression is available. The current recommended dosage is 0.25 g to 2.0 g/kg of a 20% solution

by intravenous infusion over 30 minutes. Electrolytes, serum osmolality, blood pressure, urine output, and ICP (when possible) should be monitored. Serum osmolality should be maintained under 310 mosm. If the cause of ICP elevation is thought to be an intracranial hemorrhage, mannitol should be used with caution, since it can result in extension of the bleed.

LOOP DIURETICS
Furosemide (Lasix) therapy is recommended in adjunct with mannitol to lower ICP with less elevation of serum osmolality or electrolyte disturbance. It has been recommended by some to be used alone in the very young or elderly. Furosemide reduces cerebral edema in the pathologic regions of the brain, where osmotic diuretics are ineffective. It also decreases CSF production and sodium influx into the CNS. The recommended dosage is 0.5 mg to 1.0 mg/kg IV push, and the onset of action is 15 to 20 minutes.

STEROIDS
Cerebral edema secondary to IN continues to be one of the most widely accepted indications for dexamethasone therapy. Initial dosage is 10 mg IV push, followed by 4 mg every 6 hours for 48 hours, with tapering over the next 5 to 7 days. Dexamethasone has a delayed effect in decreasing cerebral edema.

MISCELLANEOUS
Barbiturate coma, using pentobarbital or thiopental, to control elevated ICP is typically done as a last resort by the neurosurgical-anesthesiology team in the intensive care unit and is not recommended in the ED.

DISPOSITION

ROLE OF THE CONSULTANT   Neurosurgical consultation is mandatory in all patients with IN. A stat consult is warranted with status epilepticus or suspected ICP elevation. Those without significant ICP elevation and with stable vital signs may be admitted to a nonmonitored bed, while those who require hyperventilation or osmotic agents require intensive care monitoring.

TRANSFER CONSIDERATIONS   In rural or community-based facilities it may be necessary to transfer patients to a hospital where neurosurgical consultants are readily available.

COMMON PITFALLS

- Unenhanced CT alone cannot completely exclude IN.
- Because of the nonspecific quality of an IN headache, the diagnosis of brain tumor is often missed initially. Follow-up is essential in all patients in whom the cause of headache is not reasonably certain.
- An appropriate history and physical examination must be done on all patients, even those with primarily psychiatric symptoms.
- A careful neurologic examination must be done, no matter how trivial the chief complaint seems.
- There are no consistently reliable indicators of elevated ICP.
- Not everyone with elevated ICP has papilledema.
- Withholding mannitol and diuretics in a patient who displays signs of impending herniation while awaiting CT confirmation or neurosurgical consultation is unwise.

PART VII

Emergency Aspects of Urology

31 Urinary Tract Infections in Men

It is impossible to separate infectious diseases of the male reproductive organs from diseases of the male urinary tract. Complaints of hesitancy, urgency, frequency, and dysuria may indicate urethritis, pyelonephritis, or a disease of any of the organs connected or adjacent to the urethra, bladder, ureters, or kidney. Consideration must also be given to disease of the prostate, vasa deferens, seminal vesicles, epididymides, and testes because these organs are contiguous with the male urinary tract and may present with similar symptoms. If all forms of male-specific infections, such as urethritis and epididymitis, are included in the incidence of urinary tract infection, occurrence rates are probably equal in both sexes during the adult years, despite the classic teaching that women have more frequent urinary tract infections. If prostatitis is added to the incidence of cystitis, men probably have more UTI after the fifth decade.

GENERAL DIAGNOSIS
HISTORY

The hallmark of any UTI is dysuria. Other symptoms include increased frequency of urination with scant amounts of urine, cloudy or foul-smelling urine, hematuria, and urgency. In the male, difficulty in initiation of voiding, dribbling, or a smaller or slower urinary stream may also signify the presence of prostatism. The medical history should include information concerning the presence of fever, chills, and back, suprapubic, or perineal pain. A history of prior UTI diagnostic procedures, and urinary tract operations is important to determine. Data on the patient's sexual preferences and recent contacts, prior sexually transmitted infections, as well as significant past medical history, such as diabetes or prior transplant operations, should be obtained, if possible.

PHYSICAL EXAMINATION

General condition, vital signs, and presence of fever should be noted. Toxic patients should have intravenous lines started immediately. The abdomen and back should be examined for masses, bladder fullness, bruits, abdominal tenderness or guarding, and costovertebral angle tenderness; the scrotum should be examined for tenderness and masses; the urethra should be inspected for discharge or sores; the prepuce should be retracted and inspected; and the rectum and prostate should be examined. Specific attention should be given to the presence of sores or lymphadenopathy in the groin or on the testes or penis.

107

LABORATORY EXAMINATION

The hallmark of UTI is the presence of leukocytes and bacteria in the urine. Diagnosis in males does not require the "clean-catch midstream voided urine" technique. In males there appears to be no significant difference in numbers of contaminating organisms obtained with clean-catch versus routine sampling. A urinalysis does not reliably localize the infection within the urinary tract. If the patient has a history that is suspicious for urethritis, the emergency physician must obtain smears for Gram's stain, *Chlamydia* immunofluorescence, and culture of the urethral discharge. This is best done when the patient has not voided for several hours. Discharge should be expressed directly onto a slide for the Gram's stain and then a culture taken from a urethral meatal swab. A calcium alginate swab (Calgonate) provides the least inhibition of growth of *Neisseria gonorrhoeae* and is the most comfortable size available. A second swab should be used for the *Chlamydia* immunofluorescence smear. Cultures of the urine should always be obtained before the administration of antibiotics.

URETHRITIS

Urethritis is the most common urinary tract infection in men. Urethritis has traditionally been classified as either nongonococcal (NGU) or gonococcal (GU). With the advent of easy and accurate *Chlamydia* identification techniques, it has become obvious that this is an artificial separation, and both *Chlamydia* and gonorrhea are often present in the same patient and may be contracted from the same contact.

The Centers for Disease Control estimate that there are between 800,000 and 1 million cases of gonorrhea per year. The reported incidence in any one part of the country is strongly influenced by prevalent sexual attitudes and preferences. The organism is carried asymptomatically in as many as 7% of sexually active *homosexual* males as confirmed by screening cultures and cultures of reported contacts. Because NGU and chlamydial urethritis are not reportable diseases, an estimate of the number of affected patients for either is more difficult. The reported incidence of NGU in Great Britain currently exceeds the incidence of gonorrhea by a ratio of almost 2 to 1.

GONOCOCCAL URETHRITIS

PRESENTATION

A purulent urethral exudate noted a few days after a sexual encounter, associated with dysuria, is the most common presentation in symptomatic heterosexual men. The usual incubation period is between 3 and 5 days, but it may extend to 14 or more days.

DIAGNOSIS

A Gram's stain of the urethral exudate obtained by swabbing the urethra (in symptomatic men) is a reliable method for the diagnosis of gonorrhea. The specificity is 95% to 98%, and the sensitivity is 83% to 95% when typical gram-negative diplococci are found *within* polymorphonuclear leukocytes. Gram-negative extracellular diplococci do not carry the same high specificity and sensitivity but are still highly suspicious for GU in the male. To obtain a specimen from a male without exudate, a calcium alginate-tipped swab (Calgiswab) should be inserted 2 cm to 4 cm into the anterior urethra. Cultures on Thayer–Martin or other appropriate media should be obtained if there have been reported cases of penicillinase-producing *N. gonorrhoeae* (PPNG) strains in the community, if the patient has recently been to areas of known risk for PPNG, or if the patient's symptoms do not rapidly abate with appropriate therapy.

COMPLICATIONS

About 1% to 3% of patients with gonococcal infections develop hematogenous spread of the organism that may involve joints, meninges, heart, and skin. It is notable that those strains that disseminate are usually nonvirulent in their primary site and the original infection is often asymptomatic. In addition to the bacteremic complications, local spread may occur to the vas deferens, prostate, paraurethral glands, epididymis, and adjacent soft tissues. Late scarring may cause urethral strictures.

TREATMENT

Treatment is frequently updated by the Centers for Disease Control (Table 31-1).

FOLLOW-UP CARE

All patients with GU should be rechecked after therapy. Increasing rates of PPNG make this follow-up more important, although many patients with GU are noncompliant. If the patient is not rechecked, referral to a sexually transmitted diseases clinic is appropriate. Emphatic counseling should be given to ensure that the medication is taken and that the patient's sexual partners are also examined.

CHLAMYDIAL URETHRITIS

There is little question that *Chlamydia trachomatis* causes the majority of sexually transmitted diseases in the United States. The clinical features of chlamydial urethritis resemble those of gonorrhea but are generally less severe; the discharge is thought to be somewhat thinner and clearer, but there is sufficient overlap in symptoms and characteristics to make any clinical distinction unreliable. *Chlamydia* typically has an incubation period of 1 to 3 weeks, but it may extend as long as 45 days. The diagnosis of chlamydial urethritis should be based on a urethral smear of epithelial cells for *Chlamydia,* with immunofluorescence techniques. Isolation of *Chlamydia* requires exacting tissue culture techniques.

TREATMENT

See Table 31-1.

COMPLICATIONS

Complications of chlamydial infections include epididymitis and, possibly prostatitis. Exposure to *Chlamydia* in the male does not appear to lead to infertility.

NONGONOCOCCAL, NONCHLAMYDIAL URETHRITIS

Nongonococcal, nonchlamydial urethritis is currently a "wastebasket" diagnosis for all cases in which the cause is uncertain and the infection is neither gonorrheal nor chlamydial. As greater facility with

---

Table 31-1. Treatment of Urethritis

Current Treatment of Choice

Ceftriaxone	125 mg IM single dose

All treatment for gonorrhea should be followed by doxycycline, 100 mg two times a day for 7 days, or azithromycin, 1.0 g PO single dose, due to the high percentage of patients who are also infected with *Chlamydia.*

Alternative Treatments

Ciprofloxacin	500 mg PO single dose
or	
Norfloxacin	800 mg PO single dose
or	
Cefixime	400 mg PO single dose

---

identification and isolation of pathogenic commensal organisms is gained, more specific causes of non-gonococcal, nonchlamydial urethritis may be found. The elimination of *Chlamydia* as a cause usually occurs after an apparent treatment failure. Another 20% to 25% of NGU may be caused by *Ureaplasma (Mycoplasma) urealyticum* or *Ureaplasma genitalium.* Although *U. urealyticum* does not usually cause human disease, there is good evidence that implicates *U. genitalium* as a cause of urethritis.

TREATMENT

Doxycycline or azithromycin are the drugs of choice for the treatment of NGU in general. Recurrence rates approach 20% in those cases caused by *Ureaplasma* treated with tetracyclines. *Ureaplasma* responds poorly to the sulfonamides, but aminoglycosides appear to work better. Of those who have a recurrence, between 30% and 60% continue to have symptoms despite multiple courses of antibiotics.

After *Chlamydia, Ureaplasma,* and gonorrhea have been eliminated as the cause of urethritis, about 30% of cases remain without apparent cause. Numerous studies have failed to define the cause of NGU, although *Candida, Trichomonas, Gardnerella, Bacteroides* species, *Staphylococcus saprophyticus, Corynebacterium genitalium,* and various viruses, including herpes, are isolated on occasion. Although all types of NGU respond initially to antibiotic therapy, recurrence is found in up to 50% of cases. Initial treatment should be tetracycline or doxycycline for 14 to 28 days. Erythromycin may be used as an alternative to the tetracyclines in those patients who cannot tolerate tetracyclines.

PROSTATITIS

Prostatitis is a poorly defined but common syndrome of prostatic inflammation. It includes a wide range of pelvic, urinary, or ejaculatory symptoms with or without a tender prostate and with or without evidence of bacterial infection. With this broad symptom complex it is estimated that up to 50% of men experience a variant of prostatitis at some point in their lives. Prostatitis can be classified into three subcategories: acute prostatitis, chronic prostatitis, and prostatodynia. Both acute and chronic prostatitis are characterized by bacteriuria that can be localized to the prostate. Urine, prostatic secretions, and semen usually show evidence of leukocytes, and frequently the offending organism is cultured from these secretions. Chronic prostatitis is often further subdivided into bacterial and nonbacterial categories. In chronic nonbacterial prostatitis common urinary pathogens are not found in the urine, EPS, or seminal secretions, despite evidence of inflammation, such as leukocytes in the EPS. Prostatodynia shares many of the symptoms of bacterial or nonbacterial prostatitis but lacks signs of inflammation and is not associated with urinary tract infection.

ACUTE PROSTATITIS

Acute prostatitis is the easiest entity to both diagnose and treat. Acute prostatitis usually presents as an acute illness with fever, chills, and pain in the lower back, rectal, or perineal area. Initial signs and symptoms often include malaise, arthralgia, and myalgia. These may appear several days before the local prostatic inflammation produces symptoms of dysuria, frequency, urgency, and urine retention. The patient frequently is toxic. Acute bacterial prostatitis may be so dramatic that the diagnosis is obvious once perirectal pathology has been eliminated. The infecting bacteria are most commonly *Escherichia coli, Pseudomonas,* and enterococci.

PHYSICAL EXAMINATION

Examination of the prostate is often difficult and inadequate because it is exquisitely painful. If performed, the prostate frequently is swollen, tender, warm, and firm to touch. Massage of the prostate is contraindicated because of the possibility of hematogenous spread of bacteria, although this has not been well documented. Because the prostate surrounds the urethra, the urine will usually contain the infecting organism. Cystitis often accompanies acute prostatitis. In some patients the swelling of the acutely inflamed prostate may precipitate complete urine retention with infected urine subsequently in the bladder. This combination of obstruction and infection may rapidly progress to sepsis.

TREATMENT

Acute prostatitis is quite responsive to many antibiotics that do not normally enter the prostate. Toxicity, fever, urine retention, concurrent underlying disease, and altered immune response are indications for hospitalization and the administration of intravenous antibiotics. Parenteral ampicillin and an aminoglycoside (kanamycin or tobramycin) are appropriate empiric therapy. The subsequent choice of antibiotics is ideally made from sensitivity testing of bacteria grown from urine cultures. For the less toxic patient appropriate oral antibiotics include trimethoprim-sulfamethoxazole, ampicillin, and doxycycline. Oral therapy for acute prostatitis should be reserved for select cases and not be considered the routine. Antibiotic therapy should be continued for a minimum of 4 weeks in all patients.

Instrumentation of the urinary tract should be avoided. If the patient has acute urine retention from prostatitis, catheterization may be very painful and could potentially provoke hematogenous release of bacteria. Until antibiotics and rest allow the inflammation to subside, suprapubic needle aspiration with catheter insertion is much more comfortable. This procedure can be quickly accomplished with the Seldinger technique.

Antipyretics, narcotic analgesics, and stool softeners should be given when indicated. Nonsteroidal anti-inflammatory drugs and spasmolytics are useful for milder pain. Bed rest frequently makes the patient more comfortable. Hospitalization of the toxic patient ensures that appropriate supportive care is maintained.

PROSTATIC ABSCESS

The development of a prostatic abscess was once common after acute bacterial prostatitis but is now rare, except in immunosuppressed patients. The presence of a continued elevated temperature despite treatment, rectal symptoms, and leukocytosis suggests a prostatic abscess. Rectal examination may reveal a fluctuant mass, the hallmark of the prostatic abscess, but may also only show a firm, tender prostate. Prostatic abscesses are treated surgically. Urologic consultation is indicated. Hospitalization and administration of intravenous antibiotics are necessary for proper management of these seriously ill patients.

CYSTITIS
PREDISPOSING FACTORS

In females more than 95% of urinary tract infections occur by way of the ascending route from the urethral meatus to the bladder and kidney. In normal males the longer anatomical distance discourages this retrograde travel of organisms from the penile meatus to the bladder mucosa. Congenital anomalies such as hypospadias may allow easier entrance of the bacteria with subsequent cystitis. Instrumentation of the urethra may seed the urethra or allow the rapid spread of organisms in retrograde manner. After 3 days of indwelling urinary catheter drainage virtually 100% of patients have a urinary tract infection. Autoerogenous intraurethral insertion of foreign objects may precipitate a cystitis with an unusual bacterial flora. Likewise, trauma to the urethra or bladder may allow rapid dissemination of organisms in retrograde manner from an abnormal port of entry.

Cystitis without trauma or instrumentation is rare in men and almost always a secondary manifestation of upper urinary tract disease, chronic prostatitis, nephrolithiasis, tumor, congenital malformation, or mechanical obstruction. Of these, chronic prostatitis, prostatism, and prior instrumentation are the most common predisposing causes. Abnormalities are found in up to 80% of those males who present with a urinary tract infection without antecedent trauma or instrumentation. It is particularly important to ensure that urinary obstruction is not present, since the combination of infection and obstruction is a catastrophic antecedent to sepsis.

ETIOLOGY

E. coli is the most common causative organism, accounting for more than 90% of infections. *Enterobacter, Klebsiella, Proteus, Pseudomonas,* and species of the enterococci are also seen. *Staphylococcus aureus* infections are usually associated with blood-borne spread, and a primary source should be sought. Gram-positive organisms are unusual causative agents and may be associated with diabetes, immunocompromise, or tumors.

EVALUATION AND MANAGEMENT

Management includes a thorough examination of the genitalia, rectum, and abdomen, urinalysis, and culture of urine. Catheterization may be indicated to assess residual urine. Intravenous pyelography or ultrasonography may be indicated. If the patient is toxic or febrile, blood cultures should be obtained. Antibiotic empiric therapy specific for coliforms should be instituted. Single-dose therapy is not appropriate.

DISPOSITION

In males cystitis is closely associated with other urinary tract pathology. The evaluation must be continued beyond the emergency department. Referral and possible admission should always be considered. Those patients with a known history of instrumentation, congenital malformation, and known uncomplicated benign prostatic hypertrophy with normal voiding mechanism will have been closely followed by a urologist. Consultation with the urologist is indicated.

PYELONEPHRITIS

Pyelonephritis presents in a similar manner in both males and females. Predisposition to infection from underlying urinary tract disease or abnormality is more common in males and should prompt a thorough search for these problems.

PREDISPOSING FACTORS

Abnormal anatomy, such as ureteral ectopia, bifid ureter, or renal scarring from prior renal infections, predisposes to infection of the kidney. Other common predisposing causes include abnormal physiology from neurologic trauma, urine retention from any cause, underlying renal disease, and the presence of a foreign body, such as a stone or an indwelling catheter.

EMERGENCY DEPARTMENT MANAGEMENT

Men with symptoms of pyelonephritis should be considered for admission and parenteral antibiotic therapy because of the high frequency of obstruction or anatomical abnormalities of the urinary tract. The patient who appears toxic, is nauseated or vomiting, or has a temperature of 102°F (39°C) or higher should be hospitalized and treated with parenteral antibiotics. Urine should be obtained for culture and sensitivity before therapy is initiated. Blood cultures are indicated as well as electrolytes, BUN and creatinine. Treatment should be directed against the offending organism identified by culture. Empiric therapy should be instituted while awaiting the culture results. Consideration should be given to assessing for retention as well as the status of the upper tract. The patient who presents with flank pain and hematuria and fever and chills should be suspected of having both a ureteral obstruction and an infection. Pyelonephritis in the presence of an obstruction can rapidly progress to a renal abscess, with subsequent loss of renal

tissue and generalized sepsis. This patient requires immediate urologic consultation and evaluation. Blood cultures and urine cultures should be done, followed by either intravenous pyelography or renal ultrasound, and intravenous antibiotics.

32   Urinary Tract Infections in Women

Urinary tract infection (UTI) in women is an extremely common, often recurrent clinical problem.
Complaints of dysuria or urinary frequency result in an estimated 6 million ambulatory visits (1.6
million to EDs) per year in the United States. Three percent to 10% of women may suffer from
UTI each year. Successful evaluation and management require a thorough understanding of
appropriate specimen collection, proper use of immediately available laboratory tests for presumptive diagnosis, the limits of clinical assessment for identifying those patients with upper tract
UTI, the selection and duration of antimicrobial therapy, and the proper timing of follow-up medical care. Genitourinary disorders are second only to respiratory conditions in incidence and associated disability. The frequency of symptomatic UTI in women has two periods of increased
prevalence: during pregnancy and with the onset of sexual activity. The natural history of UTI in
women appears to be primarily limited to recurrence of symptomatic infection. Relapses are
uncommon in uncomplicated UTI; therefore, a relapse should suggest the possibility of complicated UTI or renal bacteriuria. Thirty to 65% of patients may spontaneously clear their bladder
bacteriuria. Rarely does *uncomplicated,* untreated UTI lead to renal failure, hypertension, or
death, although there may be progression to pyelonephritis. Although untreated asymptomatic
bacteriuria in pregnancy can lead to subsequent pyelonephritis, only a small number of premature births can be directly attributed to UTI. Complicated forms of acute or chronic pyelonephritis may lead to perinephric abscess, emphysematous pyelonephritis (particularly in diabetes
mellitus), or infection with unusual organisms, such as *Cryptococcus* or *Candida.*
    The pathogenesis of UTI in women is most commonly related to the ascent of micro-organ-
isms that are present in the vagina. Alternatively, hematogenous or lymphatic pathway spread
may account for a small number of UTIs. The Enterobacteriaceae account for 80% to 95% of
micro-organisms associated with UTI, with *Escherichia coli* representing 80% of this group.
Klebsiella, Proteus, and *Enterobacter* occur less commonly. *Pseudomonas, Staphylococcus
saprophyticus,* and group D streptococci account for the remainder of micro-organisms in uncomplicated UTI.1 *Serratia, Morganella, Staphylococcus aureus,* and *Candida* account for a small, but
important percentage of micro-organisms associated with complicated UTIs.
    Complicated UTI is defined as a UTI in which an underlying neurologic or structural abnor-
mality coexists, such as renal calculi, postvoiding residual bladder urine, other mechanical obstruction, or instrumentation or foreign body (i.e., Foley catheter) of the urinary tract. Also, patients who
have urinary tract symptoms lasting longer than 6 days, clinical signs of septicemia, immunosuppressive disorders (including drugs and immunologic deficiencies), diabetes mellitus, pregnancy,
and relapse should be considered to have complicated UTI. Other UTIs are considered uncomplicated. *Upper tract versus lower tract UTI* is terminology generated as a result of bacterial localization studies, which attempt to differentiate bacterial infection superior to the bladder (renal
parenchymal or upper tract infection) from that of the bladder and urethra (lower tract infection).
    The potential problems prevalent in unselected ED patients are a higher incidence of
vaginitis, pelvic inflammatory disease, and sexually transmitted diseases; delayed presentation of

UTI; limitations of appropriate follow-up; and perhaps a higher incidence of complicated or "upper tract" UTI when compared with other outpatients, especially among the inner-city population. Issues include the indications for a pelvic examination in a woman with dysuria, the clinical differentiation of lower tract from upper tract UTI, the value of microscopic examination of the urine specimen, the efficacy of urine dipstick screening, the identification of the complicated UTI, the indications and timing of urinary cultures, the indications for sensitivity testing, the timing of follow-up, antimicrobial therapy (agents, dosage, and duration), and disposition.

CLINICAL PRESENTATION

The patient with **acute bacterial cystitis** typically is between 16 and 45 years of age. These patients complain of a brief period of dysuria, frequency, urgency, and, sometimes, hematuria, and mild suprapubic abdominal or back pain, although the latter is usually not well localized. Constitutional symptoms are usually lacking. A temperature in excess of 38.5°C is distinctly uncommon, although low-grade fever may occur. Physical examination is typically normal, except for mild suprapubic tenderness. Microscopic examination of urine shows leukocytes, bacteria, and often erythrocytes. Urine dipstick testing may reveal proteinuria, hematuria, leukocyte esterase activity, and nitrite positivity. Hemorrhagic cystitis occurs in patients with bacterial cystitis.

Acute bacterial pyelonephritis is recognized in a previously healthy woman who has had dysuria and frequency for several days, and who develops chills, fever, prostration, and unilateral loin or costovertebral angle pain. The history of dysuria and frequency may be lacking in some women. Typically, the past medical history is unremarkable, although attempts to elicit a history of previous UTI, diabetes mellitus, urologic abnormalities, immunologic abnormalities, and pregnancy should be vigorously sought. The physical examination is usually remarkable for an ill-appearing person, with temperature higher than 38.5°C, without hemodynamic compromise. Most often there is unilateral costovertebral angle tenderness, although it may be lacking. Microscopic examination of the urine shows an abundance of leukocytes, bacteria, and, occasionally, erthrocytes. Leukocytosis, with a left shift, is almost always present. Complications are uncommon in treated patients but include sepsis, septic shock, perinephric abscess, and transient renal insufficiency.

The **acute urethral syndrome** (now most often referred to as "low count infection") may account for >50% of cases of dysuria and frequency in young, sexually active women. Their symptoms and signs are nearly identical with acute cystitis. However, they have either sterile urine or <105 cfu/mL on urine culture. The presence of pyuria is associated with the isolation of *Chlamydia trachomatis* in >60% of cases. The absence of pyuria is associated with sterile urine or with sexually transmitted diseases other than a chlamydial infection. Colony counts >102/mL should be treated as low-count UTI.

The recognition of **asymptomatic bacteriuria** is important to identify in pregnant patients (4%–6%), in patients with immunosuppressive abnormalities or indwelling urinary catheters, and in the elderly (10%). Microscopic examination of the urine specimen demonstrates variable degrees of pyuria and bacteriuria. Urine culture demonstrates significant bacteriuria.

Women who are at greatest risk for **urosepsis** include those with indwelling urinary catheters, immunosuppressive disorders, untreated bacteriuria, and obstructive or incomplete bladder emptying. Typically, these patients present from an adult nursing facility with fever, alteration of mental status, tachycardia, tachypnea, and signs of dehydration. The history may be limited by either acute or chronic mental status deterioration but may usually be obtained from family members or the nursing home staff. If the patient is more alert, she may complain of poorly localized back or abdominal pain, thirst, or difficulty breathing. Physical examination usually demonstrates early signs of compensated shock, although moderate dehydration is the rule. Body temperature, although usually elevated, may be depressed. Delayed or advanced presentations may present with hypotension or septic shock.

DIFFERENTIAL DIAGNOSIS

The woman with classic lower urinary tract symptoms (frequency, dysuria, and urgency) or acute pyelonephritis presents little challenge in diagnosis. Patients with asymptomatic bacteriuria are discovered only by obtaining a urine specimen. Commonly, however, patients who present to the ED have a less specific illness. The patient with *dysuria* may have vulvovaginitis, pelvic inflammatory disease, or herpes genitalis. Patients with vulvovaginitis also complain of a vaginal discharge or external dysuria. Pelvic examination and appropriate wet-mount slides and cultures should be obtained. Patients with pelvic inflammatory disease usually complain more of lower abdominal pain, fever, and an associated vaginal discharge. Physical examination shows lower abdominal tenderness, often with guarding but rarely with frank peritonitis. A purulent discharge from the cervical os, cervical motion tenderness, and bilateral adnexal tenderness are usual. There may be fever and leukocytosis.

Herpes genitalis is associated with severe genital pain during a primary infection, with painful shallow ulcers or vesicles present intravaginally or on the external genitalia. Severe cases with urethral involvement may lead to urine retention. Diagnosis is based on the characteristic lesions, a positive Tzanck test, and viral cultures. Patients with unilateral costovertebral angle tenderness should be examined for evidence of renal calculi, trauma, perirenal abscess, local osteolytic processes, or musculoskeletal strains or contusions. If there is any question of a coexisting abnormality, plain-film radiography, ultrasound, intravenous pyelography (IVP), or contrast-enhanced abdominal computed tomographic scan may be diagnostic. Urinary frequency is associated with increased urine output, as might occur with pregnancy, diuretic use, diabetes insipidus, renal calculi, congestive heart failure, and overflow incontinence.

Renal calculous disease is easily recognized in the acutely writhing patient with a soft abdomen and hematuria. Less often patients present with vague abdominal or back pain, with or without dysuria and hematuria. Appendicitis may be associated with dysuria, although more often migratory abdominal pain, anorexia, low-grade fever, and right lower quadrant tenderness. Ovarian cysts, adnexal torsion, tumors, tubo-ovarian abscess, and endometriosis may present with dysuria, but most commonly they present with lower abdominal pain and pelvic findings on examination, without vaginal discharge. The pelvic examination may reveal an ovarian mass, small nodules in the cul-de-sac, pelvic ligamental structures, or bladder peritoneal reflection. Bladder tumors are painless, unless associated with UTI. Rarer entities that may present as dysuria are abdominal trauma and vascular thrombosis.

EMERGENCY DEPARTMENT EVALUATION

The history should include information relative to dysuria (external or internal), frequency, urgency, duration of symptoms, gross hematuria, presence of an abnormal vaginal discharge, external genital lesions, back pain, fever, rigor, and sexual contact(s). A history of prior pregnancy, the birth control method used, and the timing and course of the last two menstrual cycles should be obtained. The past medical history should reflect a search for complicating problems, such as diabetes mellitus, immunodepressive disorders, incomplete voiding, urethral strictures, and recent instrumentation of the genitourinary tract.

The physical examination should include vital signs, orthostatics if dehydration or hypovolemia is suspected, an examination for costovertebral angle and suprapubic abdominal tenderness, and examination for external genital inflammation. The history and physical examination does not differentiate upper tract from lower tract UTI. Identify women with *complicated UTI* because of the implications for duration of therapy and follow-up. Relapse is 80% sensitive in predicting upper tract UTI and appears to be an effective means for identifying women who will require prolonged therapy or urologic investigation.

A urine specimen should be collected from all patients with complaints of dysuria and frequency. The method of collection depends on the patient's stability, capacity to cooperate and adhere to cleansing guidelines, obesity, and menstrual blood, copious vaginal discharge, or an anatomical abnormality present. Urethral catheterization has few complications. A midstream "clean-catch" urine collection after proper cleansing of the genitalia may reliably produce an adequate specimen for microscopic examination and culture. The presence of epithelial cells that exceed the number of white blood cells (WBCs) suggests contamination and necessitates the collection of a second urine specimen. Regardless of which urine specimen collection technique is used, the urine should be promptly refrigerated or sent immediately to the laboratory since significant numbers of micro-organisms can proliferate in unrefrigerated urine. Microscopic examination of urine obtained from all patients suspected of having UTI should be performed. The *unspun* urine Gram's stain reliably predicts patients with >105 cfu/mL of urine when one or more *bacteria* per high-power field are seen. Examination of the urine sediment, after centrifuge and removal of the supernatant, is somewhat less specific for significant bacteriuria than Gram's stain but may be more sensitive, particularly for patients with low-count UTI. The identification of >10 bacteria per high-power field correlates closely with the presence of UTI, whereas the presence of a significant number of WBCs (>10/high-power field) is less specific. The presence of pyuria and bacteriuria on microscopic examination of urine has a 75% to 85% accuracy for UTI.

Several rapid dipstick chemical tests are available that may be used to screen for UTI, including nitrite, leukocyte esterase, glucose oxidase, tetrazolium reduction, and catalase. The nitrite test depends on bacterial reduction of nitrate, normally in urine, to nitrite, which is measured colorimetrically. The test is more likely to be positive with first morning urine and and more likely to show gram-negative bacteria. The nitrite test may be falsely negative with dilution, antimicrobial therapy, and frequent voiding. The leukocyte esterase test depends on the conversion of indoxyl carboxylic acid ester by WBCs to an indoxyl moiety, which turns blue when oxidized by air. When compared with microscopic detection of pyuria (>10 WBC/mm3) there is a more than 90% sensitivity and specificity. False-positive results have been reported with *Trichomonas*. Those with a negative dipstick test and urinary complaints should have a pelvic examination. The indications for urine culture in women are controversial, but include acute bacterial pyelonephritis, fever without focus, relapse of UTI, recently treated documented UTI, symptoms of cystitis but no pyuria, fever and neutropenia, indwelling bladder catheterization, and sepsis. The value of sensitivity testing in uncomplicated UTI in women is poor, since >95% of cases are cured with standard antimicrobials. Additional serologic and hematologic studies should be performed on patients with urosepsis or acute bacterial pyelonephritis and certain patients with complicated UTI. Routine studies should include a complete blood count with differential; electrolytes, blood urea nitrogen, and creatinine; and blood cultures. Pelvic wet-mount slides and cultures for *Candida albicans, Trichomonas vaginalis,* and *Gardnerella vaginitis* should be obtained. Cultures for *Neiserria gonorrhoeae* and *C. trachomatis* should be obtained if there is a suspicion of vaginitis, salpingitis, or pelvic inflammatory disease. A human chorionic gonadotropin beta-subunit assay may be indicated.

Radiologic imaging of the woman with uncomplicated UTI is virtually never indicated. Women with complicated UTI may require urgent radiologic evaluation, primarily for determination of infected renal calculi. Ultrasound may be just as sensitive and less risky than IVP for determination of obstruction.

EMERGENCY DEPARTMENT MANAGEMENT

Appropriate antimicrobial agents are seen in Table 32-1 (see pp 118–119). Patients at risk for urosepsis are those with complicated UTI, including elderly women with indwelling Foley catheters, immunosuppressed patients, and patients with renal calculi, obstructive lesions of the urinary tract, and serious underlying medical problems. After appropriate cultures have been collected, intravenous antimicrobials should be administered as rapidly as possible, particularly for patients with sepsis and pyelonephritis.

The great majority of women with presumptive UTI who have no systemic signs of toxicity may be treated with oral antimicrobial agents as outpatients. The currently accepted duration of treatment for complicated UTI is a minimum of 10 days.

DISPOSITION

ROLE OF THE CONSULTANT   Consultants are seldom required for uncomplicated UTI in women. Patients with lower tract UTI or acute pyelonephritis may be referred to primary care physicians for subsequent management. Women with complicated UTI may require urologic consultation.

INDICATIONS FOR ADMISSION   Patients with complicated UTI and pyelonephritis are candidates for hospital admission, particularly if there are signs of sepsis, bacteremia, hemodynamic instability, complicating medical conditions, moderate to severe dehydration with inability to maintain a normovolemic state, and inability to take oral medication. Patients who require intravenous hydration and antimicrobials are seldom candidates for outpatient treatment. The young, nonparous, otherwise healthy woman with acute, uncomplicated pyelonephritis may respond within 6 to 8 hours of initiating appropriate therapy and be subsequently managed as an outpatient, assuming that adequate follow-up is available within 24 hours. Patients with urosepsis and serious underlying medical problems may require critical care admission if they are hemodynamically unstable, require mechanical ventilation, or have complicating medical conditions. All other women admitted with UTI may be managed in routine, acute care floor beds.

After therapy, women should be re-examined and a urine culture obtained in 3 to 4 days after treatment. If these patients remain symptomatic or the urine culture is positive, traditional 10- to 14-day antimicrobial therapy is indicated.

COMMON PITFALLS

- Failure to perform a pelvic examination: A speculum and bimanual pelvic examination is warranted for women who have external dysuria; vaginal discharge or pyuria; a recent change in sexual partner or exposure to sexually transmitted disease when associated with pyuria; external genital lesions; suspicion of concurrent pregnancy; and trauma.
- Failure to collect an adequate urine specimen
- Misinterpretation of the urine microscopic examination
- Failure to process the urine specimen in a timely fashion
- Failure to identify the patient with a complicated UTI
- The lower the ratio of leukocytes to squamous cells in the urine specimen, the more likely it is that the leukocytes are vaginal contaminants. If a predominance of squamous cells is seen, a second urine specimen must be collected.
- False-positive urine cultures usually result from delays in transport (more than 60 minutes) on unrefrigerated urine and from contaminated specimens.
- Failure to consider the diagnosis in a septic patient
- Failure to ensure appropriate, timely follow-up

Table 32-1. Treatment Regimens for Bacterial Urinary Tract Infection

Condition	Characteristic Pathogens	Mitigating Circumstances	Recommended Empirical Treatment*
Acute uncomplicated cystitis in women	E. coli, S. saprophyticus, P. mirabilis, Klebsiella pneumoniae	None	3-day regimens: oral trimethoprim–sulfamethoxazole, trimethoprim, norfloxacin, ciprofloxacin, ofloxacin, lomefloxacin, or enoxacin†
		Diabetes, symptoms for >7 days, recent urinary tract infection, use of diaphragm, age >65 yr	Consider 7-day regimen: oral trimethoprim–sulfamethoxazole, trimethoprim, norfloxacin, ciprofloxacin, ofloxacin, lomefloxacin or enoxacin†
		Pregnancy	Consider 7-day regimen: oral amoxicillin, macrocrystalline nitrofurantoin, cefpodoxime proxetil, or trimethoprim–sulfamethoxazole†
Acute uncomplicated pyelonephritis in women	E. coli, P. mirabilis, K. pneumoniae, S. saprophyticus	Mild-to-moderate illness, no nausea or vomiting —outpatient therapy	Oral‡ trimethoprim—sulfamethoxazole, norfloxacin, ciprofloxacin, ofloxacin, lomefloxacin, or enoxacin for 10–14 days
		Severe illness or possible urosepsis—hospitalization required	Parenteral§ trimethoprim–sulfamethoxazole, ceftriaxone, ciprofloxacin, ofloxacin, or gentamicin (with or without ampicillin) until fever gone; then oral‡ trimethoprim–sulfamethoxazole, norfloxacin, ciprofloxacin, ofloxacin, lomefloxacin, or enoxacin for 14 days
		Pregnancy—hospitalization recommended	Parenteral§ ceftriaxone, gentamicin (with or without ampicillin), aztreonam or trimethoprim–sulfamethoxazole until fever gone; then oral‡ amoxicillin, a cephalosporin, or trimethoprim–sulfamethoxazole for 14 days

| Complicated urinary tract infection | E. coli, proteus species, klebsiella species, pseudomonas species, serratia species, enterococci, staphylococci | Mild-to-moderate illness, no nausea or vomiting—outpatient therapy | Oral‡ norfloxacin, ciprofloxacin, ofloxacin, lomefloxacin, or enoxacin for 10–14 days |
| | | Severe illness or possible urosepsis—hospitalization required | Parenteral§ ampicillin and gentamicin, ciprofloxacin, ofloxacin, ceftriaxone, aztreonam, ticarcillin—clavulanate, or imipenem–cilastatin until fever gone; then oral‡ trimethoprim–sulfamethoxazole, norfloxacin, ciprofloxacin, ofloxacin, lomefloxacin, or enoxacin for 14–21 days |

*Treatments listed are those to be prescribed before the etiologic agent is known (Gram's staining can be helpful); they can be modified once the agent has been identified. The recommendations are the authors' and are limited to drugs currently approved by the Food and Drug Administration, although not all the regimens listed are approved for these indications. Fluoroquinolones should not be used in pregnancy. Trimethoprim–sulfamethoxazole, although not approved for use in pregnancy, has been widely used. Gentamicin should be used with caution in pregnancy because of its possible toxicity to eighth-nerve development in the fetus.

†Multiday oral regimens for cystitis are as follows: trimethoprim–sulfamethoxazole, 160–800 mg every 12 hours; trimethoprim, 100 mg every 12 hours; norfloxacin, 400 mg every 12 hours; ciprofloxacin, 250 mg every 12 hours; ofloxacin, 200 mg every 12 hours; lomefloxacin, 400 mg every day; enoxacin, 400 mg every 12 hours; macrocrystalline nitrofurantoin, 100 mg four times a day; amoxicillin, 250 mg every 8 hours; and cefpodoxime proxetil, 100 mg every 12 hours.

‡Oral regimens for pyelonephritis and complicated urinary tract infection are as follows: trimethoprim–sulfamethoxazole, 160–800 mg every 12 hours; norfloxacin, 400 mg every 12 hours; ciprofloxacin, 500 mg every 12 hours; ofloxacin, 200–300 mg every 12 hours; lomefloxacin, 400 mg every day; enoxacin, 400 mg every 12 hours; amoxicillin, 500 mg every 8 hours; and cefpodoxime proxetil, 200 mg every 12 hours.

§Parenteral regimens are as follows: trimethoprim–sulfamethoxazole, 160–800 mg every 12 hours; ciprofloxacin, 200–400 mg every 12 hours; ofloxacin, 200–400 mg every 12 hours; gentamicin, 1 mg per kilogram of body weight every 8 hours; ceftriaxone, 1–2 g every day; ampicillin, 1 g every 6 hours; imipenem–cilastatin, 250–500 mg every 6–8 hours; ticarcillin–clavulanate, 3.2 g every 8 hours; and aztreonam, 1 g every 8–12 hours.

Used with permission (pending): Stamm W, Hooton TM: Management of Urinary Tract Infections in Adults. NEJM. 329: 18, pp 1328–1334, 1993.

33   Calculous Disease of the Kidney

CLINICAL PRESENTATION AND EVALUATION

The presentation is often characteristic. Although pain is usually present, hematuria and symptoms of urinary tract infection are also common complaints. The history should include: age, family history of stone disease, fluid intake, history of prior stone disease, history of urinary tract infections, and the character of the pain. Stone disease is rare in children and, when encountered, is an indication of a genetic disorder or an overt metabolic disorder.

A family history of stone disease is common. A history of prior urinary tract infections, especially with urea-splitting organisms, may be an important diagnostic clue and a harbinger of a true urologic emergency—an obstructing stone associated with infection. In the case of obstruction, the pain of renal colic is due to acute distention of the renal pelvis and upper ureter. Renal colic is often waxing and waning and localized to the flank, but may also be referred to the ipsilateral testis or labia. As the stone nears the bladder, frequency and urgency may be manifested. Nausea and vomiting are frequently present.

The physical examination usually shows a patient writhing in pain, unable to find a comfortable position. Patients with peritonitis typically lie quietly, as any movement aggravates their pain. A temperature above 38°C usually implies a concomitant UTI and the possibility of urosepsis. The abdominal examination may disclose costovertebral angle tenderness secondary to an acutely hydronephrotic kidney. Auscultation may disclose diminished bowel sounds, as ileus commonly accompanies renal colic. Peritoneal signs can occur if pyelonephritis is present, but they usually signify surgical causes of abdominal pain such as appendicitis, pelvic inflammatory disease, diverticulitis, or a perforated viscus. The testes should be examined to rule out other causes of testicular pain. Rarely, a large distal ureteral calculus may be palpable transvaginally. It is vital that an obstructive calculus does not coexist with urinary infection, since such patients are at significant risk for the development of urosepsis.

The most important initial laboratory examination is the urinalysis. The patient with urolithiasis almost always has hematuria. In rare instances a patient with a completely obstructed renal unit may not have hematuria. The urinalysis may reveal the presence of crystalluria. A pH greater than 7.5 in a fresh urine specimen indicates infection with urea-splitting organisms. Culture of the urine should always be performed. Electrolytes are usually normal; however, prolonged vomiting may lead to metabolic alkalosis. Hyperchloremic metabolic acidosis occurs with renal insufficiency or distal renal tubular acidosis. Serum creatinine levels are usually normal but can be slightly elevated in cases of complete obstruction. Hypercalcemia (>10.2 mg/dL) almost invariably signals the presence of primary hyperparathyroidism. Leukocytosis is common due to demargination of white blood cells caused by the stress of renal colic.

DIFFERENTIAL DIAGNOSIS

The differential diagnosis is protean (Table 33-1).

EMERGENCY DEPARTMENT EVALUATION

Radiologic studies are essential in establishing the diagnosis of urolithiasis. Approximately 90% of urinary calculi are radiopaque and are visible on the kidney-ureter-bladder (KUB) radiograph. Radiolucent stones include uric acid, xanthine, triampterene, and matrix stones. Calcium-contain-

TABLE 33-1. Diseases That Simulate Urolithiasis

Urologic Disease	Nonurologic Disease
Upper Urinary Tract	Intra-abdominal
Renal infarct	Peritonitis (esp. appendicitis)
Renal parenchymal tumors	Biliary colic
Urothelial tumors	Intestinal obstruction
Papillary necrosis	
Pyelonephritis	Vascular
Hemorrhage (blood clot)	Abdominal aortic aneurysm
	Superior mesenteric artery occlusion
Ureter	
Urothelial tumors	Retroperitoneal
Hemorrhage (blood clot)	Retroperitoneal fibrosis
Prior surgery (e.g., stricture)	Tumor
Metastatic tumors	
	Gynecolgic
Lower Urinary Tract	Cervical cancer
Urinary retention	Endometriosis
	Ovarian vein syndrome
	Musculoskeletal

ing calculi must be at least 2 mm in diameter to be visible on plain radiographs. Intravenous pyelography (IVP) is necessary for the diagnosis of urolithiasis. In the absence of a concomitant urinary tract infection IVP may be delayed until the daytime. If an obstructed nephrogram is visualized, it is important to delay the next film in the sequence to avoid unnecessary films. Extravasation occasionally occurs with complete obstruction and subsequent rupture of a calyceal fornix; it is usually self-limited and benign if the duration of obstruction is short and infection is absent. Although IVP remains the gold standard in diagnosis, it should not be considered a routine study. It is important to identify patients with prior contrast reactions and preexisting renal insufficiency before IVP. Good alternatives to excretory urography in patients with renal insufficiency and serum creatinine levels greater than 2 or a history of severe contrast reactions, such as laryngospasm and cardiovascular collapse, include ultrasound and CT scan. Ultrasound detects both lucent and opaque renal stones as well as hydronephrosis. Most ureteral stones cannot be easily identified using ultrasound. CT scanning provides excellent demonstration of urinary calculi, including radiolucent calculi, and gives information about hydronephrosis.

EMERGENCY DEPARTMENT MANAGEMENT

The goals are to make the proper diagnosis and provide relief of the pain. If the pain is typical colic, or if the patient has had similar pain with previous stones, then pain medication should be administered immediately without waiting for the results of IVP. If the pain is atypical and an intra-abdominal process is suspected, pain medication is usually withheld until the correct diagnosis is established. Once significant delay in function is noted on the initial films of an IVP, the patient should be medicated appropriately, as it may take hours to obtain delayed films. Morphine and meperidine (Demerol) are the usual parenteral narcotics used in treating colic, and large and repeat doses of either may be necessary to relieve the initial pain. Anticholinergic, spasmolytic, or anti-inflammatory medications have not been found to be useful. Nausea and vomiting are common with ureteral colic, and can be exacerbated by narcotics. In such patients administration of an antiemetic agent is appropriate, as is vigorous fluid replacement if dehydration has occurred.

DISPOSITION

Proper disposition should be made in conjunction with the consulting urologist who will be responsible for the patient's ultimate care (Table 33-2). The most common factor that necessitates patient admission is pain refractory to oral pain medications. Once the patient has been made comfortable with parenteral narcotics, an oral agent (codeine, oxycodone [Percodan], meperidine, hydromorphone [Dilaudid], or pentazocine [Talwin]) should be given for any recurrence of pain. If pain relief is inadequate, admission will be necessary for pain control. Persistent nausea and vomiting, urinary extravasation, and hypercalcemia that requires treatment are other indications for admission.

Infection in the presence of an obstructing stone is a urologic emergency that necessitates not only admission, but also immediate urologic intervention. This situation represents an abscess, and therapy for this is drainage. The obstruction can be drained either by passage of a ureteral catheter or by placement of a percutaneous nephrostomy tube. Both procedures can be accomplished under local anesthesia. Antibiotics alone are not adequate therapy as the patient can suffer from continued bacteremic showering, progression to frank urosepsis, and rapid destruction of the involved kidney until drainage is achieved. Stabilization of ongoing sepsis and vascular instability should not take precedence over drainage in these patients, as their status usually does not improve until the septic source is removed.

Other factors deserve consideration in determining the disposition. Patients with high-grade obstruction by IVP are more likely to require intervention and admission. Patients with a solitary kidney or underlying intrinsic renal disease are more likely to suffer from a significant decrease in overall renal function with any degree of obstruction; therefore, the threshold for admission of such patients is lower. In addition, the likelihood that the patient will be able to pass the calculus without intervention should be considered. Factors to weigh in this regard include the duration of symptoms and size of the obstructing stone. Ureteral calculi <5 mm usually pass spontaneously, whereas those >8 mm rarely do.

Most patients who present will not meet any of these criteria for emergent admission and may be discharged. These patients should be given sufficient oral narcotic agents and an oral antiemetic agent. Prophylactic antibiotics are not used. The patients should be instructed to strain their urine and save any solid material for analysis. They should be told to return or seek attention for recurrent severe pain, persistent vomiting, or the onset of fever. Outpatient urologic follow-up should be arranged within 2 weeks.

TABLE 33-2. Indications for Admission

Obstruction with infection*
Persistent pain
Persistent nausea and vomiting
Urinary extravasation
Hypercalcemic crisis

Relative Indications for Admission

High-grade obstruction
Solitary kidney
Intrinsic renal disease
Size of obstructing stone
Duration of symptoms
Social situation

---

*Potential urologic emergency.

34   Urinary Retention

Urinary retention must be distinguished from anuria. Anuria represents the cessation of urinary *production* or *delivery* to the bladder, and therefore implies a parenchymal, vascular, or obstructive process involving the kidneys or upper drainage system either bilaterally, or unilaterally in the case of a single functioning kidney. Urinary retention is the inability to void. Not all cases of urinary retention are acute. Acute urinary retention is an uncomfortable state, often with writhing restlessness and exaggerated by manual pressure suprapubically. Chronic retention is seen in the senile or otherwise compromised patient characterized by overflow incontinence, a uriniferous odor, and an apparent indifference to the distention or to applied Credé pressure. In less extreme circumstances discomfort is modest, and the dominant feature is urinary frequency or stress incontinence. Most causes are obstructive. Additional data that contribute to diagnosis include irritable or obstructive voiding dysfunction, neurologic abnormalities, lumbosacral cutaneous eruptions, systemic illness, exposure to pharmacologic agents, recent surgery, and emotional or psychological factors (Table 34-1).

Prompt establishment of bladder drainage is the first priority, after which establishment of cause will dictate subsequent management and specialty consultation. In the absence of trauma, urinary retention in the adult is encountered most often as a consequence of obstruction at the level of the vesical outlet or posterior urethra. Most instances are attributable to benign prostatic hypertrophy or prostatic carcinoma. Other pathologic processes are less common. Benign prostatic hypertrophy is characterized by insidious progressive onset in the late sixth decade of life of hesitancy, nocturia, postvoid dribbling, a sensation of incomplete emptying, and diminution in size and force of the voided stream. Digital rectal examination typically reveals a symmetrical, firm prostatic enlargement of homogeneous consistency.

In contrast, the malignant prostate is characterized by variable degrees of nodular induration. Symptoms of benign prostatic hypertrophy in a younger patient are commonly the result of fibromuscular obstruction at the bladder outlet (median bar). Clinical features may include a history of enuresis, epididymitis, and nocturia. The physical nature of the obstruction may defeat straight catheterization and require coudé or mandrin techniques. A patient in the same age group who abruptly develops isolated symptoms of outlet obstruction must be considered to have prostatic carcinoma. Infectious obstructions most commonly include urethritis and prostatitis, and normal voiding is usually restored after antibiotic therapy during interval catheter drainage. Postinflammatory (gonococcal) urethral stricture persists as a potential cause of urinary obstruction; more commonly, stricture disorders result from traumatic injury or iatrogenic instrumentation. Urinary retention is not characteristic of nongonococcal (chlamydial) urethritis.

Bladder access assumes the dual purposes of achieving relief of obstruction and maintaining urinary drainage until diagnosis and therapy can be instituted. Several of the available methods are preferably limited to physicians with urologic experience and may require formal operative facilities. If doubt exists about the nature of obstruction or the advisability of nonurologic management, and if circumstances permit, intervention should await urologic consultation. Most episodes are amenable to well-lubricated #13 to #16 French urethral catheterization by straight (Robinson) catheter for simple decompression or by balloon (Foley) catheter for retention. Mechanical obstructions include urethral stricture (from prior trauma, instrumentation, or infection), urethral false passage (from prior or concurrent instrumentation), vesical outlet contracture, benign or malignant prostatic or urethral obstruction, and extrinsic compression from local nonurologic processes.

TABLE 34-1. Drugs That Contribute to Urinary Retention

Beta-Adrenergic Stimulation (Detrusor Relaxation)
Isoproterenol (Isuprel)
Progesterone
Atropine

Alpha-Adrenergic Stimulation (Vesical Outlet Contraction)
Ephedrine sulfate
Pseudoephedrine HCl (Sudafed)
Phenylephrine HCl (Neo-Synephrine)
Phenylpropanolamine HCl (Ornade, appetite suppressants)
Imipramine HCl (Tofranil)
Estrogen, estradiol
Levodopa, dopamine, epinephrine
Antihistamines
Bromocriptine (Parlodel)
Mercurial diuretics
Nortriptyline HCl (Aventyl, Nortylin)
Phenothiazines
Testosterone
Amphetamines
Amitriptyline HCl (Elavil, Triavil)
Benztropine mesylate (Cogentin)
Hydralazine (Apresoline)
Isoniazid
Morphine sulfate

Musculotropic Detrusor Relaxation
Propantheline (Pro-Banthine)
Methantheline (Banthine)
Belladonna
Oxybutynin HCl (Ditropan)
Flavoxate HCl (Urispas)
Dicyclomine HCl (Bentyl)
Hyoscyamine (Cystospaz)
Imipramine HCl (Tofranil)
Estrogen
Emepronium bromide
Diazepam (Valium)
Terbutaline
Indomethacin
Nifedipine

Obstruction at the level of the vesical outlet or prostatic urethra may obstruct straight-catheter passage, but may be traversed by angulated (coudé) catheter. An alternative maneuver uses a malleable semirigid mandrin inserted within the catheter and then molded into a suitable configuration for manipulation. The mandrin technique should be restricted to experienced personnel.

Urethral strictures and false passages frequently coexist and may not permit routine catheterization. Isolated false passages (without accompanying stricture) may be bypassed by the mandrin catheter technique. An alternative maneuver particularly suited to urethral stricture disease with or without false passage uses a combination of flexible filiform guides that are maneuvered across obstructions and false passages into the bladder. Progressively larger follower catheters may then be attached for sequential dilatation and drainage. Follower catheters do not include balloon retention, and therefore must be replaced by a Foley catheter or otherwise secured. The mandrin and filiform-follower maneuvers are best restricted to experienced personnel. Failure of these maneuvers warrants urologic consultation for use of endoscopic or operative methods.

An intermediate temporary solution—in the absence of qualified urologic consultation—is the suprapubic percutaneous introduction of a small catheter, secured to the skin and attached to drainage. This maneuver is ideal for providing relief while awaiting urologic consultation. Requirements for percutaneous cystostomy include a palpable bladder and the absence of prior suprapubic surgery. If there is doubt about bladder distention, as in the obese patient, sonographic confirmation is advisable. The procedure requires a simple midline needle puncture one fingerbreadth above the symphysis pubis, with the needle directed slightly caudally and then advanced until urine is returned. The catheter is then advanced, the needle is withdrawn, and the catheter is secured in position.

35 Cutaneous Lesions of the Male Genitalia

Sexually transmitted diseases are prevalent and may cause genital ulceration in males. In general, agents cause either local primary genital lesions or a syndrome of genital ulcerations and regional lymphadenopathy (ulcer-node syndrome). Primary genital lesions are caused by trauma, scabies, pediculosis, or genital warts. The prevalence of primary genital lesions is uncertain, but the following most likely occur in decreasing order of frequency: genital warts, pediculosis, and scabies. The syndrome of genital ulceration(s) and regional lymphadenopathy (ulcer-node syndrome) may be caused by lymphogranuloma venereum (LGV), chancroid, herpes simplex virus (HSV), and syphilis. HSV is the leading cause of genital ulcers with regional lymphadenopathy among males in the United States. In decreasing order of prevalence are syphilis, LGV, and chancroid. Of the six classic venereal diseases (gonorrhea, syphilis, genital herpes, chancroid, LGV, and donovanosis), only gonorrhea is **not** characterized by cutaneous erosion or ulceration; **all** are commonly associated with regional lymphadenopathy.

CLINICAL PRESENTATION AND MANAGEMENT OF PRIMARY GENITAL LESIONS

The causes of genital ulceration, cellulitis, maculopapular eruption, abscess, eschar, and vesicular lesions are legion. Genital warts, pediculosis, and scabies all cause primary genital lesions (Table 35-1). A history of trauma to the genitalia may or may not be present. After exposure to an infected partner there is an incubation period of 2 to 3 months for genital warts, 3 days for pediculosis pubis, and 1 month for scabies. The risk of acquiring these infections is not as well defined as for some of the more venereally transmitted agents. However, the incidence of genital human papilloma virus (HPV) is increasing, and it may currently be the most common viral sexually transmitted disease.

PEDICULOSIS PUBIS

Pediculosis pubis (*Phthirus pubis*) causes lesions that are frequently erythematous and pruritic. The occurrence in a communal living situation is well described. Although the lesions are generally erythematous papules, they may appear hemorrhagic. Intense itching often results in excori-

TABLE 35-1. Characteristics of Primary Genital Lesions

Disorder	Feature
Genital warts	Multiple verrucous papules found on shaft, foreskin, or glans; small, multiple, sessile, "fine-reticulate" in appearance
Phthirus pubis pediculosis	Typical dermatitis Found only in male pubic area and eyebrows
	"Crabs"
	Severely pruritic erythematous papular lesions around hair follicles; excoriations
	Secondary infection not uncommon
	Often outbreak of infection within circle of common sexual contacts
	May be associated with blepharitis if eyebrows involved
Scabies	Intensely pruritic linear burrows on penis, perineum more often than in pubic region

ations that predispose to secondary bacterial infection. Although largely confined to the pubic region, the parasite may migrate to other hairy parts of the body, particularly the eyebrows and eyelids (blepharitis). A hand lens should be used to search for the lesions. Treatment consists of the application of Rid (pyrethins with piperonyl butoxide) for 10 minutes, followed by bathing.

GENITAL WARTS

Genital warts are verrucous-like eruptions caused by HPV. Condyloma acuminatum is a hyperplastic papilloma and the most common manifestation of genital HPV infection. Genital warts from HPV have recently been linked to the development of squamous cell genital (penile and anal) cancer. Patients with genital warts frequently have other sexually transmitted diseases, as do immunocompromised hosts. The lesion, condyloma acuminatum, typically appears as raised or flat wart-like papules, usually multiple. A large wart may show "satelliting," a phenomenon in which the large wart is surrounded by smaller lesions. Lesions of condyloma acuminatum are usually painless and nonpruritic. Although podophyllin is widely used in the treatment of genital warts, many authorities believe that cryotherapy is preferable. Laser therapy may be preferred for extensive or recurrent warts. Atypical or persistent warts should be biopsied.

SCABIES

Scabies are caused by the itch mite, *Sarcoptes scabiei*. The infection produces intense itching and areas of excoriation in a characteristic pattern on the penis, scrotum, axillae, buttocks, elbows, and interdigital web space. The incidence of scabies has increased in the United States since 1974. Conditions of poverty, poor hygiene, overcrowding, malnutrition, and sexual promiscuity are contributory factors. A history of intense nocturnal itching associated with penile and scrotal pruritic vesicles, pustules, or papules is the typical clinical presentation. Scabies are often seen as intensely pruritic, linear burrows that involve the penis and scrotum more commonly than the pubic region. The mite burrows into the skin and lays eggs in tunnels that, over a 1- to 4-month period, cause a characteristic pruritic skin eruption through sensitization. Reinfection is possible, and if left untreated, scabies may persist for decades. A nodular variant of scabies occurs in a small percentage of patients with pruritic, reddish brown nodules on the scrotum,

TABLE 35-2. Characteristics of Ulcer-Node Syndrome Pathogens

Disorder	Ulcer	Nodes
Genital herpes 2	Painful, small, discrete vesicles; confluence to ulcerations; recurrent	Bilateral, painful, nonfluctant
Syphilis	Papule first; painless, large "jagged" ulcer with raised base	Bilateral (70%); less painful
Lymphogranuloma venereum	Painless, transient ulcer	Unilateral, moderately painful, prominent suppurative nodes; inguinal sinus tract often initial finding
Chancroid	Prominent "flat" painful ulcer (like syphilis but more painful); most chancroid is herpes simplex virus	Unilateral, painful, suppurative; bubo and rupture common

penis, and axillae. Usually there is no prominent lymphadenopathy. Treatment consists of the application of topical 1% gamma benzene hexachloride treatment (lindane [Kwell]) to the pubic region for 8 hours, followed by a thorough cleansing.

CLINICAL PRESENTATION AND MANAGEMENT OF THE ULCER-NODE SYNDROME

The ulcer-node syndrome may be caused by genital herpes, LGV, chancroid, or syphilis. Any genital ulcer may be accompanied by regional lymphadenopathy. The primary lesion of most genital ulcers is a papule, vesicle, or excoriation. Unfortunately genital herpes, syphilis, LGV, and chancroid may appear identical. Adenopathy is similarly of minimal diagnostic help.

Table 35-2 provides a summary of the most common features.

GENITAL HERPES (HERPES VIRUS HOMINIS TYPE 2)

Genital herpes is by far the most common cause of genital ulcers. Eighty percent to 95% of cases occur in adolescents and young adults. Systemic symptoms (e.g., fever, myalgias, and headache) usually coincide with the onset of the genital lesions. In men painful vesicular lesions on an erythematous base usually appear on the glans penis or the penile shaft. It is important to distinguish between genital herpes that has ulcer-like features late in the course and syphilis. Both may be present or other causes of genital ulcer with regional lymphadenopathy may also be present. Dysuria and urinary retention may result from urethral involvement with genital herpes. Herpetic sacral radiculomyelitis may also develop from genital infection, with urinary retention, neuralgias, and obstipation. Diagnostic tests for HSV infection have become more rapid and specific. Laboratory confirmation is important in the setting of atypical ulcerations or doubt about the diagnosis. For the immunocompetent host acyclovir (Zovirax) may be given orally (200 mg five times a day for 10 days) for primary infection. Complicated cases that involve the central nervous system, dissemination, or a compromised host may require hospitalization.

LYMPHOGRANULOMA VENEREUM

LGV, a systemic infection that affects the genital lymphatic tissue, is caused by *Chlamydia trachomatis*. The genital ulcer is seen in only 5% to 25% of patients. More often the initial lesion is a painless papule or vesicle. The second stage follows in 3 to 4 weeks and is characterized by bubo formation (inflammatory swelling of a lymph node). Systemic symptoms and progressive enlargement of unilateral inguinal lymph nodes are distinctive. The buboes undergo fluctuant changes with acute spontaneous drainage. A draining sinus tract is often the initial finding. A distinctive feature is the suppuration and drainage of the inguinal sinus tract. Among homosexual males the initial presentation may be that of acute proctitis or proctocolitis. Homosexual men should be evaluated for other causes of proctitis (gonorrhea, genital herpes, syphilis, Crohn's disease, and ulcerative colitis) and proctocolitis (*Campylobacter* species, *Shigella,* and *Entamoeba histolytica*). Buboes may be strikingly fluctuant, and aspiration with an 18-gauge needle should be considered. Incision and drainage should be avoided. The diagnosis of LGV requires special LGV complement fixation test. Treatment of LGV includes azithromycin (1 g PO), tetracycline (500 mg four times a day for 21 days), erythromycin (500 mg four times a day for 21 days), or doxycycline (100 mg twice a day for 21 days).

CHANCROID

Haemophilus ducreyi is the causative agent in chancroid. It appears to be increasing in incidence in the United States. The typical picture is prominent, painful genital ulceration with regional bubo formation. Aspiration of painful nodes may be necessary, but incision and drainage should be avoided. Chancroidal ulcers may be difficult to distinguish from syphilis, but they tend to be deeper and more painful with ragged margins and tender unilateral adenopathy. Indeed, chancroid and syphilis may coexist. Genital herpes may also mimic chancroid; most "apparent" chancroid is due to HSV. The primary isolation of *H. ducreyi* is difficult and requires selective media. Erythromycin (500 mg four times a day for 7 days) and ceftriaxone (250 mg IM single dose) are the drugs of choice for the treatment of chancroid. Ciprofloxacin has demonstrated some therapeutic promise. Serologic tests should be done to exclude syphilis. If both chancroid and syphilis are suspect, empiric treatment with erythromycin plus penicillin G benzathine (2.4 million units I.M.) may be indicated. Although erythromycin is effective for chancroid and most cases of syphilis, 10% of cases of early syphilis will persist with erythromycin, thus masking early syphilis.

SYPHILIS

Caused by *Treponema pallidum,* syphilis is the most important disease that presents as a genital ulcer. Urban syphilis is five times higher than overall rates. The diagnosis should be considered in the patient with multiple sexually transmitted diseases or a history of homosexual contacts. Characteristically, the ulcer (chancre) is painless, indurated, and nonexudative with a smooth base and raised, firm borders. Inguinal lymphadenopathy consists of moderately enlarged bilateral (70%) or unilateral painless lymph nodes. The rash of secondary syphilis may appear before the chancre is healed (6–8 weeks). Syphilis is common among homosexual patients; one should search for anal and oral lesions, since only 20% of primary syphilitic lesions among homosexual patients may be visible. Every patient with genital ulceration should be tested for syphilis with an RPR (rapid plasma reagin). Up to 30% of patients with primary syphilis have a negative RPR or VDRL so these studies should only be confirmatory. Treatment with penicillin G benzathine (2.4 million units I.M.) is indicated with a follow-up VDRL to document cure at 3, 6, 8, and 12 months. The titer should decrease fourfold at 3 months and eightfold at 6 months. Alternative drugs in the presence of a well-documented penicillin allergy include erythromycin (500 mg four times a day for 15 days) and tetracycline (500 mg four times a day for 15 days).

DISPOSITION

Distinguishing primary genital lesions (genital warts, scabies, and pediculosis pubis) from genital ulcers has important therapeutic implications. Most often the emergency physician will not have definitive bacteriologic or virologic tests available. All patients with ulcers or inguinofemoral lymphadenopathy should have serologic testing for syphilis.

Indications for admission include fever, systemic signs and symptoms, disseminated infection, and the need to surgically drain or incise a bubo.

COMMON PITFALLS

- Failure to search for other STD's in patients with one STD
- Failure to distinguish LGV or chancroid from syphilis and genital herpes
- Failure to distinguish between syphilis and genital herpes
- Failure to admit patients with complications (dissemination, node excision, and central nervous system involvement)
- Failure to obtain infectious disease consultation for complicated or toxic-appearing patients
- Obscuration of syphilis with partial treatment
- Inguinal buboes that are large, extremely painful or unresponsive to antibiotics require aspiration, not I & D. Admission may be necessary.
- Failure to treat sexual contacts

---

36   The Acute Scrotal Mass

The three main diagnostic categories of the acute scrotal mass are torsion of the spermatic cord, torsion of an appendage testis, and acute epididymitis. (Less common entities include orchitis, acute hydrocele, spermatocele, varicocele, and hernia.) Vascular occlusion makes sudden scrotal pain a true surgical emergency. A careful history and physical examination narrow the possibilities. The acute scrotum should be examined. Both testes are compared for size and consistency. All masses should be transilluminated with a flashlight. The epididymis is a soft, comma-shaped structure posterior to the testis. The 1×3-mm testicular and epididymal appendages are not readily palpable, but are most common near the upper pole. The vas deferens feels like a thick rubber band within the 1-cm diameter cord.

TESTICULAR TORSION

Torsion of the testis has an incidence of 1 per 4000 males. It can occur at any age but is most common during puberty and the second decade of life; the average age of affected patients is 17.5 years. Testes predisposed to torsion have an abnormally high attachment of a voluminous tunica vaginalis. This is referred to as the "bell clapper" deformity. Initially, the testis and cord twist within the tunica vaginalis, causing occlusion of the venous system; arterial flow is decreased by the compression of twisting and edema. Damage relates to the duration and extent of vascular obstruction. Partial arterial flow may persist with less than 540 to 720 degrees of rotation. The degree of torsion varies, and an absolute time limit for testicular viability after the onset of pain is hard to establish. Testicular salvage has been correlated with the time of onset to detorsion. Continuous pain for 24 hours is usually associated with an infarcted testis. A salvage rate of 100% with surgical detorsion in <6 hours is a standard gauge. Contralateral testicular damage due to ipsilateral torsion is a subject of current investigation but probably is not a significant factor contributing to male infertility.

CLINICAL PRESENTATION

Testicular pain and swelling of sudden onset is the classic history. However, the history can be nonspecific. Pain is always present and can be acute or insidious and mild to excruciating. A history of milder incidents can be elicited in 47% of patients. About half report the onset during sleep. Cold weather, sexual arousal, and trauma are described as inciting factors. Nausea and vomiting are common. Voiding symptoms such as dysuria, urgency, and hesitancy are only occasionally described. Often the pain is abdominal. Scrotal pain with radiation to the abdomen or inguinal region occurs in 50%.

On physical examination a painful testis is found, elevated cephalad in the scrotum by the twisted and shortened cord. Instead of its usual vertical orientation, the testis often lies horizontally in the scrotum. The epididymis may be malrotated anteriorly. The cord is thickened in the area of torsion. Frequently the classic findings are not present, and the entire hemiscrotum is swollen, tender, and firm. A reactive hydrocele may have formed. Scrotal tissues rapidly develop redness and edema, and within a few hours the testis and epididymis may no longer be differentiated. In one series, 42% of patients presented with swelling sufficient to obscure palpation of the intrascrotal contents. Eventually the hemiscrotum becomes an amorphous painful mass referred to as "missed torsion." A useful clinical finding is the ipsilateral loss of the cremasteric reflex with torsion. The reflex is preserved in most cases of epididymitis (100% correlation between the presence of the ipsilateral cremasteric reflex and the absence of testicular torsion). The reflex, mediated by T-12 to L-2, is a contraction of the cremasteric reflex manifested by elevation of the testis. It is initiated by stroking the skin of the inner aspect of the ipsilateral thigh in an upward motion. The reflex sign is unreliable in severe epididymitis with substantial swelling. One third of patients have a leukocytosis of more than 10,000 white blood cells per millileter, and almost all have a normal urinalysis.

DIFFERENTIAL DIAGNOSIS

The differential diagnosis includes acute epididymitis, orchitis, torsion of the appendices of the testis and epididymis, tumor, hernia, and traumatic hydrocele or hematocele. Acute epididymitis, the most common misdiagnosis of testicular torsion, is rare before puberty. Epididymitis has a more gradual onset. A history of painful voiding, a urethral discharge, or an indwelling urethral catheter favors the diagnosis of epididymitis as does urinary infection. A history of similar episodes of testicular pain is suggestive of a diagnosis of torsion. Nausea with vomiting is more commonly found in torsion. Pathognomonic physical findings are found in only 8% of patients with torsion. Torsion is remarkable for global testicular pain. Scrotal erythema and tenderness of the testis occur in torsion three times more often than in epididymitis. In contrast, posterior testicular discomfort or perhaps only a tender epididymis is seen primarily in epididymitis, especially if seen early. In epididymitis a normal cord can be palpated above the testis; in torsion, an edematous cord or mass is often found. After swelling occurs the physical findings may be obscure. Fever is equally common to torsion and epididymitis, but the patient's temperature is higher in the latter case and leukocytosis is greater in epididymitis. A third to half of patients with epididymitis have pyuria.

Orchitis seldom occurs without concurrent spread from the epididymis. In primary orchitis, a history of mumps orchitis and manifestations of a systemic illness should be present. The onset of testicular pain and swelling is more gradual. The epididymis should be identified posterior, and the orientation of the testis should remain vertical. The cord is tender but without induration or thickening.

Torsion of a testicular or epididymal appendage on its narrow pedicle can cause venous engorgement with subsequent arterial occlusion and infarction. Torsion of an appendage is seen in the same age group as torsion of the spermatic cord. Sudden scrotal pain without radiation is the most common presentation. The onset of pain is not as rapid as in testicular torsion and may occur as intermittent with progressive worsening over 3 to 5 days. The symptoms are usually less severe than in testicular torsion. Nausea and vomiting are more commonly found in torsion of the cord. Occasionally, early on, the appendage may be palpated as a tender mass at the head of the testis. The "blue dot" sign is a small, tender, blue pea-like structure seen through the skin. Most often localized tenderness in the head of the testis without a palpable mass or erythema of the scrotal skin is found in appendiceal torsion. Excision of the torsed appendage is the standard treatment, although observation has been successful, since autoinfarction is the only consequence.

Carcinoma of the testis is the most common cancer in boys and men between the ages of 15 and 34 years, a similar age period for torsion. The initial diagnosis of a scrotal mass that proves to be cancer is wrong 25% of the time, and the most common misdiagnosis is epididymitis. About 10% of patients with testicular tumors present with a history of rapid swelling. Symptoms from tumors normally have a more gradual onset. Pain is not a major complaint, although hemorrhage can cause the sudden onset of pain. The testis may be generally enlarged, but more often a distinct intratesticular mass is palpated. The scrotum has less erythema and edema than in torsion, but in a delayed presentation it can appear similar to missed torsion. Ten percent of testicular tumors have a reactive hydrocele.

An incarcerated scrotal hernia may present with a history similar to that of torsion and accounts for approximately 2% of acute scrotal masses. Abdominal and groin pain are usually present. The scrotal hernia can be palpated into the groin, and the testis is displaced lower in the scrotum.

A traumatic hydrocele and hematocele should be considered, since a trauma history accompanies 5% to 10% of cases of torsion. The testis is usually not as painful as in torsion, and the epididymis and cord can be palpated in their normal positions. With significant swelling, ancillary tests or exploration is necessary to rule out torsion.

EMERGENCY DEPARTMENT EVALUATION

Rapid consideration of testicular torsion should be made based on the history and physical findings. The presentation is variable, and the scrotum develops erythema from many causes; consider torsion in the patient 12 to 30 years old. Ancillary studies (urinalysis and testicular scan) make the differentiation of torsion from other causes of the acute scrotum more accurate. Radionuclide scanning has an 89%–100% accuracy in determining testicular blood flow and is **the ancillary test of choice** in the diagnosis of torsion. Ultrasonography is the **ancillary test of choice** to evaluate a testicular mass or possible epididymal abscess. Ultrasonic Doppler detection of testicular arterial pulsation (the ultrasonic probe against the lower pole of the testis wall) has also been advocated. In practice, Doppler results have merely substantiated the original clinical impression and have not influenced the surgical decision-making process. Although nuclear scanning and ultrasonic Doppler are helpful, an aggregate clinical impression is more important. Ancillary tests should never change an otherwise positive impression of torsion or delay operative exploration. They may be obtained only during an anticipated and reasonable wait for an operative suite. It is not unreasonable to make the diagnosis at surgical exploration if torsion remains in the differential.

EMERGENCY DEPARTMENT MANAGEMENT

After the history and physical examination, a urinalysis should be obtained and a urologist notified. Manual detorsion should then be attempted, and is successful in 30% to 70% of patients. Spontaneous or manipulative preoperative detorsion results in a 100% testicular salvage rate. The maneuver is initially attempted from within outward, since most cases of testicular torsion occur from without inward. It can be attempted with the patient standing or supine. The testis is rotated 180 degrees in one direction and maintained in position. Rotation is continued as necessary. If the twisting increases the pain, the detorsion should be attempted in the opposite direction. One to three turns is usually sufficient. The rotation is stopped when the anatomy is restored and the pain relieved, both occurring promptly. If significant swelling is present, the maneuver is more difficult and there is much less chance of detorsion. Intravenous analgesics and spermatic cord block facilitate the detorsion maneuver. Although spermatic cord block eliminates pain relief as a criterion in judging the success of detorsion manuevers, the cord blockade does allow multiple detorsion attempts and experimentation with direction. Manual detorsion is followed by exploration to confirm success, as relief of pain with persistent ischemia has been reported. However, no patient has had recurrence of torsion in the interval between manual detorsion and orchiopexy.

DISPOSITION

ROLE OF THE CONSULTANT   The urologist is obligated to make the final diagnosis and perform immediate detorsion. Ancillary tests are coordinated so as not to delay surgery. An infarcted testis must be removed to prevent persistent pain and allow resolution of the inflammatory process. Contralateral testicular damage from antibody formation remains a source of controversy. Bilateral orchiopexy is required, since the predisposing anatomical defect is present bilaterally.

INDICATIONS FOR ADMISSION   All patients suspected of having torsion should be admitted by way of the operating suite. Observation or serial examinations are seldom useful. Patients should have preoperative laboratory studies and consent to expedite surgery. If manual detorsion is successful, arrangements for delayed orchiopexy can be made between the consultant and the patient. Medicolegal considerations make it imperative that the urologic consultant assume ultimate responsibility for any planned delay in scrotal exploration and orchiopexy.

COMMON PITFALLS

- Misdiagnosis and delays in detorsion are the most common pitfalls.
- The history and physical examination can be misleading: erythema and swelling tend to confuse the diagnosis with epididymitis.
- Ancillary tests may result in unnecessary delay. Waiting for a consultant or an operating suite is also a source of delay.
- Manual detorsion by the emergency physician is the most rapid means of salvaging a torsed testis.
- The missed diagnosis of torsion can be a source of malpractice litigation. The time between the patient's presentation and the time of surgery is most often scrutinized to assess the salvage potential.

ACUTE EPIDIDYMITIS

Inflammation or infection limited to the epididymis that causes acute pain and swelling of rapid onset is termed acute epididymitis. Epididymo-orchitis implies extension of the inflammation or infection into the testis. Epididymitis is the most common cause of the acute scrotal mass. It is primarily a disease of adults and seldom occurs before puberty; it most often results from infection caused by retrograde spread of organisms up the vas deferens. In men <age 35, the organisms most often responsible are those that cause urethritis, (Chlamydia trachomatis and Neisseria gonorrhoeae). In men > age 35, bacteriuria caused by obstructive urinary disease is more common, involving (Escherichia coli, enterococci, Pseudomonas, and Proteus). In the prepubertal patient coliform bacteria predominate.

CLINICAL PRESENTATION

The onset of scrotal pain and swelling gradually peaks over a period of 3 to 24 hours. Pain can be sharp and often radiates to the groin. Often the only complaint is a dull, aching scrotal discomfort. However, the pain may be of sudden onset (51%) or gradual (49%). Irritative voiding symptoms, such as frequency, dysuria, and urgency, occur in 10% to 20% of patients. A history of fever is common, and on occasion a patient presents in sepsis. A recent diagnostic cystoscopy, an indwelling urethral catheter, or a history of urinary tract infections or genitourinary surgery may be present, especially in older men. Nausea is unusual. Often the entire epididymis is involved, and the distinction between the testis and the epididymis is less evident due to edema and a reactive hydrocele. The involved testis hangs low in an erythematous and edematous scrotum. A urethral discharge is present in 10% of patients. Nearly a third of patients have an admission temperature higher than 101°F. Progression of the infection leads to epididymal abscess formation. Scrotal wall fixation to the underlying testis and epididymis is a hallmark of impending epididymal suppuration. More commonly an erythematous edematous scrotum overlies an amorphous tender mass.

DIFFERENTIAL DIAGNOSIS

See the differential diagnosis of testicular torsion.

EMERGENCY DEPARTMENT EVALUATION

A urinalysis and urine culture should be obtained. A urinalysis shows pyuria or bacteriuria in 50%; a smaller number have a urethral discharge. The white blood cell count is commonly, but not always, elevated. A nuclear isotope scan determines testicular blood flow. Ultrasonic imaging is accurate in evaluating the epididymis for abscess formation and testicular parenchyma for tumors. If sepsis is suspected, blood cultures are obtained and intravenous fluids and broad-spectrum antibiotic therapy are started.

EMERGENCY DEPARTMENT MANAGEMENT

See Table 36-1.

Antibiotics, analgesics, bed rest, warm tub soaks, and scrotal elevation are key in the management. Antibiotics should be prescribed in all cases; cultures of the urine and urethral discharge are frequently negative despite an infectious cause. Men >35 suspected of having epididymitis associated with a UTI caused by enteric gram-negative bacilli or *Pseudomonas* should be treated on the basis of the results of a urine culture. Empiric treatment for gram-negative rods and gram-positive cocci should be initiated with a sulfonamide or fluoroquinolones. An anti-inflammatory agent (ibuprofen or indomethacin) should be prescribed. Urology follow-up is arranged within several days.

TABLE 36-1. Treatment of Epididymitis

All Cases

Gram's stain of urethral swab or urine sediment
Culture for gonorrhea, and immunofluorescence for *Chlamydia*
Look for concurrent sexually transmitted diseases.

Ceftriaxone, 250 mg IM followed by
Azithromycin, 1 g PO once

Presumed E. coli or Pseudomonas species

Trimethoprim-sulfamethoxazole, twice a day for 14 days or
Ciprofloxacin, 500 mg PO bid for 10 days
Urine culture and Gram's stain; immunofluorescence for *Chlamydia*
Look for predisposing genitourinary pathology

Optional Therapy (All Cases)

Scrotal support or athletic supporter
Nonsteroidal anti-inflammatory drugs

DISPOSITION

ROLE OF THE CONSULTANT   Outpatient management of epididymitis is appropriate in most cases. Urologic consultation should be obtained within a few days. Immediate consultation should be obtained if torsion is considered. Consultation is required for severe cases that require hospitalization or if an abscess is suspected. All pediatric cases require immediate consultation.

INDICATIONS FOR ADMISSION   Adult patients with severe constitutional symptoms, including intractable pain, nausea and vomiting, require hospitalization and parenteral antibiotics. Patients who present with signs of early sepsis (fever, chills, severe malaise) should be admitted. Patients for whom the physical examination and ultrasonography are equivocal for the finding of abscess should be admitted.

COMMON PITFALLS

- The assessment of a patient with delayed presentation of the acute scrotal mass may cause confusion between epididymitis and torsion.
- Torsion and testicular tumors must always be considered.
- The most common misdiagnosis of a testicular tumor is epididymitis.
- Because bladder outlet obstruction may be the underlying cause of epididymitis, all patients should be examined for urinary retention, especially older men.

OTHER DISORDERS PRESENTING AS A SCROTAL MASS

Infectious disorders of the scrotum and urethra can present as an acute scrotal mass. Primary abscesses of the scrotal wall occur from infections of the hair follicles or sweat glands. These are common, and similar to abscesses anywhere else on the body. This type of abscess is limited to the superficial layers of the scrotal skin. Deep scrotal infection usually arises from infection of the lower urinary tract or perirectal disease. Commonly they originate from extravasation of infected urine as a result of urethral instrumentation or from lower tract infection that has spread to the periurethral glands. Infection also originates from perirectal and ischiorectal abscesses. Often the source is not clear. These abscesses are rooted deep in the perineum and may spread extensively by the time they cause obvious cutaneous lesions. Fournier's gangrene, or idiopathic synergistic necrotizing fasciitis, is a rapidly spreading infection that presents as massive scrotal swelling with progression to necrosis of the scrotal wall within 24 hours. The average age of affected patients is 55, and diabetics have a higher incidence. Steroid use, chronic ethanol abuse, and a history of prior skin infections are all contributing factors. The typical organisms include hemolytic streptococci, staphylococci, *Bacteroides fragilis, E. coli,* and *Clostridia* species.

CLINICAL PRESENTATION

Superficial scrotal abscesses seldom cause difficulty in diagnosis. A localized area of erythema with a smaller area of suppuration is found. The patient is afebrile, without constitutional symptoms, and the urinalysis and white blood cell count should be normal. Superficial abscesses may be incised and drained in the ED.

   Deep scrotal abscesses and early Fournier's gangrene can present as generalized scrotal swelling. The onset usually follows several days after instrumentation of an infected urethra. An indwelling urethral catheter may be present, or the patient may have a history of perirectal disease. Pain is usually intense. Fever and other constitutional symptoms are often present. A diabetic may present in ketoacidosis. The scrotal contents cannot be palpated because the entire scrotum is edematous, red, tense, and warm. Frequently no localized area of fluctuation is detected.

DIFFERENTIAL DIAGNOSIS

Scrotal edema from congestive heart failure or lymphatic obstruction can occasionally appear similar. Concomitant anasarca or edema of the lower extremities shifts the differential away from an infectious cause. Occasionally edema of the scrotum occurs as a result of an allergic reaction. The scrotum should not be tender to palpation and the erythema is considerably less. Constitutional symptoms, including fever, are absent. Cellulitis of the scrotum may present with significant edema. This is rare without an underlying abscess. Less tenderness should be found in an otherwise healthy patient, but the distinction from a deep abscess may be difficult. Epididymo-orchitis that has progressed to suppuration and skin fixation can cause a scrotal swelling similar to that seen with a deep scrotal abscess. Often indistinguishable on examination, both require surgical drainage.

EMERGENCY DEPARTMENT EVALUATION

Rapid diagnosis and treatment of sepsis and shock are the principles of initial management. If the diagnosis remains in question, ultrasonography detects abscess cavities within fascial planes and is helpful in differentiating cellulitis from a deep abscess. A plain pelvic radiograph occasionally demonstrates subcutaneous air. A urethral catheter should be placed in the bladder. If obstruction is encountered, an immediate urethrogram should be obtained. The rectum should be carefully examined for perirectal disease.

EMERGENCY DEPARTMENT MANAGEMENT

A deep scrotal abscess and Fournier's gangrene require aggressive therapy. Urine and blood cultures are indicated and intravenous fluids with broad-spectrum antibiotics started. Urologic consultation is requested. If perirectal disease is the suspected cause, a general surgeon should also be consulted.

DISPOSITION

ROLE OF THE CONSULTANT   Surgical drainage with wide debridement and antibiotic therapy must be accomplished rapidly, as the mortality of severe infection approaches 50%.

INDICATIONS FOR ADMISSION   Patients with severe scrotal abscesses should be admitted through the operating room. Cellulitis of the scrotum is often difficult to distinguish from a skin reaction secondary to a deeper infection. Cellulitis requires intravenous antibiotics and serial examination.

COMMON PITFALLS

- The most common mistake is underestimating the severity of an infection. With scrotal gangrene, a delay of 4 to 8 hours can make a great difference in morbidity.
- In the early stages, most of the serious infections can look like cellulitis, and the clinician may be tempted to treat the problem on an outpatient basis with oral antibiotics.

PART VIII

Emergency Aspects of Obstetrics

37   Pregnancy Testing

The diagnosis of pregnancy is established by detecting the presence of human chorionic gonadotropin (hCG). The beta subunit is specific to hCG, and therefore represents a highly specific indicator of pregnancy. After implantation of the ovum in the endometrium trophoblastic cells initiate placental development with rapidly rising levels of hCG. The major biologic effect of hCG is maintenance of the corpus luteum. Serum hCG levels double every 1.4 to 2.1 days, until they peak at 60 days. Thereafter, hCG levels plateau and remain detectable until approximately 2 weeks after delivery or termination of the pregnancy. hCG can be detected as early as 6 to 9 days after implantation. Levels of 50 IU/mL may be reported as early as 1 week after implantation, although much individual variation exists. This represents the lowest level of hCG to which most urine pregnancy tests are sensitive. One day after a missed menses the levels are generally in excess of 100 IU/mL. Thirty percent of circulating hCG is cleared by the kidneys. Urine hCG levels closely parallel serum values.

Only two types of pregnancy test should be considered: the beta-specific hCG radioimmunoassays (RIAs) for serum and the beta-specific enzyme-linked immunosorbent assay (ELISA).

False-positive results are seen in both urine and serum pregnancy tests. Pregnancy tests detect hCG and do not *per se* test specifically for pregnancy. Trophoblastic cells are not the only cells that are capable of secreting hCG. hCG has been secreted by a variety of tumors, including gastrointestinal neoplasms, lymphoma, leukemia, myeloma, sarcoma, breast carcinoma, bronchogenic carcinoma, adrenocortical carcinoma, renal cell carcinoma, and melanoma. More important, normal tissues such as ovary, pituitary gland, lung, liver, kidney, spleen, and stomach contain biologically inactive hCG. As lower levels of hCG are detected by both urine and serum tests, more false positives are expected. Drugs such as phenothiazines and methadone can produce false-positive pregnancy tests. Several mechanisms have been proposed, although none has been proved. The newer beta-selective tests have reduced false-positive results. Proteinuria produces false-positive results when older urine pregnancy tests are used. False-negative urine pregnancy tests have also been noted in patients with ectopic pregnancy when hCG levels are generally less than expected for dates.

The measurement of serum progesterone levels using a direct RIA kit has shown promise in discriminating normal and abnormal gestations. Because there is a clear distinction between normal and abnormal values, the diagnosis of abnormal gestation can be made in a single visit. Serum levels below 15 ng/mL are indicative of abnormal gestations.

Transabdominal ultrasonography can be used to determine the presence of an intrauterine pregnancy. A gestational sac should be detectable at approximately 6 weeks when the serum hCG level is above 6500 IU/mL. Other imaging techniques include vaginal ultrasonography and magnetic resonance imaging.

38   Drugs in Pregnancy

TERATOGENIC EFFECTS ON THE EMBRYO AND FETUS

During the first 2 weeks after conception but before implantation (to menstrual age 4 weeks) the embryo is relatively insensitive to teratogenic effects. The most sensitive time of development is during the next 8 weeks (to menstrual age 12 weeks). During this period organogenesis occurs and histogenesis begins. Teratogenic drugs acting at this time may produce characteristic multiple malformations or syndromes. Throughout the remainder of pregnancy there is continued histogenesis and functional maturation of the fetus. Drug effects during this period can cause generalized growth retardation usually secondary to decreased uterine blood flow. Toward the end of pregnancy and during delivery direct pharmacologic effects on the fetus and neonate can occur and may complicate postnatal care of the newborn.

FDA DRUG CLASSIFICATION SCHEME

All drugs ingested by pregnant women represent a potential hazard to the fetus. The U.S. Food and Drug Administration (FDA) has established five categories indicating a drug's potential for causing birth defects:

CLASS A   Controlled human studies have failed to demonstrate a risk to the fetus during pregnancy; the possibility of fetal harm seems remote.

CLASS B   Either (a) animal reproduction studies have not demonstrated a fetal risk, but there are no controlled human studies; or (b) animal studies have shown an adverse effect on the fetus that was not confirmed in controlled human studies.

CLASS C   Either (a) animal studies have shown an adverse effect on the fetus, but there are no controlled human studies; or (b) there are no studies in humans or animals. Drugs should be given only if the potential benefit justifies the potential risk to the fetus.

CLASS D   There is positive evidence of human fetal risk, but the benefits may outweigh the risks in certain situations.

CLASS X   Studies or experience has shown fetal risk that clearly outweighs any possible benefit. The drug is contraindicated in women who are or may become pregnant.
In an attempt to reduce the risk of fetal harm to an absolute minimum the following principles should be followed:

1. No drug should be prescribed for a pregnant woman without a clear and special need for it. A distinction needs to be made between medications that are essential and those that will merely alleviate symptoms.
2. The exposure should be decreased by giving the minimum effective dose for the shortest time possible.
3. Well-known preparations should be chosen over newer drugs about which less is known.
4. The physician should be aware of the multiple components of many formulations.

ANALGESICS

Acetaminophen is the analgesic and antipyretic of choice during all phases of pregnancy. Although it readily crosses the placenta, acetaminophen is not associated with any adverse effects on the fetus when it is used in standard therapeutic doses. Aspirin is the most frequently used drug during pregnancy. It readily crosses the placenta. Because of its inhibition of prostaglandin synthesis, aspirin causes an increased average length of gestation, an increased rate of postmature deliveries, and an increased mean duration of spontaneous labor. Chronic or intermittent high-dose therapy may lead to premature closure of the ductus arteriosis and still-birth. The use of aspirin during pregnancy should be avoided whenever possible.

Only a few of the other nonsteroidal anti-inflammatory agents (fenoprofen, ibuprofen, indomethacin, naproxen, and phenylbutazone) have been used in pregnant women, mainly as tocolytics. Any drug in this class has the potential to inhibit labor and prolong the duration of pregnancy due to the inhibition of prostaglandin synthetase. Premature closure of the ductus arteriosis may occur when these agents are administered after the 34th or 35th week of pregnancy. The use of these agents during pregnancy should be avoided if possible. The cautious use of either morphine or meperidine appears to be safe during pregnancy and has not been associated with teratogenic effects. The use of codeine also seems to be safe, and no evidence has been found to suggest a relation to large groups of birth defects. A possible association with respiratory malformations and other defects has been noted, although the significance of this association is unknown.

The use of other oral opiates, such as hydrocodone, hydromorphone, oxycodone, and oxymorphine, is not widespread, and there are no data regarding their safety in pregnancy. Neonatal respiratory depression can occur with the administration of any narcotic analgesic to the mother and may be safely reversed in the infant with naloxone. The short-term intermittent use of a 50:50 mixture of nitrous oxide and oxygen for pain relief appears to be safe during pregnancy. Chronic occupational exposure in pregnant health care workers, however, may pose a risk to the fetus.

ANTIASTHMATICS

The usual first-line drugs for the treatment of an acute attack of asthma are the adrenergic agents, mainly epinephrine, terbutaline, metaproterenol, and albuterol. Except for epinephrine, these are not known to have any teratogenic effects. Epinephrine is only relatively contraindicated and may be used when other drugs are failing. Theophylline compounds have not been shown to have any adverse fetal effects. Oral corticosteroids are not known to be teratogenic; prednisone and prednisolone cross poorly into the fetal circulation. They may be used in the pregnant asthmatic, although lower doses of aerosolized steroids are preferred.

ANTIMICROBIALS

The penicillins, including the semisynthetic derivatives, are considered safe for use during pregnancy. They cross the placenta readily, allowing simultaneous treatment of infections in both the mother and fetus. The use of erythromycin base is a safe and effective alternative for the penicillin-allergic pregnant woman. However, the *estolate* form of erythromycin is associated with an increased incidence of cholestatic hepatitis in the mother and should *not* be used. Cephalosporins have not been reported to cause birth defects or adverse fetal reactions. The sulfonamides should be avoided in the third trimester, since they compete with bilirubin for albumin binding sites and increase the risk of kernicterus. Because of theoretical concerns regarding their antifolate activity and its effect on fetal development in the first trimester, it is prudent to avoid their use, if possible. The tetracyclines are not recommended during pregnancy because of effects on both the fetus and the mother. The chelating properties of tetracycline lead to discoloration of the teeth and depressed bone growth in the fetus, while the mother has an increased risk of hepatotoxicity. Metronidazole (Flagyl): human studies have led to conflicting conclusions regarding its safety in pregnancy. Metronidazole should be used only if other therapies have failed, and then only in the latter half of pregnancy.

CARDIOVASCULAR DRUGS

Digitalis preparations may be used to treat a variety of supraventricular arrhythmias and congestive heart failure during pregnancy. Although it crosses the placenta by passive transfer, it has no teratogenic effects. The dosage used is identical in pregnant and nonpregnant patients. Most of the standard antiarrhythmic agents—atropine, isoproterenol, lidocaine, procainamide, and quinidine—have not been demonstrated to be teratogenic and are safe for use during pregnancy. Phenytoin is associated with congenital anomalies, notably the fetal hydantoin syndrome, and its use should be avoided during pregnancy. Data on other agents such as amiodarone, bretylium, disopyramide, mexiletine, tocainide, timolol, and verapamil are scarce, and their safety during pregnancy has not been established. Of the antihypertensive agents, hydralazine, labetalol, methyldopa, and the thiazide diuretics are not teratogenic and may be safely used during pregnancy. Hydralazine increases uteroplacental blood flow in animals and is considered the drug of choice for the treatment of hypertensive emergencies during pregnancy. The beta-adrenergic blocking agents are used safely during pregnancy and have not been shown to be teratogenic. The exception is propranolol, which may be associated with premature labor, fetal growth retardation, and neonatal hypoglycemia, bradycardia, and respiratory depression. Nitroprusside is not known to be teratogenic and has been used successfully in pregnant women; however, concern about the potential for fetal cyanide toxicity should limit its use to short-term administration for severe hypertension.

COLD PREPARATIONS

The antihistamines (chlorpheniramine, diphenhydramine, pheniramine, and tripelennamine) have not demonstrated teratogenicity and are probably safe for use in the pregnant patient. Only brompheniramine has been shown to cause birth defects and should not be used. Sympathomimetics are commonly used as decongestants and administered in combination with other drugs to alleviate the symptoms of allergy and upper respiratory tract infections. Although they are not considered to be teratogenic in humans, there is an association between the first trimester use of sympathomimetics and minor malformations, inguinal hernia, and clubfoot. The use of this class of drugs, especially in the first trimester, is not without risk.

GASTROINTESTINAL MEDICATIONS

Most antacid preparations are well tolerated during pregnancy. Only the use of sodium bicarbonate is contraindicated because it is well absorbed and may alter the pH of the mother and fetus. Drugs with a high sodium content should be avoided, especially if the woman has pre-existing hypertension, preeclampsia or is prone to fluid retention. The use of antiemetics should be considered only after more conservative measures to control nausea and vomiting have failed. Neither trimethobenzamide (Tigan) nor the phenothiazines prochlorperazine (Compazine) and promethazine (Phenergan) have been found to be teratogenic in large studies and are probably safe for use during pregnancy. Because of the small risk of hypotension and resultant placental insufficiency associated with the phenothiazines, their use should probably be restricted to cases of hyperemesis gravidarum or when trimethobenzamide has failed.

IMMUNIZATIONS

Vaccines that contain toxoid or inactivated virus and immune globulins may be given whenever they are indicated during pregnancy. In nonemergency situations it is advisable to wait until after the first trimester because of theoretical concerns over possible teratogenesis. Live virus vaccines (measles, mumps, rubella, and polio) should not be given to pregnant women or those likely to become pregnant within 3 months. Commonly used immunizations and immunoprophylactic agents that may be given to pregnant women include tetanus toxoid, tetanus-diphtheria toxoid, tetanus immune globulin, rabies human diploid cell vaccine, rabies immune globulin, hepatitis B vaccine, hepatitis B immune globulin, and pooled immune globulin.

COMMON PITFALLS

All drugs administered to the pregnant woman represent a potential harm to the fetus. Medications should not be prescribed to alleviate minor symptoms. There should be a clear medical indication. Only the minimum effective dose should be used, and it should be prescribed for the shortest time possible to decrease the fetus's exposure. Drugs that can be considered safe for use in pregnancy include acetaminophen, the penicillins, and the cephalosporins. Drugs that are absolutely contraindicated include brompheniramine and the tetracyclines.

39   Hemorrhage in Early Pregnancy

Bleeding in the first trimester of pregnancy is seldom a life-threatening event, but it is essential to accurately diagnose the cause of vaginal bleeding to ensure adequate and timely obstetric evaluation. Bleeding in the first trimester of pregnancy occurs in up to 20% of pregnancies. These patients may be divided into three groups: (1) normal intrauterine pregnancies, (2) ectopic pregnancies, (3) nonviable pregnancies (complete, incomplete, or inevitable abortions). Ectopic pregnancy is addressed elsewhere. Abortion is defined as the termination of pregnancy before 20 weeks' gestation, counting from the first day of the last menstrual period. If the expelled fetus, whether liveborn or stillborn, weighs less than 500 g, this situation has been defined as an abortion. An early abortion is one that occurs before 12 weeks' gestation. A late abortion is one that occurs between 12 and 20 weeks. Spontaneous abortion is premature expulsion of the products of conception from the uterus and is classified as threatened, inevitable, incomplete, missed, and complete abortion. Spontaneous, threatened, inevitable, incomplete, and complete abortions account for first trimester bleeding in 10% to 15%. of all pregnant women; 20% of patients with threatened abortion eventually progress to abortion.

Ectopic pregnancy is the leading cause of maternal death in the first trimester. As many as 4% of patients with first trimester bleeding may have an ectopic pregnancy. Approximately 50% of patients with first trimester bleeds have normal intrauterine pregnancies. The cause of bleeding is probably due to the normal implantation process. The cause of abortion is seldom determined. Causes of spontaneous abortion include chromosomal aberrations; defective uterine environment; external factors such as drugs, virus, chemicals, and radiation; maternal factors (severe systemic acute infections such as pneumonia, pyelonephritis, and influenza); and certain surgical procedures (e.g., excision of corpus luteum and appendicitis). Uterine malformations, tumors (i.e., intramural leiomyoma), trauma, defective sperm, and psychogenic causes play minor roles in the pathogenesis of abortion.

CLINICAL PRESENTATION

Vaginal bleeding can be classified as major or minor by the rate of visible blood loss and the patient's hemodynamic status. Patients with resting tachycardia, postural hypotension, or instability of vital signs have evidence of major bleeding. The main causes of hemorrhage in early pregnancy are as follows:

THREATENED ABORTION

Bleeding is variable.

Os is closed.

Mild transient cramps and bleeding are present.

No passage of fetal tissue.

Uterus is enlarged, consistent with time from last menstrual period.

Pregnancy test is positive.

Fetus remains viable.

INEVITABLE ABORTION

As with threatened, but os is dilated and effaced.

Patient may have persistent cramps and moderate bleeding.

Although the bag of waters may rupture, there is no passage of tissue. The nitrazine pH test differentiates vaginal secretions (acidic) from amniotic fluid (alkaline), but if there is any bleeding, the test is unreliable.

COMPLETE ABORTION

Entire contents of uterus are expelled.

There is little or no bleeding or cramps.

Cervix is closed; uterus is firm, normal sized, and nontender; all signs and symptoms of pregnancy disappear.

INCOMPLETE ABORTION

Clots and fetal tissue pass through the endocervical canal and are visible in the cervical os or vagina.

Os is open.

Cramps and bleeding are persistent and excessive.

MISSED ABORTION

Uterus fails to expel dead fetus for 2 months after the pregnancy has terminated.

Os is closed.

Uterus is firm and smaller than expected.

Fetal heart tones are absent.

Diagnosis is made by history, physical examination, and the conversion of a positive pregnancy test to negative. Ultrasound is diagnostic.

Septic abortion, ectopic pregnancy and gestational trophoblastic disease are discussed elsewhere.

DIFFERENTIAL DIAGNOSIS

Non-pregnancy-related causes of vaginal bleeding in the first trimester must be excluded. These include cervical lacerations, inflammation (acute or chronic cervicitis), cervical polyps and ulcers, cervical carcinoma, vaginitis, vaginal trauma, nonuterine bleeding from the urethra or rectum, and trauma. These non-pregnancy-related causes of vaginal bleeding can usually be identified through a history and physical examination.

EMERGENCY DEPARTMENT MANAGEMENT

ABCs are essential in cases of major hemorrhage; special emphasis should be placed on limiting and reversing hypoxemia. Hypoxemia may cause fetal injury or death as well as contribute to increased maternal morbidity. Supplemental oxygen should be administered even in the absence of respiratory distress or cyanosis. Once the airway is secured, the degree of hypoxemia must be frequently assessed by pulse oximetry, as well as monitoring the fetal heart rate. Fetal heart tones by Doppler are heard as early as the 10th week and consistently by the 12th week. Two large-bore peripheral intravenous lines should be established for crystalloid and potential blood replacement. Blood should be drawn for a complete blood count, electrolytes, blood urea nitrogen, and glucose, type and crossmatch, serum pregnancy test, and Rh.

The pelvic examination involves inspection for bleeding sites. Products of conception in clotted blood are important to identify in an incomplete abortion. For the inexperienced it may be difficult at first to distinguish blood clots from fetal tissue. Clots usually disintegrate easily when squeezed through gauze pads, whereas tissue or products of conception do not. Any tissue or products of conception found in the vaginal vault should be sent to the pathology department for analysis.

The next step is to confirm pregnancy with a urinary pregnancy test that can detect 40 mIU/mL to 50 mIU/mL of B-hCG; this test becomes positive at about 1 week gestation. The gold standard, however, remains radioimmunoassay, which can detect as little as 1 mIU/mL to 10 mIU/mL of hCG. The next step is to determine whether the pregnancy is intrauterine or ectopic. If an ectopic pregnancy is suspected, ultrasonography is indicated. If intrauterine pregnancy is established, treatment depends on whether the patient has a threatened abortion or has progressed to an inevitable abortion. Unless the patient with a threatened abortion has severe pain or bleeding, she may be sent home.

Inevitable and incomplete abortions require intravenous oxytocin to promote uterine evacuation or suction curettage. Oxytocin (Pitocin), 20 units in 1000 mL saline solution, is given at a rate of 20 mU/min and titrated to diminish the rate of bleeding and to contract the uterus for curettage. Once the patient is stabilized, the obstetrician should perform a curettage to remove all products of conception from the uterus. Patients who are Rh negative and unsensitized (without circulating anti-Rh antibody) are given 50 µg Rh immunoglobulin if the uterus is 12 weeks in size or less and 300 µg if larger. The patient with a missed abortion who is stable may be sent home if close follow-up is ensured. Most patients spontaneously abort within a few weeks. Evacuation of the uterus is indicated with any laboratory or clinical suggestion of disseminated intravascular coagulation or in those women who are emotionally distressed from the condition.

Often overlooked during the emergency treatment of a woman with bleeding during pregnancy are the psychological effects of the situation. Depression and severe anxiety are frequent problems experienced by pregnant women with vaginal bleeding.

DISPOSITION

ROLE OF THE OBSTETRIC CONSULTANT

Suspected ectopic pregnancy
Completed abortion
Failure to visualize a gestational sac by ultrasonography
Performance of culdocentesis
Any pregnant patient with unstable vital signs
Penetrating pelvic trauma
All patients who require admission or suction curettage

INDICATIONS FOR ADMISSION

1. Inevitable and incomplete abortions. Patients may be admitted for uterine evacuation or suction curettage, or suction curettage may be performed in the ED or outpatient surgery setting.
2. Hypovolemia, need for blood transfusion, or marked anemia.
3. Diagnosis of complete abortion. This is a difficult diagnosis to make unless the patient has brought in the products of conception. If doubt exists, or if bleeding continues, the patient should be hospitalized.
4. Missed abortion. Evacuation of the uterus by curettage is indicated with laboratory or clinical suggestion of a coagulopathy or in those women emotionally distressed from the condition.

5. Patients with or suspected of having gestational trophoblastic disease (GTD).
6. Hemodynamic instability in any pregnant patient, regardless of diagnosis.
7. Patients with threatened abortion who experience continuing severe abdominal pain, tenderness, cramps, as well as severe vaginal bleeding.
8. Ruptured ectopic pregnancy. (See Chapter 46.)

DISCHARGE CRITERIA
1. *For threatened abortion:* Patients with mild or moderate bleeding, little or no pain, normal hematocrit, and no orthostatic changes may be safely discharged with the following instructions:
   a. Avoid strenuous activity. There is no evidence that strict bed rest or sedation is helpful, so this restriction is unnecessary. After a 24-hour rest period the patient may resume normal activity as tolerated.
   b. Douching and intercourse should be avoided while the bleeding is present but are not otherwise contraindicated.
   c. The patient should be seen by her obstetrician in 24 to 72 hours, although she should seek immediate medical attention if increased bleeding or abdominal cramping occurs, if products of conception begin to pass, or if temperature exceeds 100.4°F (38°C).
   d. Any tissue passed should be brought in.
2. *For complete abortion:* The management of complete abortion is controversial. If the uterus is well contracted and the cervix tightly closed, some recommend observation and reserving curettage for recurrent bleeding or cramps. Others believe that it is better to perform curettage on all such patients, since it is a relatively low-risk procedure and may spare the patient a subsequent hemorrhage or infection.
3. *For missed abortion:* Patients with missed abortion who are stable may be sent home if close follow-up is ensured.

COMMON PITFALLS

- Failure to recognize significant blood loss in a patient with normal vital signs. The difficulty arises from two conditions of pregnancy: (1) the maternal blood pressure is normally low during pregnancy, with the average 110/70 mm Hg, and (2) there is normally a 35% increase of blood volume during pregnancy. This increase in blood volume means that a 30% volume loss must occur before vital signs change. This may mask significant blood loss.
- Failure to administer oxygen to the mother due to lack of recognition of the danger of hypoxemia to the fetus.
- Failure to diagnose an ectopic pregnancy is a medicolegal risk.

---

40   Hypertensive Disorders of Pregnancy

Hypertensive disease of pregnancy is the most common cause of perinatal morbidity and mortality. It is a disease with preventable complications. The pathophysiology of hypertension during pregnancy is unclear, but there is consensus that aggressive treatment is warranted to prevent complications to both fetus and mother. Fetal growth retardation, abruptio placentae, and still-birth are more common in hypertensive pregnancies.

CLASSIFICATION

Gestational hypertension
Preeclampsia (pregnancy-induced hypertension)
Eclampsia (pregnancy-induced hypertension)
Chronic hypertension
Chronic hypertension with superimposed preeclampsia or superimposed eclampsia

Table 40-1 provides the diagnostic criteria for hypertension in pregnancy.

HIGH-RISK GROUPS FOR PREECLAMPSIA AND ECLAMPSIA

The following groups of patients have an increased risk for preeclampsia and eclampsia. Multiparas become high risk in the presence of those conditions marked with an asterisk (*).

Primigravidas or nulliparous
Familial history of preeclampsia and eclampsia

TABLE 40-1. Diagnostic Criteria for Hypertension in Pregnancy

| | Period of Onset | Blood Pressure (mm Hg) | | Central Nervous System |
		Systolic	Diastolic	
Gestational Hypertension	Second half of pregnancy	140	90	None
Preeclampsia				
Mild	After 20th wk of gestation	140 >20 above baseline	90 >15 above baseline	None
Severe		160	110	Altered mental status; blurred vision
Eclampsia	Third trimester	160 (variable)	110 (variable)	Convulsions or coma
Chronic Hypertension	Before pregnancy <20 wk of pregnancy	140	90	None
Chronic Hypertension				
Superimposed Preeclampsia	Both can occur earlier than the 20th wk of gestation	140–170 Sharp increase >30	90–110 Sharp increase >15	Same as preeclampsia
Superimposed Eclampsia		Same or variable	Same or variable	Convulsions or coma

(cont'd.)

*Plural gestations (risk increases sixfold)
*Chronic hypertension
Hydatidiform mole or extensive molar degeneration of the placenta
Fetal hydrops
Extremes of age
Lower socioeconomic status (infrequent or nonexistent medical care)
*Diabetes mellitus
Rheumatic heart disease
Coexisting renal disease
Alpha thalassemia
*Rh sensitization
*Multiple fathers (multiparas with multiple paternities)

CLINICAL PRESENTATION AND EMERGENCY DEPARTMENT EVALUATION

The evaluation requires a comprehensive obstetric history, a pertinent review of systems, and an examination with particular attention to the target organ systems. The obstetric history should address gravidity, character of prior pregnancies, and current gestational age. A history of chronic hypertension,

TABLE 40-1 (cont'd.).

Pulmonary	Hepatic	Renal	Hemato-poietic	Other
None	None	Proteinuria <300 mg/24°	None	0–trace dipstick BP of 125/75 before 32 wk associated with increased fetal risk
None	None	Proteinuria	None	Edema of hands and face; wt gain > 2 lb/wk; +1 to +2 dipstick
Pulmonary edema	Marked dysfunction	Proteinuria >5 g/24°	Thrombocyto-penia	Generalized edema; wt gain > 6 lb/wk; +3 to +4 dipstick
Pulmonary edema (variable)`	Marked dysfunction (variable)	Same as preeclampsia (variable)	Same as preeclampsia (variable)	Eclampsia can present with only minimal elevation in blood pressure
None	None	Proteinuria < 300 mg/d	None	
←———— Same as preeclampsia ————→				
←———— Same as preeclampsia ————→				

headache, visual disturbances, change in mentation, abdominal pain, renal disease, diabetes, or illicit drug use should be noted. On physical examination vital signs should be recorded, including temperature. Mental status should be assessed. Tremulousness or obtundation may indicate impending eclampsia. A fundoscopic examination should be done, noting arteriolar spasm, papilledema, or hemorrhages. The cardiovascular system should focus on signs of pulmonary edema (jugular venous distention, tachycardia, gallops, tachypnea, and rales). The abdominal examination may reveal hepatic tenderness, epigastric tenderness, or signs of hemoperitoneum. The uterus should be assessed for fundal height to rule out intrauterine growth retardation. Fetal heart tones should be monitored and recorded. Bimanual examination may be done to assess for cervical effacement and dilation. The neurologic examination may reveal hyperactive deep tendon reflexes, but this finding is not predictive of imminent eclampsia. The presence of ankle clonus, however, is indicative of impending eclampsia.

COMPLICATIONS

Complications of preeclampsia and eclampsia may be life-threatening. Pregnancy-induced hypertension in older gravidas can induce heart failure. Circulatory collapse may occur before, during, or after delivery. Pulmonary edema is also seen, the cause of which is uncertain. Liver function is impaired, proportional to the severity of hypertension. Thrombocytopenia occurs in the absence of other coagulation abnormalities, often in association with hemolysis. The major cause of death in pregnancy-induced hypertension is intracranial hemorrhage.

EMERGENCY DEPARTMENT MANAGEMENT AND DISPOSITION

The goal is the successful termination of pregnancy with minimal maternal-fetal morbidity. The efficacy of treatment must be weighed against the side effects. Drug therapy is usually reserved for severe preeclampsia and chronic hypertension. Antihypertensive agents are withheld if the blood pressure is mildly elevated (diastolic 90 mm Hg). Antihypertensive agents are used if the diastolic blood pressure is >95 mm Hg in the second trimester and >100 mm Hg in the third trimester. The drug of choice is methyldopa (Aldomet), although beta blockers and hydralazine are relatively safe and efficacious. Table 40-2 contains guidelines for severe pregnancy-induced hypertension, preeclampsia and eclampsia. Pregnant women with hypertension should not be placed on a low-sodium diet or receive diuretic therapy. The only indication for diuretic therapy during pregnancy is the presence of pulmonary edema or congestive heart failure. Rest promotes a fall in blood pressure and is advocated in all forms of hypertension.

Specific treatment depends on the level of blood pressure elevation, protcinuria, and premonitory signs of eclampsia. Initial laboratory studies in the ED include blood urea nitrogen, creatinine, electrolytes, and glucose; hematocrit; platelets; transaminases; urinalysis; and 24-hour urine for protein. If imminent delivery is anticipated, the patient should also receive a complete type and crossmatch of blood. Frequent blood pressure readings and aggressive fetal maturation determination should be done.

Severe elevations of the blood pressure constitute a medical emergency. Hydralazine (5 mg to 10 mg IV every 20 to 30 minutes) is the drug of choice to maintain the diastolic pressure at 90 mm Hg. A precipitous drop in pressure should be avoided. If hypertension is refractory to hydralazine, sodium nitroprusside is an alternative. Oral antihypertensive agents, such as labetalol and nifedipine, are being used with good results; however, long-term side effects to the fetus have not been fully delineated.

The definitive treatment of eclampsia and severe preeclampsia, depending on gestational age, is delivery. Lowering the blood pressure and terminating the seizure activity are the highest priority before delivery. Magnesium sulfate should be administered prophylactically in severe preeclampsia and for seizure control in eclampsia. It has the advantage of seizure control without sedative properties. If seizures are not controlled with repeated doses of magnesium sulfate, sodium amobarbital and diazepam are alternative choices, but both may induce

TABLE 40-2. Treatment Protocol for Hypertension in Pregnancy

Gestational Hypertension	Preeclampsia		Eclampsia	Chronic Hypertension
	Mild Preeclampsia	Severe Preeclampsia		
Observe for at least 6 h.	**Without proteinuria** Decrease activity at home or work.	**>36 wk** Hospitalize with bed rest in the left recumbent position (ICU).	**Eclamptic seizures** 2–4 g $MgSO_4$ over 5–10 min IV.	**Mild** Methyldopa (drug of choice), hydralazine, or labetalol.
Discharge if less than 90 mm Hg diastolic for follow-up in 2–3 days.	24-hour urine for protein.	Foley catheter; maintain urine output to >30 ml/h.	Follow with 5 g IM in each buttock.	
Home blood pressure monitoring.	Follow-up with Ob-Gyn in 2–3 days with home blood pressure monitoring.	Magnesium (seizure) prophylaxis: 1. 2–4 g $MgSO_4$ IV (loading dose); over 5–10 min (20 ml 10% solution or 4 ml 50% solution = 4 g).	If seizures persist >15 min, 2 g of $MgSO_4$ IVP., and then 5 g of $MgSO_4$ q 4 h IM or 1 g/h in continuous infusion. Stop 24 h after delivery.	**Superimposed preeclampsia** Treat blood pressure as above.
	With proteinuria Hospitalize for bed rest.	2. Follow with 5 g of $MgSO_4$ in each buttock. 3. Maintenance dose of 1 g/h continuous infusion.	For seizures resistant to $MgSO_4$: 1. Sodium amobarbital 250 mg or phenobarbital 200 mg IVP. slowly.	Treat as a preeclamptic, depending on clinical findings and severity of hypertension.
	24-hour urine for protein.	Blood pressure control: 1. Hydralazine 5–10 mg IVP. q 20–30 min to maintain diastolic BP 90 mm Hg; if refractory, use:	or 2. Diazepam 5–10 mg slowly IVP. q 15–30 min.	**Superimposed eclampsia** Treat blood pressure as above.
	Ob-Gyn consult.	2. Nitroprusside or labetalol (if delivery within 30 min).	Consult Ob-Gyn for immediate delivery.	Treat as eclamptic.
		Delivery if indicated	Treat hypertension same as a severe preeclamptic.	
		<36 wk See treatment for eclampsia.		
		Delivery as per Ob-Gyn.		

Important Points:

1. $MgSO_4$ toxicity may cause respiratory depression and arrest, bradycardia, and heart block. Calcium gluconate, 1 g IVP. slowly will correct.
2. When using $MgSO_4$ follow deep tendon reflexes; if absent, discontinue drug, since therapeutic endpoint has been attained. Adjust dose to urine output or serum levels; stop if levels >4–6 mEq/L, or if urine output <25 mL/h.
3. Provide $MgSO_4$ prophylaxis before pelvic examination in severe preeclampsia.
4. Laboratory workup should include CBC, electrolytes, BUN, creatinine, liver function tests, urinalysis, magnesium, arterial blood gases, and type and crossmatch.
5. Watch for respiratory depression when giving diazepam and barbiturates.
6. Provide a quiet, dark environment during hospitalization.

147

maternal and fetal depression. Phenytoin is thought to be too slow in onset to be of value in eclampsia.

COMMON PITFALLS

- All pregnant women with newly diagnosed hypertension have pregnancy-induced hypertension until proved otherwise. Even mild hypertension compromises intervillous perfusion and predisposes the patient to eclampsia.
- Eclampsia can occur rapidly even with minimal symptoms.
- When diagnosis is uncertain and compliance is questionable, the patient should be admitted.
- Obstetric consultation should be sought early in the emergency management and always before discharge.
- The physician should be aware of the side-effects and therapeutic endpoints of all drugs used in the treatment guidelines.

---

41   Asthma in Pregnancy

Asthma occurs in 0.4% to 1.3% of pregnant women. Fetal mortality has been associated with severe asthma. Congenital malformations are not increased among infants of asthmatic mothers.

DIFFERENTIAL DIAGNOSIS

The differential diagnosis of asthma in the pregnant patient is the same as in the nonpregnant patient. Specific to pregnancy, the differential diagnosis of severe respiratory distress includes recurrent pulmonary emboli, acute left ventricular heart failure with pulmonary edema due to peripartum cardiomyopathy, and amniotic fluid embolism. Peripartum cardiomyopathy is associated with the onset of congestive heart failure among women with no prior history of heart disease. Although it can occur during the last month of pregnancy or within the first 5 months postpartum, most cases are first seen in the first 3 months postpartum. It is more common among older black multiparas, frequently with a history of preeclampsia. The presence of mural thrombi with resulting pulmonary embolism is not uncommon. The cause is unknown. Amniotic fluid embolism normally presents with severe respiratory distress, cyanosis, shock, and disseminated intravascular coagulation. The onset of symptoms is sudden and catastrophic. An important feature in the diagnosis is that bronchospasm is rare with this entity.

EMERGENCY DEPARTMENT EVALUATION

The evaluation is essentially the same as for a nonpregnant patient. Physical examination should include level of consciousness, use of accessory muscles of respiration, pulse and respiratory rates, auscultation of the lungs, and measurement of FEV_1. The following findings may indicate severe airway obstruction and the need for hospitalization: altered sensorium; tachycardia >120–130 beats/min; respiratory rate of >30 breaths/min; or $FEV_1 < 1$ L.

LABORATORY EVALUATION

Laboratory evaluation for an acute asthmatic attack may include a complete blood count with differential, sputum analysis, arterial blood gas (ABG). Severe hypoxia or hypercapnia, both potentially detrimental to the fetus, should be rapidly detected and treated. Probably the most reliable indicator of severity of airway obstruction and response to treatment is the FEV_1. An FEV_1 of <1 L can be an indication of severe airway obstruction. Repeat ABG is often of little value when the FEV_1 is greater than 1 L.

CHEST RADIOGRAPHY

Chest films should be done if pneumonia or pneumothorax is suspected and for patients who do not respond to standard therapy. Proper shielding of the abdomen is important. Exposure of the developing fetus to radiation can lead to birth defects, fetal growth retardation, microcephaly, and mental retardation when such exposure is excessive. An exposure of 5 rad or less is thought to be safe for the developing fetus.

EMERGENCY DEPARTMENT MANAGEMENT

The management of asthma is essentially the same as in nonpregnant patients. Treatment with beta agonists and corticosteroids should not be withheld because of pregnancy. The control of asthma is essential to improve maternal and fetal outcome (Table 41-1). Oxygen by nasal cannula at 2 L to 3 L/min should be administered after an initial ABG analysis is obtained.

EPINEPHRINE   Epinephrine in pregnancy is controversial. Some authorities favor subcutaneous epinephrine as the treatment of choice during pregnancy: others advise that epinephrine is best avoided during pregnancy because of its ability to decrease uterine blood flow and a reported increase in congenital malformations. Selective $beta_2$ agonists, on the other hand, cause either no change or an increase in uterine blood flow. There are no advantages, and there are possible disadvantages to the use of epinephrine over the more selective $beta_2$ agonists.

CORTICOSTEROIDS   Most patients respond to a beta agonist. Corticosteroid therapy is recommended if the attack is moderately severe (125 mg methylprednisolone every 6 hours) is preferred. Cortisol and other corticosteroids freely cross the placenta, but they are rapidly converted by the fetoplacental unit into an inactive form, cortisone. After maternal ingestion, prednisone is rapidly converted to its active form, prednisolone. However, prednisolone is poorly transferred across the placental barrier, and fetal levels are considerably lower than maternal levels. Beclomethasone dipropionate permits significant reduction or discontinuation of prednisone in corticosteroid-dependent asthmatic patients.

ANTIBIOTICS   Bacterial pneumonia and bronchitis can initiate an acute asthmatic attack. Ampicillin or erythromycin (500 mg PO every 6 hours) or cephalosporin such as cefaclor (Ceclor; 250 mg PO every 8 hours for 10 days) are recommended. Patients with pneumonia or a febrile respiratory tract infection would benefit from intravenous antibiotic treatment.

DISPOSITION

During pregnancy patients who develop pneumonia or require intravenous therapy for an acute asthmatic attack should be considered for hospital admission. The same patients could benefit

---

Table 41-1. Drugs Used to Treat Acute Asthma in Pregnancy

Beta Agonists	Dose	Comment
Terbutaline (subcutaneous)	0.25 mg	After 15–30 min a 2nd dose of 0.25 mg may be given.
Albuterol	1–2 puffs (90 µg/puff)	Repeat every 4–6 h
Metoproterenol	2–3 puffs (0.65 mg/puff)	Repeat every 3–4 h

from consultation with maternal–fetal medicine, pulmonary specialists, or internal medicine. The obstetrician should be notified.

COMMON PITFALLS

- Judging the severity of an asthmatic attack based on physical findings may be misleading.
- Appropriate treatment with beta agonists and corticosteroids should not be withheld because of pregnancy. Control of asthma is essential to improve maternal and fetal outcome.
- Epinephrine use should probably be replaced by the more selective $beta_2$ agonists.
- Fetal toxicity to theophylline can occur in the absence of maternal toxicity due to increased fetal sensitivity and slower elimination of the drug. To avoid fetal toxicity, if used, the dose of intravenous aminophylline should be reduced.
- Oxygen, even with mild asthma in pregnancy, should be used to reduce hyperventilation.

42 Sickle Cell Disease in Pregnancy

Sickle cell anemia is associated with a significant increase in maternal and perinatal morbidity and mortality. With improved prenatal care maternal mortality has declined to the current rate of about 2%. Maternal mortality is primarily due to complications of sickle cell anemia, including congestive heart failure (2% to 20%), pulmonary embolism (20% to 40%), and a significant increased risk of preeclampsia. The overall fetal wastage is approximately 30%, due to an increased risk of spontaneous abortion, stillbirth, prematurity, and intrauterine growth retardation. This increase in fetal wastage is probably related to thrombotic events in the placenta. The frequency and severity of sickle cell crises vary greatly. Many authors believe that pregnancy worsens the disease with an increase in vaso-occlusive crises, especially during labor and the postpartum period. Prompt recognition and intervention are vital for optimal maternal and fetal outcome. Sickle cell–thalassemia disease and sickle cell–hemoglobin C disease are treated similarly to sickle cell disease in pregnancy.

CLINICAL PRESENTATION

During pregnancy most crises are vaso-occlusive and occur most often in the latter half of pregnancy. They follow the usual pattern of recurring attacks of sudden pain, most often affecting the extremities, abdomen, chest, and vertebrae. Although infrequent in pregnancy, hemolytic crisis is characterized by the sudden onset of severe anemia and a low reticulocyte count. Aplastic crisis is usually self-limited and associated with infection. This has proved fatal in pregnancy when sensitization from prior blood products prohibits transfusion.

DIFFERENTIAL DIAGNOSIS

When a known sickle cell anemia patient presents with pain, the physician must determine whether it is the usual vaso-occlusive crisis. If so, is it associated with an infection, or is the pain caused by a surgical or obstetric disorder. The diagnosis of vaso-occlusive crisis is one of exclusion. Consultation with a perinatologist or hematologist is essential. A reason for the pain crisis should always be sought. Infection will be discovered in about 25% of parturients and is associated with one third of all deaths in sickle cell patients. In pregnancy the most common infections are pneumonia, cystitis or pyelonephritis, and osteomyelitis. After delivery endometritis should always be considered. Gram-negative sepsis with *Escherichia coli* and *Salmonella* replace pneumococci as the major offending organisms. *Mycoplasma* should also be considered with pneumonia.

EMERGENCY DEPARTMENT EVALUATION

Laboratory tests include complete blood count with reticulocyte count, clean-catch urinalysis with culture, and hemoglobin electrophoresis for percentage of hemoglobin A. Crisis is unlikely if the hemoglobin A percentage is higher than 40% to 50%. Other laboratory tests should be based on potential organ complications. Hemodilution of pregnancy normally causes a relative lowering of the hematocrit. The white blood cell (WBC) count may increase to 10,000 to 16,000/μL in the absence of infection. Both total and segmental leukocytes increase during pregnancy as well as with infection and vaso-occlusive crisis. However, a substantial rise in the WBC count with an increase in band (nonsegmented) leukocyte level above 1000/μL is often seen with significant bacterial infection. A complete physical examination is mandatory. Ultrasonography is recommended if the differential diagnosis includes pregnancy-related complications. After initial evaluation, continuous electronic fetal monitoring is indicated if the pregnancy has reached a gestational age of about 28 weeks.

EMERGENCY DEPARTMENT MANAGEMENT

All pregnant women with sickle cell disease should be admitted to the hospital if there is any suspicion of crisis or infection. If necessary, the patient should be stabilized and transferred to the nearest perinatal center with maternal–fetal medicine and hematology subspecialists. Management of sickle cell disease in a pregnant patient is similar to that in a nonpregnant patient, and involves rest, adequate nutrition, hydration, and analgesia.

1. The patient should be admitted to the hospital and transferred to the appropriate center when indicated.
2. Hydration, in the absence of congestive heart failure, should be provided (D_5LR 1000 mL over 2 hours and then 125–150 mL/h).
3. Acetaminophen is the preferred analgesic for milder pain. If narcotics are required, satisfactory results can be achieved with a combination of meperidine (50–100 mg) or butorphanol (1–2 mg) in combination with promethazine (25 mg given IV or IM).
4. Prophylactic antibiotics are not indicated, but appropriate antibiotics should be initiated immediately if infection is suspected or diagnosed.
5. Oxygen should be delivered by nasal cannula at 2 L to 4 L.
6. Unless the patient has severe preeclampsia or congestive heart failure, invasive central monitoring and Foley catheterization are to be avoided to minimize the risk of iatrogenic infection.
7. Partial exchange transfusion is the cornerstone of management for the prevention as well as treatment of crisis during pregnancy. Crisis should begin to improve within 1 to 2 hours after partial exchange. This is not an ED procedure. Simple blood transfusion is used when the initial hematocrit is less than 15% or for women in active labor with crisis.

The routine use of partial exchange transfusion during pregnancy to decrease the incidence of vaso-occlusive crisis as well as improve pregnancy outcome is controversial but appears to be gaining support. If the hematocrit is less than 25% or vaso-occlusive crisis or severe infection develops, exchange transfusion is performed before 28 weeks. The goal is to maintain a hemoglobin A level higher than 40% and a hematocrit higher than 30%. Repeat partial exchange is advised if (a) hemo-globin A is less than 20%, (b) hematocrit is less than 25%, or (c) vaso-occlusive crisis occurs.

DISPOSITION

ROLE OF THE CONSULTANT   It is appropriate to consult the obstetric service. Consultation with maternal–fetal medicine or hematology is then at the obstetrician's discretion.

INDICATIONS FOR ADMISSION   Any pregnant woman with sickle cell disease who is suspected of having a crisis or infection should be admitted to the hospital.

TRANSFER CONSIDERATIONS   Care is best done at a center with appropriate subspecialists experienced in the management of sickle cell disease. If such subspecialists are not readily avail-able, strong consideration for transfer is indicated. Hydration, oxygen, and appropriate analgesics should be initiated before transfer. Because of the decrease in oxygen tension with altitude, ground transportation is ideally suited for most transports. Helicopter flight is at about 2000 feet above ground level for flights less than 100 miles and 3000 to 5000 feet for flights over 100 miles. Fixed wing aircraft are theoretically pressurized to ground level.

43   Diabetes in Pregnancy

Maternal mortality is that of the general population and perinatal loss has decreased to 3% to 5%. The incidence of major malformations is three to four times higher among infants of diabetic women, accounting for almost half of all fetal loss and the major cause of perinatal death.

CLASSIFICATION   The classification is based on (a) duration of disease, (b) age at onset, and (c) underlying vascular involvement.

DIABETIC KETOACIDOSIS   Diabetic ketoacidosis (DKA) during pregnancy is associated with a 50% fetal loss rate. Early recognition and treatment improve both maternal and fetal outcome. Dur-ing pregnancy DKA may develop with relatively low blood sugars of only 200 to 300.

DIFFERENTIAL DIAGNOSIS

HYPOGLYCEMIC COMA   Onset is usually rapid, without other symptoms that are associated with DKA. Blood sugar is low.

NONKETOTIC HYPEROSMOLAR COMA   Dehydration is the major problem, with a blood urea nitrogen level greater than or equal to 70 mg/dL commonly found. Hyperglycemia is marked with levels as high as 1000 mg/dL.

ALCOHOLIC KETOACIDOSIS   These patients are usually not diabetic, but often are alcoholics with poor nutrition. Ketosis is present, but blood glucose is normal.

STARVATION KETOSIS   The differential diagnosis between starvation ketosis and DKA is made difficult because of the accelerated starvation ketosis seen during pregnancy. The accelerated metabolic response to starvation in pregnancy results in blood ketone levels that are up to four times higher than in the nonpregnant state. The presence of ketonemia or ketonuria with low or normal blood glucose levels suggests starvation ketosis rather than DKA. Treatment consists of increasing dietary or intravenous carbohydrates.

EMERGENCY DEPARTMENT EVALUATION

It is important to identify an infectious site that could precipitate DKA. Most patients have an altered sensorium. Other physical findings include evidence of dehydration and a rapid, shallow respiration, often with a fruity breath odor owing to acetone. Because home glucose monitoring is standard care for the diabetic woman during pregnancy, a careful review of recent glucose control is beneficial.

LABORATORY TESTS

Complete blood count, serum glucose, electrolytes, bicarbonate, blood urea nitrogen, creatinine, and ketones; arterial blood gas analysis; and urinalysis with culture should be obtained and repeated every 2 hours during the initial phase of treatment. Other laboratory tests and cultures should be obtained as indicated.

EMERGENCY DEPARTMENT MANAGEMENT

Regular insulin (6–10 units) should be administered by IV push and then a continuous insulin infusion of normal saline (500 mL) with regular insulin (50 units [1 unit/10 mL]) begun at 6 to 10 units per hour. If blood sugar does not fall by 30% in 2 hours, the insulin dose should be doubled. When blood sugar reaches 250 mg to 200 mg/dL the insulin infusion rate should be cut in half. The intravenous fluids should be changed to dextrose 5% in sodium chloride 0.45% when blood sugar is less than 200 mg/dL. When blood sugar falls to less than 150 mg/dL and the serum ketone level is decreasing, insulin should run at a basal rate of 1 to 2 units per hour. If pH remains less than 7.30 and is not rising, the insulin dose should be increased despite a falling blood sugar. Dextrose 5% in water should be infused at 200 mL/h to avoid hypoglycemia and possibly cerebral edema. If serum hyperglycemia is reversed too rapidly, cerebral edema may be precipitated. This is usually irreversible and fatal.

Because patients in DKA are generally behind by 3 to 6 L of fluid, 1000 mL sodium chloride 0.45% should be given over the first hour and then 300 mL to 500 mL/h. When blood sugar is less than 200 mg/dL the intravenous fluid should be changed to dextrose 5% in sodium chloride 0.45%. Rapid correction of acidosis in the pregnant woman is important because of the tremendous fetal risk. In utero fetal resuscitation may occur with correction of maternal hyperglycemia and acidosis.

For mild acidosis (pH greater than 7.10) bicarbonate should not be given. If pH is less than 7.10, 88 mEq sodium bicarbonate in 1000 mL sodium chloride 0.45% should be administered. DKA is accompanied by a shift in the potassium from intracellular to extracellular. A normal serum potassium level before initiation of treatment may mask the total body potassium depletion. Once the acidosis is corrected, hypokalemia may become obvious. After 3 to 4 hours of treatment potassium chloride (40 mEq/L) should be added to the intravenous fluids. DKA has been associated with sudden fetal death. When the fetus has reached a viable gestational age (25 weeks) continuous electronic fetal monitoring is generally used. If the fetus appears compromised, cesarean delivery should be delayed until the mother is metabolically stable.

DISPOSITION

ROLE OF THE CONSULTANT   Under optimal conditions consultation with a maternal–fetal medicine physicians should occur. In most hospitals care is divided between endocrinology and an obstetrician.

TRANSFER CONSIDERATIONS   Patients with DKA should not be transferred until therapy has begun and the condition is stable or improving. Continuing care should be at a facility that has an obstetrician or maternal–fetal medicine physician available to assess fetal status.

OTHER PROBLEMS ASSOCIATED WITH DIABETES

URINARY TRACT INFECTION OR PYELONEPHRITIS   Urinary tract infections are more common during pregnancy among diabetic women. Early diagnosis and treatment of bacteriuria and cystitis can prevent the development of pyelonephritis. Pyelonephritis requires hospital admission for administration of intravenous antibiotics.

PREECLAMPSIA   The frequency of preeclampsia is greatly increased among women with diabetes. Compared with a 5% to 8% incidence in the normal population, up to 25% of pregnancies in diabetic women are complicated by preeclampsia. Patients may present with asymptomatic hypertension or with complaints such as headache, epigastric pain, visual disturbance, and eclamptic seizures. The combination of preeclampsia and diabetes significantly increases the risk of fetal loss. Immediate consultation with the obstetric service is advised if blood pressure elevation is detected.

YEAST VULVOVAGINITIS   Vaginal pruritus caused by yeast infection is frequently seen among diabetic women during pregnancy. Presenting complaints include vaginal itching, dysuria, and dyspareunia. The diagnosis is confirmed by culture or microscopic identification of mycelia or pseudohyphae on direct microscopy in a potassium hydroxide 10% preparation. During pregnancy miconazole nitrate 2% cream (Monostat) applied daily for 7 days provides prompt resolution in most patients.

SIGNIFICANT DECREASE IN FETAL MOVEMENT   Pregnancy among diabetic women is associated with an increased risk of stillbirth. Decreased fetal movement may be an early warning sign for impending fetal demise. Any pregnant woman who perceives a significant decrease in fetal movement after the 28th week of pregnancy should be evaluated. Immediate consultation with the obstetric service for antepartum fetal heart rate testing is mandatory.

MYOCARDIAL ISCHEMIA (HEART FAILURE)   Any diabetic woman with complaints that suggest myocardial ischemia should be thoroughly investigated. Ischemic heart disease is unusual among diabetic women during pregnancy, but it carries a grave prognosis. Most patients have been at least 30 years of age. Because of the poor prognosis, termination of pregnancy with permanent sterilization is recommended for any diabetic woman with ischemic heart disease.

VISUAL LOSS DUE TO DIABETIC RETINOPATHY   All women with diabetes should have ophthalmic examinations annually for early detection of diabetic retinopathy. Diabetic retinopathy is not affected by pregnancy. However, macular edema has been recognized during pregnancy among diabetic women, usually associated with hypertension and proteinuria. Many of these women also have proliferative retinopathy. Delivery is indicated if progressive visual loss occurs.

PREMATURE LABOR   Beta-sympathomimetic drugs used to treat preterm labor, (ritodrine and terbutaline) can cause extreme elevations in blood glucose levels and even DKA in diabetic women. If treatment of preterm labor is necessary, intravenous magnesium sulfate has no effect on blood glucose and is the drug of choice.

BLOOD GLUCOSE CONTROL   The ability to make frequent blood glucose measurements at home has reduced both maternal and perinatal mortality and morbidity and is an important part of prenatal care for diabetic women. Blood sugar determinations are made at home one to four times daily, depending on the recent glucose control. When patients present to the ED the physician should inquire as to the recent blood sugar levels by home glucose monitoring.

DISPOSITION

ROLE OF THE CONSULTANT   Diabetes in pregnancy is a high-risk situation for mother and baby. Optimal prenatal care requires either a maternal–fetal medicine physician or an obstetrician experienced in the management of diabetes in pregnancy. If such a subspecialist is not available, the combined efforts of an obstetrician and an internist to assist in insulin adjustments is advised.

INDICATIONS FOR ADMISSION   Admission is indicated when poor glucose control remains uncorrected after 3 to 4 days of home glucose monitoring and insulin adjustment and when complications are present, including diabetic ketoacidosis, preeclampsia, pyelonephritis, dehydration, and febrile illness (viral or bacterial).

COMMON PITFALLS

- The major cause of fetal loss among diabetic women is major birth defects. This can only be reduced by achieving euglycemic control at the time of conception and throughout the first 7 to 10 weeks of pregnancy.
- During pregnancy DKA can occur with blood glucose levels as low as 200 mg to 300 mg/dL.
- Ketones in the urine and blood can occur with normal blood glucose levels as a result of accelerated starvation ketosis.

44   Urinary Tract Infection in Pregnancy

Urinary tract infections (UTIs) are one of the most common medical complications in pregnancy and a frequent cause of ED visits. The physiologic changes of pregnancy further enhance the risk for UTI and render the upper tract more susceptible to infection. In pregnancy the bladder has decreased tone and increased capacity, causing increased stasis and risk of vesicoureteral reflux. The ureters are physiologically dilated in pregnancy due to a decrease in ureteral muscle tone and peristalsis secondary to progesterone. In addition, there is ureteral compression by the enlarged pregnant uterus and the enlarged ovarian veins. The typical microbiologic isolates are similar in pregnant and nonpregnant patients. *Escherichia coli* accounts for 50% to 75% of all isolates. Other gram-negative aerobes such as *Klebsiella* and *Proteus* are commonly isolated. Both enterococci and group B streptococci have been implicated in UTI. *Staphylococcus saprophyticus* is also an important uropathogen.

CLINICAL PRESENTATION

In pregnancy urinary infection may be divided into asymptomatic bacteriuria, cystitis, and pyelonephritis. Both untreated asymptomatic bacteriuria and cystitis may progress to upper tract (renal) infection. Approximately 4% to 7% of all pregnant women have bacteria without symptoms. If untreated, 20% to 40% develop pyelonephritis during the pregnancy. *All* pregnant patients should be screened at their perinatal visit for asymptomatic bacteriuria. A urinalysis or urine culture performed on pregnant women with no prenatal care during an ED visit for any complaint would probably be prudent. Pregnant patients with an uncontaminated urinalysis with bacteria and leukocytes should be treated. Eradication of asymptomatic bacteriuria will prevent progression to pyelonephritis. Cystitis commonly presents with urinary frequency, urgency, and dysuria. Suprapubic discomfort and tenderness may also be seen. Bladder infection does *not* customarily result in fever or costovertebral angle tenderness.

In symptomatic patients, a concentration of >100 colonies/mil is sufficient to confirm the diagnosis and warrant treatment. Appropriately treated patients respond quickly and have a good prognosis. Inadequate or delayed therapy may result in progression to pyelonephritis with its possible complications. Pyelonephritis is always a serious infection, but it can be more so in the pregnant patient. Pregnant patients may develop septic shock, premature labor, or preterm delivery. Classically, patients present with chills, fever, flank pain, nausea, vomiting, urinary frequency and urgency, and dysuria. The presence of fever or costovertebral angle tenderness with a positive urinalysis or urine culture is strongly suggestive of pyelonephritis. Pyelonephritis may have serious consequences in pregnancy. From a fetal perspective, there is an association between pyelonephritis and preterm labor and delivery, and fetal wastage.

EMERGENCY DEPARTMENT EVALUATION AND MANAGEMENT

Pregnant patients with no prior prenatal care should have a urinalysis to exclude asymptomatic bacteriuria. A clean-catch urinalysis can be obtained; however, vulvovaginal contamination is common in pregnant women, and special attention is needed to proper collection technique. Catheterization should be avoided if possible. In an uncontaminated urine specimen (no or few epithelial cells) the presence of bacteria with leukocytes indicates asymptomatic bacteriuria. Urine should be sent for culture for confirmation. Treatment should not await the culture and consists of 7 to 10 days of ampicillin (500 mg PO every 6 hours), nitrofurantoin (100 mg PO three to four times per day), or a short-acting sulfonamide. Because both nitrofurantoin and sulfonamides displace bilirubin from its albumin binding sites, with resultant neonatal hyperbilirubinemia, these two drugs should be avoided in the third trimester. Ampicillin is the drug of choice in the third trimester. In areas where E. coli shows resistance to ampicillin, cephalexin (500 mg PO every 6 hours) is an acceptable alternative.

Patients with symptoms of cystitis should have a clean-catch urinalysis and culture. In symptomatic patients, only >100 colonies/mil are required to demonstrate an infection. Although catheterization should be avoided, it may be necessary in symptomatic patients from whom an uncontaminated specimen cannot be obtained. Treatment of cystitis is the same as that of asymptomatic bacteriuria.

Pyelonephritis requires prompt attention. The diagnosis of pyelonephritis is most commonly made with the finding of a positive urinalysis, fever, and costovertebral angle tenderness. Because of the possible complications of renal infection, pregnant patients with pyelonephritis should be hospitalized. Many are dehydrated. Management includes intravenous hydration, intravenous antibiotics, antipyretics, and close observation for septic shock and renal dysfunction. Because the predominant pathogens are gram-negative aerobes, ampicillin (2 g IV every 6 hours) is a good initial drug. However, if E. coli show resistance to ampicillin, Cefazolin (1 g IV every 6 hours) is the drug of choice. With the exception of patients who appear septic, are allergic to the initial therapy, or are not responding to the initial therapy, aminoglycosides should be avoided because of the high prevalence of transient renal dysfunction. If the patient appears septic, therapy with ampicillin or cefazolin plus an aminoglycoside (1.0 mg to 1.5 mg/kg every 8 hours) should be initiated. All pregnant patients who receive aminoglycosides should have a serum creatinine to exclude renal dysfunction and monitor aminoglycoside levels. Antibiotics appropriate to culture and sensitivities or intravenous pyelography or ultrasonography may be needed if there is a poor response to therapy.

DISPOSITION

Patients with cystitis or pyelonephritis are at risk for premature labor and delivery so they should be evaluated for contractions with an external fetal monitor and have their cervices checked. The presence of any contractions should prompt an obstetric consult to evaluate the patient for preterm labor. Likewise, an effaced or dilated cervix should be evaluated. The presence of preterm labor is an indication for admission and treatment with terbutaline, ritodrine, or magnesium. An important consideration for pregnant patients with any urinary infection is follow-up. Pregnant patients with a prior UTI have a high rate (60%) of recurrence. If asymptomatic bacteriuria is subsequently found, it should be treated as outlined. Because close monitoring or suppression is commonly necessary, the obstetrician following the patient should be notified of the infection, or arrangements made to ensure prenatal care and appropriate follow-up.

45   Infections in Pregnancy

Infections in pregnancy affect not only the patient, but the fetus and the course of the pregnancy. The stage of pregnancy influences the physician's choice of therapy. Physicians often need to choose more aggressive management, since infections are tolerated less well in pregnancy. The choice of drug therapy is also guided by teratogenicity and toxicity to the fetus. The presenting signs and symptoms of infection in the pregnant patient are usually identical to those in the nonpregnant patient. However, special considerations regarding diagnostic procedures and management are key to resolving infections with the least morbidity to the pregnant patient and fetus.

RESPIRATORY TRACT INFECTIONS

There is no evidence that pregnancy places the mother at increased risk for acquiring a respiratory tract infection. Therefore, pregnant patients presumably encounter the same risks as nonpregnant patients in comparable health. Cough, sputum production, and fever are the hallmarks of pneumonia. Physical examination often reveals a mildly ill patient with fever. Auscultation and percussion confirm the presence of infiltrates or lobar consolidation. Evaluation should consist of sputum for white blood cells, Gram's stain, and culture. Blood cultures should be performed. The diagnosis is supported by a chest radiograph with abdominal shielding to evaluate the extent of infiltrates. For the fetus there is minimal radiation (usually less than 1 rad) with an anteroposterior, lateral, and the occasional oblique chest film. Lobar consolidation is more consistent with bacterial infection, while patchy infiltrates are seen with a viral infection. The two most common organisms that cause pneumonia in this population are *Streptococcus pneumococcus* and *Mycoplasma pneumoniae.*

Normal physiologic changes of pregnancy decrease functional residual lung capacity; because of less reserve, hospitalization for most pregnant patients with pneumonia is prudent. Although there are no studies indicating that pregnant patients with pneumonia tend to become septic, pregnant patients with other febrile infections may become overtly ill and are at risk for developing septic shock and acute respiratory distress syndrome. Optimal therapy for pneumococcal pneumonia (penicillin V potassium [Pen Vee-K.], 500 mg PO four times daily for 7 days) differs from therapy for mycoplasmal infection (erythromycin, 250–500 mg PO four times daily for 14 days). The most important consideration in the pregnant patient with an upper respiratory tract infection is to maintain adequate oxygenation. Maternal hypoxia affects fetal oxygenation. Although some recommend that all pregnant patients with pneumonia undergo PO_2 assessment, clinical judgment must be used in deciding which patient does *not* need an arterial blood gas.

VIRAL INFECTIONS

Viral syndromes in pregnancy pose variable risks to the unborn fetus. Maternal morbidity and mortality are rare. Therefore, ED management involves supportive care and prevention of communication to other potentially pregnant women (including personnel and other patients). The acronym

TORCH [Toxoplasmosis, Other (hepatitis B virus, varicella zoster), Rubella, Cytomegalovirus, and Herpesvirus] is discussed below.

Varicella (chickenpox) is associated with a pathognomonic vesicular outbreak. Rubella (German measles) is rare but may cause malaise and generalized fatigue. Viremia and transmission by respiratory droplets can occur before a rash develops for varicella (10–21 days) and after exposure in rubella infections (10–21 days). Diagnosis of both varicella and rubella is made by a fourfold rise in IgG serum titers or IgM specific tests. Serum for IgG should be drawn initially and a second specimen 2 to 3 weeks later, with both serums run simultaneously to assess increasing IgG titer over time. Infection in early pregnancy (first trimester) causes the most fetal harm, and can result in congenital abnormalities of the cardiac, neurologic, and ophthalmic systems. These patients should be referred to an obstetrician for counseling and follow-up. It is critical that the patient call her obstetrician before entering the office to avoid exposing other patients to the virus.

Infection in late pregnancy by either virus seldom affects pregnancy outcome. In the immunosuppressed state of pregnancy, however, evolution of *varicella pneumonia* should always be considered. Varicella pneumonia in pregnancy increases the risk of maternal complications and death. Admitting the patient suspected to have varicella pneumonia is wise because acute respiratory distress syndrome develops rapidly in these patients. Infection that occurs within 4 days of delivery places the fetus at high risk since passive transmission of protective maternal antibodies to the disease has not yet occurred. In addition, premature labor is always a concern, particularly in the presence of infection. Attempts should be made to determine if the patient is in labor by asking about contractions (abdominal tightening and back pain). Patients who are suspected of being in labor should be sent to the labor and delivery room for evaluation.

Most adults infected with cytomegalovirus (CMV) are essentially asymptomatic. Unfortunately it is the most common cause of intrauterine infection. Documented in 0.5% to 2.5% of all deliveries, CMV infection has a wide range of effects, from rare but significant neurologic damage in the fetus to simply producing an asymptomatic carrier state accompanied by viral shedding. In light of the difficulty of diagnosis due to its asymptomatic presentation and low incidence of fetal morbidity, clinicians will only be able to help pregnant patients suspected of being exposed to CMV by obtaining laboratory data and confirming seroconversion.

Toxoplasmosis, a protozoan infection, is usually asymptomatic but rarely the patient may present with a mononucleosis-like picture. Most infections are self-limited without significant complications. Many neonates are asymptomatic. No increase in fetal demise is observed. If toxoplasmosis or CMV infection is suspected in pregnancy, the patient should be referred for counseling and serology testing.

Mumps virus, a paramyxovirus, is transmitted by respiratory secretions. Typically, the patient presents with fever, malaise, myalgia, and anorexia followed by parotitis in 24 hours. Treatment of mumps is supportive, and there is no increase in maternal morbidity or mortality. Mumps infection in the first and second trimester may be associated with increased fetal loss. However, there is no fetal congenital disorder clearly associated with maternal mumps infection.

Herpesvirus infection in pregnancy raises concern for neonatal transmission associated with vaginal delivery. Five percent of infants who are delivered through the infected birth canal acquire the infection, and more than 50% of those infected die of disseminated disease. Patients often complain of pain from acute lesions of the perineum. Accurate ED diagnosis is critical for management in later stages of pregnancy by the patient's obstetrician. A herpes culture should be obtained from suspicious lesions. Accurate documentation of the status of the membranes is paramount. If uterine contractions and rupture of the membranes have occurred, the patient should be transferred to the labor suite immediately. The emergency physician should provide supportive care, including analgesics and suggestions about hygiene (e.g., Burow's soaks to the perineum). There is a growing body of information about the safety of oral acyclovir use in pregnancy.

GASTROINTESTINAL INFECTIONS

Nausea and vomiting can occur any time in pregnancy, although morning sickness typically occurs in the first trimester. If accompanied by diarrhea or malaise, the differential diagnosis includes viral gastroenteritis (rotavirus, Norwalk virus) and bacterial food poisoning. Nausea, vomiting, and chronic fatigue may also suggest the possibility of hepatitis. Gastroenteritis is similar in pregnant and nonpregnant patients. Viral gastroenteritis has a variable incubation period, is brief and self-limited. Symptoms include nausea and vomiting with or without a low-grade temperature. Therapy is usually supportive with fluids and rest. Of major concern in pregnancy, however, is dehydration and the ability to maintain oral intake. Hospitalization may be recommended for intravenous supplementation and correction of electrolyte imbalance.

Bacterial gastroenteritis (*Salmonella, Shigella, Campylobacter, Staphylococcus, Bacillus cereus, Clostridia,* or *Vibrio* spp) may occur in pregnancy. Symptoms begin abruptly with nausea and crampy abdominal pain often followed by diarrhea. High fever (temperature higher than 38.5°C) and chills are often present. The volume of diarrhea may be large. Mucus and blood may be present. Diagnosis is made from fresh stool cultures. Dehydration may be significant, and hospitalization is often necessary. Antibiotics for *Salmonella* and *Shigella* infections are not standard in the healthy adult nonpregnant population but should probably be initiated in pregnant patients who are moderately to severely affected. Therapy may decrease the duration of symptoms. Ampicillin (500 mg PO four times daily for 5 days) is recommended.

Viral hepatitis in pregnancy follows the same disease course as in nonpregnant patients. Fetal morbidity and mortality are not increased. Diagnosis is made by serologic identification of specific viral antigens and antibodies. Therapy for pregnant patients is similar to that for nonpregnant patients. Hospitalization is recommended for the patient who is unable to maintain fluids or who is severely debilitated. All patients with elevated coagulation studies (prothrombin time, partial thromboplastin time) require hospitalization. For pregnant women at high risk for hepatitis B, immune-specific vaccine and globulin can be given safely. The usual dose for hepatitis B vaccine is 1 mL intramuscularly, immediately at 1 month and 6 months later. Placental transmission is not a risk. Prophylaxis given at the same time as the vaccine can be administered as an intramuscular injection of hepatitis B-specific immunoglobulin.

BREAST INFECTION

Breast symptoms of infectious cause (mastitis and breast abscess) must be differentiated from engorgement in the postpartum period. Engorgement (breast congestion with milk) usually occurs within the 1st week after delivery. Breasts become firm and warm, and patients complain of diffuse tenderness. Low-grade fever may accompany engorgement. In contrast to bilateral breast engorgement, mastitis is unilateral, painful, and often accompanied by a high fever. Caused by coagulase-positive *Staphylococcus aureus* transmitted from the neonate's oropharynx, treatment includes cephalexin (Keflex, 500 mg) or dicloxacillin (500 mg PO four times daily for 1 week). Continued breastfeeding is allowed. Symptomatic relief of pain can be achieved by warm showers, expression of milk, use of a supportive bra, and analgesics. Nipples may be lubricated with lanolin agents to prevent fissure formation. Abscess formation should be suspected when focal fluctuance and increased tenderness are found. Incision and drainage and antibiotic therapy are needed. Incision and drainage of these lesions should not be attempted in the ED since such lesions often dissect deeply. Breastfeeding should be deferred until the abscess is cleared.

VAGINAL, CERVICAL, AND LOWER GENITAL TRACT INFECTIONS

Lower genital tract discharge is most often vaginal in origin but may be due to cervicitis. Evaluation of the vagina and cervix should include a speculum examination, testing of the pH of vaginal secretions with phenaphthazine paper (Nitrazine), wet mount (placement of vaginal secretions in normal saline solution and potassium hydroxide [KOH] 10% preparation for microscopic examination at 10× and 40× power), and cultures of the cervix for the presence of sexually transmitted diseases such as gonorrhea and chlamydial infection.

The differential diagnosis for a vaginal discharge in a pregnant patient should also include one other entity: rupture of membranes. This condition should be suspected in all pregnant patients, and a careful history should be obtained. Was a gush of fluid present? Is clear fluid present? Are contractions present? If there is suspicion of ruptured membranes, an assessment should be performed. Pregnancy may be accompanied by a vaginal discharge that is physiologic or abnormal. A physiologic vaginal discharge occurs in pregnancy due to increased hormonal status; it is normally white and nonirritating, and may drain onto the undergarments. Wet-mount evaluation is remarkable for an acidic pH (less than 4.5) and numerous epithelial cells.

Pathologic vaginal irritations are caused by *Trichomonas vaginalis* infection, *Candida* vaginal infection, and bacterial vaginosis (previously called nonspecific vaginitis or *Gardnerella vaginalis*). It has been suggested that *T. vaginalis* may play a role in the pathogenesis of preterm labor. At this point, however, no consistent recommendations exist. Treatment for *T. vaginalis* may be initiated for patients who are symptomatic with annoying malodorous, copious discharge. Motile organisms can be seen on microscopic analysis of secretions and pH higher than 4.5. Metronidazole is the only bactericidal agent available that is effective against *T. vaginalis*. Dosage of 500 mg twice daily or 250 mg four times daily for 3 to 5 days is effective. The treatment of pregnant women with metronidazole (when used after 12 weeks of pregnancy) results in no increased risk of complications.

T. vaginalis or bacterial vaginosis may suggest that the patient has a concomitant sexually transmitted disease (gonorrhea or chlamydial infection); culture for these at the same visit. *Candida albicans* is normally present in 10% to 20% of patients. In physiologic quantities its presence causes no symptoms. With overgrowth, the chief complaint is often pruritus with or without notable discharge. The vulva may also be irritated and result in extreme itching. Hyphae and buds on the wet-mount KOH slide confirm the diagnosis. The vaginal pH is less than 4.5. Antifungal vaginal cream (clotrimazole [gyne-lotrimin] or miconazole nitrate 2% [Monistat], one applicator per vagina at bedtime for 5–7 nights) is recommended. Nystatin is not recommended because of its poor efficacy. However, if no other agent is available, it is not contraindicated, but must be used twice daily for 14 days. Candidal vaginal infections are not associated with obstetric complications. Only symptomatic patients need to be offered treatment.

More than half of all patients with bacterial vaginosis are asymptomatic. Symptomatic patients present with a chief complaint of a fishy, foul odor instead of vulvar or vaginal pruritus or discharge. Examination is remarkable for the lack of inflammation of vulva or vagina, hence the name vaginosis. Diagnosis is confirmed by (a) positive amine test when KOH is added to a slide with vaginal secretions, (b) wet mount showing "clue" cells (epithelial cells studded with bacteria), (c) *Lactobacillus* morphotypes less than background bacteria, and (d) pH > 4.5. Symptomatic patients may be offered treatment, the same regimen as for *T. vaginalis* infections. For asymptomatic patients, treatment options are left to the judgment of their obstetricians. Evidence currently suggests that patients with bacterial vaginosis may be at increased risk for premature rupture of membranes, preterm labor, and postpartum endometritis.

Gonorrhea and chlamydial infections cause both symptomatic and asymptomatic cervicitis and either may present as a yellow-green cervical discharge. However, both gonorrhea and chlamydial infection may produce no mucopurulent discharge. A finding of excessive white blood cells on the wet-mount examination in the presence of no visible pathogens should alert the clinician to the possible presence of a sexually transmitted disease. Although 75% to 90% of women with gonorrhea are asymptomatic, aggressive diagnosis and treatment are important. Obstetric complications include premature rupture of membranes, preterm delivery, and chorioamnionitis (infection of the uterine cavity with a fetus *in utero*). Women with other venereal diseases (trichomoniasis, bacterial vaginosis, and chlamydial infection), patients with mucopus or complaints of a vaginal discharge, and patients with known exposure to gonorrhea should be cultured in addition to culturing all pregnant women at the beginning of their pregnancies. All partners of culture-positive women need to be identified and treated.

The ED evaluation includes a Gram's stain of endocervical material for gram-negative diplococci. Culture provides the definitive diagnosis; it is positive in 80% to 90% of patients with gonorrhea. Simultaneous chlamydial cultures should be performed as well, since 50% of all patients with gonorrhea have concomitant chlamydial infection. Treatment in pregnancy includes ampicillin (3.5 g P.O.) or amoxicillin (3 g P.O.) and probenecid (1 g) before the β-lactam antibiotic. Ideally, one should await a positive *Chlamydia* test before initiating treatment, which in pregnancy consists of erythromycin (500 mg four times daily for 10 days). Tetracycline for *Chlamydia* is contraindicated in pregnancy because of its effect on bone development. Penicillin and cephalosporins are ineffective against *Chlamydia*.

If awaiting results is not possible, initiating treatment is appropriate. However, the effect of *Chlamydia* on obstetric outcome is less clear. The major objective with cervical chlamydial infection during pregnancy is to prevent neonatal transmission. This occurs in 60% of neonates born to infected mothers and is manifested as conjunctivitis (50%) or late neonatal pneumonia (10%). It is important to eradicate chlamydial infections in patients close to delivery. If a patient far from term demonstrates a chlamydial infection, treatment may also be offered at this time.

Syphilis in pregnancy is diagnosed either from a positive screening nontreponemal antibody test (i.e., VDRL [Venereal Disease Research Laboratory test] or rapid plasma reagin [RPR] test) followed by a positive FTA-ABS (fluorescent treponemal antibody absorption test) or when serologic tests are ordered because of clinical suspicion (painless lower genital tract lesions). The CDC recommend penicillin G benzathine (2.4 million units I.M.). Subsequent treatment depends on the duration and stage at diagnosis. Transmission to the fetus is possible at any gestational age. Fetal complications include intrauterine demise, preterm labor, development of early congenital syphilis (rash, lymphadenopathy, snuffles, hepatosplenomegaly, and chorioretinitis), and signs of late congenital syphilis (Hutchinson teeth, saddle nose, and mulberry molars). Treatment should be initiated as early as possible, and all pregnant patients should have a screening test for syphilis.

INFECTIONS RELATED TO PREGNANCY

All fevers in pregnancy need to be explained. It is extremely important to exclude chorioamnionitis, an infection of the amniotic cavity with the fetus *in utero*. If the diagnosis is not made, complications occur, including premature rupture of membranes, preterm labor, maternal sepsis, fetal sepsis, and maternal or fetal death. The diagnosis is suggested by fever and uterine tenderness without contractions. Fetal tachycardia may be present due to maternal fever. Leukocytosis is often present. If the membranes are ruptured, the fluid may be foul-smelling. If chorioamnionitis is suspected, an obstetrician should be notified to admit the patient for antibiotic therapy, amniocentesis, or delivery. Laboratory studies include complete blood count, urinalysis or urine culture, blood cultures, and cervical cultures for gonorrhea and chlamydial infection.

Episiotomies may become superficially infected, or the fascia may become involved in more extensive infection. For superficial infection with local erythema and tenderness the perineal incision should be opened to allow drainage and spontaneous healing. No attempt should be made to repair the infected wound. Sitz baths and warm water are helpful for cleaning and symptomatic relief. If an abscess is suspected, the patient should be referred for incision and drainage. Necrotizing fasciitis, a deep infection involving the fascia, is a serious process. Spread along fascial planes occurs quickly and results in sepsis and sometimes death. The key to diagnosis is the appearance of cool, necrotic skin, often with a serosanguineous exudate. If this condition is suspected, an obstetrician or surgeon should be notified and plans made for admission, antibiotic therapy, fluid and electrolyte support, and immediate debridement in the operating room.

Postpartum endometritis is associated with fever, uterine tenderness, and foul lochia. It may occur after vaginal or cesarean delivery. Urinary tract infection needs to be excluded. Complete blood count, urinalysis, and blood cultures may be helpful. An obstetrician should be consulted.

46   Ectopic Pregnancy

One of the leading causes of maternal morbidity and mortality in the United States is ectopic pregnancy. It is also a major factor in decreasing the patient's future fertility. The frequency of ectopic pregnancies in the United States has tripled since 1970. It is estimated that out of 100 women with a history of ectopic pregnancy, approximately 50% will be infertile, 35% to 40% will subsequently have a successful pregnancy, and 10% to 15% will experience a second ectopic pregnancy. Ectopic pregnancy is the result of implantation of a fertilized ovum at a site other than the endometrium of the uterine cavity (Figure 46-1). The most frequent site of implantation is the lateral two thirds of the fallopian tube (80%). Interstitial and abdominal implantations carry the greatest risk of mortality because of their hemorrhagic tendencies. Combined intrauterine and extrauterine gestations are rare and are estimated to occur 1 in 30,000 pregnancies. The most common predisposing factors include intrinsic or extrinsic abnormalities of the fallopian tube and abnormal development of the embryo itself.

Abnormalities of the fallopian tube are believed to be the most important cause of ectopic pregnancies. The most common source of tubal pathology is pelvic inflammatory disease (PID). The risk of ectopic pregnancy is known to be several times more likely among women with a history of salpingitis. All pathogens, including *Chlamydia* and gonococci, are believed to cause tubal distortion and scarring. Subacute infection with less virulent organisms may actually increase the amount of residual tubal pathology because diagnosis and treatment may be delayed.

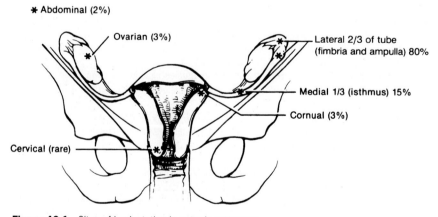

Figure 46-1. Sites of implantation in ectopic pregnancy.

There are multiple risk factors for developing an ectopic pregnancy: (1) Age is a relative risk factor, with ectopics increased with maternal age. (2) Fourteen percent of all pregnancies in women currently wearing an intrauterine device (IUD) are ectopic. (3) PID is universally accepted as the major causative factor. Major risk factors for PID are age in the 20s, divorce, and marital separation. Rates for nonwhite women are 2.5 times higher than those for white women. (4) Tubal sterilization: 16% of women who become pregnant after tubal sterilization have an ectopic gestation. (5) Elective abortion within the preceding 2 weeks and symptoms referable to the genital tract suggests an undiagnosed ectopic pregnancy. Confirmation of the products of uterine extraction are necessary to exclude ectopic pregnancy.

The major life-threatening condition associated with an ectopic pregnancy is intra-abdominal hemorrhage, the cause of death in approximately 85%. Misdiagnosis by physicians contributes to 50% of the fatalities.

CLINICAL PRESENTATION

Any patient with lower abdominal pain or vaginal bleeding with a positive pregnancy test in the first trimester should be suspected of having an ectopic pregnancy. The "classic" triad of amenorrhea, vaginal bleeding, and abdominal pain is neither sensitive (15%) nor specific (14%) for ectopic pregnancy. Abdominal pain is the most common symptom (97%). Abnormal vaginal bleeding is present in 55% to 86%. A "normal" menstrual history is obtained in 15% to 30% of patients. Abdominal pain occurs *without* bleeding in 33%. The quality, character, and location of the pain are highly variable. Flank or lower back pain may be noted, or tenesmus from rectal irritation caused by blood in the cul-de-sac. The pain may be localized to either lower quadrant or may be generalized, suggesting hemoperitoneum. Profuse vaginal hemorrhage occurs in the minority of cases and suggests rupture of a cornual implantation. Vital signs are often normal except in significant blood loss (orthostatic hypotension, tachycardia, or frank shock). Any woman of childbearing age who presents with signs of hemorrhagic shock without evidence of trauma has a ruptured ectopic pregnancy until proved otherwise. Fever is seldom present. Tenderness on pelvic examination is the most common sign and is present in 83% to 97%. The physical findings depend on whether intraperitoneal irritation has occurred from leakage or rupture of the ectopic gestation. Palpable masses are nondiagnostic and may even be felt on the side opposite the ectopic gestation.

DIFFERENTIAL DIAGNOSIS

The differential diagnosis of ectopic pregnancy is broad: PID, threatened or incomplete abortion, corpus luteum or follicular cyst, ovarian cyst with a twisted pedicle, endometriosis, dysfunctional uterine bleeding, and mittelschmerz. PID is the diagnosis most commonly confused with ectopic pregnancy. The signs and symptoms may be identical and the same population is at risk. A significant percentage of normal intrauterine pregnancies are associated with pelvic pain and vaginal bleeding in the first trimester, as are almost all cases of nonviable intrauterine pregnancies. Rupture of a corpus luteum cyst of pregnancy is associated with a positive pregnancy test, pain, and a tender pelvic mass, symptoms identical to an ectopic pregnancy. Gastrointestinal disorders include appendicitis, diverticulitis, irritable bowel syndrome, and gastroenteritis. Nephrolithiasis should also be considered. Patients with a history of tubal ligation, an IUD in place or recently removed, or a recent history of an elective or spontaneous abortion are at *increased risk of mortality* because of the failure to consider ectopic pregnancy.

EMERGENCY DEPARTMENT EVALUATION

Emphasize the patient's reproductive past, menstrual history, risk factors and review of the symptoms. A physical examination should focus on changes associated with normal pregnancy and signs of peritoneal inflammation or significant blood loss. Uterine size, adnexal masses, appearance of cervix and os, and rectal examination should be noted. Pelvic examination should be repeated only as necessary because overly aggressive palpation may precipitate rupture. Laboratory studies include a urinalysis and a pregnancy test. A hematocrit and a blood bank specimen may be necessary. Other laboratory tests are nonspecific and seldom useful. Sensitive urine pregnancy tests with a human chorionic gonadotropin (hCG) threshold of 50 mIU/mL should be used as a screening test for possible ectopic gestation. It allows detection of pregnancy at 1 week postconception (3 weeks' gestation).

Almost all patients with an ectopic pregnancy will have a positive pregnancy test if the threshold for hCG is 50 mIU/mL. A patient suspected of an ectopic who has a negative urine pregnancy test should have a serum beta-hCG radioimmunoassay. Stable patients may benefit from quantitative serum hCG level determinations. Serum beta-hCG levels rise exponentially during the first 6 weeks of gestation and peak at approximately 100,000 mIU/mL. A single quantitative serum beta-hCG serves as an objective substitute for a menstrual history (i.e., it dates the pregnancy). This becomes important because 1/3 of patients with an ectopic pregnancy cannot recall the date of their last menstrual period.

Serial quantitative serum beta-hCG levels double every 2 days in early *intrauterine* pregnancies. Abnormal gestations, both intrauterine and extrauterine, have prolonged doubling times. Patients in whom serum beta-hCG levels do not increase by more than 66% (1.66-fold increase) in 48 hours are likely to harbor an abnormal pregnancy. Serial serum quantitative beta-hCG determinations can be used in stable patients to more accurately detect a nonviable intrauterine or ectopic gestation.

The gestational sac of a normal intrauterine pregnancy becomes visible with ultrasonography at 5 to 6 weeks' gestation, corresponding to a quantitative beta-hCG of 6000 to 6500 mIU/mL. This is often referred to as the discriminatory zone. However, ultrasonography is operator-dependent and has a high incidence of nonspecific findings with gestational ages earlier than 5 to 6 weeks. False-negative and false-positive results occur in up to 25% of patients. Although a positive diagnosis of ectopic pregnancy can be made by identifying an extrauterine gestation, this is a rare finding. In practice, ultrasonography is more helpful in excluding the diagnosis when it demonstrates an intrauterine pregnancy. The correlation of sonographic findings with quantitative serum beta-hCG levels increases the accuracy of diagnosis in ectopic pregnancy. This is especially true if the quantitative beta-hCG level is above the discriminatory zone. The absence of a gestational sac with a serum beta-hCG titer of 6500 mIU/mL has a sensitivity of 100%, a specificity of 96%, a positive predictive value of 86%, and a negative predictive value of 100% for the diagnosis of ectopic pregnancy.

In summary, urine hCG screens for pregnancy and ultrasonography locates it. A single quantitative serum beta-hCG is used to date the pregnancy and increase the accuracy of sonographic results, while serial quantitative levels merely tell the clinician whether or not the pregnancy is behaving in a normal biochemical manner. Because pregnancy can be biochemically detected at approximately 3 weeks' gestation but cannot be located reliably with ultrasonography until 5 to 6 weeks' gestation, a 2- to 3-week period of uncertainty exists. During this period a pregnancy can be detected but cannot be located by noninvasive means. Reliable and stable patients during the period of uncertainty are best evaluated by serial serum quantitative beta-hCG levels.

Culdocentesis may be used when ultrasonography is not immediately available or when ultrasonography results are equivocal. A positive test is one in which nonclotting blood is aspirated from the cul-de-sac with a hematocrit higher than 15%. A "dry tap" is nondiagnostic. A negative tap occurs when clear fluid is obtained. More recently, laparascopic evaluation is a diagnostic alternative.

EMERGENCY DEPARTMENT MANAGEMENT

Management is guided by the hemodynamic status and reliability for follow-up. Hemorrhagic shock is treated with a minimum of two large-bore peripheral intravenous lines and crystalloid infusion. Baseline blood samples should be obtained in addition to a clot tube for the blood bank. Transfusion with O negative, type-specific, or fully crossmatched blood should be considered after crystalloid infusion, depending on the infusion urgency and response of the patient to initial therapy. Immediate gynecologic consultation for laparotomy should be obtained.

Patients who are stable but have potential for rapid progression need two large-bore intravenous lines, complete blood count, Rh typing, typing and screening, and a sensitive urine pregnancy test. Ultrasonography should be used if immediately available. Culdocentesis is used if ultrasonography results are nondiagnostic or if ultrasonography is not available. Urgent consultation is indicated.

Patients who are stable and ambulatory pose the greatest diagnostic and management problems. The evaluation of a possible ectopic pregnancy starts with a urine pregnancy test on all women of childbearing age who present with abdominopelvic pain. **The only exception is the woman who has had a hysterectomy.** The presence of an IUD, tubal ligation, a partner with a vasectomy, or incidental trauma should not deter consideration of an ectopic pregnancy. The diagnosis should be pursued until reasonably ruled out.

DISPOSITION

ROLE OF THE CONSULTANT   There should be a low threshold for requesting consultation from the gynecology, radiology, and surgery services. Early notification of consulting services may allow early mobilization of operating room personnel.

INDICATIONS FOR ADMISSION   All unstable patients require admission. Stable patients may be discharged after consultation with gynecologic follow-up in 48 hours. The usual timing of follow-up is 48 hours, the standard sampling interval for quantitative serum beta-hCG levels. **Exceptions to this are:**

- Positive culdocentesis
- Progressive symptomatology or physical findings
- When no intrauterine pregnancy can be visualized on ultrasonography in a symptomatic patient or in a patient with a quantitative serum beta-hCG level above the discriminatory zone
- Patients unreliable for follow-up

COMMON PITFALLS

- The most common pitfall is failure to consider the diagnosis.
- Ultrasonography and culdocentesis are of limited sensitivity and specificity.
- Women who have undergone tubal sterilization, have an IUD in place or recently removed, and recent spontaneous or therapeutic abortion suffer from delays in diagnosis because the clinician may not be aware that ectopic pregnancy **does** occur in these groups and must be ruled out.

47   Emergency Delivery

CLINICAL PRESENTATION

A rather dependable sign of the approach of labor is the "show" or "bloody show." Representing extrusion of the mucous plug that filled the cervical canal during pregnancy, show consists of a small amount of blood-tinged mucus discharged from the vagina. Bloody show must be distinguished from more active third trimester vaginal bleeding, which is classified as a true emergency and in which vaginal examination is contraindicated due to the possibility of dislodging a placenta previa.

Spontaneous rupture of the membranes usually occurs during the course of active labor and is manifested by a sudden gush of clear or slightly turbid fluid from the vagina. On sterile speculum examination fluid extruding from the cervical os or present in the vaginal fornix will help to verify rupture of the membranes. Amniotic fluid may be differentiated from vaginal fluid by placing a drop of the fluid on nitrazine paper. Amniotic fluid has a pH of 7.0 to 7.5 and will turn the paper deep green or blue; in the presence of vaginal secretions only, pH 4.5 to 5.5, nitrazine paper will remain yellow. Because of its neutral pH, blood in the vaginal vault may result in a falsely positive nitrazine test. Although less common, ferning may also be used to differentiate amniotic from vaginal fluid.

Recognition of rupture of the membranes is significant for three reasons. First, labor may be imminent. Second, if the presenting part of the fetus is not already fixed in the pelvis, cord prolapse and compression are likely and may result in fetal distress. Finally, if labor does not begin within 24 hours of rupture, the pregnancy may be complicated by premature rupture of the membranes with an increased incidence of intrauterine infection. Hospital admission should be considered for any patient in whom rupture of the membranes is documented.

EMERGENCY DEPARTMENT EVALUATION

The general condition of the mother and the fetus must be quickly ascertained. If time is available, a brief obstetric history should be obtained. Information concerning gravidity, parity, estimated date of confinement, problems with the pregnancy, and recent history of vaginal bleed or loss of amniotic fluid should be obtained. In the absence of vaginal bleeding the position, presentation, and lie of the fetus as well as staging of labor are determined by abdominal palpation and sterile vaginal examination. Fetal well-being is ascertained by auscultation of fetal heart rate (FHR).

EVALUATION OF THE FETUS
The examination should begin by determining the FHR. Normal FHR ranges between 120 and 160 beats per minute. During the first stage of labor FHR should be monitored every 15 minutes and during the second stage, every 5 minutes, with particular attention to the first 30 seconds after a contraction. Any prolonged bradycardia, prolonged tachycardia or bradycardia after a contraction (late decelerations) may indicate fetal distress. When fetal distress is suspected the mother should be placed in the left lateral recumbent position, supplemental oxygen administered, and arrangements made to expedite delivery. In the absence of bleeding a vaginal examination should be performed to rule out the possibility of umbilical cord prolapse.

Prolapse allows the cord to pass ahead of the fetus, where it is susceptible to compression by uterine contractions. Usually occurring at the time of rupture of the membranes, cord prolapse is diagnosed by palpation of the umbilical cord on vaginal examination or by visualization of the cord protruding through the introitus. Treatment consists of lessening pressure on the cord and effecting delivery as soon as possible. Compression of the umbilical cord can be minimized by exerting manual pressure through the vagina to lift and maintain the presenting part away from the prolapsed cord. Simultaneously the patient should be placed in the knee-chest or deep Trendelenburg position.

LIE, PRESENTATION, AND POSITION

At or near term more than 95% of presentations are vertex and approximately 4% are breech.

VAGINAL EXAMINATION
Unless there has been bleeding in excess of a bloody show, a manual (not speculum) vaginal examination should be performed to assess the progress of labor and confirm fetal presentation and position. Cervical effacement, dilatation, and fetal station are then assessed.

MANAGEMENT OF DELIVERY

Full dilatation of the cervix signifies the second stage of labor, heralding delivery of the infant. Imminent delivery occurs late in the second stage of labor. It is characterized by uncontrollable bearing-down movements of the mother, pressure on the rectal tissue resulting in the urge to defecate, and perineal bulging with eventual crowning of the fetal head. Delivery of the infant usually occurs spontaneously. The role of the physician is principally to provide control of the process, preventing forceful, sudden expulsion or extraction of the infant with resultant fetal and maternal injury. When delivery is imminent a large-bore IV line of crystalloid should be started and the patient placed on a stretcher with her hips and knees partially flexed, the thighs abducted, and the soles placed firmly on the stretcher. A bedpan placed beneath the patient's buttocks will enhance the delivery position by providing additional space between the bed and the perineum. Although complete sterility is not a priority, when time permits, the perineum should be cleansed, the perineal area draped, and the physician's hands sterilely gloved.

VERTEX DELIVERY

Spontaneous delivery of the vertex-presenting infant is divided into three stages: delivery of the head, delivery of the shoulders, and delivery of the body and legs (Figure 47-1). Gentle, gradual, controlled delivery is desirable. As the fetal head progressively becomes visible, the physician places one hand over the occipital area, providing gentle pressure to control delivery of the head. The other hand, preferably draped with a sterile towel, may exert forward pressure on the chin of the fetus through the perineum just in front of the coccyx. The head is gently supported during subsequent delivery of the forehead, face, chin, and neck. After the head has been delivered the infant's face and mouth should be quickly wiped and the oral cavity and nares suctioned with a bulb syringe. As the neck is delivered a finger should be passed around the neck to determine if it is encircled by the umbilical cord. If present, the cord should be gently loosened and slipped over the infant's head. If this cannot be done easily, the cord should be doubly clamped and cut and the infant delivered *promptly*.

After delivery of the head external rotation occurs. In most cases the shoulders are born spontaneously. The head is then gently lifted upward to aid delivery of the posterior shoulder. The remainder of the body usually follows without difficulty. After delivery the infant should be held in a horizontal to slightly head down position at the level of the introitus to promote drainage of accumulated mucus and bronchial secretions. Additional suctioning of the nose and mouth with a bulb syringe is performed. The umbilical cord is clamped twice and cut between the clamps as soon as possible after delivery. Blood samples from the placental end of the cord are collected for infant serology, including rhesus factor (Rh). A sterile cord clamp or tie of umbilical tape is placed around the infant cord 1 cm to 3 cm distal to the navel. Immediately after cutting the umbilical cord the infant should be briefly evaluated. Maintain body temperature by placing the neonate in warm blankets and a heated isolette when available. One- and 5-minute Apgar scores should be ascertained.

DELIVERY OF THE PLACENTA

Separation of the placenta usually occurs within 5 to 10 minutes of delivery of the infant. Once the placenta has separated, it can be delivered by suprapubic uterine pressure and minimal umbilical cord traction. One hand is placed on the abdomen just above the symphysis pubis and pressure is applied in a posterior, slightly cephalad direction. As the placenta passes through the vagina, fundal pressure is stopped and the placenta is gently lifted away from the introitus. Traction should never be used to pull the placenta out of the uterus, since traction may result in uterine inversion. The placenta should be examined for completeness and saved for later evaluation by the obstetrician. After delivery of the placenta gentle massage and an oxytocic agent are used to further stimulate uterine contractions. Oxytocin (Pitocin) is the most commonly used oxy-

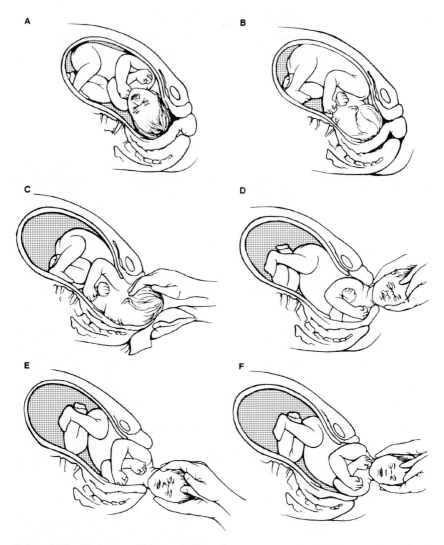

Figure 47-1. Mechanism of labor and delivery for vertex presentation. (**A**) Engagement, flexion, and descent. (**B**) Internal rotation. (**C**) Extension and delivery of the head using the modified Ritgen maneuver. After delivery of the head the infant's nose and mouth should be suctioned and the neck checked for encirclement of the umbilical cord. (**D**) External rotation bringing the thorax into the anteroposterior diameter of the pelvis. (**E**) Delivery of the anterior shoulder. (**F**) Delivery of the posterior shoulder. Note that after delivery, the head is supported and used to gently guide delivery of the shoulder. Traction should be minimized.

tocic. Typically, 20 units of oxytocin are added to 1 L of normal saline solution and given intravenously at a rate of 10 mL/min until the uterus remains firmly contracted and bleeding is controlled. The infusion rate is then reduced to 1 mL to 2 mL/min. Oxytocics should not be used before delivery of the placenta.

EPISIOTOMY

The purpose of the episiotomy is to limit maternal trauma and facilitate the second stage of labor by reducing perineal resistance. With the exception of deliveries of grand multiparous patients, episiotomies should be performed on all ED deliveries. The median episiotomy is preferred. There is general agreement that with vertex deliveries, the episiotomy should be performed when the fetal head begins to distend the perineum. Emergency anesthesia is usually limited to local infiltration with 1% or 2% lidocaine. Episiotomy is most often performed with blunt surgical scissors. Median episiotomies are performed along the median raphe of the perineum, and extend from the introitus down to, *but not including,* the anal sphincter. Once the episiotomy is completed, preparations for delivery of the head may be continued. Repair of the episiotomy is performed after delivery of the infant and placenta and after inspection and repair, if necessary, of any lacerations of the cervix and vaginal canal. An absorbable suture such as 2-0 or 3-0 chromic catgut or polyglycolic acid on a large, atraumatic needle is preferred.

DISPOSITION

In hospitals with full obstetric services, unless the patient is crowning, there is usually time to safely transfer the patient to the delivery room. In hospitals without obstetric facilities the decision to transfer the patient to another institution is a difficult one and is best made after consultation with the attending obstetrician. Factors that influence the decision to transfer include the parity of the patient, the degree of cervical effacement and dilatation, fetal station, and the distance to the receiving hospital. In high-risk pregnancies and those in which the infant is felt to be premature, delivery is usually better handled in an institution with full obstetric and neonatal facilities. When transfer is indicated, the minimal acceptable standard is a fully equipped advanced life support unit. Accompaniment by a physician for all high-risk pregnancies is desirable. In some areas, because of distance or logistics, aeromedical transport may be advantageous.

COMMON PITFALLS

- Vaginal bleeding: During the third trimester of pregnancy vaginal bleeding in excess of that of a bloody show should always be viewed as an emergency. Because of the possibility of dislodging a placenta previa and causing exsanguinating hemorrhage, pelvic examination should be deferred and the patient taken immediately to the labor and delivery area for further evaluation and management.
- Fetal distress: After ensuring stability of the mother immediate attention must be directed to the fetus by monitoring FHR, particularly during the first 30 seconds after a contraction.
- Excessive force during delivery: Delivery usually occurs spontaneously; it is the physician's role to provide gentle guidance of the birth process. Excessive or inappropriately applied traction can result in fetal or maternal injury.
- Delivery of the placenta: Traction should never be used to pull the placenta out of the uterus (uterine inversion may occur).

48   Peripartum and Postpartum Emergencies

THIRD TRIMESTER BLEEDING

Bleeding during the third trimester complicates up to 3% of all pregnancies. Placenta previa and abruptio placenta are the major causes of significant bleeding during the latter part of pregnancy and account for 50% of all bleeding episodes.

Placenta previa is placental implantation in the lower uterine segment adjacent to or over the internal os. Occurring in about 0.5% of pregnancies, its cause is unknown. Placenta previa is more common in multiple pregnancies, in patients with previous surgical scars, and in grand multiparous patients. **Abruptio placenta** refers to the premature separation of a normally implanted placenta from the uterine wall. Separation may be partial or complete. Blood dissects from the separation to the cervical os, causing external bleeding in 80%. In 20% bleeding may remain concealed behind the placental separation. The cause of placental abruption is unknown. Occurring in 0.5% to 2.7% of pregnancies, abruption tends to occur in patients with diseases that predispose to vascular injury, such as preeclampsia–eclampsia, chronic hypertension, diabetes mellitis, and chronic renal disease. Mechanical factors that contribute to placental abruption are uncommon; perhaps the most significant is abdominal trauma during late pregnancy.

CLINICAL PRESENTATION

Placenta Previa: Painless, bright red vaginal bleeding may occur in a pregnancy previously believed to be uncomplicated. Although spotting may occur during the first two trimesters, the first episode of significant hemorrhage usually begins after the 28th week of gestation and is seldom fatal. The uterus is usually soft, relaxed, and nontender. In contrast to abruptio placenta, coagulation studies are usually normal. Maternal mortality is <1%. Prematurity and maternal hypovolemic shock are major causes of perinatal mortality; the perinatal mortality rate in major medical centers ranges from 15% to 25%.

Abruptio placenta classically presents with dark red, painful bleeding. Abdominal pain is common. Examination reveals a firm, irritable uterus. The presentation varies greatly and depends on the extent of placental separation and the degree of concealment of bleeding behind the placenta. Vaginal bleeding may range from absent to heavy; pain may range from mild to severe. If abruption is extensive, fetal distress will be evident. Because of retroplacental clotting, large amounts of thromboplastin are released into the maternal circulation, depleting fibrinogen levels and leading to disseminated intravascular coagulation (DIC). Defects in blood coagulation are evident in 20% to 38% of cases. Maternal mortality is seldom >1%. Fetal mortality depends on the degree of placental separation, and may approach 35%.

DIFFERENTIAL DIAGNOSIS

The differential diagnosis of third trimester bleeding ranges from that of normal labor to that of catastrophic uterine rupture. Varying severity and presentation may make the cause of bleeding difficult to recognize with certainty. The diagnosis is often made by exclusion. Uterine rupture is an uncommon cause of vaginal bleeding, and may result from major trauma or occur during overzealous use of oxytocin for stimulation of labor. The latter situation usually occurs in multiparous patients or in those with previous uterine incisions. Presentation is similar to that of abruptio placenta, with massive painful bleeding, clinical evidence of shock, and an acute abdomen. Other causes include cervical abnormalities such as erosions, polyps, and neoplasms and lacerations of the labia and vagina. Urethral and anal bleeding may be mistaken for vaginal hemorrhage.

EMERGENCY DEPARTMENT EVALUATION

Hemodynamic stability and airway are the main priorities. Maternal blood volume increases by as much as 50% above normal during the latter half of pregnancy; 30% to 35% of maternal blood volume may be lost before clinical signs of hypovolemia develop. Early volume resuscitation is paramount. If the patient is hemodynamically stable, a brief history should be obtained: the estimated date of confinement, the presence of complicating medical conditions such as preeclampsia, an estimate of the amount of bleeding, the presence of abdominal pain, and a history of trauma or prior episodes of bleeding. Initial examination should ascertain the amount of visible bleeding. Abdominal examination determines fundal height and evaluates the uterus for firmness, tenderness, and the presence of contractions. When possible, fetal presentation should be determined. Fetal well-being is most easily assessed by the determination of fetal heart rate; (120 to 160 beats/minute); the earliest sign of fetal distress is bradycardia (<110 beats/minute).

The role of pelvic examination is disputed. Some believe that in a controlled environment, a gentle speculum examination can aid in the exclusion of local causes of bleeding such as vaginal or vulvar lacerations. In the presence of placenta previa, manual vaginal or rectal examination may dislodge the placenta and precipitate massive, catastrophic hemorrhage. Manual pelvic examination as well as sterile speculum examination should, therefore, probably be deferred to the obstetrician. If the patient is hemodynamically stable, the patient should be referred for immediate ultrasonography for placental localization.

If the patient is unstable, she should be transferred to the operating room for examination under "double setup" conditions, allowing for immediate cesarean delivery, if necessary. Ultrasonography is the initial diagnostic method of choice with third trimester bleeding and is highly accurate for the detection of placenta previa (93% to 98%). Ultrasonography has little value in the diagnosis of abruptio placenta. The main value of ultrasonography, therefore, is to exclude the diagnosis of placenta previa.

Initial laboratory studies: type and crossmatching of blood, a complete blood count, renal function studies, and a coagulation profile, including fibrinogen level. If the potential for DIC exists, type and crossmatching should include that for fresh frozen plasma.

EMERGENCY DEPARTMENT MANAGEMENT

Stabilize the patient and obtain appropriate obstetric consultation. Ensure an adequate airway and maintain ventilation and perfusion. Two large-bore intravenous lines should be inserted to infuse crystalloid. The hypotensive patient should be placed in the left lateral decubitus position to relieve vena caval compression. This simple change in position can increase cardiac output by as much as 30%. A central venous catheter will allow monitoring of fluid status. A Foley catheter is useful in monitoring urine output and the adequacy of effective circulating volume. Because large volumes of crystalloid will not prevent fetal hypoxia, early replacement of red cells after crossmatching of blood is indicated. When massive hemorrhage affects maternal hemodynamic stability and time precludes proper crossmatching of blood, type-specific blood may be used. Uncrossmatched type O, Rh-negative blood can be used if type-specific blood is unavailable. When the possibility of DIC exists fresh frozen plasma should be available.

Definitive treatment for both placenta previa and abruptio placenta requires an obstetrician and depends on the severity of hemorrhage and the gestational age and health of the fetus. In placenta previa if the fetus is immature and the bleeding slight, conservative observation and bed rest is normally used. If the fetus is mature and hemorrhage is heavy, delivery, usually by cesarean section, is indicated. Similarly, with abruptio placenta expectant management may be used when the fetus is immature, bleeding is slight, and uterine irritability is absent or minimal. In patients with more severe abruption, cesarean delivery or, in selected cases, vaginal delivery is indicated.

DISPOSITION

Unless bleeding is obviously due to local causes, all patients with vaginal bleeding during the third trimester require admission to an obstetric unit for observation, fetal monitoring, and ultrasonography. Because of the possibility of prematurity and fetal hypoxia at delivery, most patients are best managed in a facility where obstetric and perinatal services are immediately available. The appropriateness of transfer to such a facility depends on the stability of the mother, degree of fetal distress, and time and distance to the receiving center. Minimally, a fully equipped advanced life support unit is required, preferably with a physician in attendance. In certain areas distance and time constraints may make aeromedical transport the method of choice.

COMMON PITFALLS

- Because of the possibility of dislodging a placenta previa and precipitating massive hemorrhage, pelvic examination should be deferred, pending obstetric consultation and ultrasonography.
- Because the mother may not manifest clinical signs of shock until losing 30% to 35% of her blood volume, early volume replacement is essential.

POSTPARTUM HEMORRHAGE

Postpartum hemorrhage, maternal blood loss >500 mL after delivery of the fetus, is estimated to occur in 5% to 8% of all pregnancies. Accounting for up to 25% of obstetric deaths from hemorrhage, postpartum hemorrhage is divided into immediate hemorrhage (within 24 hours of delivery) and delayed hemorrhage (>24 hours after delivery). Most cases of **immediate postpartum hemorrhage (IPH)** are due to uterine atony and occur when the myometrium fails to contract. Predisposing maternal conditions include overdistention of the uterus (large or multiple fetuses), prolonged or abnormally rapid labor, high parity, and retention of placental tissue. Other causes of IPH include lacerations to the perineum, vagina, or cervix and, less commonly, coagulopathies, uterine rupture, and inversion of the uterine corpus.

Delayed postpartum hemorrhage (DPH) usually occurs 7 to 14 days after delivery. It most commonly involves retention of placental tissue and subinvolution of the placental site. Involution refers to the process by which the endometrium returns to its normal anatomical state after separation of the placenta. When retained placental tissue or necrotic debris sloughs off the endometrium, open blood vessels are exposed. Because the uterus has no stimulus for contraction and no means to tamponade the exposed vessels, hemorrhage ensues. Other causes of DPH include postpartum endoparametritis and injudicious use of hormones to suppress lactation.

CLINICAL PRESENTATION AND DIFFERENTIAL DIAGNOSIS
IMMEDIATE POSTPARTUM HEMORRHAGE

IPH is frequently characterized by steady, moderate bleeding that persists until serious hypovolemia develops, rather than by sudden massive hemorrhage. Because of the relative hypervolemia of normal pregnancy, significant changes in maternal pulse and blood pressure may not become manifest until blood loss exceeds 1500 mL. Between 75% and 90% of cases of IPH are due to uterine atony. With steady moderate blood flow, the diagnosis is suggested when uterine palpation reveals a soft, boggy uterus. Bimanual pelvic examination is frequently necessary to confirm the diagnosis. With manual massage the uterus may contract and bleeding diminish, only to relax and resume bleeding when massaging stops. Although not common, retained placental tissue and abnormal placental insertion should always be considered as a cause of uterine atony and the placenta carefully inspected for missing tissue and anatomical abnormalities.

Genital tract trauma is the second most frequent cause of IPH and must be considered when vaginal bleeding persists. Examination of the entire lower genital tract should be performed using a speculum, with particular attention paid to the cervix, a common site of lacerations. When bleeding persists and no lacerations are visualized a diagnosis of rupture or laceration of the uterus should be entertained. Diagnosis is usually made by digital examination of the uterine cavity after expulsion of the placenta. Even with manual exploration, however, these lesions may not be felt, particularly when confined to the posterior lower uterine segment. When the diagnosis is suspected provisions should be made for immediate surgical intervention.

Although rare, uterine inversion usually manifests with dramatic hemorrhage and shock. Diagnosis is made by visualization and palpation of the soft, pear-shaped fundal wall near the cervical os or extending through it. On abdominal examination no uterine fundus is felt. Treatment consists of immediate repositioning of the uterine corpus. Unless already completely separated, the placenta should be left attached during repositioning. Although blood loss with uterine inversion averages 1800 mL, with prompt replacement of the uterus the maternal mortality rate approaches zero.

Vulvar and vaginal hematomas are another source of blood loss. Usually occurring within the first 48 hours after delivery, they may appear deceptively small while actually representing dissection of blood into the paravaginal and pararectal tissues. Patients usually complain of severe pain and difficulty with ambulation and urination. Discoloration of the perineum suggests the diagnosis and vaginal examination confirms it. Small hematomas may be treated conservatively with ice packs. The treatment of larger hematomas is controversial, and necessitates consultation with an obstetrician.

Postpartum hemorrhage caused by coagulopathies is quite rare. Medical conditions such as thrombocytopenic purpura, idiopathic thrombocytopenic purpura, and von Willebrand's disease may predispose to obstetric hemorrhage. Confirmation of coagulopathies is based on abnormalities in coagulation studies, including fibrinogen levels.

DELAYED POSTPARTUM HEMORRHAGE

Most commonly occurring 7 to 14 days after delivery, DPH is usually the result of subinvolution of the placental implantation site. The most common causes of subinvolution are retained placental tissue and infection. Patients typically present with sudden, brisk, painless vaginal bleeding that may have been preceded by intermittent spotting or complaints of foul-smelling lochia. The differential diagnosis of DPH must include endometritis and withdrawal of exogenous estrogens. Abdominal examination typically reveals a large, boggy uterus that, in the absence of infection, is not usually painful. Pelvic examination reveals bleeding through the cervical os, and bimanual examination confirms the findings. The presence of fever, purulent discharge, or uterine tenderness suggests infection.

EMERGENCY DEPARTMENT EVALUATION

Evaluation should begin by assessing the degree of blood loss and hemodynamic stability. Abdominal and bimanual examination should be directed toward determining uterine size, position, and consistency. Visual examination of the cervix and vaginal canal should be performed. When available, the placenta should be examined for completeness and structural abnormalities. In all cases of IPH and when DPH is severe, laboratory studies should routinely include a complete blood count and coagulation profile, including a fibrinogen level. Blood should be drawn for type and crossmatching of packed red blood cells and, when coagulopathy is suspected, fresh frozen plasma. When the diagnosis of retained placenta is considered ultrasonography may be useful.

EMERGENCY DEPARTMENT MANAGEMENT
IMMEDIATE POSTPARTUM HEMORRHAGE

When IPH is suspected volume replacement begins with two large-bore intravenous catheters and infusion of Ringer's lactate or normal saline solution. If hemorrhage is severe, transfusion of packed red blood cells should be given. When the possibility of DIC exists fresh frozen plasma should be available. Initial management of uterine atony consists of manual massage of the uterine fundus. Uterine massage is performed with one hand placed on the abdomen to compress the posterior aspect of the uterus while the other gloved, sterile hand is used to gently massage the anterior aspect of the uterus through the vaginal wall. Packing the uterus is contraindicated in the immediate postpartum period and may result in uterine dilatation with concealed, potentially fatal hemorrhage.

Oxytocics should be administered in conjunction with massage and may be given intravenously or intramuscularly. An intravenous oxytocin (Pitocin) drip is prepared by adding 20 to 40 units of oxytocin to 1000 mL normal saline solution or Ringer's lactate and infused at a rate of 200 mL to 500 mL/h. If bleeding persists, an ergotamine preparation such as methylergonovine (Methergine 0.2 mg) may be given intramuscularly to help stimulate uterine contraction. Typically, uterine contractions occur within minutes of administration and persist for several hours. When administered rapidly oxytocin may cause hypotension, which typically resolves after discontinuation of the drug. The most serious side effect of ergot preparations is their tendency to cause vasoconstriction and severe hypertension in some patients. Ergot preparations should, therefore, be avoided in women who are known to be hypertensive.

When vaginal bleeding persists despite the presence of a firm, contracted uterus and therapy for uterine atony, the vagina and cervix should be inspected for lacerations. Bleeding from lacerations may be controlled by direct pressure or, in the case of cervical lacerations, by gentle application of ring forceps to the bleeding point. Repair of easily accessible lacerations with either 00 or 000 absorbable sutures may help to control bleeding. If lacerations are small and numerous, packing the vagina with surgical packs or sterile gauze may be attempted. Because adequate visualization of the cervix and upper vagina is difficult and repair of extensive lacerations frequently requires general anesthesia, repair of these lacerations is often better left to the obstetrician.

Management of refractory postpartum hemorrhage frequently requires operative intervention and the expertise of the obstetrician. Occasionally hysterectomy may be necessary to control persistent uterine bleeding.

DELAYED POSTPARTUM HEMORRHAGE

In the majority of cases DPH is caused by subinvolution of the placental implantation site due to retained placental tissue or infection. Initial treatment consists of administration of either oxytocin (40 units in 1000 mL Ringer's lactate or normal saline solution at a rate of 200 mL to 300 mL/h) or methylergonovine or ergonovine (0.2 mg I.M.). If bleeding is initially mild and stops with oxytocic therapy, the patient is discharged home on methylergonovine or ergonovine (0.2 mg PO every 6 to 12 hours). In such cases necrotic placental tissue is usually carried away with the onset of bleeding, and curettage is usually not necessary. Follow-up should be arranged with an obstetrician in 24 to 48 hours. If bleeding is initially severe or fails to respond to oxytocic therapy, an excessive amount of retained placental tissue should be suspected. Curettage is recommended, and generally necessitates hospital admission. When uterine infection is suspected as the cause of subinvolution, antibiotic therapy should be added to the treatment regimen.

DISPOSITION

All patients with IPH require admission. The level of care depends on hemodynamic stability and initial response to therapy. Transfer to a more specialized facility is indicated if bleeding persists and the appropriate surgical expertise is unavailable. All transfers should be made by an ALS unit.

COMMON PITFALLS

- Immediate postpartum bleeding may be due to multiple causes (e.g., uterine atony plus perineal lacerations). Care should be taken to fully evaluate all causes of bleeding.
- Uterine packing, a possibly dangerous procedure, may result in uterine distention with concealed and potentially fatal hemorrhage. Packing is advocated only in the vaginal area for temporary control of hemorrhage from lacerations that require operative intervention or for hemostasis of multiple small lacerations for which suturing is impractical.

PART IX

Emergency Aspects of Gynecology

49 Gynecologic Causes of Abdominal Pain

Abdominal pain is a common presenting complaint in women. The differentiation of pain of gynecologic origin from that of gastroenteric or urologic origin requires a thorough history and physical examination and use of laboratory tests. Not infrequently ultrasonography, culdocentesis or laparoscopy may be required to make the diagnosis. Specialty consultation is often necessary for consideration of laparoscopy or laparotomy or to provide treatment and follow-up.

CLINICAL PRESENTATION

PELVIC INFLAMMATORY DISEASE PID is discussed in chapter 50.

PERIHEPATITIS Clinical evidence of perihepatitis (Fitz–Hugh–Curtis syndrome) is seen in less than 10% of upper pelvic infections, and is frequently mistaken for acute cholecystitis. Evidence of associated PID is almost invariably overshadowed by the sudden onset of severe, sharp right upper quadrant pain. The pain may have a pleuritic component, and may be referred to the right shoulder. Nausea, vomiting, chills, fever, and generalized malaise may be present.

DYSMENORRHEA Primary dysmenorrhea occurs in adolescents, usually within 1 to 2 years of menarche. Pain occurs just before or coincident with menstruation, and is described as severe, sharp cramps in the suprapubic area.

MITTLESCHMERZ Unilateral adnexal pain at the time of ovulation can result from leakage of blood from the graafian follicle. Sharp, well-localized peritoneal irritation is usually found, with an otherwise normal physical examination. Occasionally symptoms can be severe and more generalized, but they usually resolve within 24 to 48 hours.

OVARIAN CYST HEMORRHAGE OR RUPTURE Hemorrhage into a functional or pathologic cyst can cause sudden, dull, unilateral adnexal pain. Corpus luteum cysts only rarely develop in women who are taking birth control pills, making this diagnosis unlikely. Examination demonstrates a painful adnexa with or without a palpable mass. Ovarian cyst rupture usually results in sudden onset of sharp, unilateral adnexal pain that rarely may become generalized to the entire pelvis or abdomen. Examination demonstrates signs of peritoneal irritation. Culdocentesis or laparoscopy may be necessary to confirm the diagnosis.

ADNEXAL TORSION Twisting of the adnexal structures results in poorly localized, intense, dull ischemic pain, frequently accompanied by nausea and vomiting. The pain may be unilateral, bilateral, or referred to the flank, perineum, or inner thigh. Its onset may be sudden, or intermittent over a period of days. Fifteen percent of cases occur in premenarchal girls.

ENDOMETRIOSIS   Abnormal implantation of endometrial tissue in ectopic sites can be one of medicine's great mimics, depending on the location of the implants. Endometriosis is seen in 8% to 15% of menstruating women of all ages. It causes secondary dysmenorrhea in older women, although it is also seen in adolescents. Patients may present with chronic abdominal pain, dyspareunia, abnormal vaginal bleeding, or infertility, Pelvic examination may demonstrate an immobile uterus and tender nodules in the uterosacral ligaments or rectovaginal septum. Rupture of a cystic implant may cause signs of peritoneal irritation.

UTERINE MYOMATA   Fibroid tumors of the uterus occur more frequently in the late childbearing years, and can be associated with irregular, heavy menstrual periods. These tumors may undergo ischemia, necrosis, hemorrhage, or torsion, causing dull, visceral pelvic pain that may be sudden in onset and associated with nausea and vomiting. Physical examination may demonstrate a painful, enlarged uterus without peritoneal signs. Ultrasonography may demonstrate a uterine mass.

PREGNANCY-RELATED CAUSES OF PELVIC PAIN   Ectopic pregnancy, spontaneous abortion, Braxton–Hicks contractions are covered elsewhere.

DIFFERENTIAL DIAGNOSIS

PREGNANCY-RELATED CAUSES OF ABDOMINAL PAIN
New vaginal probes can visualize the fetus and fetal heart motion at 5 and 6 weeks, respectively. Inability to localize the pregnancy in the uterus by ultrasonography suggests ectopic pregnancy.

GASTROINTESTINAL AND UROLOGIC CAUSES OF ABDOMINAL PAIN
Appendicitis is frequently confused with gynecologic causes of abdominal pain. Useful clinical features include duration of symptoms, significantly shorter in appendicitis than in PID; onset of symptoms during the first 14 days of the menstrual cycle, which is most common in PID; and the presence of nausea and vomiting, which points toward appendicitis. Anorexia, chills, and fever do not help to differentiate the two conditions. A history of venereal disease is helpful in predicting the presence of PID, whereas other gynecologic symptoms are not. Physical findings predictive of PID are cervical motion tenderness and bilateral adnexal tenderness. Isolated right lower quadrant pain is predictive of appendicitis; however, patients with other gynecologic syndromes have findings that are more like those of appendicitis than of PID. White blood cell counts and a higher percentage of polymorphonuclear cells are more common in appendicitis. Appendicitis in pregnancy carries a high morbidity and mortality for both mother and fetus. Pyelonephritis may present as abdominal pain. Percussion of the costophrenic areas and evaluation of the urine sediment lead to the correct diagnosis. Pyelonephritis occurs in 2% of all pregnancies, and must be aggressively treated.

GYNECOLOGIC CAUSES OF ABDOMINAL PAIN
Laparoscopy remains the procedure of choice to confirm the diagnosis in the patient who is acutely ill or has an uncertain diagnosis (Table 49-1). In 60%, PID was confirmed. In 20% of cases laparoscopy was normal, and in the remaining 20% other pathology was found (in order of frequency, bleeding ovarian cyst, ectopic pregnancy, appendicitis, and endometriosis).

EMERGENCY DEPARTMENT EVALUATION

Examination begins with vital signs and orthostatic vital signs in the patient with severe abdominal pain or symptoms of hypovolemia. The vast majority of women with abdominal pain require a gynecologic history and physical examination as part of the evaluation. Laboratory evaluation begins with a qualitative serum or urine pregnancy test sensitive to at least 50 IU/L. Complete blood count and urinalysis are frequently useful, although an elevated white blood cell count is

TABLE 49-1. Correlation Between Clinical and Laparoscopic Diagnosis in 100 Patients With Acute Pelvic Pain

Clinical Diagnosis	No. of Patients	Laparoscopic Diagnosis	No. of Patients
Ectopic pregnancy	36	Ectopic pregnancy	20
		Pelvic inflammatory disease	8
		Bleeding ovarian cysts	4
		Retrograde menstruation	4
Pelvic inflammatory disease	22	Pelvic inflammatory disease	8
		Normal pelvis	6
		Ectopic pregnancy	3
		Ovarian cyst complication	2
		Endometriosis	3
No diagnosis made	30	Normal pelvis	12
		Pelvic inflammatory disease	7
		Ectopic pregnancy	2
		Endometriosis	4
		Ovarian cyst complication	3
		Retrograde menstruation	2
Complication of ovarian cyst and/or endometriosis	9	Ovarian cyst complication	5
		Endometriosis	1
		Normal pelvis	2
		Pelvic inflammatory disease	1
Miscellaneous	3	Failed laparoscopy	2
		Ectopic pregnancy	1
Total	**100**		**100**

From Med J Aust. Copyright 1981. Reprinted with permission.

nonspecific. A wet mount of vaginal secretions containing predominantly leukocytes and bacteria indicates lower genital tract infection with or without salpingitis. Gram's stain of the cervix, if positive for gonorrhea, is 97% specific. Cervical cultures for gonorrhea and chlamydial infection are indicated if venereal disease is suspected. Other laboratory studies are seldom helpful. Ultrasonography is extremely useful in localizing a pregnancy.

EMERGENCY DEPARTMENT MANAGEMENT

PID management is described elsewhere. Dysmenorrhea is treated with reassurance and an antiprostaglandin agent such as ibuprofen or indomethasone. Mittleschmerz is usually a self-limited condition that requires reassurance and, occasionally, analgesics. Ovarian cyst hemorrhage or rupture is usually self-limited, with symptoms resolving in a few days. Rarely will transfusion or surgery be required. Adnexal torsion requires surgery or, on rare occasion, can be derotated through the laparoscope. Diagnosis is seldom made preoperatively, and the salvage rate of the torsed adnexia is low. Endometriosis seldom requires emergency treatment beyond analgesics and close follow-up, unless intraperitoneal bleeding has occurred. Uterine myomata may require acute surgical intervention if torsion or significant ischemic necrosis occurs.

DISPOSITION

ROLE OF THE CONSULTANT   The key to management of gynecologic pain is to determine which patients may have potentially serious acute medical or surgical conditions, to obtain gynecologic consultation for possible laparoscopic confirmation when diagnosis is obscure or when significant peritoneal signs exist, and to admit those patients to the hospital who require acute medical or surgical treatment or prolonged observation to rule out serious disease.

INDICATIONS FOR ADMISSION   Admission criteria are influenced by the diagnosis and stability of the patient's vital signs, the patient's reliability and willingness to follow instructions for treatment and follow-up, and the patient's access to medical care as an outpatient.

COMMON PITFALLS

- Failure to perform a pelvic examination in almost every woman beyond the age of menarche with abdominal pain.
- Failure to rule out ectopic pregnancy.
- Missed diagnosis of gynecologic and gastroenteric causes of abdominal pain in pregnant patients.
- Diagnosis based on history, physical examination, and laboratory tests alone. The various causes of gynecologic pain have overlapping signs and symptoms and frequently cannot be differentiated without laparoscopy. The classic error is the overdiagnosis of PID.
- Overinterpretation of ultrasonography results. Ultrasonography has limits. The physician should beware of accepting the diagnosis of intrauterine pregnancy until the fetal pole can be seen at 6 weeks.
- Failure to obtain gynecologic consultation and follow-up appropriately.

---

50   Pelvic Inflammatory Disease

Pelvic inflammatory disease (PID) is a common diagnosis; however, the term PID itself is a misnomer. The more descriptive nomenclature is endometritis, salpingitis, or parametritis. Most pelvic infections are secondary to sexually transmitted diseases. The two major pathogens are *Neisseria gonorrhoeae* and *Chlamydia trachomatis*. Other agents include *Mycoplasma* species, anaerobes, and *Haemophilus* species. Endometritis and salpingitis are more common among lower socioeconomic groups. Because the diseases are sexually transmitted, the peak incidence is during the childbearing ages, when women are most active sexually. Child abuse must be suspected in any prepubertal female with the diagnosis of salpingitis.

CLINICAL PRESENTATION

The patient with pelvic infection almost invariably presents with lower abdominal pain. Inflammation of the endometrium, fallopian tubes, and parametrial structures usually produces diffuse bilateral pelvic pain. Most women complain of dull, constant, poorly localized pain. *N. gonorrhoeae* or *C. trachomatis* cervicitis results in a vaginal discharge in >50% of patients, while involvement of the uterine lining produces abnormal vaginal bleeding in another 30%. Urinary tract symptoms are common. Almost 20% of patients with laparoscopically proven pelvic infection have irritative voiding symptoms. A temperature above 38°C (100.4°F) may be seen in only 1/3. Findings are frequently limited to the lower quadrants, unless a perihepatitis is also present.

Tenderness is present on palpation of both lower quadrants, although one side may be more tender. Rebound tenderness indicates a severe infection, and true peritoneal extension

TABLE 50-1. Criteria for Diagnosis of Acute Pelvic Infections

All Three of the Following Should Be Present:
1. Lower abdominal tenderness
2. Cervical motion tenderness
3. Adnexal tenderness (may be unilateral)

plus

One of the Following Should Be Present:
1. Temperature ≥38°C
2. White blood cell count ≥10,500/µl
3. Purulent material obtained by culdocentesis
4. An inflammatory mass present on bimanual pelvic examination or sonography
5. Erythrocyte sedimentation rate >15 mm/h
6. Evidence of the presence of *N. gonorrhoeae* or *C. trachomatis* in the endocervix
    *   Gram's stain reveals gram-negative intracellular diplococci
    *   Monoclonal antibody for *C. trachomatis*
7. Presence of >5 white blood cells per oil-immersion field on Gram's stain of endocervical discharge

Labadie LL: Obstetric and gynecologic emergencies. Emer Med Clin North Am 8: 452, 1987.

should be considered. Speculum examination may reveal a vaginal discharge. If present, discharge supports the diagnosis; when absent, it does not exclude it. A markedly inflamed purulent cervix is indicative of an acute cervicitis and supportive of some degree of pelvic infection. Bimanual examination begins with testing for cervical motion tenderness. Pain with either lateral or anteroposterior motion of the cervix is strongly supportive of pelvic infection. The uterus is frequently firm but tender. Both adnexae are tender but may be difficult to delineate. An adnexal mass may be appreciated but is not a consistent finding in the absence of a tubo-ovarian abscess. See Table 50-1 for a summary of diagnostic criteria of PID.

DIFFERENTIAL DIAGNOSIS

Possible diagnoses include ectopic pregnancy, salpingitis, and appendicitis. Ovarian cyst, urinary tract infection, hernia, and ovarian torsion should also be considered. The diagnosis of salpingitis should be considered only after ectopic pregnancy has been ruled out. The coexistence of infection and pregnancy is possible but unusual because after implantation a mucous plug forms that usually prevents the spread of lower genital infection into the upper genital system. Appendicitis may be differentiated from salpingitis by its unilateral nature.

EMERGENCY DEPARTMENT EVALUATION

Cervical cultures should be done on all patients. In those patients in whom the diagnosis is suspected on clinical grounds alone, a gonococcal culture should be taken and empirical treatment for both *N. gonorrhoeae* and *C. trachomatis* be given. Urinalysis, complete blood count, and a urine or serum pregnancy test should be done. In toxic patients with severe unilateral symptoms pelvic ultrasonography may help to confirm a tubo-ovarian abscess, although laparoscopy is more accurate. Serum samples for syphilis and AIDS may be indicated.

EMERGENCY DEPARTMENT MANAGEMENT

The goal of treatment is to prevent infertility, ectopic pregnancy, and chronic infection. Selection of the appropriate antimicrobial combination depends on the current recommendations of the local

TABLE 50-2. Indications for Admission

Appearance of toxicity, regardless of other findings
Temperature greater than 39°C
Suspected tubo-ovarian or pelvic abscess
Nausea and vomiting precluding oral therapy
Failure to improve with outpatient therapy within 72 hours
White blood cell count greater than 11,000/µL
Evidence of spread outside pelvis (Fitz-Hugh-Curtis syndrome)
Pregnancy
Adolescence
Peritonitis
Unclear diagnosis—need for laparoscopy
Intrauterine device
Adolescents, nulligravidas

public health department and the CDC. Because concomitant infection with *N. gonorrhoeae* and *C. trachomatis* is possible and it is clinically difficult to distinguish one type of infection from the other, begin empiric treatment with antibiotics that are active against both pathogens. Ceftriaxone (250 mg IM) may be used. Chlamydial coverage is provided with 10 days of doxycycline (100 mg twice daily) or azithromycin (1 g PO once).

DISPOSITION

All patients should receive follow-up care in 2 to 3 days after discharge, at which time the patient's cultures should be available. Admission criteria are summarized in Table 50-2. Most admitted patients are treated with anaerobic coverage: Metronidazole, clindamycin and gentamicin. Cefoxitin and doxycycline are also used.

COMMON PITFALLS

- The most serious problem is the *overapplication* of the diagnosis pelvic infection to every female patient with abdominal pain.
- If the clinical picture suggests pelvic infection, it is better to initiate treatment early, especially for nulligravida patients.
- Be diligent in ruling out an early ectopic pregnancy or appendicitis.

51   Vaginitis

TRICHOMONIASIS, BACTERIAL VAGINOSIS, AND VULVOVAGINAL CANDIDIASIS

Features of clinical presentation are shown in Table 51-1. Treatment modalities are given in Table 51-2. Vaginitis in pregnancy is discussed elsewhere.

TABLE 51-1. Features of Vaginal Discharge

Discharge	Normal	Candidiasis	T. Vaginalis	Bacterial Vaginosis
Color	Clear, white	White	Gray, green-yellow	Gray, white
Consistency	Floccular	Clumped, adherent to vaginal mucosa	Homogenous, occasionally frothy	Homogenous, occasionally frothy
Quantity	Variable; usually scant	Scant to moderate	Profuse	Moderate
pH	≤4.5	≤4.5	≥5.0	≥4.5
Amine Odor With KOH	Negative	Negative	Usually positive	Positive
Wet Mount	Epithelial cells, lactobacilli	WBCs, epithelial cells, spores, mycelia, or pseudohyphae Recommend KOH to dissolve nonfungal cellular elements	WBCs, motile trichomonads	Few WBCs, clue cells

TABLE 51-2. Treatment of Vaginitis

Disorder	First Line	Alternative	Partner	In Pregnancy
T. vaginalis	Metronidazole 2 g PO	Metronidazole 500 mg bid for 7 days	Same as patient	After 1st trimester, 2g metronidazole
Bacterial Vaginosis	Metronidazole 500 mg bid for 7 days*	Metronidazole 2g PO once	Exam for STD No Rx if normal	Clindamycin vaginal cream (1st trimester) or Metronidazole (later pregnancy)
Candidiasis	Butoconazole 2% cream 5 g intravaginally for 3 days	Clotrimazole 1% cream 5g intravaginally for 7–14 days (OTC)	Candicidal cream if dermatitis present.	Clotrimazole

*Not an FDA-approved indication.

COMMON PITFALLS

- A chief complaint of vaginal discharge is seldom a high priority; the most common pitfalls are a hasty history and failure to do a methodical examination.
- Noninfectious causes of vaginal irritation are often overlooked in the differential diagnosis. Chemical irritants (bubble bath, feminine hygiene products, intravaginal contraceptives, and soaps and detergents) or atrophic vaginitis in postmenopausal women should be considered when microscopy does not reveal the cause.

- Because noncompliance and possibly reinfection contribute significantly to recurrence, patients should receive instructions to complete the medication.
- Patients should be advised to abstain from sexual activity until their treatment and that of their partners is completed.
- All patients should receive a referral for further care.

52   Gynecologic Cancers

Approximately 71,000 new invasive cancers of the female reproductive tract are diagnosed annually in the United States. These cancers eventually result in approximately 23,000 annual deaths. The prevalence of these diseases is increasing. An increased incidence of human papillomavirus infection will result in an increase in cervical dysplasia and, possibly, cervical cancer, particularly if cytologic surveillance is not aggressively encouraged. The most frequently diagnosed cancer of the female reproductive tract is endometrial, followed by ovarian, cervical, and vulvar cancer and, less frequently, gestational trophoblastic neoplasia and tubal and vaginal cancer.

VAGINAL BLEEDING

Patients with vaginal bleeding secondary to a gynecologic malignancy probably have either cervical or endometrial cancer. Rarely, the cause is advanced vulvar cancer. Women who present with vaginal bleeding from cervical cancer are between 40 and 45 years. This mean age has recently decreased. Essential points in the history are:

Painless vaginal bleeding, exacerbated or caused by coitus
Lack of previous cytologic screening, or a history of prior abnormal findings on cytologic screening
Lower socioeconomic status
Multiple sexual partners

Physical examination should assess extrapelvic spread of disease, such as supraclavicular or inguinal adenopathy. The main focus of the examination, however, should be the pelvis. When vaginal bleeding is the presenting complaint, the lesion should be visible on speculum examination. A careful inspection of the vulva, vagina, and cervical os should be performed. If there is no visible lesion on the cervix and the bleeding is coming through the cervical os, then cervical cancer is an unlikely cause. Bimanual examination as well as a rectovaginal examination will assess possible involvement of the parametrial tissues.

Laboratory studies should include a pregnancy test and a complete blood count. If the bleeding is not severe, the patient can be discharged once appropriate referral and prompt follow-up has been obtained. If the bleeding is severe or life-threatening, then supportive measures should be instituted and consultation obtained. The patient may need hypogastric artery ligation, embolization, or high-dose radiation therapy. In vaginal bleeding caused by endometrial cancers the bleeding is usually not as severe as that caused by cervical cancer. Patients tend to be older (60). Essential points of the history include use of unopposed exogenous estrogens and obesity. In younger women obesity, nulliparity, and infertility may be predisposing factors. Although vaginal bleeding is the most common presenting complaint, it is seldom of magnitude.

In women who present with postmenopausal vaginal bleeding the diagnosis should be endometrial cancer until proven otherwise. Examination should assess the size of the uterus and the presence of an extrauterine tumor. On speculum examination the bleeding will be from the cervical os. Occasionally endometrial cancer presents with a visible lesion on the cervix. The bleeding is seldom life-threatening. The patient can be discharged with prompt referral to a qualified gynecologist.

Vaginal bleeding caused by gestational trophoblastic neoplasia occurs in women in either early or late reproductive age. Gestational trophoblastic neoplasia occurs in 1 out of 1200 pregnancies in the United States, but it is much more common in Asia and Latin America. Vaginal bleeding is the most common presentation. Salient points in the history include uterine enlargement greater than expected for gestational age, absence of fetal movements, repeated visits to medical facilities for bleeding (often the diagnosis is threatened abortion), and hypertension in early pregnancy. Physical examination reveals a large-for-gestational-age fundal height; speculum examination shows bleeding coming from the os. Vesicular material also may be seen extruding through the os. The diagnosis is made by ultrasonography (distinctive multiechogenic pattern). The patient with gestational trophoblastic neoplasia should be admitted.

Bleeding caused by vulvar cancer is rare. Women with this entity usually have an advanced lesion, are over age 60 and have other signs of neglect.

BOWEL EMERGENCIES
COMPLICATIONS OF NONRADIATED BOWEL

The most common bowel emergencies are bowel obstruction, colostomy problems, fistula formation, and perforation.

BOWEL OBSTRUCTION

Small-bowel obstruction, not in the perioperative period, is usually due to internal adhesions secondary to a previous surgical procedure or to gynecologic malignancy. In ovarian cancer approximately 5% of patients have small-bowel obstruction as the presenting complaint. Ovarian cancer spreads on the serosal surfaces of the bowel and can cause either adhesive or bulk obstruction. Two important points are unique to gynecologic cancer: (1) in elderly patients with no history of prior abdominal surgery small-bowel obstruction is a harbinger of ovarian cancer, and (2) in patients with a prior history of pelvic malignancy small-bowel obstruction may be the first sign of recurrence. In both situations appropriate consultation should be obtained. Large-bowel obstruction can occur by direct extension of a cervical malignancy that blocks the rectum. It is also seen when a large tumor in the omentum causes compression at either the splenic or hepatic flexure. Management should include prompt consultation with a gynecologist. The most critical aspect is to rule out overdistention of the cecum; if >10 cm diameter, prompt surgical decompression is necessary.

COLOSTOMY EMERGENCIES

Colostomy complications occur in approximately 30% of patients. These are stenosis of the stoma, peristomal hernia, wound infection, and prolapse. Most problems can be managed by a stomal therapist. Peristomal herniation of bowel requires admission for prompt surgical correction. Surgical or gynecologic consultation should be obtained and the bowel should be kept moist. Mucosal prolapse of the stoma can be reduced by gentle digital pressure, but expeditiously to prevent infection and stomal damage.

FISTULA FORMATION

Bowel fistulas are usually enterocutaneous, enterovaginal, or rectovaginal. Rarely, these fistulas are the presenting sign of a gynecologic malignancy. More often they occur secondary to therapy. The patient with a new fistula should be admitted so that prompt evaluation can be done.

COMPLICATIONS OF RADIATED BOWEL

Radiation therapy is most frequently used for the advanced cervical cancer or cervical cancer in patients who are not operative candidates. It is also used with increasing frequency as adjuvant therapy for endometrial cancer or consolidation therapy in ovarian cancer. Two stages of complications result from radiation therapy: early and late.

An early bowel complication is radiation proctitis enteritis with diarrhea. This injury can be seen during therapy or shortly after completion. Patients with severe diarrhea secondary to radiation enteritis or proctitis can usually be treated conservatively and seldom need to be admitted. The diarrhea can be managed with diphenoxylate (Lomotil). The patient can be treated and discharged.

Late complications of radiation injury to the bowel are caused by endarteritis and progressive sclerosis of the smaller vessels. This leads to several complications, including ulceration, infarction, enteroentero fistulas, necrosis, and stenosis. Usually the patient presents with either intestinal obstruction or severe intractable abdominal pain. The patient must be managed with fluid resuscitation, nasogastric suction, prompt gynecologic or surgical consultation, and admission.

Another common presentation is rectal bleeding from radiation proctitis. If the bleeding is minimal, the patient can be discharged on Cort enemas (hydrocortisone) and a low-residue diet. Prompt arrangements should be made for follow-up. When the bleeding is severe or symptoms of shock exist, fluid resuscitation, transfusion, and prompt consultation should occur.

UROLOGIC EMERGENCIES

URETERAL OBSTRUCTION

Ureteral obstruction most often presents as nonspecific flank pain, occasionally radiating to the pelvis and groin. Urinary infection is common, and may result in urosepsis. In rare cases where there is bilateral obstruction, anemia and azotemia may result. Ureteral obstruction can occur at any time after surgery or radiation therapy, but it is usually seen during the first post-treatment year. It may be the first presenting sign of late recurrence of genital malignancy. It can also be an initial sign of cervical cancer. The diagnosis is made on intravenous pyelography, computed tomography, or ultrasonography. Management depends on the severity of the obstruction. In patients with urosepsis, hospitalization should be arranged and antibiotics started after specimens for blood and urine cultures have been obtained. In patients who are stable and have insidious signs of ureteral obstruction, discharge may be contemplated once arrangements are made for continuing follow-up.

UROLOGIC FISTULAS

Urinary fistulas occur either because of extensive primary disease or secondary to radical hysterectomy for cervical or endometrial cancer. Surgical fistulas occur from 7 to 21 days after surgery. Occasionally fistulas occur secondary to radiation therapy, and are diagnosed 6 to 12 months after completion of treatment. The incidence of fistula formation after radical hysterectomy is approximately 1%. There is a threefold to fourfold increase in this rate when radiation is given in conjunction with surgery. Fistulas that occur in patients after radical surgery are usually diagnosed by the patient's surgeon and seldom present to the emergency department. However, in inner-city situations, it is possible that the presenting sign of the malignancy may be vesicovaginal fistula secondary to spread of the disease into the trigone of the bladder.

Fistulas can be diagnosed either by direct observation of urine in the vagina or by injecting indigo carmine intravenously and placing a tampon in the vagina.

HEMORRHAGIC CYSTITIS

Hemorrhagic cystitis can be due to either radiation therapy or chemotherapy. Hemorrhagic cystitis is not uncommon after radiation, and the pathophysiology is similar to that of radiated bowel.

Management can usually be done in the ED with a three-way catheter and irrigation. Once clots are removed and if the bleeding is not severe, the patient may be discharged with follow-up. In severe hemorrhage the patient will need to be admitted. Urologic and gynecologic consultation are necessary.

URINARY CONDUIT COMPLICATIONS

Urinary conduits are either ileal or transverse colon conduits. Complications include blockage of the uretero-conduit anastomatic site with ureteral obstruction and possibly urosepsis; conduit necrosis; stomal necrosis secondary to avascularity; stomal problems; and electrolyte imbalance. Management is supportive. Admission depends on electrolyte balance, urinary obstruction, and ability to return for follow-up care. Intravenous pyelography or ultrasonography usually defines the problem. If urinary obstruction has resulted in urosepsis, emergency percutaneous nephrostomy is necessary. Appropriate consultation with the radiologist and gynecologist needs to be obtained.

POSTOPERATIVE COMPLICATIONS

The emergency physician is most likely to be involved with three types of postoperative complications: (1) bowel obstruction, (2) urologic fistula, and (3) postoperative infection. The first two have been discussed earlier. In the vast majority of cases postoperative infections are diagnosed while the patient is still in the hospital. The postoperative infections most likely to be seen by the emergency physician are wound infection, wound dehiscence, and wound evisceration. Wound dehiscence occurs 5 to 7 days after surgery. The patient can usually be managed with debridement and dressing changes. The patient's surgeon should be consulted. In situations where home care is inadequate the patient may need to be admitted.

If signs of necrotizing fasciitis (skin discoloration, skin necrosis, and crepitus) are present, the patient needs to be admitted for surgical debridement. If there is fascial separation (evisceration), the patient must be admitted. The wound should be covered with sterile, moist towels and arrangements made for the operating room.

The other common infections are vaginal cuff cellulitis and cuff abscess. Vaginal cuff cellulitis occurs in 8% of those who receive antibiotic prophylaxis before a hysterectomy. The most common cause is a mixed infection of anaerobes endogenous to the vagina. The patient should be admitted and broad-spectrum antibiotic coverage started (metronidazole, ampicillin-sulbactam, and ticarcillin-clavulanate). If an abscess is identified, gynecologic consultation should be obtained and arrangements made for drainage.

Complications secondary to outpatient therapy such as colposcopy, conization, and laser therapy may be seen. The most common problem is postoperative cervical bleeding. This can usually be managed by the application of Monsel solution or packing the vagina with a Neosynephrine- or epinephrine-impregnated pack. Occasionally the cervix needs to be sutured. Gynecologic consultation should be obtained. If the patient is not severely bleeding and the bleeding is controlled with the procedures outlined above, the patient may be sent home and told to avoid intercourse and to follow up promptly with her primary physician.

COMPLICATIONS OF CHEMOTHERAPY

Chemotherapy is used primarily in ovarian cancer and gestational trophoblastic disease and as an adjuvant in endometrial cancer. The most commonly used drug is cisplatin. Complications caused by cisplatin are nausea and vomiting which occurs during the day of administration. Occasionally the vomiting can be severe enough that the patient may come to the ED the day after chemotherapy. The patient can often be managed by intravenous antiemetic medication as well as metoclopramide (Reglan). If nausea and vomiting are unremitting, the patient needs to be admitted for hydration.

Other drugs that are commonly used in gynecologic oncology are cyclophosphamide, methotrexate, fluorouracil, doxorubicin, dactinomycin, vinblastine, and etoposide. The most common complication is bone marrow suppression. If the patient presents with a neutropenia of <500 granulocytes and fever, she should be admitted for antibiotic therapy. If the platelet count is <20,000 with spontaneous bleeding, the patient needs to be admitted for transfusion as well as platelet therapy. Bleomycin, another commonly used drug, may cause pulmonary fibrosis. The patient may present with dyspnea, cough, and bibasilar rales. A chest radiograph usually shows basilar infiltrates. The patient needs to be admitted.

COMPLICATIONS OF TOTAL PARENTERAL NUTRITION (TPN)

As home infusion services increase, it is more common to see complications of TPN. The most likely complications are infection and metabolic derangements. Sepsis should be managed aggressively and the patient promptly admitted. Metabolic complications include acid-base and abnormalities in glucose metabolism as well as hypokalemia, hypomagnesemia, hypophosphatemia, and hypocalcemia. Patients may present with muscle weakness, hyporeflexia or hyperflexia, lethargy, and mental status change. It is imperative to obtain adequate laboratory studies.

ORGAN FAILURE

Renal failure can occur from ureteral obstruction, conduit anastomosis problems, or urosepsis. It may represent a primary presentation of cervical cancer with bilateral ureterovesical junction obstruction. Liver failure is most frequently due to metastasis from ovarian cancer and less frequently from gestational trophoblastic neoplasia and endometrial, vulvar, or cervical cancer. Pulmonary metastasis is seen most frequently in endometrial cancer or cervical cancer; parenchymal pulmonary metastasis is seen less frequently in ovarian cancer. It is not infrequent, however, to see pleural effusions secondary to ovarian cancer in association with ascites. Brain metastasis is rare in gynecologic malignancies except for gestational trophoblastic neoplasia. In gestational trophoblastic neoplasia, headache, seizure, visual disturbance, or mental status change should be evaluated with a CT of the head.

COMMON PITFALLS

- In the presence of vaginal bleeding, pregnancy should be ruled out.
- If the cecum is dilated to 10 cm from large-bowel obstruction, prompt decompression is mandatory.
- Necrotizing fasciitis requires prompt surgical debridement and admission.
- If any amount of ureteral obstruction is diagnosed, urosepsis must be ruled out before discharge.
- Febrile neutropenic patients must be admitted.

53   Sexual Assault

Most state statutes define rape as the unlawful carnal knowledge of a woman by a man forcibly and against her will. In other words, rape is unlawful sexual intercourse without consent by force, fear, fraud, drink, or drugs. In 1985 more than 87,000 rapes were reported; only one in five attempts is reported. Defendants charged with rape and other sex-related crimes are four times less likely to be convicted than defendants charged with any other crime. Sexual assault is the fastest-growing violent crime in the United States, and it is estimated that one in every six women will be a victim of rape during her lifetime.

CLINICAL PRESENTATION

The sexual assault victim may present immediately after the event. She may have visible physical trauma and be emotionally distraught. Or it may be hours or days later before she presents. The victim may feel guilt, shame, humiliation, and embarrassment. She may not be immediately able to share her experience with anyone and may delay seeking treatment. The victim with physical trauma, such as airway compromise, severe laceration, or fracture, is most likely to obtain early medical intervention.

EMERGENCY DEPARTMENT EVALUATION

The first duty is to evaluate for any life threat. The ABCs—airway, breathing, and circulation—must be addressed appropriately. Care must be taken not to destroy or alter any evidence. The patient should be placed in a private room. If the hospital has a special sexual assault team, the team should initiate involvement. Once consent has been obtained, obtain history necessary for treatment and for the collection of evidence, including time, date, and place of the event. This information may be important when trying to relate physical findings, such as a bruise, to the assault, or when looking for corroborating evidence, such as sand if the assault occurred at the beach. Threats of violence or reprisal made by the assailant should be noted. If any type of weapon, restraints, foreign bodies, alcohol, or drugs were involved, these facts should be noted, as well as the number of assailants.

It should be noted whether vaginal, oral, or anal penetration was attempted, and if ejaculation occurred. If ejaculation occurred, seminal deposits must be carefully sought on clothing as well as on the patient. The patient should be asked if she has douched, bathed, urinated, or defecated since the assault. If she has, some evidence may have been destroyed. A pertinent gynecologic history should include gravidity, parity, last menstrual period, contraceptive history, date of last consensual intercourse, history of recent sexually transmitted disease, and any recent gynecologic surgery. If the victim is taking birth control pills, she should be asked if she has missed taking any pills. All this information will assist in deciding what type of medical treatment is necessary.

The chain of evidence should not be broken. Most departments have specific protocols and prepared forms. It is important that the physician be understanding, supportive, and caring. The purposes of the physical examination are to determine the need for medical treatment, to gather specimens for analysis, and to make and document observations for corroboration of the assault. If the police are present and if the victim is wearing the clothes she wore during the attack, the police may want to take photographs before she undresses. Paper bags are used because plastic bags do not "breathe" and may promote molding of blood and seminal stains. The skin should be inspected for scratches, lacerations, abrasions, contusions, and bite marks; special attention should be paid to the neck, mouth, breasts, wrists, and thighs. When the mouth is being examined for trauma, a saliva sample should be obtained. The sample can be used to determine the patient's status as a blood group antigen secretor or nonsecretor.

The teeth should be swabbed for acid phosphatase and sperm analysis. The presence of any foreign material such as hair, blood, or semen should also be noted. Foreign material should be scraped from under the fingernails and placed in the appropriate envelope. This material may reveal bits of the assailant's hair, blood, or skin, if the victim was able actively to resist. Semen may appear as lightly crusted areas. A Wood's light can help to identify these areas because they fluoresce in ultraviolet light. Semen can be removed with a water-moistened swab. If photographs are not taken, the physician must be even more careful to document the findings.

The pelvic examination should be performed next. The external genitalia should be checked for trauma and evidence of semen. If semen is present on the upper inner thighs, it can be swabbed. If it is present on pubic hair, the hairs should be trimmed. The patient's pubic hair should be combed to find strands of the assailant's hair, which can be analyzed to help identify the assailant's race and hair color. In order to differentiate it from the victim's hair, some of her pubic hair must be plucked for analysis also. Each specimen should be placed in the appropriate envelope. Small vaginal lacerations can be identified with the use of toluidine blue. The hymen should be inspected to determine if it is present, intact, absent, or traumatized with bleeding or fresh clots. The speculum should be lubricated only with water; other lubricants may affect the acid phosphatase determination and sperm motility.

The vaginal wall should be inspected for lacerations and for evidence of the penetration of any foreign objects. Any secretions that have pooled in the posterior fornix should be aspirated and placed in a sterile receptacle. These secretions can be used to determine the presence of sperm, acid phosphatase, and blood group antigens. If no secretions are present, the vagina should be washed with 5 mL to 10 mL of nonbacteriostatic sterile saline solution and followed with aspiration. If washing is not necessary, the posterior fornix should be swabbed with a cotton-tipped applicator and secretions smeared on two glass slides. One more swab should be obtained for wet-mount examination. A Papanicolaou smear should be obtained from the cervix to help determine the presence of nonmotile sperm (the smear is useful up to several days after the assault).

Cultures for gonorrhea, chlamydial, and herpes should be obtained, if indicated. A bimanual examination should be performed and uterine size, adnexal masses, and tenderness noted. The rectal area should be carefully examined, especially if anal intercourse took place. Signs of trauma, semen stain, blood, and lubricant should be noted. Anal and rectal swabs can be obtained through the lumen of a water-lubricated anoscope and are used to determine the presence of motile and nonmotile sperm and acid phosphatase. Blood should also be drawn for ABO analysis, syphilis serology, drug and alcohol screen, and beta human chorionic gonadotropin (hCG). If the test result is negative initially and positive at a follow-up visit, the pregnancy probably originated at the time of the assault.

The oral, vaginal, and rectal swabs obtained for the identification of sperm must be examined microscopically for motile and nonmotile sperm. Sperm are not usually found motile after 12 hours. The presence of motile sperm is a reliable indication that the assault occurred in the 12 hours before the examination, provided consensual intercourse did not also take place in that time period. Nonmotile sperm may be present for 72 hours or longer. The acid phosphatase enzyme may also indicate sexual contact. This enzyme is present in vaginal secretions but is found in much greater quantities in prostatic secretions. A high concentration of acid phosphatase is an excellent indicator of the presence of seminal fluid, even in the absence of sperm. The presence of acid phosphatase correlates better with the time since intercourse than does the presence of sperm.

A major seminal plasma glycoprotein produced in the prostate, p30, has been identified as another semen-specific marker. The forensic laboratory will also develop a specific genetic profile of the assailant to compare with that of the victim. Genetic typing can determine the blood group and type of both parties. Three genetic markers found in semen are phosphoglucomutase (PGM), the peptidase-A (Pep-A) enzyme marker, and the ABO blood group antigens. Reference markers for the victim must be obtained at the initial evaluation; these markers are also in vaginal secretions but in lower concentrations. DNA typing or fingerprinting is the newest method used to identify the assailant. This method involves the extraction of DNA from a small sample of blood, semen, or other DNA-bearing cells. Through various procedures a specific "DNA fingerprint" is developed. This "fingerprint" can be analyzed and compared with the assailant's to establish a positive identification. The chance that two unrelated persons have the same DNA fingerprint is one in a quadrillion.

EMERGENCY DEPARTMENT MANAGEMENT

Physical trauma experienced by a sexual assault victim is treated like trauma in any other patient. In addition, the possibilities of psychological trauma, pregnancy, and venereal disease must be addressed.

Efforts to decrease the victim's distress can begin with her arrival. She has just experienced a threat to her life and must be helped to feel safe and secure. It is often helpful to have a rape crisis volunteer present to provide additional support and to make sure the patient understands the procedures explained to her by the physician and nurse. The emotional trauma often can be described as a post-traumatic stress disorder. It is estimated that pregnancy occurs in 1% of rape victims. Pregnancy should be ruled out before prophylactic treatment is considered. The "morning-after pill" can be administered if prophylaxis is desired. Diethylstilbestrol (DES; 25 mg PO twice daily for 5 days) must be administered within 72 hours of sexual contact to be effective. If conception occurs despite DES prophylaxis, a female fetus is at risk for vaginal adenosis and cancer, and a male fetus is at risk for penile and testicular lesions. Birth control pills may be used. A regimen that includes norgestrel or ethinyl estradiol (two pills initially and two pills 12 hours later) is acceptable. Ethinyl estradiol (0.5 mg daily for 5 days) may also be used. Premarin (25 mg), an oral conjugated estrogen, may be administered daily for 5 days. Good results and less nausea have been reported with the use of intravenous Premarin (50 mg for 2 days).

If the initial pregnancy test result is negative and a follow-up test result is positive, counseling is indicated, after which the patient may want to have a suction curettage or a therapeutic abortion.

The risk of contracting a sexually transmitted disease as the result of sexual assault is hard to estimate; the incidence of positive gonorrhea cultures taken at the initial examination is 2%–9%. Patients are usually treated as if they had been exposed to gonorrhea and Chlamydia.

DISPOSITION

A gynecologist may be called during the initial examination if necessary, especially if operative intervention is needed. The emergency physician should strongly recommend that the victim seek follow-up care from a gynecologist or family physician. Most hospitals have rape crisis volunteers available to consult with the victim during the first 24 hours after the assault. Encourage the patient to seek counseling with psychologists or psychiatrists if indicated. Admission to the hospital may be required in the case of significant physical trauma. As a rule, the sexual assault victim may be discharged with relatives or friends. Follow-up care for the victim must be arranged before discharge. She will need to return after 2 weeks and after 6 weeks to be re-evaluated for pregnancy and venereal disease. Any physical injury such as a laceration will need follow-up care. Psychological trauma may necessitate long-term treatment. "Rape trauma syndrome" consists of a two-phase reaction. The short-term phase, characterized by disorganization, may last from a few days to a few weeks. During this time the victim may exhibit a wide range of emotional behavior, from being quiet and subdued to demonstrating anger and fear. The long-term phase, characterized by reorganization, may last for months or years. Many victims experience depression, flashbacks, anxiety, and sexual dysfunction. Eighty percent of rape victims end primary relationships within 1 year of the rape. Because the rape victim may have a large spectrum of psychological needs and concerns, be certain that follow-up evaluation will address them.

COMMON PITFALLS

- Be certain that the collection, disposition, and transfer of all specimens are documented at every stage, from collection to introduction into the courtroom. This legal protocol is the chain of evidence and safeguards the rights of the accused during the judicial process. All specimens must be correctly collected and labeled. Documentation must be made of each person who takes possession of the evidence—the physician or nurse who gathers the evidence, the police officer who transfers it to the forensic laboratory, and laboratory technicians. No break must occur in this process or the evidence will not be admissible in court. Each institution and state may have some variation in their requirements and protocol, so the emergency physician must be familiar with the sexual assault kit and the forms and procedures of his or her institution.
- Follow-up: Up to 94% of rape victims do not return for their follow-up visits. Some member of the medical team, such as a social worker, should contact the victim after discharge, to address concerns that arise later and to encourage follow-up care.

SECTION II

TRAUMA

54   General Principles of Trauma

CLINICAL PRESENTATION

Trauma is the leading cause of death in the first three decades of life. Patients assessed by pre-hospital personnel as having a major mechanism of injury, or those arriving on their own who are recognized as having potential for serious injury should be triaged immediately to a suitable treatment area capable of a major resuscitation. Details regarding the mechanism of injury are important clues in predicting potential injuries (Table 54-1).

EMERGENCY DEPARTMENT EVALUATION AND MANAGEMENT

The approach to the multiple trauma patient begins with a rapid initial examination requiring no longer than 1 minute and is accomplished while vital signs are being assessed. The patient is stripped of all clothing. The patency of the airway is immediately ascertained. The neck is exam-

---

TABLE 54-1. Important Details About Mechanism of Injury

I. **Blunt Trauma**
    A. Motor Vehicle Accident
        1. Estimated speed of both vehicles on impact
        2. Orientation of the vehicles (head-on, broadside, etc.)
        3. Trajectory and extent of damage to patient's vehicle
        4. Was there an explosion or fire?
        5. Was the patient restrained?
        6. Was the windshield intact?
        7. Was the steering wheel intact?
        8. Was there an initial loss of consciousness at the scene?
        9. Was any alcohol or drugs recovered from the patient or car?
      10. How long did it take to extricate the patient?
      11. What is the ambient temperature (potential for hypothermia)?
    B. Fall
        1. Estimated height?
        2. Possible reason for fall (electrocution, explosion, etc.)
        3. Was there an initial loss of consciousness at the scene?
        4. Were any alcohol or drugs recovered from the patient or scene?
        5. How long was the patient down?
        6. What is the ambient temperature (potential for hypothermia)?

II. **Penetrating Trauma**
    A. Stab Wound
        1. Description of the weapon (length, width, etc.)
        2. See 4 and 5 under I-B
    B. Gunshot Wound
        1. Description of the weapon (including caliber)
        2. See 4 and 5 under I-B

ined for direct trauma, carotid pulsation, tracheal position, and character of neck veins. The chest is quickly observed for sucking wounds or paradoxical motion, palpated for crepitus, and auscultated for the absence of breath sounds or presence of adventitious sounds. The extremities are palpated. If they are cool, moist, or pale, shock must be presumed. In the absence of any contraindications the patient is rolled from side to side to ensure that there are no wounds on the back.

In the ED an attempt should be made to auscultate the systolic and diastolic pressure. It should also be remembered that the location of a palpable pulse tells one much about the perfusion pressure. For example, if a radial pulse is present, the patient must have a systolic blood pressure of at least 80 mm Hg. A palpable femoral pulse indicates a systolic blood pressure of at least 70 mm Hg, and a carotid pulse, a systolic blood pressure of 60 mm Hg. At the time intravenous lines are placed blood is drawn for a hematocrit and type and crossmatch. Additional blood is set aside for other tests as indicated. The cervical spine must remain immobilized until it is radiographically cleared of injury. Hyperextension or flexion of the neck should be avoided if neck injury is suspected or if the patient is unconscious from a head injury.

Supplemental oxygen should be administered. If the patient needs active airway management because of secretions, the kind of injuries present, or respiratory distress, the airway should be secured. Major trauma victims often need active airway management even if they are breathing spontaneously. Many patients have injuries that distort their airways (e.g., a gunshot wound of the neck). It is preferable to intubate before anatomy becomes so distorted that it will be impossible to carry out an intubation. There is often some degree of head injury in the patient with multiple trauma, and it is well worthwhile to try to prevent or contain cerebral edema by hyperventilation. Finally, because few trauma patients have an empty stomach at the time of injury, there is always a risk of vomiting and aspiration that intubation can help prevent. It may be safest to follow the standard of nasotracheal intubation or cricothyrotomy until the cervical spine has been radiographically cleared, but one should be willing to modify this approach, depending on the circumstances.

External hemorrhage is controlled by direct pressure only. Blind probing and clamping deep within a wound risk further injury to vessels and nerves.

Shock can be defined as inadequate perfusion of the tissues. Cool, pale, moist skin indicates shock. A Foley catheter is needed to monitor renal perfusion. A central venous catheter is also helpful in monitoring central volume. Vascular access is critical. Two large-bore (14 to 16 gauge) percutaneous catheters should be placed, avoiding, if possible, injured extremities. It is best to insert a minimum of two large-bore peripheral lines. A Ringer's lactate or normal saline solution are the preferred initial resuscitation fluid, although new research suggests that hypertonic saline–dextran mixtures may be very useful. Older patients may require a higher hematocrit because of underlying cardiorespiratory disease. When massive transfusions are necessary, remember the need for additional platelets and other clotting factors. Blood should be warmed.

In all cases the amount of fluids administered will depend on continued losses. These should be minimized through proper splinting, bandaging, and avoidance of probing large soft-tissue wounds. It is often forgotten how much a soft-tissue injury, especially to the scalp, can bleed, and the best treatment of hypovolemia is to locate the source of bleeding and stop the blood loss. The degree to which long bone and pelvic fractures bleed is also not generally appreciated, and it is far more effective to begin the administration of blood as soon as these injuries are recognized than to await the clinical presentation of severe shock.

The neck veins are valuable in identifying the cause of shock. If the neck veins are collapsed, hypovolemia must be presumed. If they are distended, then cardiogenic shock, tension pneumothorax, or pericardial tamponade must be excluded. Most trauma patients in shock are hypovolemic. Tension pneumothorax causes shock by increasing intrathoracic pressure, shifting the mediastinum, and compressing the great veins, thereby preventing venous return. The diagnosis is suspected in any patient in shock who has distended neck veins and an increased resistance to bagging. An ipsilateral decrease in breath sounds may be noted as well as a contralateral tracheal shift. Unfortunately these physical findings are often not present in the acute trauma situation, and the only clues to the presence of a correctable cause of patient collapse may be a sudden rise in pulse, a drop in blood pressure, and an increased resistance to ventilation. Even the neck veins may not distend if the patient is concomitantly hypovolemic.

Time should not be wasted in obtaining radiographic confirmation of a suspected tension pneumothorax, as the patient may well arrest while the film is being obtained. Thoracostomy should be performed by inserting a large-bore chest tube in the fifth intercostal space, in the midaxillary line. This will evacuate any blood that is present as well as any air.

Cardiac causes of shock must not be overlooked. Pericardial tamponade is rare with closed chest injuries, and another source for the patient's shock should probably be sought. It must always be considered with penetrating injuries, even if the entrance wound appears anatomically remote. The physiologic response to tamponade is to compensate for the fall in cardiac output by raising the pulse rate. The classic physical findings may also be absent in the acute situation. If the patient has lost vital signs or has suddenly become bradycardic, then an immediate thoracotomy should be performed.

Myocardial contusion, most commonly from blunt trauma, may cause arrhythmias, often within the first hour after injury. An electrocardiogram (ECG) should be obtained in those patients with significant anterior blunt chest trauma. Continuous ECG monitoring is indicated. Myocardial infarction may occur as a result of the stress associated with blood loss and catecholamine release, or it may have preceded the traumatic injury. Coronary arterial air embolization occurs with penetrating neck and chest trauma or serious rib fractures after intubation and positive-pressure ventilation. Air passes from the airway into the pulmonary veins and embolizes to the arterial circulation, often involving the cerebral and coronary arteries. If air embolization is suspected, the patient should be immediately turned to the left lateral decubitus position (i.e., right side up), fluid infusion increased, and immediate thoracotomy with bypass arranged. It may be possible to salvage some of these patients with immediate femorofemoral bypass while preparing the operating room.

Possible sources of significant blood loss causing hypovolemic shock include the chest, abdomen (including pelvis and retroperitoneum), and thighs. Head injuries seldom cause hypovolemia, and other sites of occult blood loss must be excluded in a head-injured patient with shock. Spinal cord trauma with loss of sympathetic vascular tone can be assessed by rectal examination and examination of peripheral reflexes.

The diagnosis of intra-abdominal hemorrhage is often difficult. Abdominal examination may be totally normal despite significant intra-abdominal pathology. The pulse may not be rapid, especially if the bleeding has been sudden and profound, or if the patient has alcohol or other drugs in his system. Bowel sounds may be present, and no abdominal tenderness or guarding may be seen. Distention is a late finding that may be present even if there is no abdominal pathology, and does not predict the degree of blood loss. The patient may also have other problems that interfere with an accurate diagnosis (e.g., intoxication, head injury, or competitive pain from another major injury). Few patients can perceive more than one major source of pain at a time. Unfortunately the pain they may focus on may not be from the most serious injury. The hemoglobin and hematocrit may not dilute, and be normal right up to the time the patient arrests from hypovolemia. A diagnostic peritoneal lavage may be indicated if the patient had a significant mechanism of injury. There is enthusiasm for the use of computed tomography (CT) of the abdomen. Unless one is willing to operate on all unstable patients, which leads to too many unnecessary laparotomies, aggressive diagnostic peritoneal lavage is mandatory.

Military antishock trousers (MAST) are of limited value in the treatment of hypovolemia. They are of particular value in the temporary control of hemorrhage from pelvic fractures or in the splinting of lower-extremity fractures. Most of the problems associated with the use of the garment occur with inappropriate deflation, which may cause not only serious hypotension, but also arrhythmias.

Collection and reinfusion of blood from a traumatic hemothorax can provide a useful and safe source of blood. After reinfusion of autologous blood there is a transient coagulopathy that resolves after several days. Platelet function is also depressed. Because increased bleeding may result, this procedure should be reserved for more serious hemorrhage and when banked blood is not readily available.

If the patient has a cardiac arrest from hypovolemia or pericardial tamponade, or has evidence of coronary air embolization, immediate emergency thoracotomy is indicated. Thoracotomy offers the only chance for salvage. The best results are obtained in the presence of penetrating injury to the chest, particularly the heart. It is probably of no benefit to perform a thoracotomy unless the surgical expertise and institutional resources for the rendering of definitive care are readily available.

Surgery is part of the resuscitation of the unstable trauma victim. In the patient who cannot be resuscitated from shock and who has no obvious source of blood loss, immediate exploration is indicated. A chest film determines whether the chest or the abdomen is the site of initial exploration.

In the patient who stabilizes during resuscitation the next priority is the secondary survey. This includes repeat cardiopulmonary, maxillofacial, abdominal, neurologic, and orthopedic examinations, as well as checking for occult blood loss. If the patient is unconscious, determination of the level of brain stem function and the presence of a herniation syndrome are paramount. Most trauma victims die of central nervous system-related injuries. Immobilization of the neck must be maintained in trauma patients until the cervical spine is cleared of injury. Open fractures should be gently irrigated and splinted to prevent further injury and reduce pain and bleeding. Open fractures should be covered with clean dressings and intravenous antibiotics commenced with an antistaphylococcal drug; however, their definitive care must await the diagnostic elimination or the surgical treatment of more serious, life-threatening injuries.

If the patient remains unstable, the single most useful diagnostic study is the chest film. Intravenous pyelography, retrograde urethrography and cystogram are indicated if GU trauma is suspected.

There are multiple indications for arteriography. These include penetrating neck injuries, possible thoracic aortic tears, dislocation of the knee, fractures associated with abnormal pulses, a kidney that is not visualized by intravenous pyelography, and selected pelvic fractures.

RADIOLOGIC STUDIES

The sequencing of radiologic studies should be prioritized in the same manner as the other components of the resuscitation. Because the patient's airway is the primary concern, the cervical spine should be assessed if active airway management is indicated and the patient is stable. If the airway has already been secured in the field, then the cervical spine can be immobilized while other, more pressing studies are obtained (e.g., chest and pelvic films). However, if the patient is unstable and an airway has not been secured, then immediate airway management is indicated.

In victims of blunt trauma, chest and pelvic films should be obtained next. Patients with penetrating wounds of the chest (stab or gunshot wounds) should have chest radiographs taken either before resuscitative procedures are performed (if stable) or afterward (if unstable). Abdominal series are of low yield in the evaluation of stab wounds, but are useful in localizing gunshot fragments. Two other studies that need to be prioritized are the CT scan of the head and aortography. In unstable patients with positive peritoneal lavages these studies must await laparotomy and definitive care of the abdominal wounds. If the patient has a concomitant herniation syndrome, burr holes may be made while the patient is undergoing laparotomy. A CT scan of the head may be obtained once the patient is stabilized. Victims of blunt trauma who have sustained thoracic aortic tears and survive long enough to present to the ED can await aortography until the head and abdominal injuries have been cared for.

DISPOSITION

The stable trauma patient may spend a number of hours between the ED and radiology during the completion of diagnostic tests. There is a finite period of time that it takes to completely exclude multiple occult injuries, and this time period will also allow an observation period to recognize the development of neurologic, cardiac, or pulmonary pathologies. Someone from either the trauma service or the emergency department will have to monitor the patient during these procedures to ensure that instability is not occurring and that a quick transfer to the operating room has not become necessary. It must be remembered that any patient who has had a significant mechanism of injury is likely to develop areas of pain and dysfunction that are not predictable in the ED. It is therefore prudent (although not mandatory) to provide 24 to 48 hours of observation and care in the hospital.

Transfer of the patient to another institution depends on multiple factors, but the principle to be followed is that the patient will be stable, or if unstable, transfer will be to achieve a level of medical care that cannot be obtained at the original treating facility. It may be necessary to care for a life threat (e.g., remove or salvage a torn spleen) and then transfer the patient for more sophisticated neurosurgical or thoracic observations and treatment.

COMMON PITFALLS

- Failure to ascertain details or ignoring the severity of the mechanism of injury
- Ascription of positive physical findings to a benign cause
- Failure to set up for the patient before his arrival
- Failure to have a visible trauma captain throughout the resuscitation
- Failure to utilize a well thought out, systematic approach to the patient
- Chaotic and inefficient resuscitation because of poor use of team members or because of too many physicians trying to give orders
- Focus on subspecialty need at the expense of real or potential life threats
- Overemphasis on diagnostic tests in an unstable patient

55 Airway Management in the Trauma Patient

Airway management in trauma is a unique challenge. Associated cranial and cervical trauma usually prevent the use of standard elective approaches to secure an airway. Facial fractures such as comminuted mandibular symphysis fractures, flail mandibular, and bilateral rami fractures may obstruct the airway even in a conscious patient by removing the tongue's skeletal support. As the mandible collapses, the genioglossus is unable to advance the tongue out of the hypopharynx. The airway may also be compromised by dentures and bony fragments. The major factor that determines the airway approach is the likelihood of an unstable cervical spine fracture (Figure 55-1).

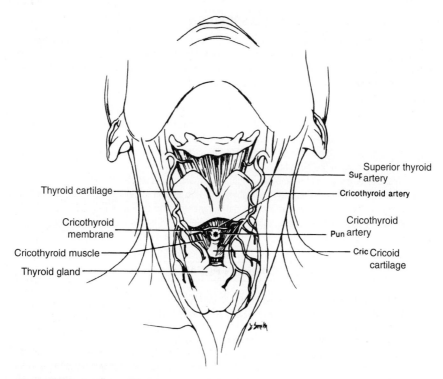

Figure 55-1. Anatomy of the airway.

AIRWAY TRAUMA

Prompt recognition of laryngotracheobronchial (LTB) injuries, appropriate airway management, and early surgical repair are essential. The true incidence is unknown, since most patients expire at the scene. Blunt airway disruption is often caused by neck hyperextension coupled with a direct neck blow to the dashboard or steering wheel. The cartilagenous trachea can also be crushed against the vertebral column. Blunt chest trauma may generate excessive intratracheal pressure when the glottis is closed. Lastly, rapid deceleration may shear the tracheobronchial tree, which is relatively fixed at the cricoid and carina. Tracheal transection and cricotracheal separations are also seen in a variety of "clothesline" injuries.

In contrast to blunt mechanisms of trauma, penetrating injuries are easier to diagnose and often result in combined airway and vascular compromise. There are numerous symptoms of LTB injuries, including aphonia, cough, dysphagia, dysphonia, dyspnea, hoarseness, laryngeal pain, and odynophagia. Suggestive signs include anterior cervical ecchymosis, hemoptysis, and cyanosis. The inability to palpate normal laryngeal landmarks, especially in a male, implies the presence of a fracture. When the larynx is fractured the voice is more often muffled than hoarse. One should assume that cervical subcutaneous emphysema is not simply from gastrointestinal tract perforation, since it is more often encountered with disruption of the respiratory tree. An intralaryngeal hematoma or edema can develop over several hours and produce ominous stridor.

EMERGENCY DEPARTMENT EVALUATION

If the patient is apneic, initiate ventilation with a bag–valve–mask or demand valve and mask unless major intraoral hemorrhage is present. This may be ineffective, since the head is not in the sniffing position.

BASIC AIRWAY CARE

Simple measures to open a compromised airway may be lifesaving, inasmuch as such obstruction, rather than airway damage itself, tends to be the major cause of morbidity. Application of the chin lift or jaw thrust in the victim may be sufficient to overcome obstruction.

NASOTRACHEAL INTUBATION

Blind nasotracheal intubation (BNI) is an essential skill and is often the most practical emergency airway control option. Directional tip control endotracheal tubes (Endotrol) are very helpful when the cervical spine has not been "cleared" and the head cannot be extended. Relative contraindications to BNI include major maxillofacial fractures, coagulopathies, and tracheobronchial injuries. Intracranial passage of a nasotracheal tube has been reported only once, and resulted from poor technique in the setting of obvious massive head trauma.

ORAL ENDOTRACHEAL INTUBATION

Oral intubation with manual cervical immobilization is considered an option in apneic trauma patients. When there is no time for lateral cervical radiography, the emergency physician may attempt percutaneous translaryngeal ventilation, BNI, or cricothyrotomy. The use of a transillumination technique with a lighted stylet for endotracheal intubation may also prove useful.

PERCUTANEOUS TRANSLARYNGEAL VENTILATION

In apneic patients percutaneous translaryngeal ventilation (PTLV) is the quickest invasive temporizing maneuver. It is most valuable in patients with severe maxillofacial trauma or probable cervical spine injuries. PTLV buys time until nasotracheal intubation or cricothyrotomy is accomplished or cervical spine radiographs are obtained. With correct technique, adequate oxygenation and ventilation can be maintained for more than an hour. Alveolar ventilation, however, may be inadequate with PTLV if thoracic compliance is altered from a crush injury or pulmonary compliance is decreased with post-traumatic respiratory insufficiency.

Either a 50-psi wall source with a flowmeter set on flush or an oxygen cylinder may be used as an oxygen source. A first-stage regulator drops the pressure to 50 psi. With the larynx stabilized with one hand, the inferior aspect of the cricothyroid membrane should be punctured at a caudal angle using a 12- to 14-gauge kink-resistant, over-the-needle plastic intravenous catheter. Easy withdrawal of air by means of a small syringe confirms correct placement. Bag–valve devices and demand valves that are limited to 50 cm H_2O do not provide sufficient driving pressure (70 cm H_2O = 1 psi).

If exhalation remains inadequate after 4 or 5 seconds of ventilation, a second venting catheter should be inserted adjacent to the first one. If the chest wall still does not fall, immediate cricothyrotomy is indicated. The only absolute contraindication to PTLV is complete airway obstruction. Laryngeal injuries or foreign bodies are relative contraindications, as are any of the contraindications to translaryngeal anesthesia. Massive subcutaneous emphysema occurs with interstitial tissue insufflation. Minor subcutaneous emphysema from air leakage around the catheter may occur. Barotrauma usually results from overzealous insufflation in the setting of inadequate exhalation. PTLV may result in pneumothorax, pneumomediastinum, and central air embolization when complete airway obstruction is present.

CRICOTHYROTOMY

If less invasive airway maneuvers are not feasible because of massive facial injuries, an unstable cervical spine, or uncontrollable intraoral hemorrhage, the emergency physician should proceed with cricothyrotomy.

TRACHEOSTOMY
The initial airway management of patients with LTB injury is determined by the degree of respiratory distress. The need for prompt intervention must be anticipated if stridor is present. "Blind" attempts to insert an endotracheal tube can convert incomplete tracheal tears into complete separations. If the patient's respiratory status decompensates, airway management should be predicated on the emergency physician's technical expertise. Ideally, in these circumstances the airway is secured with a low tracheotomy through the fourth or fifth ring. Tracheostomy has largely been replaced by various endotracheal intubation techniques and cricothyrotomy as a method for establishment of an emergent airway. The amount of time required, the risk of hemorrhage, and the degree of surgical dissection involved all constitute significant limitations of this procedure.

PERCUTANEOUS TRANSTRACHEAL VENTILATION
Intubation is frequently difficult in LTB trauma cases with significant hemorrhage. Percutaneous transtracheal ventilation below the injury site is the simplest temporizing option. This procedure may be performed without moving the neck by introducing a catheter percutaneously into the trachea. Aspiration of air indicates entry into the tracheal lumen. Complications include subcutaneous and mediastinal emphysema.

NEUROMUSCULAR BLOCKADE

Neuromuscular blockade may be required with succinylcholine. Succinylcholine mimics acetylcholine, causing persistent end plate depolarization. In contrast, vecuronium and pancuronium are nondepolarizing agents similar to curare. Succinylcholine has a more rapid onset (30–45 seconds) and shorter duration of action (5 minutes) than vecuronium or pancuronium. Maximal paralysis occurs in 2 to 3 minutes, and the usual adult dosage is 1 mg/kg IV. Succinylcholine increases intragastric pressure, which predisposes to aspiration in traumatized patients. Muscle fasciculations may displace long bone fractures. Neuromuscular blockade with vecuronium or pancuronium is far more useful as an adjunct for mechanical ventilation. Paralysis can improve oxygenation and ventilation and help to control intracranial hypertension. The preferred agent is vecuronium, which is one third more potent than pancuronium, with a duration of action one third to one half as long. It does not cause nearly the degree of tachycardia seen with pancuronium. The dose of vecuronium is 0.08 mg to 0.1 mg/kg IV. Paralysis occurs in 3 to 5 minutes and lasts for 25 to 30 minutes. See chapter 57 for Rapid Sequence Intubation Protocol.

COMMON PITFALLS

- Cervical spine immobilization without traction is difficult to maintain during some airway maneuvers.
- Recheck endotracheal tube patency frequently—cuff overexpansion, tube displacement, and thrombotic occlusion are common.
- Overzealous positive-pressure ventilation decreases venous return in hypotensive multiple trauma patients.
- Peritracheal fascial sleeves may initially maintain a patent airway until a hematoma occludes it or the distal trachea retracts into the mediastinum.
- LTB injuries are initially often difficult to diagnose.

56   Traumatic Shock

CLINICAL PRESENTATION

The presentation of the patient at risk for traumatic shock is a function of where on the spectrum of progression he lies. Because external blood loss is notoriously poorly estimated and internal blood loss is occult, the body's response to shock is still the best method of assessment.

EMERGENCY DEPARTMENT EVALUATION

The evaluation of the patient is directed toward assessment of the degree of shock and identification of the source of bleeding or the other few causes of shock. This consists of a systematic approach to the trauma patient as well described elsewhere. Assessment of the degree of shock guides the vigor of fluid resuscitation. Identification of a bleeding source guides the planning and timing of surgery. Identification of cardiac tamponade or tension pneumothorax also mandates specific management. Peripheral blood pressure is often maligned as a means of assessing shock, but it can be useful and is among the most accessible of parameters. A normal blood pressure indicates either no significant blood loss or a compensatory response. The primary pitfall is assuming the former. The presence of associated tachycardia or delayed capillary refill indicates that the normal blood pressure is in fact compensatory.

The moderately hypotensive patient should be assumed to have begun the progression into shock and be aggressively managed. The profoundly hypotensive patient has similarly declared himself. Because blood loss is the cause in most cases of traumatic shock, it is extremely important to quantitate it. Barring obvious external blood loss, occult bleeding of a magnitude to cause shock almost always occurs in the chest or abdomen, secondary to pelvic or femur fractures or some combination. Available diagnostic maneuvers to confirm such bleeding include a chest radiograph, tube thoracostomy, peritoneal lavage, and abdominal computed tomography (CT). Diagnostic studies must not impede or delay other critical aspects of resuscitation. Unstable patients should not be sent to CT scanners or to other areas that lack monitoring and resuscitative capabilities.

The spun hematocrit is the best way to quantitate blood loss. Acute blood loss theoretically does not affect the hematocrit until there has been adequate time (usually several hours) for fluid to shift from the extravascular to the intravascular space. A low hematocrit suggests a major bleed, whereas a normal hematocrit cannot rule one out and must be repeated at frequent intervals. Hematocrit is also affected by the administration of intravenous fluid, and this potential dilutional effect can be difficult to interpret; the safest course is to attribute minimal significance to dilution.

Other parameters described are less useful. Mental status reflects cerebral blood flow, but a number of other factors, including concomitant head injury, intoxication, fear, and pain, make it an ancillary parameter at best. Tachypnea is, likewise, a fairly nonspecific response. Urinary output is a fairly valid indicator of renal perfusion, but it is useful primarily over a longer course. Central venous pressure (CVP) can be a valuable and accessible extrapolation of preload, assuming normal pre-existent cardiac function. This is usually a safe assumption in the typical young trauma patient, but it must be made judiciously. A low CVP confirms hypovolemia and serves as a useful guide to fluid resuscitation, whereas an elevated CVP may be the first sign of progressing cardiac tamponade or tension pneumothorax.

Pulmonary capillary wedge pressure is more accurate than CVP, but the technical difficulties involved in catheterization may impede other critical resuscitative measures. Oxygenation and acid–base status assessed by means of arterial blood gas sampling can be extremely useful, although major discrepancies in arterial and venous values in low-flow states suggest simultaneous sampling, and comparison may be more meaningful. Cutaneous and conjunctival oximeters may also prove to be of value. Hypoxia and acidosis, particularly if more profound than the clinical picture suggests, may be early clues that shock is progressing at the microcirculatory level.

DIFFERENTIAL DIAGNOSIS

The differential diagnosis of traumatic shock is limited. The traumatized patient who is hypotensive or showing the compensatory responses should be assumed to have sustained or be sustaining a significant bleed. The other entities that may be implicated—cardiac tamponade and tension pneumothorax—should be considered when the mechanisms of trauma are consistent with these injuries or when significant blood loss has been ruled out. Central nervous system injury should also be considered. More common is the occurrence of head injury and hemorrhagic shock concurrently, in which case the management of shock must take precedence. Spinal shock can occur after major injury to the spinal cord and result in loss of peripheral vascular tone and relative hypovolemia. The absence of a tachycardic response or an actual bradycardic response helps to differentiate it from hemorrhagic shock.

EMERGENCY DEPARTMENT MANAGEMENT

The goals are dictated by the degree of shock. In less severe shock the goal is to halt the progression of shock in hopes of precluding the multisystem failure. In more severe shock, the goal must be to prevent imminent cardiac arrest. The two immediate objectives are restoration of circulating volume and hemostasis. Vascular access must occur simultaneously with basic airway management. Multiple large-bore intravenous lines must be placed. Crystalloid solutions are the initial fluid of choice. Hypertonic saline shows promise. If blood loss is severe, it must rapidly be replaced, starting with low titer type O or type specific, if crossmatched blood is not immediately available. With massive transfusions consideration must be given to restoration of clotting factors and to warming of blood.

The availability of large-bore intravenous catheters and even larger-bore tubing coupled with pressure bags makes it possible to deliver extremely high volumes of fluid in very short periods of time. However, complications such as fluid overload, extravasation from central veins, and hypothermia may occur and must be considered. Life-threatening hemorrhage can frequently not be controlled and early surgical intervention should be the goal as soon as the patient can be stabilized. In some cases such stabilization is not possible. Fluid, particularly blood, must be forced into the vascular system at maximal rates. Unless there is an immediate response to such fluid, emergency thoracotomy is the only possible recourse. Although mortality is high, a few lesions are manageable by way of this procedure.

Experience has shown that utility of ED thoracotomy may be limited to sudden deterioration in a patient with penetrating chest trauma. Cardiac tamponade and isolated cardiac wounds are the two settings in which the yields have been highest, and the ideal candidate is the patient with refractory hypotension (systolic less than 90 mm Hg) and a reasonable likelihood of such injuries but who has not yet arrested. Where actual blood loss has been excessive, aortic cross-clamping is also indicated. The advanced cardiac life support protocols for bradycardia are of questionable value in this setting; the same can even be said for cardiopulmonary resuscitation. The utility of the MAST suit, once routinely recommended, is now in question. The most qualified physician present must proceed to emergency thoracotomy.

COMMON PITFALLS

- Failure to recognize or underestimating the severity of impending shock. This translates into a lack of aggressiveness in resuscitation (too few, too small intravenous lines, too little fluid, and delay in starting blood).
- Failure to recognize and intervene in specific entities (cardiac tamponade, isolated cardiac injuries, and tension pneumothorax).
- Delay in obtaining surgical consultation and getting the patient to the operating room when appropriate.

WOUND MANAGEMENT

A summary guide to tenanus prophylaxis of the wounded patient is outlined in Table 56-1.

COMMON PITFALLS

- Failure to detect any sensory, motor, or vascular complications or injuries to specialized tissues (e.g., lacrimal or parotid duct) is one common error.
- Vasoconstrictors in anesthetic agents should not gain access to the wounds.
- Removal of hair by a razor is damaging to the skin.
- Antiseptic agents or surgical scrub solutions should not contact the wound.
- Drainage should not be used as a replacement for meticulous hemostasis, and should be reserved for removal of harmful collections of fluid.
- Dead space closure by even the least reactive suture should never be undertaken.
- Treatment of patients with contaminated wounds with **oral** antibiotics is unwarranted and should not be considered an appropriate substitute for immediate treatment with intravenous antibiotics.
- The use of either surgical needles manufactured from relatively weak stainless steel alloys or natural fiber sutures for closure of wounds should be avoided.
- Tetanus toxoid adsorbed should not be administered indiscriminately to all patients with traumatic wounds, but should be considered part of the recommended tetanus prophylaxis regimens for the patient with traumatic wounds.

TABLE 56-1. Tetanus Prophylaxis

History of Adsorbed Tetanus Toxoid (doses)	Tetanus-Prone WoundsWounds		Nontetanus Prone Wounds	
	Td*	TIG†	Td*	TIG‡
Uncertain or <3	Yes	Yes	Yes	No
3 or more§	No‖	No	No**	No

*For children under 7 years old, diphtheria and tetanus toxoids and pertussis vaccine adsorbed (DIP), (diphtheria and tetanus toxoids adsorbed [DT], if pertussis is contraindicated) are preferred to tetanus toxoid alone. For patients 7 years old or older, tetanus and diphtheria toxoids adsorbed (for adult use) (Td) are preferred to tetanus toxoid alone.
†TIG: Human tetanus immune globulin.
‡When TIG and Td are given concurrently, separate syringes and separate sites should be used.
§If only three doses of fluid toxoid have been received, a fourth dose of toxoid, preferably an adsorbed toxoid, should be given.
‖Yes, if more than 5 years since last dose. (More frequent boosters are not needed and can accentuate side effects.)
**Yes, if more than 10 years since last dose.

57   Head Injuries

In dealing with head injuries the only organ of concern is the brain. Any damage to the covering tissue over the brain—for instance, the scalp and skull—is of secondary importance, provided the brain and its functions are intact. The intracranial compartments are delineated by the rigid and unyielding skull. This anatomical arrangement characterizes the uniqueness of any intracranial injury. Any insult of sufficient severity directed at the brain would be reflected in raised intracranial pressure (ICP). If the injury results in increasing brain swelling or hematoma formation, the only egress or exit is downward toward the foramen magnum. The intracranial cavity can be depicted as a funnel. The tough tentorium effectively divides this funnel into the supratentorial and infratentorial compartments. Progressive rise in ICP in the supratentorial compartment results in the herniation of the uncus, which is adjacent to the tentorial edge. The progressive herniation of the uncus past the tentorial edge causes pressure on the adjacent third nerve with ipsilateral dilatation of the pupil. Further herniation impinges against the cerebral peduncle with decerebration, and the posterior cerebral artery with corresponding ischemic changes and infarction.

Unremitting and uncorrected rise in ICP results in shift of the contralateral cerebral peduncle against the edge of the tentorium and pressure against the adjacent third nerve and posterior cerebral artery on the other side. There is then impingement of the same structures against the tentorial edge. This progressive scenario results in dilatation of the contralateral pupil and cessation of spontaneous respiration because of bilateral functional or physiologic interruption of pathways found in the cerebral peduncles. This is the end stage, and the patient is considered unsalvageable. When similar conditions prevail in the infratentorial compartment the cerebellar tonsils herniate and compress against the medulla. The physiologic results are changes in the respiratory pattern and cardiac arrhythmia. The end result is respiratory and cardiac arrest. The emergency physician must institute aggressive corrective measures, including prompt and appropriate consultations.

CLINICAL PRESENTATION

There is a wide spectrum of head injury presentation, from subtle threshold injuries with temporary loss of consciousness to obvious penetrating gunshot wounds.

SCALP LACERATIONS   The scalp is extremely vascular. Any laceration can cause profuse bleeding, enough to deplete the blood volume and cause shock. Debridement followed by suturing should be carried out. In every case the depth of the wound or laceration should be determined by palpation with gloved fingers to rule out a depressed skull fracture.

DEPRESSED SKULL FRACTURE   A depressed skull fracture requires prompt neurosurgical attention. All such cases require skull films or computed tomography (CT) with bone windows for diagnostic confirmation. CT can also rule out an underlying hematoma.

LINEAR SKULL FRACTURE   Victims of linear skull fracture should be observed as inpatients, especially in cases where the fracture crosses the vascular grooves of the meningeal vessels.

BASAL SKULL FRACTURE   Basal skull fractures require inpatient observation and bed rest to prevent a chronically occurring cerebrospinal fluid leak. The use of antibiotic therapy is debated.

EPIDURAL HEMATOMA Epidural hematoma is one of the few true emergencies. When a patient is suspected of harboring an epidural hematoma immediate surgical intervention for diagnosis and eventual therapy is mandatory. No time should be spent on diagnostic measures. If necessary, trephination and rongeuring for decompression should be initiated in the ED by one trained to do so. The evolving events are the rapid and expanding accumulation of hematoma due to the tear of a meningeal artery, rapid rise of ICP, ipsilateral uncal herniation, and third nerve and peduncle compression. Salvageability depends on prompt intervention before this point, not when both pupils are dilated. Epidural hematomas are curable if diagnosed and treated in a timely manner.

SUBDURAL HEMATOMA Acute subdural hematoma is usually caused by torn cortical vessels either from cortical laceration or severe contusions. The evolutionary changes may rival those of an epidural hematoma in rapidity. Because of the cerebral contusion or laceration, edema is a frequent complicating factor, and the ultimate prognosis is guarded. Chronic subdural hematoma is a distinct entity from the acute type. It is usually secondary to tearing of bridging veins after even minor head trauma. The veins are stretched and more susceptible to tears in older patients because of cortical atrophy. The evolving process is slow. It may be weeks before the consequences of the mass effect become apparent. The clinical course is subtle, initially involving headache, personality change, forgetfulness, and lethargy. When cerebral decompensation occurs, stupor and hemiparesis may ensue. Seizures may hasten the process. Drainage of the hematoma is indicated; the prognosis is good when drainage is performed in a timely manner.

INTRACEREBRAL HEMATOMA Traumatic intracerebral hematomas are not as common as the spontaneous variety. They are usually located in the frontal, temporal, and, less frequently, occipital poles, sites that bear the brunt of impact injury. The diagnosis is made by CT scan, and the treatment is surgical evacuation. The prognosis is quite good because the hematoma is frequently situated away from the vital structures.

PENETRATING WOUNDS OF THE SKULL Of most concern is the presence of mass effect either from swelling or from hematoma formation. This problem will cause shift of the midline structures and can be readily seen on CT scan. Swelling should be treated promptly. Any hematoma greater than 4 cm should be surgically evacuated. Impaled objects should be left in place. The extent of injury caused by gunshot wounds is unpredictable; trajectory as well as the energy created by the mass and velocity of the missile determine the damage. Bleeding and swelling soon follow, and infection may develop later. If the missile traverses only one lobe, the prognosis may be better. If two lobes are involved, the prognosis is worse. The worst injuries involve both hemispheres and the deep-lying structures (diencephalon or rhombencephalon). A CT scan together with knowledge of the entry and exit wounds will give a fairly accurate picture of the extent of injury. Neurosurgical intervention is indicated only to debride necrotic brain tissues, remove depressed or penetrating bone fragments and bullet fragments (if accessible), and evacuate a sizable hematoma. Broad-spectrum antibiotics should be given.

MASS EFFECT When the CT scan shows a shift of the midline structures either from edema or from hematoma collection the important prognostic factor is obliteration of the cisterns. The obliteration of the cisterns in the presence of marked shift denotes a grave prognosis, and usually indicates herniation. If these cisterns are discernible, the prognosis may be quite good, even in the presence of considerable shift of midline structures. Haste in the management of such injuries may, however, be more imperative.

DIFFERENTIAL DIAGNOSIS

COMA The availability of imaging scanners simplifies the diagnosis of coma. This modality should be used to its fullest potential. The Glasgow Coma Scale should be used to establish a common denominator for communication.

DEPRESSED SKULL FRACTURES   One should not diagnose a depressed skull fracture without the benefit of skull films (preferably with tangential views) or CT scans with bone windows. A subgaleal hematoma may feel like a depressed skull fracture. Even palpable or visible depression through an open wound may actually be an indentation at a suture line or comminuted fractures of only the outer table.

CHRONIC SUBDURAL HEMATOMA   Patients with chronic subdural hematoma are usually seen during the state of cerebral decompensation, when the patient displays neurologic deficit in the form of seizures, hemiparesis, and lethargy. A CT scan will unmask the diagnosis. Some of these lesions may have the same radiologic density as cerebral tissues (isodense). Contrast scan may be required to make the diagnosis.

EMERGENCY DEPARTMENT EVALUATION

A CT scan remains the most effective diagnostic tool. In general, the following statements hold true:

- All unconscious patients with evidence of head injury should have a CT scan, including intoxicated patients and those who are in a coma of metabolic cause.
- All patients with linear skull fractures that cross the meningeal vascular groove should have a CT scan to rule out an incipient or developing epidural hematoma.
- All patients with depressed and basal skull fractures should have a CT scan.
- A Glasgow Coma Scale score of ≤8 denotes a serious condition and necessitates a CT scan. Recent work indicates minor head trauma and a GCS of 13 may require CT scan as well.
- In patients with multisystem trauma, including head trauma, the presence of low systemic blood pressure and shock indicates depletion of blood volume. Intracranial pathology is seldom the cause. In fact, a rise in ICP inevitably results in a rise in systemic blood pressure to ensure an adequate blood supply to the brain.

EMERGENCY DEPARTMENT MANAGEMENT

The vital signs, the Glasgow Coma Scale, the open wound, and coexisting injury should be known. The prime consideration is to prevent the rise of ICP and to lower it, if possible. The following steps or medications combat such an eventuality and to treat coexisting conditions. First, an airway should be maintained with endotracheal intubation (Table 57-1). One can then institute hyperventilation to lower the ICP or prevent it from rising. Usually a tidal volume of 800 mL or above with a frequency of 12 to 14 per minute will maintain PCO_2 at 25 to 30 mm Hg.

Hyperosmolar agents should be administered. Mannitol is a potent and rapidly acting hyperosmolar agent. The dose is 25 g to 50 g intravenous push, with another 25 g at 4-hour intervals, not to exceed 200 g in a 24-hour period. Be aware that the diuresis may deplete the intravascular compartment. Adequate replacement is essential, based on the urinary output. Plasma protein fraction (Plasmanate) helps to lower ICP by virtue of its hyperosmolality and is given at 30 mL/h. Other agents include: Dexamethasone (Decadron) is administered in doses of 10 mg to 20 mg intravenous followed by the same dose at intervals of 6 hours intravenously. Dexamethasone is not as potent as mannitol, but it may be beneficial in treating severe intracranial hypertension. Diuretics may be used. Lasix is given intravenously (40 mg repeated every 4 to 6 hours as necessary). Electrolytes, blood urea nitrogen, and creatinine serum and urine osmolality should be measured as a baseline. To prevent shock or dehydration, a central venous pressure line should ideally be placed and the central venous pressure should be maintained at 8 to 10 mm Hg preferably.

Barbiturates are potent anti-brain-swelling agents, but also offer some protection to damaged neurons. For short-term purposes, and when rapidity is essential, one should use a short-acting type such as thiopental sodium (Pentothal Sodium), in an initial dose of 300 mg followed

---

TABLE 57-1. Technique for Rapid-Sequence Intubation of the Acutely Head-Injured Patient

---

1. **Preoxygenation**
   100% oxygen for 5 minutes or four vital capacity breaths
2. **Pretreatment**
   Vecuronium (0.01 mg/kg IV)
   Lidocaine (1.5 mg/kg IV)
   Fentanyl (3 to 5 µg/kg IV)
3. **Wait 2 to 3 Minutes (If Possible)**
   Continue preoxygenation
4. **Paralysis and Sedation**
   Thiopental (3 to 5 mg/kg IV; 0.5 to 1 mg/kg IV if hypotensive)
   Succinylcholine (1.5 mg/kg IV)
5. **Intubation With Cervical-Spine Immobilization**
6. **Immediately After Intubation, Institute Positive-Pressure Ventilation and Consider Longer-Term Neuromuscular Blockade and Sedation**

From Walls R: Ann Em Medicine 22:6, June 1993 with permission.

by 100 mg every hour. When there is actual or potential contamination, Oxacillin (1–2 g IV) or vancomycin (500 mg) plus tobramycin (60–80 mg IV) may be used. A subarachnoid ICP measuring device can be readily placed in any ED setting, and is indicated in any case of serious head injury in order to accurately monitor ICP.

DISPOSITION

Whenever doubt exists neurosurgical consultation should be obtained.

COMMON PITFALLS

- The intoxicated patient with a possible head injury should have a CT scan. To ensure some degree of cooperation, appropriate sedation may be used.
- A subgaleal hematoma can simulate a depressed skull fracture. Skull films or a CT scan should be done.
- In all instances of hypotension with evidence of head injury a systemic cause should be sought. Intracranial injury alone does not result in hypotension or shock.
- In cases of unconsciousness with a probable metabolic cause with evidence of head injury, or unexplained unconsciousness without any evidence of head injury, a CT scan should be performed.
- Isodense subdural collection should be suspected when there is a shift of the midline structures. A contrast scan is indicated.
- In the presence of shifts of midline structures the existence of unilateral obliteration of perimesencephalic or ambien cisterns denotes the possibility of uncal herniation. The condition is potentially catastrophic and demands prompt corrective measures.

58 Neck Injuries

Injuries to the neck are difficult to evaluate. Regardless of how benign they may appear, injuries to the neck may quickly and catastrophically deteriorate. Neck injuries must be rapidly and thoroughly evaluated.

NECK STRUCTURES

The neck is divided into three anatomical zones (Fig. 58-1). The line of demarcation between zones one and two is not well accepted. The most logical line is probably the top of the clavicles because this is where a standard neck incision ends. Zone three is protected by the face and mandible anteriorly, and hence is more difficult to injure. Injuries to this region are often ascending, and may involve the structures of the face or skull. Zone two contains the cervical spine and a complex series of muscles that wrap around the deep structures of the neck. The most important of these is the sternocleidomastoid, which extends from the sternum and clavicle to the mastoid process.

The sternocleidomastoid divides the neck into two triangles. The anterior triangle is covered by the platysma muscle; immediately below this lies the cervical branch of the facial nerve. Then come the facial artery, the submandibular gland, portions of the thyroid gland, part of the external carotid artery and the internal carotid artery, the interior jugular vein, and the glossopharyngeal and vagus nerves. In the posterior triangle lie the external jugular vein, the dorsal scapular nerve, thoracic nerves, and the accessory nerve. Deep to these lie the brachial plexus and the proximal portion of the subclavian artery. The front of the neck includes a portion of the thymus gland (in children), the thyroid gland, and the branches of the external carotid and subclavian arteries that supply them. Between and lateral to the trachea and esophagus lies the recurrent laryngeal nerve. The hypoglossal nerve runs through zone three. The brachial plexus

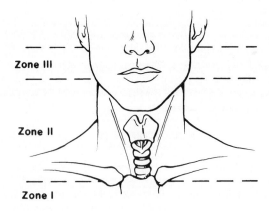

Figure 58-1. Zones of the neck.

should be examined by testing arm and hand motion. The patient should be asked to move the tongue to test the glossopharyngeal nerve and the shoulders to test the accessory nerve.

CLINICAL PRESENTATION

Injuries to the neck may damage any of the structures described. The physical examination should focus on each structure, preferably in order of their importance. The neck should be examined in a linear manner, starting with the airway and progressing to the blood vessels, spinal cord, peripheral nerves, and esophagus. Injuries to the trachea are common, and should be suspected when there is hemoptysis, if blood appears during suctioning, or if hoarseness or subcutaneous emphysema occurs. The latter conditions may also indicate esophageal injury. Vascular injuries may result in arterial bleeding or rapidly expanding hematoma. They may also result in arteriovenous fistula, aneurysm, air embolus, or infarction of distal tissues.

The patient may be hoarse due to direct laryngeal trauma or trauma to the laryngeal nerves. Penetrating trauma to the laryngeal nerve is particularly important because the nerve runs closely between the esophagus and the trachea. Concomitant injury to one or both of these structures may be present. Esophageal injuries are among the most difficult to evaluate. They are also dangerous because they often show up late and may cause serious infection and death days after the injury. Esophageal injuries from external penetrating trauma are usually associated with injuries to the trachea or the nerves that parallel it; these injuries require surgical exploration for evaluation. Injuries from instrumentation or foreign bodies, however, may be evaluated by endoscopy or barium swallow.

EMERGENCY DEPARTMENT MANAGEMENT

Airway management in patients with laryngotracheal injuries may constitute an extremely challenging problem. If the airway can be maintained through suctioning and positioning alone, this should be done. In the patient with a more serious injury a choice must be made between endotracheal intubation or a surgical procedure for airway management. In the patient with severe injury to the thyroid cartilage, intubation may be impossible, and a tracheostomy may be the only option. When the injury is below the level of the thyroid cartilage attempted tracheostomy may complete a partial injury, and endotracheal intubation would be preferable. Intubation should be done in Trendelenburg position to avoid air embolus.

In the patient with airway compromise and altered anatomy, intubation may be extremely difficult or impossible. The procedure may be rendered complicated by the presence of airway displacement due to massive hematoma or by laryngotracheal fracture or separation. In this situation direct visualization by way of endoscopy may be necessary, or a surgical airway (cricothyrotomy or tracheostomy) may be necessary.

All patients with neck trauma should have two large intravenous lines, a baseline hematocrit and blood banking. Antibiotics have been of little benefit in penetrating neck injuries. If antibiotics are administered, they should be effective against *Staphylococcus aureus*.

If there is clear injury to major blood vessels, as indicated by active bleeding or expanding hematoma, if the injury has occurred in a manner that implies extensive damage (for example, from a high-powered rifle), or if the wound is grossly contaminated or there is obvious structural damage, further evaluation is best performed in the operating room. If no obvious signs of structural damage exist, particularly if the injury is to zone one or three (which are difficult to explore), further evaluation may be warranted. The airway above the vocal cords can be evaluated with direct or indirect laryngoscopy. If there is bleeding below this point or subcutaneous emphysema is present without an obvious source, endoscopy must be performed. If there is a possibility of injury to major blood vessels, angiography (preferably digital subtraction angiography) should be performed. Although these do not completely rule out the possibility of an injury, a negative result makes observation safer, and a positive result will identify the area that requires surgical exploration.

DISPOSITION

Injuries that require immediate exploration are the most straightforward. The following cases call for immediate operation: a wound caused by a high-velocity bullet, an expanding hematoma, obvious structural damage, open contaminated wounds, and injury to one of the peripheral nerves, airway, or esophagus. The surgeon should be contacted while the evaluation of the patient is taking place. The situation becomes more complex as the injury becomes less obviously serious. A cautious examination of a presumably superficial laceration is warranted; however, if the wound penetrates the platysmas, a surgical consultation should be obtained immediately. It is controversial whether it is safer to take these patients and those with similar injuries from low-velocity bullets to the operating room immediately or to observe them; however, observation is warranted only in a facility that has the ability to do immediate surgery. Blunt trauma to the neck is perhaps the most difficult to assess because arterial injury may present late and the airway may be compromised by delayed bleeding. If the mechanism implies a significant absorption of energy, the patient should be admitted for observation.

COMMON PITFALLS

- Application of a collar may make evaluation of neck injuries impossible. If there is reason to believe that the neck may be injured, stabilization of the neck should occur without obscuring it.
- The incorrect assumption that a patient who is stable and has no signs of obvious injuries initially will remain so. Observation and transfer of patients with neck injuries are hazardous and may result in a catastrophic deterioration.
- There should be no blind probing of wounds.
- Procedures that may stimulate the patient to gag or cough should be avoided so as not to break loose a clot.

---

59   Maxillofacial Injuries

Most facial injuries are sustained as a result of altercations, sports injuries, or motor vehicle accidents. Falls and industrial accidents are responsible for the remainder. General principles include:

- Any patient who has sustained a blow sufficient to cause a facial fracture should be suspected of having a cervical spine injury. All maneuvers to establish an airway should be done with the neck immobilized in the neutral position.
- Cricothyrostomy is recommended if an airway cannot be provided by intubation or other airway maneuvers.
- In patients suspected of having severely comminuted midface injuries (Le Fort II, Le Fort III, and nasoethmoidal fractures) extreme care must be taken when nasal endotracheal or nasogastric tubes are passed.

- Facial hemorrhage is controlled by direct pressure, moist gauze packing, and ligation of obviously bleeding vessels. Rarely external carotid or internal maxillary artery ligation will be necessary.
- It is important to have the consultant involved early.
- Because facial lacerations may involve important structures, (branches of the facial nerve, the parotid duct, or nasolacrimal apparatus) all lacerations should be thoroughly explored before closure. If injuries to these structures are suspected, the wound should be thoroughly irrigated and packed with moist sterile gauze for evaluation by the consultant.
- A thorough ophthalmologic examination is mandatory if there has been significant trauma to the midface region.
- Facial fractures are usually not treated definitively until the patient has been fully assessed and other life- and limb-threatening injuries have been stabilized. Closure of "clean" or thoroughly irrigated facial wounds may be delayed up to 24 hours. As a rule, the earlier the injury is treated, the better the result and postoperative course. If the patient is not stable, definitive treatment may be delayed as long as 2 to 3 weeks.
- The examiner should obtain an accurate history of the mechanism of injury. It is equally important to determine whether the patient was wearing a dental prosthesis. Dentures and teeth that are unaccounted for at the time of injury may show up later, obstructing the patient's airway.

NASAL FRACTURES

Nasal fractures are the most common facial bone injury. They are common both as isolated fractures and in combination with multiple facial fractures. The patient usually complains of local pain, epistaxis, nasal deformity, and obstructed nasal breathing. Physical examination is performed by external inspection for deviation or deformity; palpation for crepitus; evaluation of dorsal or intranasal lacerations; and inspection of the septum by nasal speculum (with vasoconstriction, if necessary) for a hematoma, which must be urgently drained to protect the blood supply of the cartilaginous septum. Failure to drain a septal hematoma may lead to an unsightly saddle deformity.

Radiographic evaluation of nasal fractures is controversial; much can be gained from physical examination alone. If ordered, views include right and left nasal views, and nasal views in the posteroanterior skull and Waters projections. Definitive treatment is usually delayed for 7 to 10 days due to edema. Acute management may involve suturing of intranasal or extranasal lacerations; drainage of a septal hematoma by a small vertical incision and nasal packing; and anterior or posterior nasal packing to control epistaxis. Posterior nasal packing may be quickly effected by using a Foley balloon-tipped catheter. Supplemental misted oxygen by face mask should be administered to guard against hypoxia as posterior packs are in place.

MANDIBULAR FRACTURES

Mandibular fractures are common. Because of the mandible's U-shape, it is unusual for the mandible to break in only one place due to the contrecoup effect of a blow to the lower jaw. More than 50% of mandibular fractures are multiple. It is incumbent to search for more than one fracture. Many fractures are open or compound and communicate directly with the mouth between the teeth. Common areas of involvement are the subcondylar, angle, parasymphysis, and symphysis regions. Occasionally unstable segments may contribute to airway embarrassment, since the tongue musculature attaches to the mandible and may be displaced posteriorly.

Common symptoms of mandible fractures include localized facial pain; complaint of dental malocclusion or "my bite is off" (very sensitive); a numb lower lip; hemorrhage from between the teeth; dysphagia or trismus; and a grating sound transmitted to the ear when the mandible is moved. Physical examination may show local swelling; hemorrhage; separation of teeth interspaces with bimanual palpation across the fracture site; dental malocclusion with "step-offs"; localized floor of the mouth ecchymosis or edema (pathognomonic); inferior alveolar and mental nerve paresthesia or anesthesia; limitation of mandibular motion secondary to pain; loose or missing teeth; "step-offs" on palpation of the inferior border; and inability to feel movement of the mandibular condyles when the examiner palpates with the fingers in the external ear canals.

Radiographic evaluation should include posteroanterior and lateral skull films (for the mandible); right and left lateral oblique views to include the mandibular condyles; a Townes view to include the mandibular condyles; and a panoramic radiograph if available (best single view).

Initial treatment is usually limited but may involve airway management; accounting for missing teeth or dentures to prevent airway compromise; and making sure that patients with fractures through tooth-bearing bone are placed on prophylactic antibiotics to prevent infection. Penicillin is preferred, or an appropriate alternative in penicillin-allergic patients. Definitive reduction of mandibular fractures may involve closed reduction by placing the patient's teeth together in proper occlusion for 4 to 6 weeks with application of arch bars and intermaxillary fixation. Open reduction with wires, plates, or screws, with or without the need for intermaxillary fixation, may also be indicated. Occasionally external pin fixation devices or dental prosthetic splints are used when the dentition is compromised.

COMMON PITFALLS

- Failure to check for more than one fracture
- Failure to recognize potential or real cause of airway embarrassment, such as avulsed teeth, dislodged dentures, and loss of tongue support due to fractures of the symphysis
- Failure to account for missing teeth or dentures
- Inadequate radiographs that fail to show the mandibular condyles, thus resulting in missed fractures

MAXILLARY FRACTURES

Maxillary fractures are usually the result of blunt trauma, massive crush injuries, and, occasionally, penetrating injuries. Traditionally, they are named according to the Le Fort classification of midfacial fractures. Patients who have sustained significantly displaced maxillary fractures are usually severely traumatized, with other injuries being present. Physical examination of their facial fractures is done during the secondary survey and may show a massively swollen face with periorbital ecchymosis; epistaxis or CSF leaks; associated mandibular fractures; palpation that reveals "step-offs" in the frontozygomatic, zygomaticomaxillary, or frontonasal regions; separation of the lines of fracture under the palpating finger when the head is stabilized by an assistant and the anterior maxilla is grasped and "pumped" up and down; gross malocclusion with anterior "open bite"; elongated or "dished in" facial appearance caused by the midface fracture sliding inferiorly and posteriorly on the cranial base; and ocular injuries.

Radiographic examination should include a facial series with attention to the Waters projection. If the patient needs a CT scan to rule out intracranial injury, this is an ideal time to obtain cuts through the midface region. Definitive evaluation of the extent of the facial fractures is performed by the use of "bony window" CT scans in axial and coronal planes when the patient has been stabilized and the cervical spine is cleared. If greater anatomical detail is needed, three-dimensional reformatting of the standard CT scan data can provide excellent detail.

Immediate attention must be given to assure an adequate airway, since displaced midface fractures usually compromise the nasal airway with clotted blood and secretions. The airway may be compromised by massive swelling, associated unstable mandible fractures, and foreign bodies such as teeth and dentures, which must be cleared. An airway may be secured by one of the following maneuvers, proceeding from simple to complex management and keeping in mind that a cervical spine injury may be present: nasopharyngeal airway that is carefully placed parallel to the palatal plane; intubation (oral preferred); cricothyrostomy or tracheostomy (elective) if long-term airway compromise is anticipated. The patient should be placed on 100% oxygen and ventilated. Further management may require nasal packing to control epistaxis; careful passage of a nasogastric tube to clear the stomach of swallowed blood; urgent CT scan for intracranial injuries; and urgent evaluation of ophthalmologic injuries.

COMMON PITFALLS

- Failure to secure the airway with adequate attention to cervical spine control;
- Failure to exercise care when nasal tubes are passed due to the possibility of entrance into the cranial cavity;
- Overlooking ophthalmologic injuries due to the massive facial edema that hinders examination.

ZYGOMATICOMAXILLARY COMPLEX FRACTURES

Zygomaticomaxillary (ZMC) fractures are usually sustained from a blunt blow to the zygomatic prominence (cheekbone). The bone is commonly displaced inferiorly, posteriorly, and medially into the maxillary sinus. The fracture line always crosses the orbital floor and varies in its extent of injury. However, isolated zygomatic arch fractures may occur with no intraorbital involvement. Symptoms of ZMC fractures include local pain; paresthesia or numbness of the infraorbital nerve distribution (lateral nose, anterior maxillary teeth, and gums); loss of zygomatic prominence with depression; epistaxis; pain with eye movement; diplopia, if significant orbital floor involvement is present and inability to open the mouth (significant or isolated arch depression impinges on the coronoid process of the mandible and temporalis muscle tendon).

Physical examination may reveal local pain to palpation at the fracture sites; paresthesia or anesthesia of the infraorbital nerve; crepitus; "step-offs" in the infraorbital rim and zygomaticofrontal suture lines and at the zygomatic buttress area intraorally; epistaxis; decreased extraocular movement; subconjunctival hemorrhage (a reliable sign); canted pupillary line with enophthalmos; periorbital ecchymosis and edema; depressed zygomatic arch with limitation of jaw opening; and ecchymosis of the zygomatic buttress area intraorally.

Radiographic examination should include Waters view (to show fractures and air–fluid levels in the maxillary sinus); posteroanterior and lateral skull projections; a submentovertex view (especially good for evaluating depression of the zygomatic arch); and oblique orbital views. CT scans are optional if significant orbital floor involvement is present.

ED management consists of assessing possible injury to the globe, keeping the patient's head elevated and applying ice to reduce edema; arranging referral to the facial consultant and hospital admission in selected cases; and administering prophylactic antibiotics to cover sinus pathogens. A nasal spray and decongestant should be prescribed to promote drainage and lessen the chance of infection of blood trapped in the maxillary sinus.

ORBITAL BLOWOUT FRACTURES

Orbital blowout fractures are sustained by two mechanisms. First, this fracture can occur when a blunt object >5 cm in diameter strikes the globe (e.g., fist, tennis ball, or dashboard). Smaller objects tend to cause penetrating injuries. The globe theoretically expands in the bony orbit and results in a "blow out" of the thin orbital floor (maxilla) or the lamina papyracea (ethmoid) of the medial orbital wall. Second, a fracture can occur by buckling of the orbital floor when an object deforms the infraorbital rim. This force is transmitted to the much thinner orbital floor, which fractures.

Symptoms associated with orbital blowout fractures include blurred vision or decreased visual acuity; diplopia (may be the only sign) usually in primary or upward gaze; paresthesia of the infraorbital nerve (55%); epistaxis (maxillary sinus involvement); and ocular pain with movement. Physical examination may reveal periorbital ecchymosis, edema, or emphysema; enophthalmos or, occasionally, proptosis (postseptal hematoma); subconjunctival hemorrhage (a reliable sign); intraocular injury by ophthalmoscopic examination (i.e., dislocated lens or retinal tear or detachment); iridoplegia (indicating sphincter muscle injury); decreased sensation in the infraorbital nerve distribution; entrapment or paresis of extraocular muscles leading to decreased motion; a depressed pupillary line best seen by checking for discrepancies of the light reflected back from the pupil as viewed straight on (Hirschberg's reflex); and corneal abrasion.

Radiographic examination should include Waters view and posteroanterior and lateral skull films initially. These may show an opacified maxillary sinus or the classic "teardrops" sign of fat herniated into the sinus. Definitive radiographic examination may be performed by coronal CT scan (preferred) or anteroposterior orbital tomograms. Treatment depends on the severity of the injury. Significant ocular involvement may be present in up to 30% of cases; immediate ophthalmologic consultation may be warranted. Definitive treatment of orbital blowout fractures is controversial. Unquestionable signs of entrapment or enophthalmos deserves orbital exploration and placement of a bony or alloplastic implant to prevent irreversible sequelae. Questionable cases are observed for resolution of edema and diplopia. Ophthalmologic consultation is mandatory at some point during the early care of the patient.

COMMON PITFALLS

- Failure to appreciate that the edema of injury may falsely elevate the globe, thereby masking the enophthalmos and diplopia
- Failure to appreciate that even significant blowout fractures sometimes do not show limitation of globe motion due to decompression into the maxillary sinus
- Failure to adequately assess intraocular structures or the possibility of an evolving postseptal hematoma

NASOETHMOIDAL FRACTURES

Nasoethmoidal fractures usually occur from a blunt injury to the nasal region. They are serious in that they involve the nose, the frontal process of the maxilla, and the lacrimal and ethmoid bones of the medial orbit. The medial canthal tendons attach to the lacrimal crests and may be detached or displaced with this injury, leaving the patient with a disfiguring telecanthus if unrecognized. Injury to the nasolacrimal duct system may occur, with resultant epiphora. Basilar skull injury with a dural tear may also be present.

Symptoms associated with nasoethmoidal fractures may include epistaxis; local pain; clear fluid leaking from the nose; pain with eye movement; nasal obstruction; complaint of wide flat nasal bridge; and epiphora. Physical examination may reveal comminuted nasal fracture with loss of dorsal nasal projection; telecanthus with detached medial canthal tendons (i.e., intercanthal distance greater than the width of one eye); obstruction of the nasolacrimal apparatus; epistaxis or CSF leak; nasal or frontal crepitus to palpation; subconjunctival hemorrhage; and limited ocular motion secondary to pain.

Radiographic examination should include Waters view, posteroanterior and lateral skull films; and nasal views. Coronal and axial CT scans are helpful. ED management is usually limited to diagnosis; careful control of epistaxis by nasal packing; and ice packs. If significant epiphora is present, nasolacrimal duct injury may be established by instilling ophthalmic fluorescein eyedrops; and with the aid of a black light, checking for their appearance intranasally at the duct's drainage point under the inferior turbinate. Definitive treatment of nasoethmoidal fractures centers around re-establishing the correct intercanathal distance with reattachment of these canthal tendons or repositioning of their fractured bones with wires or plates. The lacrimal apparatus may also require cannulation with polyethylene tubing to ensure its patency.

COMMON PITFALLS

- Misdiagnosis as a simple nasal fracture.
- Failure to check for patency of the nasolacrimal apparatus.

FRONTAL SINUS FRACTURES

When a blow is received in the frontal skull area the patient may sustain a depressed frontal sinus fracture. This can lead to considerable deformity and possibly mucopyocoele or epidural empyema. The patient usually complains of local pain; epistaxis or CSF leak from the nose; and supraorbital depression of the frontal skull. Physical examination is usually hampered by edema; these injuries are notorious for appearing insignificant until the edema resolves. Judicious palpation of the frontal region with nasal speculum and examination for blood or CSF coming from high in the nasal cavity should lead the examiner to entertain this diagnosis.

Radiographic examination consists of Waters, posteroanterior, and lateral skull films to confirm the diagnosis. However, a "bony window" axial CT scan of the frontal sinus is mandatory to fully assess the injury and to determine if there is significant posterior table involvement and possibly a dural tear.

ED management is limited to arranging for consultation, controlling epistaxis, and applying ice packs in the neurologically intact patient. More extensive workup and neurosurgical consultation may be necessary if intracranial injury is present or suspected. Nasal spray (only for patients with no significant posterior table involvement) and decongestants may be prescribed, as well as broad-spectrum antibiotic coverage for sinus and skin pathogens if significant injury is sustained. Definitive treatment of frontal sinus fractures is controversial and depends on the extent of the injury. Treatment ranges from simple elevation and reconstruction to obliteration procedures with free fat grafts or bone. Late sequelae of mucopyocoele formation and epidural empyema occur.

60   Dental Injuries

Dental injuries are commonly the result of motor vehicle accidents, sports injuries, falls, and altercations. Child abuse is a rare, but important source of dental injuries and should not be overlooked. The anterior maxilla is the most commonly injured area, with the central incisors of male patients being frequently involved. Treatment of dental injuries depends on the type and severity of the injury, whether primary or permanent teeth are involved, and whether there is significant bodily injury.

EMERGENCY DEPARTMENT EVALUATION

Determine the exact time and mechanism of the injury. In addition, any missing teeth or dental prostheses must be accounted for, to prevent airway compromise or being retained in soft-tissue wounds. Medical history determines if tetanus immunizations are up-to-date and whether prophylactic antibiotics are necessary before any dental manipulations.

INTRAORAL EXAMINATION

Assess soft-tissue injuries from the outside in. Lips, buccal mucosa, vestibules, floor of the mouth, tongue, gingiva, and palate should be systematically scanned for lacerations or ecchymotic areas. Next, each tooth should be inspected for cracks, chips, or loose pieces and then percussed on its occlusal surface with a tongue blade to check for sensitivity. Proceeding with the aid of one tongue blade on the buccal tooth surface and one on the lingual surface, an attempt should be made to rock each tooth back and forth in its alveolar socket to check for abnormal mobility. If this is found, the exact tooth identification should be noted. If a whole segment of teeth moves, an alveolar fracture should be suspected. Lastly, a gloved hand with fingers grasping the alveolus should be used to check for less obviously mobile teeth and dentoalveolar segments. The cheeks and floor of the mouth should be bimanually palpated for foreign bodies or tooth fragments.

RADIOGRAPHIC EXAMINATION

Dental radiographs, such as panoramic, occlusal, or periapical films, are helpful. Standard mandible or facial films may be useful in certain circumstances.

EMERGENCY DEPARTMENT MANAGEMENT OF DENTAL INJURIES

The treatment of dental injuries varies according to the facilities available and the expertise of the examiner.

CONCUSSED TEETH

Concussed teeth are teeth with no obvious injury by examination other than a sensitivity to percussion. These teeth may have sustained a sufficient injury to cause later pulpal (nerve) death and necrosis. Treatment should consist of advising the patient to go on a soft diet and arranging for a dentist to provide follow-up care.

DISPLACED TEETH

Subluxated or partially avulsed teeth are recognized by obvious malalignment or abnormal mobility of the tooth in the socket. The patient may complain of not being able to bite all the way into his normal occlusion. Displaced teeth may be apically and centrally repositioned in their alveolar sockets with the aid of a gloved hand and a gauze pad. The patient may help in this process by firmly biting down on a folded 4 × 4-in gauze pad. If gentle attempts at these maneuvers are too painful to the patient, dental anesthesia by infiltration around the buccal aspect of the root surface, or nerve block anesthesia may be necessary. Dental consultation at this point may be helpful. Once reduced, splinting for 1 to 8 weeks is advisable; analgesics and dental follow-up should be provided. A soft diet should be prescribed.

INTRUDED TEETH

Occasionally teeth sustain a blow sufficient enough to intrude or embed them into the alveolar bone. These teeth are usually not mobile and present no interference to the patient's occlusion. These patients should be referred for follow-up dental care as soon as practical. Permanent teeth may be allowed to re-erupt on their own, or may require orthodontic or surgical eruption with stabilization. Subsequent root canal therapy is often required. Primary teeth are allowed to re-erupt or are extracted. Warm saline rinses four times a day may promote gingival healing.

AVULSED TEETH

Anterior incisors are the most frequently avulsed teeth. A permanent tooth that has been totally avulsed or knocked out of its bony socket represents a true dental emergency. The prognosis for recovery is greatly enhanced by prompt intervention. Primary teeth are usually not replanted.

The object is to ensure replantation of the tooth at the earliest possible moment. This will help to prevent or lessen the process of root resorption. Although early replantation is viewed as a temporary measure, it has been shown that teeth replanted within 30 minutes have a 90% retention rate without significant root resorption for up to 5 to 10 years. Conversely, 95% of the teeth replanted beyond 2 hours show root resorption. Proper handling of the tooth is important to ensure the long-term survival of the tooth and the periodontal ligament remnants. These remnants are sensitive to damage by drying, and successful replantation depends on their survival.

Patients, parents, or EMTs should be told the following:

- The root portion of the tooth should not be touched. Handling should be done by the crown only.
- If the caller is confident in his ability to replace the tooth in its exact location, have him do so after thoroughly rinsing the tooth with tap water. (Close the drain first.) Debris **should not** be scrubbed from the root surface.
- If replantation in the field is unsuccessful or impractical, have the caller transport the tooth by placing it under the injured person's tongue, if that person is a coherent, responsible adult. Alternatively, the tooth may be wrapped in moist gauze or placed in a cup of saline solution, saliva, milk, or ice. If successful replantation was accomplished in the field, the physician should check for proper alignment as well as degree of mobility. As a rule, most teeth will require some form of stabilization. Successfully replanted teeth are usually splinted for 1 to 4 weeks.

If replantation must be accomplished in the ED, follow these guidelines:

- The alveolus or socket from which the tooth was avulsed should be checked. If it is intact, replantation should be attempted.
- The tooth should be handled by the crown only. Using a pulse action from a syringe with an 18-gauge needle, saline solution should be used to irrigate debris from the root.
- The socket should then be irrigated or swabbed free of clot. The socket should not be curetted, since this damages the remaining periodontal ligaments attached to its walls.
- The tooth should be inserted into the socket using gentle pressure with the aid of gauze to provide a positive grip on the crown. Once the tooth is inserted, the patient should bite down slowly on the gauze, which will gradually seat the tooth into its proper position.
- If possible, the position of the tooth should be checked with a dental radiograph.
- The dental consultant can proceed with splinting if there is significant mobility.
- Tetanus immunization should be provided as needed.
- Arrangements should be made for follow-up care.

COMMON PITFALLS

- Delays in immediate replantation in the ED which adversely affect the long-term prognosis
- Improper handling and transportation of the avulsed tooth.

FRACTURES OF THE ENAMEL
These teeth may show minor chipping of superficial enamel surfaces, causing sharp edges that may be irritating to the patient. Referral to a dentist for follow-up care and smoothing of rough edges should be arranged.

FRACTURES OF THE ENAMEL AND DENTIN
Fractures through enamel (white) and the underlying dentin (pale yellow) also expose dentinal processes that communicate directly with the central nerve or pulp. This should be recognized on careful inspection. The patient experiences pain to touch or percussion, and frequently the exposed free nerve endings cause exquisite pain when air passes over them. The usual treatment is to cover the exposed dentin with a layer of calcium hydroxide, which is an inert substance that seals the dentinal tubules, commonly eliminating the pain. This is then covered by a composite dental material. ED treatment is limited to arranging for dental consultation or follow-

up as soon as possible. The patient should be instructed to go on a soft diet and avoid hot or cold foods.

FRACTURES OF THE ENAMEL AND DENTIN WITH PULP (NERVE) EXPOSURE
When a pink or red color or fleshy substance is noted within the surrounding dentin (pale yellow) on inspection of a fractured tooth, a fracture involving the pulp (nerve) should be suspected. The patient usually exhibits pain from manipulation of the tooth, exposure to air, or ingestion of hot or cold fluids. Most fractures that involve pulp exposure require root canal therapy as soon as possible to prevent later abscess. More conservative measures of pulp capping, or covering the exposure with calcium hydroxide, followed by restoration may be indicated in small exposures of healthy teeth. A dental consultant should be contacted to see the patient. As an alternative, referral to a dentist's office for initial and follow-up care should be arranged as soon as possible.

ROOT FRACTURES
Teeth with root fractures are difficult to diagnose by clinical examination alone. The only outward sign may be abnormal mobility or sensitivity to percussion. Dental films are mandatory to confirm the diagnosis. Immediate dental consultation is advisable. Significantly displaced teeth must be reduced to their proper position and stabilized with a splint, which will provide adequate fixation for 6 to 12 weeks. Early intervention may allow retention of the teeth without the need for follow-up root canal therapy in up to 80% of cases.

COMMON PITFALLS

Don't assume that the tooth is just loose, and will tighten up with a soft diet.

DENTOALVEOLAR FRACTURES
Fractures that involve the alveolus or tooth-bearing portion of the jaws vary in their degree of displacement, mobility, and comminution and in the number of teeth affected. The patient usually complains of malocclusion, mobile teeth or alveolar segments, and local pain on biting down. The examiner usually notes a displaced alveolar segment or group of teeth, a mobile segment on palpation, and malocclusion on biting down. Dental radiographs or facial films should be ordered. These may show fracture lines running between or just apical to the roots of the teeth. Treatment of dentoalveolar fractures usually involves bodily repositioning of the displaced segment, possibly under local anesthesia or intravenous sedation; stabilization of the segment with rigid splinting for 4 to 6 weeks; and routine follow-up care. Urgent consultation should be sought from a general dentist or maxillofacial surgeon.

ORAL SOFT-TISSUE INJURIES
Oral soft-tissue injuries consist mainly of lacerations and puncture wounds. For the most part, lacerations should be thoroughly irrigated and simple closure performed with resorbable 3-0 or 4-0 suture. Puncture wounds should be thoroughly irrigated, but may not require closure. It is imperative that the wound be carefully and thoroughly explored for foreign bodies and tooth or denture fragments before closure. Dental radiographs of the cheek, tongue, and floor of the mouth may be helpful in this regard. Salivary flow should be confirmed from both Wharton's ducts (submandibular and sublingual glands) in the floor of the mouth and both Stenson's ducts (parotid glands) near the maxillary molars in the buccal mucosa to rule out injuries. If suspected, these injuries require immediate consultation from an oral and maxillofacial surgeon for possible repair.

DENTAL SPLINTING

The method used to provide stabilization for dental injuries depends on the injury and the duration of time that stabilization will be required. This care is provided by a general dentist or maxillofacial surgeon in the acute setting.

DISPOSITION

Any significant injury to the teeth or oral structures requires follow-up care. Because many dental injuries may cause pulpal necrosis and possible abscess, sometimes years after the original injury, it is imperative that the emergency physician document that the patient was appropriately referred to a dentist for continuing evaluation. The dentist usually sees the patient at intervals to test the vitality of injured teeth and perform radiographic studies to check for pulpal (nerve) death. If this occurs, the injured teeth may require root canal therapy (endodontics) versus extraction

61   Eye Injuries

The equipment required for evaluation of an acute eye injury includes the following: visual acuity charts, a penlight with blue filter or Wood's lamp, topical anesthetic and cycloplegic drops, saline irrigating solution, eyelid retractors, and fluorescein strips. A pinhole occluder, a foreign body spud, and an electric foreign body remover are also helpful. The slit lamp is a valuable instrument.

EMERGENCY DEPARTMENT EVALUATION AND MANAGEMENT

VISUAL ACUITY

All patients with eye injuries (except those for whom intervention must be initiated without delay, such as patients suffering caustic burns) should have their visual acuity tested before any diagnostic evaluation is made. If the patient wears glasses, the acuity should be determined with the glasses in place. A pinhole occluder can be used if the patient has not brought corrective glasses or is unable to wear contact lenses. Each eye should be tested independently and the results noted in the medical record. The standard Snellen eye chart may be used, and the smallest line discernible by the patient recorded. If the patient is unable to read even the largest figures on the chart, he should be asked to count the number of fingers the examiner holds in front of him, to detect finger movement, and to perceive light, in that order.

Examination of the eye should include a funduscopic examination and evaluation with the slit lamp. Tonometry should be performed with the Schiøtz tonometer if increased intraocular pressure is suspected. The instrument should first be zeroed on the plate provided. After the instillation of topical anesthetic the tonometer is lowered onto the eye until the footplate rests on the cornea. The patient should be instructed to maintain gaze fixation on the ceiling and not to move the eye. The reading on the tonometer is converted by means of the table that accompanies the instrument.

PENETRATING INJURY

The portal of entry in penetrating injury can be obvious in some cases and almost microscopic in others. The circumstances under which an accident occurred can yield valuable clues to the presence of a penetrating injury. Small corneal or scleral lacerations may not affect ocular function, and patients may maintain good vision. Usually, however, visual acuity is decreased, and the view of the fundus may be obscured. Corneal lacerations are often plugged by a portion of the iris, with resulting pupillary deformation. Scleral laceration or rupture often presents with chemosis or hemorrhagic chemosis in addition to poor vision. If there is suspicion of penetrating eye injury, manipulation of the globe may expel ocular contents. Evaluation should, therefore, be carried out with care, and Schiøtz tonometry is **contraindicated.** Any straining or Valsalva maneuver on the part of the patient should be avoided. Radiographs may be obtained to identify a radiopaque intraocular foreign body. Large injuries should be examined in the operating room. The injured eye should be shielded. The patient should be given nothing by mouth, broad-spectrum systemic antibiotics should be started and tetanus toxoid administered. Succinylcholine is to be avoided during anesthesia, since it increases extraocular muscle tone.

CORNEAL ABRASION
Pain and photophobia are the primary symptoms of corneal abrasion. The eye may be injected. Application of fluorescein stain and illumination with the blue light of the Wood's lamp or slit lamp is the ideal method of examination. Treatment includes patching and instillation of topical antibiotics and cycloplegics.

FOREIGN BODIES
The large majority of foreign bodies that lodge in the eye are stopped by the surface layer of the cornea or conjunctiva. Corneal foreign bodies can be removed with a spud or a sterile 25-gauge needle. A cotton-tipped applicator may be used to remove conjunctival foreign bodies. Prior instillation of several drops of topical anesthetic will facilitate the procedure.

CHEMICAL BURNS
Offending agents are most commonly detergents, cleaning solutions, and strong acids or alkali (such as lye). Alkaline substances typically cause greater injury than acidic substances of comparable strength. Alkalis penetrate the cornea and enter the anterior chamber, whereas acids precipitate protein and usually do not enter the eye. When the pH of a substance is not known poison control centers or manufacturers can usually provide information regarding pH. The eye is red and painful. Minor injuries produce corneal epithelial damage, mild stromal reaction, and no conjunctival blanching. More severe injuries produce coagulation of conjunctival vessels, causing blanching. Corneal haziness or complete corneal opacity may also be present.

The condition must be recognized promptly and immediate lavage instituted with normal saline solution. Lavage at the site of injury is preferable. A topical anesthetic and a lid speculum facilitate lavage, which is performed with standard intravenous tubing. A continuous flow contact lens may be used alternatively. Lavage should continue for at least 30 minutes with 1 L to 2 L of saline or until the conjunctival pH is neutral. The pH should be checked with litmus paper immediately after completion of lavage and again 5 to 10 minutes later.

Remaining particulate material must be removed by swabbing the cul-de-sac with a cotton-tipped applicator. This is particularly important when chemosis is present. Moderate and severe burns produce iritis and painful ciliary spasm. Cycloplegics (e.g., 0.25% scopolamine or 2% homatropine) should be administered. Ophthalmologic consultation should be obtained in all but the most minor of burns.

BLUNT TRAUMA
Blunt orbital trauma can produce a variety of injuries, including contusion of the eyelids, bony facial fracture, subconjunctival hemorrhage, and hyphema.

HYPHEMA
Blood in the anterior chamber most commonly follows blunt trauma to the orbit with an object small enough to fit between the orbital bones. Fists, bottles, and small balls (e.g., racquetballs) are common injuring objects. Complications usually follow rebleeding and include glaucoma, delayed-onset glaucoma, optic atrophy, and corneal blood staining. Glaucoma is a particular danger in blacks with sickle cell trait. The blood usually layers out in the inferior chamber angle, where it can be seen as a meniscus. Before settling, hemorrhage in the aqueous obscures the view of the iris. Small hyphemas can be easily missed (particularly in brown-eyed people) if the

inferior chamber angle is not carefully inspected. The diagnosis may also be missed if the blood has not yet layered inferiorly and the entire anterior chamber is filled with blood. In this case, the typical meniscus is not seen and the pupil is obscured.

Determine whether or not there are associated injuries, such as corneal abrasions and facial bony fractures. Intraocular pressure should be measured with an applanation tonometer, as the weight of the Schiøtz instrument indents the eye and could cause further injury. Pupillary dilatation is usually not necessary, and manipulation of the eye is contraindicated. A metal shield should be applied to protect the eye from inadvertent injury. A sickle cell prep should be obtained for black patients. Coagulation studies are indicated for patients receiving anticoagulants. Patients should be advised against the use of aspirin. Ophthalmologic consultation should be obtained in all cases.

Management is directed at preventing recurrent bleeding. There is considerable controversy about optimal management. Most authorities agree on the use of a metal shield and on bed rest, with or without a patch, although most ophthalmologists no longer patch both eyes. Some authorities advocate keeping children at home resting in bed, whereas others hospitalize all patients. Antifibrinolytic agents (epsilon-aminocaproic acid, 50 mg to 100 mg/kg up to 5 g every 4 hours) are generally prescribed for adults. Epsilon-aminocaproic acid can cause nausea, vomiting, and hypertension. It is contraindicated in pregnant patients and in patients with coagulation disorders. Some authorities advocate prescribing systemic steroids.

COMMON PITFALLS

- Deferring visual acuity examination.
- Neglecting the eye examination because of the presence of other injuries or an inability to easily visualize the eye.
- Allowing ocular manipulation or Valsalva maneuver, which may increase damage in penetrating injury.
- In chemical burns, not lavaging the eye immediately or not removing particulate material from the cul-de-sac.
- In hyphema, not examining the inferior chamber angle and failing to obtain a sickle cell prep in black patients.

62   Acute Spinal Cord Injuries

The incidence of acute spinal cord injury is 30/million population, with perhaps another 20/million dying before they reach the hospital. In light of the potential for disability, maximal spinal cord protection should be a primary goal in the field and hospital treatment of trauma victims. Motor vehicle accidents account for 47.7% of spinal cord injuries, followed by falls (20.8%), acts of violence, including gunshot and knife wounds (14.6%), and sports accidents (14.2%). Diving injuries constitute two thirds of the sports-related spinal cord injuries. Football, snow skiing, surfing, and gymnastics account for the bulk of the remainder. About 14% of vertebral column injuries result in neurologic deficits. Conversely, 17% to 37% of deficits occur in the absence of plain radiographic signs of injury.

In 3% to 25% of cases of spinal injury, cord damage does not develop immediately after the primary insult, but may occur in the field or hospital setting. Therefore, the possibility of spinal injury must be considered in all patients who sustain injury to the head, face, neck, or back, have altered sensoria, or present with neck or back pain, sensorimotor deficits, or hypotension. Sixty percent of cervical spine fractures occur in the setting of associated major trauma, whereas in only 16% of cases is no associated injury present. Facial fractures have a 4% to 8.6% incidence of association with cervical spine injuries. The vertebral column is frequently injured at multiple, nonadjacent levels.

CLINICAL PRESENTATION

Cervical spine injury accounts for more than half of all spinal cord injuries. Fracture-dislocations are the most common injuries that produce cervical spine injury. The most common sites of injury are C-4, C-5, and C-6, the most mobile segments of the spine. The patient with cervical injury usually presents with occipital or neck pain and tenderness, muscular spasm, and a varying degree of motor or sensory deficit. Decreased sensation to pinprick, temperature, or proprioceptive stimuli may occur, as well as paresthesias or dysesthesias. On the other hand, fractures of the cervical spine may occur without significant physical findings, most commonly seen in patients with altered sensoria or in the presence of concomitant trauma.

The thoracic and lumbosacral levels account for 35.6% and 10.1% of cord injuries, respectively. Injuries in the T-2 to T-10 region are frequently complete neurologic lesions because of the relatively poor blood supply to this area. The degree of injury may also reflect the substantial amount of force required to fracture the relatively immobile thoracic spine. The most commonly injured area of the thoracic and lumbar spine is the thoracolumbar junction. The T-12 level accounts for 7.5% of all spinal lesions. The presenting findings differ from those of injuries higher because the cord usually terminates around the L-1 level. Presentation is frequently loss of bowel and bladder function and saddle distribution hypoesthesia.

EMERGENCY DEPARTMENT EVALUATION

Airway and cervical immobilization are critical. If the airway is patent, attention should be directed toward respiratory function. Injury at or above C-4 will typically produce respiratory arrest due to paralysis of respiratory muscles. Cervical injury below this level may spare the diaphragm, though vital capacity is typically decreased. The vital capacity may fall to 30% of normal in patients with cervical lesions below C-4. The intercostal muscles may be weak or paralyzed in thoracic spinal injuries. Respiratory motion will appear paradoxical because the rib cage expands passively on expiration and collapses during inspiration. Acute injury to the spinal cord produces a state of spinal shock that consists of the absence of neurologic function below the level of injury. Deep tendon and autonomic reflexes, voluntary motor power and all sensation are abolished.

The examiner should carefully determine the presence of an anal wink or bulbocavernosus reflex in the patient who appears to have a complete cord deficit. Any evidence of voluntary sphincter contraction or sensory function in the perianal region indicates that the lesion is incomplete and improves the prognosis for functional recovery. Although the sensory examination requires patient cooperation, some indication can be determined with respect to sensation in the unconscious patient by observing for withdrawal, localizing or posturing to painful stimuli. The awake patient should be tested for sensation to pinprick and proprioception (see Table 62-1). The motor examination consists of evaluating muscular tone and strength. Reflexes (including abdominal, anal and bulbocavernosus reflexes) and cranial nerve function should also be assessed.

Serial neurologic examinations are important to identify the patient who develops an ascending paralysis and may require increased ventilatory support or emergent neurosurgery. If there is any suspicion of abdominal injury, the patient should undergo diagnostic peritoneal abdominal lavage or abdominal CT. The patient with spinal cord injury with hemoperitoneum may complain only of nausea or shoulder pain because of diaphragmatic irritation.

The standard trauma cervical spine series consists of lateral, anteroposterior (AP) and

TABLE 62-1. Motor, Sensory, and Reflex Tests by Nerve Root Levels

Nerve Root Level	Motor	Sensory	Reflex
C3	Lower neck		
C4	Diaphragm	Clavicular area	
C5	Deltoid, biceps	Lateral upper arm	Biceps
C6	Extensor carpi radialis	Thumb and lateral forearm	Brachioradialis
C7	Triceps, wrist flexors, finger extensors	Middle finger	Triceps
C8	Finger flexors	Little finger	
T1	Hand intrinsics	Medial forearm	
T4	Intercostals	Nipples	
T10	Abdominals	Umbilicus	
T12		Suprapubic area inguinal ligament	
L1 L2	Iliopsoas	Upper thigh	
L3 L4	Quadriceps	Lower anterior thigh Medial calf	Quadriceps
L5	Extensor hallucis longus	Dorsal foot	
S1	Gastrosoleus, flexor hallucis longus	Little toe	Achilles tendon
S2 S3 S4	Anal sphincter Bladder	Perineum	Bulbocavernosus Anal wink

From Trafton PG: Surg Clin North Am 62:64, 1982. Reprinted with permission.

open-mouth odontoid views. Obtain a lateral view showing all seven cervical vertebrae and ideally, the C-7–T-1 junction. A swimmer's view may be necessary to accomplish this. The spine should be evaluated for alignment, bony changes (fractures, dislocation or subluxation), maintenance of intervertebral spaces and soft tissue injury. No single view "clears" the cervical spine. CT has the advantage of offering superior imaging of bony details and the ability to demonstrate soft tissue injury. CT may be useful in clarifying suspected injury if plain radiographs are inadequate.

Patients who exhibit neurologic deficit but no apparent plain radiographic abnormalities should be treated with the presumption that a cord disruption exists. CT or MR imaging may be utilized to delineate the extent of the injury. In patients with negative plain radiographs without neurologic deficit but in whom injury is nevertheless suspected, flexion and extension views may be obtained. These should be done under the direct supervision of the treating physician.

EMERGENCY DEPARTMENT MANAGEMENT

Oxygenation is a high priority. All patients with spinal injury should have supplemental oxygen applied by face mask. Cricothyrotomy is indicated if nasotracheal intubation is unsuccessful or contraindicated. Hypotension may be due to hypovolemia or neurogenic shock. The first step in hypotensive patients is to rule out life-threatening hypovolemia, since neurogenic shock is a diagnosis of exclusion. Patients with neurogenic shock are those with cervical or high thoracic lesions that interrupt sympathetic outflow. The result is flaccid paralysis, hypotension, vasodilatation and a normal or slow heart rate. If normal circulation is maintained in the face of a slow heart rate, no further treatment for bradycardia is necessary. Occasionally, bradycardia will require the administration of atropine or the insertion of a temporary pacemaker.

Moderate crystalloid infusion (500–1000 mL of Ringer's lactate) is generally adequate to stabilize patients with neurogenic shock. If shock is refractory to these measures, vasopressor administration may be required. Administration of pressor agents with alpha-agonist activity (high-dose dopamine, 10–20 µg/kg/min, or phenylephrine, 10 µg/min) should be instituted. Disruption of sympathetic pathways in the quadriplegic patient may produce deficits of temperature regulation. The patient must be carefully monitored. Acute gastric dilatation and paralytic ileus are common in spinal cord injuries. A nasogastric tube should be inserted, the return checked for blood, and the tube connected to low intermittent suction.

The patient frequently has an atonic bladder and will require a urinary catheter. A Foley catheter should be inserted in the initial resuscitation period, but intermittent catheterization every 6 hours is advocated after the patient is stabilized. Corticosteroids have been found to have a positive effect on neurologic outcome in experimental settings. Early administration of dexamethasone (10–20 mg intravenously or intramuscularly every 4–6 hours) or methylprednisolone is widely advocated. Local cryotherapy, hyperbaric oxygen, and administration of naloxone and thyrotropin-releasing hormone are other therapies that have displayed some experimental benefit in spinal cord injury.

SPECIFIC SPINAL CORD LESIONS

Cord deficits are characterized as being complete or incomplete. Patients with complete cord lesions initially display a flaccid, areflexic paralysis and loss of all sensory modalities below the level of the lesion. Only 6.7% of patients with complete cervical lesions and 11% of patients with thoracic lesions regain any lost motor function within a year of injury. In an incomplete lesion some motor function or sensation is retained below the lesion. The presence of even the slightest retained function may signify potential for neurologic recovery. In one study, 47% of patients with incomplete sensory findings and 87% of patients with incomplete motor findings at 72 hours post-injury were functionally ambulatory one year later.

Common incomplete lesions include the anterior and central cord syndromes and the Brown–Séquard syndrome. The anterior cord syndrome is the most common incomplete lesion. It is often the consequence of flexion injuries, usually involving the cervical spine. It results from compromised flow in the two anterior spinal arteries that supply the ventral two thirds of the cord. The anterior horn cells, corticospinal tracts and spinothalamic tracts are involved, but the dorsal columns are spared. Therefore, the patient will lack sensation to pain and temperature below the level of injury, but retains proprioception. Voluntary motor control is absent. These patients require emergent CT, and those with cord compression require immediate surgery. Almost half of patients do not regain leg function sufficient to achieve free ambulation.

Brown–Séquard lesions classically involve a cord hemisection, but partial sections are more common. The cervical cord is the most commonly involved area, and penetrating trauma is the usual etiology. The patient has absent proprioception and motor paralysis ipsilateral to the lesion. The patient also has contralateral loss of pain and temperature sensation. A band of hypoesthesia exists at the level of the lesion. Brown–Séquard lesions have a fair prognosis. Surgery is rarely required, except to remove foreign bodies from the canal.

Central cord syndrome commonly results from hyperextension injury. Paralysis of the upper extremities exceeds that of the lower. Prognosis is fair. Many patients eventually become ambulatory, but have only a 50% chance of regaining useful hand function.

DISPOSITION

Patients with obvious cervical fractures require neurosurgical consultation, immobilization and reduction. Closed reduction is achieved with traction devices such as Gardner Wells tongs or halo traction. Postreduction radiographs must be checked by the physician applying the traction device. If other life-threatening conditions have been stabilized, patients with spinal cord lesions should be referred to a regional spinal center. Personnel involved in the transport must perform thorough neurologic examinations before and after transfer. Patients with cervical fractures should be immobilized in tongs or a halo device prior to transport. Respiratory function should be carefully assessed prior to transport. A nasogastric tube and Foley catheter should be in place. There should be awareness of the potential temperature fluctuation during transport. Intravenous fluids should be infused at low maintenance levels.

COMMON PITFALLS

- Failure to consider possible spinal cord injury
- Failure to consider the possibility of injury at multiple vertebral levels
- Failure to visualize all seven cervical vertebrae and the C-7–T-1 junction
- Failure to assist ventilation in high cervical and thoracic lesions
- Failure to consider hypovolemic shock in spinal cord injury
- Failure to diagnose intra-abdominal injury by DPL or CT
- Failure to perform serial neurologic examinations and recognize ascending paralysis
- Failure to assess sacral sensory sparing

---

63   Pulmonary and Pleural Injuries

Although only about 10% of thoracic injuries require surgery, many others (such as those that produce pericardial tamponade and tension pneumothorax) can rapidly be fatal if not immediately treated.

SIMPLE PNEUMOTHORAX

Pneumothorax may occur spontaneously, but more often is associated with either blunt or penetrating trauma. Although air may enter the pleural space externally through the chest wall (open pneumothorax), most of the pleural air (even with penetrating trauma) originates internally through injuries to the trachea, bronchi, or lungs.

CLINICAL PRESENTATION

Dyspnea and pleuritic chest pain are typical symptoms. Physical examination reveals diminished breath sounds, tympany to percussion, and sometimes subcutaneous emphysema.

DIFFERENTIAL DIAGNOSIS

Tension pneumothorax causes similar symptoms and signs, but with breath sounds essentially absent on the affected side and often diminished on the opposite side as well. Neck vein distention and tracheal deviation are present only with tension. Hemothorax results in diminished breath sounds and often dullness to percussion. Splinting from pain may also cause diminished breath sounds.

EMERGENCY DEPARTMENT EVALUATION AND MANAGEMENT

If the patient is able to sit, an upright chest film is more sensitive than a supine film in detecting small amounts of pleural air. If signs of tension are present, however, pleural decompression should be achieved before radiography. Simple traumatic pneumothorax is relieved by tube thoracostomy. A chest tube (#36–#40 French) is inserted through the fourth to sixth intercostal space and connected to water-seal and continuous suction (20–30 cm water pressure). Minimal (<10%) pneumothorax without other significant injury is sometimes managed by close observation.

DISPOSITION

Surgical consultation should be obtained, and all patients with traumatic pneumothorax should be admitted to the hospital. Otherwise healthy people with **spontaneous** pneumothorax may be discharged home with a unidirectional (e.g., Heimlich) valve device in place. Because of associated injuries, transfer should be avoided unless surgical backup is insufficient. However, the pneumothorax should be treated first, and interhospital personnel must be able to detect and deal with development of tension from a malfunctioning thoracostomy device.

COMMON PITFALLS

- Mistaking diminished breath sounds due to splinting for pneumothorax.
- Not recognizing the progression of simple to tension pneumothorax due to (a) worsening of the underlying condition, (b) malfunctioning suction device, or (c) positive pressure ventilation.

TENSION PNEUMOTHORAX

If more air enters the pleural space during inspiration than escapes during expiration, intrapleural pressure rises so high that the lung completely collapses, the mediastinum is pushed to the opposite side, the opposite lung is compressed, and hypoxia becomes extreme. Moreover, increased intrathoracic pressure may sufficiently diminish transthoracic blood flow to cause shock.

CLINICAL PRESENTATION

Extreme dyspnea and often cyanosis and hypotension are present. Breath sounds are absent on the injured side and usually diminished on the opposite side. The trachea is deviated to the opposite side due to mediastinal shift, which may also cause the heart to be similarly displaced. Neck veins are distended because increased intrathoracic pressure leads to diminished venous return to the right atrium. However, neck vein distention may not occur in tension pneumothorax if there is significant hemorrhage from associated injuries.

DIFFERENTIAL DIAGNOSIS

Simple pneumothorax causes diminished breath sounds on the injured side only, neck veins are not distended, and there are no signs of mediastinal shift. Pericardial tamponade may also cause shock with distended neck veins, but breath sounds are normal, and the trachea and heart are not displaced.

EMERGENCY DEPARTMENT EVALUATION AND MANAGEMENT

Tension pneumothorax should ideally be diagnosed by physical examination. The patient may be too unstable for radiographic studies. Tension pneumothorax is an emergency and immediate pleural decompression is mandatory. A large-bore needle is inserted through the second intercostal space in the midclavicular line followed by tube thoracostomy.

DISPOSITION

The disposition of tension pneumothorax is the same as for simple pneumothorax.

COMMON PITFALLS

- Waiting for a radiograph before decompression
- Not recognizing the progression of simple to tension pneumothorax
- Not recognizing that positive-pressure ventilation has converted a previously small—or even undiagnosed—simple pneumothorax into a tension pneumothorax
- Not realizing that hemorrhage may prevent neck vein distention, and thus recognition that tension is present

HEMOTHORAX

The principle complication of significant bleeding into the pleural space is hypovolemia. However, hemothorax is often accompanied by pneumothorax. Thus hypovolemia may be compounded by hypoxia.

CLINICAL PRESENTATION

Significant hemothorax causes hypotension along with diminished breath sounds and dullness to percussion, unless pneumothorax is also present.

DIFFERENTIAL DIAGNOSIS

Large pneumothorax, especially if under tension, may mask underlying hemothorax. Pericardial tamponade may also cause hypotension, but neck veins are distended with tamponade and flat with hemorrhage of any cause, including hemothorax.

EMERGENCY DEPARTMENT EVALUATION AND MANAGEMENT

Hemothorax may be difficult to detect on a supine chest film, being reflected only by subtle haziness. However, an upright film should reveal any significant amount of fluid at the lung base. A chest tube will drain the hemothorax and accompanying pneumothorax if one is present. However, the major problem produced by hemothorax is hypovolemia. Fluid replacement is thus crucial, using large-bore intravenous lines with crystalloid and blood.

Whereas most cases of pneumothorax and even hemothorax require only tube thoracostomy, continued (250–500 mL/h) or significant (1500 mL initially) bleeding into the pleural space may require thoracotomy. Surgical consultation is warranted. Transfer should be considered only if surgical backup is unavailable.

COMMON PITFALLS

- Not recognizing pleural blood on supine radiograph
- Underestimating the amount of pleural bleeding because the chest tube is not draining adequately

PULMONARY LACERATION AND CONTUSION

Pulmonary lacerations may cause significant bleeding into the airway. Pulmonary contusion generally progresses over several hours, and ventilation may become impaired as blood and fluid accumulate in the alveoli. Most localized contusions resolve within several days.

CLINICAL PRESENTATION

Major lung laceration results in hemoptysis and obvious airway impairment. With lung contusion, dyspnea may be present initially and often increases over time. Auscultation reveals increasingly prominent rales, which may be absent initially.

DIFFERENTIAL DIAGNOSIS

Congestive heart failure also causes rales, but the rales of pulmonary contusion are more localized under the area of injury. Adult respiratory distress syndrome (ARDS) can follow significant trauma to the lung or other organs. But the rales of ARDS are also more generalized than those of pulmonary contusion, and develop more gradually over 1 to 2 days. In contrast with failure, both ARDS and pulmonary contusion are associated with normal central venous pressure (neck veins) and pulmonary artery pressure.

EMERGENCY DEPARTMENT EVALUATION AND MANAGEMENT

Significant pulmonary laceration may be indicated by the presence of active hemoptysis. Signs of pulmonary contusion may be subtle at first. An initial chest radiograph usually reveals an infiltrate underlying the area of trauma, but this sign may become more obvious after a number of hours. Significant bleeding into the airway requires endotracheal intubation and operative intervention. If hypoxia is present ($PO_2 < 60$), the patient with pulmonary contusion may also require intubation and positive-pressure ventilation, which may help prevent alveolar collapse and the development of ARDS.

DISPOSITION

Significant pulmonary lacerations are repaired in the operating room. Patients with severe lung contusions are treated with early endotracheal intubation and positive-pressure ventilation. These patients are admitted to the hospital, and transferred only if critical care facilities are not available.

COMMON PITFALLS

- **For laceration:** Airway control may be difficult, and blood may impair ventilation through the lower airway and even the endotracheal tube.
- **For contusion:** Overly vigorous fluid resuscitation predisposes to alveolar fluid collection. The accumulation of alveolar fluid may be overlooked without frequent re-examination.

64   Cardiac Injuries

CARDIAC CONTUSION

Blunt cardiac trauma is not only a relatively common clinical entity, but it can also be an important cause of morbidity and mortality in the trauma patient. The most common mechanism of injury is the sudden deceleration of the chest wall against the steering wheel, followed by the subsequent deceleration of the heart and great vessels against the sternum. Because the right ventricle is the most anterior structure of the heart, it absorbs the greatest impact against the sternum.

CLINICAL PRESENTATION

There are usually 3–4 other injuries in patients with myocardial contusion. Chest pain may, therefore, not be a prominent complaint. Find out if the steering wheel is broken, or if the chest made an imprint on the dashboard. If there is significant chest pain, it can mimic that of myocardial infarction, or be pleuritic. A chest trauma victim without chest pain does not have a myocardial contusion so long as that patient is not intoxicated and does not have a distracting injury.

Bruising of the sternum should be considered supportive evidence of significant blunt chest trauma, but 27% may not have external signs of trauma. The physical examination is not a sensitive indicator of myocardial contusion. Rhythm disturbances are common among myocardial contusion patients. It is important to question the EMTs since they may spontaneously resolve by the time the patient reaches the ED. With an elderly patient it may be difficult to determine whether or not premature ventricular contractions (PVCs) are pre-existing, but they must be presumed abnormal in a young chest trauma patient.

CHEST RADIOGRAPHY
A chest radiograph is essential in the thoracic trauma victim, with rib fractures and hemopneumothorax the most common chest film abnormalities. Sternal fracture is relatively rare, suggesting that myocardial contusion does not require inordinate kinetic energy.

ELECTROCARDIOGRAPHY
There are no pathognomonic electrocardiographic (ECG) findings other than ST segment changes seen in myocardial infarction, but this ECG pattern is relatively rare. The static ECG suggests myocardial contusion 17% to 38% of the time. This is due to the fact that the 12-lead ECG looks largely at left-sided rather than right-sided forces. T-wave peaking or flattening has not proved to be useful in the diagnosis, and neither has a prolonged QT interval. Right bundle-branch block is associated with myocardial contusion, but it also lacks adequate sensitivity.

EMERGENCY DEPARTMENT EVALUATION

Patients who were wearing seat belts and shoulder harnesses at the time of accident seldom suffer significant blunt cardiac trauma unless the steering wheel or dashboard is broken or deformed. Alert patients not under the influence of drugs must have chest pain in order for the physician to entertain the diagnosis. The only modifying factor would be a separate injury causing pain significant enough to mask chest pain. Those patients with arrhythmias or new cardiac conduction defects should be given a presumptive diagnosis of myocardial contusion. In those patients in whom there is a strong suspicion but no direct clinical evidence of cardiac contusion, first-pass radionuclide angiography (RNA) or two-dimensional echocardiography (2-D echo) can assist in establishing the diagnosis.

RADIONUCLIDE ANGIOGRAPHY (RNA)   Intravenous radioactive technetium-99m pertechnetate allows an ejection fraction to be calculated and is considered the gold standard.

TWO-DIMENSIONAL ECHOCARDIOGRAPHY   2-D echo can also detect wall motion abnormalities and seems as useful as RNA.

EMERGENCY DEPARTMENT MANAGEMENT

Hypotension occurs relatively frequently, but is usually transient and responds to volume loading because the right ventricle responds well to increased volume. Pressors such as dopamine and dobutamine can be used, but the patient's central venous pressure (CVP) should be monitored to ensure adequate venous capacitance. If there is a question about volume status with a CVP line, a Swan–Ganz monitor should be used. Those patients who are hypotensive despite adequate volume should undergo 2-D echo to rule out myocardial, septal, or valvular rupture.

All patients should remain monitored from the prehospital phase until discharge or admission. Arrhythmias usually occur within the first 4 hours. Supraventricular arrhythmias should be treated by cardioversion if the patient is hemodynamically unstable despite adequate intravascular volume. Verapamil should be avoided in atrial fibrillation and flutter because of its myocardial depressant effect. Lidocaine is not instituted unless there are frequent PVCs, multifocal PVCs, or couplets. Ventricular tachycardia and fibrillation are treated per ACLS protocol.

DISPOSITION

All patients with hypotension or arrhythmias resulting from blunt cardiac trauma should be admitted for 24 hours of observation. Those patients who have no other significant injuries that require admission should undergo 2-D echo or RNA to determine whether they should be admitted. If the 2-D echo or RNA is normal, then the patient can be discharged. In addition, patients with prehospital arrhythmias that resolve can also be spared admission if they have a normal scan. The trauma surgeon should be consulted on all potential admissions.

COMMON PITFALLS

- Consider myocardial contusion in blunt chest trauma victims.
- Aggressive fluid management is essential.

PENETRATING CARDIAC INJURY

A penetrating wound to the heart causes either massive blood loss or pericardial blood accumulation leading to cardiac tamponade. The areas of the heart injured (in decreasing order of frequency) are the right ventricle, left ventricle, right atrium, great vessels, and coronary arteries.

EMERGENCY DEPARTMENT EVALUATION

The only relevant data in a penetrating chest wound are the size, length, and width of the object to estimate the potential depth of penetration. Knowledge of the caliber and type of firearm, and its distance from the victim will help to determine the amount of kinetic energy imparted to the heart.

Clinical appearance and vital signs are the most important clues. Once a stab or gunshot wound is discovered, its location and estimated trajectory in the thorax is important. The jugular venous distention characteristic of cardiac tamponade may not appear until the patient is adequately fluid resuscitated, and is not reliable. Electrical alternans is not seen in acute traumatic tamponade. Diagnostic 2-D echo may be used in the stable patient.

EMERGENCY DEPARTMENT MANAGEMENT

Two large-bore intravenous lines should be started after control of the airway. A chest film is obtained if the patient's condition permits. Bullet wounds more commonly cause exsanguination, and stab wounds more commonly present with tamponade. Those patients with diminished breath sounds and in respiratory distress should have a chest tube placed before any radiograph. If the patient remains hypotensive or there is continuous chest tube drainage, there should be vigorous resuscitation with blood. The patient who continues to deteriorate despite adequate volume resuscitation should undergo immediate pericardiocentesis or thoracotomy. Some authors believe that pericardiocentesis may cause increased mortality by **delaying** a lifesaving thoracotomy. Cardiopulmonary bypass surgery may be needed, and may be indicated for air or bullet embolus and for coronary artery lacerations.

Emergency thoracotomy is indicated in penetrating trauma victims who are moribund or who arrest either in the ED or en route to the hospital. Those patients without vital signs in the field have a grim prognosis. The most qualified individual should perform the thoracotomy. The stable patient may have the thoracotomy performed in the operating suite.

DISPOSITION

All patients with penetrating cardiac wounds should undergo definitive repair by a surgeon. Occasionally a patient presents with a potential penetrating cardiac wound and is stable with no hemopneumothorax on the chest films. These patients should undergo 2-D echo while a surgeon is being called for urgent consultation. Chest wounds should be observed for drainage, but **not probed.**

COMMON PITFALLS

- Emergency thoracotomy is indicated for deteriorating patients.
- All penetrating thoracic wounds should be considered potential cardiac wounds.
- The emergency physician should be competent to do a thoracotomy.

---

65   Bony Thorax and Diaphragm Injuries

DIAPHRAGM

Traumatic injury of the diaphragm may result from either penetrating or blunt trauma to the chest or abdomen. The absence of distinct symptoms combined with the high incidence of serious and more obvious associated injuries may lead the physician to overlook these injuries. Missed diaphragmatic ruptures may lead to devastating sequelae acutely or years later. There are no reliable data to suggest the true incidence of this entity, since many cases may go undiagnosed. However, it is estimated that diaphragmatic injuries are present in 3% to 5.8% of patients who undergo emergency surgery for thoracoabdominal trauma.

The relative frequency of blunt versus penetrating injuries varies greatly with published reports. Stab and gunshot wounds may affect any portion of the diaphragm. However, there is a higher incidence of stab wounds to the left hemidiaphragm, theoretically because of the greater number of right hand dominant assailants. Blunt trauma also has a predilection for the left hemidiaphragm, because the right hemidiaphragm is partially protected by the liver. In addition, the posterolateral portion of the left leaflet is structurally the weakest portion of the diaphragm.

Blunt trauma typically produces defects greater than 10 cm on the average versus an average of less than 2 cm for penetrating trauma. Blunt injuries have a higher mortality rate, which is directly related to their high incidence of serious associated injuries. Ruptures of the diaphragm, regardless of size, are unlikely to heal spontaneously because of the pleuroperitoneal pressure gradient. The stomach herniates most often; thereafter, the spleen, colon, small bowel, and omentum follow in variable order.

CLINICAL PRESENTATION

The signs and symptoms are variable, depending on the size of the defect, the mechanism, the herniated viscus, and the degree of cardiopulmonary compromise. Common symptoms include cough, dyspnea, nonspecific chest or abdominal pain radiating to the shoulder, and the perception of peristalsis in the chest. Signs include an immobile left hemithorax, decreased breath sounds, and tympany or borborygmi in the left chest. However, in the absence of herniation, a diaphragmatic tear may be completely asymptomatic and without overt signs. Abdominal viscera may herniate into the thoracic cavity and dilate rapidly, resulting in severe respiratory distress. This condition may be difficult to distinguish from a tension pneumothorax. Great care should be exercised when performing a thoracostomy, always verifying a free pleural space before inserting the chest tube. Herniation has been reported in the immediate post-traumatic phase or as long as 40 years after the initial diaphragmatic injury. Delayed presentation is associated with a mortality as high as 20% after visceral incarceration, increasing to 80% after strangulation occurs.

EMERGENCY DEPARTMENT EVALUATION

Serial examinations looking for signs of obstruction, strangulation, or cardiopulmonary compromise are important. Baseline arterial blood gas measurements should be obtained. The chest radiograph is the single most important diagnostic tool. Although frequently nonspecific, it is often the chest radiograph that arouses the initial suspicion of diaphragmatic disruption. Significant findings include lower rib fractures, pleural effusion, and a high hemidiaphragm. If herniation has occurred, one may see an intrathoracic abdominal viscus, mediastinal shift, atelectasis, or the nasogastric tube positioned above the diaphragm.

Barium studies, liver and spleen scans, and computed tomography have also been used. Due to the decreased sensitivity of diagnostic peritoneal lavage in the diagnosis of isolated diaphragmatic injuries, some authors advocate lowering the red blood cell count considered positive to 5000/µL when evaluating injuries at high risk for diaphragmatic injury (i.e., lower chest or upper abdominal penetrating wounds).

EMERGENCY DEPARTMENT MANAGEMENT

If the diagnosis of herniation is suspected, a nasogastric tube should be placed for decompression as well as to aid in the diagnosis. The physician should beware of the dilated intrathoracic abdominal viscus masquerading as an atypical pneumothorax, and should place a chest tube only after careful digital verification of the free pleural space. Any patient suspected of having a diaphragmatic rupture should be hospitalized. The definitive treatment is surgical repair.

BONY THORAX

SIMPLE RIB FRACTURES

Simple rib fractures account for more than 50% of nonpenetrating chest trauma. Fractures typically occur at the site of impact or posterior angle, where the rib is structurally the weakest. Fractures are more common in adults because of the relative inelasticity of the mature thorax. Although the fourth through ninth ribs are the most commonly involved, fractures of ribs nine through eleven deserve special concern, as there is an increased incidence of abdominal injuries due to their location. Seven or more rib fractures are associated with a 50% incidence of intrathoracic injury. Clinical findings include point tenderness intensified by deep breathing or coughing, ecchymoses, crepitus, and muscle spasm. Compression over the rib posteriorly produces referred pain to the fracture site.

The diagnosis of rib fractures should be made on clinical grounds, since 50% of these injuries are missed on the initial chest radiograph and 10% will not visualize radiographically for 7 to 14 days post-injury, regardless of the views taken. A chest radiograph is valuable, however, when looking for complications of rib fractures, such as hemothorax, pneumothorax, and pulmonary contusion. The goals in the treatment of simple rib fractures are pain control and maintenance of adequate pulmonary function. The patient should be encouraged to breathe deeply. Binders are not recommended, as they decrease ventilation and promote atelectasis.

Mild to moderate pain relief may be achieved with oral pain medications such as 30 mg to 60 mg of codeine every 4 hours as needed. The most effective relief for moderate to severe pain is attained using a long-acting anesthetic such as bupivacaine (Marcaine) in an intercostal block. Hospitalization may be indicated for elderly patients and for those with pre-existing pulmonary disease to ensure adequate pulmonary toilet while controlling pain. Although delayed hemothorax or pneumothorax may develop 6 to 24 hours post-injury, most rib fractures heal uneventfully within 3 to 6 weeks. Patients should be discouraged from vigorous contact sports during that time. Rarely, the long-term course is complicated by post-traumatic neuroma or costochondral separation.

FIRST THROUGH THIRD RIB FRACTURES   Ribs 1–3 deserve special note, as they are harbingers of severe thoracic trauma. A great amount of force is required to fracture any of the initial three ribs, and such fracture should alert one to aggressively search for other injuries. There is a 15% to 36% mortality related to associated injuries. Expeditious angiography is indicated if (a) there is brachial plexus injury, (b) there is displacement of the rib fracture, (c) more than one of the first three ribs are fractured, (d) there is a widened mediastinum initially or on subsequent chest radiographs, or (e) there is a significant, unexplained change in pulse or blood pressure. All patients with fractures of the first through third ribs should be admitted for observation.

STERNAL FRACTURES

Sternal fractures usually result from direct trauma to the anterior chest wall and most commonly are related to motor vehicle accidents in which the chest strikes the steering wheel, dashboard, or shoulder strap at high velocity. A tremendous amount of force is necessary to fracture the sternum, and consequently these injuries should be viewed as harbingers of severe thoracic trauma. There is a 25% to 45% mortality associated with sternal fractures, which is directly proportional to the high incidence of myocardial contusion, cardiac tamponade, aortic trauma, pulmonary contusion, and other serious intrathoracic injuries. The diagnosis is suspected in the patient with a compatible history who is complaining of point tenderness over the sternum intensified with respirations. External signs of trauma, such as crepitus, ecchymoses, swelling, or abrasions, need not be present.

The lateral radiograph of the chest is the most useful diagnostic test. Care should be exercised not to misdiagnose the nonossified intrasternal cartilage of young patients as a fracture. In the ED these patients should have intravenous access, oxygen, and cardiac monitoring. Isolated sternal fracture is not an indication for active airway management; however, it should be undertaken if there are signs of respiratory compromise from associated injuries. A widened mediastinum should alert one to an associated aortic injury.

Mechanical ventilation using positive end-expiratory pressure has been used as internal fixation for grossly unstable fractures. Operative fixation is often unsatisfactory. All patients should be admitted for serial EKG and monitoring for myocardial contusions. If transfer is necessary, ALS personnel should accompany the patient with continued oxygen, cardiac monitoring, and intravenous access. Particular attention should be paid to the possibility of arrhythmias, pneumothorax, and pulmonary compromise.

FLAIL CHEST

A flail chest is a free-floating section of chest wall resulting from three or more adjacent ribs fractured in two or more places or rib fractures in combination with either sternal fractures or costochondral separations. This is a serious injury that carries an 8% to 35% mortality directly related to associated injuries, of which pulmonary contusions are the most common. These patients often present with pain, crepitus, and ecchymoses over the chest wall. Paradoxical movement of the flail segment refers to its unexpected movement inward during inspiration and outward during expiration in response to the intrathoracic pressure changes during the respiratory cycle. However, the paradox may not be seen initially because of muscle splinting, only to become dramatically apparent hours later as the underlying contused lung decreases in compliance and the patient physically tires. Muscle splinting with subsequent hypoventilation may result in focal atelectasis, decreased tidal volume and vital capacity, hypoxemia, pulmonary arteriovenous shunting, and decreased cardiac output.

The diagnosis is made clinically. The patient's thorax should be inspected and palpated in search of areas of tenderness and crepitus. A careful search for other injuries should be made, and baseline arterial blood gas measurements and chest radiographs obtained. Tube thoracostomy is indicated if intrapleural air or blood is present or, prophylactically, if the patient is mechanically ventilated, as such patients are at high risk for developing a tension pneumothorax. The mere presence of a flail chest is not an indication for endotracheal intubation. There is debate regarding which patients benefit from mechanical ventilation.

The following guidelines are to be used in conjunction with the patient's overall status. Intubation should be considered if one or more of the following are present: shock, three or more associated injuries, previous pulmonary disease, the fracture of eight or more ribs, age greater than 65 years, or a PaO$_2$ less than 60 mm Hg on 100% oxygen at sea level. All patients with a flail chest should be admitted to an intensive care unit for aggressive pulmonary toilet, pain control, observation, and monitoring.

66   Great Vessel Injuries

Nonpenetrating disruption of the thoracic great vessels is almost always caused by a rapid decelerative injury. The advent of high-speed automobile transportation has been accompanied by a marked increase in chest trauma as a cause of death and disability. In the USA more than 40,000 highway deaths occur annually and 25% are directly caused by chest trauma. In an additional 50% chest trauma is a major factor leading to death. The major cause of death in people who sustain blunt chest trauma is disruption of the thoracic aorta. Although a large percentage of victims of great vessel disruption do not reach the hospital alive because of rapid exsanguination, prompt and correct intervention may lead to the survival of a significant number of patients who do. However, delay or incorrect diagnosis may contribute to morbidity or mortality among these victims.

Disruption of a great vessel is usually due to rapid deceleration, such as is incurred during a high-speed motor vehicle accident, a fall from a height, or an airplane crash. The descending aorta is held in a relatively fixed position, whereas the ascending aorta is relatively mobile. On impact the ascending aorta tends to continue to move forward while the descending portion is held stationary, thus producing a shearing force at the aortic isthmus (the weakest and most susceptible portion of the aorta) just distal to the origin of the left subclavian artery. The site of rupture is in the area of the ligamentum arteriosum (just distal to the left subclavian artery) in 80% to 90% of cases. Other less common sites of involvement include the distal descending aorta at the diaphragmatic hiatus, the midthoracic descending aorta, and, rarely, the origin of the left subclavian artery.

Injury to major branches of the thoracic aorta is not uncommon and may occur concomitantly with aortic injury in up to 25% of cases. The most frequently involved vessels are the innominate and subclavian arteries. The aortic tear is transverse in 80% to 90% of patients, and extends through all layers of the vessel on the anteromedial border of the aorta. In most patients with complete disruption death is instantaneous secondary to rapid exsanguination. Of the remaining 10% to 20% who survive, the tear usually extends only through the intima and media. The adventitia, mediastinal pleura, and surrounding tissues contain the blood temporarily by the formation of a false aneurysm. If untreated, the thin-walled aneurysm follows an unpredictable course and may rupture in hours, days, weeks, or even years after the initial episode of trauma. In one review, only 20% survived more than an hour after the injury. Of those surviving at least 1 hour, 30% died within 6 hours, 49% died by 24 hours, 72% by 8 days, and 90% by 4 months.

CLINICAL PRESENTATION

Historical data that should alert one to suspect the diagnosis include any major decelerative incident—most notably a motor vehicle accident with speed more than 30 to 45 mph, but also falls from a height and airplane crashes. Symptoms are nonspecific or may be lacking. The most commonly reported complaints are chest pain (26%), dyspnea (25%–30%), and back pain (14%). Less frequently encountered are dysphagia, hoarseness, and symptoms of ischemia to the spinal cord or upper extremities.

Physical findings of importance include ecchymosis or the imprint of an automobile steering wheel on the anterior chest. The acute onset of upper extremity hypertension, especially in the face of a difference in pulse amplitude between the upper and lower extremities or despite continued blood loss, should suggest the diagnosis. Upper extremity hypertension is reported in 31% of patients with aortic disruption. Unexplained blood loss or hypotension may also suggest the diagnosis. A harsh systolic murmur over the precordium or interscapular area is present in 26% of cases.

Other less frequently encountered physical findings include hoarseness or stridor, diminution of the left radial pulse, transient anuria, paraplegia, and swelling of the base of the neck due to extravasation of blood from the mediastinum. The clinical manifestations of aortic rupture are usually deceptively meager. One third to one half of patients with aortic rupture have no external evidence of chest injury at the time of initial physical examination. Associated central nervous system, bony, facial, and abdominal injuries are often present and may be more obvious, diverting attention from the more lethal aortic rupture. Transection of the aorta has been termed "the consistently most dramatic and lethal missed diagnosis in blunt chest trauma."

EMERGENCY DEPARTMENT EVALUATION AND MANAGEMENT

The chest radiograph is the single most helpful entity, especially if used in conjunction with a compatible history. The standard upright posteroanterior chest film is often recommended in the evaluation of aortic laceration. If the study is performed in the sitting position, it is recommended that the patient lean forward 5 to 10 degrees. Such films will demonstrate the anatomy of the superior mediastinum well. However, the severely traumatized patient often cannot sit or stand for an upright posteroanterior film, and the supine anteroposterior film must be interpreted for abnormalities suggestive of the diagnosis. Such a film is often more difficult to interpret.

The radiographic features include widening of the superior mediastinum >8 cm at the level of the aortic knob in an upright study; a mediastinal–chest width ratio of more than 0.25; deviation of the trachea or endotracheal tube to the right; narrowing of the carinal angle; depression of the left mainstem bronchus below 40 degrees; irregularity of the aortic knob contour, and left apical cap. Other radiographic features include obliteration of the medial aspect of the left upper lobe apex; hemothorax; fracture of the sternum or first rib; displacement of the left or right paraspinous stripe; opacification of a clear space between the aorta and pulmonary artery (the "aortic pulmonary window"); and deviation of the nasogastric tube (representing the esophagus) to the right.

Mediastinal widening may not develop immediately, or disruption may occur without mediastinal widening. Conditions other than aortic rupture may also cause mediastinal abnormalities on the chest radiograph. Additionally, mean mediastinal widths overlap between the nontraumatized person (6.1 cm average, range 3.5 cm–8.5 cm), the traumatized patient with a normal aorta (7.8 cm average, range 6 cm–10 cm), and the patient with chest trauma and a ruptured aorta (average 9.7 cm, range 8 cm–12 cm). Mediastinal widening appears to be a sensitive, but not specific indicator of aortic rupture. Reliance on any single radiographic criterion is not only potentially misleading, but also dangerous. Multiple abnormalities are usually present on the chest film, and should be sought.

Because the risk of complete rupture and exsanguination is present for those surviving the initial injury, repair of the rupture is in order as soon as the diagnosis is confirmed. If aortic rupture is suspected, aortography should be performed regardless of the appearance of the chest radiograph. Aortography is not without risk but is the procedure of choice to confirm the diagnosis. It is important that the entire aortic arch, the proximal great vessels, and the aortic root be visualized during the procedure. The procedure should not be terminated once a single disruption is identified because multiple injuries are reported in up to 20% of cases, and lesions may not be visualized intraoperatively. The blood pressure must be kept under control during the procedure. Intra-aortic hypertension may increase stress on the pseudoaneurysm and promote rupture, while hypotension may not allow for sufficient cerebral perfusion. Hypertension is best controlled with an intravenous vasodilating agent such as sodium nitroprusside. Hypotension usually indicates bleeding and should be managed with volume replacement.

DISPOSITION

Traumatic disruption of the great vessels is a surgical emergency, and as soon as the diagnosis is suspected, consultation with a surgeon competent in vascular repair should be initiated while aortography is being arranged. If appropriate personnel or technology to confirm the diagnosis or to definitively manage the injury are not available at a facility, preparations for transfer must be made immediately. The patient should be taken to the operating room for definitive repair as soon as possible after stabilization and complete delineation of injuries allow. Significant (16%–33%) mortality and morbidity (including chronic thoracic aneurysm, renal failure, and paraplegia) are reported.

COMMON PITFALLS

- Suspect in significant decelerative injuries
- Allowing more obvious injuries to delay pursuit of or obscure the diagnosis
- Delaying aggressive radiologic confirmation of diagnosis
- Failure to transfer promptly if facilities and personnel necessary to diagnose or treat the patient are not readily available at the initial treating facility

67   Esophageal Injuries

Because of the deep and well-protected location of the esophagus, trauma to the thoracic esophagus is a rare occurrence (1 in 8000). Injury can arise from blunt and penetrating trauma, swallowed foreign bodies, ingested caustic substance, and iatrogenic mechanisms, including esophagoscopy, passage of various tubes and dilators, and operative misadventures. About 18% result from external trauma, and of these about 50% involve the thoracic esophagus. The mechanism of injury for penetrating trauma is straightforward. Gunshot wounds are predictably more complex than stab wounds, and can result in extensive disruptions and injury extending proximal and distal to the actual point of penetration. Blunt injuries can occur from two mechanisms. A sharp blow to the upper abdomen can force air and gastric contents into the esophagus. The usual site of perforation is identical to that seen with a spontaneous rupture associated with vomiting (Boerhaave's syndrome). It occurs in the left side of the distal esophagus, a physiologically weakened area. Falls and motor vehicle accidents account for most injuries by this mechanism.

The second mechanism is a rapid deceleration of the mid anterior chest. Compression of the esophagus against the spine can produce longitudinal tears in the upper thoracic esophagus. These lesions are frequently accompanied by a laceration in the membranous (posterior) portion of the trachea, resulting in a traumatic tracheoesophageal fistula. These injuries can go undetected for days in critical patients who are intubated if the inflated endotracheal tube cuff seals off the trachea below the level of perforation. On the other hand, large rents in the distal trachea that communicate with an esophageal defect are readily diagnosed when air forced into an endotracheal tube exits the mouth.

CLINICAL PRESENTATION

The clinical presentation varies with the mechanism of injury but is never specific. Because of the proximity of the esophagus to other structures, isolated esophageal injury is almost impossible. Consequently concomitant injuries often account for the clinical symptomatology or, even worse, overshadow and obscure the esophageal lesion. Regardless of the cause, pain is the dominant symptom and is present in nearly all cases of thoracic esophageal rupture. Other frequently seen signs and symptoms include subcutaneous emphysema, dyspnea, cyanosis, pneumomediastinum, pneumothorax, pleural effusion, and hematemesis. Because of the nonspecific nature of these findings, it is easy to overlook esophageal perforation. The rarity of the injury, particularly from a blunt mechanism, also contributes to missed and delayed diagnosis. One must consider the diagnosis whenever the trajectory of a wounding implement is proximate to the esophagus. In addition, whenever injury to an adjacent organ is apparent, esophageal injury should be presumed and investigated.

EMERGENCY DEPARTMENT EVALUATION

Thoracic esophageal injury can be suspected but not diagnosed on clinical grounds alone. Suspicion can be confirmed by esophagography, esophagoscopy, and exploration. A plain chest film should be performed on all victims of suspected esophageal trauma, looking for subcutaneous and mediastinal air and concomitant chest wall and respiratory tract injuries. Furthermore, in gunshot victims plain radiographs can be helpful in determining the risk of esophageal trauma. The diagnosis should be suspected and pursued whenever a transmediastinal trajectory is identified. Once the diagnosis is entertained and the patient's condition permits it, esophagography, the diagnostic study of choice, should be performed. The study should be performed with a water-soluble contrast material, such as Gastrografin, since barium leaked into the mediastinum can worsen mediastinitis. However, if the study is negative, it should be repeated using dilute barium, which more accurately detects less blatant perforations. Some authors recommend esophagoscopy if the contrast studies are unrevealing. Esophagoscopy is less reliable and should not be chosen as the initial diagnostic study.

EMERGENCY DEPARTMENT MANAGEMENT

Management consists of supportive care. Cardiorespiratory instability may result from associated injuries that are invariably present and should be addressed by appropriate stabilizing measures. Nasogastric intubation should be performed, and may be of diagnostic help if blood is recovered on aspiration. Antibiotic therapy is the only specific management required in the ED. Antibiotic coverage should be chosen in conjunction with the consulting surgeon. Infections that arise from esophageal perforations are normally polymicrobial with gram-negative rods, *Streptococcus, Staphylococcus,* and oral flora being the dominant organisms. The antibiotic regimen chosen should be broad in spectrum and include anaerobic coverage.

DISPOSITION

All patients with confirmed esophageal perforation require admission. Surgical consultation should be obtained. Nearly all patients with thoracic esophageal perforation require surgical intervention. The majority require mediastinal drainage with esophageal repair and temporary esophageal exclusion. Patients should be transferred to an appropriate facility if resources for care are unavailable locally.

COMMON PITFALLS

- The most common pitfall is failure to make the diagnosis. This usually happens because the diagnosis is overshadowed by more pressing injuries and is not considered.
- Unexplored blunt or penetrating trauma may go undiagnosed, and this significantly worsens morbidity and mortality. Many authorities quote a twofold increase in mortality when diagnosis is delayed beyond 24 hours.
- Performing an inadequate contrast study, with failure to follow a negative water-soluble contrast study with barium can result in a missed diagnosis.

68   Blunt Abdominal Trauma

Blunt abdominal trauma is responsible for approximately 20% of all civilian injuries that require surgery. The vast majority result from motor vehicle accidents. Seat belts or seat belt–shoulder harness combinations are effective in preventing or reducing serious injuries from frontal impacts. Blunt intra-abdominal injuries are due to decelerative forces of variable energy and origin. Injury to the spleen and liver is more likely from a blunt than from a penetrating mechanism.

EMERGENCY DEPARTMENT EVALUATION AND MANAGEMENT

Management begins with the assessment of more immediately life-threatening conditions. Once airway and respiratory management, circulatory stabilization, and venous access for fluid resuscitation have been accomplished, the abdomen should be assessed. In the patient with circulatory instability unresponsive to fluid resuscitation, causes of shock other than hypovolemia must be ruled out (e.g., tension pneumothorax, pericardial tamponade, and neurologic shock). In the exsanguinating patient the highest priority should be given to rapid localization of bleeding site(s) and operative therapy.

In the hypovolemic multiple blunt trauma victim it is clinically difficult to establish the intraperitoneal cavity as the source of instability. A rapidly performed diagnostic peritoneal aspiration and lavage (DPL) will discover this site or, if negative, redirect attention toward other potential causes of blood loss. In the majority of patients assessment of the abdomen can be accomplished within the secondary survey, using physical examination, DPL, and specific laboratory and radiologic tests. The appropriate use of diagnostic and therapeutic options (e.g., immediate laparotomy versus diagnostic peritoneal lavage [DPL] versus computed tomography [CT]), therefore, depends on the clinical circumstances and available technical resources and personnel. In the rare circumstances when intra-abdominal hemorrhage is obviously massive and is accompanied by physiologic instability, immediate operative hemostasis is mandatory.

HISTORY

Knowledge of the amount and direction of the forces applied to the body may aid in injury diagnosis: body position at impact, patient location in the car, and seat belt type and usage can provide important information about the potential mechanism of injury. Helpful evidence obtained about the mechanism of injury includes "starring" of the windshield, deformed steering column, extrication requirements, injury status of other victims, and signs of massive external blood loss.

PHYSICAL EXAMINATION

Abdominal examination is preceded by exposure and visualization of the entire body. The examination should be as formal and complete as time permits during the secondary survey. Inspection of the abdomen for distention, contusion, abrasion, or laceration provides clues about the mechanism and extent of injury. Evidence of lower thoracic injury should lead one to consider cardiac, pulmonary, hepatic, and splenic injury. Auscultation should be carried out to determine presence or absence of bowel sounds. Palpation is done to search for signs of peritoneal irritation. Pelvic fracture can be assessed by bi-iliac compression, pubic symphysis compression, and hip position and range of motion. Absence of discomfort in the alert patient or instability on performing these maneuvers usually rules out pelvic fracture.

On rectal examination sphincter tone, integrity of the rectal wall, and the presence of blood or subcutaneous emphysema should be noted. Rectal examination may support a diagnosis of prostatomembranous disruption, especially in the setting of pelvic fracture, if a nonpalpable or high-riding prostate is found. Both flanks and the back should be examined and palpated. Until spinal injury has been ruled out, the patient must be logrolled for examination of the back.

Physical examination is an important component in the overall workup of the patient with multiple blunt trauma. However, its unreliability in the evaluation of blunt abdominal trauma has been frequently cited. It is important that intra-abdominal pathology be considered in patients with major mechanism or multisystem injury, *despite* the absence of clinical signs. Coincident head injury, intoxicant usage, spinal cord injury, or severe pain at extraperitoneal sites can further obscure clinical manifestations. Special diagnostic studies, including DPL and CT scan, must be considered in patients with suspected intra-abdominal injury.

RADIOGRAPHIC EXAMINATION

The place of plain films is limited. Free or retroperitoneal air as well as fractures or abnormal fluid collections can be detected; their presence may affect management. Contrast gastroduodenography is indicated if pancreaticoduodenal injury is suspected in the stable patient. Endoscopic retrograde cholangiopancreatography (ERCP) is specifically indicated if pancreatic ductal injury is suspected and laparotomy is not otherwise planned. Selective usage of contrast barium enema may be useful in diagnosing colorectal perforations.

LABORATORY TESTS

Laboratory parameters seldom alter initial management, but they may be helpful for later reference. Serial measurement of serum hematocrit is valuable only to establish a trend in the event of continued hemorrhage. Serum amylase level is an insensitive and nonspecific marker of pancreatic trauma. In the setting of suspected pancreatic or proximal small-bowel trauma, if initial or persistent elevation in the serum amylase level is found, laparotomy may be indicated for inspection of the duodenum and pancreas, depending on further clinical events and diagnostic findings (e.g., contrast duodenography, CT, and ERCP).

DISPOSITION

ROLE OF THE CONSULTANT   Consultation with a trauma surgeon or qualified general surgeon should begin once the arrival of the multiply injured patient is anticipated or has occurred in the ED. A few patients with blunt injuries are obviously exsanguinating into the abdomen, and immediate laparotomy is required. As such, in patients in profound shock who are unresponsive to initial resuscitative measures, ED transthoracic aortic clamping should precede laparotomy. Other specific operative indications are present in about 5% of patients. These include presence of free or retroperitoneal air, radiographic or clinical evidence of ruptured diaphragm, significant gastrointestinal hemorrhage, and overt abdominal wall disruption.

In the absence of these findings DPL is valuable in deciding whether laparotomy is indicated. It is a safe, rapid, and cost-effective test with exceptional sensitivity in the detection of intraperitoneal bleeding. It should be performed after abdominal examination, optimally in concert with the consulting surgeon. DPL is indicated in level I trauma patients with suspected intraabdominal injuries based on mechanism of trauma or presence of significant external injuries to the torso. It is particularly useful in patients with unreliable examination, in multiple trauma patients who will require general anesthesia for associated injuries, or when there is unexplained hypotension in the field or ED.

Contrast-enhanced abdominal CT scan complements DPL. CT may be able to detect low levels of intra-abdominal hemorrhage and their source, allowing nonoperative management in certain cases. CT scanning of the abdomen is a particularly useful adjunct under the following circumstances: (a) DPL is positive by red blood cell count criterion only and the patient is stable; (b) in the presence of pelvic fracture when DPL red blood cell count results may be falsely elevated; (c) DPL results are equivocal; and (d) in the evaluation of certain retroperitoneal injuries. The accuracy and availability of CT scanning vary substantially with each institution.

INDICATIONS FOR ADMISSION   Continued evaluation is the theme of all multisystem trauma care. Victims of multisystem injury must be admitted for 12 to 24 hours of continued observation despite normal diagnostic studies such as DPL and CT scan. Patients who require operation are admitted for appropriate perioperative management.

TRANSFER CONSIDERATION   It is imperative that a patient be urgently transferred to a capable institution after close communication with the receiving physician.

COMMON PITFALLS

- *Reliance* on physical examination is to be *avoided*.
- Overlooked or delayed diagnosis of retroperitoneal injury is more likely to occur than overlooked or delayed diagnosis of intra-abdominal injury.

69   Penetrating Abdominal Trauma

Stab wounds result from low-velocity penetration or impalement by a sharp, narrow instrument. Tissue damage is confined to the projectile tract, and the resultant injury depends on depth of penetration and the organ or type of tissue traversed. Abdominal stab wounds enter the peritoneal cavity in two thirds of the patients but cause serious intra-abdominal injury in <50%. Thus only one in four patients with an abdominal stab wound requires laparotomy. Stab wounds may be managed in a selective manner (Fig. 69-1).

Gunshot wounds produce tissue injury along the missile tract as well as injury radial to the tract. The wounding potential of the blast or shock wave effect depends on muzzle velocity, bullet caliber, bullet mass, bullet expansibility, and bullet fragmentation, as well as the specific gravity of the target tissues. Because of deeper penetration with greater energy impacted and resultant blast effect of a bullet, serious intra-abdominal injury occurs in more than 95% of gunshot wounds that violate the abdomen. In contrast to a stab wound, laparotomy is mandatory for a penetrating gunshot wound, regardless of whether evidence for peritoneal irritation is present.

CLINICAL PRESENTATION

The external appearance of a stab wound or gunshot wound does not correlate with the degree or location of intra-abdominal injury. Penetrating wounds to the lower chest (nipple line anteriorly and the tip of the scapulae posteriorly) must be suspected of entering the abdomen. The incidence of abdominal involvement is 15% after stab wounds and 50% after gunshot wounds to this area. Similarly, a knife or bullet can enter the chest or retroperitoneum from a wound of entry anywhere in the abdomen. An increase in the respiratory rate may indicate violation of the pleura, while an unexpected rise in the central venous pressure suggests a cardiac wound. Hollow organ injury is more likely after penetrating abdominal wounds because the intestine takes up the largest intra-abdominal volume and thus is more likely to be struck.

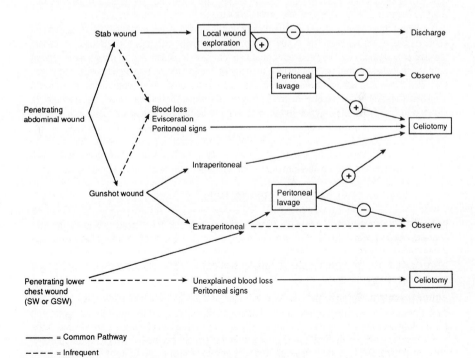

Figure 69-1. Selective management of penetrating abdominal wounds.

EMERGENCY DEPARTMENT MANAGEMENT

Figure 69-1 outlines management of penetrating abdominal wounds. Time of injury, patient position, weapon type, depth of knife penetration, and direction of missile path are important clues. Location, character, and radiation of pain should be determined from the patient, if possible. The priority is resuscitation. Immediate airway control is essential for patients who are in profound shock. Volume restitution is begun with Ringer's lactate administered by way of large-bore, upper extremity intravenous lines. Type-specific blood is transfused if more than 50 mL/kg of crystalloid infusion is required. In the event of cardiac arrest thoracotomy with internal cardiac massage and temporary clamping of the descending thoracic aorta are performed.

Physical examination should begin with a thorough visual inspection of all areas of the body, including the back, by logrolling the patient. Wounds in the perineum and axillae are easily overlooked. All entrance and exit wounds should be carefully examined and bullet trajectory estimated. Examination of the abdomen is conducted systematically in the same manner as that for blunt injuries with two exceptions: (1) avoid further wound contamination; (2) consider local wound exploration for selected cases of anterior stab wounds. Physical signs after penetrating abdominal injuries are largely unreliable, particularly in the inebriated patient. The physical examination for posterior and flank stab wounds that involve retroperitoneal structures has the same potential drawbacks.

In the seriously injured a portable chest film is taken to exclude another penetrating thoracic wound or combined thoracoabdominal injury as well as to confirm final positions of the endotracheal tube, central venous pressure lines, and thoracostomy tubes. Portable anteroposterior and lateral abdominal views are taken to identify free intraperitoneal air or retroperitoneal gas as well as to locate the missile or retained knife. The position of the bullet and pathway outlined by fragments may determine the order and extent of intraoperative evaluation.

When there is no exit site on the patient and the bullet is not identified by the abdominal films, missile embolization must be considered. In such cases extremity radiographs are essential, and arteriography may be required. Computed tomography scanning may miss hollow visceral perforation. Initial laboratory tests include hematocrit, blood type and crossmatching, and urinalysis. The admission hematocrit may not reflect acute blood loss; serial determinations are more valuable. The question of alcohol or other drug abuse should be evaluated. A Foley catheter is inserted to determine urine output and the presence of hematuria. A nasogastric tube is passed and serves to decompress the stomach and detect gastroduodenal blood. Blood revealed by rectal examination must be evaluated by sigmoidoscopy to search for penetration of the rectosigmoid colon. Tube thoracostomy is warranted preoperatively for a knife or missile injury that enters the pleural space because positive-pressure ventilation may rapidly produce a pneumothorax.

DISPOSITION

ROLE OF THE CONSULTANT   Immediate laparotomy is indicated for all patients who sustain gunshot wounds that penetrate the abdomen (the exception is that subset of patients with obvious tangential, nonpenetrating wounds). Immediate laparotomy is also indicated with evisceration, unexplained blood loss, continued systemic hypotension despite appropriate resuscitation, or overt signs of peritoneal irritation.

INDICATIONS FOR ADMISSION   For patients with anterior abdominal stab wounds who do not have signs of intra-abdominal injury, the first step is to determine whether the stab wound entered the peritoneal cavity. This is done by performing wound exploration under local anesthesia. If the stab wound is clearly superficial to the peritoneum, the patient can be discharged after appropriate wound care. DPL is done if the stab wound is known or suspected to have entered the peritoneal cavity. Peritoneal lavage will miss important injuries in about 5%. Therefore, despite a negative lavage, these patients should be hospitalized for 24 hours and operated on if abdominal symptoms ensue. Patients who have sustained a tangential, nonpenetrating, low-energy abdominal gunshot wound, even if it appears superficial to the peritoneum, should undergo DPL. Hospitalization for 24 hours is required despite an unremarkable lavage effluent. High-energy gunshot wounds can cause serious intra-abdominal injury without entering the peritoneal cavity. The safest policy is to perform an exploratory laparotomy.

TRANSFER CONSIDERATIONS   Penetrating wounds to the torso may cause life-threatening abdominal or thoracic injury with little external evidence of trauma. If the initial receiving hospital has no trauma surgeon transfer to a level I or level II trauma center is imperative.

COMMON PITFALLS

- Penetrating wounds to the chest or abdomen may cause life-threatening intraperitoneal or retroperitoneal visceral or vascular disruption with little external evidence of injury.
- Multiple penetrating wounds are common, and mandate complete inspection and examination of the patient.
- Penetrating entrance sites in the back may be easily overlooked, and yet involve the aorta, vena cava, or colon. Bullets and knives may traverse the diaphragm, resulting in major visceral injury at some distance from the skin wound. Conversely, wounds that enter the upper abdomen may inflict fatal intrathoracic injury.

---

70   Upper Genitourinary Tract Injuries

Most renal injuries are managed with observation. There are two major mechanisms of injury in blunt renal trauma: direct impact in the vicinity of the kidneys and severe deceleration of the body as a whole. A diseased kidney is more vulnerable to injury, and a significant percentage of several renal conditions (polycystic kidney and hydronephrosis) are first diagnosed after blunt injury. Concurrent renal disease should always be considered when kidney injury occurs with minimal trauma. The kidney can sustain either simple disruption in penetrating trauma or diffuse blast injury if in or near the trajectory of a high-velocity missile. Associated nonrenal injury is extremely common and usually of greater immediate concern. Always consider upper tract urinary injury in a patient with penetrating lower chest and abdominal trauma.

CLASSIFICATION
The most relevant system is one based on management, whether or not the injury will require exploration. Minor injuries (managed by observation) include minor parenchymal lacerations or contusions with small subcapsular hematomas (65% to 85%). Major injuries include renal rupture (global disruption of parenchyma), calyceal and pelvic lacerations (producing gross extravasation), and renal pedicle laceration or thrombosis (usually secondary to direct penetration or severe acceleration). Renal artery injury is an unusual (5%) but severe injury associated with a high rate of nephrectomy or late hypertension after repair. The mechanism is secondary to deceleration of the mobile kidney with sudden traction at the aortorenal junction, causing intimal disruption and thrombosis. Because the success of revascularization drops precipitously with time (being rare after 18 hours), early diagnosis and preparation for repair are essential. Approximately 25–50% present with no hematuria.

CLINICAL PRESENTATION

The care of other injuries almost always takes precedence; nonrenal injuries are a more common cause of death and morbidity. Hemorrhage and renal ischemia (from vascular pedicle injuries) are the only two emergent conditions of isolated renal trauma. Severe acceleration is seen: (a) falls from a significant height (e.g., >15 ft), (b) thrown from a vehicle, (c) intrusion of the passenger space, and (d) extrication from a vehicle. Persistent flank pain after deceleration without direct trauma should raise suspicion of vascular injury, with ischemic pain. Prior renal disease increases the risk for parenchymal injury. Vital sign alteration and other clinical indicators of shock usually arise from nonrenal associated injury.

EMERGENCY DEPARTMENT EVALUATION

The most widely used screening test for kidney trauma is the urinalysis. Catheterization does not produce hematuria from the urethral trauma of insertion. The IVP is an excellent screen for blunt injury. In penetrating trauma, IVP has a high false-negative rate. IVP is the diagnostic modality of choice for definitive evaluation of all blunt renal injuries other than those of the vascular system and for proximity penetrating renal injury. CT is indicated when IVP is abnormal or indeterminate.

Indications for IVP: (1) gross hematuria with blunt trauma, (2) any degree of microscopic hematuria with penetrating injury, and (3) microhematuria and shock (BP < 90). Renal angiography is the best modality for defining a vascular injury. Arteriography should be considered when IVP suggests significant unilateral hypoperfusion or nonfunction. If arteriography shows unilateral perfusion with only one renal artery visible, renal venography or CT can then be used to confirm the existence of bilateral kidneys.

Ureteral trauma is often an iatrogenic complication that occurs during abdominal surgery; however, it also occurs in trauma and can be easily missed. Hematuria should not be relied on to rule out ureteral laceration or transection. Penetrating injury along the course of the ureter mandates IVP. Blunt ureteral injury is virtually always associated with other intra-abdominal injuries, and is often diagnosed intraoperatively.

EMERGENCY DEPARTMENT MANAGEMENT

Urologic consultation is indicated for patients with genitourinary trauma.

71   Lower Genitourinary Tract Injuries

Lower genitourinary tract injuries (bladder, prostate, urethra, and genitalia) are most frequently seen in association with automobile accidents or crush injuries of the pelvis. The bladder is the most frequently injured. The incidence of intra-abdominal organ injury associated with pelvic fracture varies from 8.2% to 21.5%. The bladder and spleen are the most common abdominal organs injured in association with pelvic fracture. Urethral injuries occur in 2% of cases. Fractures that result in displacement of the pubic ramus are particularly prone to produce injury to the bladder and urethra; lateral compression fractures and shearing force fractures of the pelvis are less likely to result in injury. However, any fracture of the pelvis can be associated with urologic injury (Figure 71-1). The presence of pelvic fracture is indication for urologic evaluation regardless of the presence or absence of hematuria. Most patients have hematuria with significant lower urinary tract injury.

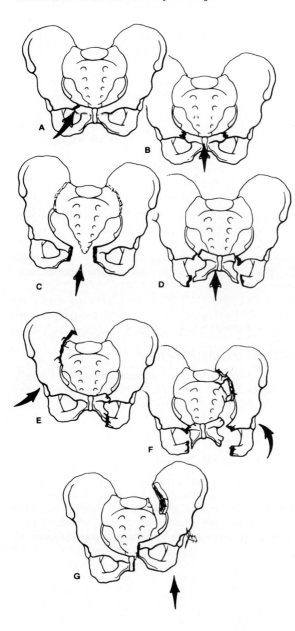

Figure 71-1. Pelvic fractures. (**A**) Simple fracture pubic ramus. (**B**) Bilateral fracture. (**C**) Open-book fracture pubic. (**D**) Butterfly fracture. (**E**) Lateral compression. (**F**) Lateral compression with rotation. (**G**) Vertical shear. (From Guerriero WG: Pelvic fracture. In Guerriero WG, Devine CJ Jr [eds]: Urologic injuries, p 12. Norwalk, CT, Appleton-Century-Crofts, 1984.)

BLADDER INJURY

Bladder injuries may be classified as extraperitoneal or intraperitoneal. Disruption of the male urethra in its membranous portion is almost universally the rule when the bladder is displaced by pelvic fracture. Extraperitoneal rupture of the bladder is more common than intraperitoneal rupture. The most frequent signs of bladder rupture are gross hematuria, lower abdominal tenderness, and shock associated with pelvic fracture. The most common area of rupture is the dome in blunt trauma and the anterolateral wall with pelvic fractures. Associated organ injuries are common. Sixty-two percent of penetrating injuries and 93% of nonpenetrating injuries had associated organ injury. Mortality is a function of associated injury and the age of the patient rather than the type of bladder injury.

Retrograde cystography is the usual means of diagnosing bladder rupture in patients with blunt abdominal trauma. Perform the IVP before instilling contrast media into the bladder, as the appearance of the lower ureters and sometimes even the kidneys can be obliterated when contrast media used for the bladder study extravasates into the peritoneal cavity or retroperitoneal space. Cystography should be done when the patient has hematuria or a pelvic fracture, or when significant force has been applied to the lower abdomen. Hematuria may not be present on microscopic examination, but gross hematuria is usually seen with bladder rupture.

POSTERIOR URETHRAL INJURY

Injury to the male posterior urethra occurs most commonly in association with pelvic fracture. The patient should have retrograde urethrography performed before catheterization but after IVP. If posterior urethral disruption is present, contrast will be seen to extravasate at the level of the prostate, sometimes even obscuring the whole bladder surface. On physical examination these patients usually have a nonpalpable prostate due to hematoma in the retroperitoneal space between the prostate and the rectum.

Females may have avulsion of the urethra at the bladder neck; when this injury is suspected, exercise diligence to be sure that there is no perforation of the vagina in association with urethral injury. Urethrovaginal fistula is extremely common in this type of injury.

ANTERIOR URETHRAL INJURY

Anterior urethral injury may occur with either penetrating or blunt trauma. Diagnosis is made by urethrography. Crush injury to the urethra occurs most commonly when the patient falls astride a fence, a chair, a motorcycle, or a bicycle frame. These injuries are often treated conservatively. A catheter is placed for a few days, and the patient is then allowed to void on his own. In most cases, stricture occurs.

INJURIES TO THE MALE GENITALIA

The penis may be entrapped within encircling rings, such as hardened ball bearing rings. All-encircling objects can usually be removed by wrapping string around the distal penis and expressing the penile edema through the ring and then slipping the ring off with a little grease. One should not make an effort to remove a hardened steel ring or other metal object with an abrasive disk or cutters, as the penis may be injured. Anesthesia may be necessary to accomplish removal of these objects.

Most cases of fracture of the corpora cavernosa of the penis occur as a result of sexual intercourse. Sudden, intense pain is followed by a snapping sound and rapid detumescence of the penis with swelling of the penile shaft. Surgical intervention may be indicated when the patient presents early. Angulation secondary to scar formation may be minimized by immediate surgical intervention.

Castration injury or genital self-mutilation is occasionally seen. Entrapment injuries of the penis, such as with a zipper, are quite common. Sedation is all that is required, and the penis can be unzipped after analgesia is obtained. Power take-off or degloving injuries of the penis usually occur when the penis or testes come in contact with rotating machinery. The skin of the penis and testes is avulsed. Treatment of a degloving injury consists of analgesics to control pain, application of warm saline packs over the injured area, and administration of broad-spectrum antibiotics. The denuded penis and testes are then covered with skin within the first 8 to 12 hours after injury.

Testicular injuries are usually secondary to blunt or penetrating trauma. Debridement and closure of the testis is necessary. Swelling of the testes after minor trauma may indicate the presence of rupture. Testicular ultrasound is useful.

72   Fractures

GENERAL PRINCIPLES

1. Most orthopedic injuries can be predicted by knowing the chief complaint, the age of the patient, and the mechanism of injury.
2. A careful history and physical examination will predict radiographic findings
3. If radiographs appear negative but a fracture is suspected clinically, treat for a fracture.
4. Be familiar with proper radiographic views and do not accept inadequate studies.
5. Perform radiographs before reduction, unless a delay may prove injurious to the patient.
6. Circumferential casting in plaster is usually not mandated of the emergency physician and is best left to an orthopedic surgeon.
7. Patients must be checked for the ability to ambulate safely before being discharged from the emergency department.
8. Patients should receive explicit after-care instructions before leaving the department, including a warning to watch for signs of neurovascular compromise.
9. In the multiple trauma patient noncritical orthopedic injuries can be diagnosed and treated after airway, head, and intracavitary injuries are addressed.
10. All orthopedic injuries should be described precisely and according to established conventions.

COMPLICATIONS OF FRACTURES
See Tables 72-1 and 72-2.

COMPLICATIONS OF IMMOBILIZATION
Fractures frequently result in long periods of immobilization. This often presents serious medical problems, especially in the elderly, including deep venous thrombophlebitis, pulmonary embolism, pneumonia, urinary tract infection, wound infection, ulcers, muscle atrophy, gastrointestinal hemorrhage, and psychiatric disorders. Thus early ambulation is a major goal of optimal orthopedic care.

FRACTURE DIAGNOSIS
RADIOLOGY

Plain films are the mainstay in the diagnosis of fractures. In addition to confirming or ruling out fractures, they can identify other pathologic conditions. At least two views perpendicular to each other are necessary when examining long bones.

RADIONUCLIDE BONE SCANNING

Radionuclide bone scanning is used to detect skeletal abnormalities that are not evident radiographically. Technetium 99m components are taken up where there is reactive bone formation, and thus can reveal occult fractures or acute osteomyelitis. A limitation is that fractures must be at least 72 hours old for this test to be sensitive. Scintigraphy is also used by some as an adjunct in the evaluation of suspected child abuse patients.

TABLE 72-1. Blood Loss Associated with Fractures

Fracture Site	Amount of Blood Loss (mL)
Radius and ulna	150–250
Humerus	250
Tibia and fibula	500
Femur	1000
Pelvis	1500–3000

TABLE 72-2. Nerve Injuries That Accompany Orthopedic Injuries

Orthopedic Injury	Nerve Injury
Elbow injury	Media (especially with supra-condylar fracture) or ulnar
Shoulder dislocation	Axillary
Sacral fracture	Cauda equina
Acetabulum fracture	Sciatic
Hip dislocation	Femoral
Femoral shaft fracture	Peroneal
Knee dislocation	Tibial or peroneal
Lateral tibial plateau fracture	Peroneal

COMPUTED TOMOGRAPHY

Computed tomography (CT) is used to confirm suspicious fractures or to better define displacement, alignment, or fragmentation of fractures. CT scanning is also useful in trauma to rule out cervical spine fracture when plain films are equivocal. Even when plain films demonstrate a fracture, CT scanning is frequently used in noncompressive vertebral fractures to assess the number of fragments and their spatial relation to the spinal canal.

EMERGENCY DEPARTMENT MANAGEMENT

Splinting or other immobilization is used after diagnosis as treatment of injuries. In some cases splints are all that are needed for definitive treatment, whereas at other times these devices are temporizing while waiting for swelling to diminish or until orthopedic consultation is available.

EMERGENCY SPLINTING AND BANDAGING

Suspected or proven fractures or dislocations should be splinted to avoid damage to muscles, nerves, vessels, and the skin. Splinting may also restore blood flow to ischemic tissues by removing pressure resulting from a bony fragment resting against a blood vessel. Finally, splinting relieves pain. Conversely, movement of fracture fragments results in severe pain.

CASTS

Casts perform a function similar to that of splints; they provide stability and relieve pain. They also immobilize injured parts in order to allow healing. Casts are not mandatory for all fractures; in situations where they are, application is usually not an immediate necessity. For these reasons and because of the many problems associated with casts, many emergency physicians choose not to apply circumferential casts themselves.

CAST PROBLEMS

Patients who have had plaster casts applied may present with complaints related to their casts. These complaints are usually pain, local irritation, swelling, and numbness of the distal part. A cast that is too tight causes swelling, pain, coolness, and change in skin color of the distal parts.

Pain may also be due to the initial injury or due to local pressure, or it may be secondary to a developing compartmental syndrome or wound infection. The safest thing to do if a patient complains of pain is to bivalve the cast and inspect the extremity. This is done by cutting the plaster as well as the padding on each side and removing half the cast at a time, using the other half as a mold to keep the extremity immobile. Afterward the bivalved cast can be held together with a bias-cut stockinette until a new cast is applied.

Patients with swelling, paresthesias, or any signs suggestive of compartmental syndrome should also have their casts bivalved. If relieving external pressure does not alleviate symptoms, the diagnosis of compartmental syndrome should be seriously considered. Casts may obscure wound infections, sources of sepsis, and even tetanus. Do not hesitate to bivalve the cast and inspect the extremity when dealing with a serious medical problem.

COMMON PITFALLS

- Many anatomical variants may be mistaken for fractures on x-ray film. Knowledge of the most common will prevent misdiagnoses. Additionally, clinical correlation should be sought, and comparison films of the other side may be helpful.
- Epiphyses may be mistaken for fractures on radiographs. When such confusion exists comparison films may be useful. It is also useful to know when centers of ossification normally appear on radiographs and at what age union occurs.
- Nondisplaced fractures are not always apparent on plain radiographs. If fracture is highly suspected, either protect the part and radiograph it again in 7 to 10 days (as in carpal lunate fracture) or perform a more definitive test (as in nondisplaced hip fracture).
- The most commonly missed fracture is the second fracture. The physician should not stop reading the film once a fracture is identified.

73   Joint Dislocations

Joint dislocations are common. Some, such as shoulder dislocations, are often associated with relatively minor trauma. Others, such as dislocations of the hip and knee, are usually associated with major trauma and are often accompanied by other, serious injuries. Rapid diagnosis and reduction are important to avoid permanent injury to blood vessels and nerves and to prevent other complications, such as avascular necrosis.

CLINICAL PRESENTATION

The patient with a joint dislocation usually complains of pain in that joint and has severe pain with any movement of the joint. In addition, there is usually some degree of deformity of the joint, which is best evaluated by comparing the affected joint with the same joint on the other side of the body. However, certain dislocations, such as a hip or shoulder dislocation in a comatose patient with multisystem trauma, may be difficult to diagnose. Such patients require careful evaluation of all bones and joints, including radiographs, after stabilization. Also, the dislocation may have spontaneously relocated before the patient sought medical attention.

EMERGENCY DEPARTMENT EVALUATION AND MANAGEMENT

A neurovascular examination distal to the dislocation should be performed before administration of analgesics or anesthetics. Appropriate radiographs of the joint should be obtained. The dislocation should be reduced under adequate analgesia or anesthesia. Postreduction films should be taken to document the adequacy of reduction and to rule out fractures that might have been missed on the prereduction film. Finally, the reduced joint must be correctly splinted to prevent recurrence of the dislocation, protect surrounding soft tissues, and make the patient comfortable.

POSTERIOR ELBOW DISLOCATION   Posterior elbow dislocation is caused by a fall on the outstretched arm in extension. The elbow is usually swollen, and any range of motion is extremely painful. Radiographs reveal the posterior dislocation of the ulna and radius on the proximal humerus. Careful assessment of the neurovascular status distal to the elbow is mandatory, since injury to the median and ulnar nerves and the brachial artery is not uncommon. After successful reduction the elbow should be splinted in 120 degrees of flexion and the distal neurovascular status again checked. Orthopedic consultation is indicated.

ANTERIOR SHOULDER DISLOCATION   Anterior shoulder dislocation usually occurs with forceful abduction and external rotation of the humerus. The patient complains of severe pain in the shoulder and usually supports his arm. On examination there is loss of the normal contour of the shoulder when compared with the uninvolved side. Neurovascular status should be checked with particular attention to the axillary nerve. Anteroposterior and axillary or true lateral radiographs of the shoulder should be obtained. The dislocation is usually subcoracoid but may also be subglenoid or subclavicular. After appropriate analgesia or anesthesia several methods of reduction may be successfully and safely used.

HIP DISLOCATIONS   Hip dislocations are almost always due to large forces, as in falls from heights and in motor vehicle accidents. They are associated with other major multisystem trauma and may be overlooked. Obtaining a pelvic radiograph will prevent this oversight and reduce the incidence of avascular necrosis of the femoral head, a common complication of unrecognized hip dislocations. Although both posterior and anterior dislocations may occur, the posterior dislocation is by far the most common. Both types of dislocations are usually reduced by an orthopedic surgeon. Before any attempt at reduction the patient's neurovascular status must be documented and adequate analgesia or anesthesia administered. Posterior hip dislocation is often caused when the patient's flexed hip and knee strike the dashboard in a deceleration motor vehicle accident. It is frequently associated with a posterior acetabular fracture. The patient presents with the involved leg shortened, adducted, and internally rotated, and complains of severe pain. Radiographs reveal the femoral head to be displaced posteriorly.

KNEE DISLOCATIONS   Knee dislocation is uncommon because it requires major forces, usually falls from heights or motor vehicle accidents, to dislocate the knee. This injury is, therefore, often associated with major trauma to other systems. The tibia may be dislocated anterior (most common), posterior, medial, or lateral, depending upon the direction of the dislocating force. This injury is associated with a relatively high incidence of injuries to the popliteal artery and peroneal nerve. Reduction must be accomplished as soon as possible, since the risk of damage to the popliteal artery increases proportionately with the duration of dislocation.

PATELLAR DISLOCATIONS   Patellar dislocation is a common injury, particularly in young women. Patients are predisposed to this injury if they have a history of recurrent dislocations, patella alta, a flattening of the lateral femoral condyle, excessive external tibial torsion, or, most commonly, excessive genu valgum. Most subluxations and many dislocations spontaneously reduce, making the diagnosis more difficult. Most occur with the knee in extension when there is sudden flexion and external rotation of the tibia on the femur with simultaneous contraction of the quadriceps. The patient experiences immediate pain and often describes the knee "giving out."

On examination, if the patella is still dislocated, the diagnosis is obvious. However, the patella has usually reduced and the examiner often finds a moderate joint effusion, tenderness medial to the patella, and a positive patellar apprehension test. If the patella is still laterally dislocated, the knee should be gently extended until the patella reduces. If this does not effect a reduction or the patient complains of severe pain, analgesia or anesthesia should be administered and pressure directed under the patella, pushing it anteriorly, causing the patella to slide over the lateral femoral condyle into its normal position. Postreduction patellar radiographs should be obtained to rule out an osteochondral fracture. The knee should be splinted in a knee immobilizer for 3 to 4 weeks and the patient referred to an orthopedic surgeon for follow-up.

ANKLE DISLOCATIONS   Ankle dislocation is usually associated with large forces and, because of the bony anatomy of the ankle, is almost always associated with fractures. The most common dislocation is posterior (talus in relation to the distal tibia). If there is evidence of neurovascular compromise or tenting of the skin, the dislocation should be immediately reduced. Radiographs should be obtained before attempting reduction. Almost all ankle dislocations require ORIF.

74   Hand Injuries

Hand injuries are a significant cause of disability and lost work time. In evaluating hand injuries first obtain a history of the injury and perform an examination of the hand. Once the extent of injury has been delineated, management or speciality referral can be undertaken.

EMERGENCY DEPARTMENT EVALUATION

The patient's age, occupation, and dominant hand should be recorded. The physician needs to determine whether the injury involved sharp or crushing forces and whether it occurred in a clean or contaminated environment. The location of the injury is described as on the radial or ulnar side and on the volar or dorsal surface. The skin is examined and skin loss is noted. Evaluation of the vascular status of the injured hand should include an assessment of arterial and venous components. Often injured hands are soiled and need to be adequately cleansed to allow proper examination for color, pallor, cyanosis, and capillary refill. Examination of the nerve supply to the hand should include an assessment of motor and sensory components.

EMERGENCY DEPARTMENT MANAGEMENT

TENDON INJURY
Tendon repairs in the ED should be confined to lacerated extensor tendons in the arm, hand, or fingers and lacerations of the palmaris longus, flexor carpi radialis, and flexor carpi ulnaris tendons. These repairs are usually performed by hand surgeons. Flexor tendon injuries should be referred.

AMPUTATIONS

Amputations represent 5% of upper extremity injuries. The hand or finger is affected in 97% of the cases. About one third of the cases are sharp injuries, 1/3 result from power saw, bicycle chain, punch-press, or crushing injuries. The amputated parts should be cleaned to remove gross debris, wrapped in a moist saline sponge, and placed in a plastic container, which is then placed in ice. Direct contact of the amputated part with ice should be avoided. The amputated part can tolerate 6 hours of warm ischemia or 24 hours of cold ischemia. Fingertip amputations are best treated by the open method. Fingertip amputations at or distal to the distal half of the nail bed can be treated in the ED, but amputations proximal should be referred to a hand surgeon.

SUBUNGUAL HEMATOMA

Subungual hematoma, if symptomatic, is drained by the following method: The tip of an open paperclip is heated by an alcohol lamp until red hot and placed over the nail center of the hematoma. Gentle pressure is applied until the nail burns through and the pressure is relieved. A battery-powered device can be also used.

FRACTURES

Single metacarpal fractures may be splinted, with next-day referral. Displaced or multiple metacarpal fractures and metacarpal fractures caused by crushing injuries merit immediate consultation. Boxer's fractures and Bennett's fractures should be immobilized and seen by a hand surgeon the next day. Intra-articular distal interphalangeal joint fractures should be correctly splinted and seen by a hand surgeon within 3 to 5 days. Fractures of the proximal and middle phalanges should be splinted and referred to a hand surgeon the next day.

BOUTONNIERE DEFORMITY

Sudden forced flexion of the proximal interphalangeal joint of the finger or crushing injuries of the proximal interphalangeal joint can disrupt the central slip of the extensor tendon. With disruption of the central slip the two lateral slips gradually migrate toward the palm. Eventually the lateral slips are sufficiently ventral that contraction of the extensor muscle causes flexion at the proximal interphalangeal joint and hyperextension at the distal interphalangeal joint. This is the classic boutonniere deformity. Splinting the proximal interphalangeal joint in extension for 6 to 8 weeks is usually adequate to solve this problem.

MALLET FINGER

Mallet finger is caused by an acute flexion of the distal interphalangeal joint that ruptures the attachment of the extensor tendon to the base of the distal phalanx. Splinting the distal interphalangeal and proximal interphalangeal joints in extension for 6 weeks is usually sufficient treatment unless avulsion of the bone occurs. In this case splinting the distal interphalangeal joint in hyperextension is necessary. Consultation with a hand surgeon should be obtained if the bony avulsion involves one third or more of the joint surface.

WORK-INDUCED OVERUSE DISORDERS OF THE HAND

Repetitious joint motion under load can cause a specific subset of disorders. The symptoms of these disorders are from tendon wear and degeneration as well as tenosynovitis owing to loading or friction. This stress may also strain the joint ligaments beyond their normal working range.

TRIGGER FINGER

Another common work-induced condition is stenosing flexor tenosynovitis, also known as trigger finger. These patients may present with a finger locked in the palm that can only be extended passively with the other hand.

GANGLION CYST

A ganglion cyst is a benign tumor-like swelling that frequently occurs in the dorsum of the wrist and less commonly on the volar-radial aspect of the wrist close to the radial artery. These cysts vary in size, but may be as large as 6 cm. They are filled with a clear jelly-like material and connected to the wrist joint by a stalk. The wall of the cyst is a clearly demarcated fibrous capsule. The origin of these cysts is probably a degenerative response to injury. Indications for surgery are pain, weakness, and tenderness causing restriction of hand function. The recurrence rate after surgery is 15%.

DEQUERVAIN'S TENOSYNOVITIS

DeQuervain's stenosing tenosynovitis occurs at the first dorsal extensor compartment of the abductor pollicis longus and the extensor pollicis brevis, which pass along the radial border of the wrist to the base of the thumb. The condition is usually seen in patients who have work that causes rapid repetitious movements of the thumb and wrist. These patients are quite disabled, and when they have an acute flareup they are unable to use their hands for the most menial tasks. Finkelstein's test is elicited by gently placing the thumb in the palm and then rapidly deviating the wrist radially. The condition is treated by rest and splinting. Chronic cases require surgical release. The resting splint should not only involve thumb, but also immobilize the wrist.

75   Hand Infections

CONTAMINATED PUNCTURE WOUNDS

Cat bites show a high prevalence of Pasteurella multocida, an organism that is also present in the oral cavity of dogs. Radiographs are necessary to look for the development of osteomyelitis and fractures. Human bite of the hand occurs in a clenched fist position when a knuckle is cut or impaled on a tooth. Radiographs are needed to rule out the presence of a tooth fragment or air in the joint. Human bite wounds are to be treated with irrigation with saline solution. The wound should be infiltrated with local anesthetic, and examination should rule out tendon or joint capsule injury. If no such injury is present, the wound should be left open and splinted in a position of function. If the joint has been entered, it should be irrigated with saline solution, left open, and dressed, splinted in a position of function. The patient should be hospitalized and a hand surgeon consulted. If not treated prophylactically, most human bite injuries become infected. Gram-positive, gram-negative, fusiform bacilli, anaerobic and aerobic organisms and Eikenella corrodens all may be involved.

The most common fungal wound contaminate is Sporothrix schenckii, seen in gardeners, foresters, and other people who are apt to be punctured by thorns and wood splinters. A nodule or pustule develops followed by invasion of regional lymphatics and formation of additional nodules all in the course of lymphatic vessels. The lesions should be aspirated for culture and should not be surgically biopsied. Treatment is application of potassium iodine.

NEEDLE-INDUCED INFECTIONS

The increased use of intravenous drugs has led to a number of hand infections involving the skin, subcutaneous tissue, tendons, bones, and joints. The dorsum of the hand is a common site for such infections. They usually heal without sequelae after adequate drainage and antibiotic treatment. Intravenous injections can also lead to extravasation injuries that may become infected. These lesions occasionally occur in the dorsum of the hand or in the antecubital fascia. Forearm infection below the fascia can produce a compartmental syndrome that requires fasciotomy.

76   Elbow Injuries

Fractures and dislocations of the elbow are usually caused by indirect forces, often with associated injury of major vessels and nerves. Examination of the nerves and vascular status should be part of the evaluation and repeated at 30-minute intervals (see Table 72-2).

FRACTURE OF THE PROXIMAL RADIUS

Fracture of the head of the radius is usually due to an indirect force and is usually isolated and uncomplicated. It is important to obtain true anteroposterior and lateral views. Most can be treated conservatively with sling immobilization and early range-of-motion exercises within a few days. When the fracture is comminuted or the articular surface is involved, surgical treatment may be indicated.

FRACTURE OF THE PROXIMAL ULNA

Fracture of the ulna is often the result of direct trauma. The fracture is usually comminuted and may be associated with dislocation of the joint. Treatment depends on the degree of displacement and the amount of comminution. If the fracture is displaced <2 mm, it can be treated with closed manipulation. Open reduction is used if closed reduction is not successful or if displacement of the fragments is >2 mm. Usually the fracture fragments necessitate internal fixation.

SUPRACONDYLAR FRACTURES OF THE HUMERUS

Supracondylar fractures occur proximal to the olecranon fossa; transcondylar fractures occur more distally and extend into the olecranon fossa. In both cases the fracture does not extend into the articular surface of the humerus. The treatment of both fractures is the same. Immediate treatment is required to avoid occlusion of the brachial artery and prevent peripheral nerve injury. Minor angular displacements may be reduced by flexion of the elbow under local or general anesthesia, followed by immobilization in a posterior splint. If displacement is marked, closed manipulation may be done if the circulation is not impaired. If the radial pulse is absent or weak, arteriography is indicated to check for vascular injury.

    Continued observation after immobilization is necessary. Circulatory compromise can cause Volkmann's ischemia and eventual contracture. In cases where a supracondylar fracture has posterior displacement, traction is indicated until fragments have stabilized. Intracondylar fractures may extend into the trochlear surface of the elbow, and the articular surface must be repositioned. However, if the fragments are not widely displaced, closed reduction may be adequate. Open reduction may be indicated.

FRACTURES OF THE LATERAL CONDYLE

This fracture either involves the articular components of the condyle or is strictly a fracture of the capitellum. Undisplaced or minimally displaced fractures of the lateral condyle may be treated with immobilization for a minimum of 6 weeks. However, if the fracture is significantly displaced, closed reduction is likely to be unsuccessful. Open reduction and internal fixation may be necessary. Fractures of the capitellum may be reduced with the closed method. Kirschner wires may be necessary.

ELBOW DISLOCATIONS

Dislocations of the elbow may have associated fractures. If there is no fracture, it is almost always a posterior dislocation. Complete dislocation of the ulna and radius implies extensive tearing of the capsule of the joint. Nerve function must be assessed before treatment is instituted. In cases of posterior dislocation the ulnar nerve is the most likely to be injured. Reduction may be achieved through closed methods. Fracture of the coronoid process of the ulna is frequently seen; immobilization for 3–4 weeks is usually satisfactory. Anterior dislocations associated with fracture of the olecranon are unstable. The distal fragment of the ulna and the proximal radius are displaced anteriorly and usually cause extensive tearing of the joint capsule and the ligamentous structures. Treatment is open reduction and internal fixation.

MONTEGGIA'S FRACTURE

Fracture of the ulna near the junction of the middle and upper thirds of the shaft is usually complicated by dislocation of the radial head. The most common type of fracture is anterior dislocation of the radial head with fracture of the ulna diaphysis with anterior angulation. Injury to the radial nerve is the most common associated neurologic lesion. Ulnar fracture is usually obvious but the dislocation of the radial head is often missed, usually due to an inability to obtain a true lateral view. Internal fixation is the treatment of choice. Usually the radial head can be reduced by closed manipulation.

77   Knee Injuries

The knee joint is a synovial hinge joint with a range of movement between 0 degree (full extension) and 130 degrees of flexion. The joint is formed by the articulation of the distal femur, the proximal tibia, and the posterior aspect of the patella. The proximal fibula serves as an attachment for supporting ligaments and muscles but does not enter into the knee joint articulation. The knee joint would be highly unstable if it had to depend on its bony architecture for stability. Instead, stability is achieved by strong fibrous surrounding structures. The medial and collateral ligaments along with the posterior capsule provide stability in the valgus and varus planes. Intraarticular stabilizers of the knee are the X-configured anterior and posterior cruciate ligaments. These serve mainly to prevent anterior and posterior subluxation of the knee, as well as hyperextension of the knee. The anterior cruciate prevents excessive internal rotation of the tibia on the femur. The medial and lateral menisci serve as shock absorbers between the femoral condyles and the tibial plateaus.

CLINICAL PRESENTATION AND EMERGENCY DEPARTMENT EVALUATION

The evaluation of the injured knee should begin with a description of the mechanism of injury. Popping often signifies an anterior cruciate tear, whereas a ripping feeling may signify a meniscus tear. A click with bending the knee may also signify meniscus injury. If swelling is present, was it sudden or gradual? Rapid swelling suggests fracture into the joint or significant ligamentous disruption. Has there been locking or other limitation of motion?

The physical examination should take only a few minutes. The knee should be inspected, looking for gross deformity that suggests knee or patella dislocation. Swelling, bruising, or previous scars should be noted. A straight-leg raise will assess the integrity of the extensor mechanism. The knee should be palpated for hemarthrosis, and any crepitus or point tenderness should be noted. Unless fracture is suspected, stability in the valgus/varus plane should be checked (see Collateral Ligament Tears).

Next, the knee should be examined for meniscus injuries—using the McMurray and Apley tests—and then for cruciate ligament injuries. Plain films are almost always ordered, and may detect fractures, effusions, dislocations, loose bodies, and underlying bone pathology. Arthrography and arthroscopy are used to more anatomically define injuries. When available, magnetic resonance imaging is useful in outlining injuries to bone, articular cartilage, menisci, and ligaments.

FRACTURES AROUND THE KNEE

DISTAL FEMUR

Fractures of the distal femur are described in relation to the femoral condyles, being either supracondylar or intercondylar. Fractures above the condyles are termed supracondylar. Assess peroneal nerve function. Treatment includes immobilization, analgesics, and immediate orthopedic consultation. Surgery and skeletal traction are used.

PROXIMAL TIBIA

The tibial plateaus are most often fractured, with the femoral condyle driven into the tibial plateau, causing an impaction fracture. The lateral plateau is the more commonly involved. Ligamentous and meniscal injuries occur in about 10%. Instability of the knee may occur even when the ligaments remain intact if there is severe depression of the plateau because it can no longer support the femoral condyle. Management includes ice, analgesics, and immobilization. Nondisplaced fractures or minimally depressed (<5 mm) plateau fractures are treated with immobilization, whereas significantly displaced or depressed fractures usually require open reduction.

TIBIAL SPINES

The tibial spines serve as attachments for the anterior cruciate ligament. About 60% occur in children. Closed reduction by hyperextension of the knee followed by casting may treat this injury; otherwise, surgical repair is indicated.

PATELLA FRACTURES

Patella fractures may result from either indirect (avulsion type) or direct trauma. A significant portion arise from dashboard injuries. The most important clinical feature is whether the patient can actively extend the knee (i.e., whether the retinaculum is intact). Complete rupture of the extensor mechanism by a transverse or comminuted fracture requires surgery; otherwise, immobilization in a cylinder cast will suffice. Open fractures also mandate surgical treatment.

DISLOCATIONS OF THE KNEE AND PATELLA

See Chapter 73.

SOFT-TISSUE INJURIES

COLLATERAL LIGAMENT TEARS

The medial collateral ligament (MCL) is injured when a valgus force is applied to the knee. Often the knee is flexed and in slight internal rotation when the valgus force is applied. Tears may be partial or complete. The injury frequently occurs in combination with injury to other knee structures and is usually accompanied by swelling or hemarthrosis. If the capsule is completely torn, however, the hemarthrosis will not be contained and no effusion will be detected. Injury to the lateral collateral ligament requires varus stress; this injury is far less common.

MCL injury is the most common ligamentous injury to the knee and is more likely to occur than lateral collateral ligament strain. The ligaments should be palpated for tenderness and stressed by applying a valgus or a varus force with the knee in both full extension and 30 degrees of flexion. If an opening is detected, compare with the noninjured side, since some laxity may normally be present. The patient may require analgesia for the exam; it may be necessary to drain a tense hemarthrosis to examine the knee.

Ligamentous injuries are graded I, II, and III: in grade I there is no instability; in grade II there is mild to moderate instability; and in grade III the ligament is completely disrupted. Isolated first- and second-degree sprains can be treated with non-weight-bearing immobilization, ice, and analgesia. More severe injuries require rehabilitation through weight training and physical therapy. Treatment of third-degree tears of the MCL is controversial, and must be individualized according to the patient's age, level of activity and associated injuries that require surgery. Early referral is mandatory.

CRUCIATE LIGAMENTS

The anterior cruciate ligament (ACL) is injured much more often than the stronger posterior cruciate ligament (PCL). The ACL is usually injured from severe trauma to the knee and accounts for 70% of cases of acute traumatic hemarthrosis of the knee. It often occurs in association with other internal derangements. The "terrible triad" includes ruptures of the ACL and the MCL and tear of the medial meniscus. The PCL is often injured by a blow (i.e., dashboard) to the anterior surface of the proximal tibia. The examination usually reveals a hemarthrosis, except when the capsule is no longer intact. Several tests for ligament integrity are available, although none is completely accurate.

The simplest test for ACL injury is the anterior drawer sign. It may be necessary to evacuate an effusion, instill local anesthetic, or provide analgesia and sedation in order to adequately perform these examinations. Even when the examination is negative the patient should be referred for evaluation within 24–48 hours. Magnetic resonance imaging and arthroscopy may be necessary. If an ACL or PCL tear is suspected, the patient should be referred to an orthopedist.

MENISCUS

The medial meniscus is torn more often than the lateral meniscus. Patients complain of a clicking, localized pain, a snap or a pop heard at the time of injury, swelling, and buckling of the knee. Patients may also complain of a history of a locked knee or present with a locked knee from meniscus tissue lodged in the intercondylar notch. Examination shows tenderness along the joint line and a positive McMurray or Apley test. Unless the knee is locked, treatment is not urgent. Most patients are evaluated arthroscopically.

LOCKED KNEE

A patient may present with a knee locked in flexion. The classic and most common cause is a bucket handle tear of the meniscus that displaces into the intercondylar notch. Other causes are a loose body, an entrapped ruptured ACL, or a dislocated patella. Sometimes the patient is simply guarding with contracted hamstring, and gentle coaxing with or without analgesia will allow the examiner to passively straighten the knee. Orthopedic consultation is indicated.

QUADRICEPS AND PATELLAR TENDON RUPTURE

Knee extension requires contraction of the quadriceps muscles and an intact extensor mechanism composed of the quadriceps tendon, the patella, and the patellar tendon. Sudden violent force may rupture either tendon. Obesity, use of steroids, and degenerative diseases may predispose to these injuries. Rupture may also occur from a fall on the flexed knee. The patient will be unable to extend the knee or to perform a straight-leg raise; there is diffuse swelling, and often a defect above or below the patella, depending on the injury. Rupture of the patellar tendon may result in the "high-riding patella" on film. These injuries must be diagnosed promptly, as complete rupture of either the quadriceps or patellar tendon requires surgical repair.

BURSITIS

The prepatellar, anserine, infrapatellar, or semimembranous bursa may become inflamed from occupational overuse, acute trauma, or infection. When the prepatellar bursa is involved there may be a palpable effusion. If there is any question of infection, the fluid should be aspirated for Gram's stain and culture. If infection is present, hospitalization for IV antibiotics is needed. Aseptic bursitis can be treated with rest, ice, and nonsteroidal anti-inflammatory medications; injection with steroid and lidocaine or bupivacaine may be necessary in severe cases.

KNEE PAIN IN RUNNERS AND IN OVERUSE SYNDROMES

Most injuries are due to a malalignment of the lower extremity from such contributing factors as hills, shoes, disparate leg length, muscle imbalances, and excessive supination or pronation. Underlying conditions that must be ruled out include stress fractures, meniscus tears, osteochondritis dissecans, Osgood–Schlatter disease, and chronic ligamentous injuries. Pain under or around the patella is common. Chondromalacia patellae is a generic term for knee pain in runners. Compression of the patella into the medial femoral groove will elicit pain; movement medially or laterally often results in diagnostic crepitus. Treatment of overuse syndromes includes curtailment of activity. Other measures include quadriceps strengthening and stretching exercises. Changing shoes, wearing orthotics, eliminating hills, and changing road surfaces may be helpful. Nonsteroidal anti-inflammatory therapy and ice after exercise may also help.

COMMON PITFALLS

- Knee pain may be referred from the hip, particularly in children but also in the elderly.
- An inadequate examination may result from severe pain, guarding, or effusion. These must be alleviated to examine the patient properly.
- Knee extension must be tested for or disruption of the extensor mechanism will be missed.
- A history must be obtained to rule out subluxing patella or dislocation that has spontaneously reduced.
- Bipartite patella is also sometimes misread as a fracture.

---

78   Shoulder Injuries

Most fractures and dislocations of the shoulder are the result of bending or compression forces. Routine radiographic studies include an anteroposterior view and at least one additional projection.

FRACTURE OF THE PROXIMAL HUMERUS   This fracture occurs most often in the elderly from indirect injury, such as a fall on the hand. The diagnosis is established by radiography. Undisplaced or minimally displaced fractures of the proximal humerus require little treatment beyond a sling.

SHOULDER JOINT DISLOCATION   Refer to Chapter 73.

ROTATOR CUFF INJURY   These injuries are often associated with anterior dislocation or subluxation of the shoulder. Complete tears involve the full thickness of the tendon (usually the supraspinatus). Symptoms include pain over the tip of the shoulder, weakness, and inability to abduct the arm. A complete tear allows the humeral head to rise superiorly out of the glenoid. When pain and disability persist for >3 weeks, arthrography should be performed.

FRACTURE OF THE CLAVICLE   This fracture occurs from direct and indirect trauma; most cases occur in the middle third. Injury to the brachial plexus is rare. If the fragments are not widely displaced, immobilization in a sling or a figure-of-eight dressing is adequate. If the coraclavicular ligaments have been lacerated and extensive displacement of the medial fragment is present, treatment is similar to that described for AC dislocation (see below). Open reduction and internal fixation may be necessary when there is interposition of soft tissue or when the fracture is not reducable.

ACROMIOCLAVICULAR (AC) SEPARATION   Acromioclavicular separation usually occurs from a direct fall onto the tip of the shoulder. The acromial end of the clavicle is displaced forward and backward; the shoulder falls downward and inward. Tenderness directly over the AC joint is the most common physical finding. Anteroposterior radiographs should be taken of both shoulders with the patient erect. Displacement is more likely to be demonstrated when the patient holds a 10-lb weight in each hand. Classification of injury is rated from type I or type II (treated by a sling until pain is relieved) to type III injuries (complete tear), which includes separation of both the AC and coracoclavicular ligaments. Treatment for type III injury is controversial.

STERNOCLAVICULAR DISLOCATION   Complete dislocation of the sternal end of the clavicle can be diagnosed by examination and anteroposterior and oblique radiographs. A step-off over the joint and tenderness are the most common findings. A computed tomography scan may be necessary. Complete dislocations are not difficult to reduce. If a retrosternal dislocation does not reduce with lateral traction applied to the abducted arm, it may be necessary to grasp the medial clavicle with the fingers to dislodge it from behind the manubrium. Complications associated with retrosternal dislocation include occlusion of the subclavian artery, pneumothorax, and rupture of the esophagus. Unreduced anterior subluxation is asymptomatic.

FRACTURE OF THE SCAPULA   Fracture of the neck of the scapula is most often caused by a blow on the shoulder or by a fall on the outstretched arm. The treatment of impacted or undisplaced fractures should be directed toward the preservation of shoulder joint function. Unstable fractures require arm traction at a right angle for 4 weeks. When fracture of the body is caused by direct violence, ribs may also be fractured; 85% of patients will have associated bone and soft-tissue injuries. Treatment is directed toward comfort and preservation of shoulder function.

79   Hip Injuries

FRACTURES

FEMORAL HEAD FRACTURES   Fracture of the femoral head is uncommon and usually results from the shearing forces of a dislocated hip; 75% occur during MVAs in young adults with a high association of other major injuries. Femoral head fractures may be subtle; CT or MRI may be necessary. Posterior dislocation or fracture is commonly associated with sciatic nerve injury, whereas anterior dislocation is more likely to produce vascular injury. Reduction of femoral head fractures must be accomplished urgently. Reductions must be anatomical, and small fragments may necessitate operative removal. Avascular necrosis and degenerative hip disease may occur.

FEMORAL NECK FRACTURES   Femoral neck fractures occur in the elderly, with a female-to-male predominance of about 4:1. Often, minimal or no trauma is reported. Some believe the fracture is from recurrent stress and that the fall is the result of the fracture rather than the cause. In younger patients femoral neck fractures usually occur from MVAs. Stress fractures are also seen in runners. Management includes strict immobilization, analgesia, preoperative workup, and orthopedic consultation.

INTERTROCHANTERIC FRACTURES   Fractures through the greater and lesser trochanters are termed intertrochanteric. The majority occur in the elderly with a female-to-male predominance of about 5:1. There is usually a history of a fall. The hip is tender, swollen, painful to attempts at range of motion, and usually shortened and externally rotated. Blood loss may be up to 1500 mL and may lead to hypotension or shock. Management includes splinting with traction, fluid resuscitation if necessary, preoperative workup, search for associated injuries, analgesia, and internal fixation. Complications arise from immobilization and concurrent medical problems; 30% die within 1 year, mostly from unrelated causes. Avascular necrosis and nonunion are rare.

HIP DISLOCATION

See Chapter 73.

SOFT-TISSUE INJURIES

BURSITIS   Patients with pain around the hip may be suffering from bursitis. The most common type is trochanteric bursitis, with tenderness over the greater trochanter. Rest, ice, and nonsteroidal anti-inflammatory drugs are useful, as is avoidance of aggravating activities.

COMMON PITFALLS

- Patients with nondisplaced femoral neck fractures may be ambulatory. Older patients with hip pain and patients who are subject to stress fractures must always have x-rays. Once these fractures displace, their prognosis worsens.
- Hip injury may present as knee pain. This is especially true in children, but it can also be true in the elderly.
- Blood loss from extracapsular hip fractures may cause hypotension and shock.
- **All** patients should be observed attempting to ambulate before discharge. If the patient with hip pain cannot ambulate comfortably and plain films are negative, admit the patient for further study, such as bone scan or magnetic resonance imaging.
- Causes of hip pain are many. Once fracture is ruled out, consider osteomyelitis of the proximal femur, septic joint, neoplasm, sickle cell crisis, rheumatic fever, and juvenile rheumatoid arthritis.

80   Compartmental Syndromes

There are four requirements for a compartmental syndrome: a **limiting envelope** within which **increased tissue pressure** produces **reduced tissue circulation,** which in turn results in **abnormalities of neuromuscular** function. A compartmental syndrome may develop anywhere in the body where neuromuscular tissue is surrounded by an anatomical limiting structure or structures. However, certain anatomical areas are more prone to be involved (see Table 80-1). The anterior

TABLE 80-1. Anatomical Locations of Compartmental Syndromes

Lower Extremity	Upper Extremity
A. Leg Anterior compartment Lateral compartment Deep posterior compartment Superficial posterior compartment	**A. Hand** Interosseous compartment **B. Forearm** Dorsal compartment Volar compartment
B. Thigh Quadriceps compartment	**C. Arm** Deltoid compartment Biceps compartment
C. Buttock Gluteal compartment	

Adapted from Matsen FA: Compartmental Syndromes. New York, Grune & Stratton, 1980.

compartment of the leg is most commonly affected. IV drug abuse results in a greater frequency of compartmental syndromes involving the biceps, deltoid, gluteal, and quadriceps compartments.

DIAGNOSIS

The diagnosis is clinical, based on evidence of increased tissue pressure, inadequate tissue perfusion, and diminution or loss of tissue function. Increased tissue pressure is manifested by the complaint of a perceived tightness, fullness, or pressure in the affected part. Examination may reveal a tenseness or tightness in the local tissue. Elevated local tissue pressure may be demonstrated by direct intratissue methods. Poor tissue perfusion may cause pain out of proportion to the findings. Pain with passive stretching of the muscles may suggest increased local pressure or inadequate local perfusion. It is important to note that pulses distal to the affected compartment are most often intact.

Diminution of pulses with a compartmental syndrome suggests associated injury causing reduction in arterial flow rather than the severity of the compartmental syndrome. Doppler ultrasonography studies are of little use in diagnosing compartmental syndromes for this reason. Excellent Doppler-indicated blood flow is often present with significant compartmental syndromes. Abnormal tissue function is evidenced by muscle weakness and hypesthesia of nerves of the involved compartment. Both muscle and nerve damage may result from direct insult or injury; a significant sign of a developing compartmental syndrome is progressive deterioration of function. A compartmental syndrome can develop when tissue pressure rises within a circumscribed anatomically limited space.

EMERGENCY DEPARTMENT MANAGEMENT

Appropriate consultation should be urgently sought; admission is indicated. A compartmental syndrome, even in its earliest stage, is a limb-threatening situation. IV access, venipuncture, or arterial puncture should not be done in any limb in which a compartmental syndrome is suspected. The involved part should be splinted. Circumferential compressive dressings must be avoided. Limb elevation may be counterproductive. Slight dependency, or at least neutral posture, should be maintained. Compartmental syndromes are often seen in conjunction with other, often life-threatening medical or surgical problems.

81   Replantation

Advances in microvascular surgery allow surgical subspecialists to replant fingers, toes, extremities, ears, noses, penises, and virtually any musculoskeletal tissue that may be revascularized. Although amputations may be partial or complete, treatment for both is similar. Partial amputations have better venous and lymphatic drainage, which improves the possibility of successful revascularization. Successful revascularization may ensure tissue survival; however, neurologic, tendon, and osseous healing are critical to functional recovery. A replanted body part has little functional value if it is disfiguring or has incomplete neurologic function, cold intolerance, and pain. Be aware of the limitations and avoid encouraging unrealistic expectations.

PREHOSPITAL CARE

Incomplete amputations with partially severed vessels tend to bleed freely. Hemorrhage should be controlled by direct pressure. Completely amputated body parts often have limited bleeding, since vessels retract and spasm. The amputated parts should be recovered, wrapped in sterile gauze, placed within a watertight plastic pouch, and then put in a container of mixed ice and water. Care should be taken to avoid freezing tissue.

EMERGENCY DEPARTMENT MANAGEMENT

History should include the time and mechanism of injury, work and avocations, right- or left-handedness, last meal or drink, tetanus history, allergies, and general medical history. Physical examination should document the level of amputation, concomitant injury to the stump or amputated part, and the neurovascular examination of partially amputated parts. If replantation is anticipated, the following steps should be taken: exposed tissue may be gently irrigated with sterile saline solution and large pieces of contamination removed. *Do not scrub or apply antiseptic solution, Betadine or detergents to the wound.* Hemostats, clamps, and sutures should be avoided because of the possibility of damaging nerves and vessels.

The wound should be kept moist with a sterile saline dressing. Wrap in kling or kerlix for pressure, and elevate. Splinting of partially amputated extremities and injured stumps will protect the patient from further injury, limit pain, and maximize tissue perfusion. The amputated part should be rinsed with saline. *Do not scrub or apply antiseptic solution, Betadine or detergent to the amputated part.* Wrap it in moist sterile gauze or a towel, depending on size, and place in a plastic bag or plastic container. The part is then put in a container, preferably Styrofoam, and cooled by separate plastic bags containing ice. Radiographs are taken of the amputated part and remaining stump, including the joint above the site of amputation; the films should accompany the patient if he is transferred. The amputated body part should be cooled and protected from further injury. Tetanus prophylaxis should be given. Many practitioners advocate the use of antibiotics. Pain control may be necessary but should not preclude appropriate surgical consent.

DISPOSITION

Contact should be made with the team capable of performing replantation in the geographical area. The team must be contacted early in order to be involved in the patient's care and to prepare for surgery without delay. Successful replantation decreases after 6 hours from the time of injury.

INDICATIONS FOR REPLANTATION

Preservation of the amputated body part is generally indicated whenever replantation is being considered. The decision to attempt surgery involves many factors and must be made by the microsurgical operating team and the patient. Indications for the replantation of fingers and hands are shown in Table 81-1; however, they should not be rigidly applied to all circumstances. Usually multiple-digit amputations, thumb amputations, and transmetacarpal amputations are indications for replantation. Amputations distal to the distal interphalangeal joint are seldom replanted. Successful replantation is more likely in distal amputations or sharp "guillotine" amputations and in children, due to their regenerative capacity and adaptability to rehabilitation. Even if the possibility of replantation seems unlikely there is no contraindication in managing the amputated part and stump as if replantation will occur (Table 81-2). Tissue recovered from an amputated part may be used to restore function to other damaged parts. Contraindications to surgery are shown in Table 81-1.

COMMON PITFALLS

- Don't be distracted from treating life-threatening injuries by the amputation.
- Unrealistic expectations about replantation should not be raised.
- Further injury to remaining tissue should be avoided.

TABLE 81-1. Indications and Contraindications for Replantation

Indications	Absolute Contraindications
Young stable patient	Associated life threats
Thumb	Severe crush injuries
Multiple digits	Inability to withstand prolonged
Sharp wounds with little associated	surgery
damage	
Upper extremity	**Relative Contraindications**
	Single digit, unless thumb
	Avulsion injuries
	Prolonged warm ischemia
	Gross contamination
	Prior injury or surgery to part
	Emotionally unstable patients
	Lower extremity amputations

Dalsey WC: Management of amputated parts. In Roberts JR, Hedges JR (eds): Clinical Procedures in Emergency Medicine. Philadelphia, WB Saunders, 1985.

TABLE 81-2. Axioms for Care of Amputations

Do's	Don'ts
Splint and elevate.	Apply dry ice or freeze tissue.
Apply pressure dressing.	Place tags on tissue.
Protect from further injury or contamination.	Use sutures, clamps, or hemostats.
Provide analgesia.	Sever skin bridges or debride tissue.
Supply tetanus prophylaxis and antibiotic.	Initiate perfusion of amputated
Obtain radiographs.	parts.
Arrange early consultation.	Place tissue in formalin or water.

Dalsey WC: Management of amputated parts. In Roberts JR, Hedges JR (eds): Clinical Procedures in Emergency Medicine. Philadelphia, WB Saunders, 1985.

- If replantation is being considered, the wound should not be debrided, and the use of clamps, hemostats, and sutures should be avoided.
- Care of the patient should be coordinated early on with the surgical team.
- The amputated part should be cooled, and both the part and the stump protected from further injury.
- Freezing of any tissue should be avoided.
- Tetanus prophylaxis should be provided.
- The loss of a body part is psychologically traumatic; be sensitive to the patient's anxiety.

82   Peripheral Vascular Injuries

Penetrating trauma accounts for 85–90% of vascular injuries; blunt trauma and iatrogenic causes are responsible for 10%. Vascular injury may result from direct or indirect trauma. Direct injury may produce partial or complete transection, contusion, laceration, or arteriovenous fistula. Indirect injury may cause spasm, external compression, mural contusion, thrombosis, or aneurysm formation. The vessels most often involved are the brachial and axillary arteries in the upper extremity and the femoral and popliteal arteries in the lower extremity. Vascular damage should be suspected in penetrating trauma when the penetrating object has traversed the path of a vessel or is in proximity to one. Blunt vascular injury may be more subtle. Stretching, tearing, or shearing forces may damage a vessel, yet leave little external evidence. A complete history and awareness of the mechanics that may produce vascular injury are essential.

CLINICAL PRESENTATION

The most obvious sign of arterial injury is profuse, spurting red blood. Venous laceration may be manifested by a continuous flow of dark blood, which also may be profuse. Significant blood loss may produce shock. However, many vascular injuries, either blunt or penetrating, appear relatively innocuous at first glance. Penetrating wounds of an extremity can present with a small entrance site that harbors significant underlying vascular damage. Blunt injury may be quite misleading because of minimal external signs. The vessel wound, either arterial or venous, may produce a significant hematoma. Occasionally a pulsatile mass is felt.

The absence of a palpable pulse distal to the site of injury in a normotensive patient is pathognomonic of vessel injury. However, the presence of a pulse does not exclude a significant wound. Collateral circulation or transmitted pressure waves through a small clot or intimal flap can produce a distal pulse; 25% of patients with vascular injury have normal distal pulses. A palpable thrill or bruit suggests an arteriovenous fistula. Occasionally comparison of blood pressure in the injured and uninjured extremities can be helpful. If the blood pressures differ by >10 mm Hg, vascular injury is suggested. In addition, an arm-ankle blood pressure comparison may be useful. The ankle blood pressure should be equal to or greater than the arm (brachial) pressure.

Classic signs of arterial compromise include "the five Ps": pallor, pulselessness, pain, paresthesias, and paralysis. Additional findings include tenseness of the extremity, coolness to touch, and delayed capillary refill (>3 seconds). Paresthesias of vascular insufficiency may be confused with those of neurologic injury. Doppler examination of distal blood flow can assist in the evaluation. Pulse deficits and limb comparisons can be performed with greater sensitivity using the Doppler device.

EMERGENCY DEPARTMENT EVALUATION

The mainstay of evaluation is arteriography. Angiography should be used when the possibility of vessel injury exists. Where the peripheral pulse is absent and the location of the injury obvious, surgery should not be delayed in favor of the radiographic study. Digital subtraction angiography has also been used with success. Venography may be used for suspected venous injury, and may be performed in conjunction with arteriography.

EMERGENCY DEPARTMENT MANAGEMENT

Priorities include control of hemorrhage, fluid resuscitation, and assessment and management of other life threats. Control of hemorrhage should be accomplished by direct pressure over the bleeding site. Blind clamping of vessels deep in a wound is to be condemned. If a bleeding vessel can be identified and isolated, it may be clamped using a noncrushing vascular clamp. Fluid restoration should be accomplished. After bleeding is controlled, vascular injuries are treated after other potential life threats have been managed. Angulated fractures associated with pulse deficits should be anatomically repositioned and splinted. This action may restore perfusion to an ischemic extremity. Unless indications for immediate surgery are present, arteriography should follow. Prophylactic antibiotics are indicated for major open wounds or when vascular grafts are indicated. Tetanus prophylaxis should be provided.

DISPOSITION

Surgical consultation must be obtained as early as possible, as the amount of time elapsed from injury until operative repair is a crucial determinant for successful repair. If surgical intervention or arteriography are not available in the receiving institution, the patient should be transferred to a facility capable of providing the necessary therapy after the appropriate stabilizing procedures have been performed.

COMMON PITFALLS

- Vascular injuries may be subtle and misleading in physical examination.
- Failure to appreciate injury mechanics or vessel proximity to a penetrating wound may lead to misdiagnosis.
- Up to 25% of patients may have normal pulses distal to the site of injury and 16% may have normal physical examinations.
- Delay in diagnosis of vascular compromise may lead to permanent deficit or loss of the limb.

83 Primary Blast Injuries

Primary blast injury is the direct result of the cussive effect of the shock wave created by an explosion, most often in industrial settings, such as grain elevator and mining explosions. The worldwide escalation of terrorism has increased the incidence of civilian blast injury.

CLINICAL PRESENTATION

Primary blast injury may be overlooked in a multiply traumatized bombing victim who presents with obvious secondary fragment wounds and displacement or deceleration injuries. Primary blast injury may be present with no external sign of injury; serious pulmonary or abdominal blast contusion injuries may range from a relatively healthy-appearing patient to one in extremis with hypotension and cyanosis from pulmonary contusion or massive internal hemorrhaging. Respiratory compromise and hypoxia secondary to pulmonary parenchymal hemorrhage or pneumothorax and cardiac arrhythmias or neurologic catastrophes secondary to air embolism are the most serious immediate consequences of blast injury. It may also produce subtle, but potentially life-threatening contusion injury in the air-containing organs of the respiratory and gastrointestinal tracts. A pulmonary contusion syndrome, with or without chest wall injury, dyspnea, hemoptysis, or chest discomfort, is the most common problem.

DIFFERENTIAL DIAGNOSIS

The parenchymal consolidation and respiratory failure of pulmonary blast injury may be difficult to differentiate from other causes of ARDS in a blast injury victim, such as smoke inhalation, crush injury, and neurogenic pulmonary edema. Air emboli-induced cardiac arrhythmias or ischemia are indistinguishable from cardiac contusion, ischemic heart disease, or metabolic or hypoxemic arrhythmias. Similarly, neurologic changes may be due to CNS air emboli or to direct head trauma. In the absence of external evidence of significant injury associated with obvious neurologic, respiratory, or cardiac compromise, the possibility of primary blast injury must be considered.

EMERGENCY DEPARTMENT EVALUATION

The ABCs apply; however, some specific indicators of blast injury include jugular venous distention or hepatojugular reflux indicating mediastinal hematoma, intrathoracic hemorrhage, acute cor pulmonale, or pneumothorax caused by blast. The presence of retinal capillary air emboli confirms severe blast injury. Tongue blanching from occlusion of vessels by air emboli also implies blast injury. Oropharyngeal petechiae or signs of paranasal sinus hemorrhage may be observed. Perhaps the most sensitive indication of a strong blast wave is tympanic membrane rupture, with or without hemotympanum. Physical signs of pneumothorax or parenchymal hemorrhage may be associated with blast injury, and are harbingers of impending respiratory compromise.

Blast-induced abdominal injury may cause ileus, tenderness, distention, and percussive tympany; all are nonspecific indicators of an abdominal catastrophe. One of the first diagnostic tests should be ECG, since evidence of right ventricular strain, arrhythmia, ischemia (ST depression), or injury (ST elevation) is suggestive of cardiac contusion or intracoronary air emboli. Laboratory tests are typically nonspecific, although prolonged coagulation parameters (prothrombin time, partial thromboplastin time, and platelets) may indicate DIC from tissue contusion. An ABG may indicate the severity of pulmonary damage.

Chest radiographs may reveal a variety of problems: pneumothorax or infiltrates with various patterns (i.e., interstitial, alveolar, or consolidative). A lateral decubitus abdominal radiograph may demonstrate layered free air or distended bowel. CNS findings necessitate a head CT with special attention to opacified sinuses and areas of ischemia. Continuous monitoring of vital signs and cardiac rhythm is necessary because a blast-injured patient may become unstable at any time.

EMERGENCY DEPARTMENT MANAGEMENT

Treat for other life- or limb-threatening injuries. All patients suspected of primary blast injury but showing minimal or absent physical findings should be admitted for observation. Strict bed rest must be maintained if blast injury is suspected. If ventilatory assistance is required, remember that positive-pressure ventilation, whether manual or mechanical, may exacerbate pneumothorax or air emboli formation. The use of ventilatory support demands careful and frequent patient evaluation. If air emboli symptoms occur (neurovascular compromise or a cardiac catastrophe), emergent hyperbaric therapy may be useful. Patients submerged in water or in a confined space during an explosion require admission without exception. Blast waves propagate well in liquids, and underwater blast is capable of inducing serious injuries at much greater distance than the same explosion in air. Blast confined in a closed space causes equally serious injuries, but the mechanism of injury is poorly understood. Israeli experience and experimental work have demonstrated a high incidence of acute and delayed pulmonary and gastrointestinal complications.

DISPOSITION

Four hours of observation is sufficient time to recognize acute pulmonary or gastrointestinal problems. A patient with no discernible blast injury whose history indicates a low probability of primary blast injury (i.e., a small explosion with little surrounding structural damage or a blast significantly distant from the patient) may be discharged. Discharge instructions should stress that the patient must return at the first sign of dyspnea, hemoptysis, or abdominal pain. Reassessment in 24–48 hours is suggested but not essential for a patient who remains asymptomatic. If abdominal injury from significant blast exposure is suspected, a surgical consultation is indicated. Signs of optic or aural damage necessitate specialty consultation.

Findings of significant blast injury, such as hypoxemia, tympanic membrane rupture, pneumothorax, or chest radiograph infiltrates, necessitate admission to the ICU. Victims of blast may be admitted for other injuries; however, even slightly injured patients should be similarly monitored for at least 48 hours. Transfer for hyperbaric therapy may be necessary if signs of significant cardiac or neurologic compromise occur. If transfer is required, ground transportation with ALS personnel should be arranged. Mechanical ventilation and transportation in an unpressurized aircraft may potentiate pulmonary barotrauma and exacerbate respiratory compromise.

COMMON PITFALLS

The most common error is failure to consider blast injury in a multiple trauma patient. Pulmonary barotrauma or significant air emboli formation from mechanical ventilation or exertion may go unrecognized. The potential for delayed bowel rupture and resulting peritonitis may not be appreciated.

84   Trauma in Pregnancy

About 1:10 pregnant women will sustain some type of injury, with MVAs the most common cause. If a choice must be made, the mother's life must take precedence, but it is also important to remember that the fetus can survive (for a short time) the death of the mother.

PHYSIOLOGIC CHANGES IN PREGNANCY
A number of changes occur during pregnancy that may render evaluation difficult. The plasma volume increases by almost 50% between weeks 10–30. There is also an increase of 18–30% in the total erythrocyte mass. However, as the increase in plasma volume exceeds that of the red cell mass, a decrease in measurable red cell mass occurs (the dilutional or "physiologic anemia"

of pregnancy). Average hemoglobin drops from 13.7–14.0 g/dL to 11–12 g/dL and hematocrit, from 40% to 34% at week 30. After week 30 both rise slightly. These changes enable the patient to tolerate an acute blood loss of 10–20% of circulating blood volume and up to a 35% of gradual loss without substantial change in vital signs. During normal pregnancy changes in heart rate and blood pressure also occur. Pregnancy is a high cardiac output, low-resistance state. Basal heart rate typically increases by 15–20 beats/minute, and arterial blood pressure is lower throughout gestation. Minute ventilation increases by up to 40% during pregnancy, although respiratory rate remains constant. The extent of an injury to the pregnant woman can be underestimated because peripheral vasodilatation occurs in response to stress, rather than the vasoconstriction usually seen in shock.

CLINICAL PRESENTATION

Pregnancy is not always obvious in the early management of the traumatized female, especially if she is unconscious or in the first trimester. In a woman of childbearing age, determine pregnancy as soon as possible, especially if radiographs of the pelvis or abdomen are contemplated. The picture of the traumatized pregnant patient is not different from the nonpregnant patient in the first few weeks of the pregnancy, but with time important differences develop, particularly with blunt abdominal injury. Maternal hypovolemia triggers the secretion of catecholamines, which are potent vasoconstrictors of the uterine vascular bed. A decrease in uterine blood flow of as much as 20% can occur without any change in the mother's blood pressure. If the fetus is monitored, it may display stress even when the mother appears stable, so such monitoring must begin immediately with an external fetal transducer. Baseline fetal heart rate is 120–160 beats/minute. Fetal bradycardia of <110 beats/minute is the earliest sign of distress, and may indicate acute maternal blood loss, diminished uterine blood flow, or fetal hypoxia. The gravid uterus becomes increasingly vulnerable to injury after the 12th week of gestation, as it grows to extend out of the pelvis.

SPECIFIC INJURIES
PENETRATING INJURY

Penetrating injury to the uterus seldom causes maternal death. However, the risk of fetal death is considerable. As the uterus increases in size it becomes vulnerable to penetrating trauma. Cesarean delivery is indicated in all gunshot wounds to the uterus and should be used selectively in uterine stab wounds.

BLUNT INJURY

UTERINE RUPTURE   Rupture of the gravid uterus by blunt trauma is uncommon except late in pregnancy. Severe abdominal pain and loss of fetal movement and heart tones are seen. Vaginal bleeding may occur. The uterus may be contracted and its contour altered, and the fetal parts may be particularly prominent to palpation. Surgical exploration is indicated. Fetal survival is rare, but maternal survival of an isolated uterine injury is the rule, provided resuscitation and intervention are instituted.

ABRUPTIO PLACENTAE   Traumatic placental separation occurs more frequently than uterine rupture, characterized by abdominal pain, uterine irritability, and vaginal bleeding. This should be considered whenever vaginal bleeding follows blunt abdominal injury. If <25% of the placenta has been involved in the separation, vaginal bleeding and premature labor occur. More extensive separation threatens fetal survival, and >50% separation is usually fatal for the fetus. Uterine tetany, maternal shock, amniotic fluid embolism, and DIC are complications.

FETAL INJURIES   Most fetal problems from blunt abdominal trauma are the consequence of maternal hypotension, hypoxia, acidosis, or placental injury. Direct fetal injuries are uncommon.

EMERGENCY DEPARTMENT EVALUATION

Determine if a seat belt was used, since an improperly worn seat belt can cause severe injury (such as a ruptured uterus). History with emphasis on the pregnancy and problems associated with it should be taken. The most common injury sustained in blunt trauma in the later stages of pregnancy is abruptio placentae with injuries to the cord, amniotic sac, or fetus. Besides the usual priorities, of vital importance to the pregnant patient is the monitoring of the fetus, by stethoscope initially but with real-time sonography as quickly as possible, especially if fetal heart sounds cannot be heard or fetal distress is suspected. Supraumbilical open peritoneal lavage can be used to determine hemoperitoneum. Abdominal and pelvic examination can size the uterus and find vaginal blood or fluid. The diaphragm is usually pushed up one or two intercostal spaces by the enlarging uterus late in pregnancy; diaphragmatic rupture is seen with a sudden increase in abdominal pressure. Chest x-ray, sonography or CT may be used to diagnose a ruptured diaphram.

EMERGENCY DEPARTMENT MANAGEMENT

Resuscitative measures are the same as for any other traumatized patient. Thoracic injuries may have more significance since injuries that might be relatively insignificant to the nonpregnant patient (such as fractured ribs, subcutaneous emphysema, or a small pneumothorax) may produce significant fetal hypoxia. Positioning of the patient is important to minimize the effect of pressure of the uterus on the inferior vena cava (IVC syndrome) in the later stages of pregnancy. Unless contraindicated by spinal injury the patient should be turned on her left side. If the patient cannot be turned with the neck immobilized, manual displacement of the uterus to the left may lessen this interference of venous return. If medical antishock trousers (MAST) are used, only the leg compartments should be inflated. IV fluids must be carefully infused because of the plasma volume changes that normally occur. Larger than normal amounts of fluid are often required. Care must be taken in evaluating laboratory data because WBC elevation to as much as 20,000/µL is seen in the second and third trimesters of normal pregnancy. Other changes occur in renal chemistries and arterial blood gas analysis because increased renal plasma flow and respiratory alkalosis may alter normal values.

DISPOSITION

The patient's obstetrician should be contacted as early as possible especially if intervention is necessary to save the fetus; the consultant can assist in the diagnosis of abruptio placentae, fetal distress, or other pregnancy-related injuries. Patients should be observed because premature separation of the placenta may be delayed. Even in trivial trauma to the abdomen at least 3–4 hours of observation with fetal monitoring is indicated. If vaginal bleeding, cramping or fluid leak occurs, patients must be admitted. Fetal heart sounds should also be carefully monitored during this period.

COMMON PITFALLS

- Failure to recognize that the injured woman is pregnant
- Inadequate fetal monitoring during resuscitation
- Positioning of the patient on her back, risking IVC syndrome
- Misinterpretation of laboratory or ECG data by not being aware of changes in pregnancy
- Failure to monitor or admit a pregnant patient for observation if in doubt about the extent of the injury

85   Thermal Burns

Burns are among the most devastating of environmental injuries. Most burns result from contact with a thermal source, such as flame or scalding liquid. Although many burns are minor, it is important to recognize which patients require hospitalization and what therapy should be initiated in the ED. Survival has improved in recent decades. Children with extensive burns are particularly salvageable. Factors that have an adverse impact on overall mortality are: inhalation injury, shock, and sepsis. Although all three are treatable, shock and sepsis are preventable.

EMERGENCY DEPARTMENT EVALUATION

Initial assessment includes a search for evidence of inhalational injury: carbon deposits on the oral and nasal mucosa, carbonaceous material in sputum or on direct laryngoscopy or fiberoptic bronchoscopy, and elevated carboxyhemoglobin levels. Depression of consciousness—often out of proportion to the extent of body surface area involvement by burn—and unexplained metabolic acidosis are important clues to the presence of toxic inhalants. Smoke inhalation is the leading cause of immediate death in fire victims, with carbon monoxide the predominant gas in smoke. Hydrocyanide, the gaseous form of cyanide, should be considered a potential contributor to severe inhalational injury. Carbon monoxide and cyanide are hematologic and cellular toxins and chemical asphyxiants that displace oxygen. The presence of both or either agent may produce an unexplained metabolic acidosis secondary to impairment of aerobic metabolism. Neck and facial burns alone, without evidence of inhalational injury, may generate insidious airway obstruction over 24–48 hours. Clinical judgment must guide the decision to intubate.

Burns may be either full thickness or partial thickness. In partial-thickness burns epidermal elements are retained, and the prognosis for regeneration of epithelium is good. In full-thickness burns all skin layers have been destroyed, and there is nothing from which to regenerate epithelium. Burns are most commonly classified by the degree of tissue depth involved.

The classic first-degree burn involves the superficial epidermis. Although the skin is red, painful, indurated, and, at times, edematous, there is minimal tissue disruption. First-degree burns heal within 7 days with little scarring. The second-degree burn results from destruction of all layers of the epidermis. The dermis is preserved, thus constituting a partial-thickness burn. These injuries are characterized by a red or mottled appearance with associated swelling and blister formation. They are extremely painful to touch. The third-degree burn may appear translucent, mottled, or waxy, or the destroyed skin may have a charred, leathery texture. It represents the destruction of the "full thickness" of skin elements, including nerve fibers. It is painless. Fourth-degree burns extend to skeletal muscle and bone.

Estimation of the extent of body surface area burn involvement is most frequently performed using the "Rule of Nines," which divides the body surface into areas of 9% or multiples of 9%. This method of estimation is adequate for emergent assessment, but its common use may contribute to inaccuracies. A more precise and reproducible estimation can be achieved using the Lund and Browder chart. It corrects for changes due to growth, and is most accurate for calculation of burn area in children.

EMERGENCY DEPARTMENT MANAGEMENT

Burned areas should be covered by dry sterile dressings. Personnel must wear gowns, masks, and gloves. The early splinting and elevation of hand burns may reduce contracture formation.

Central lines should be avoided to diminish the risk of sepsis, but they may be indicated in selected patients. Adequacy of fluid resuscitation is usually judged by the hourly urine output. A Foley catheter should be inserted if the burn areas exceed 25% TBSA; an hourly urine output of 30–50 mL in adults and 1 mL/kg in children who weigh <30 kg should be sought. If burn areas are >25% TBSA, a paralytic ileus for the first 24–48 hours after thermal injury may be seen. Give nothing by mouth and insert a nasogastric tube.

Initial fluid resuscitation with Ringer's lactate at 2–4 mL/kg of body weight/% of TBSA in the first 24 hours should maintain an adequate circulating blood volume and urine output. One half of the calculated amount is given in the first 8 hours postburn. Fluid requirements should be gauged in relation to urine output. If transfer is anticipated, contact with the receiving Burn Center may provide further guidelines for initial fluid therapy. In a third-degree burn coagulated skin forms a thick eschar that may occlude flow to the distal extremity. If the thorax is burned circumferentially, restricted chest expansion may lead to ventilatory failure.

Early escharotomy of the chest wall involves the incision of the full thickness of eschar in the plane of the anterior axillary line from the second to the fourth rib. Success is evidenced by the bulging release of constrained underlying subcutaneous tissue. Rarely, the incision must be carried to the muscular fascia. Tetanus prophylaxis should be current.

The two most important components of stabilization include calculating fluid requirements and estimating the depth and extent of body surface area burn involvement. Extent of body surface area involvement forms the basis for determining the need for interhospital transfers and has been used by third party reimbursers as a criterion for delineation of payment schedules. Errors in estimation of burn size are commonplace, with most errors higher than the computed size. Burn wound estimation affects treatment options, prognosis, allocation of resources, nutritional needs, and quality of care.

Partial-thickness burns can be immersed in cool water, but ice should not be applied directly to the skin. First-degree burns can be treated with antibiotic ointment. Second-degree burns may require debridement of nonviable tissue and ruptured blisters. Intact blisters should not be ruptured, as they afford some protection to heat-damaged skin. The wound should be covered with a thin layer of silver sulfadiazine or with gauze impregnated with antibiotic ointment. Follow-up should be within 48 hours. Hot tar removal from burned skin: immediate cooling will facilitate tar removal and reduce tissue injury. Any petroleum-based solvent can be used to facilitate removal, but Polysporin, Neosporin, and silver sulfadiazine ointments may enhance antibacterial protection. Child abuse by burning may go unrecognized. Scalds are the most common mechanism.

DISPOSITION

Outpatient care is appropriate for partial-thickness burns that involve <15% of the TBSA in adults and 10% in children. Full-thickness burns that involve <2% of TBSA do well with outpatient management. Patients with full-thickness burns >10% TBSA should be admitted. Other factors that favor admission include extremes of age, involvement of hands, feet, face, or perineum, and complicating medical illness. The American Burn Association recommends the following guidelines for transfer to a specialized unit:

1. burns >25% of TBSA or 20% in children <10 years and adults >40 years
2. third-degree burns of >10% of TBSA and second-degree burns >20% of TBSA
3. all burns of the face, eyes, ears, hands, feet, or perineum and burns associated with traumatic injury.

COMMON PITFALLS

- Failure to recognize inhalation injury or insidious airway obstruction secondary to neck and or facial edema

- Failure to appreciate occult trauma, particularly in blast-induced burn injury
- Failure to appreciate constricting full-thickness burns of the extremities or thorax and associated ventilatory impairment or compartment syndrome
- Failure to maintain strict aseptic technique
- Failure to accurately calculate the area and depth of burn
- Failure to adequately estimate fluid requirements and urine output
- Failure to recognize patterns of burns associated with child abuse
- Failure to initiate appropriate tetanus prophylaxis
- Failure to rapidly triage the burn victim who requires admission to a burn unit

SECTION III

TOXICOLOGIC EMERGENCIES

86   General Evaluation and Management of the Poisoned Patient

See Tables 86-1 to 86-6.

TABLE 86-1. Manifestations of Depressant Poisoning

Severity	Signs and Symptoms
Grade 1	Lethargic; able to answer questions and follow commands
Grade 2	Comatose; responsive to pain; brain stem and deep tendon reflexes intact
Grade 3	Comatose; unresponsive to pain; most reflexes absent; respiratory depression
Grade 4	Comatose; unresponsive to pain; all reflexes absent; cardiovascular and respiratory depression

From Reed CE, et al: Ann Intern Med 37:290, 1952.

TABLE 86-2. Manifestations of Stimulant Poisoning

Signs and Symptoms
Diaphoresis, hyperreflexia, irritability, mydriasis, tremors
Confusion, fever, hyperactivity, hypertension, tachycardia, tachypnea
Delirium, mania, hyperpyrexia, tachyarrhythmias
Coma, convulsions, cardiovascular collapse

From Epstein DE. Done AK: N Engl J Med 278:1361, 1968.

TABLE 86-3. Cause of Poisoning Based on Vital Signs and CNS

Physiologic Stimulants	Physiologic Depressants	Agents With Mixed Physiologic Effects
Sympathomimetics	**Sympatholytics**	**Baclofen**
Adrenergic agonists	Adrenergic blockers	Disulfiram with ethanol
Amphetamines	Antiarrhythmics	Hypoglycemic agents
Caffeine/theophylline	Antihypertensives	Heavy metals
Cocaine	Antipsychotics	Isoniazid
Ergot alkaloids	Cyclic antidepressants	Lithium
MAO inhibitors	Imidazoline derivatives	Local anesthetics
		Salicylates
Anticholinergics	**Cholinergics**	
Antihistamines	Bethanecol	
Antipsychotics	Carbamate insecticides	
Belladonna alkaloids	Drugs for myasthenia gravis	
Cyclic antidepressants	Edrophonium	
Cyclobenzaprine	Organophosphate insecticides	
Drugs for Parkinson's disease	Physostigmine	
GI/GU antispasmodics	Pilocarpine	
Mydriatics (topical)	Nicotine	
Plants/mushrooms		
Hallucinogens	**Narcotics**	
LSD and its analogues	Analgesics	
Marijuana	Antidiarrheal agents	
Mescaline and its analogues		
Phencyclidine		
	Sedative-hypnotics	
Drug Withdrawal	Alcohols	
Antidepressants	Anticonvulsants	
Beta blockers	Barbiturates	
Clonidine	Benzodiazepines	
Ethanol	Bromide	
Narcotics	Ethchlorvynol	
Sedative-hypnotics	Hydrocarbons	
	Glutethimide	
Miscellaneous	Methprylon	
Nitrophenols	Muscle relaxants	
Strychnine		
Thyroid hormones	**Miscellaneous**	
	Carbon monoxide	
	Cyanide	
	Hydrogen sulfide	

TABLE 86-4. Agents That Cause Anticholinergic Syndrome

Medications	Plants
Antihistamines	Angel's trumpet (*Datura sawolens*)
Neuroleptics	Black henbane (*Hyoscyamus niger*)
Cyclic antidepressants	Black nightshade (*Atropa belladonna*)
	Bittersweet (*Solanum dulcamara*)
Antispasmodics	Deadly nightshade (*Atropa belladonna*)
Belladonna alkaloids	Fly agaric mushroom (*Amanita muscaria*)
Antiparkinsonian agents	Ground cherry (*Physalis heterophylla*)
	Jimson weed (*Datura stramonium*)*
Mydriatic eyedrops	Jerusalem cherry (*Solanum pseudocapsicum*)
OTC cough and cold remedies	Matrimony vine (*Lycium halimifolium*)
	Night blooming jessamine (*Cestrum nocturnum*)
OTC sleep aids	Nutmeg (*Myristica fragrans*)
	Panther mushroom (*Amanita pantherina*)
	Potato (*Solanum tuberosum*)
	Wild sage (*Lantana camara*)
	Wild tomato (*Solanum carolinensis*)

OTC, over-the-counter.
*Also known as Jamestown weed, stinkweed, thorn apple, and devil's apple.

TABLE 86-5. Anticholinergic Effects

Site of Blockade	Effects
Muscarinic synapsis	Tachycardia
	Dilated pupils
	Loss of accommodation
	Dry skin and mucous membranes
	Flushed skin
	Decreased bowel motility
	Urinary retention
	Fever
Central nervous system	Delirium
	Seizures
	Coma
	Agitation
	Psychotic behavior
	Extrapyramidal signs
	Respiratory depression
	Cardiovascular collapse

TABLE 86-6. Drugs That Produce Acute Dystonic Reactions

Generic Name	Brand Name
Well Documented	
Chlorpromazine	Thorazine
Chlorprothixene	Taractan
Fluphenazine*	Prolixin
Haloperidol	Haldol
Loxapine	Loxitane
Mesoridazine	Serentil
Metoclopramide	Reglan
Perphenazine*	Trilafon
Prochlorperazine	Compazine
Promazine	Sparine
Promethazine	Phenergan
Thiethylperazine	Torecan
Thioridazine	Mellaril
Thiothixene	Navane
Trifluoperazine*	Stelazine
Triflupromazine	Vesprin
Less Well Documented	
Amoxapine	Asendin
Azatadine	Optimine
Cimetidine	Tagamet
Diphenhydramine	Benadryl
Ketamine	Ketalar
Phenytoin‡	Dilantin
Poorly Documented	
Benztropine	Cogentin
Bethanechol	Urecholine
Carbamezepine†	Tegretol
Nifedipine†	Procardia, Adalat
Trazadone†	Desyrel
Verapamil†	Calan, Isoptin
Antihistamines and decongestants	
Chlorpheniramine and phenylpropanolamine†	
Pheniramine and phenylephrine†	

*Piperazine side-chain phenothiazines.
†Symptoms were of latent onset (tardive dyskinesias).
‡Symptoms develop at toxic serum concentrations.

87   Acetaminophen Poisoning

The first stage of APAP poisoning is a subclinical period in which APAP is being absorbed and metabolized, glutathione stores are being consumed, and hepatotoxicity is beginning. This phase lasts for approximately 24 hours. Interventions to blunt the evolving hepatotoxicity must be begun during this

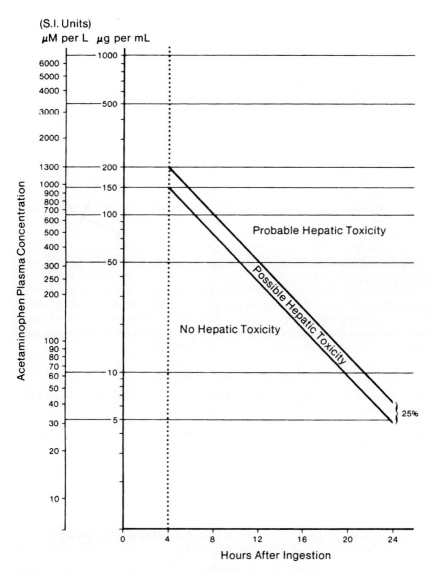

Figure 87-1. Rumack–Matthew nomogram for acetaminophen poisoning. Relationship between plasma APAP levels and toxicity correlated with time postexposure. (Rumack BH: Pediatr Clin North Am 33:691, 1986. Reproduced with permission.)

early phase. The second phase is entirely different. During this period, which begins approximately 24 hours postingestion, there is little or no APAP in the plasma. The predominant clinical picture becomes one of hepatotoxicity. There is a clear relation between the plasma levels of APAP and the potential for toxicity. This is demonstrated by the nomogram relating these levels and the potential for toxicity shown in Figure 87-1. The nomogram stratifies patients into risk categories of "probable" or "possible" hepatotoxicity. The "possible risk" category actually is a region in which toxicity would not be expected but represents a 25% margin of error to account for possible errors in establishing the time postingestion. Note that the nomogram begins at 4 hours postingestion. Plasma levels obtained before this, during the absorption and distribution phases, are not interpretable and should not be used. Based on the known volume of distribution of APAP of 0.9 to 1.0 L/kg, it can be estimated that an ingestion of 10.5 g APAP in a 70-kg adult or 150 mg/kg in a child is potentially toxic. Children with toxic plasma levels are less susceptible to APAP toxicity than are adults by a factor of five to one. The standard nomogram should be used for all age groups.

CLINICAL PRESENTATION

The evolution of APAP toxicity can be divided into four sequential stages, as shown in Table 87-1. In the first 24 hours patients may experience only nausea, vomiting, and malaise. Patients who present in stage II or III may have right upper quadrant pain, nausea, vomiting, jaundice, bleeding, encephalopathy, and symptoms of fulminant hepatic failure. Associated with this is a progressive increase in bilirubin, alanine aminotransferase (ALT), and aspartate aminotransferase (AST) levels and in prothrombin time. These liver function abnormalities can be dramatic in their magnitude, with ALT and AST levels of 10,000 to 20,000 not uncommon. In most cases these abnormalities peak in 48 to 96 hours (stage III) and gradually resolve. Liver function test results usually return to normal by 2 weeks post ingestion, and most commonly by the end of the 1st week (stage IV). The occasional patient with severe untreated APAP toxicity exhibits a pattern of rising prothrombin time and bilirubin and ammonia levels as the levels of AST and ALT decline. This pattern signifies fulminant hepatic failure. However, most patients, even with severe hepatotoxicity, eventually recover and if biopsied up to 3 to 12 months later are found to have normal livers. No chronic APAP effects on the liver have been described.

DIFFERENTIAL DIAGNOSIS

In the earliest stage of APAP toxicity the diagnosis of acute APAP toxicity is made by a history suggestive of overdose. No consistently reliable or pathognomonic signs or symptoms can be expected. Consider the possibility of occult APAP poisoning when confronted with any overdose patient. The finding of any APAP in the plasma must alert the clinician to the possibility of a toxic APAP ingestion. The patient who presents in stage II, III, or IV of APAP toxicity represents another kind of diagnostic challenge. By this time there may be little or no detectable APAP in the serum, so the diagnosis must depend on history and clinical suspicion. The differential diagnosis of hepatitis includes viral, chemical, and biliary tract disease etiologies. The correct diagnosis rests

TABLE 87-1. Stages in the Clinical Course of Acetaminophen Toxicity

Stage	Time After Ingestion	Characteristics
II	1/2–24 h	Anorexia, nausea, vomiting, malaise, pallor, diaphoresis
II	24–48 h	Resolution of above; right upper quadrant abdominal pain and tenderness; elevated bilirubin, prothrombin time, hepatic enzymes; oliguria
III	72–96 h	Peak liver function abnormalities; anorexia, nausea, vomiting, malaise may reappear
IV	4 d–2 wk	Resolution of hepatic dysfunction

From Linden CH, Rumack BH: Emerg Med Clin North Am 2:103, 1984.

on an astute history supplemented by laboratory studies. Liver function tests do not begin to rise until 1 or 2 days postingestion. Thus abnormal chemistries with a history of APAP ingestion within the preceding 24 hours should raise the suspicion of either another cause for the liver function abnormalities or misinformation about the actual time of ingestion.

EMERGENCY DEPARTMENT EVALUATION

The approach begins with the ADC's. Attention is then directed to the overdose. Thus excessive APAP ingestion should be ruled out by either a reliable history or a nontoxic APAP level. For patients who have detectable plasma levels it is essential that the time postingestion be determined as accurately as possible. If this cannot be done, the possibility of a toxic ingestion within the past 24 hours must be considered. Therefore, if there is >5 µg APAP/mL and an unknown time postingestion, acetylcysteine (N-acetyl-L-cysteine, or NAC) therapy should be instituted. If it is determined that the patient has plasma levels sufficient to warrant treatment, baseline liver function tests (AST, ALT, and total bilirubin levels and prothrombin time), serum amylase level, and renal function tests (blood urea nitrogen and creatinine levels and urinalysis) should be obtained. These same tests are necessary to evaluate existing hepatotoxicity in the patient who presents in the later stages (beyond 24 hours) of an APAP overdose.

EMERGENCY DEPARTMENT MANAGEMENT

Treatment of an acute APAP overdose includes stopping absorption and using NAC when indicated. The patient who presents early postingestion is a candidate for gastric lavage. Unless the lavage is accomplished within 1 hour postingestion it is unlikely to affect the outcome. If anticholinergic medications have been ingested, gastric emptying time may be prolonged, and it would not be unreasonable to lavage these patients even several hours postingestion. Syrup of ipecac should be used with caution, since prolonged vomiting due to both the overdose and this treatment may hinder the ability to administer either charcoal or the oral antidote. If an APAP level is not available by 8 to 10 hours postingestion, then clinical suspicion of an APAP overdose is sufficient to warrant the initiation of NAC therapy until the plasma APAP levels are known.

The most efficacious treatment for APAP overdose is NAC. NAC therapy is almost 100% effective in ameliorating APAP toxicity if it is started within the first 8 hours postingestion independent of the plasma levels. Delay in the start of therapy beyond this results in a progressive diminution of its effectiveness with toxicity ranging from 8% to 33% if it is started in the 8- to 16-hour time frame and 4% to 50% if started between 16 and 24 hours postingestion.

Three protocols are currently being used for the treatment of APAP overdoses. These are summarized in Table 87-2.

TABLE 87-2. Protocols for Mucomyst Administration

	Length	Adminis-tration	Loading Dose	Doses	FDA Approval
I	72 h	Oral	140 mg/kg	70 mg/kg every 4 h for 17 doses	Yes
II	20 h	Intravenous	150 mg/kg over 15 min	50 mg/kg over 4 h followed by 100 mg/kg over 16 h	No
III	48 h	Intravenous	140 mg/kg	70 mg/kg every 4 h	No

Patients who have overdosed on APAP should receive activated charcoal if they present within 4 hours of ingestion. Because charcoal is known to absorb NAC, causing lowered NAC blood levels, the two ought not to be simultaneously administered but separated by 2 hours. If multiple-dose charcoal is indicated for a concomitant overdose, this may be accomplished by administering the NAC and charcoal 2 hours apart, so both are given on an every-4-hours basis. It is probably unnecessary to use multidose charcoal with a pure APAP overdose when NAC therapy can be initiated within 8 hours of ingestion. APAP crosses the placenta and therefore, when a pregnant female overdoses on APAP, fetal hepatotoxicity is a possibility. Because maternal treatment with NAC appears to protect both the mother and the baby and no known fetal malformations are associated with maternal ingestion of NAC, we recommend that APAP-toxic pregnant females be treated with NAC in the standard oral manner.

A particularly perplexing patient population consists of those patients who have taken a potentially toxic cumulative amount of APAP but have done so by ingesting multiple nontoxic doses over a period of time. One approach would be to treat for potential APAP toxicity any patient who has ingested more than 10.5 g or 150 µg/kg during the preceding 24 hours. We believe that patients with a toxic plasma level according to the nomogram, based on the time since the last dose of APAP, should be treated with NAC. However, it is not clear which of these approaches may be helpful.

The management of patients with hepatic or renal failure is supportive, and consists of attention being paid to fluid balance, nitrogen restriction, treatment of coagulation defects, and dialysis, if indicated for renal failure. There is no role for NAC treatment in the patient who presents in this phase of hepatotoxicity.

DISPOSITION

Any patient who is potentially APAP toxic by the nomogram requires hospital admission and treatment. Because of the challenges and labor intensive aspects of oral NAC administration, these patients are often best served by an ICU. There is no role for outpatient NAC treatment. If an untreated APAP overdose patient presents more than 24 hours postingestion without signs or symptoms of toxicity, monitoring should consist of daily liver and kidney function studies. If there is no other reason for admission and the patient is reliable, this kind of monitoring can be prudently accomplished on an outpatient basis. For advice with regard to difficult treatment decisions and a toxicologist or regional poison center is not available, physicians may call the Rocky Mountain Poison and Drug Center, operable 24 hours a day.

COMMON PITFALLS

- Obtaining an APAP level before 4 hours postingestion
- Delaying the start of NAC treatment when indicated
- Using NAC when treatment cannot be started within 24 hours postingestion
- Nonadherence to standard protocols (Table 87-2)
- Stopping treatment prematurely when APAP levels become nontoxic or nondetectable
- Failure to consider an occult APAP overdose
- Discounting pediatric APAP overdoses

88 Acetylcholinesterase Inhibitor Poisoning

Organophosphates and carbamates are powerful inhibitors of acetylcholinesterase and pseudo-cholinesterase, the two cholinesterases that hydrolyze acetylcholine and terminate its action. Acetylcholinesterase, also known as RBC cholinesterase, occurs in the terminal endings of all post-ganglionic parasympathetic nerves, at both parasympathetic and sympathetic ganglia, at myoneural junctions, and in erythrocytes. Pseudocholinesterase, also referred to as serum cholinesterase, is formed principally in serum and in the liver. Organophosphates and carbamates inhibit both cholinesterases, with their clinical toxicity due primarily to their action as acetyl-cholinesterase inhibitors. Serum cholinesterase, along with RBC cholinesterase determinations, can be quantitated and plays a role in the diagnosis of organophosphate and carbamate poisoning.

Organophosphates phosphorylate the active site on acetylcholinesterase, rendering the enzyme inert. The resulting complex is stable, and therefore organophosphates are referred to as **irreversible** cholinesterase inhibitors. Carbamates, on the other hand, form an unstable compound as a result of carbamoylation of the active enzyme site, and are called **reversible** cholinesterase inhibitors. As a critical amount of acetylcholinesterase is inactivated, there is accumulation of acetylcholine at parasympathetic, sympathetic, myoneural, and central nervous system (CNS) synapses, with resultant signs and symptoms of toxicity.

Organophosphates and carbamates are rapidly absorbed from skin, respiratory, and gastrointestinal routes. Toxicity varies tremendously, depending on the route and degree of exposure as well as on the inherent toxicity of the specific compound. The onset of symptoms is usually most rapid after inhalation and more prolonged after skin exposure. Symptoms have been reported as early as 5 minutes after ingestion but usually occur by 12 to 24 hours. The exception to this may be some of the newer, highly fat-soluble organophosphates, such as chlorfenthion and fenthion, which undergo initial lipid storage and subsequent redistribution. The more common organophosphates and carbamates and their relative toxicities are shown in Tables 88-1 and 88-2.

Organophosphates are metabolized principally in the liver. Clinical intoxication may last for many days, and if toxic exposure is measured by RBC cholinesterase level, the effect appears even longer. Without pharmacologic intervention RBC cholinesterase concentrations may not return to pre-exposure levels for several months after organophosphate poisoning.

CLINICAL PRESENTATION

The signs and symptoms of organophosphate and carbamate poisoning result from the accumulation of acetylcholine at the muscarinic, nicotinic, and central cholinergic receptor sites. Overstimulation at the muscarinic receptors produces hyperactivity of the parasympathetic nervous system, or SLUDGE (**s**alivation, **l**acrimation, **u**rination, **d**iarrhea, **g**astrointestinal cramps, and **e**mesis). Pupillary constriction, bradycardia, and bronchoconstriction are also common muscarinic effects. Overstimulation of nicotinic receptors (sympathetic and motor) leads to tachycardia, hypertension, hyperglycemia, muscle fasciculations, and paralysis, particularly of respiratory muscle. Central nervous system effects vary from headache and slurred speech to ataxia, seizures, and coma. Death often results from central respiratory center depression. One author has described a relation between the severity of intoxication and the type of receptor activity clinically evident. Muscarinic symptoms may predominate after mild exposures, whereas more severe exposures cause more pronounced nicotinic and central effects.

TABLE 88-1. Toxicity of Selected Organophosphate Insecticides*

Highly Toxic	Moderately Toxic
Tetraethyl pyrophosphate, TEPP (Bladan, Kilmite 40, Tetron, Vapatone)	Leptophos (Phosvel, Abar)
	Dichlorvos, DDVP (Vapona, No Pest Strip)
Mevinphos (Phosdrin)	Chlorpyridos (Lorsban, Dursban)
Sulfotepp (Bladafum, Dithione)	Fenthion (Baytex, Entex, Tiguvon, Spotton, Lysoff)
Methyl parathion (Dalf, Penncap-M)	
Ethyl parathion (Parathion)	Dichlofenthion (Mobilawn, Bromex, Nemacide)
Methamidophos (Monitor)	
Bomyl (Swat)	Diazinon (Spectracide, Diazide, Gardentox)
	Trichlorfon (Dylox, Dipterex, Neguvon)
	Acephate (Orthene)
	Merphos (Folex)
	Malathion (Cythion, Karbofos, Malamar)
	Temephos (Abate, Abathion)
	Ronnel (Korlan, Trolene, Viozene)

*The common name is followed by some examples of trade names in parentheses. Agents are listed in approximate order of decreasing toxicity within each toxicity grouping. Highly toxic organophosphates have oral LD50 values less than 50 mg/kg in rats and are usually restricted to agricultural use. Moderately toxic organophosphates have oral LD50 values greater than 50 mg/kg in rats and may be sold in formulations for household use.

Adapted from Morgan DP: Recognition and Management of Pesticide Poisonings, 3rd ed. Washington, DC, US Environmental Protection Agency, 1982, and Mortensen ML: Pediatr Clin North Am 33:431, 1986, with permission.

Carbamates differ in that they are less toxic and have a shorter duration of action. Signs and symptoms have usually disappeared by 8 hours after exposure. Carbamates are more rapidly absorbed through the skin than are organophosphates. CNS effects are usually absent or minimal, due to poor penetration of the blood–brain barrier. Nonetheless, exposure to carbamates can and does result in fatalities, and serious poisoning must be managed aggressively.

The patient may present with the symptoms described above in any constellation or degree of magnitude. In addition, one must be aware of the unusual presentation or exposure to more than one class of compounds. Miosis is a classic sign of cholinesterase inhibition. Hypothermia has also been described. Chronic exposure to organophosphates at a moderate level may be indistinguishable from a flulike illness, characterized by weakness, anorexia, and malaise.

DIFFERENTIAL DIAGNOSIS

Diagnosis of organophosphate or carbamate toxicity depends on (a) a history of exposure or a high index of suspicion, (b) signs and symptoms of cholinesterase inhibition, (c) improvement of the signs and symptoms after the administration of atropine ± pralidoxime, and (d) inhibition of cholinesterase activity in the blood. (This laboratory test can usually verify organophosphate toxicity but not necessarily carbamate poisoning.) The most classic presentation is a comatose patient who is diaphoretic with pinpoint pupils, diarrhea, excessive bronchial secretions, and muscle fasciculations. However, if only the nicotinic and CNS effects predominate, without the muscarinic effects, the diagnosis can be difficult.

TABLE 88-2. Toxicity of Selected Carbamate Insecticides*

Highly Toxic	Moderately Toxic
Aldicarb (Temik)	Promecarb (Carbamult)
Methomyl (Lannate, Nudrin)	Methiocarb (Mesurol, Draza)
Carbofuran (Furadan)	Propoxur (Baygon)
Aminocarb (Matacil)	Primicarb (Pirimor, Aphox, Rapid)
Dimetilan (Snip Fly Bands)	Bufencarb (Bux)
	Carbaryl (Sevin)

*The common name is followed by some examples of trade names in parentheses. Agents are listed in approximate order of decreasing toxicity within each category. Highly toxic carbamates have oral LD50 values less than 50 mg/kg in rats and are usually restricted to agricultural use. Moderately toxic carbamates have oral LD50 values greater than 50 mg/kg in rats and may be sold in formulations for household use.

From Morgan DP: Recognition and Management of Pesticide Poisonings, 3rd ed. Washington, DC, US Environmental Protection Agency, 1982, and Mortensen ML: Pediatr Clin North Am 33:431, 1986, with permission.

Many organophosphates have a characteristic garliclike odor that can provide an initial clue to the diagnosis. Other substances with cholinergic effects to be considered are bethanechol, methacholine, pilocarpine, physostigmine, neostigmine, and edrophonium. The differential diagnosis of miosis should always be considered, including opiates, phencyclidine, phenothiazines, meprobamate, and clonidine.

When muscarinic effects are present, one must be particularly alert to the possible ingestion of certain poisonous mushrooms (Amanita muscaria, Amanita pantherina, and certain species of Boletus, Clitocybe, and Inocybe), which can present with cholinergic symptoms due to varying amounts of muscarine contained in the mushrooms. In contrast to organophosphates and carbamates, however, muscarine does not usually cause life-threatening muscarinic effects, and nicotinic effects are usually absent.

EMERGENCY DEPARTMENT EVALUATION

The history should document the amount, time, and route of exposure and the identity and type of acetylcholinesterase inhibitor involved. All patients should have cardiac and oxygen saturation monitoring. The physical examination should focus on vital signs and the assessment of neuromuscular and cardiopulmonary function. Arterial blood gases, a 12-lead electrocardiogram, a chest x-ray, and routine admission laboratory studies should be obtained on all symptomatic patients. Pulmonary function tests such as the forced vital capacity and peak expiratory flow rate are useful for assessing respiratory function in awake patients. Confirmation of the diagnosis is sought by documenting inhibition of cholinesterase activity in the blood.

Although most organophosphates and carbamates inhibit both acetylcholinesterase (RBC) and pseudocholinesterase (serum), it is the inhibition of acetylcholinesterase that explains most, if not all, of the toxicity caused by these insecticides. Thus, while both RBC and serum cholinesterase activity can be measured, RBC cholinesterase is considered to be more specific. However, serum cholinesterase determinations are often less expensive and more available, and therefore they are also used to confirm the diagnosis. Unfortunately there are several diseases and other intoxicants that can lower serum cholinesterase levels (advanced liver disease, malnutrition, chronic alcoholism, and dermatomyositis). Intoxicants that lead to false-positive results include carbon disulfide, organic mercury compounds, benzalkonium salts, and ciguatoxins. To further complicate matters, about 3% of people have a genetically determined low level of serum cholinesterase.

Enzyme depression usually occurs immediately or at least within 12 to 24 hours after a significant exposure to an organophosphate. Serum cholinesterase levels are low for a period of time ranging from several days to a few weeks. RBC cholinesterase levels may remain depressed for up to 3 months. On the other hand, in carbamate poisoning interpretation of enzyme levels can be more difficult. As reversible cholinesterase inhibitors, these compounds may exert significant clinical effect and yet enzyme levels may revert to normal within a few minutes. For both insecticides an RBC or serum cholinesterase level reduced by 25% or more of normal suggests a toxic exposure. Unfortunately this determination can be problematic because the normal RBC cholinesterase range is quite large. Although RBC cholinesterase levels that increase over several months following an exposure can be used to confirm poisoning, this kind of diagnostic confirmation is not helpful in the acute setting.

It is important to send the specimen for cholinesterase determinations **before** administering a cholinesterase reactivator (pralidoxime), which could result in a false-negative result. Finally, the diagnosis of poisoning with either class of insecticide can be confirmed by measuring alkyl phosphates, phenols, and other metabolites in the urine. These metabolites can be detected up to 48 hours after exposure and are useful in determining the specific pesticide causing the poisoning.

EMERGENCY DEPARTMENT MANAGEMENT

Attention to the ABCs is always the first priority. Patients with altered mental status should receive intravenous naloxone (Narcan), thiamine, and dextrose. Most fatalities are due to respiratory compromise secondary to a combination of bronchoconstriction, excessive secretions, respiratory muscle weakness, and central respiratory center depression. All patients should be given supplemental oxygen and one should maintain a low threshold for intubation. An often neglected management consideration is the prevention of further absorption of the insecticide by cleansing contaminated skin and hair and removing soiled clothing. Gastrointestinal decontamination procedures should be performed: activated charcoal is indicated to limit gastrointestinal absorption of remaining insecticide even in patients who have had spontaneous emesis or diarrhea.

If signs and symptoms of poisoning with either an organophosphate or a carbamate are present, antidotal therapy with atropine must begin immediately. Atropine acts by competitively blocking acetylcholine at muscarinic receptors, thereby reversing the excessive parasympathetic stimulation. It has no effect on nicotinic receptors, and therefore will not reverse the muscle weakness or the sympathetic effects. Atropine is used primarily during the first 24 hours, while the insecticide is being metabolized. Poisonings with very lipophilic agents (i.e., Fenthion) may be exceptions to this, requiring many days of atropine therapy owing to the slow elimination of these agents.

The dosing of atropine varies tremendously, depending on the severity of the poisoning. It is important to use enough atropine to achieve signs of atropinization (dilated pupils, dry mouth, flushing, and increased heart rate). This may mean using 10 to 20 times the usual therapeutic dosage. Although the average patient with a moderate poisoning requires about 40 mg of atropine per day, the use of as much as 1000 mg in a 24-hour period has been reported. In a patient who exhibits signs of atropinization after only a small dose (about 2 mg) of atropine, the diagnosis of organophosphate poisoning may be suspect.

The initial dose of atropine is 2 mg to 4 mg intravenously for an adult and 0.02 mg to 0.05 mg/kg intravenously for a child. This dose should be repeated every 10 to 15 minutes until adequate atropinization is achieved. The absolute dose and frequency depend on what amount of atropine is required to titrate the desired effect. The use of a continuous intravenous infusion has been advocated by some authors at the rate of 0.02 mg to 0.08 mg/kg/h. One caution, however: although uncommon, it is possible to induce atropine toxicity. Unfortunately the usual signs are fever and delirium, which can be indistinguishable from the signs of the original poisoning. When these occur after adequate atropinization, atropine toxicity must be considered.

After atropine has been administered, the second antidote, pralidoxime (Protopam, 2-PAM chloride) should be given to reverse nicotinic effects. In organophosphate poisoning the use of pralidoxime is clearly indicated. In carbamate toxicity its use is controversial. It is usually not necessary because of rapid spontaneous resolution of carbamate effects and is contraindicated in patients with carbaril (Sevin) poisoning. If the offending agent is unknown, pralidoxime administration is advised. Pralidoxime specifically reactivates the cholinesterase that has been phosphorylated by the organophosphate. It is much more effective for some organophosphates than for others, but should be administered in all cases. Pralidoxime reverses the nicotinic effects most effectively with less pronounced effects at the muscarinic receptors. Although it is not known to cross the blood–brain barrier, pralidoxime does seem to reverse some CNS effects.

If pralidoxime is not given within the initial 24 to 48 hours, a change may occur in the organophosphate–enzyme complex that renders the cholinesterase irreversibly inactivated. After this critical period, restoration of normal enzyme function requires total regeneration of cholinesterase molecules, a process that takes weeks. Therefore, pralidoxime should be given as soon as it is available. The recommended adult dose is 1 g to 2 g intravenously in 250 mL normal saline administered slowly over 30 to 60 minutes. The dose may be repeated in 1 to 2 hours and then at 10- to 12-hour intervals if needed. Improvement usually occurs within 10 to 40 minutes. If improvement is not noted, an intravenous infusion is indicated at a rate of 0.5 mg/h. The pediatric dose is 25 mg to 50 mg/kg. Although pralidoxime is usually not required beyond 24 hours, poisonings with certain lipophilic compounds may require several weeks of treatment.

Succinylcholine should be avoided because it promotes cholinergic stimulation. Theophylline may increase the likelihood of seizures and should be used with caution. Rarely, in severe poisoning, seizures have been described that have not responded to atropine and pralidoxime. It is important to rule out other possible causes (e.g., head trauma, mixed overdose, and hypoxia) while adding a benzodiazepine and possibly phenytoin to the regimen for seizure control.

Death from organophosphate poisoning usually occurs within 24 hours of exposure in untreated patients and within 10 days in treated cases.

DISPOSITION

Any patient with more than a trivial exposure should be observed in a monitored setting for at least 24 hours. Before a patient with an exposure by ingestion is discharged, the passage of a charcoal-laden stool should be assured. Patients seldom require transfer **if** the diagnosis is made because the two antidotes should be available at all acute-care hospitals.

Because of the relatively uncommon occurrence of cholinesterase inhibitor poisoning, it is important to alert and consult the local poison control center. There is also a 24-hour toll-free National Insecticide–Pesticide Hotline for immediate toxicologic consultation (1-800-858-7378).

COMMON PITFALLS

- The most common diagnostic error is failure to consider the diagnosis in the obtunded or comatose patient with the classic picture of SLUDGE symptoms, miosis, and muscle fasciculations.
- The diagnosis is initially a clinical one, and response to atropine will assist in confirming the suspicion. Treatment should not be delayed until serum and RBC cholinesterase levels have been determined.
- Enormous doses of atropine may be necessary in severe intoxications.
- The patient's skin and hair should be decontaminated. Health care personnel also need to protect themselves from exposure to heavily contaminated clothing and vomitus with appropriate precautions.
- The emergency physician should not be fooled into passive observation by the carbamates' reputation for lesser toxicity. There have been several reported fatalities due to carbamate poisoning.

89   Acid and Alkali Poisoning

The extent and severity of corrosive injury to the gastrointestinal tract depends on (a) the nature of the substance ingested, including its pH, pKa, concentration, and viscosity; (b) the volume ingested; (c) the duration of tissue contact; (d) the presence or absence of stomach contents; and (e) the tonicity of the pyloric sphincter. Injury, along with a marked inflammatory response, may continue over the ensuing 4 to 7 days due to the ability of lye to penetrate the layers of the esophagus and to produce vascular thrombosis and necrosis. Damage may be increased by prolonged exposure resulting from reverse esophageal peristalsis. The risk for perforation is highest during the next 2 to 4 weeks. Contraction of granulation tissue with the subsequent development of strictures begins about 4 weeks postingestion. Compared with liquids, solid formulations tend to injure the oropharynx and upper esophagus more often and are less likely to injure the stomach.

Acids produce a coagulation necrosis. Tissue penetration is limited. The antrum is the site of potential ulceration and perforation. Inflammation continues over the next few days followed in several weeks by granulation tissue formation. Ultimately scarring and strictures may develop. Short contact time with the oropharynx and esophagus limits damage to these organs.

CLINICAL PRESENTATION

Acids and alkalis can be classified as weak irritants, strong irritants, or corrosives to indicate the likelihood of potential injury (Table 89-1). Ingestion of solid alkali may severely burn the lips, mouth, hypopharynx, and upper esophagus because of its penetrating ability. Liquid alkali, however, is rapidly swallowed, producing limited damage in the oropharynx, but causing extensive damage to the esophagus or stomach. Young children may refuse to drink liquids, cry excessively, and be unable to swallow their secretions. Symptoms of such esophageal chemical burns include pain, dysphagia, odynophagia, drooling, vomiting, hematemesis, and abdominal pain. Hoarseness, stridor, aphonia, and dyspnea may indicate laryngeal edema or destruction. Chest or back pain and abdominal rigidity suggest perforation with mediastinitis or peritonitis.

The major sites of damage from acid ingestions include the distal stomach, duodenum, and jejunum. Although burns may occur on the lips, oropharynx, and esophagus, these sites are usually spared because of rapid esophageal transit and limited initial acid penetrating ability. The early presentation may include severe pain on tissue contact, retching, vomiting, hematemesis, melena, and diffuse abdominal pain. Abdominal rigidity suggests gastric perforation and peritonitis. Involvement of the oropharynx and upper esophagus produces symptoms that are similar to those of lye ingestion. Systemic complications of severe acid ingestion include metabolic acidosis, disseminated intravascular coagulation, hemolysis, hyponatremia, and shock.

Early complications of alkali and acid ingestions include hemorrhage and perforation. Infection and stricture formation are late complications. Pyloric stenosis, achlorhydria, and hourglass deformity are late sequelae of acid ingestions. The risk of cancer may be increased with corrosive ingestions.

DIFFERENTIAL DIAGNOSIS

The differential diagnosis includes foreign body ingestion, iron ingestion, pill-induced esophagitis, esophagitis, gastritis, peptic ulcer disease, esophageal varices, Mallory–Weiss syndrome, Boerhaave's syndrome, perforated viscus, infections such as epiglottitis, croup, and retropharyngeal abscess, and malignancy.

TABLE 89-1. Classification of Acids and Alkali That Indicate the Likelihood of Potential Injury

Class	Acids	Alkali

Weak Irritants (Caution)	Acetic acid (5%–10%)
	Ammonium nitrate
	Calcium chloride (anhydrous)
	Hydrochloric acid (<5%)
	Phosphoric acid (15%–35%)
		Borax
		Diethanolamine
		  (pH 10.5–11.5)
		Sodium hydroxide
		  (<1%)

Strong Irritants (Warning)	Acetic acid (10%–50%)
	Boric acid
	Glycolic acid (0.5%–10%)
	Hydrochloric acid (5%–10%)
	Nickel ammonium sulfate
	Oxalic acid (<10%)
	Phosphoric acid (35%–60%)
	Sulfuric acid (<10%)
	Zinc chloride (1%–10%)
	Zinc sulfate (5%–50%)
		Ammonia (3%–5%)
		Diethanolamine
		  (pH > 11.5)
		Ethylene diamine
		Portland cement
		Sodium carbonate
		Sodium hypochlorite
		  (3%–30%)
		Sodium silicate

Corrosives (Danger)	Acetic acid (>50%)
	Calcium oxide
	Formic acid
	Glycolic acid (>10%)
	Hydrochloric acid (>10%)
	Mercuric chloride
	Nitric acid (>5%)
	Oxalic acid (>10%)
	Phosphoric acid (>60%)
	Sulfuric acid (>10%)
	Zinc chloride (>10%)
	Zinc sulfate (>50%)
		Ammonia (>5%)
		Calcium carbide
		Calcium hydroxide
		  (dry)
		Sodium hydroxide
		  (>1%)
		Sodium metasilicate
		Sodium silicate
		Tetraethylene
		  pentamine
		Trisodium phosphate
		  (dry, concentrate)

EMERGENCY DEPARTMENT EVALUATION

The diagnosis is aided by the history of corrosive ingestion; the type, concentration, and amount of the chemical ingested; the time of injury; symptoms of oropharyngeal, thoracic, or abdominal pain; vomiting; dysphagia; respiratory distress; signs of oropharyngeal burns; and retching. Clinical manifestations are poor indicators of the presence or extent of injury. Although 2% to 20% of patients without signs or symptoms may have definite gastrointestinal injury, certain manifestations are reliable. Respiratory distress, increasing abdominal pain and rigidity, chest pain, and shock indicate airway obstruction or impending or existing perforation.

Physical examination should begin with the oropharynx. Soapy oral mucosal lesions that become brown or yellow ulcerations are characteristic of alkali exposures. Acids produce gray and white necrotic areas that are later replaced by black eschar. The absence of oral lesions, however, does not preclude the possibility of esophageal or gastric injury. Stridor is indicative of respiratory involvement. Esophageal perforation may be associated with Hamman's sign. Peritoneal signs may signify gastric perforation. Stool and vomitus should be Hemoccult-tested. Fever may be present in patients with esophageal burns.

Baseline laboratory studies should include complete blood count, determination of electrolyte, glucose, and blood urea nitrogen levels, coagulation studies, urinalysis, arterial blood gas analysis, type and crossmatch, and toxicologic drug screen. A mild leukocytosis is seen in about 30% of patients. An elevated erythrocyte sedimentation rate may also occur.

Radiographic studies should include chest and abdominal films to identify esophageal or gastric perforation. Soft-tissue lateral films of the neck should also be obtained, and inspected for swelling or perforation.

Esophagoscopy is useful because (a) it determines the extent of injury, which aids in predicting the probability of later stricture formation; (b) it is essential in determining the subsequent management; (c) symptoms do not always correlate with the extent of damage; and (d) the presence or absence of oropharyngeal burns does not correlate with burns in the rest of the gastrointestinal tract.

EMERGENCY DEPARTMENT MANAGEMENT

Prehospital care should include the immediate administration of small amounts of diluents, such as milk or water, particularly if there is residual solid caustic that requires dislodgment. Induced emesis is contraindicated because the esophagus may be re-exposed to additional corrosive. The patient should not be given excessive fluids because of the risk of vomiting or aspiration. Neutralization of the acids and alkalis should also be avoided because the heat of reaction may worsen the damage. Skin and eye exposures warrant copious irrigation with water. Rapid transport to a medical facility should be initiated for definitive care.

Initial hospital management includes stabilization of the patient's respiratory and circulatory status. If indicated, orotracheal intubation under direct visualization is preferred, but cricothyrotomy may be necessary if intubation is not possible. Blind nasotracheal intubation may be successful in patients with pharyngeal or laryngeal edema that obscures direct laryngoscopy. Intravenous access should be obtained, with administration of crystalloid solution if cardiovascular instability exists.

Because of the rapidity of damage induced by alkali ingestions and the fact that damage is probably complete by the time the patient is seen in a medical facility, dilution is unlikely to be of benefit. However, if not already done, small amounts of water may be given to patients who are able to swallow. Naosgastric or orogastric lavage is contraindicated in alkali ingestions because the rapid penetrating injury induced by these agents increases the risk of perforation. Early gastric aspiration and lavage with ice water may be beneficial after acid ingestions, as no cases of perforation occurring spontaneously or with instrumentation have been reported.

Charcoal and cathartics are ineffective in caustic ingestions, since damage occurs so rapidly; charcoal may obscure the endoscopist's view. Thus activated charcoal and cathartics are contraindicated unless the patient has coingested other, more toxic substances.

Steroids if given within 48 hours of ingestion are recommended in patients with suspected or endoscopically documented deep and circumferential esophageal burns caused by alkali. Methylprednisone is given in doses of 40 mg every 8 hours in patients over 2 years of age, and 20 mg/kg in patients less than 2 years old. The dose should be tapered over a 3-week period. Steroids are thought to be ineffective if given more than 48 hours after the injury, and hence should be started early. With acid ingestions, steroid administration is not usually indicated. Withhold antibiotics until signs of perforation or secondary infection occur. The use of prophylactic antibiotics is not advocated for uncomplicated acid ingestions.

Perforation or necrosis of any portion of the gastrointestinal tract warrants early surgical intervention. Indications for delayed esophageal replacement are (a) inability of the patient to swallow, (b) persistent strictures after sequential dilatation, (c) frequent esophageal dilatations that require extended hospitalizations, and (d) perforation during dilatation. Esophageal substitutes include the colon, most commonly, but also the stomach (reverse gastric tube) and the jejunum.

DISPOSITION

Signs and symptoms of perforation mandate early surgical consultation. A gastroenterologist or otolaryngologist should be involved early in the case, particularly if endoscopy is indicated. Psychiatric evaluation should be performed in all patients with nonaccidental ingestions. Asymptomatic older children and adults may be discharged after several hours of observation. Symptomatic patients, young children, and unreliable adults with a suggestive history should be admitted for observation and endoscopy. If endoscopy is unavailable, patients who require admission should be transferred to a facility where it can be performed.

COMMON PITFALLS

- Assuming no esophageal or gastric injury when evidence for oropharyngeal burns or symptoms is absent
- Attempting to neutralize the corrosive material with weak acids or bases, resulting in extensive heat production and further injury
- Diluting the ingested toxin with large amounts of liquids, thus increasing the risk of vomiting and perforation
- Administering emetics, charcoal, or cathartics, resulting in further injury or obscured visualization by endoscopy
- Failing to admit all symptomatic patients, to give them nothing by mouth after initial dilution, and to consult an endoscopist

90   Aromatic Hydrocarbon Poisoning

Aromatic hydrocarbons are a group of compounds that include benzene, naphthalene, and benzene derivatives such as the cresols, phenols, toluene, and xylene. The toxicity of these compounds is varied and can affect almost all organs of the human body. Benzene primarily causes hematologic and leukemic syndromes. Naphthalene, present in mothballs, when ingested can cause hemolytic anemia, and xylene can lead to gastrointestinal syndromes and dermatitis. Intoxication from these aromatic compounds frequently follows intentional inhalation, although accidental industrial and household exposures can also occur. Another indirect source of intoxication not commonly recognized is an accidental spill of aviation fuels, which contain significant amounts of aromatic hydrocarbons. Another source of toluene and benzene exposure is the ingestion of aquatic animals whose organs have concentrated these agents. Toluene inhalation also causes hyperchloremic metabolic acidosis, distal renal tubular acidosis, Goodpaster's syndrome, the formation of urinary calculi, and reversible renal failure.

CLINICAL PRESENTATION

Both acute and chronic intoxication occur when aromatic hydrocarbons are inhaled. The liquid aromatics, toluene, benzene, and xylene, if ingested, can cause aspiration pneumonia. Intoxication usually follows an intentional inhalation, but industrial exposures also occur. Fatal accidental ingestions and inhalations have been reported. The signs and symptoms of acute and chronic inhalation exposure and "sudden sniffing death" have been well described.

All aromatic hydrocarbons cause mild local respiratory tract irritation and CNS effects. Benzene uniquely affects the hematologic system, but blood dyscrasias seldom follow a single exposure to benzene. Acute exposure to very high concentrations of the solvent vapors can lead to pulmonary edema.

Acute exposures to aromatic hydrocarbons impair manual dexterity, response speed, and coordination. Ataxia and delirium may be present. A chronic inhalational abuser ("sniffer" or "huffer") may have glazed eyes, "drunkenness," and a vacant expression. Paint may be found on hands and around the nose. Visual hallucinations are more frequent than auditory hallucinations. Status epilepticus, dense hemiparesis, muscle weakness, and gastrointestinal and neuropsychiatric complaints are predominant in adult paint (toluene) sniffers. Workers who are chronically exposed to these solvents have demonstrated reduced function of peripheral nerves and adverse neurobehavioral effects. Subjective symptoms (e.g., fatigability, irritability, memory difficulty, changes in personality or mood, and impaired intellectual functions) are usually reversible.

Clinical presentations may include "sudden sniffing death" from ventricular fibrillation (usually an adolescent), inebriation (usually no alcohol odor on breath), hallucinations, memory loss, narcosis, status epilepticus, encephalopathy (particularly in children), abdominal pain and vomiting, muscle weakness, paralysis, and peripheral neuropathy. Laboratory evaluation may reveal evidence of rhabdomyolysis, anemia (aplastic anemia in benzene workers), normal or high anion gap metabolic acidosis, renal failure (e.g., renal tubular acidosis in toluene users), and profound hypokalemia.

DIFFERENTIAL DIAGNOSIS

The diagnosis of aromatic hydrocarbon intoxication is made on the basis of history and clinical findings. Laboratory studies may be supportive if they are abnormal. Blood alcohol levels should be determined because of the similarity in clinical presentations. Other causes of altered mental status and weakness such as drug or other solvent intoxication, trauma, infection, neurologic disorders, and metabolic abnormalities should be considered. Similar metabolic abnormalities may be seen in salicylates, methanol, ethylene glycol, and ethanol (ketoacidosis). Toxicologic analysis of blood and urine may be necessary to exclude these possibilities.

EMERGENCY DEPARTMENT EVALUATION

The history should include the specific identity of the offending agent(s) and the details surrounding the exposure (e.g., amount, time, duration, intent). The physical examination should focus on vital signs and neurologic and cardiorespiratory function. A detailed mental status and neurologic examination should be performed on all patients. The presence or absence of muscle tenderness should be noted. Symptomatic patients should have initial cardiac monitoring and then a 12-lead electrocardiogram. Laboratory evaluation should include arterial blood gas analysis, complete blood count, determination of serum level of electrolytes, blood urea nitrogren, creatinine, glucose, and creatine phosphokinase, and urinalysis (including myoglobin). A chest radiograph should be obtained in patients with respiratory symptoms or abnormal breath sounds. A head CT may be useful in patients with chronic exposures.

EMERGENCY DEPARTMENT MANAGEMENT

In cases of industrial or environmental accidents rescuers should be advised not to enter an area of potential exposure without adequate respiratory protection. The management of aromatic hydrocarbon intoxication is supportive. ALS measures should be instituted as necessary. If an ingestion has occurred within 2 hours, gastrointestinal decontamination is indicated. Seizures, cardiac arrhythmias, and coma are managed with standard therapy. Epinephrine should be used with extreme caution, as the myocardium may be sensitized to the arrhythmogenic effects of catecholamines. Patients with metabolic acidosis should be treated with intravenous sodium bicarbonate as an infusion (not a bolus). Volume replacement and potassium administration may be necessary. Patients who present with psychiatric symptoms should be reassured and observed in a calm, protective environment. Physical or pharmacologic restraints may be required in some patients.

DISPOSITION

Patients with arrhythmias should be admitted to a monitored bed. Those with neurologic or metabolic abnormalities that persist after 4 to 6 hours of emergency department observation and treatment should also be admitted. A neurologist should be consulted for the additional evaluation of patients with abnormal mental status or peripheral neuropathy, and a nephrologist should be consulted in cases with rhabdomyolysis, metabolic abnormalities, or renal dysfunction. Patients with persistent psychiatric symptoms may be referred to a psychiatrist or detoxification center if they are otherwise healthy. Those with hematologic abnormalities should be referred to a hematologist. Long-term follow-up is usually necessary in patients with chronic aromatic hydrocarbon exposure, particularly to benzene, which may cause leukemia. All patients should be advised to avoid re-exposure.

COMMON PITFALLS

- Misdiagnosis of aromatic hydrocarbon poisoning as psychiatric illness, alcohol intoxication, gastroenteritis, Guillian-Bárre syndrome, or dehydration
- Failure to examine blood and urine for secondary hematologic, metabolic, electrolyte, and renal function abnormalities
- Failure to refer patients for appropriate evaluation and follow-up
- Failure to warn patients to avoid re-exposure and that sudden death may occur during solvent inhalation
- Failure to perform gastrointestinal decontamination after ingestions because of fear of causing aspiration
- Failure to monitor for cardiac arrhythmias

91   Calcium Channel Blocker Poisoning

Calcium channel blockers (CCBs) are a structurally diverse group of drugs that are increasingly used in the control of supraventricular arrhythmias, hypertension, angina, heart failure, and subarachnoid hemorrhage, and in the prevention of migraine headaches. Five agents in this group are currently approved for use in the United States: verapamil, nifedipine, diltiazem, nicardipine, and nimodipine. CCBs are well absorbed after oral administration. With verapamil onset of action is noted within the first hour, and peak effects occur approximately 5 hours after ingestion. Nifedipine, nicardipine, and diltiazem, on the other hand, are more rapidly absorbed, and show peak effects in 30 minutes to 2 hours after ingestion. Peak effects may be delayed following the ingestion of sustained-release preparations. All CCBs are significantly protein bound (80%–98%), have a moderate volume of distribution (1.4–4.3 L/kg), and are extensively metabolized by the liver and excreted in the urine and bile. Only verapamil has an active metabolite, nor-verapamil, which is one fifth as active as the parent compound. The elimination half-life for all CCBs is 2 to 7 hours in therapeutic doses. After overdose the half-life of diltiazem remains unchanged.

The toxic cardiovascular effects of CCBs are due to an exaggeration of their therapeutic effects. Central nervous system effects are secondary to hypoperfusion. Hypoperfusion may also lead to lactic acidosis. Inhibition of calcium-dependent insulin release may cause hyperglycemia. It is important to note that with overdosage, drug-specific effects are often lost. Most reported toxic doses are at least two to three times the usual total daily dose. Toxicity can be seen when these agents are used in therapeutic doses with other myocardial depressants such as beta blockers and quinidine-like agents.

CLINICAL PRESENTATION

Signs and symptoms may develop in the first 30 minutes, and include hypotension, bradycardia, drowsiness, confusion, thready pulse, and peripheral cyanosis. Older patients are more likely to have chest pain and myocardial ischemia and infarction. Inadequate perfusion may also result in cerebral and renal damage in patients of all ages. In severe cases coma, seizures, and respiratory distress associated with pulmonary edema are described. Electrocardiography (ECG) often shows decreased rate and first-, second-, or even third-degree AV block, and may have changes consistent with an acute myocardial infarction. Chest radiography may show pulmonary edema. Laboratory abnormalities include metabolic acidosis and hyperglycemia. Serum drug levels are not readily available and have not proved useful in the management of these patients.

Because people ingest drugs that are readily available to them, an unusually large percentage of CCB ingestions occur in older people. Most of these are intentional, but some result from confusion or failing vision.

The duration of direct toxic effect of CCBs has been most frequently described as between 24 and 36 hours. Complications have required longer hospitalizations in many patients.

DIFFERENTIAL DIAGNOSIS

Patients with primary myocardial infarction as well as those with overdosage of β-adrenergic blockers, digoxin, clonidine, guanabenz, imidazolines, cholinergic agents (nicotine, organophosphate and carbamate insecticides, and myasthenic agents), tricyclic antidepressants, alphamethyldopa, and veratrum alkaloid-containing sneezing powders may present similarly to those with CCB ingestion. β-adrenergic blocking agents are more likely to cause hypoglycemia and CCBs, hyperglycemia. With cholingergic agents salivation, nausea, vomiting, diarrhea, and weakness dominate the presentation. Tricyclic antidepressant overdosage infrequently presents with heart block and bradycardia. The QRS complex is often prolonged in tricyclic antidepressant ingestion but is usually normal with CCB overdosage.

EMERGENCY DEPARTMENT EVALUATION

The history should include time of ingestion and all other substances ingested or available to the patient. Physical examination should focus on the pulse, blood pressure, central nervous system function, heart, lungs, and peripheral perfusion. Initial laboratory work should include ECG for all patients. In those with symptoms, abnormal vital signs, or an abnormal ECG, an arterial blood gas analysis and determination of serum electrolyte, glucose, blood urea nitrogen, and creatinine levels should be ordered.

EMERGENCY DEPARTMENT MANAGEMENT

Advanced life-support measures should be initiated as necessary. At the time of the initial assessment continuous cardiac monitoring and an intravenous infusion of normal saline solution should be started. Blood pressure should be monitored frequently. Early management should include gastrointestinal decontamination. No information exists regarding the use of multidose charcoal in the overdose setting. Mild hypotension may respond to a fluid challenge with 1 L to 2 L of saline solution (10–20 ml /kg in children). When bradycardia with or without AV block is also present, atropine (1.0 mg IV; 0.01 mg/kg in children) may be given. Hypotension and symptomatic bradycardia should be treated with calcium chloride (1 g IV slow push; 10–20 mg/kg in children). Calcium gluconate (3 g IV slow push; 30–60 mg/kg in children) may be given if calcium chloride is unavailable. This dose may be repeated up to 5 g calcium chloride in patients who show incomplete, transient, or no response. A continuous infusion at the rate of 1 g/h of calcium chloride may be used to support heart rate and blood pressure in patients with a transient response to an initial bolus.

Hemodynamically compromising bradycardia or heart block unresponsive to atropine and calcium may respond to an infusion of glucagon or isoproterenol, but a pacemaker is often required. Hypotension unresponsive to fluids and calcium should be treated with pressors. Pressors may be given without regard to the coincident presence of heart disease or acute myocardial infarction, since they are titrated to reverse the adverse pharmacologic effect of the calcium blocking agent. Dopamine, dobutamine, norepinephrine, isoproterenol, and combinations of these have been used with success. Glucagon may also be considered in this setting. Pulmonary artery catheterization may be helpful in managing these patients. The use of an intra-aortic balloon pump should be considered in patients who are unresponsive to pharmacologic therapies. Support may be withdrawn as the drug is metabolized. Enhanced elimination has been described with charcoal hemoperfusion in only a single diltiazem-overdosed patient. It should not be regarded as standard therapy. If supportive measures can maintain a pulse and blood pressure sufficient to allow hemoperfusion, there is little to be gained from the procedure. Full recovery is expected unless prolonged shock has resulted in irreversible end-organ damage.

DISPOSITION

Asymptomatic patients should be observed for 4 to 6 hours (longer if a sustained-release preparation has been ingested). Those who remain asymptomatic may be discharged or referred for psychiatric evaluation. Symptomatic patients should be admitted to an intensive care unit. A regional poison center or a toxicologist should be consulted if the physician is unfamiliar with the management of CCB overdosage. Transfer may be necessary if an intensive care unit bed is unavailable and should be arranged as soon as the ingestion is recognized.

COMMON PITFALLS

- Hypotension, bradycardia, AV block, hyperglycemia, and altered mental status suggest CCB overdose.
- Calcium is a specific antidote, and should be used early for hypotension or bradycardia.
- Priority should be given to re-establishing normal vital signs and tissue perfusion.
- Patients with myocardial ischemia secondary to hypoperfusion may require treatment with α- and β-adrenergic agents. Withholding these drugs is not warranted.
- In managing these patients a pulmonary artery catheter may be useful.

92   Carbon Monoxide Poisoning

CLINICAL PRESENTATION

The signs and symptoms of CO poisoning are highly variable and nonspecific. At low levels headache, dizziness, nausea, vomiting, and diarrhea are common. With higher levels confusion, syncope, shortness of breath, and angina pectoris may occur. Severe poisoning may cause coma, seizures, hypotension, cardiac arrhythmias, and death (see Table 92-1). Although the severity of intoxication usually parallels the CO-hemoglobin level, there are reports of patients with severe intoxication with relatively low levels, and of patients with high levels but minimal symptoms. Survivors of severe poisoning are often left with permanent neurologic injury, which may be gross (blindness, deafness, seizures, parkinsonism, or vegetative state) or subtle (memory loss or personality changes).

The physical examination may reveal cherry-red coloration of the skin, mucous membranes, and venous blood owing to the bright red color of the CO-hemoglobin complex. This finding is inconsistently noted and its presence or absence cannot be considered diagnostic. Retinal hemorrhages may be present. Neurologic examination usually reveals altered mental status, which may rapidly improve after removal from the poisoned atmosphere and the prehospital administration of oxygen. Arterial blood gas analysis and serum electrolyte levels often reveal metabolic acidosis, which is caused by tissue hypoxia-ischemia. The arterial PO_2 and hence the calculated oxygen saturation are usually normal because **dissolved** oxygen in the serum is not affected by CO. Although the oxygen saturation measured directly by co-oximetry will be less than that calculated from the PO_2 (by an amount roughly equal to the percent CO-hemoglobin), the oxygen saturation measured by pulse oximetry is falsely normal. Signs of myocardial ischemia are frequently present on the ECG, and occasionally myocardial infarction occurs. Complications also include pancreatitis and rhabdomyolysis.

TABLE 92-1. Signs and Symptoms of Carbon Monoxide Poisoning

Carbon Monoxide-Hemgloblin Level (%)	Signs and Symptoms
0–10	Usually none
10–20	Headache, dyspnea with minimal exertion, angina in patients with coronary disease
20–30	Moderate headache, dyspnea, nausea, dizziness
30–40	Severe headache, vomiting, fatigue, poor judgment
40–50	Confusion, syncope, tachypnea, tachycardia
50–60	Syncope, seizures, coma
60–70	Coma, hypotension, arrhythmias, death
>70	Rapidly fatal

DIFFERENTIAL DIAGNOSIS

Other causes of coma and altered mental status should be sought, such as hypoglycemia, head trauma, meningitis, and drug or alcohol intoxication. Many suicidal patients ingest medications and alcohol as they poison themselves with CO. Other toxic gases should be considered in any patient with smoke inhalation. Cyanide, hydrogen sulfide, agents that cause methemoglobinemia, and other toxins may produce symptoms and signs of systemic hypoxia that are similar to those of CO.

EMERGENCY DEPARTMENT EVALUATION

Evaluation should include rapid neurologic assessment and determination of the specific carboxyhemoglobin saturation. History that may be helpful in raising suspicion of CO poisoning includes being found in a car with the engine running, multiple victims found in a common room, smoke inhalation, and use of paint strippers or solvents that contain methylene chloride in a poorly ventilated area. Depending on severity, arterial blood gas analysis, routine laboratory evaluation, ECG, and chest radiography may be indicated. Patients with persistent coma should have a CT scan of the head.

EMERGENCY DEPARTMENT MANAGEMENT

ALS should be instituted as needed. Oxygen (100%) should be provided with a tight-fitting mask or a nonrebreather mask with oxygen reservoir, or by way of an endotracheal tube. If the patient is hypotensive, 1 L to 2 L of crystalloid solution should be administered. ECG, arterial blood gases, and the carboxyhemoglobin level should be monitored. Mild to moderate metabolic acidosis (i.e., serum pH 7.2–7.3) should not be treated because acidosis may facilitate oxygen delivery to the tissues by moving the oxygen-hemoglobin dissociation curve to the right. Decontamination is performed by removing the victim from the toxic environment. CO is then rapidly eliminated by application of 100% oxygen, which shortens the half-life of CO to 40 to 80 minutes. Hyperbaric oxygen (HBO), 100% oxygen provided under pressures greater than 1 atm, may further speed removal of CO to a half-life of 20 minutes or less. Some clinicians believe that HBO may also drive CO from intracellular sites, although this has not been proved.

Controversy exists about which patients should receive HBO treatment. Most hospitals do not have ready access to a chamber, which means that unstable patients may require transport over long distances at a time when arrhythmias and hypotension are most likely to occur. Proponents of HBO argue that it may provide protection against late neurologic sequelae, a claim that has never been proved. There are no controlled, prospective trials comparing 100% oxygen at 1 atm with HBO on acute or chronic outcome. Because the half-life of CO-hemoglobin in 100% oxygen at 1 atm is less than 1 hour, in most cases the level has already dropped to low levels by the time the HBO chamber is ready. Pregnant women and infants pose a special problem because fetal hemoglobin has a much greater affinity for CO than normal hemoglobin. Hence prolonged oxygen therapy and a lower threshold for HBO are recommended.

The prognosis after severe CO poisoning is unpredictable, but grim. As many as 10% of victims will have permanent obvious neurologic injury. Even more worrisome, one study suggested that 33% to 43% of survivors of CO poisoning might have subtler psychiatric changes and memory deficits. Patients with an abnormal computed tomography scan on admission appear to be at high risk for permanent gross sequelae.

DISPOSITION

All patients with loss of consciousness or with seizures should be admitted, as should those with evidence of myocardial infarction or ischemia. Infants, young children, pregnant women, and victims of methylene chloride poisoning require intensive or prolonged treatment, and should be admitted. Most authorities would also automatically admit any patient with a CO-hemoglobin level greater than 25%, regardless of symptoms. One investigator has been utilizing neuropsychiatric screening to help determine which patients with low CO levels should be admitted for aggressive therapy. The use of HBO should be considered in patients who have been comatose or who do not rapidly improve with 100% oxygen. Patients with mild symptoms who become asymptomatic after a short course (e.g., 1–2 hours) of oxygen therapy and who have a CO level less than 10%, normal physical examination, and normal arterial blood gas parameters may be discharged.

A regional poison center or medical toxicologist may provide assistance with the disposition decision and may also know the location of nearby HBO chambers. If the patient has cardiac arrhythmias or hypotension, a critical care nurse or physician should accompany the patient during transport to a HBO facility. Once the acute episode of poisoning has resolved, patients should be referred for follow-up neuropsychiatric evaluation. Those discharged should be instructed to return immediately if any signs of neurologic dysfunction develop.

COMMON PITFALLS

- Signs and symptoms of carbon monoxide poisoning are nonspecific and the diagnosis may be missed if there is no accompanying history of exposure.
- Despite common belief, the victim is seldom noted to be cherry-red.
- The arterial blood gas PO_2, calculated oxygen saturation, and pulse oximetry oxygen saturation remain normal despite severe CO poisoning.
- In smoke inhalation victims cointoxication with cyanide is not uncommon, and may mimic and aggravate CO poisoning.
- Coma may also be caused or aggravated by ingestion of alcohol or other drugs.
- Treatment errors are usually due to insufficient concentration and duration of oxygen administration.

---

93 Ciguatera and Scombroid Fish Poisoning

Ciguatera poisoning is contracted from eating fish that have been contaminated through the food chain with single-cell marine parasites known as dinoflagellates. The most notable species of this toxic-producing algae is *Ganbierdiscus toxicus*. Fish harboring this parasite are grouper, red snapper, barracuda, amberjack, and virtually any reef-feeding carnivore fish. The smaller the fish, the less likely for ciguatera poisoning. Fish that weigh <5 lb have less likelihood of ciguatera toxin contamination. Of all the sea dwellers, the eel, which lives in the reef, is considered to be the most likely species contaminated with this fish toxin. Although ciguatera poisoning is reported worldwide, in the United States, Florida and Hawaii are the most common states. Remember that with the popularity of seafood and its ability to be transported in the United States, ciguatera poisoning can be seen anywhere.

Scombroid (mackerel-like) poisoning is associated with ingestion of fish of the family Scombroidea. Included in this family are most species of tuna, mackerel, wahoo, bonito, and skipjack. Scombroid poisoning may also result from the ingestion of species from other families, such as amberjack, bluefish, dolphin, black marlin, and herring. Histamine levels in toxic fish are normally greater than 50 mg/100 g of flesh. Although signs and symptoms appear to be caused by histamine, an additional agent is thought to be present in the fish to allow the histamine to be absorbed systemically without being metabolized, since large oral doses of histamine can be given to volunteer subjects without the occurrence of signs and symptoms of scombroid poisoning. This secondary agent has not been positively identified. Scombroid toxins are heat-stable and not inactivated by cooking.

CLINICAL PRESENTATION

Signs and symptoms of ciguatera poisoning occur anywhere from 30 minutes to 30 hours after ingestion of contaminated fish tissue, but usually between 6 and 12 hours. Initial symptoms include abrupt onset of vomiting, watery diarrhea, and myalgias. Simultaneously or soon after the onset of these symptoms the patient may begin to experience circumoral numbness and tingling. The abdominal symptoms usually resolve within 72 hours, but they can persist. Muscular symptoms can persist for a number of weeks or even months. The acute gastrointestinal symptoms usually are near resolution within 1 to 2 days. The most common neuromuscular symptoms are paresthesias of the extremities, circumoral paresthesias, hot and cold sensation reversal, and arthralgia, occurring in nearly 80% of the patients.

The classic neurologic symptom associated with ciguatera poisoning is hot and cold sensation reversal. Cold objects are perceived as hot and burning, and hot objects are perceived as either not hot or actually cold. Other signs and symptoms may include ataxia, vertigo, diaphoresis, dysuria, dental or eye pain, dyspnea, nuchal rigidity, rash, and tremors. Either tachycardia or bradycardia may be present. Although acute symptoms may last for only 2 or 3 days, total resolution of the neurologic and neuromuscular features may take 8 weeks or longer; most symptoms are gone in about 3 weeks. There are no specific laboratory findings that define the diagnosis of ciguatera poisoning.

The clinical presentation of scombroid poisoning is similar to acute anaphylactic or allergic reaction. Symptoms develop quickly, usually within 30 to 60 minutes of ingestion, and include flushing and warmth of the skin (especially the head, neck, and upper chest), pruritus, urticaria (often the giant form), thirst, a burning sensation of the mouth and throat, weakness, palpitations, tachycardia, bronchospasm, and hypotension. Without treatment, symptoms usually resolve gradually over 6 to 12 hours (range 3–36 hours).

DIFFERENTIAL DIAGNOSIS

The differential diagnosis of ciguatera and scombroid poisoning includes bacterial food poisonings and gastrointestinal diseases hallmarked by vomiting, diarrhea, and abdominal pain, as well as other marine food poisonings such as paralytic shellfish poisoning and tetrodotoxin. Scombroid poisoning can usually be differentiated from true allergic or anaphylactic reactions by the history of fish ingestion. The differential diagnosis of skin flushing includes poisoning by niacin, vancomycin, rifampin, and monosodium glutamate, and disulfiram–ethanol reactions.

EMERGENCY DEPARTMENT EVALUATION

The history must include the ingestion of fish associated with ciguatera or scombroid poisoning. The symptoms and their time of onset should be noted. Known seafood allergies should also be documented. The physical examination should focus on vital signs, neurologic evaluation, and respiratory function. Patients with significant gastrointestinal symptoms should have orthostatic vital signs taken. The skin should be examined for rash, and temperature sensation should be assessed. Peritoneal signs on abdominal examination suggest alternative pathology. Laboratory evaluation should include assessment of volume status by complete blood count, electrolytes, blood urea nitrogen, creatine, and urinalysis. Unless other diagnoses are concomitantly considered, other laboratory tests are of no assistance.

The diagnosis of ciguatera poisoning is clinical. Scombroid poisoning may be confirmed by measuring histamine levels in a sample of the offending fish. State health departments often provide analytical as well as investigative assistance.

EMERGENCY DEPARTMENT MANAGEMENT

ALS should be provided if necessary. Hypotension from gastrointestinal fluid losses or histamine-induced vasodilation should be treated with intravenous crystalloids. Refractory hypotension may necessitate the use of a vasopressor such as norepinephrine. Patients with anaphylactoid reactions due to scombroid poisoning should also be given antihistamines. Type 2 histamine receptor blockers such as cimetidine (300 mg IV), famotidine (20 mg IV), or ranitidine (50 mg IV) appear to be more effective than type 1 receptor blockers (e.g., diphenhydramine 50–100 mg IV). Minor reactions, primarily nausea and protracted vomiting, may also respond to usual doses of hydroxyzine or prochlorperazine.

In patients with severe anaphylactoid reactions, epinephrine, inhaled bronchodilators, pressors, and steroids may be necessary. Mannitol (1 g/kg IV up to 50 g over 6 hours) may be effective for the neurologic symptoms of ciguatera. Other agents used with varying success include amitriptyline (antidepressant doses), antihistamines, vitamin B_{12} (hydroxycobalamin), vitamin C (ascorbic acid), calcium gluconate (1–3 g IV over 24 hours), lidocaine, and tocainide. Activated charcoal is usually the only decontamination measure necessary. This treatment should be considered in all patients who present within 4 to 6 hours of toxic fish ingestion. Patients with severe gastrointestinal symptoms and those with symptoms that last longer than 6 hours may also require antiemetic or antidiarrheal medications.

DISPOSITION

Most patients can be treated in the ED and discharged. Those with persistent hemodynamic instability and severe dehydration, anaphylactoid reactions, or neurologic manifestations should be hospitalized. The level of care and monitoring needed is determined by clinical severity. Some methods of treating persistent ciguatera neurotoxicity also require hospitalization. Consultation with a toxicologist or regional poison control center is often helpful in providing current treatments of choice. The local or state health department should be notified of all cases of suspected ciguatera or scombroid fish poisoning, since timely intervention may prevent additional exposures.

COMMON PITFALLS

- Failure to obtain a history of the ingestion of fish and its identity in patients with gastroenteritis
- Failure to consider ciguatera and scombroid poisoning in any part of the world where fresh fish is transported
- Failure to ask about reversal of hot and cold sensation in patients with paresthesias
- Failure to consider scombroid poisoning in the differential diagnosis of flushing and anaphylactoid reaction
- Failure to consider using a histamine-2 receptor blocker in the treatment of scombroid poisoning
- Failure to use fluid resuscitation as an early priority

94   Cocaine Poisoning

Cocaine is an alkaloid extracted from the leaves of the South American shrub *Erythroxylon coca*. Toxic effects from cocaine result from excessive central and peripheral sympathetic stimulation and have been termed the "caine reaction." Central nervous system and cardiovascular effects progress from an early to advanced stimulation and finally to coma and cardiovascular collapse. Nausea, vomiting, and tachypnea appear to be due to central stimulation. Hyperthermia may result from the combined effects of increased motor and metabolic activity, peripheral vasoconstriction, and hypothalamic stimulation. The onset and duration of effect varies with the dose, form of cocaine, route of administration, rate of absorption, elimination, and tolerance of the individual (Table 94-1). "Body packers" (people who attempt to smuggle cocaine across an international border by ingesting professionally wrapped packets of cocaine) and "body stuffers" (those who swallow or conceal loosely wrapped cocaine in body cavities when encountered by law enforcement agents) may become poisoned if leakage occurs. Drugs such as monoamine oxidase inhibitors, tricyclic antidepressants, methyldopa, and reserpine, which alter neurotransmitter metabolism, may also augment the toxicity of cocaine. Quantitative blood levels of cocaine or its metabolites are not clinically useful.

CLINICAL PRESENTATION

Signs and symptoms of mild cocaine intoxication include normal or minimally increased blood pressure, pulse and respiratory rate, and temperature, agitation, anxiety, euphoria, headache, hyperreflexia, nausea, vomiting, mydriasis, pallor, diaphoresis, tremors, and twitching.

Moderate intoxication may result in hypertension, tachycardia, dyspnea, tachypnea, hyperthermia, confusion, hallucinations, marked hyperactivity, increased muscle tone and deep tendon reflexes, abdominal cramps, formication, and generalized but brief tonic–clonic seizures.

Severe intoxication is manifest by hypotension, tachycardia (or preteminal bradycardia), ventricular arrhythmias, Cheyne–Stokes respirations, apnea, cyanosis, malignant hyperthermia, coma, flaccid paralysis, and status epilepticus.

The ECG may reveal sinus tachycardia or bradycardia, ventricular ectopy, tachycardia, fibrillation, or asystole. Laboratory evaluation may reveal lactic acidosis, hypoxia, and evidence of rhabdomyolysis.

Intravenous users may develop infectious complications such as cellulitis, endocarditis, hepatitis, pneumonia, and AIDS. Chronic nasal use may lead to rhinitis, septal perforation, and epistaxis. Inhalational use may result in pneumothorax, pneumomediastinum, and pneumoperi-

TABLE 94-1. Time-Course of Effects With Different Routes of Cocaine Administration

Route	Peak Effect (min)	Duration of Effect
Oral	30–60	2–4 h
Intranasal	20–30	1–2 h
Intravenous	1–2	20–30 min
Inhalation	<1	15–30 min

cardium as a result of the Valsalva maneuver or from blowing smoke into the mouth of a partner. Vascular complications from hypertension and vascular spasm (e.g., myocardial ischemia or infarction, cardiomyopathy, renal infarction, ischemic bowel, aortic dissection, placental ischemia, or abruption and subarachnoid or intracerebral hemorrhage) may follow the use of cocaine by any route. Manifestations of chronic cocaine abuse include anorexia, insomnia, formication, depression, impotency, weight loss, paranoia, and psychosis.

DIFFERENTIAL DIAGNOSIS

The differential diagnosis includes poisoning with anticholinergic agents, sympathomimetics, hallucinogens, phencyclidine, and xanthines; medical conditions such as pheochromocytoma, hypoglycemia, drug withdrawal, thyrotoxicosis, malignant hypertension, and malignant hyperthermia; and psychiatric illnesses such as mania and paranoid schizophrenia.

EMERGENCY DEPARTMENT EVALUATION

The history should include the route, amount, and time of cocaine use in relation to symptom onset. Friends (or witnesses) of confused patients should be questioned about a history of seizures or syncope and antecedent activities. New-onset seizures, epistaxis, hypertension, myocardial infarction, intracranial hemorrhage, or psychiatric illness, especially in young patients, should suggest possible cocaine use. Many patients deny such use unless approached with reassurance (of confidentiality) and compassion or confronted with a positive urine test.

The physical examination should include vital signs and examination of the cardiac, pulmonary, and neurologic systems. Rectal temperature measurement is advisable, since patients may have hyperthermia, yet the skin may be cool and clammy. When the history is clear and symptoms are mild, laboratory evaluation is not necessary. If the history is absent or unreliable or the patient manifests moderate or severe toxicity, routine laboratory evaluation should include complete blood count, electrolytes, glucose, blood urea nitrogen, and creatinine levels, arterial blood gas analysis, urinalysis, and creatine phosphokinase. Qualitative toxicologic analyses of blood and urine confirm the diagnosis and rule out other intoxicants.

A chest radiograph and ECG should be obtained on patients with chest pain or moderate to severe toxicity. Those with prolonged unexplained chest pain should have serial ECGs and cardiac enzymes to assure the absence of myocardial infarction. Persistent headache despite normalization of blood pressure requires evaluation by computed tomography scan and lumbar puncture to rule out intracranial hemorrhage. Patients with abdominal or back pain need to be evaluated for intestinal or renal infarction. Occult infections must be excluded in those with fever.

A brief seizure clearly related (temporally) to cocaine use in an otherwise healthy person does not require further work-up, provided the patient is alert and coherent, has no headache, and has a normal neurologic examination. Patients who are suspected of body packing or stuffing should be evaluated by abdominal radiographs and cavity search (i.e., digital or visual examination of rectum or vagina). Toxicity lasting for more than 4 hours suggests continued drug absorption and should prompt a similar work-up.

EMERGENCY DEPARTMENT MANAGEMENT

All patients should initially be placed on a cardiac monitor. ALS should be instituted as necessary. Those with altered mental status, seizures, or coma should be given oxygen, dextrose, naloxone, and thiamine. Patients with mild toxicity or a history of a brief seizure can be managed with observation in a quiet setting and with reassurance. They usually become asymptomatic within several hours. A short-acting benzodiazepine such as midazolam (2–10 mg IV) or triazolam (0.25–0.5 mg

PO) may be given for marked agitation, anxiety, or psychosis. Pharmacologic sedation is prefer-able to physical restraints in order to avoid hyperthermia.

Persistent or severe psychosis may require additional treatment with a neuroleptic such as haloperidol. Status epilepticus should be promptly and aggressively treated with intravenous diazepam followed by a short-acting barbiturate such as amobarbital if necessary. As in seizures caused by theophylline toxicity, phenytoin is unlikely to be of benefit. Refractory seizures may necessitate neuromuscular paralysis (e.g., pancuronium) in order to prevent hyperthermia and rhabdomyolysis. During paralysis, seizure treatment should continue as indicated by EEG moni-toring. Hyperthermia should be treated aggressively. The use of alkaline diuresis may help to pre-vent renal failure in patients with rhabdomyolysis.

Sinus tachycardia and hypertension are usually transient and can be treated expectantly or by nonspecific sedation. If severe or associated with chest pain, the alpha and beta adrener-gic blocker labetalol (10–20 mg IV every 15 minutes or by continuous infusion) may be used. Alternatively, nitroprusside in combination with esmolol or propranolol may be used. Caution is advised regarding the use of a beta blocker alone, since unopposed alpha stimulation could cause a paradoxical increase in blood pressure. Ventricular tachyarrhythmias should initially be treated with lidocaine. Propranolol or labetalol may be added if necessary. Standard therapy is recommended for asystole and ischemic chest pain. A direct-acting pressor (e.g., norepinephrine) should be used for vascular collapse.

Those who ingest cocaine should receive maximal doses of activated charcoal and per-haps gastric lavage. Because of the possibility of seizures, syrup of ipecac should be avoided. Packages of cocaine in the vagina or rectum should be removed by hand or under direct visual-ization. Asymptomatic patients who have ingested packets of cocaine should be treated with lax-atives (such as sodium sulfate, magnesium sulfate, magnesium citrate, or psyllium hydrophilic mucilage), multiple-dose charcoal, and close observation. Those who demonstrate signs or symp-toms of toxicity or who show evidence of intestinal obstruction require surgical intervention. Endoscopic removal should be avoided, since packet rupture may occur during this procedure.

DISPOSITION

Physicians who are not familiar with cocaine poisoning should consult a regional poison control center or a toxicologist for advice. Patients with mild cocaine intoxication or a single brief seizure who became asymptomatic after a 3- to 6-hour observation period may be discharged. Those with moderate or severe poisoning and those who have secondary complications should be admit-ted to an ICU. All patients suspected of ingesting packages of cocaine require ICU monitoring until a charcoal stool has passed and there is no radiographic evidence of intestinal foreign bodies. Before discharge all patients should be referred for drug abuse counseling and treatment. Intravenous drug abusers should also have AIDS and hepatitis testing.

COMMON PITFALLS

- Failure to consider cocaine intoxication as a cause of altered mental status, chest pain, seizure, hypertension, headache, palpitations, stroke, and cardiac arrest, especially in young adults
- Failure to consider body or cavity packing in patients with prolonged toxicity or those with unexplained hyperactivity after criminal arrest or incarceration
- Failure to consider secondary complications, such as barotrauma, organ ischemia or infarc-tion, sepsis, or rhabdomyolysis
- Failure to avoid the use of syrup of ipecac or endoscopy in cases of cocaine ingestion
- Failure to warn about future use and to refer for drug abuse treatment

95   Digitalis Poisoning

Toxicity results from an exaggeration of therapeutic effects. Adverse effects may also be due to coronary vasoconstriction. Excessive suppression of pacemaker function may lead to brad-yarrhythmias, and increased automaticity may lead to atrial, junctional, and ventricular tach-yarrhythmias (Table 95-1). Digoxin toxicity may be chronic or acute. In chronic ingestion there is a narrow therapeutic range, with toxic amounts being only two to three times therapeutic doses. Most instances of chronic toxicity occur in the elderly. It is frequently associated with hypokalemia, which tends to exacerbate tachyarrhythmias. Many other factors are known to pre-dispose or contribute to toxicity. In healthy adults single acute doses of less than 5 mg of digoxin seldom cause severe toxicity, with fatal doses almost always greater than 10 mg. During chronic therapy a much smaller ingestion, especially in someone with heart disease, may lead to toxicity. Chronic intoxication is associated with ventricular arrhythmias, atrial tachycardia, and junctional tachycardia.

Acute toxicity is most often associated with an accidental or intentional massive ingestion. It is more likely to be associated with hyperkalemia, owing to the massive poisoning of the sodium–potassium adenosine triphosphatase pump, leading to accumulation of potassium in the extracellular space. In this setting sinus bradycardia and varying degrees of AV block are seen, with fewer ventricular arrhythmias. Ingestion of oleander has also been reported to cause car-diotoxicity. There appears to be some cross-reactivity in the assay, but levels are not as mean-ingful as in digoxin toxicity. There also can be falsely elevated serum digoxin values in certain conditions. This digoxinlike immunoreactive substance (DLIS) has been seen in some patients with renal failure, in some women during the last trimester of pregnancy, and in some premature and full-term infants. Levels are usually low, but have been measured above 2.0 ng/mL.

CLINICAL PRESENTATION

Clinical signs of toxicity often include nausea and vomiting. In chronic toxicity there can be men-tal confusion, lethargy, depression, and fatigue. Headaches, paresthesias, weakness, scotoma, and disturbances of color vision, especially xanthopsia (yellow vision), can occur. The most com-mon arrhythmia in digitalis toxicity is ventricular premature contractions. Many types can occur. Paroxysmal atrial tachycardia with block is said to be pathognomonic of digoxin toxicity. The com-bination of tachyarrhythmias with some type of block should raise the index of suspicion. Regularization of the ventricular response to atrial fibrillation owing to AV block with a junctional escape rhythm should also suggest toxicity.

TABLE 95-1. Digitalis-Induced Arrhythmias

Bradyarrhythmias	Tachyarrhythmias
Sinus exit block or sinus arrest	Atrial tachycardia with block
Sinus bradycardia	Junctional tachycardia
AV nodal block:	Ventricular premature beats
1st degree; 2nd degree,	Ventricular tachycardia, especially bidirectional
type 1; 3rd degree	Ventricular fibrillation

Ventricular tachycardia in the setting of digoxin toxicity is associated with a 50% mortality. Overall, mortality varies with different studies but is probably about 10%. In acute ingestions poor prognostic factors have been identified as old age, a digoxin level over 15 ng/mL, and initial hyperkalemia. Complications caused by toxicity are due to inadequate perfusion secondary to significant arrhythmias. The most common morbidities constitute central nervous system and renal complications, such as hypoxic seizures, encephalopathy, loss of vasoregulation, and acute tubular necrosis.

EMERGENCY DEPARTMENT EVALUATION

Evaluation begins with the history; the timing of a single ingestion is important. Other medications taken can influence the patient's clinical course. Conditions that can influence toxicity should be recognized.

Physical examination starts with the vital signs. Hypotension is a sign of either a hemodynamically significant arrhythmia, loss of vasomotor regulation, or the presence of a coingestant. Cardiac monitoring should be routine. A 12-lead ECG should be performed. Routine laboratory studies include determination of electrolyte, blood urea nitrogen, and serum creatinine levels. A serum digoxin level also should be ordered. In an acute ingestion an initial level verifies that an ingestion occurred, but a level drawn before 8 hours after ingestion will not predict toxicity. A 2-hour level of 10 ng/mL in an acute ingestion may be associated with no significant toxicity.

EMERGENCY DEPARTMENT MANAGEMENT

Stabilization of vital signs is the initial consideration. Atropine (initially 0.5 mg IV) should be given for bradyarrhythmias. Refractory cases mandate a pacemaker. Ventricular tachyarrhythmias often respond to phenytoin, given at 25 mg/min until a desired effect is reached or until about 15 mg/kg has been given. Lidocaine can also be tried as an antiarrhythmic, and might be tried first as a bolus of 1 mg/kg. Magnesium sulfate may also be effective. Initially 2 g to 3 g are given intravenously in 1 minute followed by 2 g/h for 4 to 5 hours. It is surmised that there is hypomagnesemia at the cellular level, even if the serum magnesium level is normal. Cardioversion of ventricular tachycardia is risky in digitalis toxicity, and should be tried only after at least 200 mg of phenytoin have been given and then at reduced power settings, for example, at 5 or 10 watt-seconds.

Early lavage may be useful regardless of whether or not spontaneous vomiting has occurred. Because vagal effects associated with vomiting and gastric lavage might worsen CG toxicity, activated charcoal is the preferred method of gastrointestinal decontamination in patients with bradycardia. Repeat doses of activated charcoal are effective in shortening elimination half-life. Elimination cannot be enhanced by increasing urine flow, by peritoneal dialysis or hemodialysis, or by hemoperfusion. If hypokalemia is present in chronic toxicity and there is no evidence of heart block, replacement potassium should be given. If hyperkalemia occurs, it should be treated with glucose and insulin, sodium polystyrene sulfonate (Kayexalate), or even hemodialysis. Survival in acute toxicity correlates better with the initial potassium level than with the amount ingested.

Digoxin-specific Fab fragments (Digibind R B-W) are the treatment of choice for life-threatening arrhythmias. Fab fragments are indicated when standard therapy fails and when hyperkalemia occurs. An elevated digoxin level is useful only to confirm toxicity, and should not be used as the sole criterion for use of the Fab fragments. The effectiveness of this therapy has clearly been shown. The Fab fragments are given intravenously over 30 minutes unless the patient is in cardiac arrest, when it can be given as a bolus. The dosage (in vials to be given) is estimated by dividing the acutely ingested dose in milligrams (body load) by 0.6 mg per vial. Each vial contains 40 mg of Fab fragments, with each milligram binding 0.015 mg of digoxin. In chronic toxicity the body load in milligrams can be estimated by multiplying the steady-state serum concentration of digoxin by 5.6 times the patient's weight in kilograms divided by 1000.

Because Fab fragments cross-react weakly with other CGs, larger doses may be needed for toxicity involving digitoxin or even oleander. Hyperkalemia is rapidly reversed by the Fab fragments, bradyarrhythmias within 1 hour, and tachyarrhythmias within a few hours. Fab fragments have been used at least once for oleander poisoning. After using Fab fragments the serum digoxin level by radioimmunoassay rises owing to the drug being pulled out of tissue for binding with the antibodies. The free digoxin level can only be measured by equilibrium dialysis, and will be very low if the appropriate amount of antibodies are administered. The elimination half-life of the drug–antibody complex is about 16 hours. Even in a patient with renal failure Fab fragments have reversed digitoxin toxicity.

There is currently a limited supply of Fab fragments. Specific medical centers have been given control of this supply, and emergency availability of supplies should be ascertained by each emergency facility.

DISPOSITION

When the use of Fab fragments is considered an appropriate consultant should be sought. A poison center, medical toxicologist, or cardiologist is often the most experienced in their use. Certainly all patients with significant arrhythmias, symptoms, or elevated digoxin levels should be admitted to an intensive care unit. If Fab fragments and pacemaker therapy are not available, patients with large ingestions (greater than 5 mg) and those with signs of chronic toxicity should be transferred to the nearest center that possesses these treatment modalities using paramedic-level personnel.

COMMON PITFALLS

- Failure to appreciate the fact that a serum digoxin level drawn less than 8 hours after an acute ingestion will not reflect toxicity or need for treatment
- Failure to differentiate between acute and chronic toxicity
- Failure to use Fab fragments when hyperkalemia occurs in acute ingestions
- Failure to correct electrolyte abnormalities, especially those that involve potassium
- Failure to use low power settings for cardioversion of an arrhythmia owing to digoxin toxicity

96 Ethanol, Isopropanol, and Acetone Poisoning

The acute effects of ethanol are primarily seen on the central nervous system (CNS). Alcohol distributes into body tissues and fluids with an apparent volume of distribution of approximately 0.6 L/kg. Metabolism is primarily by hepatic enzymatic oxidation; ethanol exhibits zero-order elimination at concentrations between 20 mg and 300 mg/dL, and first-order elimination at concentrations less than 20 mg/dL or more than 300 mg/dL. The average nontolerant person metabolizes approximately 100 mg/kg/h or reduces the blood alcohol concentration by 15 mg to 20 mg/dL/h. A lethal dose is said to be 5 g to 8 g/kg in adults and 3 g/kg in children, but there is substantial interpatient variability.

Isopropanol (isopropyl alcohol) is used in the home and in industry as a disinfectant and solvent. It is an ingredient in a multitude of products, including rubbing alcohol, some radiator and fuel line antifreezes, window cleaners, animal repellants, and aftershave solutions. Unfortunately these products also frequently contain ethanol or the more toxic methanol or ethylene glycol. Isopropanol is the most commonly ingested nonbeverage alcohol despite its slightly bitter taste and distinctive odor.

Isopropanol is rapidly absorbed from the intestine after ingestion. It is also well absorbed rectally. Toxicity has been reported to occur after sponge baths with isopropanol, but the route of absorption is not agreed on. Isopropanol, like ethanol, is metabolized by alcohol dehydrogenase. The metabolite acetone is eliminated by the kidney and lungs, producing a sweet ketotic odor on the breath. Isopropanol has an elimination half-life of approximately 6 hours in nonalcoholic patients and 3 to 4 hours in alcoholic patients. A fatal dose is said to be approximately 8 oz in an adult, although, as with ethanol, much variability is seen.

Acetone is found in household and industrial cleaners and solvents, and is a major ingredient in most fingernail polish removers. In diabetic ketoacidosis endogenous production due to fat metabolism can produce acetone concentrations of 10 mg to 70 mg/dL. Acetone is rapidly absorbed after ingestion or inhalation. The major route of elimination is by way of the lungs, producing a fruity odor on the breath. The elimination half-life ranges from 20 to 30 hours. Toxicity in children is seen after ingestion of 2 mL to 3 mL/kg, but an ingested dose of 200 mL to 400 mL in an adult produces CNS depression but no serious complications.

CLINICAL PRESENTATION

Ethanol, a CNS depressant, initially produces a paradoxical CNS stimulation due to disinhibition. During this phase an intoxicated patient may appear energized and loquacious. As ethanol levels rise the patient may become aggressive, abusive, irritable, dysarthric, confused, disoriented, ataxic, and lethargic. Severe intoxication may lead to coma and respiratory depression. Aspiration pneumonia may occur, due to suppression of the gag reflex, and a tendency to vomit, due to the irritating effects of ethanol on the gastrointestinal tract. Physical examination may reveal tachycardia, hypotension, hypothermia, hypoventilation, mydriasis, and nystagmus. Hypoglycemia may be present primarily because of an inhibition of gluconeogenesis by ethanol. This may contribute to the confusion and coma. Death may result from respiratory depression.

In nontolerant people there appears to be good correlation between blood alcohol concentration and the degree of neurologic impairment, with signs of intoxication beginning to appear as blood levels reach 50 mg to 100 mg/dL. When the blood alcohol concentration approaches 200 mg/dL motor skills and speech are impaired; at 300 mg/dL equilibrium, perception, and vision are altered; at levels above 450 mg to 500 mg/dL coma, respiratory depression, and peripheral vascular collapse occur. However, people who are tolerant to ethanol have been reported to not only survive incredibly high concentrations, but also be resistant to many of the toxic effects.

Isopropanol is considered to be twice as toxic as ethanol, although the clinical applicability is unclear. The signs and symptoms of isopropanol toxicity are similar to those of ethanol toxicity with only a few exceptions. CNS depression may persist for more than 24 hours, long after levels of isopropanol are undetectable, due to the metabolite acetone, which has a very long elimination half-life (20–30 hours). Hypoglycemia, a result of altered gluconeogenesis, may contribute to the CNS depression. Pupil size varies, and both miosis and mydriasis have been reported. Gastrointestinal irritation is a hallmark of isopropanol toxicity, and may manifest as abdominal pain, vomiting, gastritis, and hematemesis, which may lead to hypotension. Hypothermia can also be seen. Tachycardia is the most common finding. Fatalities have occurred in patients who were in deep coma and were hypotensive. Coma in the absence of hypotension did not indicate a poor prognosis.

Blood levels of isopropanol do not correlate well with toxic symptoms, although toxicity is seen when levels are 50 mg to 100 mg/dL. Most comatose patients have levels >125 mg/dL, and death may be seen with levels >200 mg/dL. However, patients with levels >500 mg/dL have recovered.

The signs and symptoms of acetone intoxication are also similar to those of ethanol intoxication, with the doses required to produce toxicity similar. However, acetone has a greater anesthetic potency than ethanol. After an ingestion of acetone, nausea, vomiting, and gastric hemorrhage can be seen. Inhalation of acetone can produce coughing, bronchial irritation, and eye irritation. Pharyngeal irritation and soft palate erythema and erosions have been reported. CNS depression causes drowsiness, weakness, dysarthria, and ataxia. Lethargy can progress to coma more rapidly with acetone than with ethanol.

DIFFERENTIAL DIAGNOSIS

The differential diagnosis should include the ingestion of other CNS depressants, as well as other causes of coma such as metabolic derangements, CNS infection, head trauma, and tumors. Other causes of increased serum osmolality include ethylene glycol and methanol ingestion. Ketosis caused by isopropanol and acetone intoxication should be differentiated from that secondary to alcoholic and diabetic ketoacidosis, starvation ketosis, and salicylate intoxication.

EMERGENCY DEPARTMENT EVALUATION

The history should include the type, amount and alcohol or acetone concentration of the substance ingested, route and time of ingestion, other agents ingested, chronic use of drugs or alcohol, nature and time of onset of symptoms, and past medical history. A history of trauma or disulfiram use should be specifically elicited. The physical examination should focus on mental status, neurologic function, and gastrointestinal and cardiopulmonary systems with frequent monitoring of vital signs for tachycardia, hypothermia, hypotension, and hypoventilation. The breath odor may provide a clue to the diagnosis (e.g., the fruity odor of acetone and isopropanol). The patient should be examined for evidence of trauma.

Laboratory tests should include a quantitative serum level of the ingested agent, routine chemistries, and a blood glucose determination. Gas chromatography is the preferred testing method. A Breathalyzer may give a quick and reliable estimate of the blood alcohol concentration. Factors that interfere with the Breathalyzer include recent (15–30 minutes) use of ethanol-containing products (e.g., inhaled bronchodilators), recent belching or vomiting, obstructive pulmonary disease, and poor compliance of the patient to participate in the test. Serum ethanol concentrations are about 10% to 15% higher than whole blood concentrations, depending on the patient's hematocrit. Enzymatic methods using alcohol dehydrogenase do not differentiate among the alcohols (ethanol, isopropanol, methanol, and ethylene glycol) and should no longer be used.

Arterial blood gas analysis and serum and urine ketone measurements may be helpful. Ketonemia and ketonuria may suggest isopropanol or acetone intoxication, but their absence does not rule out these ingestions. Measuring the serum osmolality by freezing point depression (not vapor pressure) may be helpful if quantitative serum levels are not immediately available. A measured osmolality greater than that calculated from the serum levels of sodium, blood urea nitrogen (BUN), and glucose (i.e., $2 \times Na + BUN/3 + glucose/18$) of more than 10 mOsm/kg suggests the presence of a low molecular weight compound such as ethanol, ethylene glycol, acetone, isopropanol, and methanol. If the agent ingested is known, its concentration may be esti-mated from the difference between the measured and calculated osmolalities, the osmolar gap. The gap increases by about 1 mOsm/kg for each 4 mg/dL of ethanol, 5.5 mg/dL of acetone, and 5.9 mg/dL of isopropanol present.

EMERGENCY DEPARTMENT MANAGEMENT

The treatment for large ingestion of ethanol, isopropanol, or acetone is primarily supportive. Breathing must be evaluated and the patient should be endotracheally intubated as needed. The comatose patient should receive thiamine, dextrose, and naloxone. Gastric lavage can be per-formed if the patient arrives within the first hour after ingestion. A small-bore nasogastric tube is sufficient unless the patient has recently eaten or ingested additional agents. Activated charcoal is of questionable benefit, although its administration with a cathartic is probably indicated for absorption of possible coingestants. The patient should be warmed if hypothermia exists. Sodium bicarbonate may be administered if there is a substantial lactic acidosis. Fluids and electrolytes should be replaced as needed. In rare cases of hypotension unresponsive to crystalloid adminis-tration the use of vasopressors may be necessary. Patients with ethanol intoxication usually recover within 12 hours, whereas recovery from severe isopropanol or acetone poisoning may take 2 to 3 days. Hemodialysis can be used in severe cases that are unresponsive to supportive therapy to increase the elimination of all of these agents.

DISPOSITION

Patients with acute ethanol intoxication seldom require admission unless a complication such as aspiration is present. Even those who are comatose improve within hours with supportive care. Only if they cannot be treated and observed in the ED do such patients require admission. In con-trast, patients with moderate to severe isopropanol or acetone poisoning and high blood levels of these agents usually require a day or two for resolution of toxicity and should be admitted. Clinical severity (e.g., need for airway protection and mechanical ventilation) should be used to determine the appropriate level of hospital care.

COMMON PITFALLS

- The patient, not the alcohol level, should be treated. Factors such as tolerance, trauma, coingestants, hypoglycemia, and underlying disease may alter a patient's response to a par-ticular level of alcohol.
- Co-ingestions and traumatic injuries should be ruled out, particularly if the clinical severity is not consistent with the alcohol level (in light of the past and present history of alcohol use).
- Nutritional deficiencies in chronic alcoholics can also cause confusion (e.g., Wernicke's encephalopathy). Thiamine and glucose should be administered.
- Unrecognized alcohol withdrawal can be fatal. Withdrawal can occur in the presence of a positive blood alcohol concentration.
- The physician should not assume that the alcohol level has reached its peak by the time the patient is examined. Deaths have occurred when blood levels continue to rise while the patient is put in a corner to "sleep it off." If there is doubt, additional alcohol levels should be obtained.
- Acetone causes falsely elevated serum creatinine levels. Renal failure should not be the diag-nosis if the BUN is normal.
- Serum osmolality is only useful if measured by the freezing point depression method.

97   Ethylene Glycol Poisoning

The first step in the metabolism of EG is the oxidation of EG to glycoaldehyde by means of alcohol dehydrogenase. Because alcohol dehydrogenase has a much higher affinity for ethanol than for EG, when both alcohols are present, ethanol is preferentially metabolized. The presence of ethanol, therefore, inhibits the metabolism of EG and prevents the production of toxic metabolites. Another significant step in the metabolism of EG involves the generation of glycolic acid. The accumulation of glycolic acid correlates with decreased bicarbonate levels, acidotic symptoms, and increased mortality. In addition, glycolic acid causes renal tubular damage and interstitial edema. Further metabolism results in the production of oxalic acid, which rapidly precipitates as calcium oxalate crystals in various organs and tissues. Calcium oxalate precipitation in renal lumina also contributes to renal insufficiency.

CLINICAL PRESENTATION

Three distinct stages (CNS, cardiopulmonary, and renal) of EG poisoning may be seen. There is great variability, however, in the onset, progression, and confluence of these stages. Initially, CNS signs and symptoms predominate, with slurred speech, ataxia, nystagmus, and lethargy. The patient may appear drunk but lacks the odor of ethanol. Instead, a faint, sweet, or aromatic odor may be detected on the breath. As CNS depression progresses, seizures, both focal and generalized, stupor, and coma may result. At this stage the "osmolal gap" may provide a clue to the diagnosis of EG poisoning.

The difference between the measured serum osmolality and the calculated osmolality ($2 \times$ sodium + glucose/18 + BUN/3) is the osmolal gap. Normally, serum osmolality ranges from 280 to 300 mOsm/kg H_2O with an osmolal gap of <10 mOsm/kg H_2O. Low molecular weight solutes such as EG, acetone, ethanol, isopropanol, and methanol increase serum osmolality, and thus increase the osmolal gap. Osmolality measured only by the freezing point depression (not vapor pressure) method will detect these agents. EG poisoning can be confirmed by the presence of EG in serum or urine.

Cardiopulmonary signs and symptoms such as hypertension, tachycardia, arrhythmias, and pulmonary edema develop between 4 and 12 hours after the ingestion of EG. Tachypnea with Kussmaul's respirations is secondary to metabolic acidosis. During this stage an increased anion gap may suggest EG poisoning.

The normal anion gap (serum sodium minus chloride and bicarbonate) is 12 (±2) mEq/L, and represents unmeasured anions in the serum. The presence of nonvolatile acids such as formic acid, keto acid, lactic acid, or, in the case of EG poisoning, glycolic acid increases the anion gap.

Urinalysis may provide evidence of EG poisoning. Proteinuria and hematuria may be seen in up to 50% of cases. Calcium oxalate crystalluria, virtually pathognomonic of EG poisoning, is seen in 30% to 50% of patients. These crystals are needle-shaped, and may be misidentified as hippuric acid crystals. The precipitation of calcium oxalate may cause hypocalcemia with myoclonic jerks or tetanic contractions. Fluorescence of urine or gastric contents with the use of a Wood's lamp may support antifreeze ingestion, since fluorescein is added to these products. Death is most common during this stage and results from multiple organ failure and irreversible shock. The patients who survive may complain of severe flank pain and develop costovertebral angle tenderness. Acute tubular necrosis is manifested by oliguria, proteinuria, and urine with a low specific gravity and sodium content.

DIFFERENTIAL DIAGNOSIS

EG intoxication can mimic a large variety of poisonings or disease states, depending on the amount ingested and the degree of EG metabolism. Diagnostic clues include drunkeness without the odor of ethanol, increased osmolal and anion gaps, metabolic acidosis, and calcium oxalate crystalluria. Similar findings may be present in methanol intoxication, but crystalluria is absent and visual complaints and an abnormal eye examination may be present.

EMERGENCY DEPARTMENT MANAGEMENT

Aggressive supportive measures, including airway protection and respiratory and circulatory support with cardiac and hemodynamic monitoring, should be instituted as necessary. If the patient has ingested EG within 4 hours, gastric aspiration and lavage with a nasogastric tube should be performed immediately. Patients at home who are alert and have recently ingested EG should be given syrup of ipecac to induce emesis if there will be a delay of more than 20 minutes in reaching a medical facility. Activated charcoal is capable of absorbing EG and should be given after emesis or gastric aspiration.

Laboratory evaluation should include a complete blood count; electrolytes, blood urea nitrogen, creatine, glucose, calcium, and ketones; serum osmolality; arterial blood gas analysis; toxicologic screen; and a urinalysis. A quantitative serum EG level should be obtained. If results are not readily available, an estimate of the serum EG level can be made by assuming that the serum osmolality will increase 1 mOsm/kg for each 5 mg/dL of EG (and each 4.3 mg/dL of ethanol) present. Metabolic acidosis should be corrected. This may require the use of large amounts of intravenous sodium bicarbonate, given slowly in increments. The acid–base status should be frequently re-evaluated to assess the response to therapy. Serum calcium levels should be monitored. Hypocalcemia should be treated with intravenous calcium chloride or gluconate (7–14 mEq for adults and 1–7 mEq for children). The 10% chloride solution contains 1.4 mEq of calcium per mL and the 10% gluconate solution contains 0.46 mEq per mL. The 10% solution should be diluted 10:1 with intravenous fluids and infused at a rate of less than 1 mEq/min. Seizures should be treated with standard drugs (diazepam, phenytoin, or a short-acting barbiturate).

Ethanol is given to inhibit the metabolism of EG. EG can then be eliminated by urinary excretion or by hemodialysis. Indications for ethanol therapy include a history or strong suspicion of EG ingestion based on abnormal clinical or laboratory findings, a serum EG level >20 mg/dL, or acidemia (regardless of EG concentration). The theraputic goal is a serum ethanol concentration of at least 100 mg/dL. Although this can be accomplished with oral administration of ethanol, intravenous administration provides a more constant serum level. An intravenous loading dose of 10 mL/kg of 10% ethanol (with glucose to avoid hypoglycemia) followed by a maintenance infusion of 1.5 mL/kg/h will produce a serum ethanol level of slightly greater than 100 mg/dL. Serum ethanol and glucose levels should be monitored and the dose of ethanol adjusted as necessary to maintain a therapeutic ethanol concentration.

If clinical improvement does not occur with bicarbonate and ethanol therapy, hemodialysis is recommended. Hemodialysis is also recommended if the EG level is >50 mg/dL, and is required in patients with renal failure. Dialysis should be continued until metabolic abnormalities are corrected and serum EG levels are below 50 mg/dL. Ethanol treatment should be continued until the EG level is less than 20 mg/dL. During hemodialysis the infusion rate of ethanol should be increased to 3 mL/kg/h to compensate for losses. If hemodialysis is not available or technically difficult, peritoneal dialysis can be used, although this method is considerably less effective than hemodialysis.

Pyridoxine and thiamine are precursors to cofactors in the degradation of EG to less toxic products and should be given intramuscularly four times a day for 2 days (50 mg and 100 mg, respectively).

DISPOSITION

Patients with EG poisoning almost always require admission to an ICU. Early consultation with a toxicologist or local poison center is encouraged to aid in patient care and to determine the availability of EG levels. In addition, the need for hemodialysis should always be anticipated, and transfer should be accomplished if such treatment is not available.

COMMON PITFALLS

- Failure to consider EG as a cause of ethanol-like intoxication and metabolic acidosis
- Failure to treat with ethanol and to monitor ethanol and glucose levels
- Failure to correct EG-induced metabolic acidosis with bicarbonate

98   Halogenated Hydrocarbon Poisoning

Halogenated hydrocarbons are aliphatic and aromatic organic compounds that contain one or more atoms of bromine, chlorine, fluorine, or iodine (Table 98-1).

Toxicity may result from deliberate or accidental overexposure. These hydrocarbons are frequently abused by the male adolescent, and as many as 20% of high school seniors have experimented with volatile substances at least once. These agents are readily available, inexpensive, and legal, and they provide a rapid state of intoxication when inhaled. Abuse typically occurs as a group practice and involves placing the substance in a paper bag followed by inhalation (bagging) or soaking a rag and inhaling the vapors (huffing).

In industry approximately 10 million workers are exposed to organic solvents, which include chlorinated hydrocarbons. Dermal exposure is also common and may result in systemic absorption. Ingestions of solvents are infrequent and usually involve accidental pediatric cases or deliberate adult suicide attempts.

TABLE 98-1. Common Halogenated Hydrocarbons

Solvents	Refrigerants/Aerosols	Fumigants
Chloroform	Trichlorofluoromethane (Freon 11)	Methyl bromide
Carbon Tetrachloride	Dichlorofluoromethane (Freon 12)	Ethylene dibromide
Trichloroethylene (TCE)	Trifluoromonobromomethane	
Perchloroethylene (PCE)	(Freon 12-B1)	
1,1,1 Trichloroethane (TCA)*	1,2 dichlorotetrafluoroethane	
Methylene Chloride	(Freon 114)	
(Dichloromethane or DCM)*		
Trichlorotriflouroethane		
(Freon 113)		

*Also used as aerosol propellants.

CLINICAL PRESENTATION

Depression of the central nervous system (CNS) is the primary effect of the halogenated hydro-carbons. Changes in consciousness are similar to those of ether anesthesia. Initially there is euphoria in association with visual hallucinations and perceptual disturbances. An intoxicated appearance accompanied by disorientation is characteristic. In addition, there is often a feeling of omnipotence, which can result in dangerous behavior. Continued exposure results in increasing CNS depression, leading to stupor and coma. Coma may be associated with respiratory depression and seizures.

Pulmonary complaints, including cough and shortness of breath, can follow inhalational exposure. These relate to underlying bronchospasm, pneumonitis, or pulmonary edema. Nausea, vomiting, diarrhea, and abdominal pain may be prominent symptoms after solvent exposure, especially ingestion. Delayed or persistent symptoms usually reflect hepatic or renal injury.

Halogenated hydrocarbons are capable of sensitizing the myocardium to the arrythmo-genic effects of catecholamines. This is thought to account for the sudden deaths that occur after exposure in conjunction with agitation or rapid physical activity.

Exposure to some chlorinated hydrocarbons may result in distinct clinical presentations. For example, degreasers flush is a cutaneous vascular reaction characterized by red blotches on the face and trunk that sometimes occurs after ethanol ingestion in people recently exposed to TCE. Exposure to dichloromethane, which is metabolized to carbon monoxide poisoning, may produce carboxyhemoglobin levels of 5% to 50%. Although accompanying symptoms of carbon monoxide poisoning are usually mild, patients with coronary artery disease can experience angina or myocardial infarction. The apparent half-life of carboxyhemoglobin produced from DCM is considerably longer than that produced from carbon monoxide exposure owing to ongoing metabolism.

DIFFERENTIAL DIAGNOSIS

Alternate diagnoses include intoxication from psychoactive agents such as phencyclidine, lysergic acid diethylamide, mescaline, and other hallucinogens. Stimulant drugs of abuse, such as cocaine, amphetamines, and sympathomimetics, should be considered when patients present in a toxic delirium. Drugs that produce CNS depression should be considered in the lethargic, obtunded, or comatose patient (e.g., opiates, ethanol, sedative-hypnotics, cyclic antidepressants, and phenothiazines). Infectious, metabolic, traumatic, and other non-drug causes of altered mental status should also be considered.

EMERGENCY DEPARTMENT EVALUATION

Overexposure to inhaled solvents should be suspected in the adolescent with a history of bags or rags at the scene, a sweet chemical odor, and residual solvent around the face. After the history and physical examination an electrocardiogram and chest radiograph should be obtained for symptomatic patients. Determination of baseline levels of liver enzymes, blood urea nitrogen, and creatinine, as well as a urinalysis, is helpful in establishing the presence of renal or hepatic toxicity. Carboxyhemoglobin levels are important with suspected DCM exposure. Suspected halogenated hydrocarbon ingestions may be confirmed by visualizing radiopaque material layered in the stomach, on the abdominal radiographs. Serum ethanol concentration and screening the urine for drugs of abuse may be necessary to rule out other intoxications. In some cases confirmation of exposure may be documented by exhaled air sampling or measurement of urine metabolites, neither of which are usually available or practical in the emergency department.

EMERGENCY DEPARTMENT MANAGEMENT

Attention should first be directed to advanced life-support measures, since treatment is primarily supportive. Cardiac rhythm should be monitored and intravenous access established. The regional poison control center may be a useful resource for substance information and patient management issues. Decontamination measures depend on the route of exposure. The skin should be irrigated immediately with water, followed by soap-and-water washing. The eyes should be irrigated immediately with isotonic saline solution. Eye exposures should be evaluated with a slit lamp after irrigation. Antibiotic ointment and patching may be indicated if corneal erosion is present; ophthalmology consultation may be indicated.

Patients with fumigant exposures or pulmonary symptoms after inhalation should be managed as described elsewhere. Adrenergic agents should be used with caution. Gastrointestinal decontamination is indicated for all patients with ingestions. Seizures should be treated with diazepam followed by phenytoin or phenobarbital. Life-threatening arrhythmias should be treated with lidocaine or propranolol. Hepatotoxicity and nephrotoxicity are managed primarily by supportive care. Potentially beneficial treatment for chloroform or carbon tetrachloride poisoning include N-acetylcysteine (NAC), hemoperfusion, and hyperbaric oxygen (HBO). These treatments must be started early if they are to be of any benefit. NAC may be used in a dosing regimen similar to that used in acetaminophen overdose. With large overdoses, treatment may have to be extended beyond the usual 18 doses in light of continued release of solvent into the circulation from adipose stores. HBO has been reported to be useful in isolated cases that involve carbon tetrachloride ingestion. Degreasers flush may respond to propranolol (40–80 mg PO). The management of carbon monoxide poisoning is described elsewhere.

DISPOSITION

Patients with evidence of cardiac arrhythmias require admission to an ICU. Those with persistent CNS and respiratory symptoms should also be admitted to a monitored unit. Patients with potential hepatic or renal toxicity from chloroform or carbon tetrachloride or those with persistent gastrointestinal symptoms should be admitted to a floor bed for observation. Similarly, patients with DCM exposures should be admitted and have their carboxyhemoglobin levels monitored. Patients who improve rapidly and become asymptomatic after a 4-hour observation period may be discharged. Appropriate psychiatric consultation should be obtained before discharge when indicated.

Patients must be warned to avoid re-exposure. Employers and governmental regulatory agencies (e.g., Occupational Safety and Health Administration and National Institute of Occupational Safety and Health) should be notified in cases of workplace exposure.

COMMON PITFALLS

- Failure to consider the syndrome of inhalant abuse in the intoxicated adolescent
- Failure to use adrenergic drugs cautiously because of myocardial sensitization caused by halogenated hydrocarbons
- Failure to admit patients with significant chloroform, carbon tetrachloride, or DCM exposures, even if they become asymptomatic
- Failure to warn patients about avoiding re-exposure
- Failure to notify employers and governmental agencies in cases of occupational exposure

99   Iron Poisoning

There are three major iron-containing products for ingestion: hematinic preparations (ferrous sulfate, gluconate, and fumarate), prenatal vitamins, and multivitamins with iron. Multivitamins with iron contain between 12 mg and 18 mg and prenatal vitamins between 45 mg and 65 mg of elemental iron per tablet or capsule. The percentage of elemental iron in hematinic preparations is as follows: ferrous gluconate 11%, ferrous sulfate 20%, and ferrous fumarate 33%.

CLINICAL PRESENTATION

Acute iron toxicity may progress through three stages: an early stage (1–6 hours postingestion), an intermediate stage (6–48 hours postingestion), and a late stage (2 days–2 months postingestion). Early signs and symptoms of ingestion of toxic quantities of iron begin with vomiting, abdominal pain, melena, or diarrhea. Vomiting can be severe enough to result in hematemesis and diarrhea that is often black and tarry. Elevation in serum transaminase levels is evident. Early cardiovascular symptoms include hypotension owing to a reduction in vascular tone from the release of vasodepressor substances as well as a decrease in circulating blood volume from hemorrhage or loss of plasma volume. Hypotension is most often accompanied by reflex tachycardia. Increased venous stasis may result in intense vasoconstriction with peripheral cyanosis. Changes in the central nervous system range from lethargy to coma and seizures in severe cases. Metabolically, the liberation of ferric hydroxides and subsequent hydrogen ion, the poisoning of Krebs cycle enzymes, and hypotension result in a profound acidosis. Hyperglycemia may also be documented at this time.

During the intermediate stage initial clinical stabilization or improvement may be seen and then gastrointestinal signs and symptoms continue, with melena or diarrhea most prevalent. Serum transaminase levels remain elevated. Decreased cardiac output due to decreased ventricular contractility, and decreased venous return due to vascular congestion may become evident. Renal tubular damage may occur; however, the most significant change during this period involves coagulation. Coagulopathies from liver damage (hypoprothrombinemia) and an inhibition of fibrinogen to fibrin by thrombin may occur.

The final stage of iron poisoning for those who survive the initial phases primarily involves the gastrointestinal system. Segmental infarction of the small bowel and pyloric stenosis may be documented with delays as long as 2 months. In addition, fatty degeneration and diffuse fibrosis of the liver are seen.

Major complications include gastrointestinal bleeding, hypotension, metabolic complications, coagulopathies, infection, and restrictive lung changes. Gastrointestinal bleeding can be serious early (owing to local corrosive effects on the intestinal mucosal wall) or late (owing to perforation). Hypotension occurs early, but ventricular failure is late. Metabolic complications occur early and most often manifest as a severe metabolic acidosis. Coagulopathies may occur early, but most commonly appear as an intermediate finding.

DIFFERENTIAL DIAGNOSIS

Most patients present with a clear history of ingestion. The major presenting picture of acute iron toxicity is vomiting (heme positive), hypotension, metabolic acidosis, and obtundation. Other offending agents with a similar presentation would include aspirin (other nonsteroidal anti-inflammatory drugs), theophylline, caustics, and isopropyl or ethyl alcohol. Clues that would aid in this diagnosis may be the presence of radiopaque material on kidney-ureter-bladder (KUB) films and a rapid diagnostic evaluation of the gastric content.

EMERGENCY DEPARTMENT EVALUATION

The assessment of severity in acute iron overdose is made by history, clinical presentation, and laboratory parameters (Table 99-1). The least accurate method for assessing severity is the history of ingestion. Severity is based on the amount of elemental iron ingested per kilogram of weight. Although severity can be judged more accurately by clinical presentation, laboratory assessment is the most accurate method of assessing toxicity. In all cases blood should be drawn for serum iron and total iron-binding capacity assay, white blood cell count, determination of serum glucose and electrolyte levels, hemoglobin, and hematocrit. In severe cases arterial blood gas analysis, liver and kidney function tests, and clotting studies should be monitored.

A decreased hematocrit may be seen in the presence of bleeding, but an increased hematocrit caused by loss of plasma volume can also occur. Arterial blood gases may reveal metabolic acidosis in patients with significant poisoning. A white blood cell count higher than 15,000/µL and a serum glucose level higher than 150 mg/dL in patients with abdominal symptoms and a positive KUB film indicate a serum iron level higher than 300 µg/dL. The plain abdominal film (KUB) may also be useful. The potential for late-onset toxicity may be identified if radiopaque material is detected in the gut after adequate decontamination. However, the serum iron concentration, especially if determined within 6 hours of ingestion, is the most accurate way to assess severity. When serum iron concentrations cannot be determined in a timely manner, a deferoxamine challenge (25–50 mg/kg to a maximum of 1 g IM) followed by the classic *vin rose* coloring in the urine may help to identify patients with free circulating iron.

EMERGENCY DEPARTMENT MANAGEMENT

Management is based on supportive care, gastrointestinal decontamination, and chelation therapy. Supportive care is directed at maintaining blood pressure (first with fluids and then with vasopressors) and correcting acid–base disorders. Clotting dysfunction in severe overdose can be anticipated. Gastrointestinal decontamination may be achieved by ipecac syrup in alert patients or by lavage with a large-bore tube in obtunded patients. The effectiveness should be verified by KUB films. Activated charcoal does not significantly bind iron, and therefore is not indicated. To help reduce the absorption of iron that is not removed by mechanical methods, 100 mL of 1% sodium bicarbonate may be instilled. Oral Fleet's Enema preparations could lead to hypernatremia, hyperphosphatemia, and hypocalcemia, and are therefore **not** recommended.

The mainstay of therapy in iron toxicity is chelation. Ddeferoxamine (Desferal) is an iron-chelating compound and each 100 mg binds 8.5 mg of iron. Although it is not specific for iron, its affinity for iron is many times greater than for any other cation. It is most effective on free serum iron but may also bind iron from ferritin and transferrin with little effect on intracellular and probably no effect on mitochondrial stores. Therefore, early (before distribution is complete) and adequate (enough to provide chelant excess) administration is indicated. The intravenous dose is 15 mg/kg/h. Adverse effects with deferoxamine are rare and mainly involve hypersensitivity reactions. Therapy should be continued until 24 hours after the characteristic vin rose urine color has disappeared or the serum iron concentration is 100 µg/dL. Deferoxamine in pregnant patients may be associated with fetal skeletal abnormalities; however, acute short-term use (especially in third trimester patients) may be lifesaving. Deferoxamine in doses greater than 15 mg/kg/h may be used in severe overdoses as long as careful monitoring of systemic blood pressure is maintained.

TABLE 99-1. Assessment of Severity: Acute Iron Overdose

	None	Mild	Moderate	Severe
Amount of elemental iron ingested	<20 mg/kg	>20–50 mg/kg	>50–80 mg/kg	>80 mg/kg
Clinical presentation	Asymptomatic for 6 h	Vomiting, diarrhea, abdominal pain	Plus hypotension, lethargy, hematemesis, bloody or tarry black stools	Plus acidosis, coma, seizures cyanosis, shock
Laboratory Chemistry, hematology	No change	Sugar > 150 mg/dL, WBC > 15,000/µL, increased or decreased hematocrit	Plus acidosis, increased glutamic pyruvic transaminase and glutamic oxaloacetic transaminase levels	Plus increased prothrombin time
Serum iron level (2–6 h postingestion)*	<300 µg/dL	300–500 µg/dL	500–1000 µg/dL	>1000 µg/dL

*A serum iron concentration greater than the total iron-binding capacity also indicates the potential for toxicity.

DISPOSITION

Most iron ingestions are mild and can be managed in the ED. For patients in whom serum iron concentration exceeds 1000 µg/dL, consultation with surgical, gastroenterology, hematology, and toxicology specialists is indicated when signs and symptoms indicate severe toxicity, when persistent radiopaque masses are seen on KUB films, or when the patient is pregnant. Patients should be admitted to an ICU if they have moderate to severe symptoms, if they have persistent radiopaque masses, or if their serum iron level is higher than 500 µg/dL. Immediate transfer to a tertiary care unit should be instituted in patients with seizures, persistent hypotension, or coma.

COMMON PITFALLS

- Aggressive gastrointestinal decontamination is not instituted early enough to prevent absorption and distribution of iron to target organs (liver, heart, and lungs).
- Failure to inform the pregnant patient with moderate or severe toxicity of the potential problems connected with the use of deferoxamine and to advise the patient that the benefits outweigh the risks.
- Underestimation of severity.
- Failure to fully evaluate history, routine laboratory studies, radiographs, and serum iron concentrations.

100   Methanol Poisoning

In the early stage the toxic effects are due to the increasing metabolic acidosis caused by the accumulation of formic acid. In late stages, when more formate is accumulated, the toxicity is mainly caused by the histotoxic effects of formate as it inhibits the mitochondrial respiration within the cell. This leads to lactate production, which increases the acidosis and the toxicity of formate as more formate is protonated and thereby able to penetrate the blood–brain barrier.

CLINICAL PRESENTATION

Usually 6–24 hours elapse from the time of ingestion to the occurrence of symptoms. This is the time it takes for sufficient amounts of formate to be produced by methanol metabolism. This latent period may be longer, especially if ethanol is coingested, because ethanol competitively inhibits methanol metabolism by alcohol dehydrogenase. A latent period up to 90 hours has been reported when ethanol is also ingested. Methanol itself has few direct effects. Mild central nervous system depression (ethanol-like intoxication) has been reported. With concentrated methanol solutions nausea, vomiting, and abdominal pain may develop shortly after ingestion.

The first symptoms of systemic toxicity are usually a feeling of weakness, anorexia, headache, nausea, and vomiting, accompanied or followed by increasing hyperventilation as the metabolic acidosis progresses. Visual symptoms (blurred vision, decreased acuity, halo vision, tunnel vision, photophobia, and "snowfields") may appear first or with the symptoms above. Usually ocular symptoms precede objective signs, such as dilated pupils that are partially reactive or nonreactive to light and funduscopy showing optic disk hyperemia with blurring of the margins. If treatment is not initiated at this early stage of poisoning, the patient develops coma and respiratory and circulatory failure.

DIFFERENTIAL DIAGNOSIS

If quantitative methanol and formate levels are not available, other causes of metabolic acidosis should be considered. Visual complaints suggest methanol poisoning as the cause. The accumulation of formate causes a metabolic acidosis with an increased anion gap. Because of its low molecular weight and high concentration, methanol (and other alcohols) also increase the serum osmolality. This effect can easily be detected by calculating the difference between the measured osmolality (om) and the calculated osmolality (oc), where $oc = 2 \times$ sodium $+$ BUN/3 $+$ glucose/18. An osmolal difference gap of >10 mOsm/kg H_2O indicates exogenous osmoles of some kind.

In late stages of methanol poisoning all the methanol may be metabolized to formate. At this stage the anion gap will be elevated but the osmolal gap will be normal; formate detection is then the only way to confirm the diagnosis. In early stages, or if ethanol is coingested, only the osmolal gap will be elevated, as the metabolism of methanol to formate has not yet begun.

Increased anion and osmolal gaps also occur in ethylene glycol intoxication. Differentiating the two may be difficult, but the treatments are essentially the same. Hypocalcemia, seizures, and urine oxalate crystals are indicative of ethylene glycol poisoning.

EMERGENCY DEPARTMENT EVALUATION

The history should include the amount, concentration, and time of methanol ingestion, the nature and onset of symptoms, and whether or not ethanol was also ingested. Patients should be carefully questioned about the presence or absence of visual complaints, gastrointestinal symptoms, and a feeling of intoxication. The physical examination should focus on vital signs (especially respiratory rate) and the neurologic, visual, and cardiopulmonary status. Visual acuity and funduscopic examinations should be performed.

Laboratory evaluation should include arterial blood gas analysis, complete blood count, measurement of electrolytes, blood urea nitrogen, creatinine, glucose, and amylase, urinalysis, and quantitative serum methanol or formic acid level. A chest radiograph and an electrocardiogram should be obtained if clinical toxicity is pronounced. If the diagnosis is based on the osmolal and anion gaps, osmometry must be performed by the freezing point depression technique and not by the vapor pressure technique, as the latter does not detect the increased osmolality caused by volatile alcohols. A computed tomography scan of the brain may show necrosis of the putamenal areas, a finding seen late in the course of methanol poisoning.

EMERGENCY DEPARTMENT MANAGEMENT

The treatment should follow the established principles of intensive supportive care. If the patient is seen soon after ingestion, immediate gastric lavage should be performed. Emesis induction and activated charcoal alone are probably of limited value because of slow onset and limited binding, respectively. Specific treatment of methanol poisoning includes bicarbonate to combat the metabolic acidosis, ethanol to inhibit methanol metabolism to formate, and hemodialysis to remove methanol and formate. It may also be that folinic acid (leucovorin) is of value in increasing the metabolism of formate. The metabolic acidosis should be aggressively treated by infusion of sodium bicarbonate. As much as 400–600 mEq may be required during the first few hours. One should aim at a full correction of the acidosis. Bicarbonate treatment also decreases the amount of undissociated formic acid, resulting in less access of formate to the central nervous system.

Alkali treatment must be accompanied by ethanol. Otherwise, the acidosis becomes bicarbonate resistant, as more formic acid will be produced from the metabolism of methanol. Most authors recommend a therapeutic blood ethanol level of at least 100 mg/dL. However, the amount of ethanol necessary to block methanol metabolism depends on the concomitant methanol level because there is a dynamic competition for the enzyme alcohol dehydrogenase in the liver. If the blood methanol level is known, the ethanol concentrations should be at least a quarter of the methanol concentration. If a methanol level cannot readily be obtained, ethanol therapy should be started in any patient with acidosis, symptoms, or a history of a potentially toxic ingestion. Ethanol treatment should be discontinued when the methanol level drops below 20 mg/dL, provided that the acid–base status is normal and there are no complications.

A blood ethanol level of 100 mg/dL may be achieved by giving a bolus dose of 0.6 mg/kg, followed by 66 mg to 154 mg/kg/h intravenously (or orally), with the higher maintenance dose for heavy drinkers. Mixing 60 mL absolute ethanol with 500 mL isotonic glucose yields about a 10% solution if a 10% ethanol solution for intravenous use is not available. With this solution a bolus of 10 mL/kg followed by 1.5 mL/kg/h will produce the desired ethanol concentration. The maintenance infusion should be increased or decreased according to measured ethanol levels. Monitoring of the blood ethanol level is important, especially during hemodialysis, as this also removes ethanol. As a thumb rule, the maintenance dose of ethanol should be doubled during hemodialysis.

The only absolute indication for hemodialysis is visual impairment (of any degree). Other indications include severe metabolic acidosis (particularly if not responsive to bicarbonate and ethanol therapy), blood methanol level above 50 mg/dL, and ingestion of more than 1 g/kg of methanol. Hemodialysis should be continued until the blood methanol level is below 20 mg/dL and the acidosis corrected. If methanol analyses are not available, hemodialysis should be continued for at least 8 hours. Peritoneal dialysis may also remove methanol but not as effectively as hemodialysis. Hemoperfusion is not effective.

DISPOSITION

Consultation with a poison center or toxicologist may be helpful. Information on where to obtain methanol or formate levels may be provided. When the diagnosis of methanol poisoning is made or suspected a nephrologist should be consulted, as many patients ultimately require hemodialysis, especially when admitted in a late stage. If a methanol level is not available, all patients with suspected methanol poisoning should be admitted to hospital for continued clinical and laboratory evaluation. Every patient with a definite diagnosis of methanol intoxication should be admitted and have an initial and follow-up examination by an ophthalmologist. If hemodialysis is not available, the patient who needs it or will probably need it should be transferred to a facility with this capability.

COMMON PITFALLS

- Even small amounts of concentrated methanol are potentially toxic.
- Methanol poisoning should always be considered in the differential diagnosis of metabolic acidosis of unknown origin. Increased osmolal and anion gaps are supportive evidence.
- The possibility of multiple victims should always be considered when the source of methanol is unknown (or known to be contaminated ethanol).
- The lack of early symptoms does not rule out methanol ingestion. All patients must be admitted and observed until a methanol level can be obtained.
- Visual function should be formally assessed by an ophthalmologist (initially and after resolution).

101   Opioid (Narcotic) Poisoning

Narcotics may be classified as natural, semisynthetic, or synthetic. This is important clinically from the standpoint of therapeutic effectiveness (potency), side effects, and duration of action. Narcotics are rapidly absorbed by all routes except intact skin. Most narcotics are metabolized by hepatic conjugation, with 90% excreted in the urine as inactive compounds. Tolerance to narcotics is a well-known phenomenon, whereby steadily increasing dosages are required to produce the same physiologic response.

CLINICAL PRESENTATION

CNS findings may range from simple drowsiness to coma and include a paradoxical hyperexcitation. Mixed agonist–antagonists such as pentazocine (Talwin) and butorphanol (Stadol) are known to cause dysphoric reactions or even psychosis through their sigma agonist properties. Seizures are uncommonly caused by a pure narcotic overdosage with the exception of the pediatric patient and those who have taken propoxyphene (Darvon) and meperidine (Demerol). Muscle tone usually remains intact but may be increased by meperidine or fentanyl (Sublimaze). Miosis is classically described in victims of narcotic poisoning and is present in the vast majority. However, mydriasis or midrange pupils **should never** cause the care provider to rule out narcotic poisoning; instead, one should consider diphenoxylate, meperidine, hypoxia, hypoglycemia, postictal state, or cointoxicant.

Potentially lethal respiratory depression remains the hallmark of narcotic poisoning. Noncardiac pulmonary edema may be seen in significant opiate poisoning by both the parenteral and oral routes, and is thought to be a universal finding in narcotic-induced fatalities. Onset may be delayed up to 24 hours. The cause remains obscure. The patient develops copious pink, frothy sputum and rhonchi, rales, or wheezes on auscultation of the lungs in the absence of jugular venous distention or S_3 gallop. Central venous pressure (CVP) is normal or low. The chest radiograph reveals a normal-size heart and a variable pattern of pulmonary edema ranging from unilateral localized infiltrates to the classic hilar-based bilateral patchy infiltrate. Due to the CNS depressant effects of opiates, aspiration pneumonitis must also be considered as the cause of abnormal pulmonary findings on examination and x-ray film. These entities may be difficult to differentiate in the ED, and aspiration is probably the cause when the chest film abnormalities do not resolve within 48 hours of therapy.

Narcotic agents have a surprising paucity of direct effects on the cardiovascular system. Except with propoxyphene, significant hypotension suggests an alternative source, such as cointoxicant or hypovolemic shock (traumatic). A murmur in an intravenous abuser should raise the possibility of endocarditis, while cor pulmonale may stem from pulmonary hypertension resulting from the injection of contaminants or cutting agents.

The delayed gastric emptying caused by narcotics may dramatically slow drug absorption and make gastric emptying efforts fruitful as long as 27 hours postingestion. Other complications of narcotic overdose include urinary retention due to the increased sphincter tone, myoglobinuria stemming from rhabdomyolysis, hypoglycemia, and hypothermia.

EMERGENCY DEPARTMENT MANAGEMENT

All comatose or unresponsive patients should initially be assessed for airway and ventilation. Intubation can usually be avoided (and temporary ventilation provided by a bag-valve-mask) with naloxone. The patient should be placed on a cardiac monitor, intravenous access should be established, and samples drawn for determination of serum levels of electrolytes, glucose, blood urea nitrogen, and creatinine. Blood for complete blood count, prothrombin time, partial thromboplastin time, liver function tests, and toxicology screen may also be obtained for later use. If there is no response to one ampule (25 g) of 50% dextrose intravenous (along with 100 mg of thiamine), naloxone (Narcan) should be administered. A positive response to naloxone is both diagnostic and therapeutic.

If the patient is a suspected narcotic abuser or addict, it is advisable to apply four-point restraints before naloxone administration, as the patient may become uncooperative and combative. In addition, suction equipment should be set up as vomiting may occur after naloxone administration. In suspected addicts a low initial dose of naloxone (0.4 mg or less intravenous) should be administered in order to avoid precipitating a severe withdrawal reaction; this dose may be repeated every 1 minute until a total of 2 mg has been given or the patient awakens and respiratory depression is reversed.

If the patient is not a known or suspected addict, 2 mg of naloxone should be given as the initial bolus. Because some narcotic overdoses (e.g., propoxyphene) are relatively resistant to naloxone, increments of 2 mg every 2 to 5 minutes up to a total of 10 mg may be given if there is little or no response to the initial 2-mg bolus. A continuous naloxone drip may be appropriate in certain overdoses, particularly in opiates with long half-lives (e.g., diphenoxylate and methadone). One half of the original dose may need to be given as an additional bolus 15 to 20 minutes after initiation of the drip. If intravenous access cannot be obtained, naloxone may be administered into the sublingual venous plexus, or intramuscularly or endotracheally.

A partial response to naloxone requires a careful search for accompanying illness or injury. Patients who remain unresponsive should be intubated at this time. A paralytic agent (e.g., succinylcholine) may be needed in order to perform an atraumatic intubation. Chest radiography, electrocardiography, arterial blood gas analysis, electrolytes, urinalysis, and toxicology screen should be obtained, if not already done. If naloxone has been administered, the laboratory should be informed to avoid false identification of naloxone as an opiate.

Patients with oral overdoses should receive activated charcoal with or without gastric lavage, depending on the level of consciousness. Ipecac is not recommended.

Noncardiac pulmonary edema is a complication of narcotic poisoning. Endotracheal intubation is necessary in patients with hypercapnea or hypoxia despite administration of high-flow oxygen. Fluid restriction and positive end-expiratory pressure may also be beneficial, but morphine and diuresis are inappropriate in this setting.

Seizures unresponsive to naloxone administration should be treated with intravenous diazepam. Ongoing seizures should spark a search for a cause other than pure opiate poisoning.

Hypotension is usually not a prominent feature of pure narcotic overdose, and its presence should be managed initially with a crystalloid fluid bolus and an aggressive search carried out for another cause. Propoxyphene frequently causes hypotension, necessitating aggressive use of dopamine. Likewise, cardiac rhythm disturbances or cardiogenic shock should suggest that pure narcotic poisoning is unlikely (propoxyphene, once again, is the exception).

DISPOSITION

The half-life of naloxone (30–100 minutes) is shorter than almost all of the narcotic agents it antagonizes. A period of careful observation is required for any patient who has demonstrated clinical evidence of narcotic poisoning that requires naloxone administration. Intravenous narcotic overdosage should be observed for a minimum of 6 hours for evidence of relapse or the development of noncardiac pulmonary edema. Restraints may be used if the patient should attempt to leave against medical advice. Recurrence of symptoms mandates repeated naloxone administration (or a drip) and intensive care unit admission for at least 12 hours. All patients with evidence of pulmonary edema or with an oral overdose must be admitted to an ICU with cardiac and respiratory monitoring (and suicide precautions as needed) for a minimum of 24 hours and not discharged until symptom-free for 12 hours. Appropriate psychiatric and or social work follow-up must be arranged for all intentional or pediatric poisonings.

COMMON PITFALLS

- Narcotic poisoning should be considered in the patient who presents to the emergency department with any form of altered mental status, particularly seizures or combativeness.
- Ipecac should be avoided owing to the possibility of rapid deterioration (coma, seizures) after narcotic ingestion.
- Application of restraints before the administration of naloxone may prevent injury to the patient or staff.
- Because the half-life of naloxone is shorter than most narcotics and because noncardiogenic pulmonary edema may be delayed in onset, any patient who has received naloxone should be observed for at least 6 symptom-free hours.
- All patients with oral ingestions (regardless of symptoms) must be carefully observed for 24 hours owing to delayed onset of toxicity.
- Intravenous abusers are at high risk for a number of traumatic and medical illnesses, and a high index of suspicion and careful physical examination in search of these are warranted.

102   Petroleum Distillate Poisoning

Products of the fractional distillation of natural petroleum include such compounds as kerosene, mineral seal oil, gasoline, mineral spirits, naphtha, diesel fuel, motor oil, xylene, toluene, and benzene. Petroleum distillates are typically classified as either aliphatic straight chains or aromatic benzene-like rings. Aromatic compounds are discussed elsewhere. Petroleum distillates are also referred to as hydrocarbons. The term hydrocarbon describes structure rather than origin, and includes the petroleum distillates and compounds derived from plants (e.g., turpentine, pine oil, vegetable oil), animal fats, and coal. Therefore, whereas all petroleum distillates are hydrocarbons, the converse is not true. Finally, for clinical purposes, petroleum distillates are operationally divided into toxic and nontoxic.

Nontoxic petroleum distillates are those that have minimal gastrointestinal absorption and systemic toxicity. In contrast, toxic compounds, such as halogenated and aromatic hydrocarbons, may be absorbed, and produce substantial systemic effects. Toxic petroleum distillates include aromatic and halogenated hydrocarbons. The greatest toxicity of petroleum distillates is to the respiratory tract, where, if aspirated, they lead to a severe chemical pneumonitis. Petroleum distillate pneumonitis is characterized by the development of hemorrhagic bronchitis or alveolitis, respiratory failure, and death. These complications are not seen after ingestion without aspiration. Petroleum distillates are poorly absorbed and pulmonary toxicity occurs only after direct contact with the respiratory epithelium.

Many petroleum distillates have a central nervous system (CNS) anesthetic and narcotic effect. This is the basis of gasoline sniffing as a substance abuse habit. Whether inhaled, injected, or ingested such petroleum distillates lead to light-headedness, euphoria, incoordination, and impaired judgment.

Two independent physical characteristics dictate the pulmonary and CNS effects of the petroleum distillates: viscosity and volatility (Table 102-1). Viscosity (fluidity) determines aspiration risk. The lower the viscosity, the more likely a petroleum distillate will be aspirated. Substances of less than 60 SSU pose a significant aspiration risk, whereas those greater than 60 SSU do not. Volatility determines the potential for CNS effects. The more volatile a substance, the greater the likelihood of pulmonary absorption and subsequent narcosis. After exposure to volatile petroleum distillates as many as 28% of victims have lethargy, coma, or, rarely, seizures. Figure 102-1 offers an algorithm for the management of petroleum distillate ingestion.

CLINICAL PRESENTATION

Inhalation is a common method of substance abuse. The pulmonary toxicity of petroleum distillates appears to be negligible, but systemic toxicity (altered mental status, encephalopathy, and myocardial irritability) has been reported. Inhalation of leaded gasoline has also been associated with lead poisoning.

The ingestion of petroleum distillates is almost always followed by nausea and abdominal cramping. Spontaneous vomiting is also common. Vomiting increases the likelihood of aspiration. Oral pain, dysphagia, drooling, or hematemesis may also result from mucosal irritation. Additional signs of petroleum distillate ingestion include altered mental status or loss of consciousness (in up to 60% of children), fever (17%), and leukocytosis. In children intravascular hemolysis and hemoglobinuria have also been reported. Concomitant aspiration is nearly always present, making it difficult to determine the exact route of absorption (gastrointestinal, pulmonary, or both).

Aspiration leads to immediate coughing and gagging. Depending on the distillate and the amount aspirated, these symptoms may rapidly progress to tachypnea, nasal flaring, and respiratory distress. Physical examination may reveal use of accessory respiratory muscles and cyanosis, and chest auscultation may reveal diffuse wheezes and rales. In severe cases, arterial blood gas analysis shows marked hypoxia, hypercapnea, and acidosis. Radiographic findings include patchy perihilar and midlung densities. Abnormalities on chest radiograph may lag behind clinical manifestations. Pneumonitis usually worsens over 3 to 5 days and then signs and symptoms resolve. Even after clinical illness has resolved, radiographic abnormalities may persist for days to weeks. Although there are usually no long-term sequelae, some children have shown evidence of subclinical disturbances in pulmonary function 8 to 14 years after exposure.

DIFFERENTIAL DIAGNOSIS

Although gastrointestinal symptoms resulting from petroleum distillate ingestion are similar to those of corrosive ingestion, infectious gastroenteritis and food poisoning, the hydrocarbon odor of the breath or vomitus usually suggests the correct diagnosis. Similarly, although symptoms of aspiration may resemble those caused by asthma, allergic reactions, pulmonary infections, and the inhalation of irritant gases, the history and physical examination will usually disclose the correct etiology.

TABLE 102-1. Influence of Volatility and Viscosity on the Clinical Effects of Petroleum Distillate Exposure

Volatility	Viscosity	Examples	Clinical Effect
High	Low	Kerosene, gasoline	CNS, respiratory
High	High	Toluene, xylene, benzene	CNS
Low	Low	Mineral seal oil	Respiratory
Low	High	Mineral oil, motor oil	No toxicity

CNS, central nervous system.

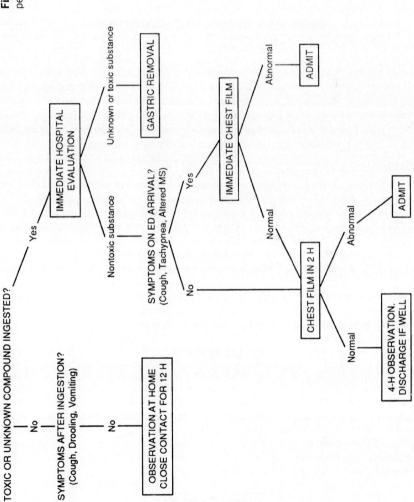

Figure 102-1. Management of petroleum distillate ingestion.

EMERGENCY DEPARTMENT EVALUATION

The history should include the identity, amount, and concentration of the petroleum distillate ingested, the time of ingestion, and any symptoms present before arrival, particularly respiratory symptoms at the time of ingestion. Because a number of different petroleum distillates may be found in a given product, all ingredients should be determined. The physical examination should initially focus on the vital signs, respiratory system, mental status, and gastrointestinal system. An arterial blood gas analysis and chest radiograph should be obtained on any patient with respiratory symptoms. Routine laboratory studies (e.g., complete blood count, determination of levels of electrolytes, blood urea nitrogen, creatinine, and glucose, and urinalysis) should also be obtained in patients with toxic petroleum distillate ingestion or evidence of aspiration. Depending on the agent ingested, other laboratory studies may also be indicated.

EMERGENCY DEPARTMENT MANAGEMENT

Management of petroleum distillate ingestion depends on whether or not the compound can cause systemic toxicity. Ingestion of a potentially toxic petroleum distillate requires gastrointestinal decontamination. Although the incidence of subsequent aspiration pneumonitis may be increased by the use of either gastric lavage or ipecac-induced emesis, either method is acceptable in an awake, alert patient. Because petroleum distillates are liquids, the use of a small-bore lavage tube is sufficient. In the patient with altered mental status gastric decontamination should be preceded by endotracheal intubation. The efficacy of activated charcoal for petroleum distillate absorption is unknown.

Because the greatest toxicity of the petroleum distillates results from aspiration and not gastrointestinal absorption, nontoxic petroleum distillates that are ingested do not require removal by gastric lavage or ipecac-induced emesis, regardless of the amount ingested. Vomiting should be prevented and activated charcoal, which may cause emesis, should not be administered.

All patients with respiratory symptoms should be given supplemental oxygen. The management of severe petroleum distillate aspiration includes early intubation and positive end-expiratory pressure to prevent alveolar collapse. Bronchodilators should be administered for bronchospasm. Cardiac monitoring is essential because these agents may aggravate myocardial irritability. Corticosteroids are ineffective in aspiration pneumonitis and may promote bacterial overgrowth. Prophylactic antibiotics may lead to the overgrowth of resistant pathogens and should be avoided. However, because petroleum distillate aspiration may cause fever and leukocytosis, antibiotics (e.g., penicillin and clindamycin) are often given empirically. Ideally, antibiotics should be given on the basis of a positive sputum culture or Gram's stain.

DISPOSITION

The disposition of patients with suspected aspiration depends on clinical, laboratory, and chest radiograph findings. If the chest radiograph or arterial blood gas analysis is abnormal, the patient should be admitted for further observation. If an early chest radiograph is normal, it should be repeated in 2 to 3 hours, since the appearance of radiographic abnormalities may be delayed. In patients who initially had symptoms suggesting aspiration but are asymptomatic on presentation, a chest radiograph should be delayed for 2 hours. If normal, the patient may be discharged after an additional 2 to 4 hours of observation. All patients with an abnormal chest radiograph or symptoms that persist for more than 4 hours should be admitted for further observation.

COMMON PITFALLS

- Failure to appreciate that only those petroleum distillates with low viscosity and high volatility represent aspiration hazards

- Failure to differentiate between petroleum distillates that cause systemic toxicity and those that do not when assessing the need for gastrointestinal decontamination
- Failure to consider the fact that gastric evaluation procedures may increase the risk of aspiration
- Failure to appreciate that radiographic evidence of aspiration may lag behind clinical findings
- Failure to admit symptomatic patients even if the chest x-ray and pulmonary examination are normal

103 Phencyclidine Poisoning

Phencyclidine (PCP) is an arylcyclohexylamine related to the "dissociative" anesthetic, ketamine.

CLINICAL PRESENTATION

The most striking manifestations of PCP intoxication are behavioral, ranging from agitation and belligerence to coma and seizures. Physical examination findings include nystagmus, ataxia, hypertension, increased muscle tone (including twitching, tremors, facial grimacing, localized dystonias, and hyperreflexia), diaphoresis, sialorrhea, and hyperthermia.

Four major and five minor clinical patterns, based primarily on the patient's sensorium and behavior, have been described. Major syndromes are coma, catatonic syndrome, toxic psychosis, and acute brain syndrome; minor syndromes are lethargy or stupor, bizarre behavior, violent behavior, agitation, and euphoria. A few patients with PCP detected in urine were asymptomatic. Variability is the most striking characteristic of PCP intoxication. When inhaled the dose is usually limited by the drug's effects, and signs and symptoms resolve over 4 to 6 hours. Ingestion of a larger dose often results in more severe and more prolonged symptoms. A patient may present with a minor syndrome, such as bizarre behavior, fairly early after an ingestion and then proceed to become comatose. The medical complications of PCP intoxication are responsible for most of the morbidity and mortality in hospitalized patients.

Rhabdomyolysis can be caused by muscle contractions, particularly in restrained patients, and may necessitate dialysis. In most cases of myoglobinuric renal failure, if vigorous renal solute flow is maintained, complete recovery of renal function is the rule. Aspiration pneumonia is the next most common complication. Hyperthermia, occasionally malignant and complicated by hepatic necrosis, has been reported. Hypertension is common during PCP intoxication, probably due to central effects that increase autonomic outflow. Fatal intracerebral hemorrhage has been reported.

The definitive diagnosis of PCP intoxication is made by detection of PCP in bodily fluids (most commonly in urine). Signs, symptoms, and laboratory studies are nonspecific.

DIFFERENTIAL DIAGNOSIS

PCP intoxication should be considered in any patient who presents with altered mental status, particularly the young patient with acute onset of bizarre behavior or psychosis, or the apparent drunk with no evidence of alcohol. Diagnostic clues include irritability and hostility, nystagmus, hypertension, sweating, hypersalivation, fever, stiffness, and dystonias. Seizures can occur. Mixed overdoses are common. PCP intoxication should be considered in trauma patients with prolonged coma, unusual rigidity, hypertension, or hyperthermia.

None of these findings is specific for PCP, although the constellation of fluctuating mental status, dystonias, nystagmus, and diaphoresis is quite suspicious, as is the combination of coma and rigidity without profound respiratory depression. In contrast to patients with PCP intoxication, those with the neuroleptic malignant syndrome have autonomic instability rather than sustained hypertension, and the limbs show "lead pipe" rigidity rather than diffuse hypertonia. Other central nervous system depressant drugs, such as sedative-hypnotics (characterized by more hypotonia and hypotension), tricyclics (anticholinergic signs and electrocardiographic abnormalities), and narcotics (pinpoint pupils, hypotension, bradycardia, and respiratory depression), should be considered.

The agitated, paranoid state of amphetamine intoxication can mimic PCP intoxication, but muscle rigidity, nystagmus, and sialorrhea are seen only with PCP. Encephalitis should also be considered. Occasionally alcohol or sedative–hypnotic withdrawal may be mistaken for PCP intoxication. A history of recent abstinence, continuous resting tremors, visual hallucinations, and lack of dystonias point to a withdrawal syndrome. In cases with coma or seizures, structural neurologic causes need to be considered, particularly since hypertension from PCP can lead to intracranial hemorrhage. Localized dystonias may be seen with PCP intoxication.

EMERGENCY DEPARTMENT EVALUATION

Careful history (including sources other than the patient), physical examination, and mental status examination form the basis of assessment for suspected PCP intoxication. Although there are no pathognomonic findings, one should look closely for focal neurologic findings as well as evidence of trauma. PCP-intoxicated patients may sustain severe injuries without awareness of pain. Evidence for aspiration pneumonia and other complications should be sought. In addition to urine toxicology testing, urinalysis (including myoglobin), electrolyte, glucose, and creatine phosphokinase levels, and renal function studies should be measured. If coma, hyperthermia, or rhabdomyolysis is present, additional workup should include arterial blood gas analysis, complete blood count, coagulation profile, liver function studies, and measurement of calcium, magnesium, and phosphorus levels.

EMERGENCY DEPARTMENT MANAGEMENT

Treatment of PCP intoxication consists of behavior control and careful supportive care. Because other drugs are commonly involved and most serious PCP intoxications are due to ingestions, oral charcoal should be given (although this may be difficult in an aggressive patient). Obtunded patients should also have gastric lavage. Ipecac should be avoided because of the risk of aspiration of gastric contents. Behavior control is best achieved with parenteral haloperidol (5–10 mg IM or IV every 20–60 minutes up to 30 mg in the first hour). Chlorpromazine (25–50 mg IM every 30–60 minutes up to 300 mg) is also effective. Although it is less likely to cause dystonias, it is more likely to lower blood pressure.

Oral diazepam has also been used successfully for agitation associated with mild intoxications, and sometimes intravenous diazepam is effective in calming obtunded patients who are struggling against their restraints. Most authors believe that diazepam is inferior to antipsychotic agents for severe behavior problems. Neuromuscular paralysis may be needed to stop muscle contractions in unusually severe cases. A quiet room with minimal stimulation is more effective in calming PCP-intoxicated patients than are attempts to "talk them down." Physical restraints are often needed to control violent behavior until pharmacologic therapy takes effect, but they clearly increase the risk of rhabdomyolysis.

Rhabdomyolysis should be treated with vigorous solute diuresis, starting with adequate intravenous volume repletion, with careful attention to electrolyte balance. Severe hyperthermia should be treated with cooling, small doses of chlorpromazine to suppress shivering, paralysis, and careful monitoring and supportive care. Hypertension usually responds to nonspecific seda-tion with antipsychotic agents or diazepam. If diastolic pressure stays >115 mm Hg or there is known coronary or cerebrovascular disease, specific treatment is indicated. Chlorpromazine may be useful because of its antipsychotic and alpha-blocking effects. Persistent hypertension can be treated with vasodilators (e.g., nitroprusside, diazoxide, or hydralazine), with the addition of a beta blocker (propranolol or esmolol) for tachycardia (over 120 beats per minute).

Physostigmine is contraindicated. Acidification of the urine is of little value, potentially harmful, and not recommended. Hemodialysis and hemoperfusion are relatively ineffective.

DISPOSITION

Patients with coma, major delirium, or the catatonic syndrome need to be hospitalized, as do patients with violent behavior, major trauma, hyperthermia (temperature >38.5°C), aspiration pneu-monia, sustained hypertension (>200/115), or significant rhabdomyolysis. All patients should be observed for at least 1 hour after all symptoms (except nystagmus) have resolved. Patients with sustained behavior problems who do not require restraints and have no medical complications should be referred to a psychiatrist. All discharged patients should have observation by friends or family, with clear instructions to seek medical assistance if behavior problems recur.

COMMON PITFALLS

- PCP intoxication should be considered as a diagnosis, particularly in psychotic young patients and in trauma patients.
- The diagnosis may be missed if a "toxicology screen" is requested because PCP is not con-sistently detected by commonly used techniques (e.g., thin-layer chromatography). When PCP intoxication is suspected a specific assay must be requested (e.g., gas-liquid chro-matography, high-performance liquid chromatography, EMIT [enzyme-multiplied immunoas-say technique], or radioimmunoassay).
- PCP should never be assumed to be the only toxin involved.
- PCP-intoxicated patients may have major trauma without apparent pain.
- Premature discharge from the ED after a brief but transient period of mental clarity is a com-mon pitfall. PCP-intoxicated patients are not competent to leave "against medical advice."
- Unproven or harmful treatments should not be used in place of good supportive care.
- Medical complications (rhabdomyolysis, aspiration pneumonia, and hyperthermia) should be recognized and treated early in their course so that permanent damage can be limited.

104   Salicylate Poisoning

Salicylate kinetics are markedly different after the ingestion of multiple therapeutic doses or a sin-gle large (over) dose. After an overdose gastric emptying is slowed, and salicylate tablets may form concretions, resulting in delayed and prolonged absorption. This is particularly true of enteric-coated and sustained-release formulations. With chronic dosing, the salicylate "half-life" increases to 6 to 12 hours, and a small increase in dose results in a much (proportionately) greater increase in serum and tissue salicylate levels with the potential for chronic intoxication. For the same rea-son, the salicylate "half-life" may increase to 20 to 40 hours after a large acute overdose.

When hepatic metabolism becomes saturated, urinary excretion becomes the major route of salicylate elimination. Alkaline diuresis increases the renal elimination of salicylate by a factor of 20 (or more).

Acute salicylate poisoning may result from a single ingestion of more than 150 mg/kg of aspirin. Ingestions of 150 mg to 300 mg/kg may cause mild toxicity, those of 300 mg to 500 mg/kg may cause moderate toxicity, and ingestions of more than 500 mg/kg may result in severe, or even fatal, poisoning. Salicylate levels may be quite high during the first 6 to 18 hours after an acute overdose without significant clinical or laboratory evidence of toxicity. Conversely, minimally elevated or even "therapeutic" salicylate levels may be seen with severe poisoning after chronic overdose or late in the course of an acute overdose. Hence the severity of poisoning is defined by clinical and metabolic abnormalities, not by the salicylate level. The salicylate (Done) nomogram is not necessary to assess severity and should never be used as the sole basis for treatment decisions.

Salicylate poisoning may also result from the topical (skin or gum) application of methyl salicylate or salicylic acid. It may occur in breast-fed infants whose mothers are chronically taking salicylates and in the fetuses or neonates of mothers who have ingested salicylates. The ingestion of salicylic acid preparations (e.g., Compound W) may also cause corrosive injury to the gastrointestinal tract.

CLINICAL PRESENTATION

Vomiting may occur shortly after ingestion as a consequence of direct gastric irritation. The early (postabsorption) phase of salicylate poisoning, which develops 3 to 8 hours after acute overdose (any time after chronic overdose), is characterized by mild dehydration, respiratory alkalosis, and alkaline urine (Table 104-1). Signs and symptoms are mild, and include nausea, vomiting, abdominal pain, headache, tinnitus (may occur at therapeutic levels), obvious tachypnea or hyperpnea (may be subtle), ataxia, dizziness, agitation, and lethargy. Mild increases or decreases in serum glucose, potassium, and sodium levels may be noted. Blood urea nitrogen (BUN), creatinine, sodium, and potassium levels may remain normal, however, despite total body fluid and electrolyte deficits.

Moderate poisoning, which usually occurs 12 to 24 hours after an acute overdose, is characterized by an increased anion gap metabolic acidosis with respiratory alkalosis, alkalemia, moderate to severe dehydration, and "paradoxical" aciduria (Table 104-1). Gastrointestinal and neurologic symptoms worsen. Fever, asterixis, diaphoresis, deafness, pallor, confusion, slurred speech, disorientation, hallucinations, tachycardia, tachypnea, and mild or orthostatic hypotension may be present. Leukocytosis, thrombocytopenia, increased or decreased glucose and sodium levels, hypokalemia, and increased BUN, creatinine, and ketone levels may be seen on laboratory evaluation.

TABLE 104-1. Stages and Treatment of Salicylate Poisoning

Stage/ Severity	Plasma pH	Urine pH	IV Solution	NaHCo$_3$ (amps/L)	Potassium (mEq/L)	Rate (mL/kg/h)
Early/mild	>7.4	>6	D$_5$NS	1	20	2–3
Intermediate/ moderate	≥7.4	<6	D$_5$ ½NS	2	40	4–5
Late/severe	<7.4	<6	D$_5$W	3	60–80	6–8

Adapted from Linden CH, Rumack BH: The legitimate analgesics: Aspirin and acetaminophen. In Hanson W Jr [ed]: Toxic Emergencies, p 118. New York, Churchill Livingstone, 1984.

Severe or late salicylate poisoning usually develops 24 or more hours after an acute overdose, and is characterized by severe dehydration, metabolic acidosis, acidemia, and aciduria. Respiratory acidosis and hypoxia may also be present in a minority of patients. Findings include coma, seizures, papilledema, respiratory depression, hypothermia or hyperthermia, hypotension, pulmonary edema, congestive heart failure, tachycardia, arrhythmias, and oliguria. Laboratory abnormalities seen with moderate intoxication become more pronounced. The chest radiograph may show pulmonary edema with a normal-size heart, and a computed tomography scan of the head may reveal cerebral edema and hemorrhage. Electrocardiographic abnormalities, other than sinus tachycardia, reflect metabolic abnormalities or the effects of coingested drugs.

Gastrointestinal bleeding, hepatic toxicity, pancreatitis, proteinuria, abnormal urinary sediment, and increased prothrombin time may be seen with therapeutic as well as toxic salicylate levels. Clinically significant bleeding, gastrointestinal perforation, blindness, and inappropriate antidiuretic hormone secretion are rare complications of acute poisoning. Chronic salicylate intoxication, especially in elderly patients, tends to be more severe than acute poisoning, and children tend to progress to moderate toxicity faster than adults. Adults appear to be more prone to pulmonary complications. Although the overall mortality rate is much less than 1%, it may be as high as 15% in patients with severe poisoning.

DIFFERENTIAL DIAGNOSIS

Occult salicylate poisoning should be considered in any patient with an unexplained acid–base disturbance. Although an increased anion gap metabolic acidosis is widely publicized, it occurs as the sole acid–base abnormality in only about 20% of patients with salicylate poisoning. Metabolic acidosis with respiratory alkalosis is actually the most common finding (in more than 50% of patients), and respiratory alkalosis alone is seen in another 20% to 25%. Other poisons that cause an anion gap metabolic acidosis include methanol and ethylene glycol, but lactic acidosis may occur in any poisoning that is complicated by hypoxia, hypertension, or seizures. A normal metabolic workup (arterial blood gas analysis and electrolytes) in a symptomatic patient with an unknown overdose rules out salicylate poisoning.

At least 25% of patients with chronic salicylate poisoning are initially (sometimes fatally) undiagnosed. These patients are often elderly, are chronically taking nonaspirin salicylates, and have serious underlying medical problems. Unless specifically questioned, the use of salicylates may not be discovered, and signs and symptoms of salicylate poisoning may be attributed to other illnesses (e.g., anxiety, cardiopulmonary disease, cerebrovascular disease, encephalopathy, alcohol ketoacidosis and withdrawal, viral meningitis, pancreatitis, Reye's syndrome, and chronic obstructive pulmonary disease).

Not infrequently patients give a history of aspirin ingestion or overdose when they actually (unknowingly) have taken acetaminophen and vice versa. Unless the agent or product ingested (or its container) is available for positive identification or the history can be confirmed by a witness, a serum level of both drugs should be obtained.

EMERGENCY DEPARTMENT EVALUATION

The history should include the time of ingestion and the amount and specific product ingested in cases of acute overdose. In all cases of intentional ingestion and in those with an unclear history, a serum salicylate level should be obtained. If the patient is symptomatic or the salicylate level is elevated, arterial blood gases analysis, serum levels of electrolytes, glucose, BUN, and creatinine, and a urinalysis should be obtained. If acid–base abnormalities are present, further evaluation should include serum calcium, magnesium, and ketone levels, liver function tests, complete blood count, prothrombin time, partial thromboplastin time, electrocardiography, and chest radiography. A toxicology screen may be useful to rule out the coingestion of other detectable poisons.

The physical examination should focus on vital signs, neurologic function, and cardiorespiratory findings. Accurate measurement of the respiratory rate and temperature is important but often done cursorily. The fundi should be examined for papilledema, and any vomitus and stool should be tested for occult blood. The presence of peritoneal signs necessitates evaluation for surgical complications. Salicylates, especially magnesium and bismuth (Pepto-Bismol) salts and enteric-coated or sustained-release formulations, may be evident on abdominal radiographs.

Because of delayed absorption, serial salicylate levels should be obtained until levels are noted to be declining. A single nontoxic salicylate level soon after ingestion is not sufficient to rule out a significant overdose. If levels continue to rise, repeat metabolic evaluation will be necessary.

EMERGENCY DEPARTMENT MANAGEMENT

Advanced life-support measures should be instituted as necessary. Patients with altered mental states should receive intravenous dextrose, naloxone, and thiamine in standard doses. Glucose administration is essential in salicylate poisoning because CNS hypoglycemia may occur with normal serum glucose concentration. Because nearly all patients with salicylate poisoning are volume depleted, treatment should begin with intravenous crystalloid administration (e.g., 1–2 L of dextrose 5% in 0.45% sodium chloride or dextrose 5% in 0.9% sodium chloride with or without sodium bicarbonate, 1/2 amp/L, and potassium, 10–20 mEq/L, over the first hour or two), provided there is no evidence of cerebral or pulmonary edema. In patients with hypernatremia a hypotonic solution should be used.

Because the immediate goal is to reverse hypotension and establish a good flow of urine, bladder catheterization is necessary for monitoring purposes. If hypotension or oliguria persists, central venous or pulmonary artery catheterization is recommended. Patients with elevated pressures should be treated with dopamine. Furosemide may also be used in an attempt to reverse oliguric renal failure unresponsive to volume replacement.

Seizures should initially be treated with standard agents (glucose, diazepam, phenobarbital, or phenytoin). If papilledema or computed tomographic evidence of cerebral edema is present, elevation of the head, hyperventilation, and administration of mannitol or furosemide and dexamethasone should be considered. Diuretics should be used cautiously, if at all, in patients with hypovolemia. Pulmonary edema should be treated with intubation and positive end-expiratory pressure ventilation. Vitamin K should be given to patients with coagulation abnormalities. Those with overt bleeding should also receive fresh frozen plasma. Underlying metabolic derangements should be corrected. Insulin is not necessary for nondiabetics with hyperglycemia and may be dangerous, particularly if there is coexisting hypokalemia. Similarly, hyperkalemia does not usually require specific therapy and usually resolves with fluid administration and correction of acidosis. Because acetaminophen is unlikely to be effective, physical measures (e.g., cooling blankets and sponging) are preferred for the treatment of fever. Tetany resulting from respiratory alkalosis may be treated with the slow intravenous administration of 10% calcium chloride or gluconate (0.1–0.2 mL/kg); it is effective and longer lasting, and can safely be given to patients with normal serum calcium levels.

Gastrointestinal decontamination should be performed in patients with accidental ingestions of more than 150 mg/kg and in all patients with intentional overdoses. Even in patients with spontaneous vomiting, large amounts of salicylate have been recovered as long as 18 hours after ingestion; hence the adage "it's never too late to aspirate [the stomach] with salicylate." Optimal decontamination may be accomplished by administering a dose of charcoal before as well as after gastric lavage. Because charcoal binds neutral agents better than ionzed ones, salicylate may desorb from charcoal in the alkaline milieu of the small intestine. At least two doses of charcoal should, therefore, be given. Charcoal alone may be preferable to ipecac followed by charcoal in patients with mild to moderate overdoses.

Salicylate elimination can be enhanced by administering repeated oral doses of activated charcoal, alkaline diuresis, and extracorporeal removal. Multiple-dose charcoal can shorten the salicylate half-life to 2 to 4 hours in patients with salicylate levels as high as 66 mg/dL after acute overdosage. It can be given to almost all patients but may be less effective in those with chronic poisoning or higher levels.

Alkaline diuresis can shorten the salicylate half-life to 6 to 12 hours in acute overdose patients with salicylate levels less than 70 mg/dL. Although urinary alkalinization alone was reported to be more effective than either diuresis alone or alkaline diuresis, patients treated by "alkalinization alone" actually received 375 mL to 500 mL/h over the treatment period. Hence alkalinization and diuresis are both important, but overdiuresis (more than 500 mL/h) may be detrimental. As with charcoal, the efficacy of alkaline diuresis is likely to be less in those patients with chronic salicylism or very high salicylate levels.

Indications for alkaline diuresis include acid–base abnormalities, the presence of symptoms, and elevated salicylate levels (more than 30 mg/dL) within 18 hours of an acute overdose. Patients who present more than 18 hours after an acute ingestion or have chronic poisoning may require treatment despite "therapeutic" salicylate levels. Contraindications to alkaline diuresis include cerebral and pulmonary edema, congestive heart failure, oliguric renal failure, and a serum pH greater than 7.55. The aggressiveness of alkaline diuresis treatment should be based on the severity of poisoning. Therapy should be individualized according to laboratory findings. The goal of alkalinization is a urine pH of 7.5 or greater. However, even during early (mild) intoxication, when the urine pH is alkaline, low doses of bicarbonate should be given to replace ongoing renal losses.

Carbonic anhydrase inhibitors (e.g., acetazolamide) should not be used to alkalinize the urine because they may also cause acidemia and enhance the distribution of salicylate. This may result in increased CNS salicylate levels and clinical deterioration. It is essential that adequate hydration and urine output be established before initiating alkaline diuresis. Because potassium reabsorption occurs at the expense of hydrogen ion excretion, it may be impossible to alkalinize the urine until potassium deficits are corrected.

Complications of the therapy include excessive alkalemia, hypokalemia, hypocalcemia, hypernatremia, and fluid overload with cerebral and pulmonary edema, particularly in the elderly and those with severe poisoning. Hence all patients treated with alkaline diuresis should have cardiac monitoring, frequent vital signs, mental status and cardiorespiratory examinations, laboratory evaluation (arterial blood gas analysis and serum electrolytes), and hourly monitoring of fluid intake, urinary output, and urine pH. If intake should persistently exceed output, diuresis may be enhanced by administering furosemide.

Hemodialysis is the treatment of choice for patients with severe salicylate poisoning. A reduction in the salicylate half-life to 2 to 3 hours can be achieved. Although hemoperfusion is slightly more effective in removing salicylate, it is technically more difficult and will not correct associated acid–base, fluid, and electrolyte abnormalities. Peritoneal dialysis (with 5% albumin added to compete with serum proteins for salicylate binding) and exchange transfusion are less effective and should be used only if hemodialysis is unavailable, contraindicated, or technically impossible (e.g., in infants or in patients with active or recent bleeding complications).

Indications for hemodialysis include coma, seizures, cerebral or pulmonary edema, renal failure, and clinical deterioration or failure to improve despite intensive noninvasive therapy. Although in acute poisoning severe toxicity is usually associated with very high salicylate levels (more than 100 mg/dL), patients with high levels without complications do not necessarily need hemodialysis. Conversely, acute or chronic overdose patients with severe toxicity or underlying cardiopulmonary disease should be treated with hemodialysis even if salicylate levels are not markedly elevated.

DISPOSITION

Patients with mild or absent clinical and laboratory toxicity after acute overdose can often be treated in the emergency department if the salicylate level is less that 60 mg/dL. Patients with chronic poisoning, higher levels, underlying medical problems, and moderate or severe toxicity should be admitted to an intensive care unit. A nephrologist should be consulted if poisoning is severe. If hemodialysis is not available, patients with severe poisoning or moderate poisoning with very high (or rising) salicylate levels should be transferred to a facility where such treatment is available.

COMMON PITFALLS

- Failure to order a serum salicylate level on patients with unexplained acid–base disturbance, particularly those with altered mental status
- Failure to obtain quantitative levels of both aspirin and acetaminophen in patients whose history cannot be verified by a third party or by examination of the drug or its container
- Failure to obtain multiple salicylate levels to rule out delayed absorption and to assess the efficacy of decontamination and elimination therapies
- Failure to treat with multiple doses of activated charcoal
- Failure to monitor for complications of both salicylate poisoning and its treatment
- Failure to recognize the limitations of salicylate levels and to treat the patient, not the level

105   Terpene Poisoning

Terpenes are a class of unsaturated, aliphatic cyclic hydrocarbons. These volatile substances are found naturally in oils and oleoresins of plants and flowers. Camphor, pine oils, and turpentine are the most common terpenes involved in poisoning. Terpenes are also present in volatile oils of plants. Camphor is a naturally occurring cyclic ketone obtained from the camphor tree or synthesized from turpentine oil. Camphor is well absorbed orally. Absorption may also occur through the skin. It is classified as very toxic, class 4, with lethal doses in humans ranging from 50 mg to 500 mg/kg. Ingestions of 10 mg to 30 mg/kg, equivalent to one swallow of camphorated oil, may result in minor symptoms. Major symptoms are uncommon below ingestions of 50 mg/kg. The acute toxic dose of turpentine has never been well defined; quantities of turpentine greater than 2 mL/kg should be considered potentially toxic. Pine oils have about one fifth the toxicity of turpentine; a suggested lethal dose for adults is 60 g to 120 g, although survival after a 400-mL ingestion is reported.

Camphorated oil was removed from the market in 1982. Turpentine is highly volatile. Vapors are easily inhaled, and aspiration of the liquid may occur during ingestion. It is well absorbed from the gastrointestinal tract. Because thickening agents are added to increase the viscosity of pine oil products, the risk of aspiration is decreased. The vast majority of ingestions are accidental and involve small amounts. It is rare to see toxicity from the gastrointestinal absorption of pine oil, but aspiration is a common problem.

CLINICAL PRESENTATION

Patients with terpene ingestion frequently have a strong odor of camphor, turpentine, or pine oil on the breath, in vomitus, or in the urine. Mild camphor poisoning results in gastrointestinal symptoms such as nausea, vomiting, and a burning sensation in the mouth, esophagus, and stomach. In some cases central nervous system (CNS) toxicity initially presents as stimulation and restlessness. Central nervous system depression with delirium, hallucinations, confusion, muscle irritability, and seizures may follow. Symptoms can occur as soon as 5 to 30 minutes after ingestion, and seizures have occurred as soon as 4 minutes after ingestion.

Turpentine causes similar gastrointestinal irritation and CNS symptoms; however, the frequency of seizures appears to be less than with camphor. Direct skin contact with turpentine can be very irritating. A single case of acute renal failure and hemorrhagic cystitis several days after ingestion has been reported. Turpentine has been implicated in the pathogenesis of thrombocytopenic purpura.

The breath odor of a patient with pine oil ingestion is characteristically violetlike from the metabolites that are excreted in exhaled air. Patients usually present with gastroenteral symptoms and respiratory symptoms from aspiration. Central nervous system toxicity (e.g., somnolence and ataxia) is usually mild. Patients with camphor poisoning may show a transient leukocytosis and modest abnormalities on liver function tests. Hepatotoxicity has also been reported after massive pine oil ingestions.

DIFFERENTIAL DIAGNOSIS

If the history is vague or unavailable, the odor of the patient's breath, vomitus, or urine may be a valuable diagnostic clue. Naphthalene, paradichlorobenzene, and other volatile oils have a vaguely similar aroma.

EMERGENCY DEPARTMENT EVALUATION

As in all toxic exposures, identification of the product, content, amount, time since exposure, and symptoms is essential. Physical examination should focus on CNS and gastrointestinal symptoms. Patients should be assessed for signs and symptoms of aspiration. Any emesis should be tested for blood. Routine laboratory studies include baseline complete blood count (CBC) with platelets, determination of electrolyte, blood urea nitrogen, creatinine, and glucose levels, and urinalysis. Arterial blood gas analysis and chest radiography should be performed if aspiration is suspected.

EMERGENCY DEPARTMENT MANAGEMENT

Because of the potentially rapid onset of seizures and pulmonary toxicity, an ambulance should be used for transport of these patients. ALS should be instituted as necessary. Patients who are symptomatic and have ingested more than 2 g or 30 mg/kg of camphor or 2 mL/kg of turpentine should have gastric emptying. Because of the risk of aspiration with CNS depression and seizures, syrup of ipecac should not be used after camphor ingestion. Gastric lavage with airway protection, or activated charcoal, is preferred. Mineral oil and vegetable oil were formerly recommended as solvents or cathartics for camphor. Because their use may increase the risk of aspiration and enhance the absorption of camphor, they are no longer recommended. Renal, hepatic, and bone marrow complications should be treated supportively. Lipid hemodialysis against soybean oil and Amberlite resin hemoperfusion have been used in patients with severe camphor poisoning. These measures are not of benefit in patients who have ingested pine oil because of its large volume of distribution.

DISPOSITION

Patients who remain asymptomatic or have only mild gastrointestinal symptoms during the 6 hours after ingestion are at low risk for serious complications and may be discharged. Patients with systemic symptoms or evidence of aspiration and those who have clearly ingested more than 3 g of camphor should be admitted for observation. Patients with seizures or CNS depression should be admitted to an ICU. Symptomatic patients should also be monitored for hematologic, renal, and hepatic complications. Patients with persistent seizures or coma after camphor ingestion should be considered for hemodialysis or hemoperfusion.

COMMON PITFALLS

- Patients who are discharged should be advised to return if any respiratory symptoms develop.
- Small amounts of camphor may be toxic (e.g., a "swallow" of 10% camphor).
- Patients with potentially toxic camphor ingestions need to have early intravenous access, since the onset of seizures can occur early and without warning.
- The risk of aspiration with syrup of ipecac or gastric lavage makes activated charcoal the preferred method of gastric decontamination.
- Symptomatic patients should have hematologic, renal, and hepatic function parameters monitored.

106   Tricyclic Antidepressant Poisoning

The tricyclic antidepressants (TCAs; amitriptyline, amoxapine, desipramine, doxepin, imipramine, nortriptyline, protriptyline, and trimipramine) are widely used for the treatment of depression, enuresis, and migraine. Up to half of all poison-related ICU admissions involve these drugs. Although the in-hospital mortality rate is <3%, the risk of death is ever present, particularly in the first 6 hours after an acute overdose.

TCAs have rapid initial absorption and an equally rapid onset of symptoms. However, as blood levels rise, anticholinergic effects cause delayed gastric emptying and a prolonged absorptive phase. It is not uncommon to recover pill fragments from the stomach 18 or more hours after an overdose. In addition, TCAs are more than 95% protein and tissue bound. This, combined with their large volumes of distribution and extended elimination half-lives (from 12 to 96 hours, depending on the drug), enhances and prolongs their toxicity.

Therapeutic doses of TCAs range from 10 to 300 mg per day, and therapeutic blood levels are 150 to 300 ng/mL. The acute ingestion of 10 mg to 15 mg/kg of a TCA is likely to cause mild to moderate toxicity, and ingestions of 20 mg to 30 mg/kg may result in severe or fatal poisoning.

The clinical effects of the TCAs on the central and autonomic nervous systems, the myocardium, and the peripheral vascular apparatus stem from their four main pharmacologic actions (Table 106-1). With the exception of amoxapine, they all have similar toxicity. Amoxapine produces fewer cardiac effects but a higher incidence of seizures. It may also cause renal failure secondary to rhabdomyolysis.

TABLE 106-1. Pharmacologic Actions and Toxicity of Tricyclic Antidepressants

Pharmacologic Action	System Affected	Clinical Toxicity
Anticholinergic effects	ANS	Dilated pupils, dry mouth, tachycardia, hyperpyrexia, urinary retention Delayed gastric emptying, decreased gastric motility
	CNS	Delerium, agitation, coma, (?) seizures
Peripheral alpha receptor blockade	PV	Hypotension
Quinidine-like effects	CV	1st-, 2nd-, 3rd-degree heart block, ventricular conduction delays, premature ventricular contractions, bundle-branch blocks, ventricular tachycardia/fibrillation, cardiogenic hypotension, asystole
Inhibition of norepinephrine reuptake at nerve terminal	CV CNS(?)	Ventricular irritability/arrhythmias ?Coma, ?seizures

ANS, autonomic nervous system; CNS, central nervous system; PV, peripheral vascular system; CV, cardiovascular system.

CLINICAL PRESENTATION

Early in the course of an overdose patients may exhibit mild anticholinergic signs, nervousness, and drowsiness. As absorption progresses (or with massive overdoses) a rapidly progressive and potentially lethal toxicity may supervene. It is not unusual for a patient to progress from mild lethargy to deep coma, hypotension, seizures, and ventricular arrhythmias within 30 minutes of presentation. For this reason any patient who presents with a suspected TCA overdose must be given the highest triage priority, regardless of his or her clinical appearance on presentation.

Major central nervous system or cardiac complications usually occur by 6 hours post overdose or not at all. Thus, determining the time of overdose is important. If major symptoms fail to develop by 6 hours or after 4 hours of observation (whichever is longer), it is unlikely that a severe overdose has occurred. There are no rapidly available blood tests that allow for ED diagnosis. Laboratory measurement of serum TCA levels may ultimately identify the offending drug, but treatment must be initiated long before those tests become available. Additionally, quantitative measurements of serum TCA levels may not be useful.

Blood levels do not reliably predict severity, and QRS prolongation often occurs with serum TCA levels <1000 ng/mL. However, limb-lead QRS duration, which is usually maximal by 6 hours post overdose, can be used to place patients into one of three specific risk categories independent of TCA levels. When the maximal limb-lead QRS duration is <0.10 seconds, patients are at negligible risk for seizures and ventricular arrhythmias. Seizures can occur at any QRS greater than or equal to 0.10 seconds, but ventricular arrhythmias are seen only in those with a QRS greater than or equal to 0.16 seconds. Seizures occur in 33% with a QRS greater than or equal to 0.10 seconds, and ventricular arrhythmias occur in 50% with a QRS greater than or equal to 0.16 seconds. These findings are not applicable to patients with amoxapine poisoning or underlying cardiac conduction defects and may not be predictive in patients with polydrug overdose.

DIFFERENTIAL DIAGNOSIS

Hypoxia, metabolic abnormalities, and intrinsic neurologic and cardiac disease should be considered. Beta blockers, propoxyphene, quinidine, procainamide, and the phenothiazines all slow cardiac conduction and widen the QRS interval. With the exception of procainamide, they can also cause seizures. Consequently, on clinical grounds alone, it may be difficult to distinguish an overdose with these drugs from an overdose with TCA. Although atropine, glutethimide, camphor, isoniazid, lidocaine, and antihistamines may cause coma and seizures, they seldom produce ventricular arrhythmias. Finally, seizures and ventricular arrhythmias can be seen after abrupt withdrawal from sedative–hypnotic drugs and in poisoning with cocaine, amphetamines, caffeine, chloral hydrate, and lithium, but with these conditions the QRS duration is normal.

EMERGENCY DEPARTMENT EVALUATION

All patients with suspected or proven TCA overdose must be regarded as potentially life-threatening emergencies, regardless of the clinical status on presentation. A medication history should be obtained. If possible, the exact time of the overdose, the total number of medications ingested, and the quantity of each should be ascertained. Vital signs and neurologic status must initially be monitored at least every 15 minutes. In addition to continuous cardiac monitoring, an immediate ECG should be obtained. The limb-lead QRS durations should initially be measured every 30 minutes. Blood and urine should be sent for toxicologic analysis. Serum TCA (parent drug plus major metabolite), electrolyte, blood urea nitrogen, and glucose levels, arterial blood gas analysis, and any other laboratory studies appropriate to the patient's underlying medical condition should be obtained. Patients with coma, hypotension, or seizures frequently have a metabolic acidosis or a combined metabolic and respiratory acidosis.

EMERGENCY DEPARTMENT MANAGEMENT

ALS should be instituted as necessary. Vigilant critical care with an eye to complications (e.g., aspiration, myocardial infarction in the elderly) must be maintained. Gastric decontamination should proceed without delay. Syrup of ipecac is contraindicated because patients can develop seizures or arrhythmias during the time interval between dosing and emesis. Lavage with a large-bore orogastric tube, preceded and followed by a dose of activated charcoal, may be optimal. Intubation for airway protection is recommended. Repeated doses of activated charcoal should be given until the patient is asymptomatic and ECG abnormalities have been resolved. The ability of activated charcoal to bind TCAs in the stomach and of repeated doses to interrupt the enterohepatic cycle cannot be overemphasized. Myoclonic jerks are common and should not be confused with true seizures.

Seizures should be treated with diazepam (5 to 10 mg IV in adults and 0.1–0.3 mg/kg IV in children, repeated as necessary) while phenytoin is being prepared for intravenous infusion. Phenytoin (17 mg/kg) should be administered by a continuous infusion in normal saline solution. Recalcitrant seizures, as seen with amoxapine overdose, may require neuromuscular paralysis (e.g., pancuronium) to prevent complications. EEG monitoring and continued seizure treatment are necessary during paralysis. Hypotension is treated initially with a crystalloid fluid bolus. Because many patients with TCA overdose develop pulmonary edema or the adult respiratory distress syndrome, norepinephrine should be used if the patient remains hypotensive after the administration of 10 mL to 20 mL/kg of intravenous fluid. Dopamine may worsen hypotension (due to unopposed peripheral vascular beta effect).

Patients with severe overdose may develop preterminal bradycardia and cardiogenic hypotension. These patients may require a temporary transvenous pacemaker if norepinephrine fails to produce a positive response. Patients usually die of ventricular arrhythmias or cardiac standstill. Prolonged resuscitation is warranted since patients who can be salvaged almost always recover completely. The optimal treatment of cardiotoxicity is controversial. Phenytoin, in the same dosage as for seizures, is the antiarrhythmic of choice for ventricular arrhythmias and conduction defects.

QRS narrowing may be observed during phenytoin infusion. However, because it takes 20 to 40 minutes to administer a full therapeutic dose of phenytoin, boluses of lidocaine and sodium bicarbonate should be given to patients with malignant arrhythmias while phenytoin is being prepared and infused. Sodium bicarbonate has the ability to reverse arrhythmias. The usual bolus dose is 1 mEq/kg. Bicarbonate should be given to normalize the pH in patients who are acidotic and a lidocaine drip can be used if phenytoin fails. Maintaining the pH in the range of 7.45 to 7.50 has been recommended for the prevention of cardiotoxicity.

Quinidine and procainamide aggravate cardiac complications and are contraindicated. The risks of physostigmine (e.g., asystole) outweigh its unproven benefits.

DISPOSITION

Consultation with a toxicologist or the regional poison control center is highly recommended. Psychiatric evaluation is necessary in all cases of intentional overdose. In the toddler or nonsuicidal elderly patient consultation with social services may be appropriate. Patients with coma, hypotension, seizures, arrhythmias, or a persistent QRS duration >0.10 seconds should be admitted to an ICU, regardless of the TCA level. In patients with severe poisoning ICU monitoring should be continued for 24 hours after signs and symptoms of toxicity have resolved. If an ICU is not available, the patient should be transferred to a center where one is available. Patients with a maximal limb-lead QRS of <0.10 seconds and serum TCA levels under 500 ng/mL who have received charcoal and remain asymptomatic after 4 hours of observation may be discharged or referred for psychiatric evaluation. Although similar patients with higher TCA levels are probably at very low risk for subsequent complications, admission to a telemetry unit or an extended period of ED observation (with a repeat dose of charcoal) may be prudent.

COMMON PITFALLS

- The most common mistake is to assume that a patient who is awake or appears stable has not taken a serious overdose.
- Failure to closely monitor the patient's cardiac rhythm and QRS duration.
- Failure to perform gastrointestinal decontamination, including administration of activated charcoal, regardless of the time since overdose.
- Failure to treat seizures aggressively in order to prevent acidosis and subsequent cardiac arrhythmias.
- Physostigmine may precipitate a cholinergic crisis, seizures, or asystole and should be used only as a last resort.

107   Theophylline and Caffeine Poisoning

Theophylline (1,3-dimethylxanthine) is commonly prescribed for the treatment of asthma, apnea of premature infants, and chronic obstructive pulmonary disease (COPD). It is available as anhydrous theophylline or as a variety of salts. Therapeutic oral doses range from 13 mg to 24 mg/kg/d, usually administered in divided doses.

Caffeine (1,3,7-trimethylxanthine) is a naturally occurring alkaloid contained in beverages such as coffee (60–180 mg/5 oz), tea (20–60 mg/5 oz), chocolate milk (2–7 mg/8 oz), cola soft drinks (45 mg/12 oz) and in chocolate candy bars (7 mg per bar). It is also contained in analgesic preparations and over-the-counter diet and "wake-up" pills in doses of 15–100 mg. Street-drug capsules that contain caffeine, phenylpropanolamine, and ephedrine are sold as stimulants. Since 1983 the marketing of products that contain combinations of caffeine and ephedrine, pseudoephedrine, or phenylpropanolamine is illegal in the United States.

Methylxanthines are rapidly absorbed after ingestion, with peak blood levels occurring in 1 to 2 hours. With sustained-release preparations peak levels are maintained for 6 to 24 hours. Absorption is prolonged and peak blood levels are delayed after overdosage, particularly with sustained-release preparations. Therapeutic serum levels are 10 μg to 20 μg/mL for theophylline. Theophylline is eliminated by hepatic metabolism (90%) and urinary excretion of unchanged drug (10%). The half-life is age-dependent and influenced by concomitant drug therapy and illnesses. It averages 20 hours in newborns, 6 to 7 hours in infants, 3 to 5 hours with age 6 months to 18 years, and 4 to 6 hours for adults. Hepatic elimination is increased by beta agonist and antiepileptic drugs (carbamazepine, phenobarbital, and phenytoin) and decreased by allopurinol, caffeine, cephalexin, cimetidine, congestive heart failure, erythromycin, fever, liver disease, nifedipine, oral contraceptives, propranolol, ranitidine, and tetracycline.

Therapeutic and adverse effects of theophylline are primarily due to the inhibition of adenosine synthesis resulting in central nervous system stimulation, reduction of the ventricular fibrillation threshold, smooth-muscle relaxation, and gastric acid and pepsin secretion. Cardiovascular effects also result from epinephrine and norepinephrine release.

Caffeine is the most potent central nervous system stimulant of the methylxanthines, and exerts its action on different regions of the brain. Caffeine stimulates the cortex (increases alertness and enhances performance). Toxic effects of caffeine are simply the result of increased pharmacologic effects. Poisoning may result from chronic (therapeutic) oral overdose, acute ingestion of more than 10 mg/kg, or excessive intravenous dosing. Fewer than 15 deaths from caffeine intoxication have been reported.

CLINICAL PRESENTATION

Initial symptoms of poisoning include nausea, vomiting, and abdominal pain. Diarrhea and gastrointestinal bleeding may develop later. Spontaneous vomiting may limit drug absorption, especially with caffeine ingestions. Additional signs and symptoms may include headache, insomnia, agitation, delirium, tinnitus, tremors, hypertonicity, jitteriness, seizures, coma, and tachyarrhythmias.

Ventricular and supraventricular tachyarrhythmias may result from a decrease of the ventricular fibrillation threshold, a nonuniform increase in the cardiac conduction velocity that favors re-entry phenomena, and the liberation of catecholamine. Hypokalemia and reduced oxygen delivery in the face of increased demand by the myocardium seen with theophylline overdoses might also precipitate arrhythmias. The arrhythmias are concentration- and age-dependent. Patients over age 40 are at greater risk of developing serious cardiac arrhythmias when serum theophylline concentrations are >35 μg/mL. In contrast, serum concentrations >50 μg/mL are necessary to induce serious arrhythmias in younger patients (age 40 or less). At low dose, theophylline induces a mild and transitory hypertension. However, at high dose, the direct effect of theophylline on the beta$_2$ adrenoreceptors reduces the total peripheral resistance, inducing a fall in blood pressure.

Seizures are usually generalized but can be focal. The neurotoxicity of theophylline seems to be dose-dependent. However, other factors also influence the development of neurotoxicity.

After an acute theophylline overdose (single ingestion), patients aged 6 months to 60 years may develop life-threatening arrhythmias or seizures when serum concentrations exceed 80 μg/mL. For the same age group serious toxic manifestations can occur with serum concentrations above 60 μg/mL with a chronic intoxication. Patients younger than age 6 months or older than age 60 years may experience serious toxic manifestations with serum concentrations above 30 μg/mL, regardless of the type of intoxication.

Some patients may present with coma, gastrointestinal bleeding, hyperventilation, polyuria, or hyperthermia. Laboratory evaluation may reveal leukocytosis, hyperglycemia, hypokalemia, hypophosphatemia, ketosis, metabolic acidosis, and respiratory alkalosis. Decreased serum calcium and magnesium levels, elevated serum amylase and uric acid levels, and evidence of dehydration (elevated blood urea nitrogen and creatinine levels) or rhabdomyolysis (elevated creatine phosphokinase level and myoglobinuria) may be noted.

DIFFERENTIAL DIAGNOSIS

Since the clinical effects of methylxanthine poisoning can be characterized as a "beta-adrenergic storm," poisoning by direct-acting beta agonists (i.e., other asthma therapies such as isoetharine, metaproterenol, and albuterol) can cause an indistinguishable clinical picture. Poisoning by amphetamines, sympathomimetics, anticholinergics, hallucinogens, MAO inhibitors, and epinephrine should also be considered. Agitated psychiatric states, drug withdrawal, and medical conditions such as CNS infections, electrolyte disturbance, hypoglycemia, hypocalcemia, pheochromocytoma, and thyroid storm may cause similar signs and symptoms.

EMERGENCY DEPARTMENT EVALUATION

The history should include the time, amount, and formulation of theophylline or caffeine ingested, past or recent therapeutic use of these agents, and routine medical history. Symptoms before arrival should be noted. The maximal serum drug level (micrograms per milliliter) can be estimated by multiplying the ingested dose (milligrams per kilogram) by 2.

The physical examination should focus on vital signs, mental status and neurologic evaluation, cardiorespiratory status, and gastrointestinal function. Vomitus and stool should be checked for overt or occult blood.

Laboratory evaluation should include a quantitative theophylline or caffeine level, complete blood count, electrolytes, glucose, blood urea nitrogen, creatinine levels, and urinalysis. Patients with elevated theophylline levels and moderate or severe clinical toxicity should also have measurements of serum amylase, calcium, creatine phosphokinase, ketones, magnesium, and phosphorus levels, arterial blood gas analysis, and measurement of urine myoglobin level. Cardiac monitoring and an ECG should be obtained on all patients. Patients with respiratory symptoms, abnormal pulmonary examination or ECG, and coma or seizures should have a chest radiograph.

EMERGENCY DEPARTMENT MANAGEMENT

ALS should be instituted as necessary. After an acute oral overdose gastrointestinal decontamination should be undertaken if the patient is seen within 2 to 4 hours of ingestion (longer if slow-release preparations have been ingested). Activated charcoal significantly reduces the absorption of theophylline. Since peak serum concentrations may not occur for many hours after ingestion (up to 24 hours with slow-release preparations), every patient with an oral theophylline overdose should receive activated charcoal, regardless of the alleged time of ingestion. A dose of 0.5 g to 1.0 g/kg of body weight should be given every 2 to 4 hours until the patient has a charcoal stool. If the patient cannot tolerate charcoal because of persistent vomiting, the administration of smaller but more frequent doses (continuous infusion by way of nasogastric tube if necessary), metaclopramide (up to 1 mg/kg), ranitidine (50 mg IV), or droperidol (2.5 mg IV) may be used. The repetitive administration of activated charcoal also enhances the total body clearance of theophylline. Serial measurements of theophylline levels are necessary until it is evident that they have peaked. Although not studied, the effects of charcoal on caffeine absorption and elimination are predicted to be similar and the same approach to gastrointestinal decontamination is recommended for patients with caffeine overdose.

The serious morbidity and mortality from seizures seem to be in direct correlation with their duration. Therefore, seizures should be stopped rapidly. Diazepam should be given first. If the seizures do not stop rapidly or recur, phenobarbital (15 mg/kg) should be administered intravenously. In the absence of an adequate response (in which seizures do not stop within 20–30 minutes), thiopental should be administered; a loading dose of 3 mg to 5 mg/kg followed by an infusion of 2 mg to 4 mg/kg/h is usually efficacious, but these doses can be increased if necessary. Phenytoin is less likely to be effective. In some patients neuromuscular paralysis (e.g., pancuronium) may be necessary to stop muscle contraction, facilitate ventilation, and prevent hyperthermia and rhabdomyolysis. EEG monitoring and continued treatment of seizures are necessary during paralysis. Permanent neurologic damage is not infrequent in patients with prolonged coma or intractable seizures.

Propranolol is the drug of choice for the treatment of both supraventricular and ventricular arrhythmias. Intravenous doses of 1 mg in adults or 0.02 mg/kg in children should be given slowly and repeated every 5 to 10 minutes until arrhythmias are stopped, or to a maximal dose of 0.1 mg/kg. Lidocaine may also be used for ventricular arrhythmias. Although propranolol is normally contraindicated in patients with asthma or COPD, it has been used in asthmatics with acute theophylline poisoning. The short-acting beta antagonist esmolol may be preferable. Bronchospasm is an absolute contraindication to the use of beta blockers.

Correction of hypoxemia, acidosis, hypokalemia, and other metabolic abnormalities is essential and should further reduce the risk of arrhythmias. Hyperglycemia is transitory and well tolerated, and usually does not necessitate insulin therapy. Hypotension should initially be treated with fluid administration. Persistent hypotension may be treated with pressors (e.g., dopamine and norepinephrine) or propranolol (because of its beta$_2$ blocking effect). Hyperthermia and rhabdomyolysis should be treated with standard measures.

DISPOSITION

Patients should be admitted to a monitored bed if their theophylline serum concentrations are >35 µg/mL. Patients with severe neurologic or cardiotoxic manifestations and serum concentrations >50 µg/mL should be admitted to an ICU. Those with levels <35 µg/mL and mild symptoms can usually be treated in the ED and discharged when they become asymptomatic.

Consultation with a nephrologist and arrangements for charcoal hemoperfusion should be accomplished for patients with the following criteria: persistently unstable hemodynamic parameters; seizures; or theophylline serum concentrations >80–100 µg/mL after an acute ingestion, 60 µg/mL after a chronic ingestion, and >40 µg/mL after an acute or chronic intoxication if age is <6 months or >60 years or there is severe underlying cardiovascular disease. Similar parameters should be used in patients with caffeine poisoning.

Although hemodialysis also enhances the removal of theophylline, it should be used only if hemoperfusion is not available. Exchange transfusion has also been used in neonates with caffeine intoxication when hemoperfusion is technically difficult. If ICU and extracorporeal treatment are not available, the patient should be transferred to a facility with these capabilities.

COMMON PITFALLS

- When interpreting theophylline serum concentrations, consider the age of the patient, the type of intoxication (acute versus chronic), and underlying diseases (previous neurologic or cardiac problems).
- Seizures must be aggressively treated in order to prevent acidosis, hyperthermia, rhabdomyolysis, and permanent neurologic damage.
- Serial theophylline levels are necessary to assess for delayed and prolonged absorption and to assess the results of treatment.
- Although beta blockers can reverse much of the toxicity caused by theophylline overdose, the risks must be weighed against the benefits in patients with asthma or COPD.
- Hypotension (not hypertension) is characteristic of significant caffeine or theophylline poisoning.

SECTION IV

ENVIRONMENTAL EMERGENCIES

108   Animal Bites

Thousands of people throughout the world are killed each year by sharks, crocodiles, pachy-derms, big cats, and other large carnivores. Ten to 20 fatal dog attacks occur in the US each year, almost always involving children. Dogs and cats inflict 95% of bites, and tend to bite the extremities of adults and older children and the face and scalp of younger children and infants. Infectious complications are often responsible for serious morbidity and mortality. Dog bites are usually crush-type lacerations with devitalized adjacent tissue. About 10% become infected. Cat bites tend to be puncture wounds with an infection rate of up to 50%.

Animal bites may inoculate the site with a host of potential pathogens, including tetanus and rabies viruses, *Staphylococcus aureus*, *Streptococcus* species, *Klebsiella*, *Enterobacter* species, and anaerobes. *Pasteurella multocida,* a small gram-negative rod that is part of the nor-mal mouth flora of many animals, has been implicated in up to 30% of infected dog bites and in 50% of infected cat bites. This organism typically produces a rapidly developing inflammatory response in the wound, often with purulent drainage, within 24–48 hours. *P. multocida* may also cause cellulitis, abscess, osteomyelitis, septic arthritis, meningitis, and septicemia. Fastidious gram-negative bacilli DF-2 can infect dog and cat bites and lead to often rapidly fatal bacteremia, DIC, or meningitis. Although most common in immunocompromised patients, these infections have been reported in normal hosts.

CLINICAL PRESENTATION

Animal bites can lead to trauma of the skin, tendons, joints, bones, major vessels, viscera, brain, and other organs. The cause of death in immediately fatal cases is usually hemorrhagic shock. Patients who present >24 hours after injury usually have signs of established local or systemic infection.

Rat bite fever caused by *S. moniliformis* typically shows sudden fever, chills, headache, and myalgias several days (range 1–22 days) after a bite by a wild, laboratory, or pet rodent or carnivore, or the ingestion of food contaminated by rat excreta. A rash (macular, petechial, pur-puric, or pustular; centripetal or generalized) and asymmetrical polyarthralgia or arthritis may also be present. Complications include soft-tissue and brain abscesses and endocarditis. Patients with *S. minus* infection usually develop relapsing fever, headache (with nausea, vomiting, and pho-tophobia), and signs of nonpurulent local infection with regional lymphangitis and adenopathy sev-eral weeks (range 1–36 days) after the initial healing of the bite wound. A rash (macular, with brown or purple hue) may be noted on the extremities.

Patients with tularemia usually present with fever, chills, headache, malaise, myalgias, ten-der hepatosplenomegaly, wound ulcer, and regional adenopathy 2 to 5 days after a bite or direct or indirect skin contact with virtually any animal (e.g., amphibians, birds, fish, or mammals). Skin inoculation most frequently results from exposure to wild rabbits (usually cottontails) during skin-ning and preparation for eating and from bites from insect vectors (e.g., ticks, deer flies, and mosquitos). Other animals that commonly harbor *F. tularensis* include beaver, cats, cattle, muskrats, sheep, and squirrels. The initial skin lesion (a bite or puncture wound or contaminated scratch) develops into a well-defined ulcer with a black base and yellow exudate. A macular rash may be present, and lymph nodes may suppurate and drain spontaneously. Contamination of the eye, throat and intestines (ingestion), or lung (inhalation) may also lead to conjunctivitis, pharyngitis, gastroenteritis, or pneumonia, and regional lymphadenopathy. Complications include endocarditis, meningitis, osteomyelitis, pericarditis, and peritonitis.

Routine laboratory findings in cat-scratch disease (see pediatric section), rat-bite fever, and tularemia are nonspecific (i.e., elevated leukocyte count and erythrocyte sedimention rate).

DIFFERENTIAL DIAGNOSIS

Envenomations should be considered in bites by lizards (i.e., gila monster), snakes, marine animals, and the short-tailed shrew. The differential diagnosis of cat-scratch disease, rat-bite fever, and tularemia is extensive, and includes infections such as plague, syphilis, lymphogranuloma venereum, sporotrichosis, anthrax, histoplasmosis, coccidioidomycosis, infectious mononucleosis, toxoplasmosis, brucellosis, bacterial adenitis, and infections with *Mycobacteria, Rickettsia, Staphylococcus,* and *Streptococcus.* Sarcoid, lymphoma, and cysts and tumors of the neck should also be considered.

EMERGENCY DEPARTMENT EVALUATION

Evaluation should include attention to basic trauma care, particularly when a small victim is attacked by a large animal. Details of the biting event include: time, offending animal, identity (wild versus domestic, immunization and health status, captured or not), and nature of the attack (provoked versus unprovoked). The health status of the victim should also be determined. The patient should be assessed for deep structure injury, particularly of the brain, vessels, viscera, nerves, tendons, joints, bones, and spinal cord. Puncture wounds are particularly prone to cause deep and often undiagnosed injuries. Wounds on the hand, wrist, foot, or joint, or on the face and scalp of an infant increase the likelihood of deep structure injury.

Local complications include wound infection, cellulitis, abscess, osteomyelitis, prosthesis infection, and septic arthritis (even when the joint is not penetrated). Local wound infections that develop <24 hours after the bite are probably caused by either *P. multocida* or streptococci. Local infections that develop >48 hours after the bite are most frequently caused by *S. aureus.* Systemic complications include bacterial sepsis, meningitis, DIC, cat-scratch disease, rat-bite fever, tetanus, tularemia and rabies. Risk of infection is high in the very young, the very old, or the immunocompromised (those with alcoholism, splenectomy, diabetes mellitus, liver dysfunction, AIDS, or those on immunosuppressive medication). Risk of infection is also high in those who have prosthetic joints or valves, or have peripheral vascular or lymphatic compromise.Other risk factors include cat bites, puncture wounds, location on a hand, wrist, foot, or joint, and treatment delay beyond 8 hours.

Although Gram's stain and culture of fresh bites are not useful, Gram's stain and culture (aerobic and anaerobic) should be obtained in infected wounds. If sepsis is suspected, Gram's stain of the peripheral blood should be examined for evidence of the DF-2 organism, and blood cultures (anaerobic and aerobic) should be obtained. CBC, BUN, glucose, electrolyte, and creatinine levels, prothrombin time, partial thromboplastin time, fibrin split products, and lumbar puncture with CSF and culture should be obtained if indicated. Extremity radiographs are useful to evaluate the possibility of joint penetration, fracture, foreign body, and osteomyelitis. Skull radiographs and head CT are indicated for infants with face and scalp bites.

The patient with fever, constitutional symptoms, and regional adenopathy should be questioned regarding animal bites, scratches, or exposures and a history of rash or skin lesions. Adenopathy, size and tenderness of lymph nodes, liver, and spleen should be noted. The patient should also be examined for endocarditis, meningitis, and other complications. Further assessment should include CBC, electrolytes, liver and kidney function studies, blood cultures, and chest radiograph. Lumbar puncture, peripheral blood smear, lymph node and skin biopsy examination, skin testing, and antibody titres (acute and convalescent) may be necessary.

EMERGENCY DEPARTMENT MANAGEMENT

Wounds should be assessed for distal function and neurovascular status before local or regional anesthesia. Local anesthetics should preferably be injected through surrounding uninvolved skin. Extremity tourniquets may facilitate exploration and repair. The most important aspect of care is copious high-pressure irrigation with sterile saline solution, 1% povidone-iodine solution (1:10 dilution of the commercial 10% solution), or Pluronic-68. Devitalized tissue should be debrided with a scalpel or fine dissection scissors. Excision of puncture wounds has been recommended but has not proven to be effective. Abrasions should be cleansed and treated with topical antibiotics.

Primary closure of animal bite wounds is controversial. When successful, the benefits are early return of function and optimal cosmetic results. As a general rule, normal hosts with relatively clean lacerations, especially of the face, can safely be sutured if seen within a few hours of injury. Alternatively, sterile skin tapes may result in a lower incidence of infection. Delayed primary closure, often an excellent alternative, and healing by secondary intention are less apt to result in infection. Buried sutures should be avoided whenever possible. All wounded extremities should be immobilized, and strict elevation should be advised.

Antibiotics may decrease the incidence of infection in high-risk situations. Because penicillin is the drug of choice for *P. multocida,* DF-2, streptococci, and most anaerobes, and the semisynthetic penicillins offer excellent coverage of *S. aureus,* the combination of penicillin (500 mg four times a day for 7 days) and dicloxacillin (500 mg four times a day for 7 days) is theoretically attractive. Amoxicillin/clavulanic acid (Augmentin "250" three times a day for 7 days) also offers an appropriately broad spectrum of activity. Semisynthetic penicillins or first-generation cephalosporins are not as effective as penicillin against *P. multocida,* DF-2,8 streptococci, or anaerobes. For penicillin-allergic patients, tetracycline (500 mg four times a day for 7 days) or doxycycline (100 mg twice a day for 7 days) is preferable to erythromycin because of better coverage of *P. multocida.* Erythromycin (500 mg four times a day for 7 days for adults; 50 mg/kg/d in two to four equally divided doses for children) can be used in penicillin-allergic patients who are pregnant, nursing, or < age 9.

IV antibiotic (i.e., penicillin G, 1,000,000 units, plus nafcillin, 1 g; or doxycycline, 100 mg; or erythromycin, 1 g) administration before wound closure, although never formally studied in bites, can produce adequate penetration of the wound coagulum and is advisable in high-risk patients. The course can be completed orally if the patient is discharged.

Septic patients with a history of recent animal bites should be given broad-spectrum IV antibiotics in the ED as soon as Gram's stains and cultures are obtained from wounds, blood, and CSF is obtained if indicated. Imipenem/cilastatin sodium (500 mg IV over 30 minutes) is a reasonable choice for initial therapy pending culture results. If CNS involvement is suspected, a combination of ceftazidime (2 g IV over 5 minutes), nafcillin (2 g IV), and metronidazole (500 mg IV) would be preferable. Abscesses and infections that involve deep structures such as tendon sheaths and joints should be referred to a surgeon for operative management.

Animal bites are tetanus-prone wounds, and immunoprophylaxis should be provided. Rabies transmission is usually by means of saliva contacting a laceration, scratch, abrasion, or mucous membrane. Postexposure prophylaxis is indicated if the offending animal is known or clinically suspected to be rabid or if it is a bat or wild carnivore (e.g., a bobcat, coyote, fox, racoon, skunk, or wolf) (Table 108-1). Livestock and unprovoked dog and cat bites should be considered individually in consultation with public health officials.

Patients bitten by healthy dogs and cats do not require immunization, provided the animal can be observed for 10 days for signs of illness. Rabbit and rodent (e.g., hamster, mouse, rat, and squirrel) bites do not require treatment unless the animal is wild and rabies is endemic in the offending species. Patients who have not been previously immunized should receive both human rabies immune globulin (20 IU/kg), with up to half the dose infiltrated at the bite site if anatomically feasible and the remainder given intramuscularly (i.e., deltoid), and human diploid cell rabies vaccine.

TABLE 108-1. CDC Rabies Postexposure Prophylaxis Guide*

Animal Species	Condition of Animal at Time of Attack	Treatment of Exposed Person†
Domestic		
Dog and cat	Healthy and available for 10 days of observation	None, unless animal develops rabies‡
	Rabid or suspected rabid	RIG^d and HDCV
	Unknown (escaped)	Consult public health officials. If treatment is indicated give RIG§ and HDCV
Wild		
Skunk, bat, fox, coyote, raccoon, bobcat, and other carnivores	Regard as rabid unless proved negative by laboratory tests‖	RIG§ and HDCV
Other		
Livestock, rodents, and lagomorphs (rabbits and hares)	Consider individually. Local and state public health officials should be consulted on questions about the need for rabies prophylaxis. Bites inflicted by squirrels, hamsters, guinea pigs, gerbils, chipmunks, rats, mice, other rodents, rabbits, and hares almost never call for antirabies prophylaxis.	

*These recommendations are only a guide. In applying them, the animal species involved, the circumstances of the bite or other exposure, the vaccination status of the animal, and presence of rabies in the region should be taken into account. Local or state public health officials should be consulted if questions arise about the need for rabies prophylaxis.

† All bites and wounds should immediately be thoroughly cleansed with soap and water. If antirabies treatment is indicated, both rabies immune globulin (RIG) and human diploid cell rabies vaccine (HDCV) should be given as soon as possible, regardless of the interval from exposure. Local reactions to vaccines are common and do not contraindicate continuing treatment. The vaccine should be discontinued if fluorescent-antibody tests of the animal are negative.

‡ During the usual holding period of 10 days, treatment is begun with RIG and HDCV at first sign of rabies in a dog or cat that has bitten someone. The symptomatic animal should be killed immediately and tested.

§ If RIG is not available, antirabies serum, equine (ARS) should be used, in not more than the recommended dosage.

‖The animal should be killed and tested as soon as possible. Holding for observation is not recommended.

DISPOSITION

Consultation with an infectious disease specialist and a microbiologist (for a careful search for organisms unique to animal bites) is advisable in cases of septicemia. A surgeon (general, hand, plastic, or orthopedic, depending on local practices) should be consulted when there is violation of a deep structure such as a joint, bone, tendon, or internal organ or extensive facial damage or tissue loss. Bites by potentially rabid animals should be reported to state public health officials. All bite wounds should be reported to local law enforcement agencies.

Patients who sustain major trauma, significant blood loss, or injuries that require operative intervention usually need to be admitted. Those who require IV antibiotics (i.e., systemic, CNS, hand, joint, or other deep structure infection or any infection in a high-risk patient) or who are unable to receive proper care as outpatients should also be admitted. All patients who do not require admission should be rechecked in 24–48 hours for signs of infection. If signs of infection develop, sutures must be removed and the wound left opened for drainage. Transfer to another institution should be arranged whenever appropriate inpatient facilities or consultants are unavailable.

COMMON PITFALLS

- Failure to diagnose deep structure or vital organ injury
- Failure to identify and admit the immunocompromised patient
- Failure to close low-risk wounds
- Failure to immobilize and elevate injured extremities
- Failure to recheck all wounds within 24–48 hours

109   Human Bites

Human bites may result in a laceration, loss of tissue, an abrasion, or a crush injury. Aerobic and anaerobic bacteria present in the mouth become embedded in the wound. The degree of injury is related to the force applied during the bite (crushing force), the depth of the wound, the amount of tissue loss, the circulation to the injured area, the victim's immune status, and the degree of contamination sustained. When a clenched fist strikes the teeth of a person with poor dental hygiene, large numbers of bacteria contained in plaque and the deposits around the teeth may be carried to deep tissue planes. Tissue layers over the trunk are thick and accessible to wound cleansing. Tissue planes over the hand are closely applied so contaminating material may become enclosed in relatively avascular spaces as the fingers are flexed to make a fist and then extended after the blow.

The patient may present with an innocuous-appearing laceration, yet soon after develop tenosynovitis, septic arthritis, or osteomyelitis if untreated. The terminal phalanges of the digits of the dominant hand are often injured in intentional bites. Damage to the fingertip may include fracture or tendon avulsion with a mallet finger. A significant degree of disfigurement may result when a portion of the ear or nose is avulsed by a bite. Human bite wounds of the hands have a significantly higher incidence of infection than wounds of the face or trunk. Bacterial infections after human bites usually become evident within 48 hours. HIV transmission secondary to a bite has not been reported.

CLINICAL PRESENTATION

A human "fight bite" should be suspected whenever a patient presents with a wound over the dorsal aspect of metacarpophalangeal joints (knuckles). Wounds of the ears, nose, tongue, nipples, fingertips, or penis should suggest a human bite. Unexplained wounds noted in children, mentally retarded, or acutely psychotic patients should also raise suspicion that the injury may represent a bite wound. Local wound infection shows erythema, swelling, warmth, or a purulence. Local infections associated with more pain than would be expected may indicate a joint, tendon, or compartmental infection or fasciitis. Accompanying lymphangitis and adenopathy indicate that local defense mechanisms have been overwhelmed and the patient is at risk for sepsis. Clusters of small vesicles or an erythematous base at the fingertip are suggestive of herpes simplex infection.

EMERGENCY DEPARTMENT EVALUATION

Ask about the circumstances that led to the bite wound. Human bites should be inspected for the depth of the wound, the involved tissue planes, whether the joint space has been penetrated, whether a tendon or nerve injury has occurred, whether a fracture has occurred, whether a foreign body is present, or whether an occult infection is present. Inspection must be performed with good lighting, anesthesia, and hemostasis. After neurovascular assessment, infiltration with 1% lidocaine may facilitate wound inspection. Tendons must be inspected through their full range of motion to detect hidden injuries.

Laboratory evaluation is of little value except in immunocompromised patients and in evidence of systemic infection. Wound cultures are helpful in identifying the infecting organisms and their antibiotic sensitivity. Most infections are due to *Staphylococcus aureus* or *Streptococcus* species. *Eikenella corrodens* and other gram-negative organisms.

Radiologic evaluation is prudent for all significant hand wounds and wounds that overlie bones and joints. It is useful when extensive infection, joint infection, or osteomyelitis are suspected. Teeth or other radiopaque materials may have become embedded or soft-tissue gas may be seen. A fracture or joint injury may be seen.

EMERGENCY DEPARTMENT MANAGEMENT

Local care includes copious irrigation with sterile saline solution and removal of foreign material. Tetanus prophylaxis should be provided as needed. Facial wounds free of infection may be closed for a satisfactory cosmetic result. The increased potential for wound infection as a result of closure should be discussed and documented. Large, uninfected wounds of the trunk may be closed if done shortly after injury and a disfiguring scar is likely if the wound heals by secondary intention. Extensive wounds of the hands and wounds with tendon injury or joint space involvement should be referred to a hand surgeon for treatment in an operating room. When a fracture is present, it should be treated as an open fracture. Amputations or wounds with significant tissue loss should be evaluated by a hand or plastic surgeon as soon as possible. Any human bite wound, sutured or not, that exhibits an accumulation of purulent material should be promptly drained.

Antibiotics are clearly indicated when infection is present. A localized infected human bite wound may be treated with oral antibiotics after incision, irrigation, and open drainage. A culture should be obtained. Amoxicillin/clavulanate potassium (Augmentin), dicloxicillin, or a first-generation cephalosporin (effective against *S. aureus*) may be used. Penicillin-allergic patients should be given erythromycin. Therapy should continue until signs of infection have resolved. If the bite wound is complicated by surrounding cellulitis, IV nafcillin, oxacillin, or a cephalosporin should be administered. *E. corrodens* is sensitive to penicillin, cefazolin, and ceftriaxone but not dicloxicillin, nafcillin, or clindamycin.

Because human bite wounds have a high incidence of infection, prophylactic antibiotics are usually given for all but superficial wounds. It may be prudent to administer an IV dose of antibiotic on presentation for wounds with extensive tissue damage. Prophylactic antibiotics should be prescribed for no more than 3 to 5 days. The value of prophylactic antibiotics in preventing infection in human bite wounds is unconfirmed.

DISPOSITION

The patient with a local infection who is reliable and healthy may be sent home on oral antibiotics, providing a follow-up visit is possible in 24 hours. An initially uninfected wound should be re-evaluated within 48 hours for infection, neurovascular compromise, or tissue necrosis. Patients with lymphangitis and adenopathy or symptoms of systemic infection such as fever, chills, and rigors should receive IV antibiotics in the ED and then be admitted for close observation and continued

IV antibiotics. Most immunocompromised patients and those with vascular insufficiency of the involved limb should be admitted for treatment of infected human bite wounds.

Those human bite wounds suitable for outpatient management should be bandaged with sterile dressing material. A wounded extremity should also be immobilized with a splint and elevated to control swelling. Dressing changes should be done daily. The patient should be instructed to return immediately if signs or symptoms of infection develop or worsen.

COMMON PITFALLS

- Failure to carefully explore a wound over the dorsum of the hand for joint or extensor tendon injury or foreign bodies
- Failure to culture an infected wound to determine the causative agent and its sensitivity profile
- Failure to arrange follow-up evaluation within 24–48 hours
- Failure to diagnose and treat suspicious wounds as bite injuries

110   Hymenoptera Envenomation

Hymenoptera envenomations include stings of bees, wasps, hornets, yellow jackets, and ants. Envenomation may result in local inflammatory reactions, immediate and delayed hypersensitivity reactions, atypical reactions, and direct systemic toxicity. Immediate (type I) hypersensitivity reactions may be either local or systemic. Delayed (type III) hypersensitivity reactions are caused by IgG and IgM antibody–antigen complex–mediated local (Arthus) and systemic (serum sickness) toxicity. Delayed atypical reactions, suspected to be allergic in etiology, include hematologic and neurologic disorders. Hymenoptera envenomation usually causes only a transient reaction at the site of the sting. Most victims develop an excessive local inflammatory response or a generalized systemic reaction. A sting in someone with no history of previous systemic reaction results in an anaphylactic reaction <1% of the time. However, because most victims of fatal stings have no history of a prior systemic reaction, a negative history does not rule out the possibility of a severe reaction in the future.

Adults with a history of a previous systemic reaction have a 60% chance of a similar reaction after subsequent envenomation. Those with a severe local reaction have about a 5% chance of a future anaphylactic reaction. Children with a systemic reaction limited to non-life-threatening urticaria or angioedema have a subsequent systemic reaction rate of <10%. Sensitization therapy can reduce the incidence of subsequent severe reactions to <10%. Depending on the size of the victim and the offending species, 10-40 simultaneous stings may be serious or fatal. Most anaphylactic fatalities are due to laryngeal edema and bronchospasm, whereas death from multiple stings usually results from vascular collapse, coma, and seizures.

CLINICAL PRESENTATION

Nonallergic local reactions are characterized by pain, wheal and flare formation, warmth, and pruritus at the sting site. Reactions to stings by winged species begin immediately and last for several hours. Fire ant stings, often in clusters, frequently develop into painful vesicles and pustules during the first 24 hours and require up to 10 days for resolution. Local allergic reactions are manifested by persistent swelling, pain, and erythema at the site of the sting. These reactions may progress to involve a large area over the first 2 to 3 days and may last for more than a week. Stings after insect inhalation or ingestion may result in swelling and obstruction of the pharynx, larynx, or esophagus. Most anaphylactic reactions develop within minutes of envenomation and peak within an hour. Recurrent reactions may occur for up to 2 days.

Mild reactions are characterized by generalized flushing and urticaria. Weakness, chest or throat tightness, nausea, vomiting, diarrhea, and generalized angioedema indicate a moderate reaction. Cyanosis, dyspnea, stridor, hoarseness, confusion, coma, and collapse are seen in severe cases. Physical findings may include hypotension, tachycardia, laryngeal and pulmonary edema, and wheezing as well as skin manifestations. Secondary complications include cerebral and myocardial infarction and coagulopathies. Delayed atypical and hypersensitivity reactions are rare. Signs and symptoms of direct systemic toxicity usually begin within minutes and include vomiting, diarrhea, generalized edema, collapse, loss of consciousness, encephalopathy, headache, muscle spasms, and seizures. Vital signs may reveal hypotension, tachycardia, and fever. Severe cases may be complicated by rhabdomyolysis and acute renal failure.

DIFFERENTIAL DIAGNOSIS

Because Hymenoptera envenomation can cause a variety of reactions, the differential diagnosis is extensive. Fortunately there is usually a history of a sting. Progressive extension of the initial reaction beginning shortly after the sting indicates an allergic reaction, whereas inflammation with fever, leukocytosis, and lymphangitis beginning 2 to 3 days after envenomation suggests infection. Anaphylactic reactions may be caused by a wide variety of proteins (e.g., pollen and food), drugs, dyes, and diagnostic and therapeutic agents. This diagnosis should be considered in any unconscious patient with hypotension and signs of airway obstruction during warm months, particularly if discovered outdoors. Direct systemic toxicity must be differentiated from anaphylaxis. Toxic reactions progress more slowly, require a large number of stings, and may produce fever. Urticaria, pruritus, and wheezing suggest anaphylaxis.

EMERGENCY DEPARTMENT EVALUATION

The history should include time and number of stings, offending species (if known), previous Hymenoptera reactions, existing medical conditions, and time of onset, progression, and nature of symptoms. The physical examination should focus on the vital signs, upper airway patency, lungs, cardiovascular system, and skin. With honey bee envenomation the stinger and venom sac may be apparent at the sting site. Patients with hypotension, chest pain, or loss of consciousness should have an ECG. Upper airway patency may be assessed by soft-tissue neck radiographs. Patients with persistent respiratory signs and symptoms should have an ABG and chest radiograph. Patients with hypotension, loss of consciousness, or more than ten stings should have measurements of CPK, BUN and creatinine levels, prothrombin time, partial thromboplastin time, and a urinalysis. A CBC may help to differentiate local allergic reactions (eosinophilia) from infection (leukocytosis with left shift) as well as detect hemolysis and thrombocytopenia.

EMERGENCY DEPARTMENT MANAGEMENT

Life support should be instituted as necessary. Epinephrine should be administered at the first sign of an anaphylactic reaction, preferably by prehospital personnel. The dose and route depend on the severity and nature of symptoms as well as the victim's underlying medical problems. An epinephrine dose of 0.3 mg to 0.5 mg (0.3–0.5 mL of a 1:1000 aqueous solution) for adults and 0.01 mg/kg (0.01 mL/kg of a 1:1000 solution) for children, given SQ and repeated every 15 minutes if necessary, is appropriate for mild to moderate reactions. Older patients with underlying cerebral or coronary vascular disease should be titrated with lower doses. Adjunctive therapy should include oral or IV diphenhydramine (0.5–1.0 mg/kg) and oral prednisone (0.5 1 mg/kg) or IV methylprednisolone (1–4 mg/kg), depending on severity and response to epinephrine.

Severe anaphylactic reactions or marked local reactions that involve the nose, mouth, and throat may require immediate airway control. Because most deaths are due to airway obstruction, early intubation may be lifesaving. Intubation should also be considered with significant central nervous system depression or severe shock. In patients with hypotension the absorption of subcutaneous epinephrine may be compromised, and IV administration may be preferable. The IV dose of epinephrine is the same, but it should be diluted 10 to 100 times (final concentration 1:10,000–1:100,000) with saline solution and administered over a period of at least 5 minutes. Aggressive volume replacement with crystalloids should proceed simultaneously in pharyngeal or laryngeal edema. Inhaled epinephrine (0.005–0.02 mL of a 2.25% racemic solution by nebulizer) may be particularly helpful. Similarly, patients with bronchospasm may respond more rapidly to an inhaled beta adrenergic agent such as albuterol. Adjunctive therapy with IV aminophylline may be helpful in severe cases. Antihistamines and corticosteroids should also be given.

The treatment of local reactions includes wound care and symptomatic treatment of pain, swelling, and pruritus with analgesics; cool soaks, ice packs, and elevation; and antihistamines. Cleansing of the puncture site and tetanus prophylaxis are routine measures. Stingers with attached venom sacs (left in the skin only after honeybee envenomation) should be removed by brushing or scraping with the sharp edge of a needle or scalpel to avoid further envenomation. Stingers without sacs may also be removed with forceps. Oral antihistamines, topical steroids, ice packs, and elevation may provide symptomatic relief. The treatment of toxic reactions after multiple envenomations is entirely supportive. Delayed hypersensitivity reactions can usually be treated with analgesics and antihistamines. Corticosteroids may be necessary in severe cases. Complications and atypical reactions should be treated by standard measures.

DISPOSITION

Patients who present immediately after envenomation should be observed for 1 to 2 hours for signs of anaphylaxis. Asymptomatic patients may then be discharged. Because milder anaphylactic reactions may be delayed, patients should be instructed to return if symptoms ensue. In asymptomatic patients with a history of previous anaphylactic reactions or severe local ones it may be prudent to prescribe a prophylactic 3-day course of antihistamines and corticosteroids, beginning with a dose before discharge. Patients with anaphylaxis should be treated and observed for 4 hours. Those who become asymptomatic may be discharged. Patients with persistent or recurrent symptoms (excluding isolated urticaria) and those with life-threatening reactions should be hospitalized. Those with ischemic complications, toxic reactions and multiple envenomations, and those without reliable home observation should be admitted.

All patients with anaphylactic reactions should be treated with a 3-day course of antihistamines and corticosteroids. Provide a prescription for epinephrine (e.g., Epipen or Ana-kit) and refer to an allergist so that they can receive instruction regarding the self-use of epinephrine and evaluation for desensitization immunotherapy. Victims of anaphylaxis should be cautioned about outdoor work and recreation and advised to avoid wearing bright colors and perfumes. The use of insect repellants may be helpful. An allergy identification bracelet is also recommended. Patients with local or delayed hypersensitivity reactions can be treated as outpatients with ED or primary care follow-up. Atypical reactions may require admission and referral to an appropriate specialist. Although the role of desensitization therapy in patients with severe local reactions is controversial, referral is advisable.

COMMON PITFALLS

- Failure to suspect anaphylaxis caused by Hymenoptera envenomation in an unconscious patient with cardiovascular collapse during an outdoor activity in warm seasons
- Failure to intubate patients with severe upper or lower airway compromise
- Failure to administer epinephrine to patients with life-threatening anaphylaxis

- Failure to prescribe antihistamines and corticosteroids for 3 days after anaphylaxis to prevent its recurrence
- Failure to prescribe an emergency epinephrine kit to victims of anaphylaxis and to refer them to an allergist

111   Crotalid Snake Envenomation

The incidence of poisonous snakebite in the US is about 7000–8000 cases/year with 9–14 deaths. Most involve the Crotalidae family and include the genera *Crotalus* (rattlesnakes), *Agkistrodon* (copperheads and water moccasins or cottonmouths), and *Sistrurus* (pygmy ratter and massasauga). The majority of bites occur in the southeast, southwest, and western regions. The incidence is greatest between March and October. Up to 25% of bites do not result in envenomation (dry bites). Most envenomations result in a combination of local and systemic effects. However, some populations of Mojave rattlesnakes have a venom (type a) that may cause presynaptic neurovascular blockade with delayed respiratory failure and mild or absent local effects. Envenomations by *Agkistrodon* and *Sistrurus* species tend to be less severe than those of *Crotalus* species. Size and species of snake, location and depth of the bite, size and health of the victim, first aid measures performed, time to definitive therapy, and type of therapy influence severity and outcome. A 24-hour Antivenin Index Service can be accessed by calling (602) 626-6016.

CLINICAL PRESENTATION

Dry bites produce no signs or symptoms other than those of a mechanical puncture wound. If envenomation has occurred, the victim typically notes sudden severe pain at the bite site soon followed by progressive swelling and sometimes paresthesias. Examination may show two puncture wounds exuding bloody fluid; scratches and single or multiple puncture wounds are also seen. Other local findings include erythema, ecchymosis, bullae, and, eventually, necrosis and ulceration. Severity can be assessed by the degree of swelling. Bites about the face may lead to airway obstruction and those of the extremities to compartmental syndromes. Because venoms contain bacteria (e.g., *Proteus, Clostridium,* and *Bacteroides*), wound infection is a potential complication.

Systemic symptoms include nausea, vomiting, diarrhea, perioral paresthesias, salivation, dysgensias, lethargy, and weakness. Severe envenomations may lead to cardiovascular collapse, coma, seizures, dyspnea, respiratory depression, and gastrointestinal and pulmonary hemorrhage. Most often vital signs show tachycardia and mild hypertension. Laboratory evaluation may reveal hemolysis, anemia, thrombocytopenia, coagulopathy (including disseminated intravascular coagulation) and blood, protein, and glucose in the urine in severe cases. The chest radiograph may reveal pulmonary edema, and the ECG may show arrhythmias or ischemic changes.

Systemic findings are also used to assess the severity of envenomation. An initially mild envenomation may progress over a period of hours to become moderate, severe, or even life-threatening. Coagulation abnormalities may peak as late as 3 days after envenomation.

EMERGENCY DEPARTMENT EVALUATION

Vital signs and a rapid survey should be performed to determine clinical stability. The time and circumstances of the bite, nature and severity of symptoms, first aid measures and allergies, medical problems, previous bites, and antivenin therapy should be noted. The bite site should be examined. Distal neurovascular status should be noted in extremity bites. Early on evaluation should be repeated every 15 minutes. The general examination should focus on the cardiovascular, pulmonary, and neurologic systems. Laboratory tests in initially minimal bites should include CBC (note red cell morphology), electrolytes, BUN and creatinine levels, prothrombin time, platelet count, and urinalysis. In severe cases or in patients with progressive worsening, creatine kinase, fibrinogen, fibrin split products, ABG and blood typing should be included. A chest radiograph and ECG should be obtained in patients with systemic signs or symptoms.

EMERGENCY DEPARTMENT MANAGEMENT

Life support measures should be instituted as necessary. Prehospital personnel should establish IV access, oxygen and transport to a medical facility that possesses antivenin. If a tourniquet has been placed, it should not be removed until IV access has been established. The limb should be maintained in a neutral position. Loose (lymphatic) tourniquets, incision and suction, and cooling an extremity are possibly effective if used within 30 minutes of envenomations, but they are not substitutes for definitive care. Local wound care and tetanus prophylaxis should be provided.

Grading of the envenomation as mild, moderate, or severe will provide a guide for appropriate administration of Wyeth equine polyvalent Crotalidae antivenin. If after several hours pain and edema remain localized to the bite site and coagulopathy is not progressing, antivenin is not necessary. Continuing observation for signs of local progression and laboratory abnormalities cannot be overemphasized. The extent of swelling should be outlined with a marking pen, and limb circumference should be measured at several sites above and below the bite. If any of these parameters should worsen, antivenin therapy is usually warranted.

A skin test should not be performed unless a definite decision to administer antivenin has been made. Unstable patients and those with obvious systemic involvement should immediately be tested. A negative skin test suggests, but does not guarantee, that an antivenin reaction will not develop. Although a positive test is an important warning, it does not absolutely preclude administration of antivenin. Those with moderate or severe envenomation who require antivenin can be pretreated with diphenhydramine, epinephrine, and corticosteroids.

Antivenin should be administered only in a critical care setting with epinephrine and antihistamines readily available. It can effectively reverse coagulopathy up to 72 hours after envenomation. Minimal envenomations with progression and moderate envenomations should receive five vials of antivenin initially. Severe envenomations require at least ten vials. Life-threatening envenomations and envenomations in children require higher dosages. Subsequent antivenin doses are guided by clinical response. Supportive care (e.g., fluids and pressors for hypotension, blood component replacement for hematologic abnormalities, and respiratory support) is extremely important but often neglected.

Fasciotomy and supportive care without antivenin have been proposed as definitive treatment; however, only in patients with documented increased intracompartmental pressure unresponsive to limb elevation, mannitol (1–2 g/kg IV), and antivenin (five to ten vials) is fasciotomy clearly indicated. Cultures and antibiotic therapy should be initiated if signs of infection develop.

DISPOSITION

Patients with dry bites may be discharged after an 8- to 12-hour observation. Severe or life-threatening bites and those receiving antivenin should be admitted to an ICU. Admission to a floor bed is appropriate for patients with mild or moderate envenomations. Mobilization of the affected extremity can begin when the progression of swelling has ceased. Discharge is appropriate when swelling is decreasing, any coagulopathy has completely reversed, and the patient is ambulatory. Outpatient follow-up may be necessary to monitor for infection and serum sickness. Nearly all patients who receive > 5-7 vials will develop serum sickness. Serum sickness may range from a mild viral-like illness to severe urticaria, rash, arthralgias, and other complications. Most cases can be treated with anti-inflammatory analgesics, antihistamines, and corticosteroids as outpatients. Physicians not familiar with snake envenomation should consult a toxicologist or regional poison control center.

COMMON PITFALLS

- Failure to diagnose envenomation from lack of history or observation of suspicious wounds of unclear cause
- Inappropriate skin testing
- Failure to monitor for allergic reactions from antivenin despite a negative skin test; failure to have epinephrine and eiphenhydramine at the bedside
- Unnecessary use and inadequate dose of antivenin
- Failure to provide supportive care as well as antivenin to patients with severe reactions
- Failure to recognize that horse serum allergy is not an absolute contraindication to antivenin administration

112   Elapid Snake Envenomations

North American representatives of the elapid family are the coral snakes. These are brightly colored snakes known for the potency of their venom. Fortunately few bites occur because these snakes are usually small, nocturnal, and shy. Coral snakes in the USA include the eastern coral snake (Micrurus fulvius fulvius), the Texas coral snake (Micrurus fulvius tenere), and the Arizona (Sonoran) coral snake (Micruroides euryxanthus). The eastern coral snake is found in the deep southeast US, while the Texas and Arizona subspecies are found primarily in the states whose name they bear. These are all brightly colored snakes with black, red, and yellow rings that entirely encircle their bodies. The red and yellow rings touch in coral snakes, but are separated by black rings in nonpoisonous snakes. A typical rhyme for identifying these snakes is "Red on yellow, kill a fellow; red on black, venom lack." Unfortunately victims may confuse the rhyme, especially when intoxicated (e.g., "red on yellow, good fellow"). Elapids lack facial pits and have nearly round pupils. Coral snakes are docile. When biting they hold on or chew, allowing them to envenomate. Their venom is discharged through grooves on two small, fixed anterior fangs. Their small size makes it difficult, but not impossible, to seriously envenomate humans. The eastern and Texas subspecies are larger and have seriously envenomated many patients. The Sonoran coral snake has not caused severe envenomation.

CLINICAL PRESENTATION

Coral snake envenomation can be difficult to diagnose and easy to underestimate. The typical bite shows little local damage and few initial systemic symptoms. Minor pain without swelling may be present. This may be followed by numbness and weakness of the affected part as the envenomation syndrome advances. Systemic symptoms may take hours to develop, and include drowsiness, apprehension, weakness, fasciculation, tremors, difficulty swallowing, dyspnea, salivation, nausea, and vomiting.

Physical examination may show fang marks and associated scratches. It is often possible to express a drop of blood. However, the history is particularly important because significant envenomation without any apparent marks, despite close examination, has occurred. In such cases injection of lidocaine under the suspected area may show minute beads of serosanguineous fluid exuding from fang punctures. Signs of systemic toxicity may be delayed in onset, and include weakness of extraocular muscles, miotic pupils, bulbar paralysis, respiratory depression, and convulsions. In severe cases arterial blood gas analysis may show hypoventilation and an elevated creatine kinase level.

DIFFERENTIAL DIAGNOSIS

The diagnosis of coral snake envenomation is usually clear because the snake frequently hangs on to the victim and has bright, identifiable coloring. When the patient cannot clearly communicate, the rapidity of onset and usually short duration of venom poisoning distinguish it from other motor neuron diseases. Laboratory testing may be necessary to rule out poisoning by agents such as botulism, heavy metals, and central nervous system depressant medications.

EMERGENCY DEPARTMENT EVALUATION

Time and circumstances of the bite, description of the snake, first aid treatment before arrival, allergies, previous bites and antivenin therapy, past medical history, and onset, progression, and nature of symptoms should be established. The physical examination should focus on neurologic assessment, particularly cranial motor nerve, and respiratory muscle function. Tidal volume, arterial blood gas analysis, and other routine studies (laboratory, chest radiograph, and electrocardiogram) should be obtained if clinically indicated. Although positive identification of the offending snake is helpful, it should not delay treatment.

EMERGENCY DEPARTMENT MANAGEMENT

Prehospital care should consist of intravenous line insertion, maintenance of airway, and timely transport to a health care facility capable of full life-support and antivenin therapy. The use of constriction bands or pressure bandages to retard venom spread may be useful.

Wound cleansing and tetanus prophylaxis should be provided. Patients who have clearly been bitten or who have developed symptoms or signs of envenomation should be given at least five vials of M. fulvius antivenin, equine by intravenous infusion. Waiting until systemic manifestations develop before administering antivenin may not always reverse them or prevent further deterioration. If symptoms progress, the dose of antivenin should be repeated. Although M. fulvius antivenin is neither effective or necessary in Sonoran coral snake envenomation, the protocol above should be followed unless a positive identification of this species has been made. The elective intubation of patients with bulbar signs or symptoms may prevent aspiration pneumonia. The prognosis is excellent. There is normally no tissue loss or permanent neurologic dysfunction. Even without antivenin treatment, recovery can be expected if appropriate supportive care is provided. Hence patients with allergic reactions to horse serum or antivenin can be successfully managed without antivenin.

DISPOSITION

All patients in whom the diagnosis of coral snake envenomation is entertained should be admitted to an ICU for at least 12 hours of monitoring of vital signs and neurologic function. This disposition applies to patients with a definitive bite, either by history or examination, regardless of whether or not they are symptomatic. Patients who have no evidence of envenomation after 12 hours of observation may be discharged. Those with severe envenomations may require several days of hospitalization.

COMMON PITFALLS

- Delaying antivenin administration until systemic signs and symptoms are present
- Failure to admit and monitor all patients with possible coral snake envenomation
- Failure to monitor for progression of toxicity after antivenin administration and to provide concomitant aggressive supportive care
- The inappropriate use of antivenin in patients with documented Arizona (Sonoran) coral snake envenomation and in those with allergic reactions to horse serum or antivenin
- Failure to take the same precautions as described for crotalid antivenin when administering coral snake antivenin

113　Cold-Induced Tissue Injuries

Soft-tissue injuries resulting from unprotected exposure to cold and wet environments include frostbite and immersion foot (trenchfoot). Frostbite is the destruction of tissue as the result of freezing. Immersion foot is tissue injury at temperatures between 32°F and 50°F with prolonged exposure to a wet environment. Frostnip is reversible cold injury caused by ice crystal formation on the skin surface. The most important factors that determine eventual tissue loss with frostbite injuries are the magnitude of temperature depression, and the length of exposure. Poor nutrition, smoking, alcohol consumption, and vascular disease all adversely affect final tissue survival and function.

CLINICAL PRESENTATION

The history given by victims of frostbite is usually sufficient to diagnose and estimate the extent of tissue damage. The patient may present with totally or partially frozen parts. Initially the skin is pale, may appear waxy white or mottled blue, and may range from rock-solid to firm on palpation. The frozen part is cold and lacks sensibility. Occasionally examination reveals a superimposed burn injury, due to attempts to rewarm the insensate part with fire or on a heater.

As thawing occurs, the frostbitten tissue takes on a different appearance that is characteristic of the depth of injury. In first-degree frostbite the thawed skin is hyperemic, warm, and sensate. Second-degree frostbite is characterized by vesicles or bullae that contain clear fluid. Third-degree frostbite bullae contain purple bloody fluid, which indicates injury to the reticular dermis and the subdermal plexus. With fourth-degree frostbite, in which subcutaneous tissues are injured, mummification occurs and muscle, tendon, or bone involvement may be present. Because only 10% to 15% of patients arrive in the emergency department still frozen, the physician must recognize the injury in numerous stages of presentation. Laboratory tests are of little assistance in the diagnosis and treatment of frostbite injury. The frostbite patient, however, may also suffer from other illness, hypothermia, or concurrent trauma.

EMERGENCY DEPARTMENT EVALUATION

The history obtained should include the exposure temperature, the duration of exposure, the extent of wetting involved, and the wind conditions. Presence of risk factors such as vascular disease, trauma, smoking history, alcohol ingestion, or other systemic diseases should be ascertained.

Physical examination should include the patient's core (rectal) temperature and a full description of the involved part. Color, the presence of blistering, temperature, consistency, capillary refill, movement, and two-point and vibratory sensibility should all be recorded. As these signs may change rapidly, multiple evaluations may be necessary. Peripheral pulses should be palpated or examined by Doppler phonogram. Rarely, cold injury to the cornea is suffered. Visual acuity and fluorescein examination should be performed when indicated. Unless other injuries are suspected or life-threatening conditions are present, further ancillary studies are unnecessary. Angiography is contraindicated owing to potential injury of the vasculature. Scintigraphy may be helpful to determine the extent of injury later in the hospital course, but it will not change early therapy.

EMERGENCY DEPARTMENT MANAGEMENT

During transportation to the emergency department there should be no rubbing, warming, or manipulation of frozen parts, as this can exacerbate a tissue injury. In the emergency department all nonadherent wet or cold apparel should be removed and the patient should be placed under warm blankets. Clothing frozen to the skin should be trimmed initially and removed only after being loosened by the rewarming procedure. Treatment of systemic hypothermia takes precedence over thawing of frostbitten extremities. Tetanus toxoid should be administered if the patient has not received such protection within the past 5 to 10 years.

Rapid thawing is the mainstay of early care of the frostbite victim. The frostbitten part should be placed in a water bath of 40°C to 42°C. Constant temperature monitoring should be instituted to maintain the bath at this temperature, as significant cooling of the bath could allow refreezing of the tissues and further tissue damage. The thawing process usually takes 15 to 20 minutes. Rubbing or manipulation should be avoided.

On rewarming, patients may complain of a painful cold feeling that gradually decreases and is replaced by numbness. A throbbing pain may develop 48 to 72 hours after thawing and continue for a number of weeks. As nerve regeneration occurs a tingling sensation may be present. Depending on the depth and extent of the injury, normal sensibility may or may not fully return. In the early post thawing period analgesia may be necessary for pain control. Elevation of the injured part and avoidance of pressure will decrease discomfort. Hemorrhage blisters should be left intact.

Aloe vera should be applied to the cold-injured tissue every 6 hours. Ibuprofen (400 mg PO every 12 hours) should be administered as a systemic thromboxane inhibitor, and ascorbic acid given (1 g PO every 12 hours). Small-vessel vasodilation and blood flow are maximized by the administration of nifedipine (10 mg PO every 8 hours) and pentoxifylline (400 mg PO every 8 hours). Smoking should be prohibited. Bed rest, elevation of the injured part, and splinting should be instituted to maximally immobilize the extremity. All patients should receive tetanus immunization as necessary. Prophylactic systemic antibiotics are not indicated. Clinical infections of the feet should be microscopically examined and cultured for fungi as well as bacteria, and treated accordingly.

There is seldom any tissue loss after second-degree or less frostbite or immersion foot that is treated appropriately. These patients, however, may suffer hypesthesia or dysesthesia for long periods of time post injury. Amputation or radical surgical debridement of tissues is reserved for wet gangrenous tissues or late gangrene. Inflicting surgical injury to marginally viable tissue by attempting early surgery may result in an extension of the tissue necrosis.

DISPOSITION

All but the most superficially injured frostbite patients should be admitted. Surgical consultation (plastic, vascular, or general, depending on local practices) should be obtained. If corneal injury has been sustained, an ophthalmologist should be consulted. All patients who have been discharged should be re-examined within 24 to 28 hours, as tissue necrosis can be progressive and infectious complication may develop. Patients with frostbite or immersion foot may have increased sensitivity and susceptibility to subsequent exposures to cold. The use of protective clothing and footwear and avoidance of future exposures should be advised.

COMMON PITFALLS

- Failure to evaluate and treat for concomitant systemic hypothermia
- Rubbing or manipulation of frozen tissue
- Failure to rapidly warm affected parts
- Failure to obtain surgical consultation and admit almost all patients for observation
- Failure to consider the adjunctive use of pharmacologic agents such as prostaglandin and thromboxane inhibitors and vasodilators
- Failure to appreciate that the extent of irreversible tissue damage may not be evident until many days after exposure
- Failure to warn patients about the hazards of re-exposure

---

114   Hypothermia

Hypothermia is defined as a core temperature less than 35°C (95°F). It may be characterized as acute (less than 6 hours' duration) or chronic (greater than 6 hours' duration); mild (32°–35°C), moderate (28°–32°C), or severe (less than 28°C); and primary or secondary. Primary or "exposure" hypothermia is usually acute and occurs in healthy people after immersion in cold water or exposure to low environmental temperatures. In contrast, secondary or "urban" hypothermia is usually chronic, and occurs in urban settings in those with predisposing illness, infirmity, intoxication, or extremes of age. Secondary hypothermia is much more common than primary hypothermia and has a very high mortality rate (approaching 100% in severe cases). Of 6460 deaths reported from 1968 to 1980, most victims were elderly and had underlying medical conditions (Table 114-1). Recovery is the rule even with moderate to severe hypothermia in young, healthy adults. Survival has been reported with a core temperature as low as 16°C (61°F).

Generalized organ dysfunction with central nervous system (CNS), cardiac, and respiratory depression occurs with core temperatures below 35°C. Respiratory and metabolic acidosis, and volume depletion resulting from cold-induced diuresis will further compromise organ function and perfusion. The threshold for ventricular fibrillation is decreased at temperatures below 28°C. Because symptoms are nonspecific, the diagnosis requires accurate measurement of the core (rectal) temperature and knowledge of predisposing conditions.

CLINICAL PRESENTATION

The symptoms and signs of mild hypothermia include apathy, confusion, lethargy, fatigue, forgetfulness, incoordination, shivering, slurred speech, withdrawal, and increased pulse and respiratory rates. A fine, at times unilateral, muscle tremor may also be present. With progressive hypothermia shivering stops and pulse rate, blood pressure, and respiratory rate are decreased. Disorientation, stupor, inappropriate behavior, polyuria, rhonchi, and wheezing may be noted. The electrocardiogram (ECG) commonly shows atrial fibrillation. Paroxsymal atrial tachycardia, interval prolongation

---

TABLE 114-1. Predisposing Factors in Hypothermia

Decreased Heat Production	Increased Heat Loss
CNS depression (metabolic or traumatic)	Environmental exposure: inadequate clothing/shelter, windchill, low humidity, perspiration, wet clothing
Immobility (age, neuromuscular disorders)	
Endocrine failure (adrenal/pituitary/thyroid)	Exfoliative skin disease
Hypoglycemia/malnutrition	Vasodilatation
	Impaired vasoconstriction
	Drugs
	Neuropathy
	Sepsis
	Shock

Hypothalamic Dysfunction	Iatrogenic Cooling
Acidosi//anoxia	Use of large volumes of cool (<35°C, 95°F) fluids for lavage or intravenous administration; overly aggressive treatment of hyperthermia
CNS hemorrhage/infarction	
Drugs (e.g., phenothiazines)	
Encephalopathy	

(PR, QRS, and QT), decreased P wave amplitude, T wave changes, premature ventricular contractions, or a humped ST segment adjacent to the QRS complex (Osborn wave) may also be seen.

Findings in severe hypothermia include coma, dilated unreactive pupils, absent reflexes, flat electroencephalogram, muscle rigidity, hypotension, weak or absent pulse, and slow, barely detectable respirations. The ECG may show marked bradycardia, asystole, or ventricular fibrillation.

Laboratory findings include respiratory alkalosis in mild hypothermia and hypoxia, metabolic and respiratory acidosis, increased amylase, glucose, and hematocrit, and leukopenia, thrombocytopenia, coagulopathy, and variable electrolyte abnormalities in moderate and severe hypothermia. The chest radiograph may disclose pulmonary infiltrates characteristic of aspiration or pneumonia.

EMERGENCY DEPARTMENT EVALUATION

The diagnosis of hypothermia may be suggested by the setting in which the patient was found (e.g., cool or cold, indoor or outdoor environment). Length and conditions of exposure, underlying medical problems, recent illnesses, and medications should be documented. Any patient with altered mental status should have a core temperature measured. The same is true for initially normothermic or hyperthermic patients treated with cooling measures or large volumes of intravenous or lavage solutions. The physical examination should initially focus on vital signs and the neurologic, cardiovascular, and pulmonary systems. In severe cases observation for 2 minutes or longer may be required in order to detect the presence of a pulse or respirations. An esophageal or rectal probe (thermocouple) or a thermometer capable of measuring low temperatures (below the usual 34°C) is required for an accurate diagnosis.

A detailed examination should then be performed, searching for coexisting pathology. An ECG and chest radiograph are usually indicated. In moderate and severe hypothermia routine laboratory tests should include arterial blood gas analysis, complete blood count, determination of amylase, electrolyte, glucose, blood urea nitrogen, and creatinine levels, coagulation profile, and urinalysis. Additional laboratory studies such as bacteriologic cultures, serum calcium, magnesium, phosphate, lactate, ketone, cortisol, and cardiac enzyme levels; liver and thyroid function tests; and toxicology screening may also be necessary to elucidate concomitant medical problems.

The interpretation of arterial blood gas analysis results in hypothermia is controversial. Because the pH increases (0.015 units per degree centigrade), and the PCO_2 (4.4% per degree centigrade) and PO_2 (7.2% per degree centigrade) decrease at temperatures below 37°C as the result of changes in gas solubility, measurement of these parameters in samples warmed to 37°C will result in "falsely" decreased pH and increased PCO_2 and PO_2 if not corrected for temperature. However, recent observations suggest that uncorrected results should be used to guide therapy for acid-base disturbances.

EMERGENCY DEPARTMENT MANAGEMENT

All patients should receive oxygen and cardiac and temperature monitoring, and have an intravenous line established. In the prehospital setting the patient should be protected from further cooling. Wet clothes should be removed, the ambulance should be heated, and the patient should be covered with blankets. If a pulse is detected, cardiopulmonary resuscitation (CPR) and endotracheal intubation should not be performed, since these procedures may precipitate ventricular tachycardia, fibrillation, or asystole. Ventilations should be assisted by a bag-mask device, and the patient should be moved as little as possible. Hyperventilation should be avoided, since it may also induce an alkalosis and result in ventricular fibrillation. Emergency department management depends on severity.

Nearly all patients require volume expansion. Normal saline solution with dextrose is preferable to lactated Ringer's, since lactate may not be metabolized during hypothermia. The volume of fluid should be determined by tissue perfusion and vital signs. Intravascular monitoring (e.g., arterial, central venous, and pulmonary artery) may be required in severe cases. Room temperature intravenous fluids are acceptable for mild hypothermia (unless the rapid infusion of large volumes is necessary [e.g., patients with bleeding or severe dehydration]). Otherwise, intravenous fluids should be warmed to 45°C. If a blood warmer is not available, a liter of room temperature intravenous fluid may be warmed in a standard microwave (high setting for 1 to 2 minutes, depending on wattage).

Patients who require intubation for airway protection, hypoxia, or respiratory depression (carbon dioxide retention) should first receive 100% oxygen, topical anesthesia, sedation, and correction of acid–base abnormalities as necessary. The prophylactic administration of lidocaine or bretylium may also be helpful. Intubation should be accomplished with as little airway manipulation as possible in order to avoid inducing arrhythmias. Nasal intubation may be preferable to the oral route if spontaneous respirations are present.

Chemical or electrical treatment of arrhythmias is usually ineffective at temperatures below 28°C; hence warming should take precedence. Supraventricular arrhythmias usually convert spontaneously during or within 24 hours of rewarming. Pulseless rhythms should be treated according to advanced cardiac life-support guidelines. Because bretylium (but not lidocaine) has been shown to increase the threshold for ventricular fibrillation and increase the success of defibrillation during experimental hypothermia, it should be considered a first-line agent for this rhythm. Although open cardiac massage in conjunction with mediastinal lavage using warm saline solution has been advocated for pulseless rhythms, its efficacy remains to be determined.

Passive (spontaneous) rewarming is appropriate for adults with mild, primary hypothermia. Warm blankets and shivering usually increase body temperature by 0.5° to 1°C per hour. Neonates and adults with secondary hypothermia should be treated by active rewarming, as should victims of moderate and severe hypothermia. Active rewarming may be accomplished by providing warm intravenous fluids; humidified air or oxygen (by mask or ventilator) heated to 42° to 45°C (mouth temperature); immersion in a 40°C water bath; peritoneal, gastric, bladder, or colonic lavage with 45°C fluid; blood warming by hemodialysis (with an in-line heat exchanger), or femorofemoral (partial) cardiopulmonary bypass pump; and pleuromediastinal lavage by way of thoracostomy or thoracotomy. Invasive (surgical) procedures should be reserved for hemodynamically unstable patients. Gastric, bladder, colonic, and pleuromediastinal lavage are less efficacious than other measures. Bath rewarming is more effective than inhalation rewarming. Cardiopulmonary bypass can support the circulation in lieu of prolonged CPR. Resuscitation should not be considered unsuccessful until the core temperature has been raised to at least 32°C.

Decreases in core temperature ("afterdrop"), acidosis and hypotension due to peripheral vasodilatation, and the exchange of cool peripheral blood for warm core blood have been noted during spontaneous, inhalation, or immersion rewarming. The magnitude and duration of afterdrop appears to be less with bath rewarming than with spontaneous or inhalation techniques. Because there are both central and peripheral thermosensors, afterdrop is theoretically possible with any rewarming technique. Metabolic rates are increased with surface rewarming but not by inhalation. It thus appears that active surface rewarming is not contraindicated (as previously speculated). The concurrent use of multiple rewarming techniques is probably most effective and safest. The use of uneven surface warming (e.g., warm packs to axilla and groin) is not recommended.

DISPOSITION

Patients with mild hypothermia should be observed until they are asymptomatic and normothermic. Those with extremes of age or coexisting underlying pathology should be admitted for further evaluation and treatment. Patients with moderate or severe hypothermia should be admitted to an intensive care unit.

COMMON PITFALLS

- Failure to diagnose hypothermia owing to lack of suspicion or accurate temperature measurement
- Failure to diligently search for underlying causes of secondary hypothermia
- Failure to recognize that chemical and electrical treatment of arrhythmias is usually ineffective at temperatures below 28°C
- Failure to appreciate that rough handling, airway manipulation, and invasive procedures may precipitate arrhythmias
- Failure to continue resuscitation attempts until the core temperature is at least 32°C
- Failure to include volume replacement in resuscitative efforts
- Failure to monitor for core temperature afterdrop and appreciate that it is theoretically possible with any rewarming technique

115   Heat Illnesses

Heat illness can be defined as the inability of normal regulatory mechanisms to cope with a heat stress. Minor heat-related problems, such as muscle cramps, edema, rash, syncope, and tetany, account for significant morbidity and are frequently confused with other common complaints. Heat exhaustion and heatstroke are major heat syndromes in that, if left untreated, organ damage or death may ensue. Among athletes heatstroke is second only to head and cervical spine injuries as a cause of death. In elderly patients mortality has been directly correlated with increased temperature (Table 115-1).

TABLE 115-1. Factors That Predispose to Heat Illness

Endogenous Factors	Exogenous Factors
Increased Heat Gain	
Infection	High ambient temperature
Drugs	Malignant hyperthermia
Stimulants	Sunlight
Hallucinogens	
Increased activity	
Exercise	
Seizures	
Drug withdrawal	
Psychosis	
Neuroleptic malignant	
syndrome	
Thyrotoxicosis	
Decreased Heat Loss	
Lack of acclimation	High temperature
Dehydration	High humidity
Hypokalemia	Restrictive clothing
Drugs	
Anticholinergics	
Neuroleptics	
Barbiturates	
Antiparkinsonism agents	
Diuretics	
Beta blockers	
Alcohol	
Extremes of age	
Skin disorders	
Cystic fibrosis	
Obesity	
Debilitated/chronic disease	
Impaired voluntary responses	

Heat cramps are due to muscle fatigue combined with water and salt depletion. Heat syncope results from vasodilation usually compounded by volume depletion or the use of drugs that interfere with cardiovascular reflexes. Heat tetany appears to be due to hyperventilation-induced respiratory alkalosis, resulting in decreased ionized serum calcium. It may be an attempt to compensate for exercise-induced lactic acidosis. Heat rash is caused by the plugging, dilation, and rupture of sweat glands after skin maceration resulting from sweating. The cause of heat edema is not known.

Heat exhaustion results from dehydration with inadequate fluid and electrolyte replacement. Water depletion, salt depletion, or a combination of the two forms may be present. Without treatment, heat exhaustion will progress to heatstroke. Heatstroke is due to severe dehydration with thermoregulatory failure, resulting in body temperatures above 40°C (105°–106°F) and a mortality rate of up to 70%.

Acclimatization is a process of physiologic adaptation to repeated heat stress occurring over a 10- to 60-day period, resulting in decreased heat production and increased heat loss for a given amount of work. Although acclimatization protects against heat illness, as the wet bulb temperature approaches 30°C (86°F) even young, well-acclimated people are susceptible during vigorous or prolonged physical activity.

CLINICAL PRESENTATION

Heat cramps are painful spasms of heavily used muscle groups, often occurring in acclimatized people, during or up to several hours after exertion. The victim often has been sweating heavily with insufficient or hypotonic fluid replacement for several days. Serum sodium levels are, however, normal.

Heat edema is manifest by ankle and wrist swelling occurring in the first few days of heat exposure and sometimes sufficient to be pittable.

Heat rash (prickly heat or miliaria rubra) most commonly occurs early in acclimatization in tropical areas where personnel are wearing tight-fitting clothing. It presents as an intensely pruritic, red, papular, occasionally vesicular dermatitis. Complications include infection and the formation of large nonpruritic plugs that take several weeks to desquamate. People with advanced heat rash are at risk for heat exhaustion or heatstroke due to loss of sweat gland function.

Heat syncope refers to a transient loss of postural tone with or without brief loss of consciousness occurring early in exposure to a new heat stress. It is often preceded by dehydration or the presence of drugs that affect the body's normal compensatory mechanisms. By the time victims are examined, vital signs are usually normal.

Heat tetany presents as carpopedal spasm, and is frequently seen in conjunction with other heat syndromes or other causes of hyperventilation. Differentiated from heat cramps, it does not involve the heavily used proximal muscles. Arterial blood gas analysis may reveal a respiratory alkalosis.

Victims of heat exhaustion are usually unacclimatized people who have been working in the heat for several days. Symptoms of the water depletion type include thirst, weakness, dizziness, anxiety, muscle incoordination, agitation, confusion, palpitations, oliguria, and elevated temperature. Those of the salt depletion variant include fatigue, weakness, headache, anorexia, vomiting, diarrhea, and skeletal muscle cramps. Thirst is absent, and the temperature is usually normal or subnormal. In both types of heat exhaustion the skin is cool and clammy, and tachycardia and hypotension are common. Most victims have a mixed-type heat exhaustion and present with a combined picture. Laboratory findings may include hyponatremia, high urine specific gravity, and mildly elevated serum creatine phosphokinase and liver enzyme levels. Without termination of the heat stressor and immediate treatment heat exhaustion may progress to frank heatstroke.

Classic heatstroke usually affects the very young or the debilitated elderly, and develops over several days, mostly during heat waves. The gradual onset may result in severe dehydration and hot dry skin. Exertional heatstroke usually occurs in an unacclimatized younger person after a few hours of severe heat stress. Victims are usually still capable of sweating.

Vital signs show hyperthermia (usually more than 40°C), tachycardia, tachypnea, and hypotension. Family or witnesses may describe a malaise or flu-like prodrome. Because a high core temperature for a short period of time can produce the same injury as a relatively lower temperature for a longer period, the presenting temperature may not predict severity or outcome.

Widespread damage to almost every organ system, especially the cerebellum, has been described. The central nervous system (CNS) is one of the first systems involved and the last to recover. Mental confusion begins with a core temperature of 38°C with cessation of function at greater than 42°C. Any CNS change from confusion and coma to seizure activity and posturing has been described.

The liver is particularly susceptible to heat injury. Serum transaminase levels may initially be in the 1000s and peak up to 2 weeks later in the 10,000s. Coagulopathies and hypoglycemia are common. The kidneys are at high risk for acute tubular necrosis. Rhabdomyolysis may contribute to renal injury in victims of exertional heatstroke. Arterial blood gas analysis usually reveals a respiratory alkalosis. Lactic acidosis may also be seen after heavy exertion. Death is usually secondary to disseminated intravascular coagulation, acute renal failure, liver failure, or acute respiratory distress syndrome.

DIFFERENTIAL DIAGNOSIS

The differential diagnosis of heatstroke includes infection, particularly meningitis, thyroid storm, drug intoxication, and the neuroleptic malignant syndrome (malignant hyperthermia). In contrast to heatstroke, those with the neuroleptic malignant syndrome have muscle rigidity.

EMERGENCY DEPARTMENT EVALUATION

The history should include duration, magnitude, and conditions of heat exposure; recent activity; nature, progression, and duration of symptoms; medications and drug use; and underlying medical problems. In young healthy victims a typical history and physical examination that reveal no other pathology are all that is necessary for a diagnosis of minor heat-related problems. Normal laboratory findings will confirm the diagnoses in questionable cases and in those with advanced age or coexisting medical problems.

In victims of heat exhaustion and heatstroke vital signs should include orthostatic pulse and blood pressure measurements as well as a rectal temperature. Depending on the severity, laboratory evaluation should include arterial blood gas analysis, complete blood count, determination of electrolyte, blood urea nitrogen creatinine, glucose, creatine phosphokinase, and liver enzyme levels, and urinalysis. Those with elevated creatine phosphokinase levels, abnormal electrolyte or liver enzyme levels, or high temperatures should also have coagulation studies; calcium, magnesium, phosphorous, and uric acid measurements; electrocardiogram; and chest radiograph.

EMERGENCY DEPARTMENT MANAGEMENT

Advanced life-support measures should be instituted as necessary. Heat cramps are treated with oral or intravenous fluid and salt replacement. Fruit juices or Gatorade by mouth is sufficient for mild cases. Intravenous normal saline solution is recommended for moderate or severe symptoms. Heat edema is self-limited and will resolve with time, elevation of the legs, and application of support hose. Patients with heat rash should keep their skin cool and dry and avoid wearing tight clothing. Antihistamines may be given for pruritus, but powders should be avoided in order to prevent further plugging of sweat glands. Desquamating agents (e.g., salicylic acid) and antibiotics effective against *Staphylococcus* may be prescribed for secondary infection. Heat syncope is treated with rest, ingestion of fluids and salt, and gradual return to activity. Heat tetany should resolve with the reversal of hyperventilation (e.g., bag breathing).

The treatment of heat exhaustion centers around replacement of fluid and electrolyte losses with isotonic saline solution. Patients who are orthostatic may require 4 or more liters of intravenous fluid. Oral fluids can substitute for or supplement intravenous fluid in mild cases. Rare cases present with severe hyponatremia that requires hypertonic saline infusion.

The cornerstone of heatstroke therapy is rapid cooling. The practice of immersion or covering the patient in ice is not recommended because skin cooling causes both vasoconstriction and shivering and could potentially increase the core temperature. The application of ice packs in the areas of large vessels such as the groin and axillae and the infusion of large volumes of cool intravenous fluids are useful for field management but insufficient for definitive cooling. Evaporative cooling and iced gastric lavage (0.2°C/min) are a more practical combination. Extracorporeal techniques (e.g., partial or complete cardiopulmonary bypass) might be considered in severe cases.

Maximizing evaporation without inducing shivering is accomplished by keeping the patient wet with lukewarm water or wet towels and blowing air over the patient with a fan. Helicopter blade fanning has also been used.

The rectal temperature should be monitored with a probe that is capable of measuring high temperatures (up to 44°C). Cooling is continued only until the temperature drops to 38.5° to 39°C, in order to avoid overshoot hypothermia. The rectal temperature monitor should be left in place, as the patient may rebound hours later and be thermally unstable for days. Along with cooling, patients will frequently need intubation and large volumes of intravenous normal saline solution. A central venous pressure line and Foley catheter are recommended to monitor fluid therapy. Acid–base, electrolyte, and coagulation abnormalities should be corrected. Alkaline diuresis may be helpful if rhabdomyolysis is present.

Shivering may be treated with chlorpromazine (25–50 mg IV) or midazolam (2.5–10.0 mg IV). Midazolam may be preferred because it does not lower the seizure threshold. Seizure activity is best treated with diazepam or phenobarbital. Phenytoin is considered to be ineffective. Dantrolene sodium has not been efficacious in canine studies.

Poor prognostic indicators are a serum glutamic oxaloacetic transaminase level of >1000 after 24 hours, more than 8 hours of coma, and a presenting temperature of 42.2°C.

DISPOSITION

Patients with minor heat-related problems may be discharged. Patients with heat exhaustion should be admitted to a floor bed if they have abnormal vital signs and laboratory findings, or remain symptomatic after fluid therapy. All patients with heatstroke should be admitted to an intensive care unit. Discharged patients should be advised to avoid conditions that precipitated their illness. Acclimatization with frequent water breaks and rest periods during hot weather activity should prevent future problems.

COMMON PITFALLS

- Failure to recognize heat-related illness and its nonenvironmental causes
- Failure to accurately measure a rectal temperature (by thermoresistor probe if necessary) in patients with suspected heat illness
- Failure to aggressively cool patients with heatstroke
- Failure to warn victims of heat-related illness about avoidance of re-exposure until acclimatization has occurred

116   High-Altitude Illness

High-altitude medical illnesses are combined in the broad category *acute mountain sickness* (AMS). This is a spectrum of disease ranging from subclinical signs to potentially lethal high-altitude pulmonary edema (HAPE) or high-altitude cerebral edema (HACE). The fraction of inspired oxygen in air remains constant at 21%, but barometric pressure decreases with increasing altitude. Therefore, PaO_2 reduction becomes clinically significant. Even a young, healthy, physically fit nonsmoker may experience PaO_2 under 60 mm Hg at 2500 m (8100 feet) and under 50 mm Hg at 4500 m (14,600 feet). Signs and symptoms occur in up to 25% of the population at 2500 m, and 75% at 4500 m. Symptomatic illness is uncommon but not impossible under 2500 m.

Pre-existing cardiac or pulmonary disease will potentiate the effects of hypobaric hypoxia at high altitude. Relative contraindications to high-altitude travel would include increasing age, chronic diseases, coronary artery disease, chronic obstructive pulmonary disease, pulmonary hypertension, sickle-cell disease, and other disease syndromes straining cardiopulmonary function.

Repeated attacks are common (about 20%), potentially limiting high-altitude activity and requiring prophylactic medications and a slow, controlled ascent.

CLINICAL PRESENTATION

Early symptoms of AMS are nonspecific and generally develop within 8 to 24 hours (range 6–48 hours). The incidence, severity, and duration of illness is proportional to the rate and height of ascent modified by individual susceptibility, physical exertion, and sleeping altitude. Symptoms vary widely but remain consistent on repeated episodes in the same patient. AMS demonstrates no sexual preference, but HAPE is more common in males.

Headache, anorexia, nausea/vomiting, malaise, insomnia, lassitude, shortness of breath, and dyspnea on exertion make up the most common symptom complex. The headache is usually throbbing, bilateral, and frontal. It is worst in the morning and worse when supine. It increases with exercise and may be poorly responsive to aspirin or acetaminophen. Sleep is generally poor and often exacerbates symptoms due to hypoventilatory hypoxia, so the patient feels worse on waking.

In mild cases, symptoms abate in 3 to 7 days as acclimatization occurs. Mild tachypnea and tachycardia attempt to compensate by maximizing oxygenation and oxygen delivery to tissues. Spontaneous diuresis reverses complicated fluid shifts but requires adequate fluid replacement to avoid dehydration and hypovolemia. Well-being at altitude is proportional to individual diuretic response. Chronic mountain sickness (CMS) or Monge's disease may develop in some patients who do not acclimatize despite prolonged altitude exposure. CMS is characterized by persistent hypoxia, polycythemia (hematocrit above 60), and development of congestive heart failure.

Worsening symptoms must not be ignored, and definitive therapy includes descent. Increasing headache, nausea, and vomiting accompanied by central nervous system (CNS) deficits such as confusion, poor judgment, or ataxia indicate rising intracranial pressure secondary to fluid shifts and herald the onset of HACE. This life-threatening complication can culminate in coma and death if untreated and may leave neuropsychological residual even if promptly recognized and treated.

HAPE is the worsening spectrum of pulmonary disease secondary to fluid shifts in hypobaric hypoxia. Worsening dyspnea, cough, hemoptysis, cyanosis, and patchy pulmonary infiltrates are harbingers of catastrophe unless recognized quickly and treated aggressively. Secondary complications of adult respiratory distress syndrome or infection may result in increasing inflammation and parenchymal damage, requiring long-term resolution. HAPE is a feared complication of AMS that recurs in susceptible individuals, thus requiring cautious reexposure.

EMERGENCY DEPARTMENT EVALUATION

Initial recognition and evaluation of AMS occurs on site at altitude. Patients may present directly to emergency departments at high elevations. A history of recent, rapid transit to high altitude should alert the physician to the potential diagnosis of AMS. A previous history of similar episodes at altitude should immediately raise suspicion.

Physical examination may reveal a dyspneic, tachypneic patient with peripheral or periorbital edema, oliguria, and rales characteristic of the antidiuretic fluid imbalance induced by hypobaric hypoxia in AMS. Despite the edema and oliguria, the patient is often dehydrated and hypovolemic, with increased hematocrit and hypercoagulable state. Petechiae may indicate disturbed vascular integrity, and papilledema may be present without raised intracranial pressure. High-altitude retinal hemorrhage (HARH) is detectable as flame hemorrhages in up to 40% of AMS patients; it is usually asymptomatic and resolves without residual unless macular involvement is present (less than 5%) and causes central scotoma. Cerebral edema may manifest itself by cerebellar dysfunction (ataxia) or cognitive impairment (confusion, disorientation).

Laboratory studies may reveal mild leukocytosis and hemoconcentration. Arterial blood gas analysis may show hypoxia, hypocapnea, and alkalosis. With HAPE, the chest radiography reveals a normal-sized heart and diffuse bilateral patchy infiltrates, in contrast to the typical butterfly distribution of alveolar edema. An ECG most often shows only sinus tachycardia, but it may show evidence of right heart strain. Pulmonary function tests indicate decreased vital capacity and peak expiratory flow rates. Pulmonary hypertension with normal left atrial pressure and normal pulmonary artery wedge pressure would be expected if pulmonary arterial catheterization becomes necessary. A kidney, ureter, and bladder (KUB) examination will often reveal increased intestinal gas.

EMERGENCY DEPARTMENT MANAGEMENT

Measures to prevent or reduce AMS in a person who is about to undergo rapid ascent to high altitude (particularly those with previous episodes) include cautious acclimatization and medication. A staged, gradual ascent is most effective to achieve acclimatization. Either remaining at 2000 m to 3000 m (6600–9800 ft) for 2 to 5 days before going higher, or ascending less than 300 m (1000 ft) per day above 2500 m (8200 ft) can significantly reduce symptomatology. Climbing high but sleeping low can also be effective in reducing the results of hypobaric hypoxia exacerbated by nighttime hypoventilation. Drinking plenty of fluids, eliminating salt intake, and limiting physical activity may restrict symptom development.

Acetazolamide induces hyperchloremic metabolic acidosis through bicarbonate diuresis that stimulates respiration to compensatory alkalosis. Pretreatment with 250 mg every 6 to 12 hours or 500 mg of the sustained-release formula each day, beginning 1 or 2 days before ascent and continuing at least 48 hours after ascent, mimics the acclimated state of acid-base balance. While some patients may not be helped, symptoms are lessened in 30% to 50% of patients. Side effects include paresthesias, gastrointestinal distress, somnolence, and dehydration if fluid intake is insufficient. Dexamethasone reduces vasogenic cerebral edema and AMS symptoms to a greater extent than acetazolamide with fewer side effects. Four mg every 6 hours should be started 48 hours before ascent and should continue 48 hours after ascent. Combining it with acetazolamide improves efficacy over either drug alone. These measures can also be used to treat mild to moderate AMS.

Severe or progressive cases require descent to below 2500 m (8100 feet), oxygen, diuretics, and fluid therapy. Depending on severity, endotracheal intubation, ventilatory support, continuous positive airway pressure, mechanical ventilation with positive end-expiratory pressure, and observation in the intensive-care unit may be necessary. If recognized early and treated aggressively, nearly all young, physically fit, otherwise healthy patients will improve quickly, often within 24 hours, with full resolution of disease symptoms.

DISPOSITION

Young, healthy patients with mild to moderate AMS may be discharged with instructions not to resume ascent until after symptoms have subsided. Medications should never be used to allow further ascent in light of persistent symptoms. Patients with HAPE, HACE, or moderate AMS and underlying cardiopulmonary or cerebrovascular disease, complications (e.g., ECG changes), or other significant medical problems should be admitted.

COMMON PITFALLS

- Minimizing or not recognizing the disease state remains the greatest danger.
- Failing to inform the patient that not descending when indicated or using medications to allow further ascent encourages disaster.
- AMS may be confused with viral illness if a history of high-altitude travel is not elicited.
- Diuretics should be used cautiously in the treatment of HAPE and HACE because coexisting volume depletion is usually present.
- Failure to improve rapidly with descent and treatment should raise the possibility of another diagnosis.

TABLE 117-1. Accepted Indications for Use of HBO Therapy

1. Arterial air or gas embolism
2. Acute blood loss anemia
3. Carbon monoxide poisoning, cyanide poisoning, smoke inhalation
4. Decompression sickness
5. Crush injury, compartment syndrome, and other acute traumatic ischemias
6. Enhancement of healing in selected problem wounds
7. Gas gangrene (Clostridial)
8. Necrotizing and mixed soft-tissue infections
9. Radiation necrosis, osteoradionecrosis, soft-tissue radionecrosis, caries in radiated bones
10. Refractory osteomyelitis
11. Selected refractory mycoses
12. Compromised skin graft or flaps
13. Thermal burns (special consideration)

---

117   Hyperbaric Oxygen Therapy

Hyperbaric oxygen (HBO) therapy is the administration of 100% oxygen to a patient who is placed in a chamber pressurized to greater than one atmosphere (1 ATA; sea level). The local application of pressurized oxygen to part of the body (generally an extremity) without the use of a chamber that completely encloses the patient is not considered HBO therapy.

Absolute contraindications to HBO therapy include untreated pneumothorax and pulmonary parenchymal damage such that the lung is unable to absorb more O_2. Relative contraindications include pulmonary bulla, seizure disorders, high-dose steroid therapy, chronic obstructive pulmonary disease, recent myocardial infarction, and claustrophobia. HBO therapy in pregnancy is controversial.

HBO therapy is the treatment of choice for decompression sickness, arterial air or gas embolism, and certain cases of carbon monoxide poisoning. See Table 117-1 for indications for HBO.

118   High-Pressure Injection Injuries

High-pressure injection injuries result from the direct injection of fluids or gases through the skin into underlying tissues via a small injection port under very high pressure (1,500–12,000 psi). On initial evaluation, they often appear benign, with only a drop of the injected material oozing from a painless entry site, but this picture belies the extreme tissue destruction and potentially severe loss of function of the extremity that commonly ensues.

The extent of injury depends on the pressure, the injected material, and the site of puncture. In the hand, the injectate tracks along the tendon sheath, bone, fascial planes, and potentially the deep spaces of the hand and forearm.

CLINICAL PRESENTATION

Although the index finger is most commonly injured, followed by the palm of the hand and the long finger, any body part unfortunate enough to be close to a high-pressure injector that discharges accidentally or a line that ruptures or leaks could sustain injury. It can happen with any fluid or gas. On initial examination there is often a small pinhole entrance wound with a drop of injectate expressible from it. The extremity or body part is often initially pain-free. This is followed by an acute inflammatory process that causes swelling and intense pain. This is the point at which patients often seek medical attention.

EMERGENCY DEPARTMENT EVALUATION

It is important to note the time that has elapsed since the injury, the material injected, the general medical evaluation of the patient, any previous care administered in other hospitals or first-aid stations, and the position and direction of the injection. The examination should be directed towards the injured part, usually the hand, and should include a peripheral neurologic examination with motor and sensory testing. All joints of the hand, wrist, forearm, and arm should be noted and their range of motion and movement assessed. A drawing or photograph of the injury can often be useful. A very careful evaluation for compartment syndrome and vascular status of the extremity should follow.

Depending on the injury, a hand, plastic, or other surgeon should always be consulted. The presence or absence of peripheral pulses, Doppler evaluation of peripheral pulses and palmar arch, as well as digital Doppler evaluation can be performed in the emergency department. In addition, the basic vascular examination, the Allen's test, should be performed in patients with hand injuries. If there is any question of compartment syndrome, compartment pressures should be measured in the ED by someone familiar with this technique.

Laboratory evaluation studies should include standard preoperative studies. Radiographic examination can be limited to plain films of the injured area and a preoperative chest radiograph. More advanced imaging has little use in this type of injury. All patients should be treated as preoperative (surgical exploration very likely) and will require admission.

EMERGENCY DEPARTMENT MANAGEMENT

The hand should be placed in a soft, bulky dressing without undue compression, splinted in a neutral position, and elevated on several pillows. There is controversy in the literature over the use of systemic steroids; there is no data to argue either way convincingly. Broad-spectrum antibiotics and tetanus toxoid should be administered, and the affected arm should not be used for insertion of intravenous lines or blood-pressure measurement. Regardless of the initial appearance, a surgeon, usually a hand specialist, should be consulted.

DISPOSITION

Because these injuries need direct and immediate surgical evaluation, observation, and nearly always intervention for drainage and debridement by someone experienced in traumatic hand problems, the simple presentation of the injury is an indication for hospital admission. The patient should be transferred if a trained hand specialist cannot be obtained to manage the case both intraoperatively and postoperatively. Future reconstruction may be necessary.

COMMON PITFALLS

- These injuries almost invariably lead to severe loss of function of the limb and are often accompanied by workmen's compensation, rehabilitation, and product liability issues.

- The major error to be avoided is failure to recognize the serious nature of the initially innocu-ous-appearing high-pressure injection injury and to underestimate its severity.
- It is imperative that the emergency physician consult a trained hand or other surgical spe-cialist or transfer the patient to a facility that can provide the appropriate care.

119 Smoke Inhalation

Smoke is a visible mixture of gases, vapors, fumes, liquid droplets, and solid carbon particles (dust) evolved during the combustion (the thermal degradation under conditions of high oxygen concentration) or pyrolysis (thermal degradation in an oxygen-poor environment) of organic mate-rial. Fire (a luminous gas) is not necessary for the production of smoke. In addition to fire and smoke, toxic products of combustion or pyrolysis (TPCs) may include heat, invisible gases, and oxygen deprivation. Hence, pulmonary and systemic toxicity due to the smoke inhalation may sometimes occur in the absence of visible warning. The nature and severity of inhalation injury and systemic toxicity from TPCs depend on the identity, concentration, and temperature of the TPCs, the particle size of soot, the length of exposure, and the victim's respiratory rate and health status. Carbon monoxide is clearly the most common TPC and is responsible for most deaths. Cyanide poisoning also appears to contribute to early mortality. This gas is present in about 54% of fires. The dose of TPCs delivered to the airways is proportional to the minute ventilation and duration of exposure.

CLINICAL PRESENTATION

Victims of smoke inhalation may present with systemic symptoms, respiratory symptoms, or both. Signs and symptoms of carbon monoxide and cyanide poisoning relate primarily to the cen-tral nervous and cardiovascular systems (e.g., ataxia, confusion, dizziness, coma, seizures, arrhythmias, tachycardia, tachypnea or bradypnea, and hypotension) and are discussed in detail in separate chapters. Nonspecific manifestations of irritant inhalation include cough, dyspnea, tachycardia, tachypnea, and cyanosis.

Signs of **upper airway injury** (eye, nose, and throat irritation) include conjunctivitis, tear-ing, rhinitis, pharyngitis, neck pain, dysphagia, drooling, hoarseness, and stridor. Fluorescein and slit-lamp examination of the eyes may reveal corneal burns. Examination of nasopharyngeal mucosa may reveal erythema, edema, hemorrhage, ulceration, or soot stains. Increased secre-tions and laryngospasm may be present. Facial burns and singed hair (head, eyebrows, or nose) are associated with the high incidence of thermal burns of the larynx and severe inhalation injury. Direct or indirect laryngoscopy may reveal laryngeal burns or soot. A lateral soft-tissue radi-ograph of the neck may show evidence of laryngeal or periglottic edema. A swollen epiglottis may be seen (irritant or chemical epiglottitis). Signs and symptoms of upper airway injury are usually immediate in onset and reach maximal severity within several hours of exposure.

Manifestations of **lower airway injury** include carbonaceous sputum production, bron-chospasm (wheezing), rhonchi, chest pain (burning or tightness), and rales (due to atelectasis). Bronchoscopic evaluation may disclose tracheobronchial findings similar to those described in upper airway mucosal injury. A pseudomembranous tracheobronchitis (mucosal sloughing) has been described. Bedside pulmonary function tests (e.g., PEFR, FEV1) may reveal decreased air flow. Flow-volume loop measurement is more sensitive than simple spirometry in detecting small changes in airway resistance. Radioisotope (^{133}xenon) ventilation-perfusion lung scans may show delayed washout of gas in areas of small airway destruction. A chest radiograph may reveal atelectasis. Arterial blood gas analysis may reveal hypoxia and hypercapnea. Severe symptoms may occur immediately, particularly in those with underlying pulmonary disease. More often, symptoms are initially mild and progressively worsen during the first 8 to 48 hours.

Pulmonary parenchymal injury causes nonspecific signs and symptoms. In contrast to localized rales from atelectasis, diffuse crackles may be heard in patients with pneumonitis or pulmonary edema. The chest radiograph may reveal patchy or diffuse infiltrates. Arterial blood gas analysis may show hypoxia and hypocapnea or hypercapnea. Unventilated areas on xenon lung scanning and decreased diffusing capacity are sensitive but nonspecific findings of parenchymal injury. Spirometry may reveal decreased lung compliance as well as increased airway resistance. Although pulmonary edema may sometimes develop immediately after irritant inhalation, it is usually gradual in onset and becomes maximal 1 to 2 days (or longer) after exposure.

Hypoxia may result in secondary complications (e.g., myocardial ischemia or infarction), particularly in patients with underlying cardiovascular disease. Although bacterial pneumonia and tracheobronchitis are common late complications, fever and leukocytosis secondary to chemically induced airway or lung inflammation may be seen in the absence of infection during the first 2 days after inhalation. Early postinhalation respiratory infections are usually due to *Staphylococcus aureus*, whereas late infections are often caused by *Pseudomonas* and other gram-negative organisms.

DIFFERENTIAL DIAGNOSIS

Patients with smoke inhalation may have concomitant dermal burns, traumatic injuries, and drug or alcohol intoxication and may be victims of arson, attempted murder, or attempted suicide. In patients with coma and shock, head CT scanning, whole blood cyanide levels, toxicology screening tests, and invasive hemodynamic measurements (e.g., central venous and pulmonary artery pressures) may be necessary to define their etiology.

EMERGENCY DEPARTMENT EVALUATION

The history should include details of exposure, symptoms, signs, and treatment prior to arrival, current symptoms, allergies, and previous illnesses (especially cardiac and respiratory problems). Important points in the exposure history include the nature of the burning material (natural or synthetic), length of exposure, open vs. closed space exposure, the presence or absence of explosion, falls, jumps, other victims (injured or dead), physical injury, steam, suicide note, mask use, and the amount, color, and odor of smoke. The likelihood of inhalation injury is greater with synthetic (plastics) fires, with closed space and steam exposures, and with exposure longer than a few minutes.

Any history of collapse or loss of consciousness also suggests a high risk of inhalation injury. Patients should be specifically questioned about respiratory symptoms, chest pain, alcohol and drug use, and suicidal ideation.

In firefighters, the type of oxygen mask used is important. With minor safety apparatus, oxygen is supplied by a demand valve requiring negative (inspiratory) pressure, and smoke inhalation can occur if the mask is not perfectly tight. With continuous positive-pressure oxygen devices (e.g., the Scott airpack), smoke inhalation is impossible unless the oxygen supply, which lasts 20 to 30 minutes depending on activity, runs out. In addition, invisible toxic gas inhalation may occur if either type of mask is removed during the the clean-up period immediately after the fire is extinguished.

After a trauma survey, the physical examination should focus on the mental status, vital signs (especially respiration), skin, eyes, nose, pharynx, and chest. Extensive burns (more than 15% of body surface area), facial burns, singed facial hair, and soot in the airways are associated with a higher incidence of inhalation injury. As with historical risk factors, however, their absence does not rule out significant inhalation injury.

Arterial blood gas and carboxyhemoglobin levels, ECG, chest radiograph, and bedside spirometry are recommended for all patients who are still symptomatic on presentation, particularly those with historical risk factors, abnormal findings on physical examination, and underlying cardiopulmonary disease. Although hypoxemia, elevated carboxyhemoglobin levels (more than 10%), abnormal breath sounds, and atelectasis or infiltrates chest radiograph are diagnostic of inhalation injury, these findings are absent in most patients who later develop respiratory complications. Since carboxyhemoglobin levels decrease with increasing time since exposure (particularly if oxygen has been given), they must be measured early in order to detect small but significant exposures. Patients who remain symptomatic should be evaluated after 3 or 4 hours, or sooner if symptoms worsen.

Patients with altered mental status should also have toxicology screening tests and a quantitative ethanol level. A whole blood cyanide level is recommended in patients with coma, acidosis, shock, and high carboxyhemoglobin levels. Although not immediately useful, it may later confirm the diagnosis of cyanide poisoning in patients who may require empiric treatment for this condition.

Laryngoscopy (indirect or direct) may be helpful in identifying mucosal damage in patients with mild to moderate upper respiratory tract symptoms, but should not delay immediate intubation in those with severe symptoms and respiratory distress. Additional evaluation for inhalation injury (e.g., bronchoscopy, ventilation-perfusion lung scanning, flow-volume spirometry) is impractical, and unnecessary for emergency department management and disposition.

EMERGENCY DEPARTMENT MANAGEMENT

Endotracheal intubation should be accomplished in patients with the following: central nervous system depression (i.e., no spontaneous or coherent verbalization); respiratory distress with stridor or drooling; cyanosis or hypoxia (PO_2 less than 60) that does not quickly improve with maximal oxygen delivery and continuous positive airway pressure (CPAP) by mask; full-thickness burns of the face (nasolabial) or neck (circumferential); pharyngeal, laryngeal or pulmonary edema; inability to clear secretions; or respiratory insufficiency (PCO_2 more than 50).

More liberal indications for early (prophylactic) intubation include less pronounced findings that progressively worsen despite treatment. In patients whose full-thickness face or neck burns restrict mandible or neck mobility and those with upper airway edema, blind nasal intubation may be successful when the larynx cannot be directly visualized. In rare cases, fiberoptic endoscope guidance, escharotomy, or cricothyroidotomy may be necessary for airway control. As always, if there is suspicion of co-existing head or neck trauma or cervical spine injury, precautions are necessary until radiographs rule out this possibility.

Aggressive suctioning of the airway to remove mucus and inhaled debris should follow intubation. Oxygen should be humidified to prevent drying of secretions. Hypoxemia despite intubation and 100% oxygen should be treated with positive end-expiratory pressure (PEEP) ventilation. CPAP and PEEP may also be helpful in the prophylactic treatment of pulmonary edema.

In patients without respiratory distress, stridor, or drooling, racemic epinephrine by aerosol inhalation may provide relief of upper airway symptoms. Bronchospasm should be treated with standard asthma medications. Chest physical therapy, incentive spirometry, postural drainage, and encouragement of coughing may help clear secretions and inhaled particles from the lower airway.

Management of carbon monoxide and cyanide poisoning are discussed elsewhere. Carbon monoxide poisoning should be treated according to usual guidelines. However, the use of the cyanide antidote kit in smoke-inhalation victims is controversial because the induction of methemoglobinemia, which decreases the oxygen-carrying capacity of hemoglobin, could be harmful in patients with hypoxemia and elevated carbon monoxide levels. Because coma, seizures, hypotension, and acidosis in the absence of alcohol, drugs, hypovolemia, hypoxemia, and carbon monoxide poisoning suggest cyanide poisoning, the use of cyanide antidotes should be considered in patients with these findings, but only if they fail to improve with supportive care. Although giving just the thiosulfate (the non-methemoglobinemia-inducing portion of the antidote kit) may be safe in patients with hypoxemia and high carboxyhemoglobin levels, the use of nitrites should be reserved for those receiving concomitant hyperbaric oxygen therapy and those in extremis.

DISPOSITION

Patients with continuing respiratory symptoms as follows should be admitted: cough and chest tightness; altered mental status; a history of loss of consciousness; abnormal lung sounds; concurrent drug or alcohol intoxication; elevated carboxyhemoglobin levels (more than 10%); abnormal arterial blood gases, chest radiograph, or ECG; facial or nasal burns; or a history of chronic cardiopulmonary disease. (These patients may be admitted simply for observation, if active treatment is not required.)

Depending on the severity of clinical findings and laboratory abnormalities and the co-existence of surface burns or traumatic injuries, intensive care unit, telemetry, or floor bed admission may be appropriate. Patients with carbon monoxide poisoning may require transfer for hyperbaric oxygen therapy, and those with significant surface burns or physical injuries may require transfer to a burn or trauma center.

Patients in good general health who are asymptomatic (on arrival or after a short period of oxygen therapy) and have a normal physical examination, arterial blood gas results (while breathing room air), ECG, chest radiograph, and carboxyhemoglobin level may be discharged, but it is generally advisable to observe these patients for at least 3 or 4 hours before making a discharge disposition. Discharged patients should be instructed to return immediately should any respiratory symptoms develop. A scheduled recheck at 24 hours may be prudent.

COMMON PITFALLS

- Failure to admit symptomatic patients despite the absence of abnormalities on initial physical examination, laboratory evaluation, and chest radiograph
- Failure to evaluate and treat for coexisting carbon monoxide poisoning, drug or alcohol intoxication, traumatic injuries, and psychiatric problems
- Failure to administer oxygen to all patients (including those with COPD) and to perform endotracheal intubation when indicated
- Failure to appropriately fluid-resuscitate patients with trauma or surface burns because of fear of exacerbating inhalation injury
- Failure to recognize the potential hazards of inappropriate corticosteroid, antibiotic, and cyanide antidote administration

---

120   Electrical Injuries

In electrical injuries, virtually all dissipated energy is converted to heat in the tissues by electrothermal transformation. Electrical power in watts is the product of voltage times current. Electrical energy in joules or watt-seconds is the product of voltage multiplied by current multiplied by the time in seconds.

When exposed to high voltage, skin will break down (char and burn), which physically removes the external barrier and allows the current to have direct access to internal tissue. Likewise, the exit point of a current path will undergo skin breakdown, usually described as an "explosive" wound. The surface area of contact, duration of contact, and the pathway of current flow are critical in assessing the potential and magnitude for hidden internal injury. Sudden death from ventricular fibrillation is three times more likely when current flows from arm to arm than from arm to leg.

Alternating current is significantly more dangerous than direct current. Tetanic muscle contractions are induced by the repeated stimulation of muscle fibers. Although all muscles will be affected, flexors tend to be stronger and predominate. This causes the "freezing" or "lock-on" phenomenon, which can prolong exposure and the severity of injury. Alternating current is also much more capable of inducing ventricular fibrillation at lower energy levels than is required for direct current. The frequency of repetitive stimuli (60 cycles per second) greatly increases the likelihood of hitting the vulnerable ventricular recovery period, analogous to the well-known R-on-T phenomenon.

It is important to understand and distinguish true conductive electrical injuries from burns associated with other electrothermal phenomena. Electrical flash burns result from the radiant heat produced by electrical arcs with temperatures ranging from 3,000°C to 20,000°C. These burns are usually localized to exposed surfaces and are treated in a manner similar to conventional thermal burns. True flame burns may also be seen as a result of ignition of clothing or other combustibles adjacent to the victim.

CLINICAL PRESENTATION

Electrocution and sudden death are usually a result of ventricular fibrillation, asystole, or other fatal cardiac arrhythmias. Sudden death may also result from direct insult to the brain stem, causing respiratory arrest. Standard ACLS protocols should be applied early and maintained for extended periods since these insults may appear refractory but eventually respond to continued resuscitative measures.

The unpredictable course of electrical current through the body makes accurate, initial clinical assessment of internal injury extremely difficult. External signs are usually limited and deceptively minor. Entrance wounds are commonly found on the hands or upper extremities and demonstrate charring, depression, edema, and inflammatory changes. Exit wounds may be multiple and varied and may have an explosive appearance. They are commonly found at the point where the body is closest to the electrical ground (i.e., the feet) or where the loop of current flow is completed. In bathtub exposures, there may be no external burns or signs of electric current entry or exit.

Cardiac arrhythmias and conduction disturbances are seen in as many as 25% of all victims with electrical injury. This is especially true for patients who have had a transthoracic current pathway. These abnormalities include ventricular fibrillation, asystole, ventricular tachycardia, sinus tachycardia, atrial fibrillation, AV block, bundle branch block, and a variety of atrial and ventricular ectopic beats.

Although nonspecific ST-T changes are common, true myocardial infarction is uncommon. This diagnosis is often confused by the fact that electrically injured skeletal muscle will produce significant elevation of CK-MB that is not of cardiac origin. Nevertheless, patients receiving conductive electrical injury through the thorax require at least 24 hours of continuous ECG monitoring. If arrhythmias persist or if other clinical factors suggest true myocardial infarction, further ECG monitoring is indicated.

Neurologic injuries are seen in some form in virtually all victims of electrical injury. Acute central nervous system manifestations include amnesia, altered mental status, irritability, depression, emotional lability, motor deficits, seizures, respiratory center depression, and coma. These acute changes are usually transient and excellent recovery may be seen.

Spinal cord injury usually has a delayed onset from a few days to several months. These manifestations are typically incomplete and predominately motor. The deficits may continue to progress with time and in general carry a poor prognosis for recovery.

Peripheral nerve injuries are common and usually result from direct electrothermal injury along the path of current. Vascular injury and compartment syndromes may also contribute to peripheral nerve deficits.

Acute renal failure is a major concern and must be addressed early in emergency management. The mechanisms of renal insult include decreased renal profusion from hypovolemia, along with the deposition of myoglobin and hemoglobin pigments released from massive muscle breakdown and hemolysis. Maintaining intravascular volume and brisk urine output are essential to prevent renal failure from these mechanisms.

Vascular and muscle damage can be extensive and severe. These tissues bear the brunt of destructive electrothermal forces. Extremely high temperatures and heat dissipation result from large current densities that will flow through these highly conductive tissues. Coagulation necrosis and vascular thrombosis are responsible for the enormous immediate and delayed devastation to these tissues. The net effect is an injury pattern more closely resembling a severe crush injury than a burn. Delayed rupture of injured blood vessels may be responsible for significant and catastrophic hemorrhaging.

A wide variety of skeletal fractures and dislocations may be seen from effects of tetanic muscular contractions or from the fall often associated with an electrical injury. Long-bone fractures, shoulder dislocations, and spinal compression fractures are common.

Electrical injury in pregnant women has been associated with fetal death and abortion. The amniotic fluid provides a rich electrolyte medium that will efficiently transmit electrical current to the fetus, creating a high risk of cardiac arrest and death.

EMERGENCY DEPARTMENT EVALUATION

Victims of electrical injury should be approached in a manner similar to multiple-trauma patients. Initial assessment and stabilization of airway, breathing, circulation, and cervical spine are appropriate, immediate priorities in these patients. As soon as possible, supplemental oxygen, large-bore intravenous lines to initiate fluid resuscitation, and ECG monitoring should be established. A careful history should be taken to determine the nature and potential severity of an electrical injury. This should include a determination of voltage, type of current (AC or DC), current pathway, and duration of exposure.

Consider other associated trauma (especially falls) as potential concurrent mechanisms of injury. A thorough and complete physical examination is mandatory to uncover potential multisystem injury. However, many important internal injuries may be missed on emergency department evaluation. A paucity of external physical signs may belie the severity of hidden internal tissue damage.

Indications for radiographic studies are established by the history and physical examination, but (as is the case in multiple trauma) special attention should always be given to the cervical spine and chest.

A complete ECG and continuous ECG monitoring are mandatory. Arterial blood gases, urinalysis, CBC, electrolytes, calcium, BUN, creatinine, cardiac enzymes, coagulation studies, and type and cross-match studies are necessary and appropriate for the early emergency department evaluation and management. An indwelling urinary catheter will allow urine to be monitored continually for volume output and for the presence of myoglobin.

EMERGENCY DEPARTMENT MANAGEMENT

Many unnecessary deaths and injuries have occurred in the field when first responders try to aid an electrical-injury victim before the electrical hazard is safely controlled. Definitive measures to ensure safety must be employed before assistance or extrication is provided.

Appropriate attention and priority should be given to the ABCs, including attention to and stabilization of the cervical spine. Use standard ACLS and ATLS protocols as indicated. For victims with cardiopulmonary arrest, resuscitative measures should be maintained for extended periods, since ultimate recovery may be achieved in cases that initially appear refractory.

Continuous ECG monitoring with arrhythmia recognition and management will be needed for at least 24 hours in all cases of transthoracic conductive injuries.

Aggressive fluid resuscitation is mandatory to prevent hypovolemia and renal failure. Extensive internal tissue damage causes large intravascular fluid losses that will greatly exceed the fluid replacement values usually calculated using formulas based on the percent of body surface area burned. Fluid requirements should instead be established to maintain brisk urine output and to prevent myoglobin nephropathy. A urinary catheter is mandatory to monitor urinary volume continuously and to detect myoglobin. If myoglobin (or hemoglobin) is present in urine, urinary output should be maintained between 1.0 and 1.5 mL/kg/hour. Once urine is clear of myoglobin, urinary output can be maintained at 0.5 to 1.0 mL/kg/hour.

Central venous or pulmonary artery pressure monitoring may be needed in patients at risk for hemodynamic instability or congestive heart failure. Intravenous mannitol and diuretics are appropriate adjuncts to enhance and maintain urinary output. Sodium bicarbonate should be added to intravenous infusions to alkalinize the urine and further prevent myoglobin precipitation in the renal tubules.

Serial monitoring of electrolytes, calcium, and arterial blood gases is necessary to detect and treat hyperkalemia, hypocalcemia, and acidosis caused by massive tissue necrosis or renal failure. Nasogastric suction may be needed to decompress the gastrointestinal tract and treat ileus. Tetanus prophylaxis must be assured.

Initial local management of surface burns is similar to that for conventional burns. Debridement and/or fasciotomy should be done only by an appropriate burn specialist and in general should not be attempted in the emergency department. For all serious injuries, consultation and/or transfer to a burn center is essential.

DISPOSITION

All patients exposed to high-tension (greater than 1000 volts) conductive injury require admission for intensive observation and monitoring. Consultation regarding transfer to a burn center is also advisable.

Patients with low-voltage nonsystemic injuries may be discharged after appropriate evaluation, observation, and management in the emergency department. When in doubt, admission is usually advisable.

COMMON PITFALLS

- Injuries to rescuers from uncontrolled electrical hazards in the field are clearly unnecessary and should be avoided.
- Pay attention to the ABCs and never neglect cervical spine precautions.
- Emergency department evaluation should be similar to the complete multisystem approach that applies to all major trauma. Give special attention to hidden injuries that may result from secondary trauma, especially falls.
- The severity of underlying injury may be hidden and is commonly underestimated in the emergency department.
- Inadequate fluid resuscitation and circulatory volume maintenance may dispose the patient to acute renal failure.
- All children with burns to the lips or the oral commissures must have a plastic surgery consultation, no matter how benign their initial injuries may appear.

121   Lightning Injuries

Five major mechanisms of lightning injury have been proposed. **Direct strike,** which occurs when the major pathway of current runs directly through the victim, results in the highest morbidity and mortality. Injury from contact occurs when lightning current strikes an object or structure that is touching the victim. With **side flash,** current splashes or sprays from an object through the air to the victim. **Ground current,** also known as step voltage or ground potential, occurs because a victim standing near a lightning strike point creates a potential difference between his legs. If ground resistance is greater than the victim's resistance, current may enter one leg and exit through the other. (Ground current and side flash mechanisms often produce multiple casualties.)

Associated trauma may result from myotonic extremity or neck contractions, acceleration/deceleration injuries as the victim is thrown, penetrating and nonpenetrating injuries from debris, and thermal burns exacerbated by metal jewelry or clothing fasteners or caused by ignition of clothing.

CLINICAL PRESENTATION

Because of the short duration of lightning exposure, current usually passes over the outside of the body (flashover phenomenon), commonly producing superficial or partial-thickness burns in characteristic linear or arborescent patterns. Entry and exit burns and deep internal burns with resultant rhabdomyolysis and myoglobinuria are rare.

The most common cause of death in the lightning victim is cardiopulmonary arrest. Internal propagation of the lightning electrical potential acts as a DC countershock and may send the heart into asystole with subsequent respiratory arrest. Because of cardiac automaticity, a spontaneous rhythm may occur, only to deteriorate secondary to hypoxia from prolonged apnea unless the victim receives prompt ventilatory assistance. A variety of cardiac arrhythmias and electrocardiographic ST-T wave changes have been reported. Primary respiratory arrest from lightning-induced paralysis of the medullary center may also occur. Pulmonary aspiration is a possibility with loss of consciousness. Resuscitative efforts should not be abandoned prematurely.

When current passes through the brain, intraventricular hemorrhage, epidural and subdural hematomas, coagulation of brain parenchyma, and thrombosis of vessels can occur. Virtually all lightning-struck patients have altered mental status and antegrade amnesia; retrograde amnesia occurs less often. Hemiparesis, hemiplegia, lateralizing neurologic signs, flaccid paraplegia, and altered autonomic function may be present. Cervical spine fracture and associated spinal cord injury may result from associated trauma. In fact, virtually any type of neurologic deficit may result from lightning injury. Evaluation and documentation of alteration in consciousness, orientation, and memory is essential. Sensorimotor deficits must be carefully evaluated. On presentation, extremities may appear cold, mottled, pulseless, and insensitive secondary to vascular spasm and sympathetic instability. Serial observation of pulses is necessary; normal function usually returns.

Half the patients with lightning injuries have structural ocular lesions. Cataracts may appear from days to years after injury. Common ocular lesions include hyphema, uveitis, iridocyclitis, and vitreous hemorrhage. Less common findings are transient unilateral or bilateral blindness, choroidal rupture, chorioretinitis, retinal detachment, and optic atrophy. Mydriasis unresponsive to light may occur and should not be taken as a sign of death. Sensorineural hearing deficit, hemotympanum, cerebrospinal fluid otorrhea, tympanic membrane rupture (in more than 50% of victims), or basilar skull fracture may result from the thunder's concussive force.

Important historical points and physical findings that may assist with the diagnosis include:

History of thunderstorm
Outdoor occurrence of accident
History from the patient or bystanders
Partial or complete clothing disintegration
Superficial linear, punctate, or arborescent burns
Tympanic membrane rupture.

EMERGENCY DEPARTMENT MANAGEMENT

Emergency department care requires continuation of the prehospital care priorities. If historical information is available, antecedent events, temporal changes in the clinical condition, treatment rendered, and data about the patient's allergies, medications, and previous health is important.

Give the patient with altered mental status 100 mg thiamine, 25 g dextrose, and 2 mg naloxone intravenously. All patients require supplemental oxygen, intravenous access, and continuous cardiac monitoring. Choice of intravenous fluids is a matter of personal preference; however, 0.9% NaCl may be preferable if dehydration is evident or if hyperkalemia is suspected (e.g., extensive or deep burns). Obtain as soon as possible a 12-lead ECG, cardiac enzyme levels, urinalysis for myoglobin, complete blood count, and other laboratory tests. Obtain radiologic studies to evaluate suspected injuries. Patients with altered mental status, focal neurologic signs, or neurologic deterioration should undergo head CT imaging and cervical spine evaluation. Myoglobinuria (indicative of rhabdomyolysis and muscular injury) may necessitate fluid loading, osmotic agent administration, diuresis, and urine alkalinization.

Give standard burn wound care and tetanus prophylaxis, if appropriate. All patients require comprehensive and repeated physical and neurologic examination. Treat cardiac arrhythmias in standard fashion.

DISPOSITION

All patients with cardiac or neurologic abnormalities require admission for continuous cardiac monitoring for at least 24 to 36 hours, serial ECGs, cardiac enzyme analysis, repeated neurovascular assessment, and supportive care. Those with associated trauma, burns, or rhabdomyolysis may require admission for injuries.

COMMON PITFALLS

- Lightning injuries are often misdiagnosed as isolated cutaneous-thickness burns or as neurovascular or cardiovascular events.
- Patients found pulseless and apneic should receive prolonged resuscitative efforts. Unreactive pupils cannot be taken as a sign of death.
- Lightning injuries are not the same as high-voltage injuries.

122   Drowning

Drowning is defined as death from suffocation due to submersion in a fluid. **Near-drowning** implies survival, at least temporarily, after such suffocation. Drowning is thought to begin with an initial period of panic, followed by a struggle with breath-holding. Subsequently, apnea occurs, followed by swallowing of large amounts of water, which may be vomited and aspirated. The victim ultimately loses consciousness; shortly after, cardiac arrest ensues.

Cardiovascular complications may develop as a result of hypoxia and acidosis. Hypothermia may also be a contributory factor. The most common findings are arterial hypotension and cardiac arrest. Ventricular fibrillation is rare, particularly in normothermic patients. Severe neurologic damage occurs in 15% to 25% of near-drowning patients. A successful neurologic outcome is more likely in those receiving cardiopulmonary resuscitation and those with hypothermia. Neurologic injury is due to hypoxia, which is further complicated by metabolic acidosis and secondary cerebral hypoperfusion. Cerebral edema may lead to brain stem herniation and sudden death. The degree of anoxic injury depends on the duration of hypoxia, the water temperature, and the patient's underlying physical condition. Ten to twenty percent of patients presenting with coma will recover completely despite initially fixed, dilated pupils.

CLINICAL PRESENTATION

Victims of near-drowning may present in various stages of resuscitation. They may be awake, lethargic but arousable, combative, comatose, or in cardiac arrest. A history of coughing, choking, or vomiting may be given. In mild cases, the pulse, blood pressure, and respiratory rate may be elevated, but in patients with severe hypoxia, vital signs may be decreased or absent. Hypothermia may be present. Examination may reveal cool, clammy, pale or cyanotic skin. Vomitus, aspirated or regurgitated food, water, or other foreign material may be present in the mouth and airway. Rhonchi, rales, or wheezing may be audible on pulmonary examination. Gastric distention is common. In severe cases, decorticate or decerebrate posturing or flaccid paralysis with unreactive pupils and absent cranial nerve, brain stem, and deep tendon reflexes may be observed. Associated traumatic injuries may also be present. Victims of scuba-diving accidents may have evidence of barotrauma. The ECG may reveal evidence of ischemia, sinus tachycardia or bradycardia, ventricular ectopy, fibrillation, or asystole. Atrial fibrillation may also occur, primarily in patients with hypothermia. Arterial blood gas analysis may reveal acidosis, hypoxia, and hypercapnea. Although leukocytosis may be present, the hematocrit is usually normal. Except for a decrease in bicarbonate, serum chemistries are usually normal on presentation. Evidence of hemolysis, infection, rhabdomyolysis, and anoxic organ damage (e.g., liver and renal failure, disseminated intravascular coagulation) may appear hours or days after the initial insult.

The chest radiograph may reveal isolated or diffuse patchy infiltrates or frank pulmonary edema. An initially normal radiograph may reveal these findings if repeated several hours later.

EMERGENCY DEPARTMENT EVALUATION

The history should include details such as submersion time, submersion medium and temperature, events surrounding the accident and level of consciousness, vital signs at the scene, and signs, symptoms, and treatment prior to arrival. For children who fall into pails of liquid (e.g., detergent, insecticide), the contents and its potential toxicity should be ascertained. An accident near rocks, in heavy surf, or while diving, or an unwitnessed event, should suggest the possibility of head or spinal injury.

The physical examination should focus on vital signs, cardiopulmonary status, and neurologic findings. To rule out hypothermia, a rectal temperature should be taken. Look for evidence of associated barotrauma, physical trauma, or chemical injury. In children, the possibility of abuse or neglect should be considered. The Glasgow Coma Scale is helpful in monitoring progress. In all symptomatic patients, an initial cardiac rhythm and subsequent ECG and chest radiograph should be obtained. Baseline laboratory evaluation should include an arterial blood gas analysis, CBC, platelet count, serum chemistries (electrolytes, glucose, BUN, creatinine), coagulation profile, and urinalysis. Seriously ill patients should also have liver function test, calcium, magnesium, and CPK measurements. Obtain cardiac enzymes in victims who require CPR or who have arrhythmias or ECG evidence of ischemia.

EMERGENCY DEPARTMENT MANAGEMENT

Rapid prehospital response and early initiation of resuscitation is the most important factor influencing morbidity and mortality. Although artificial ventilation can be started immediately in unconscious patients, cardiac compression is impractical and ineffective while the victim is still in the water. Hence, rapid extrication is essential. All victims should receive high-flow oxygen and endotracheal intubation if clinically indicated. Wet clothing should be removed to prevent cooling and allow for inspection of traumatic injuries. In patients who remain obtunded, cyanotic, or hypotensive despite intubation and fluid resuscitation, or who present with cardiac arrhythmias, acidosis is often present and $NaHCO_3$ (1–2 mg/kg) should be given empirically. Naloxone and 50% dextrose should also be given to the unconscious patient.

In the emergency department, the treatment of hypoxia is of utmost importance. Patients with an arterial PO_2 less than 50 mm Hg or PCO_2 greater than 50 mm Hg while receiving 100% O_2 by mask should be intubated. If only hypoxia is present, continuous positive airway pressure by mask (CPAP) may be useful. In intubated patients with persistent hypoxia, mechanical ventilation with positive end-expiratory pressure (PEEP) will decrease the amount of intrapulmonary shunting, reduce ventilation/perfusion mismatch, and increase the functional residual capacity, resulting in an increased Pa_2. The use of PEEP may also prevent secondary drowning due to ARDS. Aggressive suctioning and bronchoscopy may be necessary. Bronchospasm can be treated with aerosolized bronchodilators. Prophylactic antibiotics have not been proven useful in preventing infection after aspiration.

The initial therapy for hypotension is intravenous fluid replacement with an isotonic crystalloid solution. Progressive central venous or pulmonary artery pressure readings, as well as urinary output via Foley catheter, may be necessary to guide fluid resuscitation. Adequate fluid resuscitation should be achieved before vasopressors are used. Volume status must be carefully monitored so that the patient is not overloaded with fluid, which may worsen cerebral edema. Severe or persistent metabolic acidosis should be treated with intravenous sodium bicarbonate.

Early gastric decompression via nasogastric tube is recommended in any symptomatic near-drowning victim in order to prevent vomiting, aspiration, and further respiratory compromise.

Cerebral resuscitation primarily depends on rapid stabilization and correction of metabolic abnormalities. Treatments such as mild dehydration, controlled hyperventilation, induced moderate hypothermia (30°C), barbiturate coma, and paralysis are unproven. In children with increased intracranial pressure (ICP), the use of hyperventilation, elevation of the head, osmotic and loop diuretics, barbiturates, and steroids may be used with the goal of keeping ICP less than 20 mm Hg and cerebral perfusion pressure greater than 50 mm Hg. Pharmacologic treatment of agitation and seizures may also be necessary.

DISPOSITION

Admit patients who have been apneic or unconscious, those with extremes of age, those with hypoxia, arrhythmias, ECG evidence of ischemia, or an abnormal chest radiograph, and those whose symptoms persist after emergency department evaluation and treatment. The level of care (floor vs. intensive care) depends on the severity and progression of clinical and laboratory findings. Patients who are asymptomatic or become so after 4 to 6 hours of observation and have a normal physical examination, room air arterial blood gas analysis, and chest radiograph may be discharged home with a responsible relative or friend. They should be instructed to return immediately if any symptoms (e.g., cough, wheezing, dyspnea, fever) develop.

COMMON PITFALLS

- In all near-drowning victims, the possibility of occult traumatic injuries, cerebral air embolism, drug intoxication, hypothermia, and medical illness should be considered.
- The Heimlich maneuver is used to clear the upper airway of particulate matter but is of little use in removing aspirated fluid. Its inappropriate use may result in vomiting and aspiration of gastric contents.
- Patients who initially appear moribund may recover completely, and those who present with milder symptoms may later deteriorate.
- Despite the absence of abnormal findings on emergency department evaluation, patients with symptoms suggesting near-drowning should not be discharged until after being observed for 4 to 6 hours.
- Early evaluation and treatment of hypoxia is necessary to prevent permanent neurologic damage.

SECTION V

MEDICAL EMERGENCIES

PART I

Resuscitation

123 Resuscitation

The vast majority of patients suffer cardiac arrest outside a hospital, and most patients who die of myocardial infarction succumb to arrhythmias within the first hour after the infarction. The function of CPR is to provide some blood flow to vital organs until more definitive treatment, such as defibrillation, can be initiated. It is important to remember that CPR itself usually does not resuscitate patients from cardiac arrest. CPR must be accompanied by the early institution of advanced life-support.

AIRWAY In approaching the victim of cardiac arrest one must assess unresponsiveness, activate the system for initiating advanced life-support, and position the patient on the floor or a backboard to assess the airway. The tongue may fall back and obstruct the airway. Rescuers may open the airway by using the head tilt/chin lift maneuver. The head tilt/chin lift maneuver should not be used if neck injury is suspected. In patients with possible neck injury the jaw thrust maneuver is used.

BREATHING Once the airway is open, the rescuer looks, listens, and feels for an exchange of air. If the patient is not breathing, mouth-to-mouth respirations are administered. The current recommendations stress the need for taking a full 1 to $1^1/_2$ seconds for each breath to ensure adequate ventilation. The patient should be intubated and ventilated with oxygen as soon as it is practical.

OBSTRUCTED AIRWAY If the rescuer has optimally positioned the jaw, chin, and tongue and still cannot detect adequate air exchange, one must be concerned about an obstructed airway. The Heimlich maneuver is the recommended procedure for clearing the obstructed airway of a foreign body.

CIRCULATION The rescuer determines pulselessness through palpation of the carotid. If no pulse is detected, chest compressions should be instituted. CPR provides 10% to 30% of normal cardiac output. Mechanical resuscitators are available that deliver standard CPR.

ADVANCED CARDIAC LIFE-SUPPORT Because the recommended treatment protocols are based on the patient's underlying rhythm, it is important that electrocardiographic (ECG) monitoring occurs early and is followed throughout the resuscitation attempt. If the patient is in ventricular fibrillation, immediate defibrillation is recommended even before CPR, intubation, and other interventions. As soon as possible the patient is endotracheally intubated and an intravenous line placed. Central lines should be placed in the internal or external jugular veins. Peripheral lines should not be placed in the lower half of the body. (See Appendix for ACLS algorithms.)

PRESSOR AGENTS Epinephrine, a mixed alpha and beta adrenergic agent, is the pressor drug of choice for use in patients with cardiac arrest. The recommended dose is 1 mg every 3–5 minutes during the arrest, but the optimal dose has not been established.

ANTIARRHYTHMICS   Both lidocaine and bretylium raise the fibrillation threshold, and thus are useful in preventing recurrent ventricular fibrillation. Lidocaine should be the initial antiarrhythmic.

Atropine   Atropine is a parasympatholytic drug that may be useful in some patients with asystolic cardiac arrest who have an excess of parasympathetic stimulation. Accepted dosage
is 1 mg every 3–5 minutes. Atropine is useful in symptomatic bradycardia.

CALCIUM   The use of calcium should be restricted to patients who are suspected to have
hyperkalemia, hypocalcemia, or calcium channel blocker toxicity.

PACEMAKERS IN CARDIAC ARREST   Pacemakers cannot be recommended for routine use in asystolic cardiac arrest, but continue to have a role in the management of symptomatic bradyarrhythmias refractory to drug therapy.

INVASIVE CPR

Invasive CPR improves hemodynamics, resuscitation, and the chances of surviving cardiac arrest.
It has also been demonstrated that when invasive CPR is applied late in the treatment protocol
(after more than 15–20 minutes of total arrest time) there is no improvement in resuscitation. At
present, these techniques should not be used as last-ditch efforts for patients who do not respond
to standard ACLS protocols.

PROGNOSIS

The prognosis for survival after cardiac arrest depends on several factors, including initial rhythm,
cause of arrest, and the amount of time that elapses until BLS and ACLS are implemented. Time
is the most crucial determinant of successful resuscitation. The longer the patient remains in cardiac arrest, the poorer the chances for successful resuscitation. The presenting rhythm is the
most important factor in overall prognosis. Ventricular tachycardia and ventricular fibrillation have
a relatively good prognosis, whereas asystole and EMD usually have poor outcomes. Another factor is the time that elapses before CPR is initiated. Finally, the cause of the cardiac arrest is
another factor important for prognosis. In cardiac arrest due to extracardiac causes such as pulmonary embolism and hypovolemia the prognosis is very poor. In addition, specific entities such
as complete thrombosis of the left main coronary artery have poor prognoses because providing
adequate coronary blood flow is impossible.

COMMON PITFALLS

- It is important to remember that resuscitation efforts require a well-disciplined team. Often
cardiac arrests are managed in a chaotic, undisciplined environment that is not conducive
to optimal patient care.
- After the placement of an endotracheal tube, bilateral equal breath sounds should be heard
in the axilla. Breath sounds heard anteriorly may be transmitted from the stomach. Breath
sounds should be checked repeatedly during the resuscitation. Asymmetry of breath sounds
mandates prompt evaluation.
- Intracardiac medications should be avoided; epinephrine, atropine, and lidocaine (but not
bicarbonate) can be administered through the endotracheal tube.
- Hyperkalemia should be suspected as the cause of cardiac arrest in any patient with renal
failure. The ECG may show a characteristic sine wave pattern, which should not be mistaken
for ventricular fibrillation. Bicarbonate and calcium are indicated.
- Most patients in ventricular fibrillation can be defibrillated.
- Torsades de pointes can be mistaken for ventricular tachycardia or fibrillation. The ECG
reveals cycles of QRS complexes "twisting around" the isoelectric point of the ECG. It is

associated with a congenital or drug-induced prolonged QT interval, most frequently due to quinidine. Electrical cardioversion is usually successful. Magnesium may be useful.

- There are no good parameters to assess the effectiveness of CPR or to guide treatment during the resuscitation effort. Femoral pulsations may reflect venous rather than arterial blood flow. Carotid pulsations may reflect some blood flow but cannot be used as a guide to decision making during resuscitation.
- The longer the patient remains in cardiac arrest, the worse is the prognosis for resuscitation. After 30 minutes of resuscitation attempts the prognosis is very poor. No clear guidelines can be given as to when resuscitation efforts should be stopped.
- In patients who are hypothermic, as in near-drowning victims, resuscitation efforts should continue until the patient has been adequately warmed. Strong consideration should be given to cardiopulmonary bypass.

PART II

Cardiovascular Emergencies

124 Cardiogenic Shock

Cardiogenic shock is hypotension with evidence of impaired perfusion in the setting of acute myocardial infarction (AMI). Specifically, a blood pressure <90 mm Hg with confusion, cold moist skin and cyanosis, and oliguria defines the syndrome. About 10%–15% of all patients admitted with AMI develop cardiogenic shock; it remains a lethal complication of acute myocardial infarction with little improvement in mortality. A variety of causes, such as myocardial contusion, myocarditis, and cardiomyopathy, can produce cardiogenic shock, but the majority of cases result from coronary artery disease and AMI.

AMI can cause shock in several ways. Papillary muscle dysfunction or rupture can result in severe mitral insufficiency. An infarcted interventricular septum can rupture, resulting in a significant left-to-right shunt. A transmural infarct can cause rupture of the ventricular wall into the pericardium with cardiac tamponade. Finally, a right ventricular infarction can be extensive enough to impair left ventricular filling.

The main cause of cardiogenic shock, however, is extensive myocardial necrosis. When 40% of the left ventricle is infarcted the ability to maintain the systemic circulation is impaired. Catecholamine release produces tachycardia, vasoconstriction, and increased cardiac contractility, all of which increase the work load of the left ventricle and increase myocardial oxygen consumption, with extension of the infarct and compromised left ventricular function.

CLINICAL PRESENTATION

In many instances the presentation is clear: shock associated with characteristic pain and associated symptoms of AMI. In some patients the diagnosis may be obscured; for example, when the patient has an altered sensorium and cannot communicate effectively or when chest pain is not severe or is overshadowed by other symptoms. Physical findings vary from minimal signs of shock to stupor, cyanosis, and pulmonary edema. Signs and symptoms vary and can also rapidly deteriorate. Close observation and repeated examinations are indicated when the diagnosis is suspected.

DIFFERENTIAL DIAGNOSIS

Massive pulmonary embolus complicated by hypotension should be considered. Cyanosis and tachypnea could support either diagnosis. The absence of auscultatory findings favors pulmonary embolus over a cardiac etiology. Arterial blood gas analysis is probably not helpful in distinguishing the two but an electrocardiogram (ECG), a chest radiograph, and an echocardiogram are valuable. Thoracic aortic dissection may be mistaken for cardiogenic shock; however, hypertension is the rule with dissection. Hypotension can occur if the dissection extends retrograde into the pericardial sac and causes tamponade or if dissection ruptures into the chest or abdominal cavity. A chest film and ECG should help to distinguish the two diagnoses; ultimately an aortic angiogram or CT confirms or rules out dissection.

Esophageal perforation can cause many of the signs and symptoms of cardiogenic shock, including retrosternal chest pain, diaphoresis, and respiratory distress, but shock is not universally present. When shock does occur it is due to septic complications, which can occur within hours but are usually more delayed in onset. Absence of pulmonary edema and the presence of a fever and precordial crunch favor esophageal perforation over cardiogenic shock. Pleural effusion with or without pneumothorax also supports the diagnosis. Pericarditis complicated by effusion and tamponade can mimic cardiogenic shock. The more insidious course of pericarditis, the absence of pulmonary edema, and the typical ECG findings help to distinguish it from cardiogenic shock. An echocardiogram can establish the diagnosis.

Acute bacterial endocarditis complicated by severe mitral or aortic insufficiency is also a potential diagnosis. Fever and a more indolent course support endocarditis, but distinguishing the two entities may be difficult. An echocardiogram showing valve vegetations can establish a diagnosis of endocarditis, but normal findings do not rule it out. Shock of any etiology that results in coronary insufficiency and ischemic chest pain could be mistaken for cardiogenic shock. Similarly, noncardiogenic pulmonary edema with hypoxemia and secondary myocardial oxygen deprivation could be suggestive of an early phase of cardiogenic shock before hemodynamic decompensation has occurred.

EMERGENCY DEPARTMENT EVALUATION

Diagnostic evaluation proceeds synchronously with stabilization. Depending on the degree of decompensation, a variety of diagnostic tests are indicated. A history and physical examination, however, are important. Pain consistent with AMI supports cardiogenic shock, with expected physical findings of pulmonary congestion, jugular venous distention, a mitral insufficiency murmur, decreased level of consciousness, and poorly perfused skin. An ECG, chest radiograph, arterial blood gas analysis, CBC, electrolytes, cardiac isoenzymes are indicated. The ECG is helpful if diagnostic of AMI, but it may show only a nonspecific pattern. The chest film may show early changes of congestive failure or a more fulminant picture of pulmonary edema. Arterial blood gas can gauge the severity and progression of decompensation. Of great diagnostic help is a portable echocardiogram. Identification of an akinetic or dyskinetic area of the left ventricle that corresponds to an area of ischemia or infarction on the ECG supports a diagnosis of cardiogenic shock. Conversely, a normal result all but rules out AMI and cardiogenic shock. The ECHO can also diagnose correctable causes of cardiogenic shock such as ruptured ventricular septum or ruptured papillary muscle.

EMERGENCY DEPARTMENT MANAGEMENT

The management of cardiogenic shock consists of three components: prevention, supportive care, and myocardial reperfusion. Tachyarrhythmias, symptomatic bradycardia, and hypertension increase myocardial oxygen consumption and should be aggressively treated. Routine use of atenolol and metoprolol is also of proven value in limiting infarct size and improving survival. Active airway management may be necessary to assure oxygenation.

Maintenance of an adequate blood pressure is a far more complex issue. The measures normally used to restore pressure can adversely affect myocardial oxygen consumption, and thus worsen the problem. Measurements of cardiac output and left heart pressures are usually not available in the ED. The clinician must decide between empiric therapy that could be deleterious, taking the time to place a Swan–Ganz catheter, or transferring an unstable patient to an ICU. The patient's condition, however, may mandate immediate treatment without benefit of hemodynamic measurements. It is reasonable to attempt volume expansion by administering small boluses of normal saline. Some patients in cardiogenic shock have normal or low left ventricular end-diastolic pressures, and although most do not respond to volume expansion, it is nevertheless acceptable to initiate careful incremental saline infusions as a first step. If fluid challenge is ineffective, a vasopressor should be used.

Dobutamine has the advantage of increasing cardiac output and lowering left ventricular filling pressure while not increasing the pulse rate or otherwise increasing oxygen demand. Dobutamine also decreases vascular resistance, improving cardiac output without increasing blood pressure. If the blood pressure remains low despite adequate doses of dobutamine, dopamine should be added to the regimen. Both vasopressors should be titrated to the desired clinical effect. Vasodilators (intravenous nitroglycerin and nitroprusside) can be added to decrease afterload and left ventricular work and oxygen consumption. Extreme caution must be exercised when using these drugs because of their hypotensive effects. All hemodynamic parameters must be monitored continuously and drugs titrated carefully.

Furosemide and morphine may also be of help. The anxiolytic effect of morphine relieves apprehension and may help to reduce tachycardia. However, the preload and afterload reduction caused by morphine, although potentially helpful, may be detrimental. Similarly, furosemide may cause deterioration by reducing preload excessively through venodilatation and diuresis. Because of these hazards, it is probably wise to avoid these drugs. Unstable patients may benefit from an intra-aortic balloon pump. The majority of such patients do poorly and cannot be weaned from the pump.

Re-establishing coronary perfusion after AMI has proved to be beneficial, but choosing the most appropriate reperfusion modality is complicated. Options include thrombolytic therapy, percutaneous transluminal coronary angioplasty (PTCA), and surgical revascularization. A large amount of data in hemodynamically stable victims of AMI indicate that thrombolysis, alone or in combination with PTCA, is most advantageous, with emergency surgery reserved for patients in whom PTCA is not feasible. Preliminary data on the use of streptokinase show no overall improvement in survival, but in patients in whom recanalization is successful, survival rate is doubled (84% versus 42%). Data on PTCA in cardiogenic shock are also preliminary, but more favorable. Emergent surgical revascularization may be of benefit in patients in whom PTCA has failed, provided it is applied within several hours of the onset of shock. The treatment of cardiogenic shock remains unsatisfactory.

DISPOSITION

The role of the cardiology consultant is crucial. Difficult decisions must be made quickly about additional resuscitative efforts, invasive monitoring, and the feasibility of coronary angiography and reperfusion. Therefore, once the diagnosis is seriously considered, consultation should be requested immediately. The patient should go to either the CCU or directly to the cardiac catheterization laboratory. Transport must be expeditious, monitored, and accompanied by appropriate resuscitative equipment and capable physician personnel.

Transfer of patients from one institution to another is hazardous and doomed to failure unless some hemodynamic stability has been achieved. Transport should be carried out by a specialized team. Transport under less favorable conditions carries a significant risk.

COMMON PITFALLS

- Failure to promptly diagnose cardiogenic shock in its early stages is the most significant error in management. Not recognizing the diagnosis until decompensation is severe may preclude any meaningful intervention.

- Failure to recognize right ventricular infarction or surgically correctable causes of cardiogenic shock is also a serious error. The former condition requires more volume expansion; the latter ones require surgery. The prognoses for both entities are better than for shock related to extensive left ventricular necrosis. Failure to diagnose these conditions results in adverse patient outcome.
- Liberal use of morphine and diuretics may produce untoward hemodynamic effects. These drugs should be used cautiously, preferably while monitoring left heart pressures and cardiac output.
- Medical antishock trousers (MAST trousers) to treat cardiogenic shock should be avoided. MAST trousers cause an increase in afterload that further taxes the compromised left ventricle.

125 Ischemic Heart Disease, Angina Pectoris, and Myocardial Infarction

There are more than 65 million Americans with cardiovascular disease, including hypertension, coronary artery disease, rheumatic heart disease, and stroke. Approximately 45% of all deaths in the USA are due to cardiovascular disease, and nearly half of these deaths are in patients under age 65. At least 250,000 patients with ischemic heart disease (IHD) experience prehospital cardiac arrest each year. IHD most commonly presents in one of three ways: chest pain (angina pectoris), acute myocardial infarction (MI), or sudden cardiac death. The anginal IHD syndrome can be very broadly separated into two categories: stable versus unstable coronary artery disease. This classification is the most useful from a diagnostic and therapeutic standpoint, particularly with the advent of thrombolytic therapy and percutaneous transluminal coronary angioplasty (PTCA). The determinants of myocardial oxygen supply and the factors that determine myocardial oxygen demand are listed in Table 125-1.

Medical management of chronic stable angina includes oral nitrates, beta blockers, and calcium channel blockers; these either increase myocardial oxygen supply or decrease demand.

Unstable coronary artery syndromes encompass unstable angina pectoris and acute MI. The occurrence of chest pain is thought to result from intermittent flow limitations caused by platelet or fibrin thrombi, an increase in coronary vasomotor tone (i.e., vasospasm), or a combination of both, in the area of the unstable arterial plaque. Such patients may present with a prior history of chest pain and may previously have had a normal exercise stress test, or coronary

TABLE 125-1. Determinants of Oxygen Supply and Demand

Oxygen Demand	Oxygen Supply
Frequency of pressure development (heart rate)	Diastolic time
	Extravascular resistance
Rate of pressure development (contractility)	Perfusion pressure
	Collateral resistance
Ventricular volume (preload)	Coronary arterial tone
Pressure developed (afterload)	

angiography that demonstrated noncritical coronary obstruction. Myocardial ischemia can also occur in the absence of coronary atherosclerosis. Common causes of nonatherosclerotic myocardial ischemia are listed in Table 125-2.

CLINICAL PRESENTATION
HISTORY

No single presenting symptom is uniformly diagnostic of IHD. Chest pain or chest discomfort is the most common chief complaint of patients with IHD. Such pain or discomfort may be described as a burning, tightness, squeezing, or heaviness, and as dull, sharp, or knifelike in character. Substernal or retrosternal chest pain may radiate to the left shoulder or to the arm, neck, or jaw; patients may also complain of abdominal discomfort. Chest pain that can be localized with a fingertip is unlikely to be of ischemic cardiac origin. Chest pain caused by IHD usually occurs abruptly, increases in intensity over time, and reaches peak intensity within 2 to 5 minutes. If the pain occurs during or immediately after exertion, it typically resolves gradually within minutes of cessation of physical activity. Chest discomfort that lasts for only seconds is unlikely to be due to IHD. Similarly, chest pain that is constant and lasts for hours to days is not consistent with IHD. Patients with IHD, particularly in diabetes mellitus or hypertension, may present with symptoms other than chest pain and often have "silent" MI. They may complain of dyspnea, early fatigue, or declining exercise tolerance—symptoms that are due to diastolic myocardial dysfunction.

A group of clinical or historical findings has been proposed to help identify patients with acute MI: chest pain; difficulty in breathing; upper abdominal pain, nausea, or both; fainting, dizziness, or both; palpitations; pedal edema; unexplained tiredness, weakness, or both; unexplained irritability; and pain in arms, shoulders, neck, or throat. One or more of these findings has been shown to be present in greater than 90% of all patients with IHD who seek medical care, but although sensitive, these clinical signs are not specific for IHD. Patients with a prior history of chest pain or with known controlled angina pectoris may present with new symptoms (chest pain at rest, chest pain associated with previously tolerated levels of exertion, chest pain unrelieved by a previously effective dose of a nitrate preparation, or chest pain of increasing severity, duration, or frequency). Unstable angina should be considered. This group also includes new-onset chest pain that is typical of angina.

Coronary artery vasospasm may produce symptoms that are atypical for classic angina pectoris. Episodes of chest pain or discomfort may occur at rest; pain may persist longer than is common for typical angina; and symptoms more commonly occur during the early-morning hours. They may also relate no risk factors for IHD. The symptoms of an acute MI may not be distinguishable from those of a severe stable anginal episode or of unstable angina, although patients with acute MI usually have chest pain of typical anginal quality for at least 30 minutes. Based on a number of epidemiologic studies, major and minor risk factors for IHD have been identified. These are enumerated in Table 125-3 and must be elicited.

TABLE 125-2. Causes of Nonatherosclerotic Myocardial Ischemia

Valvular Heart Disease	Congenital Heart Disease	Nonatherosclerotic Coronary Disease
Aortic stenosis	Congenital valvular disease	Coronary artery spasm
Aortic regurgitation	Coarctation of the aorta	Coronary artery embolus
Pulmonary stenosis	Cyanotic heart disease	Congenital coronary
(RV ischemia)		disease
Mitral stenosis with pulmonary		Coronary ostial occlusion
hypertension		(aortic dissection)
(RV ischemia)		Coronary artery vasculitis

TABLE125-3. Risk Factors for Ischemic Heart Disease

Major Risk Factors

Factors	Minor or Questionable
Family history (MI in 1st-degree relative age <55)	Obesity*
	Hyperuricemia
Smoking*	Hysterectomy/oophorectomy
Hypertension*	Hypothyroidism*
Hypercholesterolemia*	Steroid use
Diabetes mellitus	Type A personality*
Male sex	

*Modifiable risk factor

TABLE 125-4. Physical Signs That Occur During Myocardial Ischemia

Physical Sign	Underlying Pathophysiology
Soft S_1	Decreased LV dp/dt or 1st-degree AV block
Paradoxically split S_2	
S_3 and/or S_4	Prolonged LV ejection time
Mitral regurgitation	Decreased LV diastolic compliance
Palpable precordial systolic bulge	Papillary muscle ischemia
	Anterior or lateral dyskinesis
Bibasilar rales	Increased preload

LV, left ventricular; dp/dt, rate of rise of pressure; AV, atrioventricular.

PHYSICAL EXAMINATION

Most patients with chest pain caused by IHD have one or more abnormal physical findings, but these are not specific for IHD and may occur in patients with valvular or congenital heart disease, or cardiomyopathy. If the finding of an S4 is excluded, about 25% of patients with symptomatic IHD have a normal physical examination. Common physical signs during myocardial ischemia are noted in Table 125-4. The clinician should also seek evidence of risk factors for IHD, hypercholesterolemia and hypertension.

DIFFERENTIAL DIAGNOSIS

Common diseases that may be confused with IHD include pneumonia, pulmonary embolism or infarction, mitral valve prolapse, pericarditis, aortic dissection, esophagitis, esophageal spasm, peptic ulcer disease, and chest wall pain.

EMERGENCY DEPARTMENT EVALUATION
ELECTROCARDIOGRAPHY

The initial ECG may be normal even during AMI. The initial ECG in patients with chest pain has a sensitivity of only 48%. In the ED, the initial ECG may be highly specific for acute IHD, but has a low sensitivity (i.e., a negative ECG does not eliminate IHD as the cause of chest pain). Several studies have shown that the ED ECG alone has little impact on the disposition of patients with chest pain. Common ECG findings in patients with IHD include evidence of prior MI (pathologic Q waves, T wave inversion, or poor R wave progression in the anterior precordial leads), intraventricular conduction defects (right or left bundle-branch blocks), evidence of chamber enlargement (e.g., left atrial and left ventricular hypertrophy) caused by either systemic hypertension or prior infarction with resulting ventricular dilatation, and ventricular ectopy.

The most frequent ECG findings in chronic IHD are nonspecific ST segment and T wave changes, usually defined as ST segment depression or elevation of less than 1 mm, and T wave flattening or inversion. ST segment elevation of more than 1 mm in two contiguous leads is seen in acute *transmural* MI. ST segment depression of more than 1 mm and symmetrical T wave inversion may be seen during acute *subendocardial* infarction. The latter findings may also be seen during an episode of unstable angina in the absence of myocardial necrosis but are not specific for an acute coronary syndrome.

Because in 90% of patients the right coronary artery supplies the inferior wall of the left ventricle (LV) as well as the right ventricle (RV), a right precordial electrogram should be done to detect RV infarction in the setting of inferior MI. RV infarction occurs in about 60% of patients who suffer an inferior MI, and is detected by ST segment elevation of more than 1 mm in lead V_{3R} or V_{4R}, or both. Although RV infarction commonly accompanies infarction of the inferior wall of the left ventricle, it becomes hemodynamically significant in only about 10% (arterial hypotension and distended neck veins, but clear lung fields).

CHEST RADIOGRAPHY

The most common chest film abnormality in patients with IHD is cardiomegaly, usually associated with prior infarction or chronic arterial hypertension; other findings include pulmonary venous hypertension, Kerley B lines, and chronic pleural effusions. The primary value is the detection of other causes of chest pain (e.g., pneumothorax and pneumonia).

CARDIAC ENZYMES

Serial analysis of plasma CK-MB provides the most sensitive and specific method for diagnosing acute MI. LDH and GOT are of limited value. Plasma CK-MB activity is elevated within 4–6 hours of the onset of symptoms. Peak levels are reached between 10 and 36 hours, and activity returns to normal within 48–72 hours. In subendocardial infarction CK-MB levels peak at about 15 hours; after transmural infarction the peak occurs at about 28 hours, reflecting the difference in the amount of myocardial necrosis. It is recommended that measurement of CK-MB be performed serially at 4–6 hour intervals for 24 hours. The diagnosis is usually evident within 8 to 12 hours. The value of a single isoenzyme determination is questionable. However, sequential measurements at least 6 hours apart may be of value.

NONINVASIVE ASSESSMENT OF LV FUNCTION

AMI depletes adenosine triphosphate stores, resulting in contractile dysfunction and ventricular wall motion abnormalities. Two-dimensional echocardiography and radionuclide cardiac scanning are both sensitive in detecting wall motion abnormalities, and both have been used in the screening of patients with chest pain and suspected IHD. However, neither technique can differentiate prior infarction from a new cardiac event.

EMERGENCY DEPARTMENT MANAGEMENT

Initial management should include low-flow oxygen, vascular access, and continuous cardiac monitoring.

THE UNCOMPLICATED PATIENT

If the patient is felt to be suffering an acute ischemic event (i.e., unstable angina or acute MI) and is having continued chest discomfort, attention should be directed toward pain relief. Discomfort usually resolves after administration of one or more sublingual nitroglycerin tablets (1/150 gr). If chest discomfort has not resolved after 4–5 nitroglycerin doses, an intravenous nitroglycerin drip should be considered (50 mg of nitroglycerin in 250 mL of dextrose 5% in water). The initial infusion rate is 10 µg to 20 µg/min, and can be increased in increments of 5 µg to 10 µg/min at 5- to 10-minute intervals until chest discomfort resolves or mean arterial pressure decreases by 10%. Most patients respond to infusion rates of 50 µg to 200 µg/min. At low doses nitroglycerin acts principally as a venodilator and decreases LV filling pressure, thereby lowering myocardial oxygen demand. At high doses intravenous nitroglycerin acts as an arterial vasodilator as well. Nitrate therapy may also directly affect the myocardial oxygen supply by producing coronary vasodilatation. The major complication of nitrate therapy (SL or IV) is hypotension. Ventricular ectopy should be treated with lidocaine (1 mg/kg IV followed by an infusion of 1 mg to 4 mg/min). The major side effect of lidocaine is neurotoxicity, manifested as altered mental status and seizures. If the patient's 12-lead ECG is compatible with an acute transmural infarction and the symptoms are <6 hours, or if chest pain and ST segment elevations persist after 6 hours, the use of thrombolytic agents should be considered (see Table 125-5).

COMPLICATIONS OF ACUTE ISCHEMIA OR INFARCTION

ARRHYTHMIAS

Rhythm disturbances are common during unstable angina or acute infarction; most commonly of ventricular origin. PVCs are noted in 80–100% of acute MIs. Brady- or tachyarrhythmias that compromise systemic or myocardial perfusion require immediate therapy.

CONDUCTION DISTURBANCES

Second- and third-degree AV block may occur during either inferior or anterior infarction. In inferior MI these conduction disturbances are normally associated with an increase in vagal tone, are usu-

---

TABLE 125-5. Thrombolytic Therapy in Acute MI

Indications

Chest pain >30 min and <6 h duration
Patient age <70
ECG evidence of ST elevation of ≥1 mm consistent with acute inferior or acute MI
    2 of 3 inferior leads
    2 of 6 precordial leads
    Leads I and AVL

Contraindications

History of CVA, known intracranial aneurysm, AV malformation, or CNS neoplasm
Spinal or intracranial surgery within 2 mo
Severe, uncontrolled hypertension (systolic >200 mm Hg, diastolic >120 mm Hg), even if controlled
    in the emergency department
Known bleeding diathesis or chronic anticoagulant therapy
Active internal bleeding within previous 3 wk (*e.g.*, GI)
Recent (within 3 wk) trauma or major surgery at a noncompressible site (*e.g.*, intra-abdominal
    surgery)
Women known or suspected to be pregnant
Prolonged and traumatic CPR during current MI
Diabetic hemorrhagic retinopathy

Relative Contraindications

Recent (within 10 days) puncture of a noncompressible vessel
Cardiogenic shock (consider PTCA)

CVA, cerebrovascular accident; AV, arteriovenous; CNS, central nervous system; CPR, cardiopulmonary resuscitation; PTCA, percutaneous transluminal coronary angioplasty.

ally transient and responsive to atropine. The abrupt occurrence of complete heart block is rare. In anterior MI high-degree AV block is due to ischemia of the conduction pathways, and complete heart block may occur abruptly. Bundle-branch blocks are usually associated with anterior infarction. The indications for temporary artificial pacing in the setting of acute ischemia are listed in Table 125-6.

LV pump failure begins to occur when approximately 40% of the ventricular muscle mass has been lost, with severe contractile dysfunction.

PERSISTENT CHEST PAIN

In persistent chest pain not responsive to nitroglycerin therapy, beta adrenergic blockers should be considered, especially in those who have abruptly discontinued beta blocker therapy. In other patients ED use of beta adrenergic blockers may be beneficial in reducing the work load. Containdications to beta blockade include high-degree heart block and LV failure. Propranolol may be administered in doses of 1 mg IV every 5 minutes and titrated to response until a total dose of 0.1 mg/kg has been given. Esmolol is a short-acting beta blocker (esmolol) that may be infused. Although morphine has traditionally been used to treat IHD chest pain unresponsive to nitrate therapy, usual clinical doses have little effect on cardiovascular hemodynamics and the determinants of myocardial supply-demand balance. Thus, although morphine may relieve IHD chest pain through CNS effect, it has minimal effects on the pathophysiology of acute IHD.

THROMBOLYSIS IN ACUTE MI

It is clearly established that acute transmural MI is associated with complete occlusion of the infarct-related vessel by thrombus. Dissolution of the thrombus by intravenous thrombolytic agents has been shown to reduce mortality and to improve myocardial salvage. Three thrombolytic agents are currently available: r-TPA, streptokinase, and urokinase. The first two are used most commonly. TPA has the shortest half-life, has no allergic side effects, and is clot-specific. The indications for and contraindications to thrombolytic therapy for acute MI are noted in Table 125-6. Patients with contraindications should be considered for emergency PTCA. The use of thrombolytic agents in unstable angina and subendocardial infarction is under investigation.

DISPOSITION

All patients with suspected AMI should be admitted to the hospital (ICU or CCU). Low-risk patients identified by clinical and ECG findings could be cared for in an intermediate care unit. When AMI

TABLE 125-6. Indications for Prophylactic Pacing in Acute Infarction

Indicated	Not Indicated	Controversial
Mobitz II AVB	1st-degree AVB	New LBBB
Complete AVB	Wenckebach 2nd-degree	New RBBB in inferior
New RBBB in anterior	AVB	MI
MI	Old LBBB	
RBBB + LAFB	Old RBBB	
RBBB + LPFB		
LBBB + 1st-degree		
AVB		
Symptomatic		
bradycardia		

AVB, atrioventricular block; LBBB, left bundle-branch block; RBBB, right bundle-branch block; LAFB, left anterior fascicular block; LPFB, left posterior fascicular block.

is suspected the cardiologist should be contacted as soon as possible to facilitate interventional therapy, if indicated. Patients who are not candidates for thrombolytic therapy may benefit from PTCA. Patients in the acute phase of infarction or with unstable angina should not be transferred to another facility unless definitive care cannot be given. In this situation, transfer by ACLS personnel is required after stabilization. Patients having an AMI can be safely transported to a referral center for thrombolytic or interventional therapy.

Patients discharged from the ED with a diagnosis of stable angina or atypical chest pain should be referred to a cardiologist for further evaluation as indicated (e.g., exercise stress test and ambulatory ECG monitoring).

COMMON PITFALLS

- Missed AMI is the 4th most common cause for malpractice suits against emergency physicians, but 1st with respect to monetary awards.
- For patients with uncertain diagnosis, the threshold for admission should be low. Due to limited diagnostic tools in the ED, only about 50% of patients admitted with "rule out MI" actually "rule in."
- A single ECG or CK-MB determination cannot be used to rule out the diagnosis of AMI.
- If the patient meets appropriate criteria, thrombolytic therapy should be administered as soon as possible.

---

126 Congestive Heart Failure and Cor Pulmonale

CONGESTIVE HEART FAILURE (LEFT HEART FAILURE)

Congestive heart failure (CHF) is not a disease but a symptom complex in which abnormal cardiac function is responsible for failure of the heart to pump blood at a rate commensurate with the requirements of the metabolizing tissues. CHF is associated with increasing age. Prognosis after onset of CHF is poor; 5-year survival after diagnosis is about 50% for all NYHA classes, and 1-year survival for NYHA classes III and IV is about 35%. The vast majority of cases of CHF are due to left heart failure (LHF). The symptoms and signs of LHF are produced by a variety of primary heart diseases as well as systemic diseases that affect left ventricular (LV) contractile function. The causes of LHF can be broadly grouped and subclassified as shown in Table 126-1. With the advent of effective therapy for hypertension, ischemic heart disease (IHD) has become the major cause of acute or chronic LHF in the USA. LHF caused by IHD may be of multifactorial origin: loss of ventricular muscle, intermittent ischemia and contractile dysfunction (e.g., papillary muscle dysfunction), ventricular aneurysm formation with paradoxical expansion and increased wall stress, and decreased ventricular diastolic compliance.

A decreased output (CO) at normal LV filling pressures is the hemodynamic hallmark of LHF. When CO falls, there are compensatory mechanisms that maintain perfusion. Manipulating the compensatory response to a fall in CO has become a therapeutic focus in managing chronic CHF (e.g., vasodilators and angiotensin converting enzyme inhibitors).

TABLE 126-1. Functional Classification and Causes of CHF

Contractile Dysfunction
Ischemic heart disease
Idiopathic cardiomyopathy
Myocarditis

Systolic Pressure Overload
Aortic stenosis
Systemic hypertension

Systolic Volume Overload
Aortic regurgitation
Mitral regurgitation

Restricted Diastolic Filling
Mitral stenosis
Left atrial myxoma
Hypertrophic cardiomyopathy

High-Output States
Hyperthyroidism
Anemia
Arteriovenous fistula

CLINICAL PRESENTATION

The typical patient presents with shortness of breath (dyspnea) at rest, decreased exercise tolerance, orthopnea or paroxysmal nocturnal dyspnea, ankle swelling and weight gain. In acute LHF (acute pulmonary edema) dyspnea is the major presenting symptom. Clinical findings usually include (a) rales (b) a 3d heart sound due to decreased LV compliance; (c) a 4th heart sound caused by forceful atrial contraction (not heard in atrial fibrillation); (d) peripheral edema and (e) jugular venous distention (JVD). None of the findings listed can distinguish LHF from cor pulmonale or intrinsic lung disease.

DIFFERENTIAL DIAGNOSIS

Common causes of LHF are listed in Table 126-1. Constrictive pericarditis and cardiac tamponade also impede diastolic filling and can mimic LHF caused by IHD. Common causes for sudden worsening of symptoms in patients with chronic stable CHF are listed in Table 126-2.

EMERGENCY DEPARTMENT EVALUATION

There are few diagnostic aids available in the ED. The CxR is usually useful but radiographic progression is not always seen. In addition, the chest radiograph may not correlate temporally with the patient's immediate condition, with as much as a 12-hour lag with onset of LHF and a post-therapeutic lag of up to 4 days after clinical resolution. The earliest finding is redistribution or "cephalization" of flow. When pulmonary capillary wedge pressure (PCWP) increases to 12–18 mm Hg, flow to the lower lung fields is reduced and flow to the upper lung fields increases. When the PCWP is 18–25 mm Hg, fluid accumulates in the interstitial spaces producing Kerley B lines, and the pulmonary vessels are enlarged and their shadows blurred. Alveolar edema occurs when the PCWP acutely rises to >25 mm Hg and is recognized by the classic butterfly pattern of bilateral perihilar infiltrates. In all stages the cardiac silhouette is enlarged (CT ratio >50%). In chronic LHF pleural effusions are common.

TABLE 126-2. Exacerbation of Chronic CHF: Precipitating Factors

Lack of medications (noncompliance)
Dietary indiscretion (increased sodium intake)
Arrhythmias
Myocardial infarction
Infection (increased metabolic demand)
Pulmonary embolus
Anemia
Thyroid disease

The ECG is of limited value. In chronic LHF the ECG usually shows enlargement or hypertrophy of one or more chambers, intraventricular conduction defects are frequent, and secondary ST-T wave changes caused by ventricular hypertrophy or bundle-branch block often preclude accurate diagnosis of acute ischemia or infarction. Arterial blood gas analysis predictably shows hypoxemia from ventilation-perfusion mismatch, and is of no value in diagnosis and of limited use in guiding therapy. Other blood tests show typical but nondiagnostic abnormalities.

EMERGENCY DEPARTMENT MANAGEMENT

All patients should receive oxygen, an IV line, monitor, and the head of the bed elevated. Drug therapy and acute intervention may vary, depending on the severity. Treatment is directed toward reducing LV preload or filling pressure and secondarily toward improving myocardial contractility or decreasing afterload. With mild to moderate LHF (normal or hypertensive, and rales, JVD, 3d and 4th heart sounds, and pedal edema), IV furosemide (80 mg) will decrease preload and induce diuresis, and SL (0.8–1.2 mg) or oral (20–40 mg) nitroglycerin will increase venous capacitance and lower preload. Urine output and blood pressure should be monitored carefully.

If a supraventricular tachyarrhythmia other than sinus tachycardia is present, the ventricular rate should be controlled to facilitate ventricular filling, decrease preload and improve CO. The most common supraventricular tachyarrhythmia encountered in LHF is atrial fibrillation. Cardioversion is usually not indicated; the ventricular response rate can be controlled with Cardizem, Adenocard or Digitalis. If PVCs are present, lidocaine can be given (1 mg/kg IV bolus followed by continuous infusion at a rate of 1 mg/min). A low infusion rate is recommended because of depressed CO and decreased hepatic clearance. Aggressive afterload reduction (e.g., nitroprusside infusion) is usually required only when acute CHF is the result of a hypertensive crisis.

Acute pulmonary edema is LHF in its most extreme form, and is a life-threatening emergency. The typical patient is anxious, severely dyspneic, diaphoretic, pale, cool, and clammy. Inspiratory rales and wheezes may be heard over all lung fields. A summation gallop may be heard on cardiac auscultation, and JVD is common. Hypertension is usual, and caused by intense vasoconstriction. Pedal edema and hepatomegaly may be present if acute decompensation is superimposed on chronic LHF. Immediate therapy should include furosemide (80 mg IV) and sublingual nitroglycerin (0.8–1.2 mg initially and repeated if needed at 5-minute intervals to a maximum dose of 4.0–4.8 mg). Nitroglycerin paste/patch should not be used because of limited skin perfusion. Morphine sulfate in small IV doses (2-mg increments) is time-honored therapy although its venodilation capacity is in question. Beta agonists may be helpful if wheezing is prominent. If blood pressure remains severely elevated, afterload reduction with nitroprusside can be used. If the patient is hypotensive at the time of presentation, inotropic agents should precede the use of venodilators and diuretics. Dopamine (initial infusion rate of 10 µg/kg/min) or a combination of dopamine and dobutamine (each infused at an initial rate of 7.5 µg/kg/min) can be used. If a sustained supraventricular tachyarrhythmia (e.g., atrial fibrillation) is present and thought to contribute to the hypotension, cardioversion should be attempted. Itubation may be required if the level of consciousness deteriorates.

DISPOSITION

ROLE OF THE CONSULTANT   Acute pulmonary edema is a medical emergency, and therapy should be instituted immediately and before consultation. Initial therapy and symptomatic response should be carefully documented to assist the admitting physician in planning further therapy. In the patient with mild to moderate LHF early consultation after initial assessment is appropriate.

INDICATIONS FOR ADMISSION   All patients with acute pulmonary edema should be admitted to the ICU. Hemodynamic monitoring may be required. Patients with chronic LHF and a mild worsening of symptoms who respond to diuretics may be discharged after adjustments in the chronic drug regimen, consultation with the patient's physician, and assurance of follow-up within 24 to 48 hours. Patients with more severe symptoms or other complicating factors (e.g., new rhythm disturbances, poorly controlled hypertension, or a suspected AMI) should be admitted for evaluation and optimization of drug therapy. All patients with new-onset LHF of uncertain origin should be admitted for evaluation. If a transfer is required for any reason, transfer should occur only after initial stabilization.

COMMON PITFALLS

- The signs and symptoms of cor pulmonale and acute respiratory failure are similar to those of LHF; it may not be possible to distinguish between them on physical examination alone.
- Central venous pressure (CVP) monitoring is of limited, if any, value in the management of LHF since the CVP does not reflect PCWP or LV filling pressure in patients with underlying heart or lung disease.
- RV infarction should always be considered in the patient with acute inferior wall infarction with clear lung sounds, JVD, hypotension, and a normal heart rate and rhythm. RV infarction can be diagnosed with a right precordial ECG. ST segment elevation is typically seen in leads V_{3R} and V_{4R}.
- If the cardiac silhouette is not enlarged but other radiographic findings of LHF are seen, failure is most likely to be of acute onset and caused by valvular disease (e.g., aortic insufficiency from endocarditis, papillary muscle rupture, valvular dysfunction with prosthetic valves, or AMI). Noncardiogenic pulmonary edema should also be considered.

CHRONIC COR PULMONALE (PULMONARY HEART DISEASE)

Chronic cor pulmonale has been defined as a combination of RV hypertrophy and dilatation caused by increased resistance, or hypertension of the pulmonary circulation caused by intrinsic pulmonary disease, inadequate function of the chest bellows, or inadequate ventilatory drive from the respiratory centers. This definition excludes congenital heart disease and LHF as causes. Although cor pulmonale may be acute (most commonly caused by pulmonary thromboembolism) or chronic, this section focuses only on the chronic form. In the USA, chronic bronchitis and emphysema are the major causes of chronic cor pulmonale. Cor pulmonale is estimated to occur in 40% of patients with emphysema or bronchitis. The hemodynamic hallmark of cor pulmonale is pulmonary hypertension (elevated pulmonary artery pressure), manifested at rest and worse with exercise or occuring only during exercise. Hypoxemia is a potent pulmonary vasoconstrictor, and concurrent hypercapnea and acidemia are synergistic. Most cases are accompanied by these gas exchange and acid–base abnormalities.

CLINICAL PRESENTATION

The clinical manifestations are determined by the underlying disease process; symptoms of pulmonary dysfunction most often precede manifestations of right heart failure. Symptoms include dyspnea at rest or with minimal exertion, weight gain and ankle swelling, and, in severe cases, abdominal swelling from ascites. Physical signs usually include bibasilar crackles and scattered wheezes from lung disease; the pulmonic component of the 2d heart sound may be palpable; the jugular veins may paradoxically fill during inspiration or exhibit no respiratory fluctuations; and tricuspid insufficiency may be present.

DIFFERENTIAL DIAGNOSIS

The signs and symptoms of cor pulmonale may mimic those of LHF, constrictive pericarditis, and cardiac tamponade. Severe and advanced mitral stenosis may present with predominant right heart failure. When symptoms are of abrupt onset, acute pulmonary embolism should be considered.

EMERGENCY DEPARTMENT EVALUATION

The chest radiograph usually shows only evidence of the underlying pulmonary disorder, but it may be helpful in diagnosing the cause of an acute exacerbation (e.g., pulmonary infiltrate). The ECG is not a sensitive test for detecting RV hypertrophy or dilatation, but some findings are reasonably specific: P-pulmonale pattern (P wave amplitude ≥ 2.5 mm in lead II), right axis deviation, R:S amplitude ratio in V_1 of >1, low voltage QRS, and right bundle-branch block pattern. Failure to detect radiographic or ECG evidence of RV hypertrophy or dilatation does not rule out the diagnosis. Arterial blood gas analysis usually shows some combination of hypoxemia, hypercapnea, and acidemia. Liver function tests may be abnormal because of passive hepatic congestion. Pulmonary function tests are abnormal, with an FEV_1 of <1 L.

EMERGENCY DEPARTMENT MANAGEMENT

The vast majority of patients with an acute exacerbation have acute respiratory failure due to worsening or progression of the underlying lung disease. Therapy should be directed toward reversing reactive pulmonary vasoconstriction (i.e., improving oxygenation, decreasing hypercarbia, and normalizing pH); therapy is similar to that of acute respiratory failure from emphysema or chronic bronchitis. Therapy includes oxygen, inhaled bronchodilators, corticosteroids, and antibiotics, as indicated.

DISPOSITION

ROLE OF THE CONSULTANT   An acute worsening of chronic cor pulmonale is usually due to acute respiratory failure. Acute respiratory failure is a life-threatening emergency, and immediate treatment should be instituted before consultation.

INDICATIONS FOR ADMISSION   Indications for admission for exacerbation of chronic cor pulmonale are usually the same as for acute respiratory failure.

COMMON PITFALLS

- The clinical symptoms and signs of LHF and cor pulmonale overlap. Administering high-flow oxygen to a patient with suspected LHF who has cor pulmonale may result in worsening of clinical status due to suppression of the hypoxic drive and worsening of hypercapnea.
- The diagnosis of cor pulmonale should not be ruled out because of the absence of ECG or radiographic findings of RV hypertrophy or dilatation.

- Treatment should be directed toward improving pulmonary function and decreasing pulmonary vascular resistance, rather than toward alleviating signs of right heart failure (e.g., aggressive diuresis may decrease RV preload and worsen left heart outflow).

127   Bradyarrhythmias

The cardiac conduction system consists of pacemaker cells, conducting cells, and contractile cells. *Pacemaker cells* possess the capacity to spontaneously depolarize. The sinus (SA) node, the predominant pacemaker of the heart, has an intrinsic basal rate of 60–100 beats/min. The atrioventricular (AV) node can also function as a pacemaker with an intrinsic rate of 45 to 60 beats/min. It fires in the absence of sinus node impulses, or may itself usurp control from the sinus node. Other cells in the bundle branches and Purkinje network can function as pacemakers as well, but their intrinsic rate is quite low (30–40 beats/min). Electrical impulses travel over a network of *conducting cells*. Impulses normally originate in the sinus node.

The electrocardiographic (ECG) P wave represents atrial depolarization. The P–R interval (normally 0.12–0.20 seconds in the adult) reflects intra-atrial, AV nodal, and His–Purkinje conduction. The QRS complex, representing ventricular depolarization, has a normal duration of 0.04 to 0.10 second, and the T wave represents ventricular repolarization.

Two basic mechanisms underlie the production of both tachyarrhythmias and bradyarrhythmias: disorders of impulse formation and disorders of impulse conduction. Depressed *automaticity* may result in bradyarrhythmias such as sinus bradycardia or sinus arrest. If sinus node automaticity is sufficiently depressed, escape rhythms originating elsewhere in the heart may assume control. Depressed impulse conduction may lead to AV or fascicular blocks.

EMERGENCY DEPARTMENT EVALUATION AND MANAGEMENT

The urgency and means of treating bradyarrhythmias depend on how symptomatic the arrhythmia is, the clinical setting in which the arrhythmia occurs, the propensity for the arrhythmia to progress, and concurrent drug therapy. Bradyarrhythmias may produce light-headedness, dizziness, fatigue, syncope, or seizures. Prompt therapy is required for these symptoms and for hypotension, CHF, mental status changes, or angina. However, many arrhythmias are asymptomatic and require no treatment. An arrhythmia that occurs during an AMI usually mandates a different approach to treatment than an arrhythmia that is incidentally discovered on routine physical examination.

Electrolyte disturbances and the use of certain drugs (e.g., digitalis, beta blockers, and calcium channel blockers) may also be the cause of bradyarrhythmias, and each has its own implications for treatment. Specific drug therapy or artificial cardiac pacing are also required in many instances. The cornerstone of drug therapy is atropine sulfate, a vagolytic agent that enhances sinus node automaticity and AV nodal conduction. The usual adult dose is 0.5 mg IV push, repeated up to a maximum dose of 2.0 mg as necessary. Atropine is effective when administered by the endotracheal route: 1 mg to 2 mg diluted in 10 mL of sterile saline solution.

Because it can increase myocardial oxygen consumption, atropine should be used with caution in the presence of myocardial ischemia. Adverse effects include sinus tachycardia, ventricular tachycardia, or ventricular fibrillation, as well as manifestations of anticholinergic toxicity. Isoproterenol markedly increases myocardial oxygen demand, and may cause ventricular tachycardia or fibrillation. Cardiac pacing is preferred.

DISORDERS OF IMPULSE FORMATION
ATRIAL BRADYARRHYTHMIAS

Sinus arrhythmia is a physiologic finding commonly seen in healthy young people; no treatment is indicated. *Sinus bradycardia,* defined as sinus rhythm <60 beats/min, may be the result of organic heart disease and may cause symptoms, but it is also a common finding in healthy patients. When associated with symptoms, treatment with atropine is usually successful. The *sick sinus syndrome* encompasses a spectrum of conditions, including severe sinus bradycardia, sinoatrial block, sinus arrest, and the bradycardia–tachycardia syndrome. The latter refers to the intermittent occurrence of bradyarrhythmias and tachyarrhythmias (such as atrial fibrillation, flutter, or paroxysmal supraventricular tachycardia) in the same patient. Bradyarrhythmia typically occurs immediately after resolution of an episode of tachycardia. Syncope or chest pain may result from either tachycardia or bradycardia. Effective pharmacologic therapy for tachycardia can exacerbate the bradycardia, so cardiac pacing must often be initiated before pharmacologic therapy.

ATRIOVENTRICULAR NODAL BRADYARRHYTHMIAS

An *AV junctional rhythm* may be a physiologic escape rhythm initiated by the AV node in the absence of an adequate sinus stimulus, or it may result from an abnormally rapid AV junctional focus that usurps control from the sinus node (e.g., accelerated junctional rhythm). Junctional rhythm usually exhibits the same QRS morphology as the patient's sinus rhythm. The P waves are usually inverted if they are conducted in a retrograde manner, and can fall before, during, or after the QRS complex, depending on the location of the focus within the AV junction and the degree of retrograde AV block.

   AV junctional escape beats occur singly or multiply in the absence of stimuli arriving at the AV node. Their hallmark is occurrence *after* an interval longer than the dominant cycle. The underlying disorder may be sinus bradycardia, sinus arrest, sinus exit block, or AV block; digitalis or beta blocker therapy may also be responsible. Junctional escape rhythms are an incidental finding in some otherwise healthy people with increased vagotonia. Treatment is not indicated for asymptomatic patients. If symptoms occur, the underlying rhythm should be treated rather than attempt to obliterate the escape beats; it involves withholding offending drugs or using atropine or pacing.

VENTRICULAR BRADYARRHYTHMIAS

A ventricular rhythm with a rate <50 beats/min is termed a *ventricular escape* rhythm, or idioventricular rhythm. Ventricular escape rhythm represents a physiologic safety mechanism in the absence of stimuli from above. Most patients are symptomatic, since the heart rate is low. Treatment is directed at the underlying arrhythmia (i.e., atropine or pacing). Lidocaine, which may abolish the ventricular rhythm, is contraindicated, since it has the potential of causing cardiac standstill. Also known as idioventricular tachycardia or slow ventricular tachycardia, *accelerated idioventricular rhythm* has a rate of 50–100 beats /min. It may be associated with AMI but may also be seen in otherwise healthy patients. In the absence of symptoms specific therapy is not warranted.

DISTURBANCES OF CONDUCTION
DISORDERS OF SINOATRIAL CONDUCTION

The tissue surrounding the sinus node may delay or prevent conduction of sinus node impulses to the atria and AV node, termed sinoatrial block and classified in a manner analogous to AV block. However, because of the limitations of the surface ECG, their precise diagnosis is more difficult. In *first-degree sinoatrial block* there is a delay in the propagation of the sinus node impulse out to the atrial myocardium. Every beat is transmitted, however, and no abnormality is detected on the surface ECG. *Second-degree sinoatrial block* may be divided into types I and II.

In *type I* (Wenckebach) there is a progressive delay in conduction from the sinus node to the atria, until conduction is totally blocked and a P wave is dropped (Fig. 127-1). The P–P interval progressively shortens before the dropped P wave. In *type II* second-degree sinoatrial block there is intermittent failure of the sinus impulse to reach the atria, resulting in a missing P wave and a sudden lengthening of the P–P interval. The resulting P–P interval is usually a multiple of the previous one (ie, doubled in the case of 2:1 block). (See Fig. 127-2.) *Third-degree sinoatrial block* is the failure of any sinus node impulses to be conducted to the atria.

DISORDERS OF ATRIAL-VENTRICULAR CONDUCTION

Traditionally, AV blocks have been divided into first, second, and third degree. However, AV block is a relative phenomenon and the physiologic delay normally present in the AV node is one end of a continuum. For example, in the patient with atrial flutter "normal" AV conduction usually results in 2:1 block. In addition, the degree of block is rate dependent. One patient with mild AV disease may exhibit second-degree block at a particular supraventricular rate, while another patient with more advanced AV nodal disease may exhibit 1:1 conduction if the supraventricular rate is slower.

A P–R interval of more than 0.20 second defines *first-degree AV block*. All P waves are conducted, 1:1 AV conduction is maintained, and the P–P and R–R intervals are consistent. Most commonly, the delay in AV conduction is within the AV node, and the QRS complex is of normal duration. Delays within the His bundle or His–Purkinje system are less common and are usually associated with widened bundle-branch block QRS patterns, but can be diagnosed conclusively only by intracardiac recordings.

First-degree AV block may be associated with electrolyte disturbances or the use of digitalis, beta blockers, or calcium channel blockers. It may be a finding during acute myocardial infarction, particularly inferior myocardial infarction. Treatment includes correction of electrolyte abnormalities or removal of an inciting agent. During acute myocardial infarction close observation is warranted to detect progression to higher degrees of block. Otherwise, specific treatment is not indicated.

Second-degree AV block can be divided into Mobitz types I and II. Wenckebach distinguished between these two in the pre-ECG era, using only physical observation. *Mobitz type I (Wenckebach)* second-degree AV block is characterized by repeated cycles of progressively slowing AV conduction until conduction is totally blocked. This pattern is manifested electrocardio-

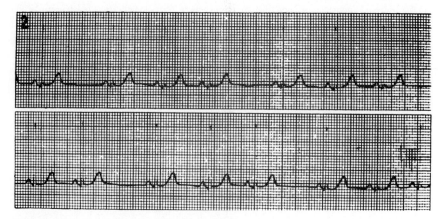

Figure 127-1. Type I (Wenckebach) sinoatrial block.

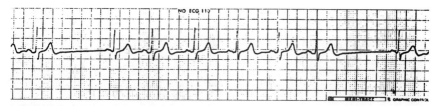

Figure 127-2. Type II sinoatrial block 2:1.

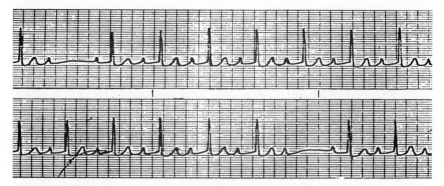

Figure 127-3. Type I (Wenckebach) second-degree AV block.

graphically by a progressive prolongation of successive P–R intervals, until there is a nonconducted P wave, after which the cycle repeats itself (Fig. 127-3). The cycle is referred to by the ratio of P waves to QRS complexes (i.e., 4:3, 3:2, and so on). Classically, the R–R interval shortens as the P–R interval lengthens.

Type I block usually results from conduction delay in the AV node. The QRS complex is usually of normal duration. Type I block may be associated with inferior AMI or the use of digitalis, beta blockers, and calcium channel blockers. It is usually transient and asymptomatic, and has a good prognosis. If symptomatic, atropine can be used but pacing is usually not necessary.

Mobitz type II second-degree AV block is less common. The site of blockage is almost always within the His–Purkinje system, and thus a bundle-branch block QRS pattern is usual. In type II block the P–R intervals are constant until single or multiple beats are suddenly dropped (Fig. 127-4). Type II block is usually symptomatic, with high likelihood of progressing to complete AV block. If associated with acute anterior MI, it carries an ominous prognosis. Most authorities agree that Mobitz type II second-degree AV block requires permanent cardiac pacing. Because atropine or isoproterenol may be ineffective, temporary pacing is often necessary as a stabilizing measure. A particular clinical problem is presented by the patient with 2:1 AV block. Although assumed than type II block is present, type I block can and does present as 2:1 block, and in fact is more common than type II. The distinction is important, given the difference in prognosis and treatment. The following principles may aid in the clinical distinction:

Type I block is more common than type II.

A narrow QRS complex usually reflects a type I block (although not all type I blocks have a narrow QRS complex). Type II block almost always has a wide QRS complex.

Coexistent acute inferior myocardial infarction suggests type I block. Acute anterior MI suggests type II.

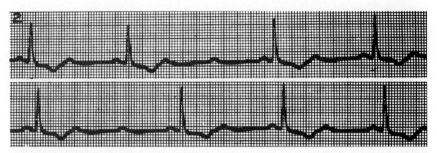

Figure 127-4. Type II second degree AV block.

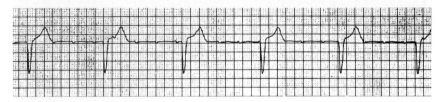

Figure 127-5. Third degree AV block.

Digitalis, beta blocker, or calcium channel blockers tend to be associated with type I block. Other areas of the rhythm strip may reflect other patterns of type I conduction, such as 3:2 or 4:3.

In *third-degree (complete) AV block* no atrial impulses reach the ventricles, and a subsidiary, escape pacemaker usually emerges. AV dissociation, with constant but independent P–P intervals and R–R intervals, results. The P–R interval is variable, and P waves have no discernible relation to QRS complexes (Fig. 127-5). The site of block may be within the AV node, His bundle, bundle branches, or Purkinje system; in general, the lower the site of block, the more severe the symptoms. Third-degree AV block may be intermittent or self-limited. If caused by digitalis, beta blocker, or calcium channel blocker therapy, it usually resolves on withdrawal of the drug. It may be associated with AMI but occasionally it is an asymptomatic.

The emergent treatment depends on symptoms and clinical setting. Symptomatic patients may improve with atropine, particularly if the block is within the AV node; if unresponsive to drugs, emergent pacing is indicated. Stable patients with acute inferior infarction may require only a prophylactic pacemaker. Acute anterior infarction complicated by third-degree AV block is more ominous and requires emergent pacing. The term *AV dissociation,* although it is commonly used interchangeably with the term third-degree AV block, encompasses a much broader range of rhythms. AV dissociation implies that the atria and ventricles beat independently, a situation that includes not only complete AV block, but also accelerated junctional and idioventricular rhythms (including ventricular tachycardia).

ARTIFICIAL PACEMAKERS

Temporary cardiac pacemakers are used in emergent circumstances, whereas permanent pacemakers are most often placed electively.

TEMPORARY PACEMAKERS

Cardiac pacing is indicated in any hemodynamically unstable bradycardia that fails to response to pharmacologic therapy. In addition, prophylactic emergent cardiac pacing may be indicated, even without symptoms, for patients with AMI in the following circumstances:

First-degree AV block with new-onset bundle-branch block
Second-degree AV block type II
Third-degree AV block
Right bundle-branch block with left anterior fascicular block or left posterior fascicular block (either new or old)
Left bundle-branch block (old or new) and placement of a Swan–Ganz catheter (because of the risk of inducing right bundle-branch block, and hence complete block).

Preliminary data suggest that emergent pacing may also be indicated in bradyasystolic cardiac arrest. Pacing is of no benefit if it is initiated >20 minutes after arrest.

Transcutaneous cardiac pacing involves the application of cutaneous electrodes to the chest and the delivery of electrical impulses through the chest wall to the myocardium. It is the technique of choice for emergent pacing in the ED and is the only option available for prehospital use. The advantages are ease and speed of use and the absence of serious side effects. Its disadvantages are non-capture in some patients and the discomfort to conscious patients. Transcutaneous pacer should still be considered a stabilizing device, to be replaced by another pacing technique as soon as possible.

Transthoracic pacing involves the placement of a pacing wire through the skin directly into the right ventricular cavity. Because significant complications, such as pericardial tamponade, pneumothorax, and coronary vessel injury, have been reported, transthoracic pacing should be considered only if transcutaneous pacing is unsuccessful or unavailable.

Transvenous pacing involves the placement of the pacing electrode into the right ventricle by way of a central vein, often the subclavian or internal jugular. It thus carries the risks of central venous catheterization, but it is the temporary modality that most closely approximates the function of a permanent pacemaker. It does not involve painful muscle contractions or the hazard of direct cardiac puncture, and it can be used for relatively prolonged periods. Unfortunately transvenous pacemaker placement in the ED is often a lengthy and unsuccessful procedure; it is ideally done with fluoroscopic guidance. With the advent of transcutaneous pacing, transvenous pacing is rapidly being relegated to those urgent situations in which fluoroscopy is possible, in which stabilization has been achieved by another modality, or in which attempts at transcutaneous pacing have been unsuccessful.

PERMANENT PACEMAKERS

Most permanent pacemakers currently in use are of the VVI type (pace the ventricle, sense intrinsic ventricular activity, and inhibit pacemaker output if ventricular complexes are sensed at a rate greater than that of the pacemaker setting). Increasingly common are AV sequential (DDD) units and units that are externally programmable. Due to improvements in pacemaker design and function, pacemaker malfunction requiring emergency intervention is now uncommon, but it occasionally occurs. Pacemaker malfunction can be classified as failure to pace, failure to capture, or failure to sense.

Failure to pace is indicated by a lack of appropriate pacer spikes on the ECG. Apparent failure to pace may be caused by the presence of a faster intrinsic rate than the pacemaker rate or by problems with the recording ECG equipment. True failure to pace is the result of battery or lead wire problems or of oversensing (e.g., sensing T waves as QRS complexes).

Failure to capture is indicated by appropriate pacer spikes without corresponding QRS complexes. This may be due to fibrosis about the electrode tip, local myocardial changes (such as infarction), migration or displacement of the lead tip, or battery or lead wire malfunction.

Failure to sense is indicated by the inappropriate delivery of pacer spikes, usually during the patient's intrinsic cardiac complexes. This may be due to battery or lead failure or to a decrease in the intrinsic QRS amplitude, as may occur with infarction or electrolyte disturbance. Most pacemakers may be temporarily converted to the unsynchronized firing mode by placing a magnet directly over the subcutaneous generator. This maneuver is particularly helpful when pacemaker malfunction is suspected when the intrinsic rhythm is fast enough to suppress pacemaker activity.

DISPOSITION

Virtually all patients with symptomatic bradyarrhythmia require admission to the hospital. Patients with type II second-degree AV block and complete AV block warrant admission even if asymptomatic. Admission should be to a monitored bed capable of initiating emergent pacing. If transfer to another facility is necessary, pacing should be initiated first if indicated and available; cardiac monitoring, transcutaneous pacing capability, ACLS personnel are indicated.

COMMON PITFALLS

- Automatically assuming a 2:1 second-degree AV block is of the Mobitz type II variety, possibly leading to unnecessary treatment and intervention
- Not taking rate into account when evaluating AV and fascicular blocks
- Misdiagnosing blocked premature atrial contractions as significant AV block, possibly leading to unnecessary treatment and intervention
- Mistakenly blocking an escape rhythm, with the potential for causing cardiac standstill

128   Tachyarrhythmias

It is important to emphasize the need to focus first on the clinical effects produced by the arrhythmia. Second, hemodynamic abnormalities are more typically dependent on the heart rate produced by any arrhythmia than they are on the arrhythmia's source. Third, the configuration of the QRS complexes during an episode of tachycardia is less important as a clue to the origin of the rhythm disturbance than as a guide to choosing between several possible therapeutic approaches.

TYPES OF TACHYARRHYTHMIAS

Tachycardias can be generated from any primary focus in the heart, since all cardiac tissue has intrinsic pacemaker activity. Supraventricular tachycardia (SVT) will not generate a ventricular response of greater than 180 beats/minute because of the damping effect of the atrioventricular (AV) node. In the presence of a bypass tract, however (e.g., the bundle of Kent found in Wolff–Parkinson–White [WPW] syndrome), faster rates (200 or more beats/minute) may be attained. Ventricular tachycardia (VT), particularly the variety produced by a circus movement mechanism, may occasionally reach rates as high as 250 to 300 beats/minute.

Tachycardias that originate below the AV node produce wide QRS complexes; therefore, any tachycardia with a narrow QRS complex can be presumed to originate from the AV node or above. On the other hand, supraventricular and nodal tachycardias can produce wide QRS complexes in a number of circumstances: underlying bundle-branch block, rate-related bundle-branch block induced by the tachycardia itself, and anterograde conduction from the atrium to the ventricle through a bypass tract that circumvents the AV node. Thus wide-complex tachycardias can be of either ventricular or supraventricular origin. VT is more likely than SVT to produce decompensation and to initiate an episode of ventricular fibrillation (VF). However, VT is not always immediately life-threatening, nor is every episode of SVT benign. VT tends to be more worrisome because of the generally greater ventricular response rate it produces. It is critical to remember, however, that very rapid atrial or junctional tachycardias can certainly produce hemodynamic instability.

ELECTRICAL CARDIOVERSION

Any tachycardia that produces significant end-organ hypoperfusion can be treated in the same manner, regardless of its mechanism. Patients with tachyarrhythmia and hypotension, altered mental status, significant chest pain, or significant congestive heart failure require cardioversion. The amount of electrical energy used depends on the mechanism: both atrial fibrillation (AF) and VF normally require significantly more energy than tachycardias, such as SVT or VT. Atrial flutter is the most sensitive rhythm, and usually responds to 10 to 50 watt-seconds. SVT and VT respond in at least 80% of cases to energies of 10 to 20 watt-seconds; an initial energy of 50 watt-seconds achieves successful conversion >90% of cases. AF and VF often require 100 to 200 watt-seconds or more. Initial doses should be small. Failing conversion, energy levels can be increased until cardioversion is achieved.

ANTIARRHYTHMIC AGENTS

Drug therapy is reserved for clinically stable patients. Lidocaine is the drug of choice in the acute treatment of ventricular arrhythmias. It is used in the treatment of VT in clinically stable patients, for prophylaxis against recurrent VF after resuscitation, and in the treatment of significant ventricular ectopy in the setting of acute ischemia. Lidocaine is very safe when used appropriately; toxicity, primarily central nervous system, can be almost entirely avoided if appropriate total doses (225 mg in adults) are given at rates no faster than 50 mg/min for the initial 1 mg/kg bolus and 50 mg/5 min for further loading doses.

Beta blockers have little role in the acute treatment of tachycardias. Bretylium has been relegated to a second- or third-line position in the recent advanced cardiac life-support guidelines. Calcium channel blockers, including verapamil, are the mainstay of therapy for tachycardias that involve the AV node. These drugs decrease conduction through the AV node, thus slowing the ventricular response in conditions such as AF and interrupting re-entry in paroxysmal supraventricular tachycardia (PSVT). Verapamil is indicated in the treatment of all PSVT associated with narrow QRS complexes but is contraindicated when the QRS complex is wide (see below).

Calcium channel blocking agents are major vasodilators and negative inotropes; they can cause significant hypotension and are contraindicated in severe hypotension or significant congestive heart failure. They are also contraindicated in sinus and AV nodal disease. They should be used cautiously in the presence of oral beta blockade, and are relatively contraindicated when IV beta blockers have recently been used. These agents are also relatively contraindicated in the presence of digitalis toxicity because of its effect on the AV node.

Digitalis slows conduction through the AV node, and is therefore useful in the control of the ventricular response in chronic AF. Magnesium has antiarrhythmic effects in a variety of circumstances in which repolarization abnormalities exist. Clinically and empirically, magnesium substantially decreases life-threatening tachycardias in acute ischemia, and has been particularly successful in treating torsades de pointes. Magnesium may also have a role in the treatment of a variety of other tachycardias, including multifocal atrial tachycardia.

EMERGENCY DEPARTMENT MANAGEMENT

Management of tachycardias should be based first on their hemodynamic consequences. When cardioversion is not required, decisions can be based on the duration of the QRS complex. Narrow-complex tachycardias are supraventricular in origin, whereas wide-complex tachycardias can be of supraventricular, nodal, or ventricular origin.

NARROW QRS COMPLEX TACHYCARDIAS

SINUS TACHYCARDIA

Therapy should be directed at the rhythm's underlying cause rather than at the rhythm itself. An exception to this is when a rapid heart rate increases myocardial oxygen demand that may lead to significant myocardial ischemia. Beta blockers may be extremely useful. In the absence of contraindications, patients with AMI and significant sinus tachycardia are candidates for these agents. Beta blockers are also important in thyroid storm. In cocaine overdose beta blockade may be appropriate for control of heart rate, provided it is used in conjunction with simultaneous alpha blockade, to avoid the greater danger of unopposed alpha adrenergic stimulation.

PAROXYSMAL SUPRAVENTRICULAR TACHYCARDIA

PSVT usually presents with narrow QRS complexes, whether or not the patient has WPW syndrome. Patients with PSVT who have signs of end-organ hypoperfusion should be cardioverted; >90% will convert with very small doses (10–50 Joules). Patients who do not require cardioversion can almost always be treated easily and successfully with adenosine. Vagal maneuvers should be tried first (carotid massage, the Valsalva maneuver, and ice-water immersion). An initial dose of adenosine of 6 mg IV is usually effective, with most patients converting to sinus rhythm within 2 minutes. A second dose of 12 mg IV push may be necessary. Adenosine is now the first line therapy for narrow complex tachycardias and second line after lidocaine for wide complex tachycardias (see algorithms). Adverse effects (such as transient hypotension, heart block, and sinus node arrest) dissipate so quickly that they have little clinical significance.

ATRIAL FLUTTER

Atrial flutter is the most electrosensitive tachycardia, and electrocardioversion is the treatment of choice in almost all cases. Diltiazem, Verapamil and digitalis are capable of slowing the ventricular response in atrial flutter. Unless cardioversion is contraindicated, however, drug therapy should be considered a secondary approach. Cardioversion occasionally produces AF rather than sinus rhythm, in which case further therapy is required.

ATRIAL FIBRILLATION

Although many patients with AF are seen in the ED, not all require emergency therapy. Patients with chronic AF with controlled ventricular rates require no specific treatment. Extremely rapid heart rates, associated with hemodynamic deterioration, may require emergent cardioversion, regardless of whether the AF is new or old. Because chronic AF is much less likely to convert to (or remain in) sinus rhythm, control of the ventricular response rate with drugs is extremely important. Although digitalis has long been considered the drug of choice to slow ventricular response in AF, it does so slowly. Diltiazem and Verapamil slow ventricular responses within the first hour of therapy.

New-onset AF has many causes, ranging from benign to serious. It has long been standard practice in the USA to admit patients with new-onset AF to rule out AMI. Recent evidence suggests that AMI is infrequently (5%–10%) the cause of new-onset AF, and that when it is, other clinical findings point clearly to AMI. It remains reasonable, however, to admit most patients with new-onset AF. Patients with *chronic* AF should be admitted if they have any signs of hemodynamic decompensation that require cardioversion, or if hemodynamic effects and rapid ventricular response are not easily and quickly controlled.

MULTIFOCAL ATRIAL TACHYCARDIA

Multifocal atrial tachycardia (MFAT) occurs primarily in patients with chronic lung disease, and within this group it is most common in patients with high or toxic levels of theophylline. MFAT is characterized by P waves of varying morphologies and by changing P–R intervals; because it originates in the atria, it is associated with narrow QRS complexes, except in the presence of underlying bundle-branch block. MFAT is thought to be due to the hypoxic effects of underlying lung disease; theophylline toxicity may also contribute. MFAT may be slowed or even converted with magnesium or verapamil. Although MFAT is itself seldom life-threatening, the ability to control it can provide significant symptomatic benefit.

WIDE QRS COMPLEX TACHYCARDIAS

Wide QRS complex tachycardias must be managed according to the hemodynamic effects they produce. They are more likely to require cardioversion, since many of them have VT with with end-organ hypoperfusion. Nevertheless, many such patients are relatively stable and respond to pharmacologic therapy. A number of clinical and ECG criteria enable clinicians to distinguish between VT and SVT. Although such criteria are relatively accurate, it is critical to understand that no single sign or combination of signs can definitively identify the origin of tachycardia. For this reason wide-complex tachycardia should virtually always be treated as though it is VT with lidocaine. Drugs that are contraindicated in VT (e.g., verapamil) should never be used to treat wide-complex tachycardia.

WIDE-COMPLEX PSVT

PSVT can manifest with wide QRS complexes when bundle-branch block (either underlying or rate-related) is present. The duration of the QRS complex is not likely to be >0.14 second, and heart rates usually range between 130–200 beats/minute. Nevertheless, it is impossible to be certain that a wide-complex tachycardia represents PSVT with bundle-branch block, and therefore treatment should almost never be based on this assumption. Wide QRS complexes can also be seen in PSVT with the WPW syndrome when antegrade conduction occurs down the bundle of Kent and retrograde conduction occurs back through the AV node. It may be possible to make this diagnosis from the ECG in patients with known WPW syndrome, although confusion with VT may still occur.

Verapamil and digitalis are both relatively contraindicated since neither slows conduction through the bundle of Kent; in some cases these drugs actually increase the speed of conduction through the bypass tract, with the potential for causing hemodynamic deterioration or even VF. Verapamil's vasodilatory and negative inotropic effect may also produce dramatic clinical deterioration. Procainamide has antiarrhythmic effects on both atrial and ventricular tissue, and could be expected to be safe and useful in wide-complex tachycardia, whether PSVT with antegrade conduction through the bundle of Kent or VT. However, procainamide is not always successful and electrical cardioversion is often necessary.

Lidocaine, the first-line pharmacologic agent for treatment of stable VT, can occasionally speed conduction through bypass tracts; thus lidocaine is less attractive than procainamide when wide-complex tachycardia is suspected to be due to WPW-related PSVT. Current recommendations include the use of lidocaine initially, followed by adenosine (see Appendix for ACLS Protocols).

WIDE-COMPLEX AF

A small number of patients with AF present with wide QRS complexes, due to underlying or rate-related bundle-branch block or to the WPW syndrome. In the presence of known underlying bundle-branch block, treatment can be similar to narrow-complex AF (i.e., cardioversion for unstable patients and digitalis or verapamil, or both, for rate control in stable patients). Patients with rate-related bundle-branch block often demonstrate both wide complexes (in beats that follow short R–R intervals) and narrow complexes (in beats that follow longer R–R intervals), but patients with AF and the WPW syndrome may also have both wide and narrow QRS complexes, depending on the conduction path followed by each depolarization. It is critically important to recognize this latter entity because agents that slow conduction through the AV node are contraindicated.

As in WPW syndrome with regular wide-complex PSVT, verapamil and digitalis are contraindicated in WPW syndrome with wide-complex AF, since they can actually increase the speed of conduction through the bypass tract. More important, relative blockade of the AV node causes preferential conduction through the bypass tract, resulting in much higher ventricular response rates; an extremely rapid ventricular response to AF can then deteriorate into VF. Cardiac arrest from VF has been reported with WPW-related AF treated with verapamil or digitalis. Although procainamide is unlikely to be harmful in WPW-related AF, it may not be effective. It seems reasonable to treat even stable patients with controlled electrical cardioversion.

VENTRICULAR TACHYCARDIA

VT is usually a life-threatening emergency. Although some patients have intermittent asymptomatic bouts of VT, most suffer from significant hemodynamic effects or other acute cardiac problems, including myocardial ischemia. The majority with VT will require consultation and hospital admission after therapy. Sustained VT usually causes hemodynamic deterioration because the heart rate is usually too fast to permit adequate end-organ perfusion. Cardioversion at 10–50 Joules will convert about 90% of patients. It should be performed in the synchronized mode to avoid precipitating VF. Lidocaine, procainamide, and bretylium are standard agents used to prevent recurrence after successful cardioversion, or to treat patients with recurrent VT. Magnesium may also be extremely efficacious (see Appendix).

Torsades de pointes is a special type of VT. The most common cause of torsades is class IA antiarrhythmic agents that cause prolongation of the QT interval. Other drugs (phenothiazines) and other conditions (hypocalcemia and hypokalemia) have also been associated with torsades. Most episodes are self-limited and without acute hemodynamic consequences. Torsades is still life-threatening because any episode can precipitate VF. Because torsades normally converts spontaneously to sinus rhythm, treatment is directed at prevention, often requiring withdrawal of the offending agent. In the ED, however, antiarrhythmic therapy is mandatory. Magnesium, IV infusion of 2–4 g over 30–60 minutes) is highly effective, and may be the optimal therapy for torsades. Overdrive electrical pacing can also be used.

VENTRICULAR FIBRILLATION

Ventricular fibrillation is never associated with effective cardiac pumping; it requires immediate defibrillation. When a defibrillator is available no other activity should take precedence. Defibrillation at 200 watts-seconds provides the greatest possibility of success. Lidocaine should be used after successful conversion to help prevent recurrences.

DISPOSITION

In most cases the disposition is obvious. Only in a minority is the disposition problematic. **ADMISSION** is indicated for:

1. Patients who are symptomatic after the onset of a tachyarrhythmia and who failed appropriate therapy or who responded only transiently;
2. Patients who were clinically unstable as a result of a tachyarrhythmia, including all patients who required cardioversion because of end-organ hypoperfusion;
3. Patients who were treated successfully before the development of serious symptoms, but who have potential for decompensation if the tachyarrhythmia recurs.

4. The underlying basis for the arrhythmia must also play a role: any patient with a potentially dangerous etiology for the arrhythmia (i.e., AMI) should be admitted.
5. It may be appropriate to admit a stable patient for ECG monitoring during initiation of chronic drug therapy.

COMMON PITFALLS

•   Tachyarrhythmias can cause life-threatening symptoms and are among the most acute crises faced in the ED. A systematic approach based on the clinical status allows for the best possible outcome.
•   It is critical to evaluate the hemodynamic effects of any rhythm, rather than worry about the nature of the rhythm itself. Patients who are unstable with a very rapid tachycardia require cardioversion. One must never be lured into using conservative therapy in the face of end-organ hypoperfusion by assuming that a narrow-complex rhythm is benign. Hesitancy can be catastrophic, since most patients (elderly or having underlying heart disease) cannot tolerate extremely high heart rates for prolonged periods; cardioversion may be the only way to prevent cardiac arrest.
•   Sedation with a short-acting benzodiazepine is an effective means of overcoming the patient's and the physician's aversions to the procedure.
•   Stable patients can usually avoid electrical cardioversion even if their tachycardia appears ominous.
•   Failure to appreciate the importance of QRS width can lead to catastrophic errors. Verapamil is the drug of choice for many narrow-complex tachycardias, but it can precipitate VF in wide-complex tachycardias; this is true not only for VT, but also for other wide-QRS complex tachycardias originating above the AV node (PSVT with anterograde conduction down a bypass tract in WPW syndrome).
•   When a patient is symptomatic, attention should first be paid to controlling the ventricular response rate. Rate control will usually ameliorate the symptoms.
•   Precipitating factors should be sought and corrected (hypoxemia, infectious/inflammatory processes such as endocarditis, myocarditis, or pericarditis, and endocrine–metabolic abnormalities such as thyrotoxicosis, hypokalemia or hyperkalemia, and hypomagnesemia).
•   Arrhythmias can be caused by intoxications (e.g., tricyclic antidepressants), drug abuse (e.g., cocaine and alcohol), or therapeutic misadventure with prescribed medications (e.g., digitalis and theophylline). In patients taking antiarrhythmic agents, an acute arrhythmia may result from subtherapeutic drug levels, an arrhythmogenic effect of the drug at a therapeutic or toxic level, or failure of the drug to prevent a pre-existing arrhythmia.
•   AMI should be always considered ruled out whenever it seems a likely cause or when the arrhythmia has itself produced ischemia as suggested by ECG changes or patient symptoms.

129   Valvular Heart Disease

A wide variety of common diseases and conditions can affect the heart valves (Table 129-1). Significant acute or chronic valvular dysfunction has predictable hemodynamic consequences. Regurgitant lesions (e.g., mitral or aortic regurgitation) cause volume overload of the affected atrium or ventricle. Although massive acute regurgitation can rapidly lead to shock and pulmonary edema, mild to moderate volume overload is usually well tolerated until after months or years, when the ventricle will often dilate and fail, leading to signs and symptoms of congestive heart failure (CHF). Stenotic lesions above, at, or below the valve cause pressure overload of the affected atrium or ventricle. Pressure overload is metabolically costlier to the myocardium than volume overload, and leads to myocardial hypertrophy and eventual CHF.

The combined hemodynamic effect of multiple valvular lesions is often complex. Some compound lesions (e.g., combined aortic regurgitation and stenosis) impose a tremendous burden on the myocardium by producing both volume and pressure overload of a single chamber. Other combination lesions may be "protective" of a given chamber (e.g., in aortic stenosis combined with mitral stenosis, the volume of blood reaching the left ventricle is decreased, thereby "protecting" it from CHF). However, the net effect may be to decrease forward flow, and thus net cardiac output.

Some valvular lesions produce a rapidly downhill course. For example, acute severe mitral or aortic regurgitation can rapidly lead to pulmonary edema and shock, usually remedied only by immediate valve replacement. Other lesions, such as chronic mitral or aortic regurgitation, can be well tolerated for decades. A structurally abnormal valve puts the patient at increased risk of developing infective endocarditis, which can further impair valvular function. Other concomitant diseases (e.g., coronary atherosclerosis and myocarditis), arrhythmias (e.g., atrial fibrillation), or valvular calcification can also unfavorably influence the patient's symptoms and length of survival.

CLINICAL PRESENTATION

Patients with valvular heart disease may present with a complication of previously known disease, or they may challenge the physician to evaluate a previously undetected and undiagnosed heart murmur. If complex congenital heart disease such as tetralogy of Fallot is excluded, complications of adult valvular heart disease are most often the result of left heart lesions (Table 129-2). The first question is whether the heart murmur is (a) causing, (b) unrelated to, or (c) caused by

TABLE 129-1. Most Common Causes of Valvular Heart Disease in Adults

Cause	Specific Disease	Valves Affected	Murmur
Congenital	Bicuspid valve	A	S, R
Rheumatic	Rheumatic fever	M > A > T > P	S, R
Infectious	Endocarditis	A, M (rheumatic)	R
		A, M, T, P, (I.V. drugs)	R
	Syphilis	A	R
Myxomatous degeneration	Prolapse	M > T	R
	Aortic root dilatation	A	R
Degenerative aging	Sclerosis	A	S

A, aortic; M, mitral; P, pulmonic; T, tricuspid; S, stenotic; R, regurgitant.

TABLE 129-2. Common Complications of Left Heart Valvular Disease in Adults

Valvular Lesion	Common Complications
Mitral stenosis	Pulmonary edema, atrial fibrillation, systemic embolism
Mitral regurgitation	CHF, endocarditis
Aortic stenosis	Angina, syncope, CHF, arrhythmias, sudden death, endocarditis
Aortic regurgitation	CHF, endocarditis

CHF, congestive heart failure.

---

the symptom complex. For example, if a 70-year-old man with dyspnea and moderate pulmonary edema on chest radiograph has a grade 3/6 systolic ejection murmur at the left upper sternal border and cardiac apex, the murmur may be due to aortic stenosis or mitral regurgitation, either of which could cause CHF. The patient's CHF could also be caused by an unrelated problem, such as ischemic heart disease, cardiomyopathy, myocarditis, or a congenital lesion (e.g., atrial septal defect).

Finally, left ventricular failure and dilatation could be causing a "functional" murmur due to dilatation of the mitral valve and its supporting structures (papillary muscle dysfunction). Myocardial ischemia (e.g., during angina) can also increase the murmur of papillary muscle dysfunction. "Functional" tricuspid regurgitation can be caused by right ventricular dilatation secondary to left heart failure.

In practice, sometimes it is impossible to determine the relation between the murmur and the patient's symptoms without further evaluation, such as ECHO or cardiac catheterization. The most frequent conditions are (a) mitral valve prolapse (MVP); (b) aortic valve sclerosis in the elderly with or (more typically) without significant stenosis; (c) valvular aortic stenosis due to congenital bicuspid aortic valve; (d) mitral regurgitation from papillary muscle dysfunction, rheumatic heart disease, or ruptured chordae tendineae; (e) aortic regurgitation from rheumatic fever, bicuspid aortic valve, or aortic root disease; and (f) mitral stenosis from rheumatic fever.

EMERGENCY DEPARTMENT EVALUATION

A careful examination often identifies the cause of a heart murmur (Table 129-3). A wide pulse pressure accompanied by a brisk (often bifid) carotid upstroke and a bounding (water-hammer) peripheral pulse is common in moderate to severe aortic regurgitation; a narrow pulse pressure with a slow, delayed carotid upstroke is seen in severe aortic stenosis. When a harsh systolic murmur suggesting valvular aortic stenosis is accompanied by a brisk carotid upstroke (and *no* aortic regurgitation), idiopathic hypertrophic subaortic stenosis (IHSS) should be suspected. In a young person (especially a male) hypertension in the upper extremities and a lower arterial pressure in the legs, with a weak femoral pulse and a basal systolic murmur, suggest coarctation of the aorta.

A third heart sound (S_3) is often heard in healthy children and young adults without heart or valvular disease. When the heart rate is rapid the third heart sound is usually termed an S_3 gallop; in the presence of heart disease it usually indicates left ventricular failure. A fourth heart sound (S_4) is abnormal in a young person; it can occur with hypertension or aortic stenosis. A loud S_4 accompanying mitral regurgitation indicates that the lesion is acute and substantial, the sound being caused by the left atrium's valiant attempt to cope with overwhelming volume overload.

Heart murmurs should be carefully timed as systolic, diastolic, or continuous. Innocent murmurs are virtually never accompanied by a thrill. It is interesting that although mitral valve prolapse occurs slightly more often in young women than in men, most complications (infective endocarditis, mitral regurgitation, and ruptured chordae) occur disproportionately more often in men.

TABLE 129-3. Classification of Common Murmurs by Timing

Systolic Murmurs

Aortic stenosis (valvular, supravalvular and subvalvular)
Mitral regurgitation, including mitral valve prolapse
Tricuspid regurgitation
Pulmonic stenosis
Idiopathic hypertrophic subaortic stenosis
Coarctation of the aorta
Ventricular septal defect
Atrial septal defect
Innocent systolic murmur

Diastolic Murmurs

Mitral stenosis
Tricuspid stenosis
Aortic regurgitation
Pulmonic regurgitation

Continuous Murmurs (Extending Through S_2 Without Relation to Aortic or Pulmonic Valve Closure)

Patent ductus arteriosus
Mammary souffle
Ruptured sinus of Valsalva aneurysm

Virtually all systolic murmurs, except that caused by IHSS, get softer or disappear during the strain phase of the Valsalva maneuver. Listening to murmurs with the patient in different body positions may also be helpful.

PROSTHETIC VALVES

Surgically implanted prosthetic valves present special diagnostic problems. Patients with such devices are at risk for (a) endocarditis (which may present with fever, chills, or peripheral embolic complications, including stroke), (b) embolization due to clot formation (which may present as a new stroke, transient ischemic attack, or occluded peripheral artery), and (c) prosthetic valve dysfunction caused by dehiscence of suture lines, thrombosis of the valve, valve degeneration (porcine heterografts or human homografts), hemolysis, or structural failure (ball or tilting disk devices).

Patients with prosthetic valve dysfunction may gradually develop CHF or fatigue, or may present suddenly with syncope or pulmonary edema. The sounds and murmurs heard after valve replacement vary from device to device. Mechanical ball-valve or tilting-disk valves should produce clicking or metallic opening and closing sounds. Most implanted valves are relatively stenotic compared with native valves, so it is common and permissible to have a short systolic murmur with a prosthetic aortic valve or a short diastolic rumble with a prosthetic mitral valve. Prominent mitral regurgitant murmurs should not be heard after mitral valve replacement unless there is a mechanical problem with the valve. Because severe mitral or aortic regurgitation due to prosthetic valve dysfunction occasionally produces no audible murmur, the development of CHF or the appearance of other potential indicators of valve failure always warrants immediate investigation of the valve's integrity.

Catheter balloon valvuloplasty is now performed for pulmonary, mitral, and aortic valve stenosis. After a successful procedure it is common to have a persistent stenotic murmur or a new murmur from valve regurgitation. Complications include valve regurgitation, inadequate opening of the stenosis, endocarditis, arrhythmias, embolization, and atrial septal defect (mitral valvuloplasty only).

EMERGENCY DEPARTMENT EVALUATION AND MANAGEMENT

PA and lateral chest radiograph and ECG complement the history and physical examination. Specific chamber enlargement or poststenotic dilatation of the aorta or pulmonary artery on x-ray film or chamber hypertrophy on ECG (LVH in aortic stenosis, left atrial enlargement in mitral stenosis, and RVH in pulmonic stenosis) can help to disclose the cause of a murmur. Cardiomegaly, pulmonary vascular congestion, pulmonary edema, and pleural effusions on chest radiograph can detect or confirm CHF.

ECHO with Doppler is a sensitive and precise means of detecting and evaluating the severity of valvular lesions. ECHO can detect vegetations or intracardiac thrombi in patients with suspected endocarditis and evidence of systemic embolization, and can be used to evaluate prosthetic valve motion and function.

Specific complications of valvular heart disease such as CHF, cardiogenic shock, embolization, and arrhythmias should be managed in the usual manner. Severe CHF, hypotension, and shock caused by massive acute aortic or mitral regurgitation may be refractory to medical therapy. It is often preferable to use dobutamine or low to medium doses (5–15 µg/kg/min) of dopamine, or both, rather than potent alpha vasoconstrictors (e.g., high-dose dopamine), since increases in afterload will only worsen valvular regurgitation. Intra-aortic balloon counterpulsation or other left ventricular mechanical assist devices may be required for stabilization before cardiac catheterization and surgery.

Antibiotic prophylaxis is indicated for the patient with significant valvular lesions about to undergo procedures that may result in bacteremia. It is not clear whether all patients with MVP (5% of the population) require such prophylaxis, but those patients who have a systolic murmur or ECHO evidence of mitral regurgitation are 35 times more likely to develop endocarditis than are those who have no systolic murmur or other evidence of mitral regurgitation. Thus all MVP patients with mitral regurgitation should be covered with antibiotics. Whether to provide coverage to other MVP patients is a decision that should probably be made by the patient's cardiologist.

DISPOSITION

Absolute indications for immediate consultation include (a) known or suspected valvular lesions that are accompanied by hemodynamic instability (CHF and shock), fever, arrhythmia, or embolization; (b) new onset or progression of symptoms; and (c) significant hemolysis after valve surgery or valvuloplasty. ICU admission is usually indicated for significant arrhythmias, pulmonary edema, and hypotension, and when there are life-threatening medical problems. Immediate cardiac catheterization and surgical intervention are indicated for new-onset, severe valvular regurgitation, prosthetic valve malfunction, systemic embolization in the face of adequate anticoagulation, valve ring abscess, intractable CHF, or shock.

If transfer is required, the emergency physician should consult with the receiving cardiologist. An advanced cardiac life-support team should always accompany the patient. Air transport by helicopter or pressurized fixed-wing aircraft may be indicated if the patient is in urgent need of cardiac catheterization and operative intervention. Most asymptomatic patients with a heart murmur incidentally found should be referred to a cardiologist for further evaluation. Pregnant patients with newly detected murmurs or abnormal heart sounds should be referred for further cardiac evaluation of possible structural heart disease.

COMMON PITFALLS

- It is easy to be misled by the physical findings when a patient is seen for the first time. The severity of valvular disease is always underestimated during periods of severe CHF, shock, or tachycardia, since the decreased cardiac output leads to a decrease in the intensity of heart murmurs. The elderly patient presents a special problem because the presence of atherosclerosis with rigid vessels may either mask or amplify pulse or blood pressure changes caused by valvular disease.

- A common error is to mistake a normal heart sound (physiologic S_3) or an innocent murmur in a young person for structural heart disease.
- Murmurs are difficult to evaluate during pregnancy; they may suddenly appear or disappear as the cardiac output, blood volume, and vascular resistance change during each trimester and in the postpartum period.

130   Acute Pericarditis and Cardiac Tamponade

ACUTE PERICARDITIS

Acute pericarditis is a diagnostic challenge because its presentation is similar to that of several other disorders and because it may have life-threatening complications. The management ranges from symptomatic, supportive treatment to life-saving invasive procedures. The common causes of acute pericarditis are listed in Table 130-1. In many episodes of pericarditis the cause is unclear (idiopathic pericarditis). Viral pericarditis is frequently diagnosed presumptively after a viral-like syndrome. Other infectious causes (bacterial, fungal, and parasitic) are less common, but pericarditis may occur as a complication of another systemic or intrathoracic infection.

Pericarditis is the most prominent cardiac complication of neoplastic disease. Nontraumatic pericardial tamponade is most frequently of metastatic origin. Lymphoma, leukemia, and breast or lung carcinoma cause most pericardial metastases. Pericarditis may also occur as a complication of chronic renal failure. Systemic lupus erythematosus, scleroderma, and rheuma-

---

TABLE 130-1. Causes of Acute Pericarditis

Idiopathic	**Drug-Related**
Infectious	Procainamide
Viral	Hydralazine
Pyogenic	Methyldopa
Tuberculosis	
Fungal	**Cardiac Disease**
Parasitic	Postmyocardial infarction
Malignancy	Postsurgical
	Postinstrumentation
Uremia	Cardiac trauma
Connective Tissue Disease	
Rheumatoid arthritis	
Systemic lupus erythematosus	
Scleroderma	

toid arthritis cause pericarditis. Medications, including those associated with a drug-induced lupus syndrome (e.g., hydralazine, methyldopa, and procainamide), may also be implicated.

Pericarditis can occur days to months after AMI; differentiation from Dressler's syndrome, a possible autoimmune pericarditis that occurs after myocardial infarction, may be difficult. Aortic dissection, cardiac trauma, invasive procedures that involve the great vessels and the heart (central venous pressure catheter insertion and cardiac catheterization), and intrathoracic surgery may also cause pericarditis and pericardial tamponade.

CLINICAL PRESENTATION

Most patients with acute pericarditis present with chest pain; it is usually sharp and often pleuritic, but it may also be described as dull, constrictive, or aching. It may radiate to any part of the chest and back and to the trapezius ridge. It is often eased by sitting up and leaning forward. The pain of pericarditis is frequently associated with shortness of breath. Patients may also present with hypotension and other signs of tamponade.

DIFFERENTIAL DIAGNOSIS

The differential diagnosis of pericarditis includes: AMI, CHF, pulmonary embolism, pneumonia, pneumothorax, pneumomediastinum, pleuritis, and aortic dissection. Cardiac tamponade may be confused with congestive heart failure and cardiogenic shock. Acute pericarditis is frequently mistaken for AMI. Patients with pericarditis may present with fever and typically have sharper pain that increases with body motion and varies with position. They show diffuse (rather than focal) ECG changes without reciprocal changes, do not develop the Q waves and have, at most, minimal elevation of cardiac enzyme levels. Patients with pericarditis (even with tamponade) have clear lung fields, as opposed to those with congestive heart failure or pneumonia. On the ECG, a normal early repolarization variant may mimic pericarditis.

EMERGENCY DEPARTMENT EVALUATION

Most patients with shortness of breath and chest pain should receive oxygen, IV access, monitoring, and a 12-lead ECG. The classic finding is the pericardial friction rub. The friction rub may be transient or intermittent, and can be confused with a heart murmur. The ECG can be diagnostic, with four stages: Stage 1 is the most characteristic (concave-upward ST segment elevation in most of the leads; P–R segment depression may also be seen). Stage 2: ST segments return to baseline and the T wave amplitude decreases; the P–R segment may be depressed. Stage 3: T wave flattening and then inversion in leads with previous ST segment elevation. Stage 4: normalization of the ECG.

The ECG findings in acute pericarditis are diffuse changes that are seen in most leads, rather than the focal abnormalities seen in acute myocardial infarction. Early repolarization, characterized by ST segment elevation, can be difficult to distinguish from pericarditis. If the clinical presentation suggests pericarditis, serial ECGs may be required to differentiate pericarditis from the benign early repolarization variant. However, diagnostic ECG changes may be absent in 4% to 33% of patients with clinically evident pericarditis.

Patients with postmyocardial infarction pericarditis (diagnosed by the presence of a pericardial friction rub) also frequently have no ECG changes. The chest radiograph is often normal. The cardiac silhouette may be enlarged secondary to a pericardial effusion, but radiographic enlargement is often not seen until 200–500 mL of fluid accumulates. True cardiomegaly represents significant myocarditis or other heart disease. The white blood cell count is not helpful in making or excluding the diagnosis of pericarditis. Cardiac enzyme levels are normal or minimally elevated. The erythrocyte sedimentation rate is usually elevated.

COMPLICATIONS

The major complications of acute pericarditis are pericardial effusion, potentially leading to cardiac tamponade, and chronic constrictive pericarditis. Arrhythmias are unusual in pericarditis, but they may occur in patients with associated myocarditis or other underlying heart disease.

CARDIAC TAMPONADE

Cardiac tamponade is an acutely life-threatening complication of pericarditis. The presentation of tamponade may be subtle, leading to a missed diagnosis and a poor outcome. Close attention to physical findings is essential to making the diagnosis. Tamponade results from the accumulation of fluid within the pericardial space, causing an impairment of cardiac filling and decrease in cardiac output. Tamponade is often mistaken for congestive heart failure because patients present with dyspnea, orthopnea, jugular venous distention, and hepatic enlargement. Patients with tamponade may have relatively normal ECGs.

With large effusions reduction of the QRS amplitude or electrical alternans (alternating beat-to-beat variation in QRS amplitude) may be seen. Central venous pressure measurements reveal an elevation of right-sided pressures and help to confirm the diagnosis. Decompensation can be rapid; ECHO is diagnostic, detecting as little as 20 mL of pericardial fluid. In tamponade it may demonstrate diffuse hypokinesis, and diastolic collapse of the right atrium, ventricle, or ventricular outflow tract. ECHO should be performed emergently in any patient with suspected tamponade.

Constrictive pericarditis, an uncommon complication of acute pericarditis, results when healing of acute pericarditis leads to encasement of the heart in fibrous tissue, impeding ventricular filling. Patients often present with ascites, peripheral edema, and hepatic enlargement. The presence of distended neck veins in constrictive pericarditis helps to separate these patients from those with severe liver disease. Pericardial calcification on chest radiograph and pericardial thickening on ECHO also provide clues.

EMERGENCY DEPARTMENT MANAGEMENT AND DISPOSITION

Most patients should be admitted to the hospital. The consultant can coordinate the evaluation, and obtain ECHO and pericardiocentesis. Whether **all** patients with acute pericarditis require admission is controversial; some young patients with uncomplicated idiopathic or viral pericarditis may be managed as outpatients. It should be recognized, however, that pericarditis may occur as a complication of AMI and that pericardial effusion and cardiac tamponade may be subtle. Obtaining an ECHO before discharge will assure that a pericardial effusion is not missed.

Patients who are not admitted to the hospital require close, careful follow-up. The therapy for uncomplicated pericarditis is largely symptomatic. Nonsteroidal anti-inflammatory agents give excellent results in viral and idiopathic pericarditis. Pyogenic pericarditis must be treated with admission, drainage and antibiotics. Uremic pericarditis is usually an indication for dialysis. Treatment of pericardial tamponade is pericardiocentesis with ECHO and ECG guidance if possible. However, emergent pericardiocentesis may be necessary for hypotensive patients who do not respond to volume infusion.

131 Deep Venous Thrombosis and Thrombophlebitis

Deep vein thrombosis (DVT) remains a diagnostic challenge with about 200,000–300,000 cases per year. There are 600,000 symptomatic cases of pulmonary embolism per year. Thrombi form in the following situations: stasis, vessel injury, hypercoagulability, and the capacity for fibrinolysis. Conditions that alter the balance of these factors may place patients at an increased risk for thrombus formation. These conditions are as follows: for stasis—congestive heart failure, stroke, bed rest, and pregnancy; for vessel injury—trauma and surgery; for hypercoagulable state—malignancy, surgery, and pregnancy.

Thrombi form most commonly in the lower extremities and often occur at multiple sites. The location is an important factor in determining the risk of embolization. Superficial thrombophlebitis, if unassociated with DVT, poses no risk of embolization. Isolated calf vein thrombosis and saphenous vein thrombosis above the knee present a low risk for significant embolization. The greatest risk of significant embolization arises from thrombi at or above the popliteal level.

The postphlebitic syndrome is associated with significant chronic morbidity. Once a significant thrombus forms, valve destruction commonly occurs, with chronic venous hypertension, skin hyperpigmentation, and eventual ulceration, usually around the medial malleolus. Patients with the postphlebitic syndrome are also at increased risk for recurrent DVT.

CLINICAL PRESENTATION

Although DVT can be asymptomatic, patients usually present with pain and swelling of the leg. Lower extremity swelling around one ankle has the greatest predictive value for DVT. Superficial venous dilatation, palpable cords, deep calf tenderness, difference in leg temperature, and, particularly, Homans' sign, are consistently unreliable in making a diagnosis of DVT. Risk factors (Table 131-1) must be identified, since these have been correlated with DVT. Positive impedance plethysmography (IPG) results were noted in 11% of patients with none of the first five risk factors listed in Table 131-1, 24% with one risk factor, 36% with two, 50% with three, and all patients with four or more. A history of risk factors and appropriate physical findings should identify those patients who need diagnostic testing to confirm DVT. It is useful to classify patients as low-risk (0–1 risk factors and equivocal physical findings) or high-risk (multiple risk factors and suggestive physical findings).

TABLE 131-1. Risk Factors for DVT

Age over 40
Obesity
Recent surgery
History of DVT
Malignancy
Pregnancy
Estrogen therapy
Trauma
Congestive heart failure
Myocardial infarction
Immobilization
Stroke

DIFFERENTIAL DIAGNOSIS

This potentially lethal entity must be ruled out. The differential diagnosis is extensive, and includes several disorders that are themselves risk factors for DVT (Table 131-2). Although lower-extremity edema is commonly seen in congestive heart failure, pregnancy, malignancy with venous or lymphatic obstruction, and paralysis, it is usually bilateral. Edema secondary to DVT is usually unilateral. Acute onset of leg pain is more typical after trauma or a ruptured Baker's cyst than the slower onset of symptoms caused by DVT.

EMERGENCY DEPARTMENT EVALUATION AND MANAGEMENT

If clinical evaluation clearly identifies a cause other than DVT, no further investigation may be necessary. However, if DVT remains a consideration, further steps must be taken. Up to 50% of patients suspected of having a DVT will not have the diagnosis confirmed by objective tests. This false–positive rate based solely on clinical evaluation is unacceptably high. Most, if not all, suspected DVTs should be confirmed with tests such as contrast venography, radionuclide venography, IPG, or Doppler ultrasonography.

Venography is considered the "gold standard." However, venography is invasive, often unavailable, and associated with some morbidity (chemical phlebitis and occasional hypersensitivity reactions). Radionuclide venography with technetium-labeled plasmin or microaggregated albumin has less morbidity, is almost as accurate, but has limited availability.

IPG is a noninvasive test that indirectly measures alterations in leg *volume* that occur in response to inflation and deflation of a pneumatic thigh cuff. The utility is based on the alteration of normal response patterns commonly seen in the presence of DVT. IPG is noninvasive and safe, but it is also frequently unavailable. IPG is accurate in the diagnosis of proximal DVT, but is less so for distal (calf vein) thrombosis. Hand-held Doppler ultrasonography (HHDU) is used to evaluate the *flow* of venous blood. The rationale is based on the tendency of DVT to alter venous flow in the leg. Although readily available, HHDU requires skill to perform and is slightly less accurate than IPG for the diagnosis of proximal thrombi. HHDU is relatively insensitive for the detection of distal thrombi. I^{131} fibrinogen can detect DVT, but takes 24–72 hours to complete the study, and is impractical for ED use.

To minimize the risk of embolization, treatment of DVT should be initiated as soon as the diagnosis is made. In the absence of a contraindication to anticoagulation, IV heparin should be given in the ED. Current recommendations: 5000- to 10,000-unit bolus, followed by a continuous infusion of 1000 U/h. This rate should be titrated to achieve a partial thromboplastin time (PTT) 1.5 to 2.5 times the normal value. Before heparinization, obtain a hemoglobin, hematocrit, prothrombin time (PT), and PTT, and type and hold for later crossmatch, if necessary. If heparin is contraindicated, consider an inferior vena caval interruption procedure.

The relative risks of PE and hemorrhagic complications of anticoagulation should be considered. Thrombolytic therapy with urokinase, streptokinase, or t-PA may be indicated for large proximal thrombi. Thrombectomy may be indicated for threatened gangrene due to extensive

---

TABLE 131-2. Differential Diagnosis of DVT (Common Entities)

Congestive heart failure
Pregnancy
Malignancy with outflow obstruction
Paralysis
Trauma
Ruptured Baker's cyst
Arthritis
Lymphangitis, cellulitis

TABLE 131-3. Disposition of Cases According to Test Results

Test	High-Risk Patient	Low-Risk Patient
Doppler ultrasound* – Perform venogram	+ Hospitalize and treat	Verify with venogram Discharge with clinical follow-up
Impodance plethysmography	+ Hospitalize and treat – Discharge with serial follow-up	Hospitalize and treat Discharge with clinical follow-up
Contrast venography or nuclear venoscan	+ Hospitalize and treat – Discharge with clinical follow-up	Hospitalize and treat Discharge with clinical follow-up

* Performed by a skilled operator. (+, positive; –, negative)

thrombosis. There is controversy about the need to treat isolated calf vein thrombosis with hospitalization and anticoagulation. Some authorities believe that an isolated calf DVT seldom, if ever, results in significant PE. Although proximal extension can occur with increased embolic risk, this probably occurs in only 20%. Currently, however, most patients with isolated calf vein thrombi are anticoagulated. An alternative is serial noninvasive evaluations on an outpatient basis over the course of a week to rule out proximal extension of the thrombus.

DISPOSITION

With the possible exception of isolated calf vein thrombosis, all patients with DVT need admission for treatment. Diagnosis should not be made on the basis of clinical evaluation alone. All patients with an abnormal contrast venogram, radionuclide venogram, or IPG, and all high-risk patients with an abnormal Doppler ultrasound examination should be hospitalized and treated. Because of the lower specificity of Doppler ultrasonography, an abnormal Doppler examination in a low-risk patient should be validated by contrast venography.

The patient with negative venogram or venoscan can be safely discharged. However, follow-up should be arranged after venography to identify potential chemical phlebitis. The low-risk patient with negative IPG or Doppler results can be discharged with conservative treatment and clinical re-evaluation. On the other hand, all negative IPG and Doppler examinations in high-risk patients need to be validated either by contrast venography or by serial IPG over 1 week, based on institutional capability and patient reliability (Table 131-3). There is seldom a need to transfer a patient with DVT, but if such a case arises, heparinization should be initiated before transfer.

COMMON PITFALLS

- Many problems can masquerade as DVT, some of which may be indistinguishable by clinical evaluation (Table 131-2). The physician who relies solely on clinical evaluation will make numerous diagnostic errors. A false–negative evaluation places the patient at risk for fatal pulmonary embolism, whereas a false–positive examination results in expense and morbidity of hospitalization and anticoagulation. Both extremes can be avoided with the appropriate use of diagnostic tests.
- Although noninvasive tests often supplant contrast venography because of increased availability, reduced morbidity, and lower expense, these tests are not as accurate as venography for diagnosing DVT. Furthermore, the accuracy of Doppler ultrasonography is very dependent on the skill of the person performing the test.

132   Infectious Endocarditis

Infectious endocarditis (IE) is an infection of the endothelial lining of the heart, usually including the valvular endothelium. The disease is increasing due to the dramatic surge in IV drug use and the increased utilization of prosthetic heart valves. IE is divided into two forms: an insidious, chronic disease, subacute bacterial endocarditis (SBE), and a more abrupt-onset fulminant form, acute bacterial endocarditis (ABE). SBE has become less common. "Modern endocarditis" is more likely to involve younger intravenous drug abusers (IVDAs) or older prosthetic valve patients, and is less likely to be of *Streptococcus viridans* etiology. Bacterial endocarditis may also develop on previously normal native and prosthetic heart valves.

Once endocarditis has developed on a valve, the clinical manifestations of the disease are due to (a) local destruction and malfunction of the valve; (b) invasive infection of contiguous structures in the heart; (c) continuous bacteremia with distant infections; (d) formation of vegetations that embolize; and (e) an antigen–antibody response, leading to immune-mediated complications.

It is easier to group patients with IE into four clinical groups: patients with a native valve, IVDAs, patients with prosthetic valves who develop early-onset prosthetic valve IE (PVE), and patients with late-onset PVE. Early-onset PVE is infection that presents <2 months after valve replacement surgery; late-onset PVE presents >2 months after surgery. Patients with native valve IE are most likely to develop "classic SBE," a relatively chronic infection with only left-sided cardiac involvement, often with a streptococcal organism.

The mitral valve is the most common valve to be infected; isolated mitral involvement occurs in 35–45% of cases, isolated aortic valve involvement in 15–35%, and involvement of both valves in 15-30%. Tricuspid valve IE is unusual in this group (1%–5%). Pulmonic involvement is extremely rare in native valve IE, and is seen in <1%.

Organisms that cause infectious endocarditis are shown in Table 132-1.

HIGH-RISK GROUPS FOR INFECTIOUS ENDOCARDITIS

Drug abusers have become one of the leading high-risk groups for IE, with cocaine abusers at highest risk of developing IE. The increased risk is due to injection frequency, lack of heating of the drug before injection and direct valvular damage caused by cocaine. About 50% of IVDAs develop IE of the tricuspid valve. The other half develop either mitral or aortic disease. Pulmonic valve IE is rare. IVDAs are often infected with normal skin flora: *Staphylococcus aureus* is the most common (50%) with *Streptococcus* species the next most common. Gram-negative bacilli, fungi, and diphtheroids are seen only slightly more often in IVDA IE than in native valve IE.

Patients with early PVE either have been contaminated intraoperatively or developed infection in the perioperative period. *Staphylococcus* species are the most commonly incriminated organisms, especially the otherwise rare coagulase-negative *Staphylococcus*. Gram-negative organisms and fungi are also seen more commonly in this group. Late PVE shares characteristics of nosocomial infection and native valve IE. The organisms responsible for late PVE fall midway between those seen in early PVE and those common in native valve IE. *S. viridans* and coagulase-positive and -negative staphylococci are most frequent, but gram-negative bacteria and fungi cause a significant number of infections.

Mechanical and tissue valves have an approximately equal incidence of infection (2.2%–4.4%), but mechanical valves are more likely to develop early-onset PVE. Mechanical valves tend to develop ring abscesses, myocardial abscesses with conduction delays, pericardi-

TABLE 132-1. Common Causes of Infectious Endocarditis

	Percentages
Native Valve IE	
Streptococcus	
viridans	25–43
bovis	7–15
fecalis	10–16
Staphylococcus	
Coag Pos	21–38
Coag Neg	5
Gram-negative rods	>5
Fungi >5	
Culture negative	3–15
IVDA	
Streptococcus	
viridans	5
fecalis	8
Staphylococcus	
Coag Pos	50
Coag Neg	>5
Gram-negative rods	5
Fungi 5	
Culture negative	>5
Early Onset PVE	
Staphylococcus (all groups)	10
Streptococcus	
Coag Pos	20
Coag Neg	25–44
Gram-negative rods	20–38
Fungi 10	
Diphtheroids	10
Culture negative	>5
Last Onset PVE	
Streptococcus	25–41
viridans	
Staphylococcus	
Coag Pos	3–10
Coag Neg	20–35
Gram-negative rods	15–31
Fungi	>5
Culture negative	>5

Note: Percentages are approximations based on multiple prior studies. (6, 8, 9, 20, 26, 28, 34, 35)

tis, and regurgitation due to paravalvular leaks. An acute regurgitant murmur caused by partial dehiscence of the sewing ring represents an emergency, since severe heart failure can develop rapidly or the valve can totally dehisce. Tissue valves, on the other hand, are more likely to develop leaflet tears, causing new regurgitant murmurs and heart failure. Valvular stenosis is also frequently seen with tissue valves.

CLINICAL PRESENTATION

Patients with IE may present with fulminant heart failure and sepsis, with an indolent nonspecific process, or with an intermediate syndrome. Table 132-2 lists the findings seen most often in IE.

COMPLICATIONS

CARDIAC
Cardiac complications of IE may involve any of the three layers of the heart. Endocardial damage may result in valvular destruction and CHF, with severe failure due to aortic insufficiency. Myocarditis or myocardial abscess results from infection of the myocardium. Infection involving the conduction system may cause conduction delays, bundle-branch blocks, or complete heart block. Ruptured myocardial abscesses may produce purulent pericarditis. Large emboli to the coronary arteries can cause AMI or sudden death.

CENTRAL NERVOUS SYSTEM
Central nervous system complications occur in 20%–40% and may be the presenting complaint in a significant number. Embolic cerebral infarction or stroke is the most common event (middle cerebral artery or its branches). Cerebral mycotic aneurysms may be asymptomatic or may enlarge and leak or rupture with disastrous outcome. Septic emboli give rise to cerebral abscesses or, if meningeal or cortical vessels are involved, bacterial meningitis. A syndrome of headache, delirium, hallucinations, and confusion may be seen. When accompanied by a stiff neck and cerebrospinal fluid consistent with aseptic meningitis, the patient has meningoencephalitis. The cause is unclear, but multiple microinfarcts or microabscesses may be responsible.

EMBOLI AND IMMUNOLOGIC RESPONSES
Embolization may also involve the splenic, renal, mesenteric, and extremity vasculature, resulting in endarteritis, myocotic aneurysm, local infection, and distal infarction. The immune com-

---

TABLE 132-2. Historical and Physical Findings Suggestive of Endocarditis

	History	Physical Examination
General	Fever, chills, malaise, weakness, anorexia, weight loss, back pain, myalgia, arthralgia	Acute or chronically ill appearance, fever, diaphoresis, pallor, splenomegaly, arthritis
Cardiopulmonary	Chest pain, dyspnea, edema	Murmurs, especially valvular insufficiency; signs of congestive heart failure
Neurologic	Headache, stiff neck, mental status changes, focal neurologic complaints, extremity pain or paresthesia	Meningismus, abnormal mental status, focal deficits
Other	Hematuria, abdominal pain	**Skin:** petechiae, Osler's nodes, Janeway lesions, splinter hemorrhages
Risk Factor	Intravenous drug abuse, heart disease, recent GI, GU, or dental procedure, poor dental hygiene	**Other:** pneumonia, skin abscess, urinary tract infection
		Embolic: mycotic aneurysm, visceral or extremity infarct or ischemia

plex–mediated process may cause glomerulonephritis or aseptic arthritis; most of the skin manifestations are immune-related.

EMERGENCY DEPARTMENT EVALUATION

Patients with IE have nonspecific complaints: fever, malaise, anorexia, and weakness. About 50% complain of headache, weight loss, night sweats, arthralgias, and myalgias. Back pain, rash, dyspnea, or a spectrum of neuropsychiatric symptoms is not uncommon. Clinicians seldom initially attribute these to IE. Always ask about recent dental, gastrointestinal, and urologic procedures. The elderly may not volunteer, or may forget, these high-risk activities. Young, healthy patients evaluated for the "flu" seldom volunteer information on IV drug abuse unless specifically questioned. Findings suggestive of endocarditis are listed in Table 132-2.

Patients with IE may appear acutely or chronically ill. Nearly all patients have fever. Abnormal vital signs, including tachycardia and hypotension, are not unusual. A cardiac exam is critical with 70–97% demonstrating a murmur. Those least likely to have murmurs are those with acute IE and tricuspid IE. It is rather uncommon for new murmurs to develop as a result of IE; most that do develop are regurgitant. Findings suggestive of heart failure should also be sought. Skin lesions are considered classic in IE, but they are found in only 5%–10%. Petechaie are most common; Osler's nodes (small, painful, tender, erythematous papules) are seen most often on distal extremities. Janeway lesions, small, flat, nontender red spots, are found on the palms and soles. Splinter hemorrhages, are seen in 10% but are nonspecific.

The remainder of the examination may reveal abdominal or neurologic findings. Splenomegly is a common finding, and a tender, enlarged liver is often noted. Neurologic examination may suggest meningitis, encephalitis, embolic stroke, or a leaking aneurysm. Subtle mental status changes or behavioral symptoms may be mistaken for psychiatric disease.

There are nonspecific laboratory findings in IE (Table 132-3). Normochromic, normocytic anemia is seen in 75% and microscopic hematuria in nearly one half of patients. Leukocytosis is seen in 50%; however, its absence does *not* rule out the diagnosis. An elevated ESR is typical, but it may be normal in 33%. The most important test is the blood culture for aerobic, anaerobic,

---

TABLE 132-3. Laboratory Findings in Endocarditis

Blood

Positive blood cultures
Anemia
Microscopic or gross hematuria
Possible leukocytosis
Uremia

Chest Radiograph

Cardiomegaly
Pulmonary infiltrates
Pulmonary infarcts
Pulmonary effusions
Chamber enlargement
Abnormal movement of prosthetic valve
Stimson's sign

Electrocardiogram

Conduction defect
Acute MI
Pericarditis

Echocardiogram

Vegetations
Valve dysfunction
Chamber enlargement
Pericardial effusion

V/Q Scan

Multiple pulmonary infarcts

Cerebrospinal Fluid

Purulent meningitis
Aseptic meningitis
Bloody leaking aneurysm

Computed Tomography

Mycotic aneurysm
Cerebral abscess
Subarachnoid hemorrhage

and fungal pathogens; 95% with IE have blood culture-positive endocarditis. The diagnosis of "possible endocarditis" should appear on the specimen label so that the laboratory will hold the specimen for 3+ weeks to detect slow-growing organisms. In 95%–98% of culture-positive patients, the organism is determined with the first two sets of cultures, although 3–5 sets should be drawn before initiating antibiotics.

Recent antibiotic use and infection with fastidious or slow-growing organisms are the two major reasons for culture-negative IE. The two groups most often with culture-negative IE are IVDAs and patients with prosthetic heart valves. The chest radiograph of a patient with IE is usually normal, although it may reveal CHF or pneumonia, especially in IVDA patients. Multiple pulmonary infarcts or nodules suggest right-sided disease, usually tricuspid valve endocarditis. Athough usually normal, the ECG should be examined for evidence of pericarditis, ischemia, infarction, conduction delay, or heart block. These changes may be indirect evidence for the coexistence of myocarditis, myocardial abscesses, pericarditis, or coronary artery embolism. ECHO should be done if IE is suspected. Vegetations are strong support for the diagnosis. ECHO may show valve malfunction, chamber enlargement, or an associated pericardial effusion. Because mechanical valves are too echo-dense to be evaluated by ECHO, cinefluoroscopy is the preferred modality.

EMERGENCY DEPARTMENT MANAGEMENT

Treatment continues to evolve; the standard 6 weeks of in-patient antibiotics is no longer the rule. Treatment regimens have become shorter, and newer antibiotics have appeared. In general, IE is treated with IV bactericidal antibiotics. Antibiotic(s) are best determined by culture and sensitivity. For patients with uncomplicated *S. viridans* and some strains of *S. bovis,* IE cure rates of >99% occur with 4 weeks of penicillin G (10–20 million U/d IV) given with a concurrent 2-week course of gentamicin (1 mg/kg IV every 8 hours). *Enterococcus* and other resistant *Streptococcus* species require 6 weeks of both penicillin and gentamicin. In penicillin-allergic patients vancomycin (15 mg/kg with a maximum of 1.0 g IV every 12 hours) should be used in place of penicillin. *Staphylococcus epidermidis* IE usually requires triple antibiotic therapy with vancomycin, gentamicin, and rifampin. In cases of gram-negative IE, sensitivity data should be used to guide therapy, usually with a third-generation cephalosporin. In patients with suspected IE who present with sepsis, CHF, or coexistent pneumonia, empiric therapy should begin in the ED. Table 132-4 lists the best antibiotic choices and dosages based on the patient's IE risk group.

ANTICOAGULANTS

Anticoagulation is contraindicated in patients with native valve IE because of risk of intracranial bleeding. The exception to this may be in patients who develop massive life-threatening pulmonary emboli. Patients with PVE already on anticoagulation should probably continue but be monitored for complications. Valve replacement is accepted therapy for complicated IE. There is agreement on the indications for surgery, but timing is debated. General indications for valve replacement: CHF from new valve malfunction; major embolic complications; continued infection despite appropriate antibiotics; arrhythmia or new conduction defect; or a fungal cause. It is unclear if the size of vegetations seen on ECHO affect prognosis and need for valve replacement.

DISPOSITION

Because of serious complications and use of parenteral antibiotics, all patients with suspected IE need hospital admission. Patients with overwhelming sepsis, serious embolic complications, or any degree of CHF or conduction block require admission to an ICU. ICU admission is mandatory for a PVE patient with any evidence of paravalvular leak. A cardiologist should be consulted for ECHO. Patients with PVE or a patient who may need valve replacement should have a cardiac surgeon involved early. For patients with possible brain abscess or aneurysm, a neurosurgeon should be consulted promptly.

TABLE 132-4. Empiric Therapy of Endocarditis Prior to Culture Results

Native Valve

Penicillin*	2 million units IV and Q 4 h
or	
Naficillin*	2 g IV and Q 4 h
and	
Gentamicin	1.5 mg/kg IV then 1 mg/kg IV Q 8 h

Intravenous Drug Abuser

Naficillin*	2 g IV and Q 4 h
and	
Gentamicin	1.5 mg/kg IV then 1 mg/kg IV Q 8 h

Prosthetic Valve Endocarditis

Vancomycin	1 g IV and 12 h
and	
Gentamicin	1.5 mg/kg IV then 1 mg/kg IV Q 8 h
and	
Rifampin	300 mg PO and 12 h

*Substitute vancomycin 1 g IV Q 12 h if patient is penicillin-allergic.

ENDOCARDITIS PROPHYLAXIS

The aim of antibiotic prophylaxis is to prevent transient bacteremia during procedures in patients prone to endocarditis. Unresolved are questions on whether all patients with mitral valve prolapse should receive prophylaxis, the relative merit of parenteral versus oral regimens, and, finally, how effective prophylaxis really is. Currently, all patients at risk should receive prophylaxis.

COMMON PITFALLS

- Missing the diagnosis in the elderly by attributing a cardiac murmur to chronic heart disease
- Failure to remember that IE in drug abusers usually presents without a murmur
- Failure to remember that IVDAs are at high risk for endocarditis
- Not asking about risk factors for IE in patients about to undergo a procedure prone to cause bacteremia
- Not asking about risk factors in patients who present with nonspecific symptoms consistent with endocarditis
- Not asking specifically about IV drug abuse in patients who present with nonspecific symptoms consistent with endocarditis
- Failure to consider the embolic complications of IE as the cause of stroke, meningitis, or myocardial infarction
- Failure to recognize that in patients with a mechanical valve, a regurgitant murmur is a sign of impending heart failure or valve dehiscence
- Failure to consult a cardiac surgeon in IE with only mild to moderate heart failure
- Forgetting the fact that mild degrees of heart block and conduction delays are highly suggestive of myocardial abscess or myocarditis

133   Cardiac Syncope

Syncope, *the sudden, transient loss of consciousness associated with an inability to maintain postural tone and resolving without medical intervention,* is the presenting complaint in an estimated 1%–3% of ED visits. The approach is problematic, in that the symptoms and signs have invariably resolved before medical attention is sought. Frequently, despite clinical evaluation, the problem remains unexplained. The diagnostic effort should focus on identifying patients who are likely to benefit from further inpatient evaluation and therapy. This group of high-risk patients represents only a small fraction of the population with syncope. The challenge of accurately identifying this small group is formidable. The Framingham study evaluated men and women (30–62 years); over 26 years, 3.3% reported at least one episode of "isolated syncope" (defined as syncope in the absence of prior or concurrent neurologic or cardiovascular disease). In contrast, an incidence of 23% was noted in all cases of syncope in an elderly, institutionalized population.

PATHOPHYSIOLOGY AND DIFFERENTIAL DIAGNOSIS

The mechanism common to most causes of syncope is sudden, transient reduction in cerebral blood flow (Table 133-1. This results in impaired function either in the brain stem reticular activating system or in both cerebral hemispheres simultaneously. In seizures the loss of consciousness is related to widespread bilateral electrical discharge. SVT or ventricular tachycardia may produce syncope by limiting stroke volume, resulting in systemic hypotension and a decrease in cerebral blood flow. LOC may also occur from transient bradyarrhythmias, although most are asymptomatic.

TABLE 133-1. Differential Diagnosis of Syncope

Cardiovascular Causes

Arrhythmias: Supraventricular and ventricular tachycardia, sick sinus syndrome, conduction disturbances with bradycardia, Stokes-Adams, pacemaker malfunction

Structural disease: Aortic stenosis, hypertrophic cardiomyopathy, mitral valve prolapse, atrial myxoma

Vascular disease: Carotid sinus hypersensitivity, aortic dissection, myocardial infarction, pulmonary embolism, pulmonary hypertension, air embolism

Vasodepressor or Vasovagal Syncope

Neurologic Causes:

Seizure disorder, cerebrovascular accident, central nervous system injury, subarachnoid hemorrhage

Postural Syncope:

Hypovolemia, orthostatic hypotension, drugs

Situational Syncope:

Micturition, defecation, cough, "weightlifters," postprandial

Hyperventilation and Breath Holding

Miscellaneous:

Hypoglycemia, glossopharyngeal neuralgia, subclavian steal syndrome

---

Ventricular tachycardia is responsible for more episodes of syncope than are brad-yarrhythmias. Sick sinus syndrome is associated with both tachyarrhythmias and conduction abnor-malities. Pacemaker failure may also produce syncope in a pacemaker-dependent patient as a result of either bradycardia or pacemaker-induced tachyarrhythmias. Attributing syncope to these syndromes requires documenting LOC during the arrhythmia. Exertional syncope may be the clue to aortic stenosis or hypertrophic cardiomyopathy. Mitral valve disease may also cause syncope. Severe mitral stenosis may be associated with syncope, probably most commonly during periods of rapid atrial fibrillation. A myriad of tachyarrhythmias and neuropsychiatric complaints occur in patients with mitral valve prolapse, which is frequently associated with syncope. Left atrial myxoma is a rare disease that causes an abrupt decrease in cardiac output, often when a change in posi-tion causes the tumor to occlude the mitral orifice. Again, referral to a cardiologist is necessary.

Carotid sinus hypersensitivity most commonly occurs in elderly hypertensive patients, and may produce syncope when the carotid sinus is stimulated, usually by turning the neck, shaving, or wearing tight collars. Treatment options include pacemaker implantation for the cardioin-hibitory type and measures designed to cause fluid retention (e.g., Florinef [fludrocortisone]) for the vasodepressor type. Referral is required.

AMI or ischemia may result in syncope when accompanied by cardiogenic shock or ven-tricular arrhythmia. Acute pulmonary hypertension causes functional acute obstruction to pul-monary flow, and thus abruptly decreases left ventricular preload and cardiac output. This may occur with massive pulmonary embolism. In patients with chronic pulmonary hypertension activi-ties that acutely raise intrathoracic pressure, such as coughing, or Valsalva maneuver during defecation, may produce the same phenomenon. Air embolism may interfere with blood flow any-where in the circulation, and may produce syncope by obstructing flow through the heart, lungs, or carotids, causing AMI or ventricular arrhythmias.

Vasodepressor or vasovagal syncope is a common, benign cause of transient LOC. Its def-inition requires either an emotional precipitant (typically fear, anger, or surprise), an unpleasant anatomical stimulus (venipuncture, examination of the throat, sigmoidoscopy, or sight of blood or body parts), or a typical setting (exhaustion or a hot or close environment). It usually occurs in young people, with a female predominance. The resulting bradycardia and vasodilation may pro-duce profound hypotension, and as with any cause of acute reduction of cerebral blood flow, brief seizure activity, with or without incontinence, may result. Once postural tone is lost, the victim collapses, resulting in improved cerebral flow and spontaneous recovery. Vasovagal or vasode-pressor syncope accounts for 4–58% of all episodes of syncope, depending on how strictly the criteria of precipitating phenomena are applied.

Seizures also cause transient LOC. Although distinguishing seizures from other causes of syncope is usually straightforward (Table 133-2), occasionally confusion may remain. TIA and stroke are often claimed to be the cause of syncope. However, for cerebrovascular disease to cause LOC, either both hemispheres or the brain stem must be suddenly deprived of blood flow. In a patient who has already suffered a massive hemispheric infarction, theoretically a new mas-sive infarction on the contralateral side may cause syncope; however, it is unlikely that transient, spontaneously resolving LOC would be the only result. Similarly, vertebrobasilar ischemia may cause syncope, but not in isolation. Other manifestations of brain stem dysfunction (e.g., diplopia, vertigo, or nausea) are required to make this rare diagnosis.

Neurologic causes of syncope (other than seizures) are exceedingly rare. Subarachnoid hemorrhage can be a frighteningly elusive diagnosis. It can produce syncope, presumably as a result of a sudden increase in intracranial pressure and a sudden, transient global decrease in cerebral metabolism. Headache or focal neurologic findings in the patient with syncope raises this possibility.

Other causes of syncope include postural hypotension, which is usually easily identified by history and physical examination. "Situational" syncope results from a number of mechanisms.

TABLE 133-2. Differentiation of Seizure From Other Causes of Syncope

	Seizure	Other Causes of Syncope
Prodrome	Usually absent	Common
Loss of Consciousness	Abrupt	Gradual (except in cardiac causes)
Injuries Resulting From Event	Common	Uncommon
Recovery	Gradual, postictal confusion common	Sudden
Focal Neurologic Signs	Common	Rare

Postmicturition syncope probably results from a combination of postural hypotension, Valsalva maneuver, and vasovagal stimulation. Cough syncope involves an increase in intrathoracic pressure, transient hypoxia, and vagal stimulation. In postprandial syncope splanchnic vasodilation is thought to produce systemic hypotension in some elderly patients. Hyperventilation-induced hypocapnea causes a decrease in cerebral blood flow; when it is followed by breath-holding and the Valsalva maneuver hypoxemia further contributes to LOC.

EMERGENCY DEPARTMENT EVALUATION

The cause of syncope is usually determined by history, physical examination and ECG. These alone can establish the diagnosis in 88% of cases. In addition, specific abnormalities led to the performance of other tests that established a diagnosis in another 5% of patients, resulting in a net yield of 93% from a directed ED evaluation. Head CT established a diagnosis only in patients with focal neurologic deficits. Cardiac catheterization and ECHO were useful only in patients with murmurs of aortic stenosis or hypertrophic cardiomyopathy. Blood studies identified no unsuspected causes for syncope (hypoglycemia was clinically suspected, electrolytes never accounted for the LOC, and anemia from bleeding was clinically obvious).

The history should focus on the events and sensations before, during, and after the syncopal episode. The presence, duration, and nature of warning symptoms, the patient's station, position, activity, and emotional state, and all symptoms noted during the event, the nature and timing of recovery, and past medical history should be elicited. The physical examination focuses on vital signs (including orthostatic changes) and a careful cardiovascular and neurologic evaluation. The ECG is analyzed for arrhythmias, conduction abnormalities, and signs of ischemia or infarction.

Several diagnoses require special mention. It has become common practice to consider AMI as an occult cause of otherwise unexplained syncope, and patients are frequently admitted to the hospital to "rule out myocardial infarction" when the ED workup is negative. There is little basis for this approach; there are no reports of AMI presenting solely with isolated syncope. The association of acute dyspnea or cardiovascular collapse and ECG changes with syncope is suggestive of AMI, particularly in the elderly. Syncope has been described as the initial symptom in aortic dissection, ruptured aortic aneurysm, pulmonary embolism, subarachnoid hemorrhage, and ruptured ectopic pregnancy.

Attributing syncope to transient arrhythmias is most problematic. Only a minority of cases in which tachyarrhythmias are eventually determined to be the cause of syncope are identified while the patient is in the ED. Ambulatory ECG monitoring, inpatient telemetry, or electrophysiologic studies (EPS) are often required to uncover these arrhythmias. Potentially causative arrhythmias occur in up to 64% of patients during prolonged monitoring, but establishing these as the cause of syncope requires that the two occur simultaneously; this is noted in only 2–3%.

Attributing syncope to an arrhythmic cause in an asymptomatic patient is controversial. Even malignant-appearing arrhythmias (VT) may occur in 2–4% of healthy, asymptomatic subjects. Similarly, profoundly slow ventricular rates may also be asymptomatic. Nevertheless, finding ventricular arrhythmias in patients with syncope identifies a group with an increased risk of sudden death and a higher mortality rate. For this reason, if arrhythmias are suspected, prolonged monitoring with cardiology follow-up is recommended.

Referral of the patient with unexplained syncope for EPS is even more controversial. Although abnormalities are found in 50%, these studies are performed in selected patients with increased risk for significant arrhythmias (prior AMI, CHF, valvular heart disease, or arrhythmias or conduction block). There is a reduction in recurrent syncope when treatment is directed toward arrhythmias noted during EPS, but a reduction in mortality or the incidence of sudden death has not yet been noted. Even when all potentially useful diagnostic tests are applied to all patients during an inpatient evaluation, a significantly large population will not have a cause of syncope identified.

EMERGENCY DEPARTMENT MANAGEMENT AND DISPOSITION

Understanding outcome in syncope helps the physician determine which high-risk patients might benefit from an inpatient evaluation. The Framingham Study found that patients with isolated syncope are no more likely to develop TIA, stroke, or AMI than patients without syncope. Furthermore, there was no increase in mortality, cardiovascular mortality, or sudden death associated with syncope. In contrast, syncope of cardiovascular cause is associated with a much worse prognosis, with an 18–33% mortality at 1 year. This compares with a mortality of 6–12% in syncope from other causes and a 0–12% mortality in patients in whom no cause was found. Most deaths in the cardiovascular group were sudden, whereas sudden death in the other two groups was rare.

It is convenient to divide patients with syncope into those with cardiovascular causes, those with noncardiovascular causes, and those with no cause established. The incidence of recurrent syncope (31–43% in 30 months) is similar in all three patient groups. Recurrences are not predictive of mortality or sudden death. "Major injury" (defined as fracture, subdural hematoma, or MVA) occurs with syncope in approximately 2.5% < age 60, but in 9.5% of those >60; major injury occurs with equal frequency in all etiologic groups.

Although it is not clear that appropriate management improves the outcome in subgroups with syncope, decisions regarding admission to the hospital should be based on the outcome data that are available. When a cardiovascular cause of syncope is established or suspected, the patient should be admitted to the hospital, usually to a monitored bed. Ventricular arrhythmias, bifascicular block, pacemaker malfunction, exertional syncope with an aortic outflow murmur, suspicion of aortic dissection, AMI, pulmonary embolism, or other possible cardiovascular catastrophes should prompt admission.

There are four predictors of increased mortality: (1) frequent or paired ventricular premature depolarizations on prolonged ECG monitoring; (2) the presence of CHF; (3) serum creatinine level >2.0; and (4) a sinus pause >2 seconds. These factors are consistent with the high mortality known to be associated with CHF, renal insufficiency, and other types of organic heart disease. Whether syncope adds to the independent mortality of these risk factors is unknown. Hospitalization for a noncardiovascular cause of syncope depends on the disease process. In syncope of unknown cause, it may be prudent to admit those with CHF or other types of organic heart disease, those with major injury as a result of syncope, and elderly patients who live alone. These groups account for a small minority of patients with syncope; the majority may be discharged home after follow-up is arranged.

COMMON PITFALLS

- Attribution of syncope to vasovagal or unknown cause because of failure to take a compulsively detailed history of the syncopal event.
- Attribution of syncope to incidentally found asymptomatic arrhythmia.
- Attribution of syncope to transient ischemic attack.
- Attribution of syncope to an associated finding when the causal relation is tenuous. Almost half of patients never have a cause determined, and these patients have a good prognosis.
- Failure to take seriously an aortic outflow murmur in a patient with syncope.
- Admission of patients with isolated syncope of unknown cause to the hospital to rule out AMI.
- Failure to recognize the following catastrophic scenarios—
  - Syncope with headache: subarachnoid hemorrhage
  - Syncope with chest pain: AMI, aortic dissection, pulmonary embolism, pulmonary hypertension
  - Syncope with exertion: aortic stenosis, hypertrophic cardiomyopathy
  - Syncope with abdominal pain: leaking aortic aneurysm, ruptured ectopic pregnancy.

134 Hypertensive Emergencies and Urgencies

Elevations of blood pressure may be grouped into hypertensive emergencies in which blood pressure (BP) must be lowered within hours, and hypertensive urgencies in which the BP can be lowered over a period of days. A true hypertensive emergency is a severe elevation in BP that represents a threat to life or vital organ function unless treatment is initiated immediately. Many patients with hypertension (HT) tolerate much higher levels chronically without acute end-organ damage. When the same severe elevation of BP occurs without any evidence of acute end-organ damage, the condition is called a hypertensive urgency. The diagnosis of hypertensive emergency should never be made solely on the basis of the BP measurement although most authors believe that the diastolic pressure must be >130 mm Hg. The patient's response to the BP and the immediate risk to the cardiovascular system are of major importance.

HYPERTENSIVE EMERGENCIES
CLINICAL PRESENTATION

Malignant HT is the prototype of the hypertensive emergency, seen in 2% with essential HT. It is more prevalent in young black men and those with underlying renal parenchymal or renovascular disease. The diagnosis is usually based on marked elevation of the BP and characteristic eye ground changes (papilledema is considered by most to be the *sine qua non* of the diagnosis). Flame-shaped hemorrhages occur around the optic disk due to the high intravascular pressure; "soft" exudates are due to ischemic infarction of the nerve fibers secondary to occlusion of supplying arterioles. Increased arteriolar light reflex, AV nicking, arteriolar tortuosity, and hard exudates are all chronic changes and cannot be used to establish the diagnosis of malignant HT. Commonly noted symptoms are headache (85%), visual blurring (55%), nocturia (38%), weakness (30%), and weight loss (25%).

Laboratory studies show progressive azotemia, proteinuria, microscopic or gross hematuria and cylindruria; microangiopathic hemolytic anemia, thrombocytopenia, and increased fibrin degradation products are also seen. Hypokalemia and metabolic alkalosis result from stimulation of the renin–angiotensin system. Untreated, malignant HT carries a 90% 1-year mortality, usually from uremia, cerebrovascular accident (CVA), or congestive heart failure. With treatment, 1-year survival is decreased to 85%.

HYPERTENSIVE ENCEPHALOPATHY
The most serious manifestation of acute severe HT is hypertensive encephalopathy, characterized by significant alteration in cerebral function that improves with lowering of the blood pressure. Patients complain of headache, nausea, vomiting, confusion, and blurred vision. On physical examination there is a marked elevation of BP (>130 mm Hg diastolic), altered mental status, and commonly papilledema. Focal neurologic deficits are sometimes noted, as are seizures. The differential diagnosis is vast, but no other condition resolves with lowering of the blood pressure.

Other possibilities must be differentiated from hypertensive encephalopathy. Cerebral infarction usually has a more rapid onset (minutes to hours); the headache is normally mild, and neurologic deficits are fixed. Cerebral embolism has a sudden onset, and usually causes minimal or no headache or mental status change. With intracerebral or subarachnoid hemorrhage, neurologic deficit or alteration of consciousness is also of rapid onset; sudden severe headache is also characteristic, particularly of subarachnoid hemorrhage. A head CT must be done immediately while other supportive measures are being initiated. Lowering the blood pressure is the key to management of hypertensive encephalopathy, but if it is lowered too rapidly, hypoperfusion may result. A rough guideline is that the diastolic BP be lowered only 20–30% during the first 24 hours, with close attention to the mental status. Drugs of choice include nitroprusside and labetalol. Avoid drugs with sedative effects (clonidine, methyldopa).

HYPERTENSION WITH CEREBROVASCULAR ACCIDENTS
With HT and CVA, the major concern is to avoid hypoperfusion. For a chronically hypertensive person, the mean arterial BP (MAP) necessary for maintaining cerebral blood flow is higher than normal (i.e., MAP of 120–160 mm Hg may be necessary rather than the 60 mm to 120 mm Hg in normal persons). If the BP is lowered below the lower limit of autoregulation, cerebral blood flow will fall, leading to further neurologic damage. HT is also a risk factor for intracranial hemorrhage, most often in the putamen, thalamus, pons, or cerebellum. As with thrombotic strokes, cautious lowering of the BP with a short-acting, titratable agent such as nitroprusside or labetalol is advisable. A reasonable target is a diastolic BP of 100–110 mm Hg.

AORTIC DISSECTION
Aortic dissection occurs when there is a sudden tear in the aortic intima and a dissecting hematoma propagates in the aortic media. More than 90% of patients are hypertensive even if they are not hypertensive on presentation. Therapy consists of stabilization and control of hypertension. The goal is to lower the BP to a systolic of 100–120 mm Hg over a few hours. Drugs of choice include nitroprusside (in conjunction with a beta blocker), and labetalol. Diaxozide and hydralazine should be avoided.

ISCHEMIC HEART DISEASE AND MYOCARDIAL INFARCTION
In patients with severe coronary artery disease, HT increases resistance to left ventricular emptying, leading to increased ventricular wall tension and increased myocardial oxygen demand. Excessive BP reduction should be avoided so as not to compromise coronary artery perfusion. To control ischemic pain, the usual antianginal drugs should be tried first, since they are often effective in treating the HT as well. IV nitroglycerin is an excellent agent; IV nitroprusside and propranolol are reasonable alternatives. Diaxozide and hydralazine cause reflex tachycardia and should be avoided.

ACUTE LEFT VENTRICULAR FAILURE
Untreated HT can lead to acute CHF. Therapy for pulmonary edema with HT is to treat the pulmonary edema in the usual manner; if HT persists, nitroprusside and nitroglycerin are the drugs of choice.

CATECHOLAMINE EXCESS
HT from catecholamine excess occurs with pheochromocytoma, in patients on monoamine oxidase (MAO) inhibitors who eat tyramine-containing foods or ingest sympathomimetic drugs, and in patients who are withdrawing from certain antihypertensives.
Hypertension in pregnancy is covered elsewhere.

HYPERTENSIVE URGENCIES
CLINICAL PRESENTATION

A common problem is the chronic hypertensive who has come to the ED for an unrelated reason and is found to have a significant but asymptomatic elevation of the BP. The physical examination may reveal signs of chronic HT but no evidence of acute end-organ damage in the cardiovascular, neurologic, and renal systems. On funduscopic examination there may be evidence of retinopathy, but there are no acute changes of papilledema or flame hemorrhages. It is controversial whether acute reduction of BP should occur in the ED; some authorities recommend that a diastolic BP >120–130 mm Hg be decreased to 105–110 mm Hg. Oral medications are usually sufficient for this purpose. The patient should be followed up in 2 to 3 days in order to continue chronic BP management.

RENAL DISEASE AND RENAL TRANSPLANTS
Eighty percent to 90% of patients with significant renal disease develop HT at some point with HT accelerating the deterioration of the underlying renal disease. Moderate to severe HT is also seen in patients with renal transplants, and if it persists, it can damage the small vessels of the transplanted kidney. HT may also occur during allograft rejection or with stenosis of the vascular anastomosis. The corticosteroids given to these patients for immunosuppression may also aggravate the HT.

EMERGENCY DEPARTMENT MANAGEMENT: HYPERTENSIVE EMERGENCIES

The goal of therapy in hypertensive emergencies is to control the blood pressure to a level that will prevent end-organ damage. It is important not to lower the blood pressure too quickly or to levels that produce cerebral or myocardial ischemia, especially in patients with atherosclerosis. If the patient has been hypertensive and poorly controlled for years, the cerebral autoregulation curve may be shifted, and rapid reduction of BP may not be well tolerated. A safe goal is to bring the diastolic BP to 100–110 mm Hg over a period of hours, with the higher level being more appropriate in atherosclerotic or elderly patients. The patient should be closely monitored for symptoms of cerebral or coronary insufficiency.

      True hypertensive emergencies require parenteral therapy, ideally given in an ICU with cardiac and BP monitoring. Diuretics should be avoided unless necessary to treat fluid overload. IV furosemide is a relatively ineffective antihypertensive when used alone; moreover, patients with malignant HT may be volume-contracted and may deteriorate when given diuretics. In addition, diuretics can cause hypotension, especially in the presence of vasodilating drugs. The agents most commonly used in hypertensive emergencies are either direct vasodilators (e.g., nitroprusside, nitroglycerin) or inhibitors of the sympathetic or adrenergic system (e.g., labetalol, phenotalamine, and trimethaphan camsylate). Table 134-1 provides a guide to the pharmacologic management of hypertensive emergencies as well as hypertensive urgencies.

      The agent chosen depends on the clinical situation, the availability of monitoring, and the

TABLE 134-1. Pharmacologic Management of Hypertensive Emergencies and Urgencies

Problem	Drug	Dose/Route	Pitfalls
Emergencies			
Malignant hypertension	Nitroprusside	0.2–0.5 µg/kg/min up to 8 µg/kg/min IV	Papilledema, flame hemorrhages, soft exudates must be present for diagnosis
	Diaxozide	75–150 mg Q 5 min IV or 15 mg/min IV infusion	
	Labetalol	20–80 mg Q 10 min IV or 2 mg/min IV drip	
Hypertensive encephalopathy	Nitroprusside	As above	Avoid Aldomet; exclude intracranial process
	Diaxozide	As above	
	Labetalol	As above	
	Trimethapan camsylate	1–15 mg/min	
Hypertension and CVA	Nitroprusside	As above	Lower diastolic only 20%–30% initially
	Labetalol	As above	
Aortic dissection	Nitroprusside + propranolol	As above	Avoid diaxozide and hydralazine
	Trimethaphan camsylate	As above	
	Labetalol	As above	
Myocardial infarction ischemia	Nitroglycerin	5–200 µg/min IV	Avoid diaxozide and hydralazine
	Propranolol	1–2 mg Q 15 min	
	Nitroprusside	As above	
Acute left ventricular failure	Morphine	2–5 mg IV	Treat fluid overload before hypertension
	Furosemide	20–80 mg IV	
	Nitroglycerin	As above	
	Nitroprusside	As above	
Eclampsia	Magnesium sulfate	4–6 g IV	Avoid diaxozide and trimethaphan
	Hydralazine	5–20 mg IV/M Q 6 hr	
Pheochromocytoma/MAO inhibitor	Phentolamine	5–10 mg IV	Use alpha blocker prior to beta blocker
	Phenoxybenzamine	5–10 mg PO	

(cont'd.)

TABLE 134-1. *(Cont'd.)*

Problem	Drug	Dose/Route	Pitfalls
Urgencies			
Elevated/accelerated	Nifedipine	10–20 mg SL or bite and swallow	Avoid rapid lowering
	Clonidine	0.1–0.2 mg PO then 0.1 mg Q 1 hr to 0.8 mg	
	Labetalol	200–400 mg PO	Avoid captopril and enalopril in renal artery stenosis
	Captopril	25–50 mg PO	
	Enalopril	5–20 mg PO	
Renal disease	Nifedipine	As above	
	Clonidine	As above	
	Labetalol	As above	
Perioperative	Nitroprusside	As above	Postpone nonemergent surgery
	Labetalol	As above	
Body burns	Nitroprusside	As above	Treat pain first
	Diaxozide	As above	
	Labetalol	As above	
	Nifedipine	As above	
	Clonidine	As above	
Quadriplegia	Nitroprusside	As above	Limit excessive tactile stimulation
	Diaxozide	As above	
	Labetalol	As above	
	Nifedipine	As above	
	Clonidine	As above	

physician's familiarity and experience with the drugs available. Nitroprusside is the drug of choice in many hypertensive emergencies, including malignant HT, hypertensive encephalopathy, aortic dissection (combined with a beta blocker), and hypertension-precipitating pulmonary edema or ischemic heart disease. Nitroprusside is a direct arteriovenous vasodilator that decreases both preload and afterload. Its onset of action is 1 to 2 minutes and the effect lasts for only 2 to 5 minutes after the drug is discontinued. It is given as an IV infusion starting with 0.2 µg to 0.5 µg/kg/min and increasing every 5 minutes to a maximum of 8 µg/kg/min or until the desired effect is achieved.

Monitoring of the BP and pulse should prevent inadvertent hypotension. There is no tachyphylaxis, but thiocyanate toxicity may occur if the drug is used over a period of days. Nitroprusside is light-sensitive, so bottles and tubing must be kept covered. Because there is no oral form, the patient must be switched to another antihypertensive once control is achieved. Labetalol, a combined alpha and beta blocker, has been used in certain hypertensive emergencies as an alternative to nitroprusside. It can be given either IV or orally and has the advantage of not causing reflex tachycardia. Labetalol should not be used in patients with contraindications to beta blockade.

EMERGENCY DEPARTMENT MANAGEMENT: HYPERTENSIVE URGENCIES

Hypertensive urgencies do not represent a threat to life or vital organ function, and therefore do not require therapy that is as aggressive as that for hypertensive emergencies. The patient with a hypertensive urgency should be placed in a quiet room for 30 to 60 minutes. The blood pressure should then be rechecked to assure that hypertension is still present, since many people have labile BP. Causes of an elevated BP include stress, anxiety, pain, and drug withdrawal. If the BP remains elevated, it is reasonable to lower the diastolic BP to between 105 and 110 mm Hg. It can then be brought to normal over a period of days or weeks.

There are a number of oral antihypertensive agents, preferred because of ease of administration and the ability to send the patient home on the same medication. Clonidine is a centrally acting alpha agonist used to treat any hypertensive urgency, but it is particularly appropriate for use in the clonidine withdrawal syndrome. For acute BP control, 0.1 mg to 0.2 mg orally is given initially and then 0.1 mg every hour until BP is controlled or a total of 0.8 mg has been given. A typical required total dose is 0.45 mg, with an average time to control HT of 3 to 4 hours. The drug should be avoided in patients likely to be noncompliant to avoid rebound HT.

Nifedipine, a calcium channel blocker that decreases systemic vascular resistance, has been used in both hypertensive emergencies and urgencies. Better plasma levels are obtained by having the patient bite the capsule and then immediately swallow it. The average dose is 10 mg, with onset of action at 10 minutes. Patients treated with nifedipine acutely can be continued on oral nifedipine with reasonable control. It can cause precipitous hypotension, as well as headache and reflex tachycardia.

Labetalol can be given orally for less emergent lowering of the BP. Although it is rapidly absorbed, it suffers a first-pass phenomenon in the liver. The peak effect is at 2 hours and the maximal effect at 4 hours. The initial dose is between 200 and 400 mg, depending on the level of the diastolic BP. Angiotensin converting enzyme inhibitors are useful. Captopril is rapidly absorbed and has an onset of action of 30 minutes. The usual dose is 25 mg to 50 mg. The hypotensive response is usually not excessive unless the patient is volume depleted.

DISPOSITION

All true hypertensive emergencies require admission to an ICU or a monitored bed. Close BP monitoring is indicated. Patients with hypertensive encephalopathy or CVA may require neurologic consultation. Aortic dissection requires immediate medical and cardiothoracic consultation while

BP is controlled. Eclamptic patients require emergent obstetric consultation. Patients with hypertensive urgencies do not usually require hospital admission; the BP can be controlled over a period of days, but close medical follow-up is required.

COMMON PITFALLS

- The major pitfall is to diagnose an emergency when one does not exist. Many patients who present to the ED have BP elevations related to stress, anxiety, drug withdrawal, or pain. It is important to control the underlying process first and then to determine whether HT is still present.
- Most patients with hypertensive emergencies have underlying evidence of chronic HT with retinopathy and nephropathy. In diagnosing malignant HT one should see characteristic flame-shaped hemorrhages, soft exudates, and papilledema.
- A common error is to reduce the BP too quickly or to too low a level. In patients with chronic HT whose autoregulation curve has been reset, this can lead to cerebral or cardiac ischemia.
- In patients with CHF and HT, it is important to treat fluid overload first and to treat the underlying HT cautiously afterward, thus avoiding precipitous hypotension and reduced coronary blood flow.
- Pregnant patients with BP >140/90 mm Hg or with an increase in the BP of >30/15 mm Hg during pregnancy should be considered hypertensive and treated in conjunction with obstetrical care.
- Appropriate therapy should be instituted and the patient's cerebral and cardiac status closely followed as the pressure is lowered. Decreasing the BP to an absolute number in every patient, or attempting to normalize the BP completely in the ED may result in hypotension and serious sequelae of hypoperfusion.

PART III

Pulmonary Emergencies

135 Acute Respiratory Insufficiency

From a pragmatic viewpoint, the key aspects of emergency care can be targeted from the following questions:

1. Does the patient need ventilatory support (a certain number of manual or mechanical breaths to remove CO_2)?
2. Does the patient need oxygenation support (hemorrhage control or transfusion, supplemental O_2, positive-pressure lung inflations, or even positive end-expiratory pressure), with or without circulatory support?
3. What are the potential complications of interventions (e.g., barotrauma and circulatory compromise)?

Although oxygenation and ventilation are undeniably intertwined, a critically ill or injured patient should be approached by specifically distinguishing between the need for ventilatory support and that for oxygenation support (OS). Some patients may require mechanical ventilatory support for one and not the other. In summary, respiratory support involves the preservation of adequate Hgb levels and adequate circulation, adequate lung inflation and O_2 supplementation, and appropriate clearance of CO_2.

Common reasons for inadequate ventilation are airway obstruction, high spinal cord injury, flail chest, and open pneumothorax (sucking chest wound). Underlying medical problems such as acute asthma or chronic lung disease can cause expiratory phase airflow obstruction and may also result in CO_2 retention, as may narcotic and other sedative drug overdoses, stroke, head injury, and neuromuscular disorders. Hemodynamic compromise (extreme blood loss, tension pneumothorax, and pericardial tamponade) may eventually result in ventilatory failure because of the resulting severe shock state.

OXYGENATION SUPPORT

In the absence of severe anemia or circulatory compromise, the need for tissue oxygenation support (OS) normally arises from pulmonary failure to oxygenate the bloodstream, usually when a critical number of the lung's gas exchange units fail to remain inflated. Although inadequate ventilation can lead to hypoxemia, the degree of hypoxemia usually is not great, and is readily reversible once ventilatory support or supplemental O_2 is administered. On the other hand, *hypoinflation* is more likely to result in serious hypoxemia (PaO_2 <60 mm Hg). This is a common mechanism of respiratory insufficiency in the critically ill or injured patient.

IDENTIFYING WHO NEEDS VENTILATORY AND OXYGENATION SUPPORT
In identifying which patients require ventilatory and oxygenation support, four considerations should be kept in mind: (1) Certain immediately life-threatening problems (e.g., airway obstruction, inadequate respirations or apnea, and open or tension pneumothorax) require urgent attention before other assessments. (2) Some urgent problems can be detected by repeated assessments (e.g., simple pneumothorax and flail chest). (3) The risk of late pulmonary complications (e.g., ARDS and pneumonia) can often be predicted by initial assessments. (4) Underlying conditions (e.g., asthma, COPD, heart failure, and overdose) must be promptly addressed.

DIFFERENTIAL DIAGNOSIS

See Table 135-1.
The chest radiograph is a critical tool in the evaluation of respiratory status. It usually reveals the source of any intrapulmonary shunt detected by ABG analysis (e.g., pulmonary edema, pneumonia, atelectasis, mainstem intubation, or pneumothorax). Aside from cardiac right-to-left shunts (congenital and traumatic), pulmonary emboli, and early hypoinflation, hypoxemia unresponsive to low levels of F_iO_2 (<0.3) usually can be identified by a chest radiograph. If not obvious on initial films, in most cases follow-up films show the source of infiltrate progression within a few hours. But while radiographic infiltrates are usually present in severe hypoxemia, the severity of hypoxemia does not necessarily correspond to the amount of infiltrate seen. The clinical picture, associated findings, ET secretions, ABG analyses, and response to positive-pressure ventilation can aid in delineating the causes of infiltrates.

EMERGENCY DEPARTMENT EVALUATION AND MANAGEMENT

ABG values are the immediate end-point of early respiratory support: the aim is to deliver the adV_E that will maintain normal blood pH (7.35–7.45) and to maintain adequate saturation of Hgb (preferably >97%) by maintaining adequate arterial O_2 tensions (PaO_2 >70 mm Hg). Acutely, pH rather than $PaCO_2$ should be the focus of ventilatory interventions; an abnormal $PaCO_2$ is not necessarily harmful except for its effect on pH and ICP. The usual normal range for $PaCO_2$ is 35-40 mm Hg, but in a patient in shock whose $PaCO_2$ is 38 mm Hg, the pH may be <7.10 due to lac-

---

TABLE 135-1. Differential Diagnosis of Acute Respiratory Problems

Cardiac Output Problems

Bleeding, myocardial ischemia, pericardial tamponade, tension pneumothorax, etc.

Pulmonary Problems

Airway obstruction (upper airway problems like anaphylaxis, foreign body, inflammation, infection, trauma)
Bronchial obstruction (asthma, bronchitis, COPD)
Congestive heart failure and other forms of pulmonary edema
Drug-induced (stimulants, *e.g.*, cocaine, vs. depressants, *e.g.*, narcotics)
Emboli (air, thrombi)
Fractures (with or without underlying contusions)
Gross hemoptysis (usually from bronchial circulation fed from the aorta)
Hemothorax and pneumothorax (spontaneous and traumatic)
Inhalation injuries (CO, toxic fumes, near-drowning, aspiration)
"Junky" lungs (pneumonia, cancer, empyema)
"Kompensation" for metabolic acidosis (shock, ketoacidosis, renal failure, toxins)
Lower (subdiaphragmatic) problems and restrictive breathing (tense ascites, pain, injury)
Muscle weakness (Ca^{++}, PO_4^-, K^+, Mg^{++}, myasthenia, dystrophies)
Neurologic impairment (spinal or central lesion, Guillain-Barré)

tic acid. In such cases the $PaCO_2$ should be temporarily lowered by increasing adV_E enough to return the pH toward normal.

In a patient who has received excess sodium bicarbonate (e.g., during cardiac resuscitation) or in a patient with chronic CO_2 retention, a high $PaCO_2$ should be left untreated as long as the pH is normal. Attempts to lower $PaCO_2$ acutely will raise the pH and increase the risk of life-threatening complications from alkalosis. Because misinterpretation of ABG values can have serious consequences, during the early hours after acute illness or injury, trends in PaO_2 (rather than a single result) should guide therapy. The variability of duplicate PaO_2 analysis can be as much as ±10%. If the sample is run within 10 or 15 minutes, air bubbles and failure to place the sample on ice are not significant problems.

Even without a specific indication, supplemental O_2 should be considered in all ill or injured patients, since it provides a small but possibly critical margin of tissue PO_2 in a patient with an unexpected setback (e.g., sudden airway obstruction, hemorrhage, and arrest). The basic modes of oxygen administration include nasal cannula, face mask, and ET tube. As discussed earlier, the use of ET intubation should be emphasized in critically ill and injured patients. In cases in which ET intubation or 100% inspired O_2 is not specifically indicated, low-flow O_2 (i.e., 2L/min) should be administered by nasal prongs in alert or semialert patients without obvious nasopharyngeal injury.

Patients who are short of breath often become apprehensive when their faces are covered by masks, and they tend to pull the masks off. A mask may also promote aspiration by the supine obtunded patient. Nasal cannulas can deliver up to 35% inspired O_2 at 6 L/min, a level that should suffice in most noncritical cases but may be inadequate if there is a significant intrapulmonary shunt (>15%). In cases in which a very high F_iO_2 is indicated but ET intubation cannot be readily performed, an oxygen mask should be considered along with available suction and close observation. A mask with an attached reservoir can supply nearly 100% inspired O_2 at high-flow rates. Assisted ventilation with bag–valve–mask, oral airways, and proper positioning is a mandatory adjunct to ET tube placement attempts.

136   Pneumonia

Pneumonia describes inflammatory processes within the lung parenchyma. Although pneumonia is most commonly thought of in terms of infectious causes, noninfectious causes may also result in inflammatory lung processes. It is the infectious causes of pneumonia that most commonly bring patients to the ED. Pneumonia remains the most common infection that results in death in the USA and ranks between the fourth and sixth most common disease causing death. Some patients may be immunocompromised, be elderly, or may have other, underlying diseases. Pneumonia may also affect otherwise healthy adults, respond readily to routine treatment, and resolve without long-term sequelae. The exact incidence of community-acquired pneumonia is difficult to determine, but it is estimated that 3.3 million cases occur annually in the USA.

Many pathogens are capable of infecting the lower respiratory tract. *Streptococcus pneumoniae* remains the most common organism for community-acquired pneumonia, accounting for an estimated 40–80% of all cases. In children and young adults *Mycoplasma pneumoniae* is the second most common cause of community-acquired pneumonia, accounting for approximately 15–20%. *H. influenzae* may result in community-acquired pneumonias in young children, but there is also a significant incidence among adults with COPD. The incidence of *Legionella pneumophila* and other *Legionella* species that cause pneumonia is variable; in some regions *Legionella* species may account for 15% of pneumonias. *S. aureus* and gram-negative aerobic rods account for 1–25% of community-acquired pneumonias, depending on the population studied. *S. aureus* pneumonia most commonly occurs as a secondary bacterial invader in patients with influenza; it is also commonly seen as a lower respiratory tract pathogen in patients with cystic fibrosis.

DIFFERENTIAL DIAGNOSIS AND EMERGENCY DEPARTMENT EVALUATION

Pneumonia may be divided into two broad categories. The typical bacterial-like syndrome includes fever, productive cough, and a localized infiltrate on chest radiograph. The atypical pneumonia syndrome refers to a different presentation dominated by constitutional complaints. The typical organism responsible for the bacterial-like syndrome is *S. pneumoniae*. Pneumonias caused by *S. aureus*, other streptococcal species, *H. influenzae, Klebsiella pneumoniae,* the Enterobacteriaceae, and other gram-negative aerobic rods result in a bacterial-like pneumonia syndrome.

M. *pneumoniae* is the prototypic organism causing the atypical pneumonia syndrome. Pneumonias caused by viral agents, *Rickettsia,* and *Chlamydia* also result in the atypical pneumonia syndrome. Legionnaires' disease (gram-negative rod, *L. pneumophila)* results in features of both the bacterial-like syndrome and atypical pneumonia syndrome.

Pulmonary infections caused by fungi and tuberculosis are not considered under these two broad categories; their presentations are different. Distinguishing pneumonia from other causes of fever and chills is accomplished by the chest radiograph. The difficulty in diagnosis arises in distinguishing various potential causative agents. In addition, underlying lung pathology must be excluded in patients with parenchymal infiltrates: pulmonary neoplasms, pulmonary embolus with infarction, and tuberculosis all merit consideration. COPD should be considered with frequent pulmonary infections.

THE BACTERIAL-LIKE PNEUMONIA SYNDROME
Patients with the classic bacterial-like pneumonia syndrome present with the abrupt onset of fever and chills associated with pleuritic chest pain and a cough productive of a mucopurulent sputum. Prodromal complaints are not a prominent feature. A detailed travel, social, occupational, and past medical history are important in discerning the causative agent. Patients with a recent history of viral influenza most typically have *S. pneumoniae* as the cause, but the incidence of *S. aureus* pneumonia is also markedly increased after influenza infection. Patients with COPD have a greater incidence of pneumonia caused by *H. influenzae* and *Branhamella catarrhalis.* Intravenous drug abusers are at a greater risk for infection caused by *S. aureus*. Alcoholics are at particular risk for aspiration and infection caused by anaerobic bacteria; alcoholics also have a greater incidence of pneumonia caused by *Klebsiella*. HIV positive patients or those with known risk factors of AIDS are at a marked risk for pneumonia caused by *Pneumocystis carinii,* although this pneumonia typically presents in a more insidious manner.

On physical examination there is typically fever, tachypnea, and tachycardia. Auscultation may reveal evidence of consolidation: rales, decreased breath sounds, inspiratory rhonchi, decreased vocal fremitus, and increased tactile fremitus. Leukocytosis is the most common laboratory abnormality; elevated white blood cell count with immature (band) forms also occurs. Patients with overwhelming infection, however, may exhibit leukopenia. Electrolytes, liver and kidney function tests are typically normal unless complicated by overwhelming sepsis. ABG analysis typically reveals hypoxemia with a respiratory alkalosis.

The diagnosis is confirmed by the presence of an infiltrate on the chest radiograph. The radiographic pattern is not useful in determining the cause of pneumonia; it is inaccurate in distinguishing bacterial from viral disease, as well as differentiating among the different bacterial agents. A lobar consolidation or bronchopneumonia pattern is commonly seen on the radiograph. Bulging of the major fissure is classically associated with *Klebsiella* pneumonia, but it may also be seen in pneumonia caused by *S. pneumoniae* or *H. influenzae* and in plague pneumonia.

Examination of expectorated sputum is of diagnostic importance, but one must be certain that the specimen represents organisms from the lower respiratory tract. A sputum specimen is considered adequate if there are abundant polymorphonuclear cells (>25/hpf), alveolar macrophages, and <10 squamous epithelial cells/hpf. A single dominant organism on the sputum Gram's stain strongly suggests that the sample is representative of lower respiratory tract flora. Certain organisms produce a sputum with particular characteristics. Anaerobic bacteria produce a putrid, foul-smelling sputum while the sputum of pneumococcal pneumonia is rust-colored. Dark red mucopurulent sputum (currant jelly) is noted in *Klebsiella* infections. Gram's stain of the sputum is helpful in determining antimicrobial therapy because it may reveal a predominant organism.

STREPTOCOCCUS PNEUMONIAE　The pneumococcus is the most common bacterial pathogen causing pneumonia and the most common cause of community-acquired pneumonia. At risk are patients with cardiopulmonary disease, diabetes, alcoholism, malignancies, and immunocompromising diseases. Recent influenza infection may also be complicated by pneumococcal pneumonia. About 25% of patients have a preceding URI. Symptoms begin abruptly with the onset of shaking chills or a single rigor, followed by fever and the productive cough. Pleuritic pain is common. Nausea, vomiting, headache and other constitutional complaints may be present. Bacteremia occurs in 25–33% of cases. The typical radiograph is one of lobar consolidation; most often a single lobe is involved although up to 25% of patients may have two lobes involved. Pleural effusions are not uncommon. Patients with a prior history of splenectomy or sickle cell anemia are at risk for overwhelming pneumococcal sepsis.

HAEMOPHILUS INFLUENZAE　H. influenzae, a small Gram-negative rod, is a major pathogen in children 3 months–3 years, but adults with COPD, alcoholism and debilitation are also at increased risk. Patchy alveolar infiltrates are typical on chest radiograph; however, lobar consolidation also may be seen.

STAPHYLOCOCCUS AUREUS　The clinical presentation of *S. aureus* pneumonia does not distinguish it from other causes of pneumonia. Typically a lobar or lobular consolidation is seen, and 25% of patients develop cavitation. Those with pneumonia via a hematogenous route (e.g., IVDAs) develop multiple pulmonary infiltrates. Within a few days some may cavitate.

KLEBSIELLA PNEUMONIAE　Although comprising <1% of all bacterial pneumonias, pneumonia caused by *K. pneumoniae* is more common in debilitated patients, diabetics, alcoholics, and patients with COPD; it occurs after aspiration of oropharyngeal secretions. Bacteremia occurs in 66%.

OTHER GRAM-NEGATIVE PNEUMONIAS　Gram-negative bacillary pneumonia is a major cause of death among immunocompromised hosts. Before the antimicrobial era gram-negative organisms accounted for a small minority of all pneumonia. *Klebsiella, Escherichia coli*, and *Pseudomonas aeruginosa* are the most frequent gram-negative bacillary pneumonias in immunocompromised hosts. They now account for an increased number of community-acquired pneumonias. Patients in nursing homes and other extended-care facilities suffer infection patterns with organisms similar to those acquired in the hospital environment. Up to 33% present in septic shock with other organ system disease commonly found.

LEGIONNAIRES' DISEASE

Pneumonia caused by *L. pneumophila* may occur at any age, but is most common in the sixth decade of life. About 66% of patients are cigarette smokers or have underlying cardiopulmonary disease. Immunosuppressed patients are at particularly high risk. Legionnaires' disease presents as an acute pneumonic disease with multisystem involvement. Features typical of both the bacteria-like pneumonia syndrome and the atypical pneumonia syndrome may be present. Constitutional complaints and gastrointestinal complaints are common.

Patients become progressively ill over a 2–3-day period. Malaise, anorexia, fatigue, and cough are often present early. Fever increases and shaking chills are common. Sputum is typically nonpurulent, but 33% have hemoptysis. Dyspnea and pleuritic chest pain also occur; 50% complain of watery, nonbloody diarrhea, as well as nausea and vomiting. Headache is quite common and changes in mental status, confusion, lethargy, and coma are seen. Sputum reveals a nonpurulent watery specimen with leukocytes on Gram's stain. Often a predominant organism is lacking. Chest radiographs show lobar, segmental, or patchy consolidation, and radiographic progression. Diagnosis can be made rapidly by direct fluorescent antibody examination of the sputum but the test has serious limitations.

THE ATYPICAL PNEUMONIA SYNDROME
The patient with atypical pneumonia syndrome has prominent constitutional complaints: fever, headache, malaise, myalgia, and a nonproductive cough. Physical findings are lacking, but fine rales or rhonchi may be heard. Radiography usually demonstrates an interstitial process rather than consolidation. White cell counts are only modestly elevated. Sputum analysis fails to reveal a predominant organism, and attempts at isolating a bacterial cause are unsuccessful. The most common causes of the atypical pneumonia syndrome are *M. pneumoniae* and viral etiologies.

MYCOPLASMAL PNEUMONIA
M. pneumoniae is a common cause of pneumonia in children and young adults, and accounts for 10–50% of all community-acquired pneumonias. Transmission occurs from respiratory droplets. Outbreaks among people living in close quarters are well documented. Fever, headache, and malaise precede the onset of pulmonary complaints by 2–4 days. The cough is nonproductive and hacking, although scant watery or even purulent sputum may be produced. Pleuritic chest pain is common. Sore throat and ear pain may be noted, and nausea, vomiting, diarrhea, rash, and confusion are not uncommon, but patients do not appear toxic.

Rales, rhonchi, or wheezing is usually noted. but consolidation is rare. Rash is common, especially in younger patients; macular, papular, petechial, and urticarial rashes have been described, as well as the vesicobullous lesions of erythema multiforme (Stevens–Johnson syndrome). Extrapulmonary manifestations may include aseptic meningitis, ascending paralysis, splenomegaly, pericarditis, and myocarditis. Chest radiography reveals a unilateral, segmental bronchopneumonia with lower lobe involvement in 75–90% of patients. Bilateral disease may occur in 40%. Routine lab studies are nondiagnostic, and WBC is normal or modestly elevated. Diagnosis can be confirmed by a fourfold increase in antibody titers in acute and convalescent sera. New culture techniques have been developed to diagnose *M. pneumonia* from sputum.

VIRAL PNEUMONIA
Influenza virus, adenovirus, and respiratory syncytial virus account for the majority of viral pneumonias. However, herpes viruses (varicella zoster, herpes simplex, and cytomegalic virus) and measles virus may also cause pneumonia. Coryza, sore throat, mild-moderate fever, malaise, and diffuse myalgia, as well as headache and photophobia, are common in viral pneumonia and typically precede respiratory tract complaints. Nonproductive cough becomes prominent later; dyspnea and wheezing may develop. Physical findings are scarce. Rash, pharyngitis, conjunctivitis, and inflammation of the nasal mucosa may be noted. Laboratory studies are nondiagnostic; leukocytosis may or may not be present. Sputum Gram's stain may reveal a few neutrophils but no predominant organism. Chest radiography reveals a reticulonodular interstitial pattern, often with multilobe involvement and hilar adenopathy.

EMERGENCY DEPARTMENT MANAGEMENT AND DISPOSITION

Appropriate management is determined not only by the severity of the illness, but also by the patient's underlying health status. Most patients benefit from supplemental oxygen and bronchodilators. Severely ill patients may require either high-flow oxygen by mask or endotracheal intubation. Volume depletion or septic shock require aggressive fluid resuscitation or vasopressor therapy.

Admission is indicated for the elderly and patients with multilobe disease, very high or very low WBC counts, underlying cardiopulmonary disease or other serious disease, hypoxia, or respiratory distress. Antibiotic therapy should be initiated in the ED. Young, otherwise healthy patients with pneumococcal or mycoplasmal disease may be managed as outpatients.

Antibiotic selection is governed by the following goals: (a) the regimen should treat the most likely causative agents; (b) the regimen should not fail to cover potentially dangerous likely pathogens; and (c) the regimen should be as selective as possible in order to avoid complications of drug toxicity, superinfection, and excessive cost.

Patients who present with a typical bacterial pneumonia and candidates for outpatient therapy should be treated with a penicillin; penicillin-allergic patients should receive erythromycin. Oral first-generation cephalosporins should not be routinely used, since they are less active than penicillin against *S. pneumoniae* and are significantly more expensive than penicillin.

Cigarette smokers and patients with COPD are frequently colonized by *H. influenzae* and *B. catarrhalis*. Although ampicillin and amoxicillin are frequently used for these patients, 10–40% of *H. influenzae* and up to 75% of *B. catarrhalis* are resistant to these agents. Alternative outpatient regimens include amoxicillin-clavulanic acid, cefaclor, trimethoprim-sulfamethoxazole, and ciprofloxacin.

Otherwise healthy young adults with atypical pneumonia syndrome should be treated with erythromycin, which provides adequate coverage for *M. pneumoniae* and *S. pneumoniae*, in addition to adding coverage against *L. pneumophila*. Tetracycline and doxycycline may be used as alternatives to erythromycin.

Antibiotic regimens for patients who require hospitalization are summarized in Table 136-1. Penicillins remain the drugs of choice in community-acquired pneumonia. Patients who are at risk for gram-negative infections may be treated with ureidopenicillins to provide coverage against aerobic gram-negative, gram-positive, and anaerobic organisms, as well as *P. aeruginosa*. Ticarcillin plus clavulanic acid and ampicillin plus sulbactam have activity against β-lactamase-producing strains of *H. influenzae*, *S. aureus*, *Bacteroides* sp., *Klebsiella*, and *E. coli*.

Cephalosporins also have been used extensively for community-acquired pneumonia but first-generation cephalosporins provide little advantage over penicillin. The second-generation cephalosporins (cefamandole, cefoxitin, cefonocid, cefuroxime, and cefotetan) are more active against gram-negative aerobic organisms. Cefamandole and cefuroxime are active against β-lactamase-producing strains of *H. influenzae*; cefoxitin has particular application in the treatment of anaerobic pulmonary infections. Ceftazidime is unique in its potent activity against *P. aeruginosa*. Recently, many authorities have suggested that azithromycin 500 mg PO day 1 (250 mg PO qd x 2–5 d) should be used for healthy (< age 60) adults with community-acquired pneumonia.

Patients with suspected aspiration pneumonia should be treated with penicillins combined with β-lactamase inhibitors. Clindamycin and cefoxitin are useful in the management of anaerobic lung disease.

COMMON PITFALLS

- The diagnosis of pneumonia is not usually difficult; however, failure to consider other serious causes of pulmonary infiltrates (e.g., foreign body aspiration, bronchiectasis, or tumor) can result in delays in diagnosis.
- Determination of appropriate antibiotics requires understanding risk factors and epidemiologic patterns for each pathogen.
- Failing to recognize patients who require hospitalization: very young patients, very old patients, and patients with multilobe involvement, leukopenia, leukemoid reaction, hypoxia, or an underlying immunocompromised state.

TABLE 136-1. Intravenous Antibiotics for Pneumonia

Clinical Setting	Antibiotic Regimens	Comments
Community-acquired, no underlying disease; suspect bacterial cause	Penicillin G Erythromycin or cefazolin	S. pneumoniae most probable pathogen
Community-acquired, normal host; atypical pneumonia	Erythromycin Tetracycline (doxycycline)	Covers S. pneumoniae, M. pneumoniae, and L. pneumophila Additional coverage for less common atypical pneumonia pathogens (Q fever, psittacosis)
Community-acquired, elderly patient or COPD; bacterial syndrome	Second-generation cephalosporin (cefonocid, cefamandol, cefoxitin) Ampicillin and aminoglycoside Ampicillin + sulbactam	Cefamandole provides good H. influenzae coverage Active against Haemophilus, E. coli, Klebsiella, and Bacteroides sp producing β-lactamases
Community-acquired, aspiration	Penicillin Clindamycin Cefoxitin Ureidopenicillins	All have excellent anaerobic activity
Community acquired, high risk for gram-negative bacillary pneumonia	Third-generation cephalosporin (ceftriaxone or cefotaxime) Cefazoline + aminoglycoside Ampicillin + aminoglycoside Aztreonam + clindamycin Imipenem/cilastatin	Good penetration into lung tissue; cefoperazone and ceftazidime have superior P. aeruginosa coverage Limited anaerobic coverage Need to maintain therapeutic aminoglycoside levels Aztreonam has excellent activity against gram-negative aerobes; no anaerobic activity Excellent broad-range aerobic and anaerobic, gram-positive and gram-negative coverage; reserve only for patients with suspected multiply resistant organisms

137   Mycobacterial Illness

In 1986, the first reported increase of human tuberculosis occurred; the reasons are several, and their impact may be only beginning to be felt. They include the acquired immunodeficiency syndrome (AIDS) epidemic, immigration of Third World populations to the United States, growing antimicrobial resistance patterns among native mycobacterial strains, and the latent reservoir of still undetected infection, with a predictable rate of reactivation, in middle and elder populations. Nontuberculous mycobacteria are also gaining recognition as causative agents in several forms of pulmonary and systemic illness with and without AIDS.

The physical findings of TB are varied and include manifestations of wasting illness; fever; occasionally chest findings, enlarged lymph nodes, liver and spleen, and cold abscesses; and painful or destructive lesions in such varied organs as skin, bone, and central nervous system (Table 137-1). In immunosuppressed patients, who often exhibit only fever and weight loss and have negative tuberculin tests, there may commonly be intense mycobacterial involvement, which can be demonstrated by strongly positive smears and cultures from tissue (liver or lymph nodes), stool, urine, or even blood. Pulmonary lesions may be strikingly absent, while constitutional and localized manifestations can be particularly prominent.

Distinguishing mycobacterial infection from other opportunistic infections, or from HIV infection itself, may prove quite difficult. It is important to make the diagnostic effort, however, since identification of the potentially communicable agent, M. tuberculosis var. hominis, has important public health implications. Nontuberculous myocobacteria have not been shown to have person-to-person infectivity and are quite difficult to treat and eradicate both because of antimicrobial resistance patterns and because infection may occur very late in the course of AIDS. These agents have, however, been detected in about 25% of HIV-infected patients preterminally, and may be demonstrable in as many as 50% at necropsy.

It is hoped that most new cases of TB will be identified by screening of high-risk groups (Table 137-2). About 90% of new cases of active TB each year may represent reactivation of remote infection, rather than fresh infection. Identification requires incubation of specimens for many weeks. They include M. tuberculosis var. hominis and var. bovis, and the nontuberculous mycobacteria. Of the latter, M. avium-intracellulare, often referred to as MAI or the Mycobacterium avium complex (MAC), is the most important. Before the advent of AIDS this agent was known to produce pulmonary disease in older white men, frequently in the presence of COPD. It was and is the second most commonly isolated mycobacterium in the US.

TABLE 137-1. Signs and Symptoms of Mycobacterial Disease

Pulmonary	Constitutional	Localized (Nonpulmonary)
Cough	Fatigue	Mass ("cold abscess")
Sputum production	Fever	Pain
Hemoptysis	Weight loss	Lymphadenopathy
Chest Pain	Anorexia	Organ dysfunction/derangement
Dyspnea	Night sweats	CNS (meningitis or tuberculoma)
		Pericardium
		Bowel/bladder
		Hepatic

TABLE 137-2. Risk Factors for Mycobacterial Disease

Ethnic and Demographic Risk Factors	Individual Risk Factors
Health care providers	Childhood/adolescence/senescence
Urban residents	Peripartum status
Poor socioeconomic status	Postgastrectomy
Nursing home inhabitants	Diabetes/uremia
Prison inmates	Lymphoma
"Recruits"*	Sarcoidosis
Immigrants from Third World	Steroid therapy
countries	Anthracosilicosis
Immunosuppressive therapy or	Substance abuse—alcohol/
illness, congenital or	intravenous drug usage
acquired	Immunosuppressive therapy or illness,
	congenital or acquired

*Susceptible young adults gathered for living in crowded conditions, such as military service, and recreational or work camps.

A tuberculin skin test with >15 mm of induration at 48 hours is almost invariably due to *M. tuberculosis.* Tests showing 5–15 mm of induration are consistent with mycobacterial illness, either TB or nontuberculous; those with <5 mm induration are usually considered negative, but the false-negative rate may approach 20%. Tuberculin testing has been a mainstay of screening and detection efforts for many years, but it is often unreliable in overwhelming infections in a normal host or in immunosuppressive therapy or illness. Detection is most successful if all forms of screening and testing are used liberally, including skin testing, radiography, and smear and cultural methods.

Radiographically, primary TB is characterized by involvement of the lower lobes, lymphadenopathy (either hilar or mediastinal), and occasionally by pleural effusion, but seldom is cavitation seen. In the normal host postprimary TB occurs in the lung with exudative (effusion), fibronodular, cavitary, pneumonic, or miliary. When localized, the disease is typically in the upper lobe or in the superior segments of the lower lobes. The morphology of TB is greatly modified in AIDS. TB and nontuberculous mycobacterial illness in the immunodeficient host seldom cavitates, may exhibit little beyond lymphadenopathy on chest radiograph, and frequently shows no chest radiographic abnormality whatsoever.

Mycobacteria must be sought not only from sputum and tissue specimens, but also from blood, urine, stool, and cerebrospinal fluid. Useful tissue sites are lymph nodes, bowel, bone marrow, and liver. Cultures are ten times more sensitive than smears, but are slower by 2 to 6 weeks; unfortunately this time may be critical in determining outcome. If the clinical situation warrants it, initiate empiric therapy while awaiting the outcome of cultures.

Treatment of mycobacterial illness is under continuous review; current recommendations are published by the Centers for Disease Control. All new cases of mycobacterial illness should start on therapy. If the infecting organism eventually proves to be *M. tuberculosis* var. *hominis*, short (6–9 months), intensive regimens are usually effective in the normal host, with a high prospect of sterilization and cure (Table 137-3). Treatment is hindered by noncompliance and antimicrobial resistance, so it is best directed through a public health center, an infectious disease clinic, or by a pulmonologist. In the immunosuppressed host less information is available as to the duration of therapy and potential for cure of TB.

In addition to controlling the infection, prevention of spread to susceptible contacts should be a priority. In the normal host a combination of multiple-drug therapy has achieved moderate

TABLE 137-3. Chemotherapy for Adults With Pulmonary Tuberculosis

Drugs	Doses	Duration of Treatment
Two-Drug Regimen		
Daily		
Isoniazid	5 mg/kg, maximum 300 mg	Both drugs given daily for 9 mo
Rifampin	10 mg/kg, maximum 600 mg	
Twice Weekly		
Isoniazid	15 mg/kg, maximum 900 mg	Twice weekly administration may
Rifampin	10 mg/kg, maximum 600 mg	begin after an initial 1 to 2 mo of
Three-Drug Regimen		daily therapy; total duration of treatment 9 mo
Daily		
Isoniazid	5 mg/kg, maximum 300 mg	All three drugs administered daily for
Rifampin	10 mg/kg, maximum 600 mg	2 mo followed by twice-weekly
Pyrazinamide	15–30 mg/kg, maximum 2 g	administration for remainder of 6-mo course
Twice Weekly		
Isoniazid	15 mg/kg, maximum 900 kg	All three drugs administered daily for
Rifampin	10 mg/kg, maximum 600 mg	1 to 2 mo, followed by twice-weekly
Pyrazinamide	50–70 mg/kg	administration for remainder of 6-mo course

success. Most drugs used have problem side effects and poor therapeutic ratios, necessitating the use of five- and six-drug regimens and long treatment periods. In the immunosuppressed host therapy has little impact on the course of illness, but it is not clear whether such failure is due to the treatment regimen, the advanced debility of the host, or the overwhelming effect of multiple simultaneous opportunistic infections.

COMMON PITFALLS

- It is easy to think of the diagnosis of TB when there are cavitary lesions in the lung. The many other presentations of mycobacterial illness require a higher level of suspicion, additional laboratory aids, and follow-up.
- New diagnostic techniques, including nucleic acid probes, staining techniques of greater sensitivity, and evaluation of microbe-specific metabolic processes, may shrink the diagnostic interval to a few days. Until more immediate testing is available, special administrative arrangements must be made to keep track of smears and particularly cultures that may be reported back as positive many weeks after their submission.
- Once the diagnosis has been made, the physician must know the treatment agents, their risks and complications, and the community resources available for monitoring continuing therapy and addressing public health concerns.

138   Pleural Effusion

Pleural effusions are abnormal accumulations of fluid in the pleural space due to any number of causes, many of them serious. Many effusions are chronic and have been previously diagnosed, but the differential diagnosis of a new effusion is extensive.

CLINICAL PRESENTATION

Pleural effusions are occasionally asymptomatic and are discovered on routine chest radiograph. More commonly, however, an effusion presents with symptoms caused by an underlying disease. For example, weight loss may be associated with malignancy or tuberculosis, fever with empyema or parapneumonic effusion, and orthopnea and edema with CHF. Symptoms such as cough, dyspnea, and chest pain may be caused by the effusion. A very large effusion may compress the lung, causing respiratory compromise and dyspnea. Determining whether symptoms are due to associated pulmonary or vascular disease or to the effusion itself may be difficult.

DIFFERENTIAL DIAGNOSIS

Radiographic pleural effusions should be differentiated from chronic pleural thickening, pneumonia and pulmonary infiltrates, lung or diaphragmatic tumors, and eventration of the diaphragm. Diaphragmatic rupture may also be confused with pleural effusion. There are many causes of pleural effusion (Table 138-1). Nontraumatic pleural effusions are most frequently caused by CHF, infection, or neoplasm. Parapneumonic effusions are found with pneumonia. Many agents can cause intrathoracic infection. Empyemas are far less common and are characterized by the presence of frank pus or micro-organisms in the pleural fluid. *Streptococcus pneumoniae* is most

---

TABLE 138-1. Cause of Pleural Effusions

Intrathoracic Disease	Extrathoracic Disease
Congestive heart failure	Cirrhosis
Infection	Pancreatitis
Bacterial: parapneumonic, empyema	Abscess, subphrenic or intra-abdominal
Mycobacterial	Nephrotic syndrome
Fungal	Peritoneal dialysis
Parasitic	Urinary obstruction
Mycoplasmal	Meigs' syndrome
Rickettsial	Myxedema
Viral	
Neoplasm	
Pulmonary embolism and infarction	
Collagen vascular disease	
Atelectasis	
Sarcoidosis	
Asbestosis	
Superior vena cava obstruction	
Chest trauma with vascular disruption	
Aortic dissection	
Esophageal rupture	
Drug reactions	

---

often the cause of parapneumonic effusion. Anaerobic bacteria are the most frequent pathogens found in empyemas. *Staphylococcus aureus* and *Haemophilus influenzae* are associated with both empyema and parapneumonic effusions. *Legionella* and gram-negative rods such as *Escherichia coli, Pseudomonas, Klebsiella,* and Proteus are also seen.

EMERGENCY DEPARTMENT EVALUATION

Attention should be paid to the patient's pulmonary and cardiac status. Physical exam may reveal dullness to percussion and decreased breath sounds over the involved hemithorax. A localized pleural friction rub may be heard. In cases of large effusions, there may be displacement of the trachea or cardiac impulse away from the effusion, due to shifting of the mediastinum. To help identify possible causes, search for stigmata of pulmonary, cardiac, hepatic, renal, or collagen vascular disease, as well as trauma, malignancy, or infection.

The chest radiograph is the primary study to confirm a pleural effusion. Blunting of the costophrenic angle on an upright film represents a collection of at least 175 ml of fluid. If the effusion is large, an upwardly concave meniscus may be seen. The hemidiaphragm is often obscured, and above the diaphragm a haziness may be seen that gradually becomes less dense as it progresses cephalad. Other findings may include the appearance of thickened pleural fissures, or densities located in the pulmonary periphery from loculated fluid. Findings on supine chest radiograph may include a generalized homogenous density, obliteration of the diaphragmatic silhouette, blunting of the costophrenic angle, apical capping, and a widened minor fissure.

Small effusions may be identified on a lateral decubitus view. This technique may also be helpful in determining whether an effusion is loculated or freely moving. The chest radiograph may also be able to reveal the cause of the effusion (e.g., pneumonia, CHF, malignancy, or sequelae of trauma). Ipsilateral and contralateral decubitus views allow evaluation of the underlying lung previously obscured on the upright or supine chest radiograph. Computed tomography can help to differentiate subpulmonic effusion from atelectasis or subphrenic fluid.

Additional routine workup of the effusion should include complete blood count, serum electrolyte, blood urea nitrogen levels, and urinalysis. If thoracentesis is anticipated, measurement of serum glucose, protein, lactic dehydrogenase (LDH), amylase, and creatinine levels, and prothrombin time should be ordered. An ABG may be useful to assess the degree of respiratory compromise. Severe hypoxia may suggest pulmonary embolism or infarction as a cause of the effusion. An ECG may reveal an associated pericarditis or manifestations of underlying heart disease. Additional diagnostic tests (e.g., liver or thyroid function tests, tests for collagen vascular disease, and ventilation-perfusion lung scans) may be indicated.

More specific information is obtained by thoracentesis. Effusions have been traditionally classified as transudates and exudates. Reliable characteristics of transudates are a ratio of pleural fluid protein to serum protein of <0.5; a level of LDH in the pleural fluid <200 IU/mL; and a ratio of pleural fluid LDH to serum LDH of <0.6. Exudates usually have values above these levels (Table 138-2). Empyema, hemothorax, and chylothorax have the characteristics of exudates. Urinothorax has the characteristics of either.

TABLE 138-2. Classification of Pleural Effusions

	Transudates	Exudates
Ratio of pleural fluid protein to serum protein	<0.5	>0.5
Pleural fluid LDH	<200 IU/mL	>200 IU/mL
Ratio of pleural fluid LDH to serum LDH	<0.6	>0.6
Specific gravity	<1.016	>1.016
Pleural fluid protein	<3 g/dL	>3 g/dL

LDH, lactate dehydrogenase. (From Light RW: Pleural Diseases. Philadelphia, Lea & Febiger, 1983.)

EMERGENCY DEPARTMENT MANAGEMENT

The first priority is the airway management. Treatment of a nontraumatic effusion must be directed toward the underlying process. If a diagnostic thoracentesis is required to identify the underlying cause, it is usually performed subacutely, or electively on an inpatient basis; pleural biopsy is also often indicated. For those who are toxic or who are likely to have empyema, parapneumonic effusion, or esophageal rupture, immediate thoracentesis in the ED is indicated for diagnosis and drainage. For significant respiratory or cardiovascular compromise, therapeutic thoracentesis may also be indicated. Large pleural effusions may cause a restrictive ventilatory defect and compress the lung, leading to shunting and loss of lung volume. Successful thoracentesis decreases the anatomical shunt, thereby increasing the arterial oxygen tension.

Several techniques for thoracentesis have been described. In most cases removal of the largest possible amount of effusion, up to 1500 mL, is advised. However, removing >1500 mL may increase the likelihood of the patient's developing postexpansion pulmonary edema, hypoxia, or hypoalbuminemia. After evacuation, a chest radiograph is obtained to rule out iatrogenic pneumothorax. If a moderate or large pneumothorax has been inadvertently created, or if the fluid removed was an empyema, a chylothorax, or a hemothorax, a thoracostomy tube is usually necessary. Parapneumonic effusions with low pH may resolve more effectively with thoracostomy drainage. Specimens are sent in most cases for cell count and differential, specific gravity, pH, LDH, protein, glucose, appropriate microbial stains and cultures, and cytology. Some authors suggest that only pleural fluid protein and LDH levels need to be determined if the fluid is a transudate. Additional analyses of exudates may be indicated by the clinical picture (Table 138-3).

DISPOSITION

If thoracentesis has been performed in the ED, admission is usually indicated for further treatment and observation for complications of the procedure. Patients with an effusion that was not evacuated may require admission, depending on the severity of symptoms, the underlying diagnosis, and response to treatment. Patients are usually admitted to a regular floor unless cardiovascular or pulmonary instability warrants admission to a monitored bed. It is important to communicate with the primary or consulting physician. This ensures that information about the patient's previous history can be integrated into the clinical picture and a coordinated plan for further management developed.

COMMON PITFALLS

- A pitfall often encountered is the failure to recognize an effusion by failing to order or by misreading the chest radiograph (misread as thickened pleura or infiltrate), leading to inadequate or delayed treatment. Delays are critical in empyema, esophageal rupture, or intrathoracic hemorrhage. Pulmonary embolism and infarction may also be missed if an effusion is not recognized.
- An incorrect diagnosis of the cause of an effusion, or an incorrect presumption that an effusion is old and unchanged, can likewise result in inadequate evaluation and treatment. Comparison with old x-ray films may be helpful.
- Another pitfall is the overly enthusiastic use of diagnostic thoracentesis. An incorrect diagnosis of pleural effusion may lead to an attempt to evacuate an intrathoracic mass (e.g., in diaphragmatic rupture). Furthermore, failure to recognize the potential need for pleural biopsy may lead to evacuation of fluid only making subsequent biopsy more difficult if only a small effusion remains.
- Failure to recognize complications of thoracentesis: clotting abnormalities are a major contraindication to thoracentesis. Complications include pneumothorax, laceration of the liver, spleen, and intercostal vessels; shearing of the catheter tip, infection, postexpansion pulmonary edema, hypoxia, and hypoalbuminemia.

TABLE 138-3. Diagnostic Features of Pleural Fluid

Exudates	Description	WBC	Predominant Leucocyte	Glucose	pH	Comments
Parapneumonic	Turbid	Elevated	P	Low	>7.3	If pH <7.2, may need thoracostomy tube
Empyema	Turbid, purulent	Elevated	P	Low	<7.3	Positive Gram's stain, culture
Tuberculosis	Straw color, serosanguineous	<10,000	M or P	Low	<7.3	Positive AFB stain, culture, or pleural biopsy
Malignancy	Turbid, bloody	<10,000	M	Low	<7.3	Positive cytology or pleural biopsy
Pulmonary embolism/infarction	Straw color, bloody	Elevated	M or P	Serum	7.4	Hypoxia; positive lung scan
Collagen vascular disease	Turbid	Variable	M or P	Very low	<7.3	Positive ANA
Rheumatoid arthritis	Green	Variable	M or P	Serum	<7.3	Elevated rheumatoid factor
Systemic lupus erythematosus	Yellow	Variable	M or P	Serum	>7.3	Positive LE cells
Hemothorax	Bloody	Variable	P	Serum	<7.3	Hematocrit > 50 peripheral level
Chylothorax	White, cloudy	Variable	M			Elevated pleural triglycerides; chylomicrons present; positive Sudan III stain
Pancreatitis	Turbid, serosanguineous	Elevated	P	Serum	>7.3	Pleural amylase > serum
Esophageal rupture	Turbid, bloody	Elevated	P	Serum	<<7.3	Pleural amylase elevated
Transudates						
Congestive heart failure	Clear, straw color	<1000	M	Serum	7.4	Clinical features
Cirrhosis	Clear, straw color	<500	M	Serum	7.4	Clinical features
Nephrotic syndrome/ hypoproteinemia	Clear, straw color	<1000	M	Serum	7.4	Clinical features
Transudate or Exudate						
Urinothorax	Straw color to bloody			Low		Obstructive uropathy Pleural creatinine > serum

P, polymorphonuclear cells; **M**, mononuclear cells (*i.e.*, lymphocytes, macrophages, mesothelial and plasma cells); **ANA**, antinuclear antibodies; LE, lupus erythematosus.

139   Asthma

Asthma is characterized by increased airway responsiveness to various stimuli. It is manifested by bronchoconstriction, widespread bronchial wall edema, and thick tenacious secretions, all of which can be relieved spontaneously or as a result of therapy. The characteristic that differentiates asthma from other airway diseases is its reversibility—acute exacerbations of asthma are interspersed with symptom-free intervals.

Asthma affects about 5% of the adult population of the US. About 50% of all cases are diagnosed before the patient reaches age 10, and another 33% are detected before age 40. Although the male to female ratio is 2:1 in childhood, the ratio equalizes during early adulthood.

The natural course of asthma has not been investigated thoroughly, but studies suggest that between 50–80% have a good prognosis, especially those with mild disease or disease that develops in childhood. Nevertheless, asthma has a high morbidity with 15 days of restricted activity per year and 5.8 days in bed on average. There are about 2,000 deaths/year in the US from asthma.

Asthma can be separated into two groups: allergic or extrinsic asthma, and nonallergic or intrinsic asthma. Extrinsic asthma accounts for <10% and tends to develop early in life. It is associated with a well-defined sensitivity to inhaled allergens, a family history of allergic diseases, increased serum levels of IGE, positive immediate skin tests and blood eosinophilia. It may be seasonal (trees, grasses, spores) or perennial (animal, garden, house dust), depending on the inciting agent. A good response to bronchodilator therapy is usually observed. Intrinsic asthma is the more common type of asthma. An inciting allergen cannot be identified, a family history of allergies is less common, IgE levels may be normal or low, and skin tests are negative. Intrinsic asthma is perennial, tends to be more severe than extrinsic asthma, and demonstrates a limited response to bronchodilator therapy. Many patients with asthma have components of both extrinsic and intrinsic disease. All asthmatics have hyperresponsive airways that narrow when exposed to a variety of stimuli.

Respiratory infections, particularly viral, commonly precipitate bronchospasm. Pharmacologic agents also may induce acute asthma. The agents most frequent are aspirin and nonsteroidal anti-inflammatory compounds, and beta-adrenergic antagonists. Up to 10% of adult asthmatics suffer from the triad of aspirin-induced bronchospasm, nasal polyps, and eosinophilia. Regardless of the underlying precipitant, airway narrowing, bronchial wall edema, bronchial smooth muscle contraction, and mucosal plugging ensue. These changes result in increased airway resistance, decreased forced expiratory volumes and flow rates, lung hyperinflation, increased work of breathing, and ventilation–perfusion mismatch.

CLINICAL PRESENTATION

Asthma attacks frequently occur at night. The classic triad of symptoms is cough, dyspnea, and wheezing. Chest tightness and nonproductive cough may precede dyspnea and wheezing. As airway obstruction worsens, the expiratory phase becomes prolonged. Asthmatic patients are frequently anxious, tachypneic, tachycardiac, and mildly hypertensive. Lung hyperinflation, accessory respiratory muscle use, muscle retraction, and pulsus paradoxicus may be noted. The patient may sit upright or lean forward in an effort to ease the work of breathing. These signs can be absent despite severe airway obstruction, however. The appearance of a "silent chest" indicates insufficient air movement or extensive mucous plugging and is an ominous sign. Cyanosis may appear immediately before respiratory arrest only and should not be relied on as an indication of the severity of an asthma attack.

Complications include pneumothorax, pneumomediastinum, and subcutaneous emphysema, and may require a chest tube for evacuation. Mild atelectasis may occur as a result of bronchial mucous plugging, but rarely requires intervention other than conventional bronchodilator therapy. Rib fractures and costochondral strain may occur from coughing. Arrhythmias may occur as a result of hypoxia.

DIFFERENTIAL DIAGNOSIS

Wheezing, coughing, and dyspnea are present in many conditions: pneumonia, bronchitis, croup, bronchiolitis, COPD, CHF, pulmonary embolism, allergic reactions, and upper airway obstruction from edema or foreign body. A careful history and exam should help differentiate asthma.

EMERGENCY DEPARTMENT EVALUATION

Therapy directed at relieving airway obstruction should begin. Obtain a history from family members or from the patient after airway obstruction is relieved. Important historical points include: duration and onset of current attack; identification of precipitating causes; type and amount of medications used before arrival in the ED; response to prior therapy, including current or previous use of steroid therapy; frequency of ED visits and hospitalizations; previous need for intubation; history of medications and allergies; other medical problems.

Immediate attention also should be directed to the patient's appearance, vital signs, chest and heart examination. The presence of a pulsus paradoxus should be noted. Assessing the ventilatory status and pulmonary function clinically can be difficult. The degrees of tachycardia and tachypnea often do not correlate well with the degree of airway obstruction. Pulsus paradoxus may be absent in up to one third of severe asthmatics. Furthermore, wheezing is absent if airflow is minimal. To complicate matters, these clinical parameters normalize with minimal improvement in pulmonary function.

Quantification of airway changes must be assessed using either the forced expiratory volume in 1 second (FEV_1) or the peak expiratory flow rate (PEFR). An initial FEV_1 of <1.0 L (<30% predicted) or a PEFR of <100 L/min (<20% predicted) indicates severe obstruction. Hypoxemia is a common finding during acute exacerbations. Arterial blood gases (ABGs) should be obtained only for severe or prolonged attacks. In general, hypercapnea, severe hypoxemia, or metabolic acidosis do not occur until the PEFR or FEV_1 is <25% predicted, but young children and elderly patients are exceptions. The degree of hypoxemia determined by ABG generally reflects the extent of ventilation–perfusion mismatch. A normal or increased $PaCO_2$ indicates severe airway obstruction and impending ventilatory failure.

Chest radiographs may demonstrate hyperinflation and atelectasis, but are usually nondiagnostic. A chest radiograph is necessary only if pneumonia, pneumothorax, or pneumomediastinum is suspected or if the patient fails to respond to aggressive bronchodilator therapy.

The ECG may reveal evidence of right ventricular strain, but is generally not helpful, except to rule out concurrent cardiac problems. All older patients, especially those with cardiac disease, should be monitored during therapy.

Complete blood cell (CBC) count is seldom useful; a theophylline level, however, should be obtained to guide therapy if theophylline is used.

EMERGENCY DEPARTMENT MANAGEMENT

The goal is to relieve bronchoconstriction. No ideal therapy is available, and the use of multiple drug regimens is commonplace. Bronchodilators, humidified oxygen, and oral or IV hydration are the mainstays of asthma treatment in the ED. Acute drug therapy can be grouped into four categories: beta-adrenergic agonists, glucocorticoids, and anticholinergics.

BETA-ADRENERGIC AGONISTS

Beta-adrenergic agonists produce bronchodilation through stimulation of beta receptors, resulting in the formation of cyclic AMP. Drugs in this category include catecholamines, resorcinols, and saligenins (Table 139-1). The catecholamines available in the US include epinephrine, isoproterenol, and isoetharine. Epinephrine is a nonselective alpha- and beta-adrenergic agonist given via inhalation (nonprescription medication) or subcutaneously. The usual subcutaneous dose in adults is 0.3 mL to 0.5 mL of a 1:1000 solution, repeated every 20 minutes up to a total of three doses. Side effects include increased myocardial irritability, arrhythmias, and nervousness. Although recent studies suggest that epinephrine may be safely used in patients over 40 years of age, extreme caution should be exercised in those with coronary artery disease. Sus-Phrine via SQ lasts up to 6 hours. Isoproterenol is a potent selective beta-adrenergic agent available in aerosolized form, metered-dose inhaler, and IV. The duration of action is 3 hours with inhalations repeated every 3 hours. IV isoproterenol should be reserved for dire emergencies and must be accompanied by strict monitoring of heart rate, rhythm, and blood pressure.

Resorcinols and saligenins include metaproterenol, terbutaline, albuterol (salbutamol), and bitolterol mesylate. Aerosolized forms are available for metaproterenol and albuterol. Metaproterenol, bitolterol mesylate, and albuterol are available in metered-dose inhalers. Both aerosolized agents and metered-dose inhalants are rapidly acting, are theoretically long lasting, and may be repeated every 3 to 4 hours in the acute situation. Albuterol, metaproterenol, and terbutaline also are available in oral form. Finally, terbutaline is available for subcutaneous injection.

Inhaled or aerosolized administration is preferred over parenteral administration of beta-agonists, because the inhaled agents rapidly promote bronchodilation, are theoretically longer lasting, and cause fewer side effects. Recent studies suggest that more frequent administration of smaller doses is more effective in improving and maintaining pulmonary function. The resorcinols and saligenins are highly $beta_2$ selective and virtually devoid of cardiac side effects when administered in inhaled or aerosolized form.

GLUCOCORTICOIDS

Steroids are thought to exert their effect on acute asthma by reducing airway inflammation. A loading dose of 4 mg/kg of IV hydrocortisone (or its equivalent dose of methylprednisolone) is appropriate. An infusion of 3 mg/kg/hr may follow. Patients who receive glucocorticoids early in the ED visit require fewer hospital admissions and sustain fewer relapses after ED discharge. Steroids should be given if there is poor response to 1–2 doses of beta-agonists. Because the effects are not noted for 4 hours, it is essential to continue vigorous concomitant bronchodilator therapy.

ANTICHOLINERGIC AGENTS

The use of aerosolized atropine sulfate (1–3 mg in 4 mL of saline) has been limited by its side effects. Metered-dose inhaled ipratropium bromide (2 puffs at 36 µg/puff), a nonabsorbable quarternary ammonium compound, has fewer side effects and is a good bronchodilator. Bronchodilation peaks within 1 to 2 hours, at which time ipratropium inhalation may be repeated.

MAGNESIUM

Magnesium sulfate has been demonstrated recently to be an effective bronchodilator by direct inhibition of bronchial smooth muscle contraction. Both aerosolized magnesium (0.66 g in 10 mL of saline) and IV magnesium solutions (0.5 mmol/min infused over 20 minutes) have been used experimentally to treat asthma, although neither use is approved in the US. Bronchodilation is observed within 2–5 minutes but disappears rapidly. Additional bronchodilator therapy must

TABLE 139-1. Adrenergic Agents Used to Treat Acute Bronchospasm

Preparation	Dosage	Dosing*	Side Effects
Epinephrine Hydrochloride	0.3–0.5 1:1000 aqueous solution, subcutaneous injection	Every 20 min up to a total of 3 doses	Myocardial irritability, arrythmias, nervousness, hypertension, tremor (CNS)
Epinephrine in Thioglycolate	0.15–0.25 ml 1:200 aqueous solution, subcutaneous injection	Every 6 hr	Myocardial irritability, arrythmias, nervousness
Isoetharine	1% solution, 0.5 ml diluted in 1.5 ml saline, aerosolized inhalation	Every hr	Uncommon
	2 puffs (34 mg per puff), metered-dose inhaler	Every 3 hr	
Isoproterenol	0.5% solution 0.5 ml in 2.5 ml saline, aerosolized inhalation		Paradoxical bronchospasm
	2 puffs (131 µg per puff), metered-dose inhaler		Paradoxical bronchospasm
	0.5–5 µg per min, 1 mg 1:5000 diluted in 500 ml 5% dextrose solution, intravenous drip	Every 3 hr	Myocardial necrosis, arrythmias, hypotension
Terbutaline Sulfate	0.25–0.50 mg, subcutaneous injection	Every 30 to 60 min, up to a total of 3 doses	Tachycardia, hypertension, tremor (CNS)
Metaproterenol	5% solution, 0.3 ml diluted in 2.5 ml saline, aerosolized inhalation	Every 3–4 hr	Uncommon, tremor
	2 puffs (0.65 mg per puff), metered-dose inhaler	Every 3–4 hr (possibly more frequently)	Uncommon, tremor
Albuterol	5% solution 0.5 ml diluted in 2 ml saline, aerosolized inhalation	Every 3–4 hr (possibly more frequently)	Uncommon, tremor
	2 puffs (90 µg per puff), metered-dose inhaler	Every 3–4 hr (possibly more frequently)	Uncommon, tremor
Bitolterol Mesylate	2 puffs (370 mg per puff), metered-dose inhaler	Every 3–4 hr	Tremor (musculoskeletal)

*Dosing frequencies during acute exacerbation, maintenance dosing intervals may vary from the acute situation.

accompany the use of magnesium. A slight decrease in PaO_2 has been noted after magnesium. Side effects include hypotension, malaise, and a warm sensation. Cardiac rhythm, blood pressure, pulse, neurologic status, and renal function must be monitored closely.

When the patient deteriorates or fails to improve, intubation must be considered. Although there are no absolute criteria besides respiratory arrest and coma, the following patients should be considered for intubation and mechanical ventilation: worsening pulmonary function tests despite vigorous bronchodilator therapy; decreasing PaO_2, increasing $PaCO_2$, or progressive respiratory acidosis; and declining mental status or increasing fatigue. Intubation of the asthmatic patient is fraught with difficulty. Ketamine is a potent bronchodilator with rapid onset of action and short half life. Ketamine is contraindicated in patients with ischemic heart disease, severe hypertension, preeclampsia, or increased intracranial pressure, and hallucinations are a frequent side effect. Close monitoring of heart rate, blood gases, and blood pressure is essential; consultation with an anesthesiologist may be required.

DISPOSITION

Several asthma scoring indices have been proposed to predict a patient's need for hospitalization, but all have proven disappointing. Many factors must be considered but the following patients should be considered for hospital admission: those whose condition deteriorates in the ED; those who return for further therapy within several days after ED discharge; dyspneic patients with significant hypoxemia ($PaO_2 < 60$), hypercapnea, or acidosis; patients with a pretreatment FEV_1 <1.0 L (<30% predicted) or PEFR <100 L/min (<20% predicted), and a post-treatment FEV_1 <2.1 L (60% predicted) or PEFR <300 L/min (<60% predicted); patients who remain subjectively dyspneic after aggressive therapy; patients with continued abnormal vital signs after therapy; and patients who are unreliable.

Even patients who improve enough to be discharged have residual airway obstruction for up to several weeks after the acute episode subsides. Early follow-up and continuous bronchodilator therapy treatment should be arranged. Either a beta$_2$ adrenergic metered dose inhaler or a long-acting theophylline preparation should be prescribed. Instruction in the proper use of the inhaler is essential. If oral theophylline is used, the serum level must be monitored. In addition, a 1-week course of high-dose, rapidly tapering steroids may be considered.

COMMON PITFALLS

- A common error is withholding beta-agonist therapy because of beta agonist use at home.
- Failure to consider pulmonary function measurements, in addition to clinical and subjective parameters of dyspnea, when judging the adequacy of bronchodilator therapy.
- The patient's age, concurrent medical problems, and medications must be considered.
- Glucocorticoids should be initiated if there is poor response to 1–2 doses of beta agonists.
- Chest radiograph, CBC and ABG are unnecessary, unless one suspects pneumonia, pneumothorax, or pneumomediastinum.
- Failure to recognize a silent chest or a normal $PaCO_2$ as a sign of severe obstructive disease may result in respiratory arrest.
- Failure to appreciate the potential morbidity and mortality (2000 people still die in the US each year from asthma).

140   Chronic Obstructive Pulmonary Disease

Chronic obstructive pulmonary disease (COPD) is a spectrum of conditions characterized by irreversible limitation of airflow. It is the 5th leading cause of death in the US. Excluding asthma, the two most common disorders of obstruction of airflow are chronic bronchitis and emphysema. Chronic bronchitis produces a chronic productive cough due to excessive bronchial mucus production and airway inflammation. Pulmonary emphysema, in contrast, is defined by an irreversible abnormal enlargement of the alveolar air spaces with associated destruction of the alveolar wall and pulmonary capillary bed. Some patients demonstrate nearly pure forms of each condition, but in most patients there is marked overlap. The predominant cause of COPD is cigarette smoking. Other risk factors include environmental pollution, industrial or occupational exposure, and recurrent pulmonary infections. Occasional asthmatic patients with long-standing severe disease develop a COPD-like clinical picture in older adulthood. The abnormalities of COPD may be reversed after cessation of smoking; continued tobacco use causes irreversible changes.

The natural course of COPD is one of progressively worsening dyspnea, hypoxemia, and diminished exercise tolerance, with recurrent exacerbations. Chronic hypoxemia leads to cor pulmonale, which worsens diminished lung function; recurrent episodes of respiratory failure and death result.

CLINICAL PRESENTATION

All patients with COPD exhibit airflow obstruction; with emphysema, there is a tendency to hyperventilate to compensate for the decreased ability of the lungs to oxygenate the blood. These are the classic "pink puffers"—working hard to maintain a more normal pO_2, they appear dyspneic and tachypneic. They are barrel-chested and use pursed-lip breathing to effect positive end-expiratory pressure and decrease early airway closure. Breath sounds are diminished with a prolonged expiratory phase. In contrast, patients with chronic bronchitis tolerate hypoxemia well and make no effort to hyperventilate. Chronic hypoxia induces a secondary polycythemia that, combined with marked desaturation of hemoglobin, produces the picture of the "blue bloater." These patients tolerate an elevated pCO_2 and the less labored respiratory pattern accounts for the plethoric appearance without tissue or muscle wasting. Lung examination reveals rhonchi, rales, and variable wheezing.

The majority with an acute exacerbation of COPD do not fit either picture precisely. Patients typically complain of dyspnea and chest tightness and note a change in the character of their sputum. Physical examination reveals tachypnea and a variable degree of respiratory distress as evidenced by accessory muscle use, retractions, and cyanosis. On auscultation there may be diminished breath sounds, a prolonged expiratory phase, wheezing, rales, or rhonchi. Signs of cor pulmonale should be sought—a centrally displaced point of maximal impulse (PMI), heart gallop, tricuspid murmur, peripheral edema, jugular venous distention, or hepatomegaly and hepatojugular reflux. Cor pulmonale, a complication of longstanding disease, is associated with substantial mortality.

Exacerbations may have many causes. These include upper respiratory infection, noncompliance with medications, changes in weather, exposure to certain drugs (e.g., sedatives, beta blockers), and environmental exposure to pollens, fumes, or other irritants. Patients typically present with a gradual, but progressive, deterioration over hours to days.

Some critical events cause acute decompensation. The COPD patient with spontaneous pneumothorax, pulmonary embolism, or acute CHF requires prompt treatment. Spontaneous pneumothorax in COPD patients carries a significantly higher complication and mortality rate. The chronic bronchitic is predisposed to embolic and thrombotic phenomena because of hyperviscosity associated with polycythemia. Other illnesses or disorders that affect the work of breathing (e.g., pneumonia, pulmonary edema, uremia, acidosis, or hepatic failure) may overtax the COPD patient's limited reserves, resulting in respiratory failure.

DIFFERENTIAL DIAGNOSIS

COPD is a clinical diagnosis; some patients with shortness of breath, cough, or wheezing may have pneumonia, and COPD may become apparent only after resolution of the acute pneumonic process. Pulmonary embolism also causes dyspnea and hypoxemia. Because wheezing and cough also may be present, the diagnosis must be considered, especially if the onset of symptoms was abrupt with pleuritic chest pain. The older patient with dyspnea and cough commonly has CHF; orthopnea and nocturnal dyspnea associated with cardiomegaly supports the diagnosis. Unfortunately, the physical examination does not reliably distinguish between CHF and COPD, because both may be associated with wheezing and rales. JVD is not uncommon in COPD, particularly when cor pulmonale is present, and a cardiac gallop may not be heard. The chest radiograph often aids in clarifying the clinical picture, but it may be prudent to initiate therapy for both conditions.

EMERGENCY DEPARTMENT EVALUATION

If the respiratory status allows a brief history, determine the rate of onset and duration of symptoms, medications, and precipitating factors. The examination should focus on mental status, the extent of respiratory distress and cardiac and pulmonary auscultation; search for concomitant diseases. Repeated examinations after therapy are mandatory to monitor the response. Be vigilant for signs of fatigue and CO_2 narcosis; confusion, irritability, or somnolence are manifestations of this ominous condition. Because signs of hypoxemia and hypercapnea are variable, ABG analysis is crucial in the acutely ill COPD patient. The $PaCO_2$ reflects the adequacy of ventilation. Hypercapnea with a normal pH and an elevated serum bicarbonate level suggests chronic CO_2 retention, whereas hypercapnea with acidemia signals acute respiratory insufficiency. The PaO_2 and oxygen saturation address the adequacy of oxygenation; a PaO_2 of <60 mm Hg is of concern, but some patients maintain this degree of hypoxemia chronically. Previous records should be consulted for baseline values. The chest radiograph (CXR) is another useful tool; it should be portable, unless the patient is stable. Chest radiography is most useful to rule out other diseases, such as pneumothorax, atelectasis, infiltrate, or CHF.

Measurements of air flow may be useful in judging the response to therapy (FEV_1 and PEFR). However, spirometric testing does not usually demonstrate a marked response to therapy, because bronchospasm is not the major component of dysfunction in the COPD patient.

Laboratory studies in COPD patients are of limited value, but a serum theophylline level must be obtained in patients taking the drug. Although recent dosing is associated with a higher likelihood of a therapeutic theophylline level, this is not a consistent finding.

An ECG may suggest right arterial enlargement or right ventricular hypertrophy or strain (cor pulmonale). Acute ischemic patterns must be sought, since an AMI may be triggering or complicating an exacerbation of COPD.

EMERGENCY DEPARTMENT MANAGEMENT

Management depends on rapid estimation of severity, aggressive therapy, frequent reevaluation, and recognition of treatable entities that have precipitated or complicated the patient's course. Patients must be monitored because arrhythmias are common in COPD, especially in patients with concomitant pulmonary edema, cor pulmonale, or hypercapnea. IV access is indicated. Oxygen must be given, since hypoxemia is the major immediate threat to life. The PO_2 should be maintained at >60 mm Hg if possible (O_2 saturation of about 90%). The Venturi mask can deliver a precise oxygen concentration ranging from 24% to 50%. In patients who cannot tolerate a mask, oxygen (2–4 L/min) by nasal cannula may be acceptable. Although the concern of eliminating the hypoxic drive in CO_2 retainers is genuine, most COPD patients are not at risk of this; further, the benefits outweigh the risks in the patient who is cyanotic, acutely dyspneic with acute respiratory failure. Adjustments in oxygen delivery must be guided by ABG results. Endotracheal intubation is the final option if an adequate PO_2 or the work of breathing cannot be met.

Sympathomimetic drugs are useful. Although oral and parenteral forms are available, inhaled preparations are used most commonly because they produce a rapid onset with minimal side effects. Inhalation therapy given by hand-held nebulizer or metered-dose inhaler coupled with a reservoir may be equally effective. Many beta-adrenergic agonists are available; metaproterenol, 10 to 15 mg (0.2–0.3 mL) and albuterol 1.25 to 2.5 mg (0.25–0.5 mL) are widely used as inhaled agents. Although most data support a 4–6 hour dosing interval, many physicians find that repeating initial treatments as often as every hour is efficacious in the very ill patient. The severity of obstruction and its degree of improvement with therapy must be balanced against the risk of drug toxicity in determining the most prudent interval. Undesirable effects of sympathomimetic drugs include tachycardia, hypertension, increased cardiac work, and nervousness.

The methylxanthines are also used in obstructive lung disease, although they are weak bronchodilators and the efficacy in the acute setting is limited. The usual loading dose is 5.6 mg/kg of aminophylline IV over a 30 minutes. Patients who are already taking theophylline preparations need a drug level. A concentration of 10 to 20 mg% is considered therapeutic; if the level is found to be lower, a loading dose may be based on the assumption that a 1 mg/kg bolus will raise the serum level by 2 mg%. An infusion of 0.5 mg/kg/hr is appropriate as an initial maintenance dose.

Another class of bronchodilators is the anticholinergic. Ipratropium bromide is a synthetic congener of atropine that has minimal systemic absorption when given in inhaled form. Bothersome anticholinergic effects are not seen. Ipratropium is as effective or more at bronchodilation than beta-adrenergic agents in patients with COPD. In the acute setting, however, its addition to other agents has not been demonstrated to result in greater bronchodilation than when either is used alone.

Corticosteroid therapy is not as useful in COPD as in asthma; however, a short course of high-dose IV steroids has been shown to be efficacious in improving the FEV_1 values of patients with acute respiratory insufficiency. In addition, patients with a history of recent or current steroid use may have suppression of the adrenal–pituitary axis, and thus require steroids with the stress of acute illness. Methylprednisolone, 0.5 mg/kg every 6 hours, is one suggested regimen.

The decision to intubate the patient with COPD for mechanical ventilation depends on the severity of ventilatory compromise. The patient with grossly ineffective respiratory effort, clouded consciousness, and severe hypoxemia is a candidate for assisted ventilation, especially in the setting of profound acidosis. These patients are admitted to an ICU and require consultation with a pulmonary specialist.

An acute exacerbation of COPD associated with the production of purulent sputum is treated with an oral broad-spectrum antibiotic such as ampicillin, trimethoprim–sulfamethoxazole, erythromycin, or a first-generation cephalosporin. If pneumonia is suspected, a sputum sample should be collected for Gram's stain and culture. Admission and parenteral broad-spectrum antibiotics are advisable for the seriously ill patient.

DISPOSITION

The majority of patients with an acute exacerbation of COPD require admission to the hospital. This is in contrast to most asthmatic patients and reflects the modest reversible component of airway disease in COPD. For a patient who responds promptly to therapy and has no pneumonia, however, consideration of discharge is appropriate if the vital signs and respiratory function are approaching baseline status and if adequate follow-up can be assured. The discharged patient should be continued on a bronchodilator regimen that may include one or several of the following: a sustained-action theophylline product (e.g., Theo-Dur); an oral beta-adrenergic agent (e.g., terbutaline, metaproterenol, or albuterol); and hand-held metered-dose inhalations of metaproterenol or albuterol. If acute bronchitis is suspected, a broad-spectrum antibiotic should be prescribed. Close follow-up within several days is imperative. The patient should be instructed to return immediately if breathing worsens or vomiting, fever, or chest pain complicates recovery.

Patients requiring further inpatient therapy may be admitted to a general medical floor, a specialized respiratory care unit, or a medical ICU. Trends in ABG results and pulmonary function tests, estimation of patient fatigue, and degree of supervision needed in each setting are important factors to consider in making a safe disposition.

COMMON PITFALLS

- The COPD patient is different from the asthmatic patient; the course, degree and reversibility is much slower.
- Patients with an acute exacerbation must have a thorough evaluation of identify precipitating causes or complicating events. If CHF is suspected, one should treat both conditions initially.
- A chest radiograph and ABG are necessary to fully evaluate and properly identify the more seriously ill patient.
- Adequate oxygenation is paramount when treating the acutely dyspneic patient who is struggling to breathe; do not withhold oxygen because of concern over its potential respiratory depressant effect.
- Pulmonary function must be supported by pharmacologic intervention and mechanical ventilation if necessary.

141   Pulmonary Embolism

Pulmonary embolism (PE), the occlusion of pulmonary arteries by venous thrombi, is a potentially lethal condition. It occurs in patients predisposed to thrombosis because of venous stasis, damaged vascular endothelium, hypercoagulability, or a combination. In the US, annual deaths from PE are estimated at 200,000. The Urokinase Pulmonary Embolism Trial (UPET) in 1975 was the first large series in which all patients underwent pulmonary arteriography for confirmation of the diagnosis of PE. An overall early mortality of 8% was found in angiographically documented PE.

CLINICAL PRESENTATION

The presentation depends on the degree of pulmonary vasculature occlusion and pre-existing cardiopulmonary disease. Healthy patients with small PEs are frequently asymptomatic, whereas patients with underlying COPD or CHF who suffer occlusion of a lobar artery can present with syncope or cardiopulmonary arrest. Patients with no immediately life-threatening events commonly complain of either dyspnea or chest pain. In documented PE, the most common symptoms are dyspnea (81%), pleuritic chest pain (73%), and cough (60%). The association between deep venous thrombosis (DVT) of the lower extremities and PE is well documented; therefore, particular attention should be paid to signs of DVT in the legs of patients with complaints suggestive of PE. Unfortunately, 50% of patients with lower extremity DVT have no clinical signs apparent to the physician.

The most useful information is the presence of predisposing factors that cause venous stasis, endothelial damage, or hypercoagulability (Table 141-1). Oral contraceptives are a real but weak risk factor in otherwise healthy women.

DIFFERENTIAL DIAGNOSIS

The differential diagnosis is extensive and depends on the patient's presenting complaint. In patients who present with chest pain, acute myocardial infarction (AMI) must be considered. Although a pleuritic character of the chest pain lessens the likelihood of AMI, the pain of PE is often steady in character and retrosternal in location. In young (age <40) and healthy patients with acute onset of pleuritic chest pain pulmonary infections (pneumonia and pleurisy) should be considered. The *absence* of risk factors for venous thrombosis, with no physical signs of lower extremity DVT, and no pleural effusion on chest radiograph (CXR) strongly diminishes the possibility of acute PE. Seventy percent of patients with acute PE have abnormal radiographs although most are nonspecific effusions and infiltrates.

EMERGENCY DEPARTMENT EVALUATION

Evaluation (Fig. 141-1) begins with risk factors assessment. Patients with significant risk factors for venous thromboembolism should be evaluated initially with ABG, ECG, and CXR. The chief value is to eliminate other possibilities such as AMI and CHF; these tests cannot diagnose pulmonary embolism, however. ECG and cardiac isoenzyme determinations may be helpful. Significant thrombosis of the pulmonary capillary bed elevates pulmonary arterial pressures; one would expect the ECG to show right heart strain. Unfortunately, few patients have ECG findings specific for right-sided heart strain. An abnormal alveolar–arterial oxygen gradient is no more a *sine qua non* than an abnormal pO_2 in identifying patients with PE.

Because of these limitations, the necessary next step is radionuclide ventilation–perfusion (V–Q) scanning. The distribution of pulmonary blood flow can be visualized. The distribution of pulmonary ventilation is also revealed after the patient inhales a radioactive gas. Areas of ventilated, but nonperfused, lung are suggestive of PE. The interpretation of V–Q scans is complex, however.

Based on V–Q scan patterns, patients can be classified into risk groups for PE. A completely normal scan is useful because it eliminates PE. A "low probability" (matched ventilation and perfusion defects) V–Q scan result does not reliably eliminate PE. PE has been found at angiography in 25-40% of patients with "low probability" V–Q scans. It is imprudent to withhold treatment for a strongly suspected PE because of a low probability V–Q scan. Such patients may need pulmonary arteriography. Others have suggested noninvasive venous studies as an alternative to pulmonary arteriography in patients with low probability V–Q scan patterns (impedance plethysmography; IPG).

TABLE 141-1. Risk Factors for Pulmonary Embolism

Immobility (bed rest, traction, etc.)
Heart disease
Cancer
Estrogen therapy
History of deep venous thrombosis
History of PE
Hypercoagulability or abnormal physiologic thrombolysis

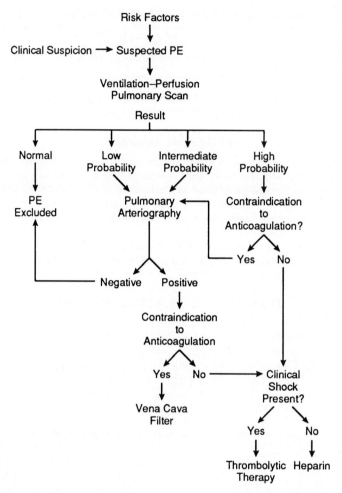

Figure 141-1. Evaluation and management of suspected pulmonary embolism.

Since proximal DVT requires heparin anticoagulation, pulmonary arteriography is rendered unnecessary in this subgroup.

Management of a suspected PE, a low probability V–Q scan, and negative venous studies remains controversial. Some feel these may be safely followed by serial IPG. One study of both IPG and pulmonary arteriography found PE in 47% of patients with an initially normal IPG.

The patient with an "intermediate probability" V–Q scan needs pulmonary arteriography to establish or rule out PE and avoid unnecessary and potentially dangerous anticoagulation. A high probability V–Q scan in a patient with strong risk factors for pulmonary thromboembolism is sufficient justification for initiation of anticoagulation, unless the patient has contraindications to heparin therapy.

Pulmonary arteriography remains the gold standard. Mortality is about 0.3%, largely limited to patients with pulmonary hypertension. Morbidity is 4% and consists of contrast reactions, cardiac arrhythmias, and cardiac perforations.

EMERGENCY DEPARTMENT MANAGEMENT

The goals of treatment are the removal of emboli and prevention of recurrent embolization. Therapeutic alternatives include physical removal of thrombus, heparin anticoagulation, thrombolytic agents, and vena cava filters. Surgical embolectomy is invasive and complex, and no consensus on indications exists. Embolectomy is likely to be used in special circumstances only (e.g., ICU patients suffering massive PE with readily available thoracic surgeons). Heparin anticoagulation is the standard treatment. In the absence of progressive thrombosis, normal thrombolytic mechanisms dissolve *in situ* emboli and restore pulmonary blood flow. In the UPET trial, heparin-treated patients had a mortality of 8%, an early recurrence rate of 22%, and a complication rate (chiefly hemorrhage) of 27%. In clinical practice, complication rates of 5–10% are seen. Heparin is given by 5000- or 10,000-unit IV bolus followed by an infusion at 1000 U/hr. The infusion rate is adjusted to maintain the activated PTT at 1.5 to 2.0 times control.

Thrombolytic therapy actively dissolves formed thrombi, rather than merely halting progressive thrombosis. The standard agents are streptokinase and urokinase. In the UPET trial with urokinase acute mortality was about 8%, recurrence rate 17%, and the complication rate (chiefly hemorrhage) 45%. Urokinase complication rates of 10% are more common in clinical practice.

The excellent results with heparin and the perception that thrombolytic therapy involves a higher rate of complications has limited the use of the latter. Thrombolytic agents may be more effective than heparin in the preservation of pulmonary capillaries, and therefore may be of greater long-term benefit. t-PA is "thrombus specific"; no thrombolytic activity occurs unless it is bound to formed thrombi. Patients in shock are likely to benefit more from thrombolytic therapy than from heparin. There is a high risk for complications in active internal bleeding or recent (<2 months) stroke, other intracranial disease, surgery, organ biopsy, trauma, childbirth, or gastrointestinal bleeding.

Patients with a documented PE with these or other contraindications to heparin or thrombolytic drugs, or who experience recurrent PE during therapy, may be protected from further embolization by vena cava barriers. The Greenfield filter is easily placed percutaneously and reduces the rate of PE recurrence to <5%.

DISPOSITION

THE ROLE OF THE CONSULTANT   Prospective protocols are useful for issues of thrombolytic therapy (indications, doses, monitoring) and noninvasive vascular studies (IPG, doppler ultrasound) in the management of the patient with a "low probability" V–Q scan. Consultation with the admitting physician should be sought after demonstration of PE by "high probability" V–Q scan. Patients with "low" or "intermediate" probability V–Q scans frequently have acute PE; thus, consultation with a pulmonologist is indicated to discuss immediate pulmonary arteriography; admission and heparin therapy pending elective pulmonary arteriography; or close follow-up with sequential noninvasive vascular studies of the lower extremities.

INDICATIONS FOR ADMISSION   All patients requiring heparin or thrombolytic therapy must be admitted to the hospital. Patients with "intermediate probability" V–Q scans have a risk of acute PE sufficient to make hospital admission for further evaluation mandatory.

COMMON PITFALLS

- Diagnostic evaluation for acute PE can be initiated only if the patient at risk is identified (e.g., immobility, cancer, heart disease, inherited disorders of coagulation).
- The presentation is nonspecific. Only a minority of patients with acute PE manifest the so-called "classic triad" (hemoptysis, pleuritic chest pain, dyspnea). Chest wall tenderness does **not** eliminate the possibility of acute PE. The chest radiograph and electrocardiogram are frequently abnormal, but the abnormalities are not specific.

- A pO_2 of >90 torr or normal A–a gradient on ABG does not eliminate the possibility of acute PE.
- A "low probability" ventilation–perfusion scan does not rule out acute PE.
- A "high probability" ventilation–perfusion scan is not diagnostic of acute PE; in patients without strong risk factors or in those with significant contraindications to anticoagulation, even "high probability" scans should be followed by pulmonary angiography.

PART IV

Gastrointestinal Emergencies

142   Upper Gastrointestinal Bleeding

Upper gastrointestinal (UGI) bleeding is a common complaint in the ED. Appropriate management depends on accurate assessment of the severity and rate of bleeding and knowledge of the diagnostic and therapeutic resources available to deal with it. The major causes of upper GI bleeding differ according to the population being considered (i.e., pediatric, healthy young adult, alcoholic, elderly, etc.). Knowing this, the clinician can focus on the most likely and serious causes (Table 142-1). Despite improvements in endoscopic therapy, the mortality rate is still 8%, prominently in variceal bleeding and the elderly. Arterial bleeding is the least common but carries the highest early mortality (e.g., aortoduodenal fistula, erosion of posterior duodenal ulcer into the gastroduodenal artery). Capillary bleeding is seen in erosive gastritis (aspirin or alcohol); it has an excellent prognosis. Variceal bleeding, although venous, has a poor prognosis, because the vessels are under high pressure and such bleeding is frequently associated with medical illnesses and coagulopathies.

Orthostatic abnormalities indicate a loss of intravascular volume of >10%; although the elderly may present only with postural symptoms and narrowed pulse pressure. The hematocrit does not reflect acute blood loss and should not be used to judge the extent of blood loss. Morbidity and mortality result from the myriad complications of acute hemorrhagic shock.

DIFFERENTIAL DIAGNOSIS

The major causes of upper GI bleeding are listed in Table 142-1. Table 142-2 summarizes the major causes by historical and clinical features. Patients with known esophageal varices often bleed from nonvariceal causes as well (about 50%). Aortoduodenal fistula is an uncommon but frequently fatal cause of upper GI bleeding, generally originating from an aneurysm or a synthetic aortic graft. In some patients a "herald" bleed of modest volume is noted to have occurred within the week before the massive bleed.

CLINICAL PRESENTATION

Chronic upper GI bleeding presents as anemia (microcytic) or occult bleeding in the stool with no other findings. Acute bleeding may be classified as occult, overt, or massive. Blood per rectum is a common sign. The gross appearance cannot localize the site of bleeding. Melanotic stool suggests only that blood has remained in the bowel for some time and has been exposed to acid. Although melana is a sign of peptic ulcer, it does not exclude other sources. About 10% of GI

TABLE 142-1. Causes of Upper Gastrointestinal Bleeding

Esophageal

Esophagitis
   Gastrointestinal reflux
   Infectious (candida, CMV, Herpesvirus)
   Chemical (acid, alkaline)
Ulcer
   Inflammatory
   Neoplastic (mostly squamous cell, few adenocarcinoma, rare other)
Varices

Gastric

Erosive gastritis (NSAIDs, alcohol, stress)
Peptic ulceration
Neoplasm (mostly adenocarcinoma, few lymphoma, melanoma, leiomyoma, other)
Vascular
   Arterial-venous malformation
   Osler-Weber-Rendu syndrome
   Vasculitis syndromes
   Varices
Mallory-Weiss tear
Amyloidosis
Paraesophageal hiatal hernia
Uremia

Duodenal

Duodenitis
Duodenal ulcer
Arterial-duodenal fistula

Hematobilia

Blunt trauma
Penetrating trauma and iatrogenic causes

---

bleeds that by history, stool and nasogastric tube aspirate, appear to be from the lower tract, turn out to be of upper GI origin (usually duodenal ulcer).

EMERGENCY DEPARTMENT EVALUATION

A CBC should be done and nasogastric aspiration performed. A decreased hemoglobin level indicates subacute or chronic blood loss and a decreased mean corpuscular volume indicates chronicity; neither excludes superimposed acute blood loss. The nasogastric tube is helpful diagnostically in indicating the presence, appearance, and rapidity of bleeding. A negative aspirate does not exclude upper GI bleeding. Nasogastric aspiration also makes it possible to clear the stomach before endoscopy or surgery. "Therapeutic lavage" is of no proven benefit.

Stool is evaluated for appearance and occult blood. An elevated BUN may be seen and active bleeding often results in leukocytosis and thrombocytosis. Clotting times should be done to rule out coagulopathy. A chest radiograph and abdominal films may be helpful. If occult bleeding is identified, further evaluation may be performed on an outpatient basis (internist or gastroenterologist). Overt bleeding requires admission, with urgent panendoscopy. Although early endoscopy has not decreased morbidity, it it often permits a definite diagnosis and provides a guide for decisions on admission to a critical care bed, the use of blood products, and the indications for and timing of surgery. Recent studies show sclerotherapy or coagulation therapy may improve morbidity, particularly in selected subgroups.

TABLE 142-2. Differential Diagnosis of Upper Gastrointestinal Bleeding

---

Age

Pediatric—caustic ingestion
Elderly—increased risk of cancer

Habits/Medications

Alcohol use raises the likelihood of erosive gastritis as well as the
    possibility of portal hypertension and esophageal or gastric varices
All nonsteroidal anti-inflammatory drugs may be associated with erosive
    gastritis
Anticoagulants

Previous Medical Illness

Known cirrhosis or varices
Peptic ulcer
Cancer
Surgery
Vascular disease, especially aortic or splenic artery aneurysm

Pain

Pain generally indicates inflammation and raises the likelihood of
    esophagitis, gastritis, duodenitis, and ulcer
Painless bleeding is sometimes inflammatory, but is more often due to
    varices, Mallory-Weiss tear, cancer, or vascular-duodenal fistula

Physical Examination

Epigastric tenderness (see "Pain" above)
Signs of chronic liver disease or portal hypertension (splenomegaly,
    ascites, caput medusae) make variceal bleeding more likely
Mass, lymphadenopathy, or other signs of cancer
Abdominal aneurysm

For massive bleeding, emergency panendoscopy is the procedure of choice; it yields a diagnosis in >95%. In cases where bleeding is active and the diagnosis in doubt, arteriography usually demonstrates the bleeding site. Radionuclide scan may be helpful if done quickly, as a "screening" test to determine when to do arteriography. Arteriography or radionuclide scanning should not delay surgery for massive bleeding unresponsive to initial measures. Barium studies have no role in the evaluation of upper GI bleeding.

EMERGENCY DEPARTMENT MANAGEMENT AND DISPOSITION

Initial management is based the urgency of the situation. The goal is to maintain or restore cardiac output and oxygen delivery. For *occult bleeding,* management is geared toward making the diagnosis. This can almost always be on an outpatient basis. The management of *overt bleeding* should involve urgent evaluation and prevention of circulatory compromise. Type and crossmatch and initial labs are sent. Large caliber IV access should permit the transfusion of a minimum of 2 units of blood products/hour. Crystalloids are used for immediate infusion in combination with packed red blood cells. Fresh frozen plasma should be administered if coagulopathy is identified and when clotting factors are depleted after massive transfusion.

Random-donor platelet transfusion is indicated if the platelet count is <60,000/μL. Albumin and synthetic volume expanders have little role. Oxygen, close monitoring of vital signs and cardiac rhythm should be done. Re-evaluation and serial hematocrits are essential. Early (<12 hours) panendoscopy should be scheduled to establish a diagnosis, to assess the rate of bleeding and possibly provide definitive treatment.

For bleeding ulcers, definitive endoscopic treatment includes heater probe cautery, bipolar electrocautery, and injection sclerosis. Laser cautery is effective but less practical and expensive, and is therefore seldom used. Esophageal varices are treated with injection sclerosis. Where surgical expertise is available, portacaval shunting may be necessary for varices although this is generally reserved for sclerotherapy failures. Gastric varices are difficult to manage endoscopically and often require surgery.

For *massive bleeding*, volume resuscitation takes precedence, with rapid crystalloid and blood product infusion. Endotracheal intubation may be necessary to ensure adequate oxygenation and minimize the risk of aspiration in an obtunded patient. Cardiac, pulse oximetry and blood pressure monitoring are essential. The surgical consultant should evaluate the patient at the earliest possible moment. Although endoscopy is best performed in a specialized endoscopy unit, emergency panendoscopy for massive bleeding often is performed in the ED. Its major role lies in the potential for providing specific therapy endoscopically. Arteriography is used primarily for active bleeding when endoscopy is unavailable or nondiagnostic, for guiding surgery, and if the mortality of surgery is prohibitive.

Arterial embolization is performed rarely but selective infusion of vasopressin continues to be a helpful measure; it may be used for bleeding from any site, and the drug can be given systemically as well. Specialized nasogastric tubes are sometimes useful but require experience for safe use. The Minnesota tube is a modified Sengstaken–Blakemore tube with an esophageal port permitting esophageal drainage to be performed while the esophageal balloon is inflated. When endoscopy or surgery is delayed, this device may tamponade bleeding at the gastroesophageal junction (usually varices). Although this is not definitive therapy (sclerotherapy is preferred), it may be effective as a temporizing measure, with or without simultaneous vasopressin infusion, and may allow for more effective endoscopy. There is no role for antacids, H_2-receptor antagonists, or sucralfate in acute bleeding.

Occasionally, patients with upper GI bleeding may require transfer to another facility, primarily because critical care beds, endoscopy, full blood-banking services, and surgical capability are unavailable. Adequate IV access, replacement of volume and blood products, and continuous monitoring are mandatory; oxygen and adequate airway are also critical. The usual standards regarding communication and records apply. ACLS level personnel will accompany most of these transfers. Transfer of acutely bleeding patients is to be discouraged.

Priorities for the successful treatment of GI bleeding are: recognize bleeding, determine urgency, and resuscitate. The key to a good outcome is the ability to combine rapid assessment with initial diagnostic and treatment interventions, followed by the timely application of specialized diagnostic and therapeutic techniques.

COMMON PITFALLS

- Err on the side of caution: admit the patient to a closely monitored setting if necessary. The inpatient physician can transfer the patient to a less acute bed when convinced it is safe to do so.
- Prompt identification of high-risk patients (elderly, alcoholic, and coagulopathies) is crucial.
- The nasogastric aspirate may not sample duodenal contents and bleeding may be intermittent. Both may result in a false-negative aspirate. A carelessly placed nasogastric tube may yield a false-positive aspirate, as well as distress the patient.
- A normal hemoglobin level does not preclude significant bleeding; an normal blood pressure does not exclude hypovolemia.

- About 10% of apparent lower GI bleeding is from the upper tract.
- There is no role for barium studies in upper GI bleeding.
- Know the options available at your institution; this includes endoscopy equipment and expertise, surgical backup (including anesthesia), Minnesota tube, vasopressin, and so forth.

143   Peptic Ulcer Disease

Peptic ulcer disease (PUD) eventually affects one of every ten Americans. There are 4–8 million active cases at any given time. There has been a significant decline in the total number of cases since the 1960s. The disease is becoming less common in developed countries while more common in developing nations. Duodenal ulcer occurs more frequently than gastric ulcer (5:1), and men are afflicted more commonly than women (1.8:1). The stereotypes of young or middle-aged affluent males developing duodenal ulcers and the elderly or poor developing gastric ulcers is grossly inaccurate. Among the elderly, gastric or duodenal ulceration is an increasing problem.

While mortality rates for PUD have declined since 1960, they remain high for the elderly— 50 to 100 times greater at age 75 than at age 35. Many factors predispose to the development of ulcers (Table 143-1). Of these, cigarette smoking plays a major role in ulcer formation and in recurrence. Aspirin and nonsteroidal anti-inflammatory drugs cause alterations of the gastric mucosa, but there is still no conclusive evidence that they actually produce ulceration. Alcohol and caffeine have not been conclusively linked to ulcer disease. Diet also is not clearly related to PUD, and at present the only reasonable dietary recommendation for ulcer patients is to avoid foods that produce symptoms.

Peptic ulcer disease continues to produce major *complications* despite the introduction of H2 blockers. The type of surgical procedure performed has changed; fewer elective procedures

---

TABLE 143-1. Risk Factors for Peptic Ulcer

Definitely Related

Family history
Associated diseases (COPD, cirrhosis, chronic renal failure)
Male gender
Advanced age
Smoking

Possibly Related

Use of certain drugs (ASA, NSAIDS, etc.)
Psychological profile

Not Related

Diet (caffeine, spicy or fatty foods)
Alcohol

(Modified from Ruoff GE. Peptic ulcer disease. The role of the primary care physician in therapeutic intervention. Postgraduate Education. 81(5):86, Apr 1987.)

are performed in the younger population, and more emergent operations are performed on older and sicker patients who are less able to tolerate surgery.

Perforation continues to occur in nearly 20% despite effective medical treatment. Perforation is heralded by a dramatic change in pain pattern: severe pain and a surgical abdomen develop rapidly, or a constant deeper pain increases gradually with a slower onset of surgical signs (this is seen in posterior penetration or a partially occluded perforation). Perforation is a surgical emergency requiring rapid diagnosis, resuscitation, and operation.

Hemorrhage is usually self-limited but occasionally is massive and life-threatening; it accounts for 20%–30% of patients who require surgery for PUD. A common complication of PUD, the presentation ranges from melena to shock.

Gastric outlet obstruction, due to scarring from repeated episodes of ulceration and fibrous healing, is usually associated with duodenal ulcer. It may also be caused by edema from an active ulcer. Fluid and gas accumulate in the stomach, causing fullness or distress that is often relieved by vomiting. Massive distention of the stomach can occur; fluid and electrolyte disturbances may be dramatic. In the ED, fluid resuscitation should be performed and the stomach should be decompressed by means of a nasogastric tube, but surgery may be necessary. Gastric outlet obstruction is responsible for 30% of ulcer operations.

CLINICAL PRESENTATION

Peptic ulcer is a chronic disease marked by periods of exacerbation and remission. Pain may develop and persist for several days or weeks, but rarely longer. Many patients do not seek medical assistance. The vast majority have a benign course with occasional symptomatic periods. However, 10%–20% develop some complication. Most patients present for relief from a constant burning, gnawing, or aching pain. The pain is primarily epigastric, but can be occur anywhere in the upper abdomen. With perforation of a posterior duodenal ulcer, pain often begins in the epigastrium and moves to the back. If pneumoperitoneum develops, pain may be referred to the shoulder.

The description and location of the pain is not as important in diagnosis as is its timing and any exacerbating and ameliorating factors. *Gastric ulcer* usually produces pain immediately after eating, when acid production increases in response to food. The pain of *duodenal ulcer* is most common between or just before meals and at night, when the upper GI tract is empty. Ingestion of food or antacids may bring rapid relief. Pain at 2 AM or 3 AM is classic for duodenal ulcer, because acid production is high and unbuffered by food.

The classic history of a repetitive pain–food–relief sequence remains one of the better clinical diagnostic clues to PUD. Asymptomatic peptic ulcer is not uncommon, with 20%–25% of all ulcers silent. Nearly 33% of patients with ulcer perforation and 20% with upper GI hemorrhage have had no previous symptoms of ulcer disease.

Uncomplicated peptic ulcer disease does not produce remarkable physical findings. Epigastric tenderness may be noted, but guarding and rebound are absent. Rectal exam may show guaiac-positive stool. The physical examination can exclude complications and other diseases rather than confirm the peptic ulcer. Heart and lungs should be examined to assess for cardiac or pulmonary disease.

Guarding, rebound, and a tense abdomen signal perforation of an ulcer. Patients usually lie perfectly still because the slightest movement produces intense peritoneal pain. In the elderly, findings may be minimal or absent, causing delays in diagnosis in the group least able to tolerate delay. Hemorrhage may cause few physical findings. A history of melanotic stools should be sought, and orthostatic vital signs should be done. Significant bleeding often presents with hematemesis; a nasogastric tube can be inserted to determine if blood is present in the stomach.

Gastric outlet obstruction usually produces some degree of bloating and a tympanitic epigastrium or succussion splash secondary to a distended stomach.

DIFFERENTIAL DIAGNOSIS

Myocardial infarction and *angina* are perhaps the most important diagnoses to consider; they may present atypically as midepigastric pain with complaints of nausea, bloating, and burning similar to PUD, but without the typical periodicity and ameliorating factors. Moreover, a substantial number of ulcer patients also have coronary artery disease. A history and ECG can usually differentiate heart disease, however. *Gastritis* usually produces a constant feeling of bloating and may not be relieved by antacids. *Gastroenteritis* produces colicky or crampy abdominal pain associated with diarrhea and vomiting. *Biliary tract disease* causes upper abdominal pain after ingestion of fatty foods, but typically there is no history of early morning pain or improvement with antacids. *Esophagitis* as a complication of *hiatal hernia* may be associated with intense pain immediately or shortly after swallowing. The constant, boring pain of *pancreatitis* frequently radiates to the back and is associated with elevated serum amylase levels. A host of *other conditions* is capable of producing pain in the upper abdomen but are often ruled out during the evaluation.

EMERGENCY DEPARTMENT EVALUATION

The history and physical remain the most important methods for evaluating uncomplicated peptic ulcer. However, because other diseases may also present with epigastric distress and because some complications of PUD may not be immediately apparent, additional diagnostic interventions are recommended.

For any patient in the age group at risk for coronary artery disease, an ECG should be done and monitoring should be utilized initially. A nasogastric tube should be passed if bleeding or obstruction is suspected, but routine use is probably not necessary. Chemical tests for the presence of occult gastric blood are available, but their value is questionable since clinically insignificant iatrogenic bleeding often accompanies nasogastric tube insertion.

The chest x-ray (CXR) is a useful adjunct for detecting free air from perforation and for ruling out thoracic disease. The patient should be placed in the upright, sitting position for 10–15 minutes prior to the x-ray to allow time for any free air to rise to the diaphragm; insufflating 100 to 200 cc of air through the nasogastric tube may enhance the chances of detecting free air. Pneumoperitoneum is seen on x-ray in <50% of perforations; the absence of free air is associated with delayed diagnosis and increased mortality. Abdominal x-rays can also be useful but are not routinely necessary. If the CXR does not show free air but suspicion of perforation is still high, an upright abdominal or left lateral decubitus view can be done.

Endoscopy in the ED for uncomplicated PUD is not warranted. A CBC is justified in most patients with abdominal pain. Low hematocrit suggests significant recent blood loss, and red cell indices may suggest anemia from chronic blood loss. A white blood cell (WBC) count is usually normal in uncomplicated peptic ulcer disease, but it may help to differentiate upper abdominal pain of other causes. Serum amylase determinations are helpful if pancreatitis is considered but are not of value for uncomplicated PUD. Electrolytes, BUN and serum creatinine are also indicated for ill patients and those who are bleeding, vomiting, or "third-spacing" fluids. Hypochloremic hypokalemic metabolic alkalosis may be noted with intractable vomiting or gastric outlet obstruction.

Relief with antacids is part of the classic peptic ulcer history but it is not diagnostic of PUD. Up to 25% may have concomitant coronary artery disease; it is may be difficult to distinguish the symptoms. The indiscriminate use of "GI cocktails" is to be discouraged.

EMERGENCY DEPARTMENT MANAGEMENT

Most patients have normal vital signs and do not require major intervention. If complications have not occurred, antacids may relieve pain. Improvement usually justifies continuing antacids. H_2 receptor antagonists reduce acid secretion and are safe and effective. Cimetidine, ranitidine, and famotidine are available: dose of 800 mg of cimetidine is equivalent to one dose of 300 mg of ranitidine or 40 mg of famotidine. Cimetidine interferes with the metabolism of diazepam, chlordiazepoxide, lidocaine, propranolol, theophylline, warfarin, and phenytoin. Sucralfate appears to heal ulcers as effectively as H_2 blockers. Patients with complications require more intensive management, including crystalloid or blood, oxygen, monitoring, and endoscopic or surgical intervention.

DISPOSITION

Patients who are critically ill, have unstable vital signs, or who are suffering from complications of PUD require prompt consultation with a specialist. Others may need admission for pain control, gastric decompression, and/or fluid resuscitation, and do not necessarily require monitoring. Cases of uncomplicated PUD may be referred to a family physician. Patients who require admission may need to be transferred to another institution for endoscopy, critical care or surgery. Potentially unstable patients should be transported by an ALS unit.

144   Gastrointestinal Foreign Bodies

Foreign bodies of the gastrointestinal tract range from the commonplace to the bizarre. The history of ingestion may be intentionally kept from the physician or may be unknown to the patient. About 1500 deaths/year occur from the ingestion of foreign bodies. Persons likely to ingest foreign bodies include those with dementia, impaired mental functioning, psychiatric illness, and alcoholism. Children, denture wearers, and prisoners also have an increased risk. Ingestion of foreign bodies may be intentional or accidental. Ingestions may be denied in the psychiatric patient or prisoner. Accidental ingestions may not be discernible because of impaired mental functioning or unawareness of ingestion as in denture wearers or alcoholics.

The physical characteristics of a foreign body are important. Objects < 5–6 cm are more likely to traverse the gut than those > 6 cm. Round objects are more likely to pass spontaneously from the gut than sharp, irregular, long, or thin objects. A foreign body that fails to pass from the esophagus into the stomach should have immediate endoscopic removal; however, > 50% pass through the esophagus, and once in the stomach have an 80–90% chance of traversing the gut without incident. The common points for esophageal impaction are the cricopharyngeal muscle, aortic arch, left mainstem bronchus, and the narrowing of the lower esophageal sphincter. Once in the stomach, common sites are the pylorus, the duodenum, ileocecal valve, and the anus.

CLINICAL PRESENTATION

The spectrum may range from asymptomatic to unstable with irritation, obstruction, bleeding, or perforation of the gut. In the esophagus, odynophagia, chest pain, bloody secretions, or dysphagia may be observed. Gastric, intestinal, colonic, and rectal foreign bodies may produce pain and other symptoms.

DIFFERENTIAL DIAGNOSIS

In the absence of an accurate history (a common occurrence), the differential diagnosis is difficult. Processes that irritate, erode, perforate, obstruct, or cause bleeding of the gastrointestinal tract should be considered: appendicitis, diverticulitis, localized abscess, neoplasm, intestinal obstruction, and cardiac disease. Chronic symptoms do not exclude a foreign body.

EMERGENCY DEPARTMENT EVALUATION

The examination should be directed toward signs of esophageal or distal obstruction, bleeding, localized inflammation or infection, and perforation. Imaging studies are most helpful since many foreign bodies are radiopaque. Barium swallow is used for esophageal foreign bodies. The remainder of the gut is evaluated with plain and contrast radiography.

EMERGENCY DEPARTMENT MANAGEMENT

Management of obstruction, bleeding, inflammation or infection, and perforation is the priority since these are serious sequelae of foreign body ingestion and will most likely result in operative intervention. Localization is pursued after stabilization. If the foreign body has direct toxic effects (ie, button battery), immediate consultation should occur with an endoscopist or surgeon. A foreign body lodged in the esophagus should be removed endoscopically, with one exception: food bolus impaction may be resolved by IV glucagon, 1 mg, and the oral administration of proteolytic enzymes such as papain. Contraindications include bones and suspected mucosal injury or perforation. If this approach is unsuccessful, endoscopy will be necessary.

The use of catheters and emetics is not appropriate. Once the foreign body has reached the stomach, it likely will pass the remainder of the gut without difficulty. In the absence of symptoms, the foreign body should take 7–10 days for spontaneous passage out of the stomach and 2–3 weeks for passage through the remainder of the gut. Cathartics and enemas should *not* be administered. Close follow-up should be arranged with this conservative management. Objects at high risk for perforation or a known history of intestinal disease (e.g., Crohn's disease) merit consultation with an endoscopist or surgeon for removal of the foreign body.

DISPOSITION

Discharge is acceptable only for asymptomatic patients without complicating intestinal disease who have foreign bodies of low perforation potential distal to the esophagus. Close follow-up by a surgeon must be arranged. All other patients need consultation on an immediate basis with an endoscopist or surgeon, depending on symptoms and location of the foreign body.

COMMON PITFALLS

- Failure to recognize a foreign body with direct toxic effects (battery)
- Blind attempts with catheters, enemas, or gas-producing substances may cause mucosal damage, further impact the foreign body, or cause perforation.

---

145   Pancreatitis

Pancreatitis has been estimated to affect up to 0.5% of the general population in the US. It can be divided into acute and chronic. Acute pancreatitis, although often a mild disease, may be life-threatening with hemorrhage and necrosis and potentially lethal manifestations in other organ systems. The mortality may be 5%. Chronic pancreatitis, recurrent episodes of acute pancreatitis superimposed on a chronically damaged pancreas, is only fatal rarely. The major causes of acute pancreatitis are shown in Table 145-1. In the US, alcoholism and cholelithiasis account for 80–90%. Pancreatitis is seen in 1–10% of alcoholics; most episodes occur after 6–8 years of heavy alcohol abuse. In nonalcoholic patients, gallstones are seen in 60%.

Severe cases of acute pancreatitis can cause cardiac dysfunction, acute renal failure, central nervous system dysfunction, DIC, pleural effusion, hypoxemia, ARDS, and hypocalcemia. As acute pancreatitis resolves, pancreatic pseudocyst or pancreatic abscess may develop. In some, pancreatic endocrine or exocrine dysfunction (i.e., diabetes mellitus, malabsorption and steatorrhea) may be prominent.

CLINICAL PRESENTATION

Although no findings are pathognomonic, abdominal pain is almost always present and often severe; it may be diffuse but is often localized to the epigastrium or left upper quadrant and back. The pain is exacerbated by recumbency and relieved by sitting up and flexing forward. Nausea and vomiting are noted in most. On examination, there is abdominal tenderness and guarding. Fever, tachycardia, and diaphoresis also may be noted. Elevated serum amylase activity may be present but amylase can also come from extrapancreatic locations (salivary glands, small intestine, and female genital tract). Reliance on the amylase level alone may be misleading.

Hemorrhagic or necrotizing acute pancreatitis is a systemic disease. Intravascular volume loss from pancreatic hemorrhage, to massive edema and exudation of fluid into the peritoneal cavity, or to systemic effects of released vasoactive substances may lead to frank hypovolemic shock. Two classic signs of retroperitoneal hemorrhage are Cullen's sign (periumbilical ecchymosis) and Grey Turner's sign (flank ecchymosis), but these are uncommon. In some cases the clinical picture is dominated by manifestations of remote organ system dysfunction or by the systemic effects of pancreatic abscess.

TABLE 145-1. Causes of Acute Pancreatitis

Metabolic	**Vascular**
Ethyl alcohol and methyl alcohol	Vasculitis
Hyperlipoproteinemias (types I, IV, V)	Atheroembolism
Drugs (azathioprine, estrogens, corticosteroids,	Surgery
tetracycline, diuretics, sulfonamides, valproic acid)	Shock
Hypercalcemia	**Infectious**
Scorpion venom	
Heredity	Coxsackie virus
Pregnancy	Campylobacter
Mechanical	Mycoplasma
	Legionnaire's disease
Biliary tract disease	Mumps
Abdominal surgery	
Trauma	
Endoscopic retrograde cholangiopancreatography	
Upper gastrointestinal endoscopy	
Carcinoma of the pancreas	
Duodenal obstruction	
Posterior penetrating ulcer	

Adapted from Geokas MC, Baltaxe HA, Banks PA, et al: Acute pancreatitis. Ann Intern Med 103:86, 1985; Nakashima Y, Howard JM: Drug-induced acute pancreatitis. Surg Gynecol Obstet 145:105, 1977; Ranson JHC: Etiologic and prognostic factors in human acute pancreatitis: A review. Am J Gastroenterol 77: 633, 1982.

DIFFERENTIAL DIAGNOSIS

The most common conditions confused with acute pancreatitis are acute cholecystitis and peptic ulcer disease, but any intra-abdominal emergency may be mimicked. The pain of cholecystitis is located more often in the right upper quadrant, tends to be more gradual in onset, and is not always constant. Ultrasound examination and radionuclide scanning are useful in establishing the diagnosis of biliary tract disease. An elevation of the alkaline phosphatase in the absence of a comparable elevation in serum transaminases also is suggestive. Although simple acute cholecystitis may be complicated by acute pancreatitis, the serum amylase may be elevated in both conditions. Gallstones should be excluded early in acute pancreatitis because their presence is associated with increased morbidity and mortality.

Alcoholic gastritis is seen with alcohol-induced pancreatitis, and distinguishing the two is often difficult or impossible. Tenderness and peritoneal signs are more likely to represent pancreatitis, but a posterior penetrating ulcer may produce features of both illnesses. Other serious disorders causing abdominal pain and elevated amylase include intestinal obstruction, ruptured ectopic pregnancy, mesenteric infarction, dissecting aortic aneurysm, peritonitis, acute appendicitis, and diabetic ketoacidosis. Myocardial infarction, pneumonia, and renal colic should also be considered.

EMERGENCY DEPARTMENT EVALUATION

The challenge of suspected pancreatitis is to make the diagnosis and to exclude other causes. The severity of the disease affects the disposition. The diagnosis is based on the history and physical examination and is *supported* by laboratory studies, notably the serum amylase level. The diagnosis should be questioned if the amylase is normal although a normal amylase may be found in 33% of patients with pancreatitis. Amylase is nonspecific. The urinary amylase/creatinine clearance (Cam/Ccr) appears to offer no advantage. There is no correlation between the severity of the disease and the degree of amylase elevation. Some patients with many episodes of acute pancreatitis may have a "burned out" pancreas that releases little amylase. Serum lipase is the confirmatory test used most widely when the diagnosis of pancreatitis is in doubt. Because the pancreas is the only major source of lipase, an increased level is very specific.

Plain radiographs of the chest and abdomen should be obtained to rule out other entities (pneumoperitoneum, small bowel obstruction, and aortic dissection or aneurysm.) The abdominal radiograph in acute pancreatitis may show regional or localized ileus ("sentinel loop"), gallstones, widening of the duodenal sweep, blurring of the left renal outline and psoas margin, elevation of one or both hemidiaphragms, or pleural or pericardial effusion. Pancreatic calcifications indicate that previous episodes of acute pancreatitis have occurred and are diagnostic of chronic pancreatitis.

Other imaging studies can be helpful. Ultrasonography can identify pancreatic edema as well as such complications as pancreatic pseudocyst or abscess. It also is useful in identifying the presence of gallstones or dilatation of the biliary tree. Computed tomographic (CT) scanning is the study of choice for visualizing the pancreas; it also identifys pseudocyst, abscess, or fistula.

Once the diagnosis is made, the next priority is to determine its severity. About 5–10% of patients develop serious complications or die from the disease. An increased risk of complications correlates with certain clinical features, the so-called Ranson criteria or their modifications (Table 145-2). Cardiopulmonary collapse or neurologic impairment are also poor prognostic signs.

EMERGENCY DEPARTMENT MANAGEMENT

Ninety percent of all cases pancreatitis may be treated with supportive measures only. Oral intake of clear liquids is not harmful in mild to moderately severe cases. Intravenous fluids should be administered as needed, and electrolyte abnormalities, such as hypokalemia, hypocalcemia, and

TABLE 145-2. Ranson Criteria for Predicting the Severity of Acute Pancreatitis

On Admission	Within 48 Hours
Age > 55 years	BUN > 5 mg/dL
WBC > 16,000/mm³	PaO$_2$ < 60 mm Hg
Blood glucose > 200 mg/dL	Serum Ca < 8 mg/dL
LDH > 350 IU/L	Hct fall > 10%
AST > 250 U/L	Base deficit > 4 mEq/L
	Fluid sequestration > 6 L

Mortality is based on number of prognostic signs as follows: 0–2, 1%; 3–4, 15%; 5–6, 40%; >6, 100%.

Adapted from Ranson JHC: Etiologic and prognostic factors in human acute pancreatitis: A review. Am J Gastroenterol 77:663, 1982; Ranson JHC: Risk factors in acute pancreatitis. Hosp Pract 4:69, 1985.

hypomagnesemia, corrected. In patients with moderate to severe pain, meperidine is the analgesic of choice because it is thought to cause less spasm of the ampulla of Vater than morphine. Anti-emetics such as prochlorperazine or hydroxyzine may be given for vomiting.

Nasogastric suction has not been shown to offer any additional benefit in mild to moderate pancreatitis if ileus is not present. Likewise, anticholinergics are of no value. Cimetidine has no benefit. About 5% of cases result in serious complications or death. These patients require aggressive fluid replacement. A CVP or Swan–Ganz catheter and urinary catheter may be needed to monitor intravascular volume status and to guide fluid replacement. In patients with ileus or intractable vomiting, a nasogastric tube should be inserted. Antibiotic administration should be reserved for those patients with evidence of established infection.

DISPOSITION

Patients with mild pancreatitis with no biliary tract disease may be managed on an outpatient basis if they are able to tolerate clear liquids and have no evidence of systemic complications. A clear liquid diet, oral analgesics and close follow-up should be arranged. Patients with alcohol-associated pancreatitis should be encouraged to stop drinking. All other patients must be admitted. If hemorrhagic or necrotizing acute pancreatitis is suspected, admission to an ICU is mandatory for monitoring of cardiac, pulmonary, and renal function.

In the patient with unremitting fulminant pancreatitis, a surgeon should be consulted for possible laparotomy to debride the necrotic pancreas and to ensure that there is no other cause amenable to surgical treatment. Prompt surgery is indicated with signs of sepsis or pancreatic abscess. For patients who do not respond to initial supportive measures, peritoneal lavage has been recommended to help remove the toxic pancreatic exudate from the abdominal cavity. Individuals with gallstone-induced pancreatitis may benefit from early endoscopic papillotomy.

COMMON PITFALLS

- No clinical or laboratory finding is pathognomonic of pancreatitis. The serum amylase is not specific for pancreatitis, nor is an elevated serum amylase a *sine qua non* of the diagnosis. Other disorders causing abdominal pain and elevated serum amylase must be excluded before the diagnosis of pancreatitis can be made.
- Underestimating the severity of an attack must be avoided. The Ranson criteria provide objective guidelines to identify the patient with a high likelihood of clinical deterioration.

146   Hepatitis

Viruses are responsible for most cases of acute hepatitis: hepatitis A virus (HAV), hepatitis B virus (HBV), the non-A, non-B viruses (NANB), and the hepatitis D virus (HDV), also called the delta agent. Epstein-Barr virus (EBV), cytomegalovirus (CMV), and other viruses are known to cause hepatitis as part of a systemic infection (Table 146-1) as will toxic and anoxic processes.

CLINICAL PRESENTATION

The clinical manifestations are protean and variable in severity, duration and ultimate outcome. The course depends on the etiology, pre-existing or underlying liver disease, and interaction between host factors and the pathogen. Classically, viral hepatitis has a characteristic picture: after a variable incubation period, a "prodromal phase" occurs, with anorexia, low-grade fever, malaise, and lassitude. Often characterized as "flu-like," symptoms are nonspecific. Gastrointestinal symptoms may predominate, and abdominal discomfort reported. Within days to weeks after the onset of symptoms, the patient with an "icteric phase" notes discoloration of the urine, followed by light (clay-colored) stools, scleral icterus and clinical jaundice if the serum bilirubin level exceeds 3 to 4 mg/dl. At this point, symptoms may begin to resolve with the convalescent phase.

Physical findings are variable: the examination may be normal or may reveal jaundice and hepatic dysfunction. Liver enlargement and tenderness are common, and splenomegaly and lymphadenopathy are seen in 15–20%. Extrahepatic manifestations are prevalent in hepatitis B and are may be due to immune-complex formation: urticaria, morbilliform rashes, arthralgias, arthritis, hematuria and proteinuria, and less often vasculitis. Occasionally a patient presents with advanced hepatic failure and no history of previous hepatitis. This occurs in progressive chronic hepatitis, a toxic insult, or acute-on-chronic hepatitis. Unexplained encephalopathy, coagulopathy, hypoglycemia, or respiratory alkalosis should prompt consideration of a hepatic disorder.

DIFFERENTIAL DIAGNOSIS OF VIRAL HEPATITIS

Acute viral hepatitis is characterized by four stages: the incubation period, the pre-icteric phase, the icteric phase, and convalescence. During the incubation period there are no clinical manifestations of disease. All hepatotropic viruses are capable of producing a similar clinical picture. It is imperative to understand the serologic markers associated with the various types.

TABLE 146-1. Viruses Known to Cause Hepatitis

Primary Hepatitis Viruses	Secondary Hepatitis Viruses
Hepatitis A (HAV)	Epstein-Barr
Hepatitis B (HBV)	Cytomegalovirus
Hepatitis D (HDV)	Herpes simplex
Non-A non-B (NANB)	Varicella-zoster
Waterborne	Rubella
Blood transmitted	Rubeola
Coagulation-factor transmitted	Mumps
	Adenovirus
	Coxsackie B
	Yellow fever

HEPATITIS A

The hepatitis A virus (HAV) is spread primarily by the fecal–oral route, although the virus can be found in the blood as well as the liver, bile, and stool late in the incubation period. The 2-week period before jaundice occurs is the time of greatest infectivity; infectivity diminishes markedly when the icteric phase begins (Fig. 146-1). Source outbreaks are the result of fecal contamination of water supplies or contaminated food. The disease also may be spread by oral–anal contact. The incubation period is 2 to 7 weeks.

The "pre-icteric" lasts 4–14 days, with nonspecific symptoms (weakness, malaise, anorexia, nausea, and vomiting). There may be pain in the right upper quadrant and a characteristic loss of taste for cigarettes. The term "pre-icteric" is presumptive, because not all patients go on to have clinically evident jaundice. Dark urine may herald the icteric phase, and often prompts medical attention. Most of the other symptoms resolve shortly after the appearance of jaundice Jaundice appears in the minority of patients infected with hepatitis A virus, but may persist for up to a month.

The convalescent period is variable; weakness and malaise may last for months. Figure 146-1 depicts the serologic and biochemical course of hepatitis A. The ALT (formerly SGPT) level begins to rise late in the incubation phase, just before the onset of symptoms. During the symptomatic period, about 4 to 5 weeks after exposure, IgM antibodies to HAV (anti-HAV IgM) begin to rise. Because this antibody usually becomes undetectable after 4 to 5 months, its presence implies recent infection; HAV itself is not measured. Antibodies of the IgG variety (anti-HAV IgG) rise a little later and remain detectable for life. The presence of such antibodies in the serum of at least 50% of adults reflects the high incidence of asymptomatic or unrecognized disease early in life and is responsible for the effectiveness of pooled serum in preventing disease in exposed individuals.

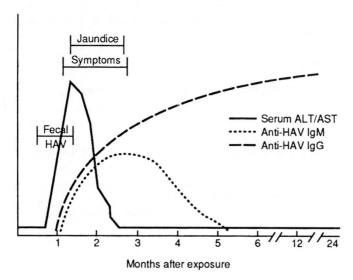

Figure 146-1. Serologic course of viral hepatitis A. Children usually have only mild symptoms with no jaundice. Adults more often develop jaundice. (Adapted from Hoofnagle JH: Serologic diagnosis of acute and chronic hepatitis. In Hepatology Update/Portal Hypertension; Viral Hepatitis [postgraduate course of the American Association for the Study of Liver Diseases]. In Hosp Med 6:26, 1988.)

HEPATITIS B

The hepatitis B virus (HBV) is spread by the parenteral route, including exposure to blood, via contaminated needles and syringes (both in drug abusers and health care workers), infected excretions or saliva; sexual contact; and perinatal contact. Its prevalence is high among homosexual men, IV drug abusers, dialysis patients, clients and staff of institutions for the mentally retarded, and in certain endemic regions of the world. Hepatitis B has an incubation period of 45–160 days. During this phase the virus is actively replicating and is present in virtually all body fluids, including blood, saliva, semen, and vaginal secretions. The implications are important—patients can transmit disease during this incubation period, biochemical and serologic markers can be measured before disease becomes clinically apparent, and immunoprophylactic measures given after exposure but before the onset of symptoms may prevent or ameliorate the disease.

Acute hepatitis B usually follows a course similar to that of hepatitis A. Jaundice is more likely to occur in hepatitis B but still occurs in a minority of cases. About 80–85% resolve completely, leaving the patient immune. One percent to 3% evolve into fulminant hepatitis, with a mortality rate of 90%; the remaining 5–10% become chronic. The serologic and biochemical course of acute hepatitis B is depicted in Figure 146-2. The first marker to appear in the serum is the hepatitis B surface antigen (HGsAg), indicating infection with hepatitis B. Next, DNA polymerase, HBV DNA, and the hepatitis e antigen (HBeAg) appear in the serum. These reflect active HBV replication and infectivity and appear well before the onset of biochemical damage to the liver. Of this group, only HBeAg can be measured easily; the presence of antibody to the HBeAG (anti-HBe) suggests low infectivity.

In patients who become symptomatic, the ALT rises and, in some, jaundice appears. Most patients seen at this time will still be HBs Ag positive. The next *important* immunologic event is

Acute type B hepatitis

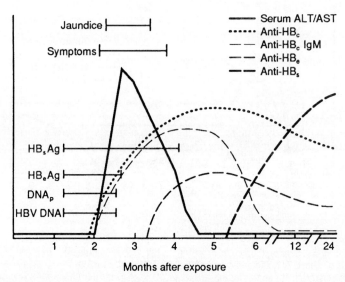

Figure 146-2. Serologic course of acute hepatitis B. This is more likely to cause jaundice than type A or non-A/non-B types. (From Hosp Med 6:33, 1988.)

the appearance of antibody to the hepatitis B core antigen (anti-HBc), first of the IgM class and then IgG. This rise precedes the rise in antibodies to the surface antigen (anti-HBs). (In Fig. 146-2, note the gap between the box labeled HBsAg and the line labeled anti-HBs.) Therefore, in some patients recently infected with HBV seen during this gap or "window," the sole specific marker of recent infection with HBV is the presence of anti-HBc IgM.

Anti-HBsAg is a neutralizing antibody and therefore its rise correlates with abatement of symptoms and the return of ALT to normal levels, and signifies immunity to HBV. Thereafter, the patient will test positively only for anti-HBs, anti-HBc IgG, and anti-HBe. The *carrier state* occurs when HBsAg remains positive for 6 months or more in the absence of clinical or laboratory features of acute infection. Some but not all carriers represent a source of infection (those with circulating HBV particles and HBeAG). The carriage rate in the USA is only 0.1–0.5%, although in some parts of the world it is 5–20%.

Chronic persistent hepatitis (CPH) and *chronic active hepatitis (CAH)* are two distinct forms of chronic liver disease that may be due to hepatitis B or other causes. Although each has distinct clinical presentations and biochemical profiles, the diagnosis can only be made histologically. Symptoms and biochemical abnormalities tend to be less severe with CPH, and the long-term prognosis is generally good. Biochemical abnormalities and clinical manifestations are more severe in CAH, and the long-term prognosis poor, with progression to cirrhosis and end-stage liver disease. Treatment with immunosuppressive agents (prednisone and azathioprine) may be beneficial in CAH unrelated to hepatitis B. Figure 146-3 depicts the serologic course of chronic HBV disease. Note that the HBsAg remains positive, antibodies (anti-HBs) are lacking, and the patient remains susceptible to further liver damage or to superinfection with hepatitis D (see below).

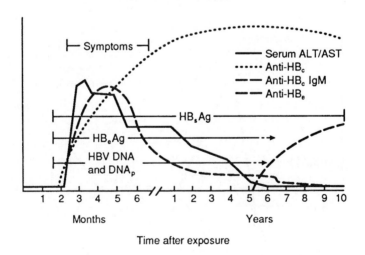

Figure 146-3. Serologic course of chronic HBV disease. (Adapted from Hoofnagle JH: Serologic diagnosis of acute and chronic hepatitis. In Hepatitis Update/Portal Hypertension; Viral Hepatitis [postgraduate course of the American Association for the Study of Liver Diseases]. In Hosp Med 6:33, 1988.)

HEPATITIS D

Hepatitis D (delta) is caused by a defective virus dependent on the presence of HBsAg synthesis. The virus consists of the delta-antigen-bearing core encapsulated by an HBsAg coat. It follows a similar transmission pattern as HPV. The clinical course of HDV depends on whether it is acquired at the same time as HBV (co-infection), or whether HDV infects a patient with chronic HBV infection (superinfection). In co-infection, the fate of HDV parallels that of HBV. Because most cases of acute HBV subsequently are cleared, HDV, which requires the presence of HBV for replication, also is cleared. The clinical course of HDV is similar to that described for hepatitis B, although it frequently is more severe. Because patients with HDV superinfection have not been able to mount an immunologic response sufficient to clear their HBV infection, HDV replication may result in fulminant hepatitis. Immunity to hepatitis B renders one immune to hepatitis D infection. Table 146-2 lists the serologic features of HBV/HDV co-infection and HBV/HDV superinfection.

NON-A, NON-B HEPATITIS

At least three viruses (other than D) with no serologic markers can cause non-A, non-B hepatitis (NANB). The lack of serologic markers makes specific screening of blood impossible and has thwarted attempts to ensure blood free of these agents. The first virus,"Waterborne non-A, non-B hepatitis," has not occurred in Western countries. The second virus is "blood-transmitted non-A, non-B hepatitis"; it develops in 5–15% of those who receive 1–5 units of blood; 71% are asymptomatic, 4% anicteric with nonspecific symptoms, and 25% icteric with symptoms similar to those seen in hepatitis B. Chronic hepatitis is common, but fulminant hepatitis is a rare sequela. "Coagulation-factor-transmitted non-A, non-B hepatitis" is the third type; it produces less severe disease than the blood-transmitted type and is less prevalent. It is seen in hemophiliacs.

DIFFERENTIAL DIAGNOSIS OF HEPATITIS FROM INFECTIOUS, NONVIRAL CAUSES

Hepatitis can accompany a wide variety of bacterial, rickettsial, and protozoal diseases.

TOXIC AND METABOLIC CAUSES

Liver injury from toxic or metabolic causes may result from direct hepatocellular toxicity or from idiosyncratic injury due to a hypersensitivity-type reaction. Toxic exposures also may manifest as cholestasis, in which elevations of alkaline phosphatase and bilirubin predominate. Pharmacologic and chemical agents are shown in Table 146-3. *Acetaminophen* may be responsible for striking liver enzyme elevations. Toxicity is dose dependent, but concomitant alcohol ingestion, chronic phenobarbital use, or chronic exposure to moderately large doses of acetaminophen contribute synergistically. Hepatitis due to *isoniazid* resembles acute viral hepatitis and may occur in 20% taking the drug; the risk and severity of injury increase with the age of the patient. Clinical toxic-

---

TABLE 146-2. Serologic Factors in HBV/HDV Coinfection and HBV/HDV Superinfection

HBV/HDV Coinfection		HBV/HDV Superinfection	
HBsAg+* anti-HBcIgM+	(implies recent) HBV infection	anti-HBcIgM– anti-HBcIgG+	
anti-delta IgM+	(implies recent) HDV infection	anti-delta IgM+	(implies chronic HBV infection)

*Unless in window period.

TABLE 146-3. Drug-Induced Hepatitis

Clinical/Morphologic Presentation	Examples
Hepatitis—acute	Alpha-methyldopa
	Isoniazid
	Phenytoin
	Chlorathiazide
	Nonsteroidal anti-inflammatory agents
	Lovastatin
Cholestasis	Anabolic steroids
	Oral contraceptive agents
	Erythromycin estolate
	Methimazole
	Chlorpropamide
	Chlorpromazine
Hepatic necrosis	Carbon tetrachloride
	Amanita phalloides mushrooms
	Acetaminophen
	Yellow phosphorous
Hepatitis—chronic	Alpha-methyldopa
	Arsenic
	Isoniazid
	Halothane

ity occurs in the first few months of therapy, but progression to fulminant hepatitis may occur at any stage.

   Lovastatin is a cholesterol-lowering agent; concomitant use of nicotinic acid (also used for hypercholesterolemia) may promote additional toxicity.Hepatotoxicity to *phenytoin* is unusual; serious toxicity is caused by toxic metabolites, a heritable metabolic defect that may predispose to a viral hepatitis-like hypersensitivity reaction within weeks of starting therapy at usual therapeutic doses.

   Hepatitis has been reported to be associated with the use of several of the *nonsteroidal anti-inflammatory drugs (NSAIDs)*. Diclofenac has been well established as a cause of hepatitis, including fatal hepatic necrosis; it is the only NSAID for which routine evaluation of liver function tests is recommended.

   Another cause of elevated transaminases (transaminitis) is *hepatobiliary disease*. Elevated ALT and AST levels should not suggest hepatitis or toxicity when the chemistry patterns suggest hepatobiliary obstruction (i.e., elevated serum bilirubin, alkaline phosphatase [Alk], and gamma glutamyl transpeptidase levels [GGTP]).

EMERGENCY DEPARTMENT EVALUATION

The first step is to make the diagnosis. If the likelihood of hepatitis is present but low, a reasonable approach is to order a serum AST (SGOT) level as a screen. The AST is released with hepatocellular injury. Although nonspecific, it is sensitive, and a normal AST virtually excludes hepatocellular disease. In the patient likely to have hepatocellular disease or with abnormal AST, more extensive laboratory testing is necessary, consisting of AST and ALT (necrosis) and Alk, total bilirubin, or GGTP (cholestasis). Although they lack diagnostic specificity, patterns may be helpful in limiting the differential.

A transaminase elevation of >10 times normal strongly suggests acute viral or toxic injury and essentially excludes chronic hepatitis. Elevation of alkaline phosphatase and bilirubin suggests intrahepatic or extrahepatic obstruction. Transaminase elevations of two to three times normal, with the AST higher than the ALT, suggest alcoholic injury.

The second step after the diagnosis of liver disease has been made is to determine hepatic synthetic function: serum protein, albumin, and glucose. These can be used in conjunction with the serum bilirubin level to assess the extent of hepatocellular dysfunction. An arterial ammonia level may be obtained if CNS dysfunction is present.

The third step defines more specifically the cause of the illness. If hepatocellular necrosis is the dominant picture, detailed serologic studies (anti-HAV IgM, HBsAg, anti-HBs, anti-HBc, and Monospot test) are warranted, as well as a search for risks for NANB, drug, or toxic exposures. If cholestasis is the dominant picture, ultrasound examination should be performed to exclude mechanical obstruction. If none is found, a search for drug or toxic exposures is warranted.

EMERGENCY DEPARTMENT MANAGEMENT

Patients with acute viral hepatitis may present with a viral-like syndrome (prostration, nausea, vomiting, and dehydration). Treatment is symptomatic and limited to IV fluids, acetaminophen, and anti-emetics. Metoclopramide (Reglan) is the anti-emetic of choice, because phenothiazines may impair hepatic function and produce cholestasis. There is no specific therapy beyond routine supportive care and symptomatic treatment. If the prothrombin time is prolonged, the patient should receive IV vitamin K. Immunoglobulin (Ig) is of no use in the patient who has already contracted hepatitis. Corticosteroids are probably harmful.

Patients who present because they have been or think they have been exposed present a different problem. (For needle-stick patients, see Chapter 168.) Immunoprophylaxis is highly effective if given under the proper circumstances. Because this treatment should be guided in part by serologic studies, it is often not initiated in the ED. If serologies are not available, therapy is empiric and based on probabilities (Table 146-4). Patients at risk for contracting hepatitis A include household and sexual contacts of persons with hepatitis A; staff/attendees at day-care centers; and staff/residents in close contact at custodial care institutions. Ig is given as a single intramuscular dose of 0.02 mL/kg as soon as possible within the first 2 weeks after exposure. Casual contacts need not be treated, needing only reassurance.

TABLE 146-4. Immunoprophylaxis or Viral Hepatitis

Type	Persons at Risk	Immunoprophylaxis
A	Household and sexual contacts* Staff, attendees of daycare centers Staff, residents of custodial institution	IG 0.02 mL/kg IM
B	Sexual contacts Percutaneous or transmucosal exposure	HBIG 0.06 mg/kg IM Begin active immunization (Heptavax or Recombivax)
D	Same as B	Protection against Hepatitis B
NANB	Percutaneous exposure to blood or certain products of patients with no serologic evidence or HAV or HBV	IG 0.06 mL/kg IM, repeat in 30 days

*Dormitories and barracks are frequently considered in this group.

Postexposure prophylaxis for hepatitis B is indicated for sexual contacts of persons with hepatitis B, or after percutaneous or transmucosal exposure to HBsAg-positive blood. Treatment is with hepatitis B immunoglobulin (HBIg) 0.06 mL/kg IM; active immunization is begun at the same time. This assumes that serologic data are available on the index patient with hepatitis, and that the immune status of the exposed patient is known. If the data are not available but can be obtained within 5–7 days, it is reasonable to wait. If not, one must make a decision based on life styles and risk factors, including sexual contacts and IV drug use.

For individuals in whom NANB exposure is suspected because of exposure to blood from a patient with hepatitis but negative serologies, Ig 0.06 mL/kg intramuscularly should be given.

DISPOSITION

Most patients with hepatitis do not require admission. Hospitalization is recommended under the following circumstances: persistent nausea and vomiting unresponsive to treatment; dehydration or electrolyte imbalance that cannot be corrected in the ED during a reasonable length of stay; or signs of hepatic deterioration, as evidenced by changes in sensorium or prolongation of the prothrombin time (50% activity is commonly used as a criterion). A fulminant course warrants admission. The absolute levels of serum transaminases should not be a criterion for admission.

Patients discharged home should be given anti-emetics and instructions on adequate caloric intake. Small meals of foods of choice often work better than the high-calorie or high-protein dietary regimens. Prolonged bed rest is of no value; indeed, most patients will limit their physical activities as needed. Alcohol consumption should be avoided. After complete recovery, alcohol consumption is no more harmful than for the general population. Estrogen-based oral contraceptives may be continued during hepatitis.

Patients should be seen by an internist or gastroenterologist for follow-up within a few days after the results of serologic tests. Patients with any prolongation of the prothrombin time are often admitted to the hospital, but those who are not should be rechecked within 24 hours. Instructions should include: return if food and fluids cannot be kept down or if there is any change in sensorium. It is the duty in many locales to notify public health authorities of cases of acute hepatitis.

COMMON PITFALLS

Diagnostic errors
- Missed toxic ingestion or exposure
- Failure to diagnose surgically correctable lesions
- Diagnosis of viral or alcoholic hepatitis as hepatobiliary disease
- Failure to recognize atypical presentations as secondary phenomena of liver disease and not primary events (e.g., coagulopathy, altered mental status, psychiatric abnormalities, hypoglycemia)
- Failure to recognize the distinction between liver tests and liver function
- Inappropriate admission of patients with uncomplicated hepatitis and markedly elevated ALT or AST without evaluation of synthetic factors or clinical status
- Inappropriate discharge of patients with early evidence of synthetic failure
- Excessive ED evaluation because of inappropriate use of strategies and preliminary laboratory results
- Failure to follow-up contacts for recommended prophylaxis
- Inappropriate restrictions: patients with hepatitis need not be excluded from school or work simply because of the diagnosis of hepatitis; education regarding precautions is indicated
- Administration of hepatotoxic drugs for symptomatic treatment in patients with hepatic injury (e.g., phenothiazines, nonsteroidal anti-inflammatory)
- Administration of hepatically cleared drugs with resultant decreased clearance and high serum levels or duration of action

147   Hepatic Failure and Cirrhosis

Although acute hepatic failure differs clinically and prognostically from an exacerbation of chronic liver failure, the emergency diagnostic and therapeutic priorities for the management of both entities are similar. Despite recent advances in the management of hepatic encephalopathy, the exact mechanism for the widespread neural inhibition continues to elude investigators. Ammonia, a substance liberated from the intestinal flora and known to accumulate in hepatic failure, has been suggested as the cause of hepatic encephalopathy, but ammonia accumulation causes an excitable state rather than neural inhibition, and the severity of hepatic coma does not correlate well with blood ammonia levels.

No single mechanism has explained all the features of this disorder. Viral hepatitis continues to be the most common cause of fulminant hepatic failure (FHF) worldwide. Acetaminophen overdose, acute and chronic ingestion of isoniazid and rifampin, and Reye's syndrome are other important causes of FHF. Less common causes include fatty degeneration of pregnancy, *Amanita phalloides* mushroom poisoning, and metastatic liver cancer. Hepatic cirrhosis most commonly is caused by alcoholism; chronic active hepatitis is the second most common cause. Progressive destruction occurs over several years with resulting fibrosis. Hepatocellular dysfunction results in impaired glycogen storage, coagulopathy, and loss of detoxifying capability. Continued fibrosis shunts blood away into the portal vein, resulting in secondary portal hypertension and esophageal varices.

CLINICAL PRESENTATION

The presentation of FHF depends in part on the etiology, but most patients have altered mentation, coagulopathy with clinical bleeding, jaundice, motor dysfunction, and fetor hepaticas. Hepatotoxic drugs such as acetaminophen may cause abdominal pain. The manifestations of hepatic encephalopathy in both FHF and cirrhosis are similar, but the onset is generally slower with cirrhosis. FHF may present with rapid deterioration of mental status over several hours from slowed responses to coma. Cirrhosis presents with euphoria, depression, or muscular incoordination, or more obvious mental status changes. Symptoms such as malaise, lethargy, fluid retention, loss of libido, and pruritus are common, and typical findings include hepatomegaly, spider nevi, ascites, and jaundice. Asterixis is a classic sign not always present. The most common precipitating factors for hepatic encephalopathy in cirrhotics are gastrointestinal bleeding, tranquilizing drugs or alcohol, overuse of diuretics, and infection.

COMPLICATIONS OF HEPATIC FAILURE AND CIRRHOSIS

The most common cause of death in FHF is cerebral edema. Hypoglycemia may be profound and recurrent. More than 50% of patients have coagulopathy, usually with gastrointestinal, nasopharyngeal, or bronchial bleeding. Hypotension from decreased systemic vascular resistance may occur in the absence of hemorrhage. Patients are tachypneic but increasing the pCO_2 toward normal leads to deterioration. Hypoxia and noncardiogenic pulmonary edema are common. Prerenal azotemia, acute tubular necrosis, or renal failure may occur. Hypokalemia and hypocalcemia are common. Infection is also seen with sepsis accounting for 11% of deaths. Because of portal hypertension and esophageal varices, death from gastrointestinal bleeding is more common with cirrhosis than with FHF.

Patients with cirrhosis have an increased incidence of pneumonia, sepsis, bacteremia, spontaneous bacterial peritonitis, and endotoxemia. In the later stages, ascites may become symptomatic and limit ventilation. The hepatorenal syndrome occurs in advanced cirrhosis and is usually fatal, despite treatment.

DIFFERENTIAL DIAGNOSIS

The differential diagnosis of jaundice includes hemolysis, obstructive jaundice, viral hepatitis, hepatotoxic ingestions, septicemia, and numerous minor causes. Mental status change and jaundice should suggest hepatic encephalopathy. Without chronic liver disease, the differential of hepatic encephalopathy includes viral hepatitis, fatty degeneration of pregnancy, Reye's syndrome, and hepatotoxic ingestions such as acetaminophen, isoniazid, rifampin, *Amanita phalloides* mushrooms, or carbon tetrachloride. Information such as pre-illness activity, previous suicidal behavior, and the presence of fever or malaise is useful. There are few clinical features to differentiate hepatic encephalopathy from other causes of acute mental status change with the exception of fetor hepaticas (commonly mistaken for halitosis).

Patients with cirrhosis may have chronic jaundice and develop mental status changes from other causes. Because alcoholic patients are at greater risk for trauma, subdural hematoma must be ruled out. Alcoholics may develop pancreatitis or alcoholic hepatitis, with dehydration and mental status changes that mimic hepatic encephalopathy.

EMERGENCY DEPARTMENT EVALUATION

Information should be sought from prehospital personnel, family, the patient's private physician, and previous medical records. The conjunctiva and skin should be examined for the presence of jaundice. The respiratory system should be assessed for possible aspiration or pulmonary edema. Although an enlarged liver is common in alcoholic liver disease, the liver is usually small in FHF or advanced cirrhosis. A rectal exam and stool guaiac should be done. A neurologic exam should focus on changes in mental status and focal findings. Asterixis, alterations in motor tone, or abnormal posturing should be noted. Hypoxemia and hypoglycemia should be ruled out. A serum ammonia level should be measured, but patients may be encephalopathic before serum ammonia is elevated. A CBC, electrolytes, and coagulation studies are required; aminotransferases, bilirubin, serologic tests, and serum amino acids may aid in diagnosis. An ECG is advisable. The diagnosis of hepatic encephalopathy is clinical; no single test confirms the diagnosis with certainty.

EMERGENCY DEPARTMENT MANAGEMENT

Endotracheal intubation is indicated if the patient is critically ill, obtunded or comatose. Patients should be monitored. Fluid resuscitation should be aggressive in hypotensive or bleeding patients and should be undertaken despite the possibility of pulmonary edema. Pulmonary capillary wedge pressure measurements may be needed. An accucheck should be done and 50% dextrose given if necessary as well as IV thiamine. Signs of increased intracranial pressure should be evaluated after stabilization with a head CT; mannitol 1 gm/kg IV may be indicated as well as hyperventilation to an arterial pCO_2 of 25 mm Hg. Fresh frozen plasma should be given when the prothrombin time is >1.5 times normal. Platelet infusions are usually not necessary.

Spontaneous bacteremia and spontaneous bacterial peritonitis are common in cirrhosis and FHF. The responsible organisms are usually gram negative; cefotaxime or a similar broad-spectrum cephalosporin is recommended. Aspiration pneumonia should always be considered. Lactulose increases intestinal motility and lowers colonic pH; it accelerates recovery from hepatic coma. Lactulose enemas are given in a dose of 200 mg; lactitol may be more effective. Oral neomycin, 2–4 gm/day, is effective, but should be withheld if an aminoglycoside is given. Exchange transfusion, extracorporeal liver perfusion, hemodialysis, plasmapheresis, hemoperfusion, and administration of branched-chain amino acids are best made by a gastroenterology consultant.

Gastrointestinal bleeding in the cirrhotic is more difficult to manage than in FHF.

Endoscopic sclerotherapy appears to be the best method to manage variceal bleeding. A porta-caval shunt to prevent rebleeding may be necessary. The patient with cirrhosis and a non-life-threatening condition should avoid medications that cause deterioration (sedatives, nonsteroidal anti-inflammatory drugs, acetaminophen). Symptomatic ascites from cirrhosis is probably best manageed with paracentesis, and not diuretics.

DISPOSITION

Indications for admission to the hospital should be liberal. Cirrhotics have limited ability to resist infection, so IV antibiotics and admission should be considered for most infections. Patients with advanced hepatic encephalopathy require admission to an ICU, and immediate consultation with a gastroenterologist is indicated. Consideration may be given to transporting the patient to a "liver center," provided such a facility is within a reasonable distance and ALS transport is available.

COMMON PITFALLS

- Patients with hepatotoxic drug ingestion may be unwilling to provide this history (aceta-minophen).
- The diagnosis of hepatic encephalopathy cannot be ruled out on the basis of a serum ammo-nia level.
- Hypoglycemia should be evaluated immediately and treated.
- It is essential to consider other causes of coma: subdural hematoma, drug overdose, and meningitis.

148   Inflammatory Bowel Disease

Inflammatory bowel disease (IBD) consists of ulcerative colitis and regional enteritis or Crohn's disease. Both are characterized by recurrent episodes of gastrointestinal disturbances separated by periods of remission, and both have a variety of systemic manifestations. IBD must be con-sidered in the differential diagnosis of patients with gastrointestinal complaints, particularly with recurrent complaints. Patients with well established diagnoses of IBD often present for manage-ment of acute exacerbations and complications. The cause of IBD is unknown. There is a bimodal distribution of the age of onset, with peaks at 15–25 years and at 55–60 years. About 30% have relatives who also are affected. Interestingly, the incidence of Crohn's disease has been rising over the past 20 years; ulcerative colitis has remained stable.

Ulcerative colitis tends to remain localized to the colon; in most patients, the disease is found in the rectum and left colon only, but the entire colon may be involved in the most severe cases. Ulcerative colitis is usually limited to the intestinal mucosa and submucosa.

Crohn's disease is found along the entire gastrointestinal tract. In 30% of patients, only the terminal ileum is involved. Twenty percent have colonic disease only, and in 50% both small and large bowel are affected. The lesions tend to involve the entire bowel wall and extend into the mesentery. Deep ulcerations commonly penetrate the bowel wall and cause fissures, fistulae, and abscesses. About 50% will manifest perianal complications (abscesses, fistulae, fissures, and skin tags).

CLINICAL PRESENTATION

The most common presentation (seen in 75–80%) of Crohn's disease includes chronic diarrhea, abdominal pain, fever, anorexia, and weight loss. However, the symptoms are nonspecific, so there is typically a long delay (weeks to months) in making the diagnosis.

The presentation of ulcerative colitis is variable and quite similar to that of Crohn's disease. In fact, separation of the two by clinical findings alone can be very difficult. In mild cases, constipation and rectal bleeding may be the only complaints. In the most severe form, many bloody diarrheal stools per day, fever, tachycardia, crampy abdominal pain, weight loss, and anemia are seen. Ulcerative colitis is more commonly associated with rectal bleeding, whereas abdominal pain, abdominal masses, and perianal lesions are more common in patients with Crohn's disease.

Ten to 20% of patients with IBD have extraintestinal manifestations; the most common are erythema nodosum, pyoderma gangrenosum, nongranulomatous anterior uveitis, polyarthritis, and ankylosing spondylitis. The extraintestinal manifestations may be the presenting complaint preceding gastrointestinal symptoms. This is particularly true in children with IBD. Ulcerative colitis and Crohn's disease may be associated with hepatobiliary disease. In Crohn's disease with small bowel involvement, malabsorption syndromes and fluid and electrolyte imbalance can occur. Calcium oxalate nephrolithiasis is common. Pneumaturia occasionally occurs in Crohn's disease from an enterovesical fistula.

Patients with well established IBD are most likely to present with complications of the disease; intractable pain, intractable diarrhea, abscess formation, massive hemorrhage, intestinal obstruction, dehydration, bowel perforation, and toxic megacolon. Massive hemorrhage and toxic megacolon are seen most often in ulcerative colitis, whereas abscess formation is far more common in Crohn's disease. Be aware that medications taken for IBD, particularly steroids, may mask the findings.

Toxic megacolon is the most dramatic complication; it's the result of a loss of muscular tone in advanced disease. The patient is toxic, with a distended, tender, and tympanitic abdomen. Fever, tachycardia, and volume depletion are noted. Other findings include leukocytosis, anemia, electrolyte disturbances, and an abdominal radiograph demonstrating a long continuous dilated segment of bowel (>6 cm wide). The mortality can be as high as 30%.

A long-term complication is colon carcinoma. Patients with ulcerative colitis have 10–30 times the risk of developing colon cancer than the general population. (Crohn's disease has a threefold increase in risk.) The symptoms of a new colon cancer may be subtle (e.g., anorexia, weight loss, occult bleeding, anemia, vague abdominal pain, constipation, and partial or complete bowel obstruction). The diagnosis can be difficult due to the overlap of these symptoms with those of IBD.

DIFFERENTIAL DIAGNOSIS

Differentiating Crohn's disease from ulcerative colitis based on clinical presentation is difficult—the diagnosis ultimately depends on radiographic and endoscopic evaluation and pathologic examination of involved tissues. One should recognize IBD as a cause of diarrhea, vague abdominal pain, malaise, or low-grade fever. Other entities present with similar complaints. Acute infectious diarrheal illness due to *Shigella, Salmonella, Campylobacter jejunii,* or *Yersinia* must be considered. Parasitic disease such as amebiasis also can masquerade as IBD. Stool cultures and examination of stool for ova and parasites are necessary. Serologic tests may rule out invasive amebiasis, but in up to 50% of cases of presumed infectious diarrhea, no pathogen is isolated.

When the symptoms primarily involve the rectum, gay bowel syndrome should be considered. Symptoms of chronic diarrhea, low-grade fever, and cachexia are consistent with HIV infection. Noninfectious causes must be sought. Antibiotic-induced colitis due to overgrowth of *Clostridium difficile* must be considered. Ischemic colitis in older patients and radiation colitis may present with a similar picture. When abdominal pain is the major complaint, IBD must be distinguished from appendicitis, cholecystitis, intestinal obstruction, abdominal aortic aneurysm, and mesenteric occlusive disease. These entities can often be distinguished from IBD on the basis of history and physical examination. Abdominal radiographs, a CBC, serum amylase and urinalysis can be helpful.

EMERGENCY DEPARTMENT EVALUATION AND MANAGEMENT

Significant complications of IBD (GI hemorrhage, obstruction, bowel perforation, and toxic megacolon) should be detected. Steroids may mask symptoms. The abdomeninal exam should assess for tenderness, rigidity, distention, rebound, and masses; stool should be checked for blood. A CBC, electrolytes and abdominal radiographs may be useful. Patients with hemorrhage, obstruction, or perforation are managed in the standard manner. Fluid resuscitation, gastrointestinal decompression, blood products as necessary, and surgical consultation are all indicated. Antibiotics for gram-negative and anaerobic bacteria are appropriate in suspected perforation. Patients maintained on steroids should receive stress-dose IV steroids to prevent adrenal insufficiency. Patients with toxic megacolon are given a 48–72 hour trial of intensive medical therapy before surgical intervention. Such therapy includes fluid administration, gastrointestinal decompression, and antibiotic coverage for bowel pathogens (enteric bacilli and anaerobes).

Patients with IBD may also present with acute or subacute exacerbation without evidence of a complication requiring surgical intervention. A history should focus on frequency of bowel movements, associated symptoms, severity of abdominal pain, and past history of hospitalizations. The physical examination should assess signs of toxicity, dehydration, and metabolic imbalance and should include an abdominal examination. Laboratory evaluation includes a CBC and chemistry profile. If there is a suspicion of liver involvement, liver function studies should be ordered. Abdominal radiographs may detect intestinal perforation or obstruction.

Those patients not requiring admission should follow-up with a gastroenterologist or internist. Management usually includes dietary adjustment, bowel rest, antibiotics, and sulfasalazine and steroids, but this should be done consultation with the patient's usual physician or a consultant. Typical outpatient medications include oral prednisone 40 to 60 mg/day, sulfasalazine 4 to 6 g/day, and antidiarrheal agents such as loperamide (Imodium) or diphenoxylate (Lomotil). Patients admitted usually require IV fluids, steroids, and sulfasalazine. The medication regimen usually includes prednisolone 60 mg/day IV, sulfasalazine 4 to 6 g/day, and in some cases, hyperalimentation; metronidazole, 6-mercaptopurine, and steroid enemas may be used.

DISPOSITION

Most cases can be managed in an outpatient setting. Admission should be considered for those with the following conditions: severe manifestations (> six bowel movements/day, severe abdominal pain, grossly bloody stool); systemic toxicity (fever, tachycardia, weight loss, cachexia); dehydration or metabolic disturbances; acute complications (intestinal obstruction, bowel perforation, GI hemorrhage, toxic megacolon); and those refractory to outpatient therapy.

COMMON PITFALLS

- Failure to suspect and refer patients with IBD can result in a delay of several months from the onset of symptoms to the time the diagnosis.
- Patients with previous episodes of similar symptoms, a family history of IBD, perirectal disease, or extraintestinal manifestations (rashes, back pain, arthritis, iritis) suggestive of IBD should be referred for endoscopic evaluation or double-contrast barium enema.
- IBD may present with severe abdominal pain, fever, tachycardia, and dehydration caused by perforation, abscess formation, and peritonitis.
- Corticosteroids can mask abnormal findings and serious complications

149   Diarrhea and Proctitis

DIARRHEA

Frequent, loose, watery stools (i.e., diarrhea) may affect 25% of all adults. A categorization of the underlying cause is usually possible at the initial visit.

CLINICAL PRESENTATION

Patients with diarrhea may actually have rectal discharge, rectal bleeding, and abnormally colored stools, or they may simply report a change in their usual bowel habits. Fecal incontinence or inability to reach the bathroom should be investigated vigorously. Diarrhea is most often associated with at least vague symptoms of discomfort or malaise, and often with pain, cramps, nausea, vomiting, bloating, or fever. Dehydration is an indication that the problem is significant and that acute therapy is needed.

DIFFERENTIAL DIAGNOSIS

There are countless causes of diarrhea; hallmarks of the common diagnostic groups are noted below.

VIRAL DIARRHEA   The most common diarrhea is viral diarrhea: hallmarks are the absence of high fever and a acute onset with several or many nonbloody stools per day. Upper GI distress with or without nausea is common, but severe abdominal pain is not characteristic. On examination there may be mild tenderness, but there are no peritoneal findings; rectal examination elicits no tenderness. Examination of the stool reveals few or no white cells.

BACTERIAL DIARRHEA   The three most common pathogens, *Shigella, Salmonella,* and *Campylobacter,* cause fever and many stools per day, often of an explosive character. WBC and RBC in the stool are noted, and abdominal distress may suggest an acute surgical abdomen.

PARASITIC DISEASES   Amebiasis and giardiasis have variable courses, but share features that suggest the diagnosis. Parasite-induced diarrheal stool is usually nondiagnostic, so the history is important. Most often, the symptoms are subacute, with previous diagnostic (stool culture, contrast studies) and therapeutic (antibiotic) interventions. Although both parasites are encountered throughout the US, (*Giardia* is ubiquitous), a history of foreign travel is an important risk factor. Because parasites are transmitted through sexual contact in homosexual males, sexual habits should be determined. When bloating or excessive flatulence is prominent, parasites, particularly *Giardia,* must be considered.

INFLAMMATORY BOWEL DISEASE (CROHN'S DISEASE; ULCERATIVE COLITIS   Undiagnosed Crohn's disease or ulcerative colitis are rare causes of acute diarrhea.

FOOD POISONING   Food poisoning is caused by the ingestion or elaboration of a bacterial toxin. The distinction between this and other diarrheas in which bacteria play a role is somewhat historical and arbitrary, since some toxin-induced diarrheas are considered bacterial enteritis (e.g., enterotoxigenic *Escherichia coli,* cholera) while others are not (e.g., staphylococcal food poisoning). Diarrhea may be a feature of virtually all food poisonings including the two most common, staphylococcal and clostridial. The distinguishing feature is not the characteristic of the diarrhea but the typical sudden onset, intense abdominal pain, and a history of ingestion of a suspicious food. Concurrent illness in others exposed to the same food is the strongest single confirmatory factor, but the absence of illness in other exposed individuals does not necessarily exclude the diagnosis.

ACUTE SURGICAL ABDOMEN   Small bowel obstruction, perforated appendicitis, diverticulitis, mesenteric infarction, and cancer can present with diarrhea. there is no substitute for a careful examination.

TRAVELLER'S DIARRHEA   Travellers' diarrhea is a common problem. Most cases from Mexico, South America, and Africa are related to the ingestion of toxigenic *E. coli,* although other causes must be considered. The onset of watery diarrhea after a few days of travel is the usual presentation. Symptoms may be delayed for up to 1 week after the trip.

ANTIBIOTICS   Although some antibiotics are more strongly associated with "pseudomembranous" colitis, virtually every antibiotic has been implicated. An overgrowth of *Clostridium difficile* caused by exposure to an antibiotic is responsible for elaborating the toxin. The onset can occur even after the antibiotic has been stopped. Although the diarrhea is toxin-induced, the colonic mucosa may be severely involved, and the stool is often bloody and positive for leukocytes. Sigmoidoscopy may be helpful but most cases do not have typical "pseudomembranes," and the diagnosis suspected from the history.

EMERGENCY DEPARTMENT EVALUATION

Determine the severity of illness and look for signs of dehydration. On physical examination, special attention is given to the abdominal exam. Note tenderness, peritoneal signs, distention or abnormal bowel sounds. The only routinely indicated study is microscopic examination of the stool for leukocytes. Place a drop of the liquid or semi-liquid stool under a cover slip and examine with the high-dry lens of the microscope. An unstained specimen is satisfactory. The normal stool has few or no visible WBC. The presence of white cells implies that there is an invasion in the lining of the gut. Although WBC are seen in many conditions, (appendicitis, IBD, infectious enteritis) this simple test can identify invasive disease that demands treatment and follow-up. Furthermore, presumed bacterial enteritis is a contraindication to antimotility agents. It is the single immediate study that can presumptively identify bacterial disease.

In the patient with hypovolemia, WBC or RBC in the stool, or an abnormal abdominal examination, further investigation is warranted and should include CBC, electrolytes, BUN, abdominal films and a urinalysis. Stool culture and sensitivity are not likely to be helpful in the absence of fecal leukocytes or a strong suspicion of bacterial enteritis. Stool parasite exam is reserved for cases suggested by history.

EMERGENCY DEPARTMENT MANAGEMENT

The routine case of enteritis without fecal leukocytes or dehydration is managed symptomatically. There is no contraindication to antimotility agents such as diphenoxylate or loperamide, and anticholinergics or anti-emetics can be judiciously administered. It is often wise to restrict lactose-containing products. The patient should expect a gradual recovery over several days to a week. Follow-up can be with a primary care provider if necessary. Presumed bacterial enteritis can be identified by history and stool examination, although the precise organism is seldom unknown. Many patients require rehydration.

Empiric antibiotic therapy is controversial. Evidence favors treatment antibiotics in sexually-transmitted enteric infections and in settings where transmission within a family is likely. Trimethoprim sulfamethoxazole (one double-strength tablet twice a day) is active against all of the most common bacterial pathogens, is inexpensive, and is relatively nontoxic. The quinolone agents also are active against the usual enteric pathogens and are a reasonable alternative.

Antimotility in presumed bacterial enteritis may predispose to the development of toxic megacolon. Dietary instructions are reasonable (avoid milk products); follow up with a primary practitioner is indicated if symptoms last longer than one week. Stool for culture and sensitivity testing varies. Admission may be necessary for toxic patients, with inadequate response to several hours of IV fluids or unable to maintain an adequate fluid intake. Inflammatory bowel disease can mimic infectious enteritis; the patient who does not improve as expected with several days of therapy may need a GI evaluation.

DISPOSITION

Almost all cases of diarrhea can be managed in the ED. The exception is diarrhea secondary to another process. For example, if there is a question of bowel infarction or obstruction, a surgical consultation is mandatory. Similarly, if examination reveals an unexpected finding (e.g., an abdominal mass), surgical consultation is necessary. It may be wise to perform GI studies in the ED, particularly with a high suspicion of inflammatory bowel disease and GI consultation is readily available, but proper practice will vary according to local resources. Patients with AIDS and diarrhea often have multiple pathogens and present special problems: parasites (*Cryptosporidium, Isospora belli, Entamoeba hartmani*, and others) for which effective treatment is difficult or impossible. The precise organism may be impossible to identify. These patients should be referred to a physician with special expertise.

COMMON PITFALLS

- Overdiagnosing viral gastroenteritis. There is a temptation to label all diarrheas of uncertain cause as viral. Particularly in older patients, the diagnosis of viral gastroenteritis is statistically less likely, and many serious causes of diarrhea are more likely. If there are WBCs or RBCs in the stool, it is unwise to attribute diarrhea to a viral cause.
- Failure to examine the stool. Examination of the stool is very useful.
- Failure to take a sexual history. The transmission of enteric pathogens is extremely common. This "gay bowel syndrome" is often distinct from AIDS, but is important to identify because of the other pathogens that must be treated for personal and public health reasons.
- Failure to consider *Giardia*. Giardiasis is common in this country; >5% have the parasites in the cyst stage with few or no symptoms. Symptoms of diarrhea, constipation and bloating may mimic other gastrointestinal diseases, especially functional bowel disease. With subacute or chronic symptoms, giardiasis should be considered. Empiric therapy is reasonable.

PROCTITIS

The evaluation of proctitis is straightforward; a history and examination will ordinarily define the diagnostic possibilities. Effective treatment is often available. The epidemiology of proctitis varies with demographics: in urban areas with homosexual males, high rates of infectious proctitis can be expected; in more elderly populations, proctitic symptoms are caused by other gastrointestinal disorders.

CLINICAL PRESENTATION

Response to rectal inflammation includes pain, discharge, bleeding, and disordered bowel function. Associated signs such as fever, weight loss, abdominal pain, nausea, and vomiting may indicate that proctitis is a manifestation of a more generalized process.

DIFFERENTIAL DIAGNOSIS AND EMERGENCY DEPARTMENT EVALUATION

First consider the possibility that the complaint may be due to perirectal abscess, rectal polyps, anal fissures, or other conditions involving the rectal area. The causes of proctitis can be classified as infectious and noninfectious. The most common infectious cause, and by far the most common in sexually active homosexual men, is gonorrhea. In other populations, no organism predominates. Gonococcal infection of the rectum occurs commonly in conjunction with gonococcal urethritis. Gonococcal infection of the female rectum is the result of anal intercourse; less often, it is caused by the spread of the organisms through vaginal secretions.

In homosexual males sexual contact is the usual route of spreading, although transmission also occurs through manual–rectal and implements used for sexual stimulation. Ten to 20% of patients with genital gonorrhea have positive rectal cultures for the organism. About 3% have rectal gonorrhea alone. Gonococcal infection in all sites is frequently asymptomatic; in symptomatic gonococcal proctitis the usual presenting complaint is rectal discharge and staining of the undergarments. Scant bloody discharge and rectal pain may be noted spontaneously or with rectal intercourse. An accurate sexual history, including a history of previous treatment for venereal disease, is important.

Anoscopy should demonstrate mucosal exudate and blood and permit rectal cultures. Gram's stain of rectal discharge may be helpful but does not definitively make or exclude the diagnosis. Urethral or cervical cultures should be taken, particularly when gonorrhea is suggested by the sexual history. A similar evaluation is appropriate for most of the other infectious proctitides.

Chlamydial proctitis should be considered in a patient with symptoms that persist after penicillin therapy for gonococcal proctitis. Chlamydial cultures and immunoassays are available. Lymphogranuloma venereum is a chlamydial infection that may present with proctitis. Although this infection is generally more severe than that caused by non-LGV strains, these two diseases cannot be reliably distinguished. Chlamydial proctitis may have a subacute or even chronic presentation with regional adenopathy, fibrosis and stricture.

Proctitis from herpes simplex virus (HSV) infection, type 1 or type 2, is a common cause of proctitis, particularly in sexually active homosexual men. Rectal pain and tenesmus are often severe enough to preclude anoscopy. Other evidence of HSV infection, vesicles in the genital or buttocks area, may be found, but this is the exception rather than the rule. Coexistence of urinary complaints, particularly urinary retention, is possibly due to involvement of the sacral ganglia. Urinary retention should always prompt consideration of HSV. Anoscopy may reveal mucosal inflammation, but herpetic vesicles are seldom seen.

Other bacteria, including anaerobes, have been implicated in proctitis, particularly with recent trauma to the rectal mucosa. In these cases proctitic symptoms may reflect perirectal cellulitis or perirectal abscess, even when fluctuance is not demonstrable. Treatment is surgical, and misdiagnosing rectal abscess as proctitis can have unfortunate results. A deep rectal infection is often of mixed flora with multiple anaerobes. A markedly elevated WBC count and proctitic symptoms favor early abscess.

Treatment and admission decisions are based on the general and anoscopic examination. Occasionally, amebic infection of the colon and rectum presents with proctitic symptoms, bloody rectal discharge, and disordered bowel function. Anoscopy and proctoscopy reveal shallow ulcerative lesions that resemble those of ulcerative colitis. Consultation with a gastroenterologist may be necessary to differentiate the two diseases. Diagnosis can be made by biopsy or direct demonstration of the parasite in stool or rectal discharge.

Noninfectious causes of proctitis should be suspected when there is no history of exposure and when microbiological studies fail to implicate them. Ulcerative colitis frequently involves the rectum and can present with localized proctitis and proctitic symptoms. Anoscopic examination reveals a cobblestone appearance of the mucosa. Bacteriologic studies and consultation may be indicated (although not necessarily emergently) to confirm the diagnosis and guide therapy.

Proctitis can be caused by direct irritation of the perirectal and mucosal tissues by a variety of substances or foreign bodies. Lubricants, sprays, and certain rectally administered medications, in particular theophylline suppositories, have been incriminated.

EMERGENCY DEPARTMENT MANAGEMENT AND DISPOSITION

ED management of proctitis is analogous to that of urethritis. If the diagnosis of proctitis is confirmed (by visible mucosal abnormalities or by WBCs in the rectal discharge), the patient should be treated, usually with standard therapy for gonococcal or chlamydial disease. Parenteral procaine penicillin G, not oral, is the preferred treatment for rectal and pharyngeal gonococcal infection, although ceftriaxone is indicated in areas where beta-lactamase producing strains are prevalent. Because infection with chlamydia cannot be excluded, oral therapy with tetracycline, doxycycline, or erythromycin should be prescribed concurrently for 10 days. Spectinomycin is used in the penicillin-allergic patient.

Empiric therapy is instituted even without proof of proctitis, especially in the high-risk setting (homosexual males, history of anal sex, known or suspected exposure to sexually transmitted disease). Resolution of symptoms can be expected within a few days. All patients should be referred for follow-up of culture results, documentation of cure, and identification of sexual contacts. Empiric treatment of sexual consorts is indicated; notification of public health authorities is mandatory in most jurisdictions. When another pathogen is suspected either on epidemiologic or clinical grounds, treatment for gonorrhea and chlamydia is still reasonable since these two usually cannot be excluded in the ED and antibiotic therapy will not compromise subsequent management.

Systemic therapy of herpetic proctitis with acyclovir is indicated when the diagnosis is suspected. In those uncommon cases in which amebic proctitis is strongly suspected, treatment with metronidazole may be instituted pending laboratory confirmation of the diagnosis. Follow-up within several days is mandatory for both of the latter conditions.

Differentiation between proctitis and perirectal disease may be difficult; admission may be necessary. If outpatient therapy is elected, the patient requires close follow-up. Worsening of symptoms or failure to improve on antibiotic therapy and Sitz baths within 48 hours mandates admission and probable surgical intervention.

The phrase "nonspecific proctitis" is without meaning. Some may be due to irritants or allergies, and Sitz baths and steroid-containing creams or suppositions may help. The role of microorganisms such as mycoplasmas, *Ureaplasma urealyticum,* and viruses is undefined, but syphilis must be considered, especially in homosexual men. Evaluation by a surgeon may disclose unsuspected pathology such as fissures, sinus tracts, rectal ulcer (e.g., secondary to Crohn's disease), or crypt abscess.

Most patients with proctitis can be managed without consultation or admission. Consultation is advisable when there is an unusual mucosal appearance, a question of perirectal infection, systemic symptoms or local signs suggesting malignancy, or a suspicion of inflammatory bowel disease. It may also be necessary when severe symptoms occur with herpetic proctitis (e.g., severe pain or urinary retention).

COMMON PITFALLS

- Failure to consider rectal chlamydia or herpes, which can occur not only in homosexual men but also in heterosexual men, women and in children
- Failure to elicit a sexual history
- Failure to question a sexual history once elicited—many patients do not at first admit to rectal intercourse

- Failure to do anoscopy to visualize the mucosa, and to examine and culture the exudate
- Failure to arrange for proper identification and treatment of contacts
- Failure to consider or identify other rectal lesions that mimic proctitis (e.g., anal fissure, fistula in ano, and perirectal abscess)

150   Lower Gastrointestinal Bleeding

The chief complaint of "rectal bleeding" may mean melena, black tarry stools, maroon stools, or dark red to bright red blood noted in or on the stool, on toilet tissue, in the toilet bowl, or on the underwear. To produce a black, melanotic stool there must be the rapid loss of at least 100 mL of blood. Rectal bleeding with symptoms (weakness, dizziness, near syncope) indicates at least a 1000-mL blood loss. About 33% of patients with syncope may not receive attention for several hours, even days. The sudden loss of 2000 mL (40% of circulating volume) can be fatal. As a general rule, if melena or black tarry stools are the complaint, the source is usually upper gastrointestinal (UGI); if maroon or dark red stools, the source is usually the terminal ileum or proximal 2/3d of the colon; and if bright red, the source is usually the descending colon, sigmoid, or anorectum. Massive lower gastrointestinal (LGI) bleeding with hypovolemia severe enough to require transfusion occurs in about 10% of LGI bleeds. Rectal trauma may cause LGI bleeding, but the patient may be reluctant to divulge the history. If rectal trauma has been established, perforation must be ruled out.

DIFFERENTIAL DIAGNOSIS

The differential diagnosis of LGI bleeding is extensive (Table 150-1).

Diverticulosis is possible in patients > age 40; its prevalence increases with age. Blood is usually dark red-brown or maroon, and pain is often mild. Leukocytosis or fever are seen with an inflammatory component; recurrent hemorrhage occurs in 50% of patients. Neoplasms do not usually cause massive LGI bleeding; change in bowel habits, pain, weight loss, symptoms of anemia, and obstructive symptoms suggest neoplasm, as should a mass on digital rectal examination. Adenocarcinoma is the most common malignancy.

Infection and inflammation are usually manifested by minor chronic blood loss, although major bleeding may occur. Shigellosis, amebiasis, and infection with *Campylobacter jejuni* are common infectious causes of bloody diarrhea and pain. Inflammatory bowel disease can cause bloody diarrhea with mucopurulent material, as well as abdominal cramps and tenesmus. Vascular ectasia (e.g., angiodysplasia, arteriovenous malformation, telangiectasia, colonic varices) can cause major, acute painless hemorrhage, which, depending upon location, can be bright-red or maroon. It is more common in older patients and associated with aortic valvular disease and portal hypertension. Rigid proctosigmoidoscopy, flexible colonoscopy, or angiography permit diagnosis.

Anorectal disorders (e.g., hemorrhoids, fissures, fistula, abscess, prolapse, proctitis, infection, impaction) usually cause minor or chronic hemorrhage. If a major bleed is present with hemorrhoids, one should suspect concurrent significant disease such as cancer or portal hypertension. Anorectal infections and abscesses rarely cause significant bleeding. Rectal prolapse may cause incontinence of bloody, mucoid stool. Radiation proctitis must be considered with a history of GI or pelvic neoplasms (testicular, prostate, cervix, uterus, or bladder). The bleeding,

---

TABLE 150-1. Common Sources of Lower GI Bleed

Adults (All Ages)	Children (0–15 yrs)
Diverticulosis	Polyps (juvenile; hereditary syndromes)
Neoplasm, including polyps	Meckel's diverticulum
Infection/inflammation	Infection/inflammation
Vascular ectasia	Fissure
Anorectal disorder	UGI source
UGI source	Non-GI source vs. unknown
Penetrating or blunt trauma	
Bleeding disorders	

---

which is usually bright red, may occur during radiation therapy or up to 6 months after the cessation of treatment; up to 50% of patients will have proctocolitis and bleeding.

Fecal impaction rarely causes significant bleeding or bloody diarrhea. The upper GI tract should be considered in patients with frank or occult melena, a previous history of UGI disorders, or when investigation fails to identify a LGI source. Penetrating, blunt, iatrogenic, or self-induced trauma may be the cause of LGI bleeding. Iatrogenic bleeding should be considered after barium enema or instrumentation. GI foreign bodies also cause bleeding. A Meckel's diverticulum can cause ulceration and bleeding. Drugs are associated with UGI and LGI bleeding (e.g., salicylates, anticoagulants, estrogens, anti-inflammatories, steroids, alcohol).

EMERGENCY DEPARTMENT EVALUATION

The priority is to identify hypovolemia and to treat it. If signs of hypovolemia or impending shock are present, fluid resuscitation must be initiated. Baseline laboratory studies should include a CBC, coagulation profile, liver function tests, chemistry profile, and a type and screen (if stable) or type and cross (if unstable) for at least 4 to 6 units of blood. Serial hematocrits can provide an indication of the severity of bleeding. The history should emphasize the duration and frequency of the bleeding, the nature and color of the stools, and the character of any pain. A history of previous bleeding or GI disorders (e.g., cirrhosis, pancreatitis), weight loss, fatigue, near syncope or syncope, alcohol use, and medications may be helpful.

Physical examination may reveal jaundice, abdominal wall varices (caput medusae), abdominal distention, or a palpable mass. Abdominal rigidity, guarding, or rebound, or absent bowel sounds suggest peritonitis or perforation. In the elderly or in cardiac patients, slow chronic blood loss may present initially as congestive heart failure secondary to anemia. A rectal examination should be performed to detect masses or other rectal pathology, and to obtain a stool specimen for guaiac testing. Black stools can be caused by iron, charcoal, bismuth, food dyes, beets, jello, Koolaid, and some antibiotic syrups. False-positive guaiac is seen with red meat, raw fruits and vegetables, and some iron preparations. False-negative results can be found in small bleeds. Visual inspection or guaiac testing of gastric aspirate from an nasogastric tube can confirm an UGI source, but a negative aspirate does not rule out duodenal bleeding when the pyloric sphincter is competent. Anoscopy and rigid proctosigmoidoscopy will reveal a bleeding source if it is within 40 cm of the anus. In general, cleansing enemas should be avoided.

EMERGENCY DEPARTMENT MANAGEMENT

Consultation will depend on availability and institutional capabilities. Continued evaluation will often involve angiography and colonoscopy. The 60-cm flexible fiberoptic colonoscope is an accurate diagnostic tool that is safe and well tolerated; trained endoscopists perform this procedure after adequate bowel preparation, not emergently. Angiography is considered by many the procedure of choice for either massive or continuous LGI bleeding or when other diagnostic modalities have failed to reveal a source.

Angiography is useful not only diagnostically, but also therapeutically. Local administration of vasopressor agents (vasopressin or epinephrine) or embolization with autologous clots or Gelfoam spheres can be done. Accuracy is enhanced if the bleeding is continuous, even at rates as low as 0.5 mL/min; 70–75% of bleeding sites can be localized. Complications are uncommon, but include local catheter problems, vessel perforation, and allergic or nephrotoxic contrast media reactions.

Radionuclide scanning with technetium-99m sulfur colloid or technetium-99m labeled red blood cells can provide valuable diagnosis and localization. Repeated imaging is possible without reinjection for 24 hours, a useful feature for intermittent LGI bleeding. Radionuclide scanning is valuable if patients cannot tolerate angiography or colonoscopy.

Barium enema (BE) is employed much less frequently now; it fails to detect the bleeding site in 50%. If a BE is done before angiography, radionuclide scanning, colonoscopy, or endoscopy, the residual barium in the bowel often makes interpretation of these studies impossible until the barium is cleared. Surgical consultation is indicated with massive bleeding, continued bleeding, when the source of bleeding has been detected and is surgically amenable, or when no bleeding source can be identified.

DISPOSITION

All cases of LGI bleeding need follow-up. Patients with abnormal vital signs, significant initial blood loss or continued bleeding, significant associated or underlying illness or injury, poor social supports, or questionable reliability for follow-up should be admitted to the hospital. The majority with stable vital signs, minor LGI bleeds due to conditions amenable to surgical or medical treatment, good social supports, and reliability for follow-up care can be discharged. Nearly 20% will prove either to have no bleeding at all, or to have bleeding from a non-GI source (e.g., nose, pulmonary tree, vagina).

COMMON PITFALLS

- Failure to appreciate the significance and volume of the initial LGI bleed, leading to delays in early, aggressive therapy.
- Failure to consider co-existing serious causes of bleeding once a benign, treatable source of bleeding has been established. Not all LGI bleeding is from hemorrhoids!
- Excessive time can be spent on identifying the exact location of bleeding, with resultant delayed therapy, consultation, or admission.
- Failure to obtain and record serial laboratory and clinical evaluations.
- Failure to recognize that it takes several hours for the hematocrit to reflect the magnitude of blood loss.
- Failure to consider LGI bleed in the presence of continued abnormal vital signs when the initial evaluation was directed at non-GI etiologies.
- Failure to consider perforation after instrumentation or foreign body insertion or removal
- Reliance on the color of the blood as an indicator of source or location of the bleed. The color is unreliable because of variability in its degradation and transit time.

PART V

Renal, Metabolic, and Endocrine Emergencies

151   Acid–Base Disturbances

Patients who present with life-threatening acid–base abnormalities are often in the advanced stages of their disease. Attention should be directed toward identification and treatment of the underlying disturbance. The body responds to a primary *metabolic* disturbance with adjustments of respiratory rate and pCO_2 *(respiratory compensation)* and to a *respiratory* disturbance by increasing or decreasing renal hydrogen ion excretion *(metabolic compensation)* (Table 151-1). When two or more acid–base abnormalities occur simultaneously, the abnormality is termed a *mixed acid–base disturbance*. Normal compensatory responses are seen in Table 151-2. Tables 151-3 and 151-4 list the causes of simple or mixed acid–base disturbances most commonly seen.

EMERGENCY DEPARTMENT EVALUATION AND MANAGEMENT

Acid–base disturbances should be suspected in all critically ill patients, those with with extreme dyspnea, abnormal mental status, or vomiting or diarrhea. Arterial blood gas and electrolytes provide enough data for the initial metabolic assessment. *Acidemia* is defined as a pH <7.38, and *alkalemia* as a pH >7.42. *Is the disturbance respiratory or metabolic?* The serum bicarbonate and arterial pCO_2 (Table 151-5) should be noted to answer this question. *Is the acid–base disturbance simple or mixed?* When the appropriate formula (see Table 151-2) is applied, deviation from the parameters of a simple disturbance indicates a mixed disorder.

SIMPLE METABOLIC ACIDOSIS
This is the most frequent acid–base disturbance; the underlying cause may be identified by considering the patient's *anion gap*, the serum sodium (chloride + CO_2 content); normal anion gap is 10–12 mEq/L. This gap represents anions present in the serum but not routinely measured. A normal anion gap in an acidotic patient indicates excess hydrochloric acid, whereas anion gaps >14 mEq/L usually indicate an excess of organic acids. Table 151-3 divides the causes of metabolic acidosis according to the presence or absence of an abnormal anion gap. A small increase in the anion gap (12–20 mEq/L) is noted in some situations in which a metabolic acidosis is not present (e.g., dehydration, alkalosis, and treatment with citrate, lactate, and certain antibiotics), whereas an anion gap >25 mEq/L is seen only with lactic acidosis, ketoacidosis, and the toxin-associated acidoses. Serum potassium must be closely monitored with suspected metabolic acidosis. The serum potassium increases with acidemia.

TABLE 151-1. Primary Disturbances and Compensatory Responses in Terms of Changes in Carbonic Acid Constituents

	Usual PH	Hydrogen Ion Concentration	Serum Bicarbonate (Measured as Total CO_2 Content)	pCO_2
Metabolic Acidosis	<7.38	Primary increase	Immediate decrease	Rapid compensatory decrease
Metabolic Alkalosis	>7.42	Primary decrease	Immediate increase	Variable compensatory increase
Acute Respiratory Acidosis	<7.38	Secondary increase	Immediate small compensatory increase	Primary increase
Chronic Respiratory Acidosis	<7.38	Secondary increase	Slow larger compensatory increase	Primary increase
Acute Respiratory Alkalosis	>7.42	Secondary decrease	Immediate compensatory	Primary decrease
Chronic Respiratory Alkalosis	7.40–7.42	Secondary decrease	Slow larger compensatory decrease	Primary decrease

TABLE 151-2. Formulas Describing Expected Compensatory Response to Primary Acid-Base Disturbances

Simple Metabolic Acidosis

Predicted decreased (pCO_2) mm Hg = 1.2 · Δ (HCO_3^-) mEq/L
Predicted pCO_2 mm Hg = 1.5 (HCO_3^-) mEq/L + 8 ± 2
Anticipated pCO_2 approximates last two digits of arterial pH

Simple Metabolic Alkalosis

Predicted increased Δ(pCO_2) mm Hg = 0.6 · Δ(HCO_3^-) mEq/L

Simple Acute Respiratory Acidosis

Predicted decreased Δ(pH) units = 0.8 Δ(pCO_2) mm Hg
Predicted increased Δ(HCO_3^-) mEq/L = .1 Δ(pCO_2) mm Hg

Simple Chronic Respiratory Acidosis

Predicted decreased Δ(pH) units = 0.3 Δ(pCO_2) mm Hg
Predicted increased Δ(HCO_3^-) mEq/L = .35 Δ(pCO_2) mm Hg

Simple Acute Respiratory Alkalosis

Predicted increased Δ(pH) units = 0.8 Δ(pCO_2) mm Hg
Predicted decreased Δ(HCO_3^-) mEq/L = .2 · Δ(pCO_2) mm Hg

Simple Chronic Respiratory Alkalosis

Predicted increased Δ(pH) units = 0.17 · Δ(pCO_2) mm Hg
Predicted decreased Δ(HCO_3^-) mEq/L = .5 · Δ(pCO_2) mm Hg

TABLE 151-3. Causes of Simple Acid-Base Disturbances

Simple Metabolic Acidosis

Elevated Anion Gap
  Diabetic ketoacidosis
  Alcoholic ketoacidosis
  Starvation
  Lactic acidosis
  Renal failure
  Methanol, ethylene glycol

Normal Anion Gap
  Renal tubular acidosis
  Diarrhea
  Early renal failure
  Carbonic anhydrase inhibitor therapy
  Hydronephrosis

Simple Metabolic Alkalosis

Vomiting/gastric suction
Volume depletion
Diuretic therapy
Corticosteroid therapy

Respiratory Acidosis

CNS lesion
Sedative therapy/overdose
Neuropathies
Myopathies
Chest wall abnormalities
  Trauma
  Kyphosis
Pleural disease
Obstructive airways disease

Simple Respiratory Alkalosis

Anxiety
Progesterone therapy/increased exogenous
  progesterone
Sympathomimetic therapy
Fever
Hyperthyroidism
Hypoxia
Liver disease

TABLE 151-4. Mixed Acid-Base Disturbances

Metabolic Acidosis–Respiratory Alkalosis

Salicylate ingestion
Liver disease
Sepsis
Pulmonary embolism or pulmonary edema with hypotension
Pulmonary-renal syndrome

Metabolic Acidosis–Respiratory Acidosis

Cardiopulmonary arrest
Pulmonary edema
Drug overdose

Metabolic Alkalosis-Respiratory Alkalosis

Critical illness
Pregnancy
Mechanically ventilated chronic hypercapnea

Metabolic Alkalosis–Respiratory Acidosis

Chronic hypercapnea with:
    Diuretic overuse
    Dehydration
    Hypokalemia

Metabolic Acidosis–Metabolic Alkalosis

Diarrhea/vomiting
Organic acidosis/vomiting
Metabolic acidosis with excessive bicarbonate administration

TABLE 151-5. Respiratory vs. Metabolic Acidosis/Alkalosis

	pH	pCO_2	HCO_3
Metabolic acidosis	Decrease	Decrease	Decrease
Metabolic alkalosis	Increase	Increase	Increase
Respiratory acidosis	Decrease	Increase	Increase
Respiratory alkalosis	Increase	Decrease	Decrease

SIMPLE METABOLIC ALKALOSIS

Metabolic alkalosis is a common condition suspected with very high values for the total serum CO_2 content. Most metabolic alkaloses are initiated by primary volume depletion, potassium depletion, or both. Patients with this disorder rarely present with a pH in the life-threatening range (> 7.60), but may require vigorous fluid or potassium administration. Metabolic alkalosis tends to be self-perpetuating if it remains untreated.

PRIMARY RESPIRATORY DISTURBANCES

Primary respiratory abnormalities are acute or chronic. Because the renal compensatory process takes 48–72 hours, patients with acute respiratory disturbances have a pH further from the normal range than those with chronic disturbances. In chronic respiratory alkalosis, compensation can be so effective that the pH may return to the normal range. The treatment includes increasing ventilation for respiratory acidosis or adding dead space to the upper airway for respiratory alkalosis. Longer term treatment involves identifying and treating the underlying cause. Avoid treatment that suddenly normalizes the pCO_2 in a chronic respiratory disturbance. Rapid normalization risks a dangerous overshooting of normal pH. Respiratory acidosis requires emergent intervention, because the pCO_2 can rise quickly to cause both a life-threatening acidosis and serious encephalopathy (CO_2 narcosis). An ABG is mandatory for **all** patients with abnormal mental status.

MIXED ACID–BASE DISTURBANCES

When a mixed disorder is present, the patient may be acidemic, alkalemic, or have a normal pH. Any two primary acid–base disturbances (other than acute respiratory acidosis and acute respiratory alkalosis) can coexist. Three of the more frequent mixed acid–base disturbances deserve mention.

Metabolic acidosis with respiratory acidosis: Alkalosis is diagnosed when the patient's pCO_2 deviates significantly from that which would have been predicted (see Table 151-2) in simple metabolic acidosis.

Combined metabolic acidosis and respiratory acidosis: This is seen in cardiac arrest or the postictal state, in which ventilation is inadequate for the degree of metabolic acidosis.

Combined metabolic acidosis and respiratory alkalosis: This is commonly noted in salicylate poisoning, in which salicylate induces metabolic acidosis and also directly stimulates ventilation in excess of that which would be induced by the acidosis.

The combination of metabolic acidosis and metabolic alkalosis often manifests with a relatively normal pH and an anion gap elevation significantly exceeding the decrease in total CO_2 content. A common setting is the patient with alcoholic ketoacidosis who has been vomiting. If combined metabolic acidosis and metabolic alkalosis occurs in a patient with a normal anion gap acidosis, however, there is no anion gap elevation to serve as a marker for the disturbance. An example would be a patient who is experiencing severe diarrhea (metabolic acidosis caused by loss of sodium bicarbonate in the stool) associated with vomiting (metabolic alkalosis caused by loss of gastric hydrochloric acid). Unless this disturbance is suspected because of the clinical setting, the presence of two acid–base abnormalities may become evident only when one of the deficits is corrected. In the vomiting–diarrhea example, rapid volume correction with normal saline but without concomitant bicarbonate replacement might unmask the normal anion gap acidosis, with the serum bicarbonate decreasing as volume is restored.

CONTROVERSIES IN MANAGEMENT

DIABETIC KETOACIDOSIS (DKA)   Authorities agree about the need for intravenous rehydration and close monitoring (and replacement) of potassium in DKA, but there is disagreement about the quantity and route of insulin administration, as well as the indications for bicarbonate. "Paradoxic central nervous system (CNS) acidosis" may occur after vigorous bicarbonate administration or cerebral edema. Bicarbonate should be given to patients with a pH <6.9.

LACTIC ACIDOSIS   This common acidosis is defined by a pH <7.35 with a serum lactate >6 mmol/L. There is both strong support for and opposition to the routine use of IV sodium bicarbonate for lactic acidosis. The most important aspect of the treatment of lactic acidosis is to identify and treat its underlying cause. Bicarbonate therapy should begin with 50–100 mEq (depending on the severity of the acidemia); the laboratory parameters should then be followed closely.

TOXIN-INDUCED ACIDOSIS   Methanol and ethylene glycol are two low-molecular-weight alcohols that can produce severe metabolic acidosis. Parenteral sodium bicarbonate is an effective interim treatment; 1 mEq/kg for a pH <7.20. The amount of further doses is guided by the response.

COMMON PITFALLS

- Search aggressively for underlying causes of significant disturbances.
- Serious respiratory disturbances demand aggressive intervention.
- Although there is controversy about the indications for sodium bicarbonate, bicarbonate should not be withheld if the patient appears critically ill and has a pH <7.1.

152   Diabetic Ketoacidosis

Diabetic ketoacidosis (DKA) is a syndrome of hyperglycemia, ketonemia, and acidosis resulting from absolute or relative insulin deficiency. It occurs as a complication of insulin-dependent diabetes (DM), but may also be seen in non-insulin-dependent diabetics or as the first manifestation of previously undiagnosed DM. DKA is common; despite advances in treatment, mortality rates remain between 6% and 10%. Death may result from metabolic derangements attributable to DKA itself, to associated illness, or to complications of treatment. Two processes are important: alterations in glucose production and disposal (causing hyperglycemia, osmotic diuresis, volume depletion, and electrolyte loss) and increased ketogenesis (causing metabolic acidosis).

CLINICAL PRESENTATION

DKA presents with nausea and vomiting, drowsiness, abdominal pain, thirst, and polyuria. Most patients are tachycardic, tachypneic, and normotensive. Kussmaul breathing represents respiratory compensation for metabolic acidosis and is present in 62% with a bicarbonate level <10 mEq/L. Patients with DKA and an underlying infection may not manifest pyrexia. On exam, dehydration is evident. The odor of acetone may be present. Abdominal pain and tenderness are common in DKA and have been attributed to gastric distension or stretching of the liver capsule. Pain often resolves promptly with treatment of metabolic abnormalities, but when pain and tenderness persist, one should suspect an underlying medical or surgical condition. Older patients are more likely to have an identifiable underlying cause of abdominal pain. Level of consciousness varies from normal (20%) to coma (10%) and closely correlates with hyperosmolality.

PRECIPITATING FACTORS

DKA is precipitated by any stress that causes the amount of insulin to be inadequate. Noncompliance with medication, infection, myocardial infarction, CVA, trauma, pregnancy, pancreatitis, or emotional stress may initiate DKA. Noncompliance with medication and infection are the two most common precipitating causes; no cause is found in many cases. A chest radiograph and urinalysis help rule out infection.

DIFFERENTIAL DIAGNOSIS

Alcoholic ketoacidosis (AKA), hyperosmolar nonketotic coma (HHNK), starvation ketosis, uremia, lactic acidosis, and toxin ingestion should be considered. The diagnosis of AKA is based on history and the absence of hyperglycemia. It is generally seen in the setting of recently diminished or discontinued alcohol consumption in a patient with a history of alcohol abuse. AKA is difficult to distinguish from DKA in a patient with ketonuria and a normal or modestly elevated glucose. Because patients with AKA may also have diabetes mellitus, DKA and AKA may coexist.

Most patients with HHNK are elderly, and many have underlying cardiovascular, renal, or other chronic diseases; 30–90% have DM but are not insulin dependent. Patients with HHNK have enough circulating insulin to suppress ketogenesis but not enough to reduce serum glucose levels. Half have an anion-gap metabolic acidosis attributed to lactate and renal failure. Mental status changes are typical in HHNK and correlate with the degree of hyperosmolality. Precipitating factors are common and should be investigated.

Starvation may also lead to ketoacidosis. However, it is unusual for serum bicarbonate levels to be <16 mEq/L or for the pH to be <7.35. Serum glucose level is not elevated. Uremia is a common cause of an anion-gap metabolic acidosis, but acidosis does not become significant until GFR is <20 mL/min and BUN and creatinine levels are >40 and 4, respectively. Importantly, ketones are not present. The anion gap in uremic acidosis increases by only about 10 mEq/L; greater increases should suggest an alternative diagnosis. Methanol, ethylene glycol, or salicylate ingestion may increase the anion gap but do not cause hyperglycemia or ketonuria. Isopropyl alcohol, which is metabolized to acetone, causes ketonemia, but does not increase the anion gap or the serum glucose. If ketoacidosis, uremia, and ingestions have been ruled out, metabolic acidosis with an elevated anion gap suggests lactic acidosis, which may be precipitated by seizures, sepsis, or hypovolemic shock.

EMERGENCY DEPARTMENT EVALUATION

DKA presents with hyperglycemia, an anion-gap metabolic acidosis, ketonemia, and ketonuria. Laboratory evaluation includes glucose, electrolytes, BUN, creatinine, ABG and urinalysis. However, a well-hydrated patient is not extremely hyperglycemic, not all patients have an anion-gap acidosis, and ketonemia and ketonuria are frequently absent early. Initial glucose levels average 675 mg/dL, but range from near normal to levels more characteristic of hyperosmolar nonketotic coma (HHNK). A normal serum glucose does not rule out the diagnosis of DKA. Very high glucose levels occur if extracellular volume is contracted causing diminished urine flow and excretion of excess glucose. Volume depletion results in an average BUN of 25–30 mg/dL. Interpretation of creatinine is complicated by the interference of acetoacetate with autoanalyzer assays, which falsely elevates measured creatinine.

Metabolic acidosis is of two types. Anion-gap acidosis results from an accumulation of organic acids and increased unmeasured anions such as AcAc and BHBA. Non-anion-gap or hyperchloremic acidosis results from the loss of bicarbonate. Although DKA is classically considered an anion-gap acidosis, the absence of an increased anion gap does not rule it out. DKA may produce a spectrum of acid–base disturbances ranging from pure hyperchloremic acidosis to pure anion-gap acidosis, the type of acidosis present on admission depending on the patient's volume status. Individuals with significant volume depletion due to osmotic diuresis and vomiting present with an increased anion-gap acidosis. This is because renal perfusion is diminished, ketoacids cannot be excreted in the urine, and the ketoacids are buffered by bicarbonate. Patients who maintain salt and water intake sustain renal perfusion and excrete ketoacids, which would otherwise be metabolized to bicarbonate during recovery. This loss of potential bicarbonate and compensatory retention of chloride results in hyperchloremic metabolic acidosis. Regardless of presenting acid–base disturbance, hyperchloremic metabolic acidosis is common during the recovery phase of DKA.

In DKA absolute levels of BHBA, AcAc, and acetone are increased. BHBA and AcAc are in equilibrium with one another, and when insulin treatment is begun, BHBA is oxidized to AcAc. Although the mean ratio of BHBA to AcAc is usually only slightly elevated in DKA (about 3:1), in some patients it may be very high. The qualitative nitroprusside test for ketones detects AcAc, but does not react with BHBA. In patients with a high BHBA:AcAc ratio, the nitroprusside test will be only weakly positive or entirely negative, and the diagnosis of DKA may be missed. As the patient improves metabolically, BHBA levels decrease, while AcAc increases. An initially negative nitroprusside reaction can paradoxically become positive, or more positive, despite clinical improvement. Acetone levels may remain elevated for up to 42 hours after blood glucose, AcAc, and BHBA levels return to normal. The nitroprusside reaction may be misleading initially and is not useful in monitoring the response of ketoacidosis to therapy.

EMERGENCY DEPARTMENT MANAGEMENT

Treatment includes correction of hypovolemia, reversal of ketonemia and acidemia, replacement of electrolyte losses, and attention to precipitating causes. The goal is gradual restoration of a normal clinical and metabolic state. Overly rapid correction may cause volume overload, cerebral edema, hypoglycemia, or hypokalemia. A large-bore IV should be inserted and normal saline begun while the results of laboratory studies are awaited. If the patient has an abnormal mental status, an accucheck should be done. Hypoglycemia is the most common cause of altered mental status in a diabetic; 25 g of dextrose to a patient in DKA is harmless.

In most patients, glucose-induced osmotic diuresis produces deficits averaging 5 L of water. Normal saline is the initial replacement of choice at a rate of 1 L/hr for the first 2 to 3 hours titrated to clinical response and urine output. Volume replacement lowers the serum glucose by increasing urine flow and glucose excretion, and by decreasing levels of counterregulatory hormones. Once hypovolemic has been corrected, half-normal saline is used to replace the large free-water deficit. Some diabetics with renal failure may not be capable of an osmotic diuresis and may not be dehydrated. Fluids alone cannot reverse ketogenesis or restore pH to normal; insulin is required for effective treatment of both hyperglycemia and ketoacidosis.

Intravenous insulin produces a more rapid fall in glucose and ketones during the first 2 hours of treatment than do IM or SQ routes. Although the latter routes can be efficacious, absorption of insulin is erratic in the face of volume depletion, so IV therapy is recommended. Continuous infusion offers advantages over bolus techniques. Since IV insulin has a 1/2 life of 20 minutes, steady-state blood concentrations in an effective range can be achieved or abolished very quickly. A loading dose is unnecessary; the risk of hypoglycemia is minimal once the infusion is discontinued. Because insulin adsorbs to intravenous tubing, 50 mL of the infusion should be allowed to run through the pump prior to administration.

A continuous IV infusion of 10 U/hr prevents a rapid fall in glucose or potassium but produces a good response in almost all patients. Blood sugar may be anticipated to fall by 75 mg to 100 mg/dL/hr. Infection may increase insulin requirements, and occasional patients show unusual resistance. If there is no fall in glucose after 2 hours, the infusion rate can be doubled. Correction of ketonemia and acidemia takes much longer than the reversal of hyperglycemia. Insulin therapy must be continued to inhibit ketogenesis, even when the blood sugar is in the normal range. To prevent hypoglycemia, the insulin infusion should be slowed to 2 to 4 U/hr and the IV fluids changed to 5% dextrose with half-normal saline when the serum glucose is 250 mg/dL. Once the anion gap has normalized, with serum bicarbonate >15, and the patient is able to eat, the glucose infusion may be stopped. Insulin infusion is continued until several hours after the patient's normal subcutaneous insulin regimen is resumed.

Osmotic diuresis produces total body deficits of potassium. Virtually all patients are total-body potassium depleted. Serum potassium levels measure the concentration of extracellular potassium, representing only 2% of total body stores and do not accurately reflect total body deficits. The initial serum potassium level may be high, normal, or low. Administration of insulin, correction of acidosis, and increased urine output with fluid resuscitation all tend to lower extracellular potassium concentration. A nadir is generally reached 1 to 4 hours after treatment is initiated. Thus, patients who present with hypokalemia can be assumed to have profound deficits and are at risk for respiratory and generalized paralysis, arrhythmias, or death from cardiac arrest. Withholding potassium from a patient with a normal serum potassium level is also potentially disastrous. If the initial potassium level is normal or low, and urine output is documented, replacement should begin immediately at a rate of 10 mEq/hr to 40 mEq/hr. These patients need continuous ECG monitoring and frequent serum potassium measurements.

Bicarbonate is controversial. There may be no advantage to bicarbonate therapy, even when the presenting pH is as low as 6.9. The patient's electrolytes should be monitored frequently (every 2–4 hours). The serum glucose level must be followed hourly. Sequential measurements of serum or urine ketones are not helpful. If the patient appears to be resistant to the usual doses of insulin, or if relapse occurs after switching to subcutaneous insulin, one should suspect an unrecognized precipitant, such as occult infection or silent myocardial infarction.

Complications of treatment such as hypoglycemia, hypokalemia, and hypophosphatemia result from overzealous use of insulin and inadequate monitoring. Another potential complication is cerebral edema. This is most likely to occur in children, 6 to 10 hours after therapy begins. Mental status deteriorates abruptly, progressing to coma and respiratory arrest due to brain stem compression. The mortality rate is 90%. There are no warning signs and no clinical predictors. Some clinicians advocate maintaining the serum glucose level above 250 mg/dL during the first few hours of therapy to avoid the osmotic gradients that may contribute to cerebral swelling. Patients with DKA are also predisposed to vascular thrombosis, especially of cerebral vessels. This has been attributed to dehydration, diminished intravascular volume, low cardiac output, and increased serum viscosity.

DISPOSITION

Most patients with DKA require admission to an ICU where vital signs, cardiac rhythm, and hemodynamic status can be closely monitored. Patients with mild DKA may be candidates for ED therapy, provided they have no underlying precipitating cause that will require prolonged intervention, such as pneumonia or myocardial infarction. Reliable patients may be discharged if, after treatment, they have normal vital signs, are able to take oral fluids, are well hydrated, have a glucose level <300, a normal pH and anion gap, and bicarbonate >15 mEq/L. Such patients need close follow-up with their primary care physicians.

COMMON PITFALLS

- Failure to diagnose DKA in patients who are euglycemic, have a negative nitroprusside test, or have a non-anion gap metabolic acidosis.
- Dextrose should be given to all diabetic patients in coma to avoid prolonged hypoglycemia
- Failure to recognize the magnitude of total-body potassium depletion and to begin replacement despite a normal serum potassium level may lead to fatal cardiac arrhythmia.
- Inadequate monitoring of glucose may result in hypoglycemia unless dextrose is added to the infusion once the serum glucose level falls to 250.
- Ketogenesis may be inadequately reversed unless insulin treatment is continued until the anion gap has normalized.
- Failure to recognize precipitating causes results in increased morbidity/mortality from underlying infection or myocardial infarction

153   Hyperosmolar Hyperglycemic Nonketotic Coma

Hyperosmolar hyperglycemic nonketotic coma (HHNC) is a syndrome of profound dehydration that develops from osmotic diuresis. It is defined by a plasma osmolarity >350 µOsm/kg water, serum glucose >600 mg/dL, and an absence of ketoacidosis in a patient with depressed consciousness. A wide range of serum glucose values is seen; the absence of ketoacidosis or ketonuria is not absolute, and ketones may be present in small amounts. The patient may also not be comatose but often drowsy or confused. HHNC carries a high mortality.

PREDISPOSING FACTORS

The patient most at risk is elderly. Diabetic-type stress precipitates the hyperosmolar state. Chronic renal insufficiency, pneumonia, gram-negative sepsis, myocardial infarction, pancreatitis, and GI bleeding are associated with HHNC and contribute to its high mortality. Drugs are also implicated in HHNC: thiazide diuretics, corticosteroids, phenytoin, propranolol, chlorthalidone, furosemide, ethacrynic acid, diazoxide, cimetidine, chlorpromazine, L-asparaginase, immunosuppressive agents, loxapine. Also involved are hyperalimentation, peritoneal dialysis and hemodialysis, cardiac surgery, stroke, severe burns, pancreatitis, and heat stroke. Two thirds of patients have no history of diabetes, while 1/3 have non-insulin-dependent DM (a small number are insulin dependent). Patients may present with serious associated illnesses. HHNC is under-recognized. The high mortality rate of HHNC (20%–60%) is thought to be due to delays in diagnosis, failure to treat aggressively, and the high incidence of serious underlying disease.

CLINICAL PRESENTATION

Most patients experience polyuria and polydipsia for days or weeks before seeking medical attention. Insidious dehydration progresses until mental status is altered. Unresponsiveness or coma is the most common presentation. The duration of symptoms before presentation is 12 days for HHNC and 3 days for DKA. Signs of dehydration (poor skin turgor, dry mucous membranes) are not reliable in elderly patients; it is not always possible to estimate fluid deficits by clinical or laboratory findings. Neither the serum sodium nor the plasma osmolarity has been found to correlate with the volume of replacement fluid required by patients with HHNC.

The advanced state of dehydration may be underestimated if urine output is maintained by osmotic diuresis. On the other hand, renal dysfunction due to diabetic nephrosclerosis or other causes may prevent polydipsia or polyuria from occurring, even with progressively increasing levels of serum glucose. The severity of mental status changes in HHNC has been found to correlate with the degree of hyperosmolarity and the rate at which hyperosmolarity develops. HHNC can also cause other neurologic findings: seizures, Babinski reflexes, bilateral or unilateral focal deficits, etc.

HHNC may be found in association with other serious illness, most commonly chronic renal insufficiency, pneumonia, gastrointestinal hemorrhage, and gram-negative sepsis.

DIFFERENTIAL DIAGNOSIS

The differential diagnosis includes diabetic ketoacidosis and other causes of altered mental status (hepatic failure, uremia, CVA and drug ingestion) and other causes of severe dehydration. In altered mental status, blood glucose must be performed immediately. Lactic acidosis is often suspected, because patients are gravely ill and display signs of shock.

EMERGENCY DEPARTMENT EVALUATION

Laboratory studies include electrolytes, glucose, BUN, creatinine (Cr), CBC, urinalysis, and ABG. Serious underlying illness should be sought. A chest radiograph, ECG, blood and urine cultures, serum amylase, liver enzymes, coagulation studies, and, in some cases, cardiac enzymes should be obtained. The blood glucose in HHNC is typically >600 mg/dL, and may be as high as 4800 mg/dL, with average values of about 1000 mg/dL. Serum sodium and potassium concentrations may be low, normal, or high, and the values do not reflect total body losses. Potassium depletion is the rule, and profound deficits may be seen. All patients with HHNC are initially azotemic due to both prerenal and renal causes. The BUN-Cr ratio may exceed 30-1 with values of BUN and Cr of 87 mg/dL and 5.5 mg/dL, respectively. After treatment the average values usually normalize.

The serum osmolarity can be calculated using the formula:

Osmolarity (µOsm/kg H_2O) = 2(serum sodium) + (blood glucose)/18 + [BUN]/2.8

Although the measured and calculated osmolarity values follow similar trends, there is not always a reliable correspondence between the values. The *effective* osmolarity should be calculated by excluding the BUN term from the equation, because azotemia may mask actual hypotonicity of the extracellular fluid. If a patient presents with hyperglycemia and a normal or low effective plasma osmolarity, it is dangerous to administer hypotonic fluids or insulin because both treatments lower the tonicity of the extracellular fluid and could induce cerebral edema. About 50% of patients in one series had mild metabolic acidosis with an anion gap about twice normal. Accumulation of lactic acid or beta-hydroxybutyric acid (not measured by Acetest or Ketostix test), or acute or chronic renal insufficiency with accumulation of acid metabolites may explain the acidosis. The CBC may show an elevated WBC suggestive of a serious underlying infection. Because of profound dehydration, hemoconcentration should be expected to elevate the hemoglobin and hematocrit. The urinalysis may show only modest (i.e., 1+) glycosuria, and ketonuria need not be absent in order to make the diagnosis of HHNC.

EMERGENCY DEPARTMENT MANAGEMENT

Priorities include volume (sodium) replacement, correction of hyperosmolarity, and identification of underlying illness. Hypotension requires immediate fluid resuscitation with normal saline since average fluid deficits are 9–12 L. One to 2 L of normal saline should be infused rapidly until the patient's blood pressure and urine output are acceptable or the central venous pressure (CVP) begins to rise. It is reasonable to switch to one half normal saline to replace 1/2 of the estimated volume deficit during the first 12 hours, and the remaining estimated deficit during the second 12 hours. All patients have total-body potassium deficits, so potassium (10 mEq/hr I.V.) should be administered if urine output is present.

Insulin may not be necessary. Blood glucose levels decrease by 25% from dilution by fluid replacement. When the volume status improves, hyperglycemia may resolve further through metabolism and renal excretion of glucose. Insulin should be given, however, if a patient is acidotic, hyperkalemic, or in renal failure. If the decision is made to initiate therapy, a low-dose regimen should be used (0.15 U of regular insulin/kilogram body weight IV initially, followed by a continuous infusion of about 0.1 U/kg/hr). This therapy should be discontinued when the blood glucose has fallen to 250 mg/dL or the osmolarity is 315 µOsm/kg H_2O. At this stage, 5% dextrose should be added to the infusion to avoid hypoglycemia. If fluid resuscitation does not improve the urine output, furosemide should be given if volume has been restored. Initial management may also involve empiric phosphate repletion, anticoagulation with subcutaneous heparin, and broad-spectrum antibiotic prophylaxis.

DISPOSITION

All patients should be admitted to an ICU.

COMMON PITFALLS

- Because of theoretical concern that treatment of HHNC with hypotonic fluids can cause cerebral edema, it is safest to initiate therapy with normal saline while monitoring central venous pressures.
- Giving insulin before fluid deficits are restored may decrease the hypertonicity of the extracellular fluid abruptly and place the patient at risk for cerebral edema, systemic hypoperfusion, and cerebral infarction. Initial therapy should be consistent with the degree of hyperglycemia and the calculated effective osmolarity.

- Iatrogenic hypokalemia may result from insulin therapy if potassium replacement is not given and serum potassium level monitored.
- Phenytoin should not be used in treating seizures associated with HHNC. It is ineffective in this setting, and inhibits the release of endogenous insulin.
- Blood sugar measurement in all patients with new neurologic abnormalities will avoid a misdiagnosis of cerebral vascular accident and a potentially lethal delay in proper treatment.

154   Alcoholic Ketoacidosis

Alcoholic ketoacidosis (AKA), characterized by an elevated anion gap from accumulation of ketone bodies, is a metabolic disorder that most commonly affects alcoholics who have recently ceased binge drinking. It is affects both men and women equally. Ketosis is attributed to multiple factors.

CLINICAL PRESENTATION

Alcoholic ketoacidosis usually occurs in persons with a history of chronic alcohol abuse. The patient is often a binge drinker who has recently stopped drinking. There may be some alcohol detectable on the patient's breath or in the serum. The cessation of alcohol intake usually is not caused by an effort to abstain from alcohol, but rather by the onset of abdominal pain, nausea, and vomiting. Anorexia and poor caloric intake are associated. There is usually no history of diabetes mellitus. The patient may complain of abdominal pain due to liver disease, pancreatitis, alcoholic gastritis, or other diseases that may or may not be related to alcohol abuse. There is a spectrum of severity.

On physical examination the vital signs may be markedly abnormal with profound orthostasis. Respirations may be deep and rapid (Kussmaul respirations). Signs of dehydration due to decreased oral intake, diaphoresis, and vomiting may be present. Mental status is often normal or slightly impaired, but severe obtundation and coma have been reported. Abdominal examination may reveal pain and tenderness suggesting liver disease, pancreatitis, gastritis, or other intra-abdominal pathology. Examination of the skin may reveal spider angiomata or other markers of liver disease. Evidence of alcohol withdrawal may also be present.

In addition to the history, the diagnosis hinges upon laboratory findings of an elevated anion-gap metabolic acidosis. Other acid–base disorders may be present as well: metabolic alkalosis due to persistent vomiting and respiratory alkalosis as a result of liver disease, alcohol withdrawal, or infection. Thus, ABG analysis may not show marked acidemia. One third of patients with AKA may be alkalemic.

Table 154-1 summarizes the characteristics of AKA. Patients with AKA are ketotic. There are three types of ketone bodies: acetone and the two acids, beta-hydroxybutyrate (BHB) and acetoacetate (AcAc). The nitroprusside reaction, commonly used to detect ketones, may be misleading in determining the degree of ketosis, because only AcAc and acetone cause a positive reaction, whereas BHB does not. The ratio of BHB to AcAc depends on the ratio of reduced and oxidized nicotinamide adenine dinucleotide (NADH/NAD). In AKA, this ratio is high. A negative nitroprusside reaction may be misinterpreted as a lack of ketones. As the patient is rehydrated and given glucose, the NADH-NAD ratio changes to favor the conversion of more BHB to AcAc, and the test for "ketones" may become more strongly positive. A similar phenomenon is seen in DKA.

TABLE 154-1. Characteristics of Alcoholic Ketoacidosis

History	Laboratory Data
Nausea	Metabolic acidosis
Vomiting	Elevated anion gap
Anorexia	Ketoacidosis
Abdominal pain	Elevated BHB/AcAc ratio
History of alcohol abuse	Nitroprusside reaction: positive, weak, or negative
Binge drinking recently terminated	Glucose: low, normal, or slightly elevated
Poor caloric intake	± Elevated liver function tests
	± Elevated plasma lactate

Adams SL, Mathews JJ, Flaherty JJ: Alcoholic ketoacidosis. Ann Emerg Med 16:93, 1987.

Although the classic presentation of AKA is one of ketoacidosis without marked hyperglycemia, the glucose may be low, normal, or minimally elevated. The serum lactate level may also be minimally elevated. Liver enzymes, amylase, BUN, and creatinine (Cr) may be elevated, not as a direct result of AKA, but because of the effects of dehydration and underlying chronic medical problems.

DIFFERENTIAL DIAGNOSIS

The differential diagnosis of AKA consists of diseases that cause an elevated anion-gap metabolic acidosis discussed elsewhere. The most common is diabetic ketoacidosis (DKA). Other entities causing a ketotic state include hyperemesis gravidarum, starvation, cyanide poisoning; isopropyl alcohol causes ketosis but not acidosis.

EMERGENCY DEPARTMENT MANAGEMENT

Treatment is straightforward. Volume repletion with saline and glucose is the basis of therapy. Saline corrects volume depletion and promotes renal excretion of the ketone bodies BHB and AcAc. Insulin is not indicated if diabetes mellitus is not present. Bicarbonate is controversial, although it may be indicated if the pH is <7.1, especially in the presence of heart disease or ventricular irritability. Thiamine, magnesium sulfate, and vitamin supplementation should be administered as indicated.

DISPOSITION

Admission is indicated for patients who cannot tolerate oral hydration because of persistent nausea and vomiting, and for significant, persistent metabolic acidosis. If the cause of abdominal pain is unclear or an associated illness complicates the picture, admission for evaluation and observation is indicated. Because uncomplicated cases usually resolve with appropriate therapy within 12 to 24 hours, overnight admission on a general medical floor or observation in a holding unit may be sufficient.

The patient should not be discharged until he has demonstrated the ability to tolerate fluids, has been volume repleted, and has shown resolution of metabolic abnormalities. Underlying or precipitating illnesses must have resolved or been ruled out. Consultation is ordinarily not necessary unless there is a question of other pathology. If the patient is stable for discharge, close follow-up should be arranged. The patient may benefit from referral to a rehabilitation program.

COMMON PITFALLS

- Lack of appreciation of mixed acid–base disorders and the limitations of the nitroprusside test for ketones may cause confusion, with failure to consider the diagnosis with a normal pH or minimal ketosis by nitroprusside test.
- Patients with ketosis, Kussmaul respirations, and minimally elevated blood glucose may be mistakenly diagnosed as having DKA.
- Isopropyl alcohol ingestion may be confused with AKA, but acidosis is not a feature of this poison.
- Hyperemesis gravidarum may present with a similar picture, although there may be no history of alcohol ingestion.
- Ethanol-induced lactic acidosis may also be confused with this disorder.
- Failure to treat with glucose and the failure to consider other causes of nausea, vomiting, and abdominal pain when the patient does not respond to conservative therapy.

155   Hypoglycemia

Hypoglycemia is defined by three criteria: a low blood glucose concentration, typical symptoms, and reversal of symptoms by the administration of glucose. The lower limit of normal for blood glucose can be arbitrarily set at 45 mg/dL ±10 mg/dL, but even lower glucose levels may not cause symptoms in some patients. Because the severity of symptoms might also depend on the rapidity of the fall, it is possible for symptoms to occur at relatively high levels as well. The typical patient with hypoglycemia is the diabetic who administers insulin (or an oral hypoglycemic agent), but either ingests insufficient calories or exercises excessively. After appropriate therapy to reverse hypoglycemia, determine whether the cause of the hypoglycemia is exogenous or endogenous (Table 155-1). Exogenous hypoglycemia usually responds rapidly to therapy. The less common endogenous or spontaneous types of hypoglycemia are caused by disease of organ systems or glucoregulatory hormones.

CLINICAL PRESENTATION

The hypoglycemic patient is symptomatic because of the lack of glucose for brain metabolism (neuroglycopenia) or because of the counterregulatory hormonal response. The more acute the fall in the blood glucose, the more prominent the adrenergic symptoms (sweating, tremulousness, palpitations, weakness, lightheadedness, and mental clouding) and signs (diaphoresis, pallor, tachypnea, tachycardia, and hypertension). If hypoglycemia has developed gradually or if treatment is delayed, the adrenergic response may not be prominent or may even be absent. The symptoms (fatigue, headache, insomnia, nightmares, visual problems, confusion, disorientation, memory loss, depression) and signs (altered level of consciousness, neurologic deficits, catatonia, convulsions, coma) of CNS dysfunction may be the sole presentation.

Hypoglycemia can result in significant complications. The tachycardia and hypertension can lead to acute coronary or cerebrovascular insufficiency, particularly in the diabetic, but also in the elderly and in those with hypertension or coronary artery disease. If hypoglycemia is not

---

TABLE 155-1. Causes of Hypoglycemia

Exogenous

Insulin/sulfonylurea (including surreptitious/suicidal/drug interactions)
Alcohol and fasting/malnutrition
Other drugs (salicylates, pentamidine, disopyramide, propranolol, lithium, phenformin, haloperidol, propoxyphene, chlorpromazine, chloroquine)
Ackee fruit poisoning

Endogenous

Postprandial (reactive): alimentary hyperinsulinism, early diabetes mellitus, idiopathic postprandial syndrome
Underproduction of glucose: Hormonal deficiency (pituitary, adrenal, catecholamine, glucagon, thyroid)
    Enzyme defects (glucose-6-phosphatase and others)
    Substrate deficiency (severe malnutrition, chronic renal failure, hypothermia, sepsis)
    Acquired liver disease (hepatic congestion, fulminant hepatitis, hepatotoxins, Reye's syndrome, cirrhosis, hepatoma, metastases)
Overutilization of glucose:
    Hyperinsulinism (insulinoma, antibodies to insulin receptors)
    Appropriate insulin levels (large extrapancreatic tumors, cachexia with fat depletion, systemic carnitine deficiency, marked hypothermia, sepsis, prolonged exercise)

---

recognized and reversed promptly, the CNS effects may become irreversible and may even lead to death from cerebral edema due to prolonged seizures or profound hypoglycemia.

EMERGENCY DEPARTMENT EVALUATION

It is prudent to consider hypoglycemia to be the cause of altered mental status or abnormal vital signs, until proven otherwise. The glucose test strip and accucheck are rapid and reliable tools. Symptomatic patients should be given dextrose before the serum glucose is available.

EMERGENCY DEPARTMENT MANAGEMENT

Immediate intervention is the key to reversing hypoglycemia. If an IV line cannot be started and the patient cannot take sugar orally, intramuscular administration of glucagon is appropriate, but its onset of action is slow. If there is any doubt as to the presence of hypoglycemia, it is best to give dextrose pending laboratory confirmation. Hyperglycemic diabetics who receive dextrose are not adversely affected. Because some patients with depleted thiamine stores may suffer adverse neurologic effects from dextrose, it is standard to administer thiamine 100 mg I.V. before giving dextrose. If the patient is alert with an intact swallowing mechanism, oral sugar may be sufficient. Patients who cannot take oral glucose should be started on an IV of D5W after D50 is given, and the infusion continued until the patient can eat. Equally important is to determine the reason for hypoglycemia. It is important to identify those who have either inadvertently or deliberately overdosed on oral hypoglycemic agents, because hypoglycemia may be prolonged, requiring days of continuous glucose infusion.

DISPOSITION

Insulin-dependent diabetics whose condition is rapidly reversed and who suffer no complications can be sent home if the reason for the hypoglycemia is apparent. Adjustment in the regimen may be required. Telephone consultation with the patient's physician is necessary in order to arrange follow-up. Admission is indicated for hypoglycemia due to oral agents or long-acting insulin; if a deliberate overdose is involved, psychiatric evaluation is indicated. Patients with no obvious cause of hypoglycemia require admission for further evaluation. A monitored setting is indicated if hypoglycemia persists despite IV dextrose or if the patient has suffered neurologic or cardiac complications.

COMMON PITFALLS

- All too often the hypoglycemic patient is allowed to languish until the laboratory calls with a "panic" value. This is most often seen in the alcoholic or the patient with chronic multisystem disease, diabetics who cannot/do not communicate about their diabetes and, the suicidal patient who willfully withholds pertinent history.
- Don't wait for the laboratory result before giving dextrose
- Failure to follow a D50 bolus with a dextrose infusion
- Failure to feed the patient after the initial response to dextrose
- Failure to admit patients who are at risk for relapse, particularly those who have taken oral hypoglycemic agents
- Failure to consider the possibility of suicidal intentions
- For discharged patients, failure to make the adjustments in insulin dosage, diet, or activity and to insure close follow-up.

156   Metabolic Disorders

HYPERKALEMIA

Because ECG changes correlate only roughly with serum potassium levels, cardiac monitoring is advisable whenever the serum potassium level is elevated, although dangerous effects usually do not occur at <6.5 mEq/L. Therapy is indicated if ECG changes are present (Table 156-1). For mild hyperkalemia (no clinical/ECG manifestations), address the most likely etiology and correct predisposing factors (discontinuing oral potassium supplements). Spurious hyperkalemia should be ruled out. If there is no reason that the potassium level will rise further, the patient can be discharged with outpatient follow-up arranged for a repeat potassium determination and further evaluation within 48–72 hours. Admission is advisable for higher levels of potassium.

When ECG or clinical manifestations are present, cardiac monitoring and therapy are indicated. These patients should be admitted to an ICU. Calcium is the principal therapy for severe hyperkalemia because its effect is almost immediate, and lasts 30–60 minutes. The dose is 5 mL of 10% calcium chloride (13.6 mEq/10 mL) or 10 mL of 10% calcium gluconate (4.6 mEq/10 mL) given over at least 2 minutes via a peripheral vein and repeated in 5–10 minutes if necessary. IV calcium should be reserved for severe hyperkalemia and cardiac manifestations requiring immediate intervention. It is relatively safe, although it has the potential of causing transient hypercalcemia. IV sodium bicarbonate has a therapeutic effect that begins within 15 minutes and lasts 1–2 hours. Like calcium, it is a temporizing measure, causing a shift of potassium without altering total body potassium. The dose is one to two ampules (approximately 50 mEq per ampule) given IV over 2 minutes and repeated after 15 minutes if necessary.

Glucose and insulin act to shift potassium from extracellular to the intracellular space but do not change total body potassium content. They provide another temporary decrease until

TABLE 156-1. Electrocardiographic Manifestations of Hyperkalemia

Early Changes	Advanced Changes
Tall peaked (tented) T waves	Absent P waves
Shortened QT interval	Marked QRS complex widening
Later Changes	Sine wave pattern
	Ventricular fibrillation
Widened QRS complex	Asystole
Increased PR interval	
Low-amplitude P waves	
Elevation or depression of ST segment	

There is only a rough correlation of ECG changes with serum potassium concentration. Life-threatening dysrhythmias can occur at even mildly elevated serum potassium concentrations.

definitive therapy can be instituted. Therapeutic effects begin within 30–60 minutes and last 4–6 hours. Glucose and insulin should always be used in combination, even in the nondiabetic. Infusion is preferred with the typical dose 500 mL of D10W with 10 units of regular insulin, infused over 30–60 minutes. Potential complications include hyperglycemia, hypoglycemia, and hyperosmolality.

Definitive therapy for hyperkalemia removes potassium from the body and decreases the total body potassium. If renal function is adequate, the most straightforward way of removing potassium from the body is by increasing renal excretion with furosemide. If renal function is inadequate, other means must be employed. Sodium polystyrene sulfonate (Kayexalate) removes potassium from the body by exchanging sodium ions for potassium ions. Kayexalate can be given orally or rectally with 1 mEq of potassium removed for each gram of orally administered Kayexalate.

By the rectal route, Kayexalate acts more quickly, but total potassium removal is less. Orally, 15–30 g of Kayexalate is given with 15–30 mL of 70% sorbitol (or 50–100 mL of 20% sorbitol) and may be repeated every 2 to 4 hours. Contraindications to the oral route include ileus, complete or partial bowel obstruction, and GI surgery. Kayexalate is given as a retention enema in a dose of 50 g in 200 mL of 20% sorbitol (or 150 mL of tap water with 50 mL of 70% sorbitol), which may be repeated every 2–6 hours. Potential complications include hypervolemia due to the sodium load and hypokalemia.

Dialysis is the most efficient way of removing potassium from the body. It is indicated when the above measures have failed, and is the definitive therapy in acute or chronic renal failure. Dialysis is most helpful when the potassium level is rising very rapidly (rhabdomyolysis). Hemodialysis is preferred over peritoneal dialysis because it removes potassium more quickly.

The patient with severe hyperkalemia requires cardiac monitoring and electrolyte levels every 2 hours until out of danger. Admission, generally to an ICU, is mandatory. If the patient must be transferred, transport must be by ALS vehicle and staff.

COMMON PITFALLS

- It is not advisable to institute vigorous therapy for hyperkalemia when the potassium is elevated but the ECG is normal and the patient has no clinical manifestations. Cardiac monitoring should continue while the potassium is repeated and possible causes of hyperkalemia are evaluated.
- Failure to recognize patients at risk for hyperkalemia (Table 156-2) and not checking the serum potassium level

TABLE 156-2. Etiologies and Differential Diagnosis of Hyperkalemia

Artifactual Hyperkalemia	Decreased Renal Potassium Excretion
Hemolysis *in vitro* or due to venipuncture	Acute renal failure
Extreme leukocytosis or thrombocytosis	Chronic renal insufficiency
Mild forearm exercise during venipuncture	Hypoaldosteronism
General exercise within 20 minutes of venipuncture	Drugs
	Nonsteroidal anti-inflammatory drugs
Laboratory error	Cyclosporine
Cold agglutinins	Heparin
Increased Potassium Loads	Angiotensin-converting-enzyme inhibitors
	Potassium-sparing diuretics
Oral or intravenous potassium supplements	**Transcellular Maldistribution**
Penicillin potassium salts	Acidemia
Massive blood transfusion	Hyperkalemic period paralysis
Intravascular hemolysis	Succinylcholine
Burns	Massive digitalis overdose
Crush injuries	Insulin deficiency
Mesenteric or muscular infarction	Beta-blockers
Tumor lysis due to chemotherapy or radiotherapy	Hypertonic agents
	Mannitol
	Hyperglycemia (endogenous or exogenous)

HYPOKALEMIA

Most authorities agree that patients with potassium levels of <2.5 mEq/L need admission since potassium of 2.5 mEq/L generally reflects a total body potassium deficit of 200 to 300 mEq. Those with mild hypokalemia (i.e., 2.5–3.5 mEq/L) can usually be managed as outpatients with gradual oral potassium repletion, if there are no cardiac dysrhythmias, ileus, muscular weakness, or other serious effects (Table 156-3). ED management should focus on determining the etiology of hypokalemia, (Table 156–4) confirming that the patient can tolerate oral potassium repletion, and excluding other serious conditions or complications. Patients who can be sent home with oral potassium supplementation should have follow-up within 48–72 hours with a potassium level and further evaluation as necessary. In mild hypokalemia, oral potassium repletion is preferred because of its ease, safety, and economy. Potassium chloride (KCl), 40–80 mEq per day, with no more than 40 mEq given as a single dose, is usually effective. KCl may be given as a liquid, in enteric-coated tablets, or in wax matrix tablets.

For more severe hypokalemia (K^+ < 2.5 mEq/L), the total body potassium deficit can be profound, and repletion is more urgent. Patients should have an IV and be monitored for rhythm disturbances. In the absence serious manifestations, repletion can be accomplished by the oral route while observation and cardiac monitoring are continued. Otherwise, repletion generally should begin with combined IV and oral KCl. IV KCl should not exceed a rate of 40 mEq per hour. At rates >10 mEq per hour, cardiac monitoring and a constant infusion pump are advisable to avoid accidental overinfusion. Simultaneous oral and IV repletion improves the level rapidly, but carries a higher risk of hyperkalemia.

Patients with persistent vomiting often develop "hypokalemic contraction alkalosis." The dehydration and metabolic alkalosis from gastric acid loss cause the kidney to conserve sodium and chloride and to increase potassium and bicarbonate excretion. In addition to potassium, these patients require rehydration, usually with IV sodium chloride, to correct the hypokalemia.

Hypokalemic patients with any of the following conditions should be admitted to an ICU: malignant cardiac dysrhythmias, digitalis toxicity, profound weakness with impending respiratory insufficiency, a serum potassium <2.0 mEq/L, rhabdomyolysis, or hepatic encephalopathy.

TABLE 156-3. Manifestations of Hypokalemia

Neuromuscular	Gastrointestinal
Weakness, areflexia, paralysis	Ileus
Respiratory insufficiency due to severe weakness	**Renal**
Rhabdomyolysis	
Paresthesia	Polyuria
	Metabolic alkalosis
Cardiovascular	Increased renal ammonia production
U wave prominence	**Endocrine**
T wave flattening or inversion	
ST segment depression	Glucose intolerance
Potentiation of digitalis toxicity	
Orthostatic hypotension	

TABLE 156-4. Etiologies and Differential Diagnosis of Hypokalemia

Decreased Potassium Intake	Transcellular Maldistribution
Increased Potassium Excretion	Alkalemia
	Insulin excess
Increased renal potassium excretion	Beta-adrenergic agonists
	Acute theophylline toxicity
Drugs	Poisoning with soluble barium salts
Non-potassium-sparing diuretics	Vitamin B_{12} therapy of
Amphotericin B	megaloblastic anemia
Aminoglycosides	Rapid malignant cell growth and
Renal tubular acidosis	multiplication
Magnesium deficiency	Hypokalemic periodic paralysis
Diuretic phase of recovery from postobstructive	
nephropathy or acute tubular necrosis	
Primary hyperaldosteronism	
Secondary hyperaldosteronism	
Hyperreninemic states	
Hypovolemia	
Nephrotic syndrome	
Congestive heart failure	
Cirrhosis	
Bartter's syndrome	
Osmotic diuresis	
Increased gastrointestinal potassium loss	
Protracted emesis or nasogastric suction	
Diarrhea	
Villous adenoma	
Chronic laxative abuse	

COMMON PITFALLS

A common error is to attempt to replete potassium too rapidly or without appropriate cardiac and laboratory monitoring, risking potentially dangerous hyperkalemia. Overshoot into hyperkalemia is more likely when hypokalemia is due to transcellular potassium shifts (hypokalemic periodic paralysis)

HYPERCALCEMIA

Primary hyperparathyroidism and malignancy (especially breast, lung, and kidney) are the most common causes of hypercalcemia (Table 156-5).

TABLE 156-5. Causes of Hypercalcemia

Endocrine Disorders	**Drugs**
Parathyroid, thyroid	Thiazides, lithium, vitamin D, vitamin A
Malignancies	**Miscellaneous**
Granulomatous Diseases	Dehydration or immobilization
Sarcoid, tuberculosis, berylliosis, histoplasmosis, coccidioidomycosis	Excess calcium ingestion Milk-alkali syndrome

CLINICAL PRESENTATION

The manifestations depend on the serum calcium level and rate of rise from normal values. With increasing calcium levels, weakness, lethargy, depression, confusion, or personality change are fairly consistent, as are anorexia, nausea, vomiting, and constipation. In the kidney, hypercalcemia results in the inability to concentrate urine; coupled with CNS and gastrointestinal effects, this leads to dehydration. Peptic ulcer disease, pancreatitis, nephrolithiasis, conjunctivitis, and ocular band keratopathy are seen in chronic hypercalcemia. The most common ECG finding is a shortened QT interval.

EMERGENCY DEPARTMENT MANAGEMENT

Symptomatic hypercalcemia or a calcium level >15 mg/dL require immediate intervention. Forced saline diuresis is first-line treatment; IV furosemide (20–40 mg or more) enhances urinary output once intravascular volume has been repleted. Calcitonin 2–4 IU/kg intramuscularly every 12 hours causes a rapid fall of the serum calcium level in most patients and is appropriate in those not responding to saline diuresis or for whom saline loading and diuresis are not possible (e.g., renal failure, severe CHF). Mithramycin is another option but dialysis may be necessary to control serum calcium levels quickly. IV phosphate should not be given because of the risks of soft-tissue calcification and possible sudden death. IV sodium ethylenediaminetetraacetic acid (EDTA) should be avoided as well. Cardiac monitoring is necessary, and serum calcium, potassium, and magnesium levels must be followed closely.

COMMON PITFALLS

- A common error is to administer a loop diuretic before intravascular volume repletion occurs; this tends to further deplete volume and may worsen hypercalcemia.
- Frequent levels of calcium, magnesium, and potassium are necessary during treatment.
- Thiazide diuretics can cause an increase in serum calcium.

HYPOMAGNESIUM

Magnesium (Mg) is essential; dietary magnesium deficiency is unusual because magnesium is found in green vegetables, meats, seafood, and grains. Serum magnesium levels are regulated primarily by changes in renal excretion. The normal serum level is from 1.5 to 2.5 mEq/L. Twelve to twenty percent of hospitalized patients and 29% of ICU patients have abnormal serum magnesium levels. Because 99% of magnesium is found intracellularly, patients with symptomatic hypomagnesemia may have normal or only minimally decreased magnesium levels (alcoholics and renal patients particularly). Most cases of hypomagnesemia are from renal loss, gastrointestinal disease, or endocrine disorders (Table 156-6).

TABLE 156-6. Causes of Hypomagnesemia

Increased Urinary Excretion	Gastrointestinal Disorders
Drugs—alcohol, diuretics, aminoglycosides, cisplatin	Malabsorption syndromes
	Chronic or severe diarrhea
Renal tubular disorders	Acute pancreatitis
Hypercalcemic states	Severe malnutrition

CLINICAL PRESENTATION

The clinical manifestations are diverse but generally mimic those of hypocalcemia, with CNS complaints dominating the clinical picture. Malaise, diffuse weakness, anorexia, nausea, and vomiting are not unusual, but more specific are Chvostek's sign, Trousseau's sign, tremor, twitching, clonus, increased deep tendon reflexes, carpopedal spasm, and frank tetany. Psychiatric symptoms are common but delirium, movement disorders, dysarthria, and seizures less common. Magnesium deficiency has been associated with both atrial and ventricular tachyarrhythmias. Magnesium deficiency is a cause of torsades de pointes. The ECG most often shows prolongation of the QT interval.

EMERGENCY DEPARTMENT MANAGEMENT

In severe hypomagnesemia, ECG monitoring is mandatory. Emergent therapy and admission are warranted if cardiac arrhythmias are present, if marked central neurologic manifestations noted, or if the patient is severely symptomatic. For seizures or malignant ventricular arrhythmias, 2 g of magnesium sulfate may be given IV over several minutes followed by 5 g IV over 6 hours. Arrhythmias may be unresponsive to usual therapy but respond well to IV magnesium. As a general rule, serum magnesium levels <1 mEq/L necessitate hospitalization because repletion takes several days, often with 1 mEq of magnesium/kg body weight IV. Mild hypomagnesemia can be treated with oral magnesium hydroxide 200 to 600 mg four times daily and an adequate diet. Treatment should also be directed toward correcting the underlying cause of the hypomagnesemia.

COMMON PITFALLS

- Deep tendon reflexes usually indicate a magnesium level <4–6 mEq/L.
- Hypomagnesemia is commonly associated with other electrolyte abnormalities (eg, hypokalemia refractory to potassium replacement may be secondary to hypomagnesemia).
- Hypomagnesemia predisposes to digitalis-induced arrhythmias.

157   Azotemia, Oliguria, and Renal Failure

Renal insufficiency or failure occurs when kidney function declines to a point at which nitrogenous wastes can no longer be cleared effectively from the circulation. This leads to azotemia, in which urea and creatinine accumulate in the blood. The serum creatinine concentration is used widely as an index of renal function, but it varies with age, sex, and body weight; creatinine production rate is lower in women and declines with age. In acute renal failure, the creatinine level does not reflect renal function accurately.

CLINICAL PRESENTATION

There is no specific syndrome characteristic of acute or chronic renal failure. Patients may be critically ill or azotemia may be detected on a routine blood test. Renal failure affects nearly every organ system. Uremia is the syndrome of detrimental effects of renal failure on other organ systems: cardiovascular (pericarditis), central nervous system (CNS) (somnolence, coma, seizures), gastrointestinal (GI) (nausea, vomiting), hematologic (anemia, coagulopathy, qualitative platelet dysfunction), immunologic (sepsis, other infections, poor wound healing), and others.

DIFFERENTIAL DIAGNOSIS

Azotemia from acute renal failure may be divided into three categories: prerenal (renal hypoperfusion states), renal (intrinsic renal parenchymal disorders), and postrenal (obstruction) (Table 157-1). *Prerenal azotemia* includes hypovolemia or intravascular depletion (vomiting, diarrhea, GI bleeding, and diuretic use); decreased *effective* intravascular volume (CHF, sepsis, cirrhosis, or vasodilator therapy). If the underlying disorder is corrected, the condition is potentially reversible.

   Intrinsic renal azotemia may be divided into disorders affecting the glomeruli (e.g., acute glomerulonephritis), the renal interstitium (e.g., acute interstitial nephritis), the renal vasculature (e.g., vasculitis, malignant hypertension), or the tubules (e.g., acute tubular necrosis). Acute tubu-

---

TABLE 157-1. Causes of Acute Renal Insufficiency

PRERENAL AZOTEMIA	POSTRENAL OCCLUSION
Volume Depletion	*Urethral Obstruction*
Hemorrhage	Prostatic hypertrophy
Excessive diuresis	Prostatic carcinoma
Diarrhea	Cervical carcinoma
Vomiting	Urethral stricture
Heat losses	
Burns	*Ureteral Obstruction*
Decreased Effective Volume	Blood clots
	Intra-abdominal tumor
Congestive heart failure	Bilateral calculi
Sepsis	Retroperitoneal fibrosis
Cirrhosis	Retroperitoneal malignancy
INTRINSIC RENAL INSUFFICIENCY	
Acute Tubular Necrosis	
Ischemic injury secondary to shock, hemorrhage	
Aminoglycosides	
Intravenous contrast agents	
Pigment nephropathy secondary to trauma	
Others	
Acute Interstitial Nephritis	
Drugs	
Systemic infections	
Idiopathic	
Acute Glomerulonephritis	
Vascular Disease	
Vasculitis	
Malignant hypertension	
Vascular occlusion	

lar necrosis (ATN) is one of the most common intrarenal causes of acute renal failure, especially in hospitalized patients, and is often reversible. Common causes include ischemic insults to the kidney (e.g., shock, hemorrhage), drugs (e.g., aminoglycosides, contrast agents), and pigment nephropathy (e.g., myoglobinuria from crush injuries or other trauma). ATN may be either oliguric or nonoliguric, with the latter having a better prognosis.

Acute interstitial nephritis (AIN) is most often due to a drug reaction, although it may occur with infection or no apparent precipitating event. The drugs involved are antibiotics, especially the beta-lactam antibiotics. Nonsteroidal anti-inflammatory agents also may cause AIN. Others include diuretics, allopurinol, and cimetidine. Patients with AIN may present with fever, skin rash, arthralgias, eosinophilia, and eosinophiluria, but may also have no findings.

Postrenal azotemia occurs from obstruction distal to the kidney. For renal failure to develop, obstruction must be bilateral (except in the case of a single functioning kidney); obstruction of only one ureter or kidney should not result in renal failure. Among the common causes are prostatic hypertrophy or carcinoma, cervical carcinoma, and urethral stricture. Ureteral obstruction may occur from blood clots, tumors, calculi, retroperitoneal fibrosis or malignancy. Patients may present with anuria, oliguria, or normal urine output. Microscopic urinalysis is essentially normal.

EMERGENCY DEPARTMENT EVALUATION

The evaluation centers on determining whether renal insufficiency is acute, chronic, or "acute on chronic" and on distinguishing among prerenal, intrarenal, and postrenal causes. Some clues may help: bilaterally small kidneys indicate chronicity. A well tolerated hemoglobin of 6–7 g/dL strongly suggests chronic renal disease. Because obstruction is potentially the most easily correctable cause, early efforts should exclude postrenal causes (ultrasound, CT). Anuria or sudden fluctuations in urine output suggest obstruction. A prostate examination or a pelvic examination are mandatory. A Foley catheter should rule out bladder outlet obstruction; the catheter should be left in place to monitor urine output. Renal ultrasonography is sensitive in identifying upper-tract obstruction. Once obstruction is ruled out, attempts should be made to differentiate between prerenal and renal causes.

A history is essential, including recent ingestion of potentially nephrotoxic agents; recent fluid loss (diarrhea, hemorrhage, ascites, etc), previous episodes of renal dysfunction, and symptoms of systemic diseases known to affect the kidneys (vasculitis, diabetes, myeloma, etc). On examination, look for signs of absolute or relative intravascular volume depletion (orthostatic hypotension, peripheral edema, poor skin turgor or color, or signs of CHF).

CBC, electrolytes, glucose, calcium, phosphorous, BUN and creatinine, urine analysis and culture should be sent. The UA in AIN may demonstrate eosinophiluria and granular and white cell casts; acute glomerulonephritis often shows red cells and red cell casts in the urinary sediment. Urinary and serum sodium and creatinine concentrations should also be measured in patients with azotemia. Urinary sodium is <20 mEq/L in prerenal azotemia. In ATN and AIN, tubular reabsorption of sodium is compromised, and urinary sodium concentration is often >40 mEq/L.

EMERGENCY DEPARTMENT MANAGEMENT

Management should be directed toward rapid identification of the cause and intervention to restore renal function if possible. If azotemia is postrenal, relief of obstruction is indicated. Bladder outlet obstruction can often be relieved by a Foley catheter. If prerenal, repletion of intravascular volume is indicated. In cases of volume loss, IV crystalloid or blood may often correct the condition. Furosemide may be used in oliguric ATN. Moderate initial doses (100–250 mg) may be doubled every 30 to 60 minutes until urine output increases or a potentially ototoxic dose (500 mg or higher) is reached. Dialysis (either peritoneal dialysis or hemodialysis) should be considered if severe metabolic abnormalities (e.g., hyperkalemia, hyponatremia, or significant acidosis) develop. Other indications for dialysis include fluid overload, bleeding complications, encephalopathy, pericarditis, and severe uncontrolled hypertension.

DISPOSITION

Surgical consultation is necessary if azotemia is secondary to obstruction. For metabolic or uremic complications of renal failure, nephrology consultation is indicated. Most patients with new-onset azotemia or oliguria must be admitted. Patients with urinary obstruction corrected by bladder catheterization may be discharged with an indwelling catheter; however, if the patient was azotemic, a post-obstructive diuresis may occur and admission is warranted in this case. Transfer should be considered if dialysis is necessary but not available since life-threatening uremic and metabolic complications can develop rapidly.

COMMON PITFALLS

- Don't forget the simple things; perform a prostate exam on all men and a pelvic exam on all women; insert a Foley catheter to rule out bladder outlet obstruction.
- Serum creatinine is not an accurate measure of renal function in acute renal failure.
- Giving diuretics to the hypovolemic oliguric patient will only increase volume contraction and worsen renal perfusion.
- Don't wait until life-threatening uremic complications occur before transferring a patient to a center where dialysis is available.

---

158   Dialysis-Related Emergencies

Patients with chronic renal failure on hemodialysis or chronic, ambulatory peritoneal dialysis (CAPD) are subject to complications. Hemodialysis and CAPD are associated with specific complications.

HEMODIALYSIS: VASCULAR ACCESS

The vascular access device is the patient's lifeline and must be treated with care to avoid causing thrombosis or bleeding, or introducing infection. Avoid blood pressure measurement in the involved arm, and a tourniquet should never be applied. Avoid drawing blood from the access or placing an IV in it. However, if no other site is available and it is absolutely essential to obtain blood samples, the fistula or graft can be used. Careful skin cleansing and sterile technique are mandatory and firm but nonocclusive pressure should be applied to the site for 10 minutes after the puncture. The presence of a thrill both before and after the procedure should be documented.

Likewise, if IV access is critical but otherwise impossible, an IV line may be placed in the access, but with similar infection precautions. Special care should be taken not to puncture the back wall of the access. An automated infusion pump is necessary to control the infusion rate. Hemorrhage from a recent puncture site is usually managed with continuous, firm, but nonocclusive pressure over the site. Thrombosis, signaled by the loss of the thrill in the access, requires immediate consultation with a vascular surgeon, who may elect to perform a radiocontrast fistulagram, to infuse a thrombolytic agent, or to revise the access surgically. Forceful irrigation attempts are inadvisable.

The most common access-related problem is access infection, more likely to occur in an artificial graft than in a native fistula. Most infections are staphylococcal; Vancomycin 1 g IV is given as a loading dose; an aminoglycoside can be used in addition if infection with a gram-negative organism is suspected. Vancomycin is not hemodialyzable and can be given only once every 5 to 7 days, an attractive choice for staphylococcal coverage; in addition, its major toxicity is renal.

Although a febrile illness may prove to be of viral etiology, it is prudent to assume bacterial illness. Not all febrile dialysis patients are invariably admitted to the hospital. After IV antibiotic loading, a reliable patient who otherwise feels relatively well and is not hypotensive may be sent home with careful instructions to return if there is any deterioration. This decision is best reached in conjunction with the consulting nephrologist.

PERITONEAL DIALYSIS: PERITONEAL ACCESS

In CAPD, the patient's peritoneum serves as the membrane across which diffusion of water and solute occurs. Sterile dialysis fluid is infused into the peritoneal cavity through a Tenckhoff catheter. The most common problem is peritonitis, presumably through contamination of the peritoneal cavity. Peritonitis is less severe than other types of peritonitis and rarely lethal. In fact, these infections are usually treated on an outpatient basis. Occasionally, if infection cannot be eradicated with antibiotic therapy, the catheter must be removed surgically and hemodialysis initiated until a new catheter can be placed.

About 66% of peritonitis cases are due to gram-positive organisms, primarily staphylococci. In the remainder, assorted gram-negative organisms are responsible; a small percentage are due to fungal infection, an indication for catheter removal. Polymicrobial infection suggests a communication with the bowel or genitourinary tract. The diagnosis is usually based on the cloudiness in the dialysate effluent at the time an exchange is performed; this is often the earliest sign. Patients are instructed to seek medical attention immediately when they notice it. Abdominal pain and fever often develop if treatment is not initiated promptly. Hospital admission becomes necessary if there is high fever, hypotension, severe abdominal pain, nausea and vomiting, or if the patient cannot carry out exchanges and administer antibiotic therapy at home.

The diagnosis is confirmed by Gram's stain of organisms of the peritoneal fluid, or of a cell count of >100 WBCs (predominantly neutrophils). Even in patients who have not noted cloudiness of the peritoneal effluent, but who have fever, abdominal pain, or vague malaise, it is advisable to obtain a sample of fluid for examination. CAPD-related peritonitis can usually be treated on an outpatient basis. Treatment decisions should be made in conjunction with the patient's nephrologist or the CAPD nurse specialist. A common regimen is cefazolin 1 g intramuscularly or IV in the ED with 250 mg injected into each 2-L bag of dialysate before infusion into the peritoneal cavity for the next 10 days. Heparin 1000 units also is generally added to each bag for the first few days to decrease the risk of fibrin obstructing the catheter.

Arrangements should be made for follow-up within 2 days to check culture results and adjust therapy accordingly. Vancomycin is an alternative to cefazolin: the dose is 1 g IV load, followed by intraperitoneal doses of 50 mg per 2-L bag for 10 days, but newer regimens that employ only intermittent IV or intraperitoneal loading have been successful. An aminoglycoside can be added to the regimen for gram-positive coverage if there is reason to suspect infection with gram-negative organisms. Important caveats should be noted. (1) Acute abdominal processes such as pancreatitis, diverticulitis, or ruptured viscus may present similarly to peritonitis and may be missed. (2) Intra-abdominal free air on radiograph may be from dialysis exchanges and does not necessarily indicate perforation. (3) Brownish or fecal material in the dialysate mandates immediate surgical consultation. (4) Grossly bloody dialysate (but with no pain) in young women on CAPD may be due to retrograde menstruation.

INFECTION

Infections are a major cause of death in dialysis patients. Vascular access infection and peritonitis are the most common infections in hemodialysis patients and CAPD patients, respectively, but other infections are seen. Most infections are from usual pathogens rather than opportunistic organisms.

HYPOTENSION

Hypotension, from rapid fluid and electrolyte shifts, occurs often during or immediately after dialysis but usually resolves spontaneously or responds readily to fluid infusion. CAPD patients are not subject to this but they too can become volume-depleted if intake does not keep up with losses through dialysis. Other serious causes of hypotension must be considered. Sepsis, drug effects, myocardial dysfunction, dysrhythmia, myocardial infarction, and pericardial tamponade are important considerations in patients on either dialysis modality; acute electrolyte disturbances, vascular instability, anaphylactoid reaction, and air embolism are considerations in hemodialysis patients.

Pericardial tamponade may develop acutely when there is bleeding into the pericardial sac or when volume depletion allows a subclinical effusion to produce significant circulatory compromise. One helpful clue is a history of a recent decrease in the requirement for antihypertensive medications, often despite weight gain. Although tamponade in this setting generally presents with the expected physical findings, coexistent cardiac or pulmonary disease may make the diagnosis difficult.

Echocardiography is useful in detecting pericardial fluid. Many dialysis patients have effusions of varying size without clinical difficulties. ECHO demonstration of right ventricular collapse is a much better indicator of tamponade. Emergency pericardiocentesis may be necessary if the condition deteriorates and tamponade is thought likely; it can establish the diagnosis and buy time until definitive therapy can be undertaken. Another temporizing measure is IV saline to raise filling pressures. Dialysis is appropriate.

DYSPNEA AND VOLUME OVERLOAD

Dyspnea is most often due to volume overload during the interval between dialyses. Physical examination is not always reliable and chest x-ray findings may be misleading. The most reliable clue is a history of recent weight gain. The definitive treatment of volume overload is dialysis, but several temporizing measures are available: oxygen, patient in the sitting position, morphine, furosemide, and sublingual nitroglycerin to reduce preload and afterload. IV nitroglycerin and nitroprusside are useful options and can be titrated to effect. Thiocyanate toxicity can result from prolonged use of the latter agent in renal failure, however. Although volume overload is the most likely cause of shortness of breath, dyspnea can be due to cardiac, hypotension, infection, pleural or pericardial effusion, or any of the other causes of dyspnea in nondialysis patients.

Another potentially adverse effect of volume overload is severe hypertension, since blood pressure is partly volume-dependent. For hypertensive crisis, therapy should include not only sodium nitroprusside but also prompt dialysis to lower blood volume. It is important not to lower blood pressure too rapidly or to too low a level.

CHEST PAIN

When chest pain occurs, an ischemic cardiac event *must* be ruled out, because most dialysis patients die from cardiovascular causes and most patients have risk factors (hypertension, hyperlipidemia, and carbohydrate intolerance). In addition, chronic anemia and intermittent or chronic volume overload increase the problem. When chest pain consistent with angina occurs, a low threshold should exist for admission. Initial interventions include attention toward correctable factors such as volume overload, hypertension, and anemia. The diagnosis of myocardial infarction by standard ECG and enzyme criteria is generally not affected by the abnormalities of end-stage renal disease although baseline CPK levels may be somewhat higher. When infarction does occur, the pattern of enzyme changes is not affected.

Hemodialysis is usually delayed if possible, when angina or infarction is suspected, to avoid the associated cardiovascular stresses. In a significant number of dialysis patients with chest pain, the degree of coronary artery narrowing is <75% (the luminal narrowing considered "critical" in limiting myocardial oxygen delivery). Dialysis patients are often anemic, hypertensive, or volume overloaded, so lesser degrees of luminal narrowing may be sufficient to limit myocardial oxygen delivery. Thus, findings on previous cardiac catheterization of "noncritical" coronary narrowing should *not* dissuade the physician from a cardiac etiology.

Chest pain may also be due to other causes, but pericarditis should always be considered. Pericarditis may occur even in well-dialyzed patients, and causes such as bleeding, viral infection, and drugs (e.g., minoxidil) should be considered. The signs and symptoms are the same as those noted in nondialysis patients, but signs of tamponade should also be sought.

BLEEDING

Bleeding is relatively common, in part related to platelet dysfunction not completely corrected by dialysis, and transient anticoagulation with hemodialysis. Because many patients have a hemoglobin level of 6–7 g/dL, small amounts of blood loss may cause abrupt cardiovascular decompensation. Increased angina or dyspnea are common presentations. It is important to determine the usual hemoglobin level. Life-threatening processes may result from occult bleeding: intracranial, intraocular, pericardial, and retroperitoneal bleeding have been reported. Treatment follows standard principles; occasionally intervention with platelet infusions, cryoprecipitate, DDAVP, or conjugated estrogens is used to correct the bleeding time and control bleeding.

ELECTROLYTE ABNORMALITIES

Although hyperkalemia is a life-threatening emergency, it is seldom a problem in the dialyzed patient. When hyperkalemia does occur it is usually due to noncompliance with dietary restrictions or to skipping dialysis treatments. It also may be the result of rhabdomyolysis, sepsis, or severe acidosis. Hyperkalemia should be considered if a dialysis patient presents in cardiac arrest; IV calcium and bicarbonate should be administered.

ADMISSION DECISIONS

A critical decision is whether emergency dialysis is necessary for patients with acute clinical problems. Some patients may have deteriorated between hemodialysis treatments or despite continuing CAPD; others may have missed scheduled dialyses. The most common indication for emergency dialysis is severe volume overload or pulmonary edema; temporizing measures can be effective. Temporizing measures may be also be used in malignant hypertension, severe electrolyte disturbances, or severe acidosis while awaiting dialysis.

Uremic symptoms (e.g., lethargy, confusion, asterixis, nausea and vomiting) indicate that dialysis is needed, but are not indications for emergency dialysis. Serum creatinine and BUN levels correlate only roughly with uremic symptoms or life-threatening metabolic disturbances and do not indicate an urgent need for dialysis. Pericarditis, with or without pericardial tamponade, is often considered an indication for urgent or intensified dialysis, but pericarditis can occur even in well-dialyzed patients; it is unclear whether there is an increased risk of deterioration if not treated aggressively.

COMMON PITFALLS

- Failing to consider vascular access infection in hemodialysis patients, or peritonitis in CAPD patients, because of lack of specific findings

- Failing to consider the diagnosis of tamponade because the patient does not demonstrate all the classic signs and symptoms
- Discounting angina because of "noncritical" stenosis on coronary angiography
- Overlooking anemia as a cause of increased angina or shortness of breath
- Failing to assess for hyperkalemia
- Inducing symptomatic hypocalcemia through bicarbonate therapy
- Failing to check with the patient's nephrologist or specialty nurse to take advantage of their expertise and to assure optimal continuity of care

159   Hematuria

Hematuria, the presence of an abnormal number of red blood cells in the urine, suggests either primary genitourinary (GU) disease or GU involvement from a systemic disorder. Gross hematuria is startling to most patients, prompting an ED visit. Microscopic hematuria requires investigation as well.

CLINICAL PRESENTATION

The most common causes of hematuria are infections, nephrolithiasis, neoplasms, and benign prostatic hypertrophy (BPH). Neoplasm is a prime concern in adults greater than age 40 and must be ruled out. Other important entities, e.g., sickle cell disease, sickle-thalassemia, and diseases associated with vasculitis, such as Goodpasture's syndrome or Henoch–Schönlein purpura, should be considered. Anticoagulant therapy may cause hematuria but most patients are found on further testing to have occult urologic pathology. BPH may result in hematuria, but an evaluation is still indicated since other associated urologic problems of potentially greater significance may also be present. A leaking abdominal aortic aneurysm may mimic renal colic. Hematuria may occur from erosion of an aneurysm into the ureter or renal pelvis.

DIFFERENTIAL DIAGNOSIS

The differential diagnoses are legion. A common error is failure to obtain a complete history. Medical problems are associated with hematuria and may support a probable cause. Dysuria, frequency, and suprapubic pain suggests hemorrhagic cystitis; severe colicky flank pain radiating to the groin may indicate a ureteral calculus; voiding disorders may be due to benign prostatic hypertrophy; fever and a history of a murmur may indicate endocarditis; recent streptococcal infection suggests poststreptococcal glomerulonephritis.

EMERGENCY DEPARTMENT EVALUATION

The urine dipstick readily detects hematuria. Dipsticks can detect levels of hemoglobin corresponding to five or fewer RBCs/hpf. Colored urine and a negative dipstick for blood suggest the presence of pigmenturia, seen in porphyria, foods such as beets or rhubarb, and with certain medications that discolor the urine. If the dipstick is positive for blood, microscopic examination should be performed for RBCs, white blood cells (WBCs), and casts. If no RBCs are noted, myoglobin or free hemoglobin is present. The latter is usually associated with a pink color of the serum. If both RBCs and WBCs are seen in the urine, an infectious process is likely. RBC casts indicate significant renal disease, usually glomerulonephritis.

In patients without protein, WBCs, or casts, further evaluation is indicated on an elective basis (except renal colic) and in consultation with a urologist or nephrologist. After renal function is assessed by BUN and creatinine, an intravenous pyelogram (IVP) or ultrasound may be done in the ED. Cystoscopy, computed tomography (CT), and renal biopsy may be indicated later. With renal colic, a plain abdominal flat plate does not identify stones; an IVP or ultrasound (to identify obstruction) are indicated. If renal artery aneurysm or embolism is considered, CT scanning is indicated although arteriography will probably be necessary.

EMERGENCY DEPARTMENT MANAGEMENT

Nontraumatic hematuria, except for renal artery aneurysm rupture or renal infarction from an embolus, rarely causes life-threatening bleeding. In the two conditions noted above, however, aggressive evaluation and management are necessary. Pain and hematuria in a younger individual suggest ureteral calculi; older adults with apparent ureteral colic must be considered to have a potential acute vascular catastrophe. If infection is the cause, uncomplicated cases in normal hosts may be treated as outpatients.

DISPOSITION

The presumed or confirmed cause of hematuria determines disposition. Patients with suspected vascular disease of the renal arteries should be admitted after diagnostic studies and consultation. Indications for admission for calculi are found elsewhere. Hematuria from infection requires hospitalization if bacteremia is suspected or if dehydration or renal failure is present. Admission should be considered for infected patients with malignancy, diabetes, indwelling Foley catheters, or known stone disease. The patient with glomerulonephritis may need admission if the diagnosis is new or if there are complications (severe hypertension, oliguria, volume overload, pulmonary edema, or electrolyte imbalance).

COMMON PITFALLS

- Malignancy should be suspected in any patient >age 40 with hematuria. Attributing hematuria to a benign condition may result in delays in evaluation and serious misdiagnosis.
- There is increased risk for radiocontrast-induced renal failure in patients with a previous history of an episode, age over 60, pre-existing renal insufficiency, diabetes, multiple myeloma, and dehydration. When an IVP is considered, careful determination must be made of potential risk *versus* diagnostic benefit. Ultrasound provides an excellent alternative, as does non-contrast CT.

160   Myoglobinuria

Myoglobin is an iron-containing, oxygen-binding protein present in skeletal and smooth muscle. Small amounts are normally present in blood and urine but at clinically insignificant levels and undetected by conventional diagnostic tests. Myoglobinuria occurs with rhabdomyolysis from severe muscle destruction or diseases that alter the cell membrane. Myoglobinuria is significant because it implies the presence of an underlying causal disorder and may result in acute renal failure.

CLINICAL PRESENTATION

The presentation depends on the underlying cause. The most frequent causes are ethanol and drug abuse, seizures, and trauma, but a reliable history is often not obtained. The mechanism of ethanol-induced myoglobinuria is not completely understood; other depressant drug ingestions allow prolonged compression of an extremity to occur. The excessive muscle activity seen in phencyclidine (PCP) ingestions or in status epilepticus may result in rhabdomyolysis and myoglobinuria. Crush injuries and compartment syndromes also cause muscle damage with release of myoglobin.

The history and physical examination may be deceptive. Neither muscle pain nor swollen, tender muscles need be present with significant rhabdomyolysis and myoglobinuria. Any patient with a history of prolonged immobilization or prolonged unusual use of any extremity should be suspected of having myoglobinuria. A triad of laboratory findings has been described: a positive urine dipstick for blood; pigmented (red or brown) granular casts on microscopic examination; and elevated serum creatine kinase (CK). Because of rapid clearance, however, myoglobin in the urine is often fleeting and may be missed. The serum myoglobin peaks at 4–6 hours post injury and returns to normal within 12 hours. An elevated creatine kinase is probably the most sensitive and specific test for rhabdomyolysis and should be performed when the diagnosis is suspected. Other laboratory tests yield important information: ABG, electrolytes, calcium, phosphorus, BUN, creatinine, and uric acid.

DIFFERENTIAL DIAGNOSIS

Once myoglobinuria is detected, identifying the cause may be difficult. Myoglobinuria may also be overlooked if the paitent is critically ill from an underlying disease.

EMERGENCY DEPARTMENT EVALUATION

Once myoglobinuria is detected, identifying the cause may be difficult. Myoglobinuria may also be overlooked if the patient is critically ill from an underlying disease.

The major complication of myoglobinuria is acute renal failure (ARF). The mechanism is unclear. All patients at risk should receive treatment aimed at preventing ARF. Abnormalities of serum chemistry values are frequently associated with myoglobinuria. Initial elevation in BUN and creatinine may occur, although a normal value does not rule out the possibility of ARF developing later. Acid–base derangements (either alkalemia or acidemia) may be present, and ABG analysis should be performed. Hyperkalemia may be seen in 50% and may require treatment. However, IV calcium may worsen muscle destruction and should only be used to treat life-threatening hyperkalemia.

EMERGENCY DEPARTMENT MANAGEMENT

Saline infusion is an accepted intervention, and aggressive fluid resuscitation is mandatory. Fluid may be "third-spaced" in injured muscle, resulting in intravascular volume depletion, prerenal azotemia, or even shock. Crystalloid (lactated Ringer's or normal saline) should be given to maintain a urine output of 100–200 mL/hour, although some prefer an output of at least 300 mL/hour. Because large volumes may be necessary, patients should have a Foley catheter and a CVP line should be considered. Forced diuresis with mannitol or furosemide offers theoretical benefit and is often advocated. Guidelines for administration are not well established, however, and remain controversial.

Some authorities give mannitol (25 g IV to a maximum of 1 g/kg) and/or furosemide (100–200 mg) at the beginning of treatment, whereas others recommend their use only if fluids fail to establish adequate urine output. No clinical studies have clearly established the effectiveness of such treatment. Sodium bicarbonate prevents the precipitation of myoglobin in renal tubules when the urine pH is maintained >6.5. Bicarbonate has been recommended by some for prevention of ARF despite the risks of exacerbating the effects of hypocalcemia encountered in rhabdomyolysis. Although improved outcome with the use of bicarbonate has not been demonstrated, it is reasonable to give it when fluids and diuretics have failed to maintain urine pH above 6.5, while closely monitoring serum calcium levels.

DISPOSITION

Patients with known or suspected myoglobinuria should generally be admitted to the hospital. An ICU is appropriate for patients in shock, inadequate urine output, or marked potassium or calcium derangements. Swan–Ganz monitoring should be considered, particularly in the elderly. Consultation with a nephrologist is indicated. Transfer may be required if dialysis is contemplated or ICU capabilities are unavailable.

COMMON PITFALLS

- Because myoglobinuria results from rhabdomyolysis, its presence places the patient at risk for renal failure and acid–base, electrolyte, and volume disturbances. Appropriate treatment should be instituted early.
- Marked electrolyte disorders may occur, but only hyperkalemia requires specific treatment.
- Underlying compartment syndrome must be suspected; early diagnosis and treatment lead to improved outcome.

PART VI

Infectious Disease Emergencies

161   Skin and Soft-Tissue Infections

CELLULITIS

Cellulitis is infection of skin and subcutaneous tissue characterized by erythema, edema, warmth, and pain. With the exception of erysipelas, lesions in cellulitis have borders with poorly defined margins, reflecting a deep inflammatory process. Fever, chills, and regional lymphadenopathy are common. Cellulitis typically follows skin trauma but may occur secondary to hematogenous and lymphatic dissemination of bacteria. It usually occurs on an extremity with the legs a common and particularly troublesome site of involvement. Common bacterial pathogens include *Staphylococcus aureus*, group A beta-hemolytic *Streptococcus*, and *Haemophilus influenzae* type B.

    Streptococcus cellulitis is usually caused by group A beta-hemolytic streptococci and associated with recent trauma or operative procedure. If untreated, it spreads rapidly and may be difficult to differentiate from its more superficial counterpart, erysipelas. Antibiotics are usually curative. Staphylococcal cellulitis is usually associated with an area of previous trauma or infection. The lesions of staphylococcal cellulitis are usually localized and contain a purulent center or abscess but do not usually cause systemic toxicity. Treatment is described below.

    Gram-negative cellulitis is caused by a variety of organisms. There may or may not be gas production. Gram-negative cellulitis tends to initiate around mucus membranes, with lymphadenitis and septicemia frequent complications. Diabetics and other immunosuppressed persons are predisposed. The diagnosis can often be made by Gram's stain and cultures. Patients should be hospitalized and started on parenteral antibiotics.

    Erysipelas is a superficial infection that involves the dermis and uppermost subcutaneous tissues. Group A beta-hemolytic *Streptococcus* is usually the cause. Erysipelas may occur at any age, although infants, young children, and the elderly are most often affected. Predisposing factors include lymphatic congestion, diabetes mellitus, arterial insufficiency, cirrhosis, and idiopathic causes. The infection typically begins with a break in the skin. Classic skin changes usually appear 2 to 5 days after the injury and occur predominantly on the face or extremities. Affected skin is erythematous, warm, and painful, with elevated, advancing margins. A "peau d'orange" appearance may be seen as a result of lymphatic involvement. Chills, fever, headache, and malaise suggest systemic toxicity. Erysipelas is diagnosed by clinical appearance. Further support is found in an elevated erythrocyte sedimentation rate, rising antistreptolysin O titers, and positive blood culture or wound margin culture results. Erysipelas should be treated aggressively because the condition is rapidly progressive and may be fatal. Beta-hemolytic streptococci are sensitive to penicillin.

COMMON PITFALLS

- The most common pitfall is failing to select the most appropriate antibiotic. Immunosuppressed patients, as well as those with suspected erysipelas or gram-negative infection, require prompt laboratory evaluation and hospitalization with prompt initiation of parenteral antibiotics.

SUBCUTANEOUS ABSCESSES

An abscess is a painful and localized collection of pus that causes fluctuant soft-tissue swelling surrounded by firm granulation tissue. Abscesses can affect any area of the body. On the skin, most result from minor cutaneous trauma, which allows bacterial pathogens to penetrate the epidermal barrier. Initial infection is rapidly followed by development of a firm, warm, erythematous, and painful mass. Purulent drainage may be noted. Healthy patients show minimal evidence of systemic toxicity. Fever suggests that the infection has become systemic.

Most cutaneous abscesses involve common pathogens indigenous to local skin. Abscesses in the perineal region usually contain anaerobic or aerobic fecal organisms. Likewise, subcutaneous abscesses of the vulvovaginal area are usually caused by anaerobes from vaginal flora. Abscesses of the head, neck, axilla, trunk, and extremities are most commonly caused by gram-positive cocci such as *S. aureus* or *Staphylococcus epidermidis.* Deeper secondary abscesses also may contain anaerobes such as *Peptococcus* and *Propionibacterium.* Four to five percent of cutaneous abscesses are sterile. Most are associated with subcutaneous or IV abuse and are usually found at needle injection sites.

In the afebrile and immunocompetent patient, optimal treatment is incision and drainage alone. One should avoid unnecessary laboratory testing; Gram's stain and culture are unnecessary, as are antibiotics. High-risk patients, however, require incision and drainage, Gram's stain of wound material, aerobic and anaerobic cultures, IV antibiotics, and hospitalization. High risk patients include those with immunocompromise, facial abscesses drained by the cavernous sinus, and fever and significant tachycardia.

A furuncle is an infected hair follicle. A carbuncle is a subcutaneous infection of a group of hair follicles. The face, axilla, neck, and buttocks are common sites for furuncles. Carbuncles affect the same areas but generally cluster on posterior neck, thigh, shoulders, back, and hips. Treatment of both infections consists of warm compresses to the affected areas, which aid in localizing and initiating drainage. Pilonidal disease generally follows puberty; the majority of affected men are obese and hirsute.

Pilonidal abscesses commonly occur at the sacrococcygeal junction. On close examination, pits can be seen in the midline sacrococcygeal area. The differential diagnosis includes furuncles, carbuncles, hidradenitis suppurativa, and perianal abscess. Although painful or fluctuant pilonidal abscesses can be drained in the ED, incision and drainage alone is generally not curative. Recurrences are common unless hair follicles and sinus tracts are excised.

Hidradenitis suppurativa is a recurrent, suppurative, and scarring disease of apocrine sweat glands. Persons of African descent have a greater incidence. The most common anatomic sites in decreasing order of frequency are the axilla (especially in females), perianal and inguinal regions (especially in males), labia majora, posterior neck, breast (areola), and periumbilical area. Predisposing factors include excessive sweating, acne, poor skin hygiene, irritation from clothing, irritating deodorants, depilatory creams, and close shaving or plucking of axillary hair. Early localized lesions must be distinguished from furuncles, carbuncles, lymphadenitis, cellulitis, Bartholin gland abscess, and pilonidal abscess.

In late or chronic forms of the disease, the differential diagnosis includes lymphogranuloma venereum, granuloma inguinale, recurrent anal fistula, and carcinoma. In the chronic phase, contiguous apocrine glands are involved and the lesions are painful, with formation of sinus tracts, multiple abscesses, and honeycombed scarring. This results in axilla and groin contractures, leading to partial immobility. Treatment of the acute phase consists of incision and drainage, antibiotics, and warm soaks applied to the affected area. Surgery is the definitive treatment and consists of surgical removal of scarred apocrine glands in the affected area.

Bartholin glands are nonpalpable secretory glands located near the labia minora. They continually secrete a mucoid solution that prevents drying and adherence of the vulva, beginning with puberty. If a Bartholin gland duct becomes obstructed, a cyst or abscess can result. Duct obstruction is most frequently caused by scarring secondary to trauma, parturition, or an episiotomy. Bartholin cysts are usually asymptomatic, although they can become large. Abscesses quickly become painful. Most contain mixed bacterial pathogens from the vaginal flora, but gonococcal infections have been implicated in 11% of cases. Incision and drainage can be performed in the ED. Without definitive surgery there will often be a recurrence. Definitive management consists of marsupialization or placement of a Word catheter for 4 to 6 weeks.

COMMON PITFALLS

- The causative organism is often bacteria indigenous to the particular region of the body.
- Immunosuppressed patients require admission, wound and blood cultures, and systemic antibiotics.
- One should differentiate abscess from cellulitis.
- Optimal treatment consists of incision and drainage.
- Some abscesses (e.g., pilonidal, hidradenitis suppurativa, Bartholin gland abscess) are recurrent and require consultation for definitive treatment

NECROTIZING FASCIITIS

Necrotizing fasciitis is a rare, rapidly progressive, life-threatening infection characterized by severe systemic toxicity and necrosis of skin, subcutaneous tissue, and deep and superficial fascia. Hemolytic streptococcal gangrene, synergistic gangrene, Fournier's gangrene, and synergistic necrotizing cellulitis appear to be the same entity. Most develop as a complication of minor trauma, surgery, or cutaneous ulcers, especially in diabetics and intravenous drug abusers; other factors include obesity, malignancy, peripheral vascular disease, malnutrition, renal failure, cirrhosis, and other chronic debilitating diseases. Most patients are elderly.

The infection is usually polymicrobial, although *Bacteroides* and clostridial species are frequently isolated. Aerobes and anaerobes may act synergistically. Enzymatic toxins probably account for the fulminant nature of the disease. Massive necrosis of subcutaneous fat and fascia quickly follows. Initially, the wound is hot, edematous, and painful. Rapid development of infection with profound prostration is highly suggestive of the disease. Late clinical features include bulla formation, crepitus over the area of involvement, wound hypesthesia or anesthesia, and skin necrosis over the affected area. In severe cases, gas may be present in the wound. Patients rapidly deteriorate with altered mental status, fever, septicemia, electrolyte abnormalities, acidosis, hypocalcemia, and hemolytic anemia. Also seen are severe hypovolemia from extracellular fluid shifts, disseminated intravascular coagulation, respiratory failure, septic shock and death.

Early necrotizing fasciitis must be distinguished from erysipelas, acute cellulitis, clostridial gangrene, diabetic gangrene, and phlegmasia cerulea dolens. Definitive diagnosis is usually made at surgery. If necrotizing fasciitis is suspected, the patient's respiratory and circulatory status should be carefully assessed. Gram's stain and aerobic and anaerobic wound cultures may identify causative organisms; blood cultures should be done. Soft-tissue radiographs will identify gas. Antibiotics must be instituted rapidly, with consideration of the polymicrobial nature (Table 161-

TABLE 161-1. Suggested Antibiotics for Necrotizing Fasclitis

Antibiotic	Adult	Pediatric
Gentamicin	3–5 mg/kg/day IV 3 div. doses	5–7.5 mg/kg/day IV 3 div. doses
+ Penicillin G	20–40 million U/day IV 4 div. doses	1.2 million–3 million U/day IV 6 div. doses
+ Clindamycin	450–2700 mg/kg/day IV 3 div. doses	1–20 mg/kg/day IV 3–4 div. doses
Penicillin-Allergic Patients		
Cephalothin	12 g/day IV 3 div. doses	80–160 mg/kg/day IV 4 div. doses
Clindamycin	450–2700 mg/kg/day IV 3 div. doses	10–20 mg/kg/day IV 3 div. doses

1). Surgical consultation is indicated for wide debridement of necrotic subcutaneous tissue and fascia. Hyperbaric oxygen treatment is controversial and insufficiently studied. Despite broad spectrum antibiotics and improvements in surgical technique, mortality still ranges from 8–67%. Poor prognostic factors include delay in diagnosis, age >50, peripheral vascular disease, diabetes mellitus, septicemia, renal failure, malignancy, and involvement of the head, neck, trunk, or perineum.

COMMON PITFALLS

- Failure to make an early diagnosis before fulminant disease occurs
- When necrotizing fasciitis is suspected, aggressive treatment with parenteral antibiotics, surgical consultation, and consideration of HBO therapy must be carried out.

162 Meningitis

Meningitis is inflammation of the leptomeninges and of the cerebrospinal fluid (CSF) bathing the subarachnoid space and brain ventricles.

Aseptic meningitis is generally self-limited with fever, headache, nuchal rigidity and characteristic CSF findings (lymphocytosis, variable protein elevation, and normal glucose); it is most often of viral origin. Enteroviruses and mumps virus cause >85% of cases. Most viral meningitides are relatively benign, with Polioviruses and herpes simplex the notable exceptions. Many nonviral causes of aseptic meningitis (e.g., syphilis, tuberculosis) cause significant morbidity and mortality. Aseptic meningitis may have other causes, however, including certain bacteria (*Mycobacterium tuberculosis, Leptospira* species, *Treponema pallidum, Borrelia* species, *Nocardia,* and partially treated pyogenic infections), fungi, rickettsiae, *Mycoplasma,* parasites, parameningeal infections, malignancy, autoimmune diseases, and miscellaneous causes (intrathe-cal injections, heavy-metal poisonings, nonsteroidal anti-inflammatory agents, and antibiotics). Chronic immunosuppression, including HIV and organ transplantation, is a risk factor for fungal meningitis. Risk factors for viral meningitis include poor hygiene, since most viral meningitis is due to enteroviruses with oral–fecal spread.

Bacterial meningitis has a mortality rate of >90% if untreated and accounts for over 2000 deaths/year in the USA, with significant neurologic deficit in survivors. Early diagnosis and antibi-otics are key to decreasing morbidity and mortality. Bacterial meningitis accounts for 1/1000 hospital admissions. Although primarily a disease of young children, 20–25% are adolescents and adults. *Streptococcus pneumoniae, Neisseria meningitidis,* and *Haemophilus influenzae* account for >90% of all cases with *S. pneumoniae* the most common in adults. *N. meningitidis* causes 30% of cases, mostly in children and adolescents, but 10% occur in those over age 45. *Listeria monocytogenes* is implicated in 5%, generally in elderly or immunocompromised individuals. Risk factors include age (the very old and the very young), sex (men > women), nasopharyngeal col-onization, chronic disease, immunosuppression, and lower socioeconomic status.

Specific host risk factors may offer a clue to likely pathogens: pneumococcal meningitis occurs with certain infectious processes (e.g., otitis, sinusitis, pneumonia), trauma (head injury), and immunocompromised states (e.g., sickle cell disease, Hodgkin's disease, immunoglobulin deficiency, renal or bone marrow transplantation). Overcrowded living conditions (e.g., college dormitories, military barracks, skid rows) and poverty increase the risk of contracting meningo-coccal meningitis. Close association with victims of meningococcal meningitis increases the risk by a factor of 500 to 800. Risk factors for Listerial meningitis include the immunocompromised state and ingestion of *Listeria*-contaminated foods. Adults who develop *H. influenzae* meningitis should be scrutinized for anatomic defects such as dermal sinus tracts, previous head trauma with CSF leaks, or infectious processes (e.g., otitis, sinusitis). Staphylococcal infection should be suspected with penetrating skull injuries or neurologic or otolaryngologic procedures. Gram-neg-ative meningitis is noted after neurosurgical procedures or in association with other nosocomial infections.

CLINICAL PRESENTATION

Fever, headache, and nuchal rigidity constitute the classic presentation; any patient with these findings warrants a prompt evaluation for CNS infection. Headache is often severe, generalized, and throbbing but is not always present, especially in the elderly or early in the course. Nuchal rigidity is seen in >80% and is the most characteristic finding; it's most marked in bacterial, fun-gal, and tuberculous meningitis and is less severe in viral meningitides. Other signs characteris-tic of meningeal irritation cannot always be elicited (Brudzinski's sign, Kernig's sign). Petechiae, purpura, and morbilliform rash are often noted in meningococcal meningitis. Similar rashes may occur with *Staphylococcus, H. influenzae,* and *S. pneumoniae,* as well as some viral meningitides, especially echoviruses.

Nausea and vomiting reflect CNS inflammation and raised intracerebral pressure and are often noted. Mental status or behavioral changes (inattention, confusion, lethargy or coma) may be the only clue in the elderly. Focal or generalized seizures occur in up to 30% and may be due to the illness or reversible causes such as electrolyte disturbances (e.g., hyponatremia), or hypoxia. Coma and seizures are most often seen in pneumococcal and *H. influenzae* meningitis and are uncommon in meningococcal meningitis. A fundoscopic exam may reveal papilledema which suggests brain abscess or encephalitis. Neurologic sequelae may occur early or late and include learning difficulties, ataxia, hearing loss, memory impairment, seizures, sensory distur-bances, spinal cord dysfunction, polyneuropathy, cranial nerve abnormalities, paralysis, and hydrocephalus.

DIFFERENTIAL DIAGNOSIS

The differential diagnosis includes infections (brain abscess and encephalitis), neurologic (migraine, other vascular headaches, postictal state, new-onset seizures), toxicologic (phencyclidine, salicylate), and behavioral disorders (psychosis, mania).

EMERGENCY DEPARTMENT EVALUATION

The majority of patients with meningitis display classic complaints of severe headache, fever, and nuchal rigidity. Up to 20% present in an atypical fashion (elderly or immunocompromised). Risk factors aid in the diagnosis and assist in antibiotic selection (the six I's):

Infection (upper or lower respiratory tract infection, sinusitis, otitis, etc.)
Immunosuppression (splenectomy, sickle cell disease, steroids, Hodgkin's disease, myeloma, organ transplant, etc.)
Injury (head trauma, neurologic or ENT procedures, etc.)
Indwelling (catheters, shunts, ventricular reservoirs, etc.)
Imbiber (alcoholic)
Identification (close contacts such as spouses, roommates, paramedics, etc.).

The physical examination should focus on likely sites of infection: oropharynx, ears, and sinuses. The chest x-ray may identify sources of infection. Rashes should be noted. Fundoscopy is mandatory; if papilledema is noted, or if a focal seizure has occurred, the stable patient should have a brain CT. If the patient is too unstable or if a mass lesion is seen on CT, blood cultures should be drawn from two sites, as well as from any obvious sites of infection, and antibiotics given without delay. In all patients, IVs should be secured and blood sent for a CBC, electrolytes, and glucose. After this, if not contraindicated, lumbar puncture is carried out.

LUMBAR PUNCTURE

Lumbar puncture confirms the diagnosis of meningitis. Clear contraindications to LP include infection at the site of the puncture and the presence of a mass on head CT. Papilledema and anticoagulants are relative contraindications.

CEREBROSPINAL FLUID PARAMETERS

GRAM'S STAIN

Visualization of the responsible organism on a Gram's stain of CSF is pathognomonic of bacterial meningitis; bacterial organisms are seen in 80–90% of culture-proved cases. CSF counts are highest for pneumococcal and *H. influenzae* meningitis. Patients with Listerial meningitis or those receiving prior antibiotics show bacteria on Gram's stain 60% of the time. Fungal meningitis requires examination of a large volume of fluid, since only a small number of fungal organisms are present in the CSF. India ink preparations for fungal elements in CSF are positive in only 50%. Similarly, acid-fast smears of CSF for TB meningitis are not consistently sensitive. Tests for fungal or TB meningitis should not be routine unless there is an indication (ie, immunocompromised).

GLUCOSE

Normally, the ratio of CSF to serum glucose concentration is 0.60. CSF glucose level of <50 mg/dL, or a CSF to serum glucose ratio of <0.50 is noted in >50% of bacterial, fungal, and TB meningitis and is not uncommon in mumps meningitis, lymphocytic choriomeningitis, and herpes simplex meningitis. Normal CSF glucose levels are usually noted in viral meningitides, as well as in the early stage of pyogenic meningitis or TB meningitis.

PROTEIN

Normal protein levels in the CSF range from 15 to 45 mg/dL. Marked elevations are seen in bacterial, fungal, and TB meningitis. Viral meningitides generally have normal or mildly elevated protein. Levels of >1000 mg/dL suggests impending or actual subarachnoid block.

CELL COUNTS AND DIFFERENTIALS

Normal CSF contains no red blood cells and has a white blood cell (WBC) count of <five cells/mm^3, all mononuclear. A single granulocytic cell in cytocentrifuged CSF is considered pathologic by many. It should be considered normal if the total CSF WBC count is <five/mm^3. Bacterial meningitis classically has CSF cell counts ranging from 100 to 10,000 cells/mm^3, with polymorphonuclear forms predominating early and lymphocytes later. Viral meningitis characteristically manifests a CSF lymphocytosis with cell counts of 10–1000 cells/mm^3. Mononuclear cells usually predominate in TB and fungal meningitis, as well as in other causes of aseptic meningitis.

Unfortunately, considerable overlap exists between bacterial meningitis and aseptic meningitis. Up to 10% of bacterial meningitis may initially demonstrate a CSF lymphocytosis. CSF in both TB and fungal meningitis may initially manifest neutrophilia, and neutrophils may predominate throughout the illness. Patients with viral meningitis occasionally demonstrate CSF leukocytosis of >1000 cells/mm^3 with > 75% neutrophils, but CSF obtained within 8–24 hours generally shows a significant decrease in the proportion of neutrophils. Several ancillary CSF tests are available to help differentiate bacterial from nonbacterial meningitis: most helpful are those that detect bacterial antigens (counterimmunoelectrophoresis, latex agglutination, or enzyme-linked immunosorbent assay). These tests should not interfere with antibiotic therapy. CSF obtained early may be devoid of cells and organisms, with no glucose or protein abnormalities. On occasion, even in normal hosts, the CSF in fulminant meningitis (especially pneumococcal) demonstrates no cells but is teeming with bacteria.

Although no single CSF value can of itself make the diagnosis when the Gram's stain is negative, patterns may correlate with certain etiologic agents. CSF neutrophilia, very low glucose (5–20 mg/dL), and elevated protein (100 mg/dL) are suggestive of bacterial meningitis. The CSF in TB and fungal meningitis generally has mononuclear cells, low glucose (20–40 mg/dL), and elevated protein. Viral meningitis usually shows mononuclear cells, normal glucose, and normal or slightly elevated protein.

CULTURES

The CSF should be cultured in all cases of suspected meningitis because the diagnosis is made only from the culture in 20% and antibiotic selection is guided by the results. Cultures are even more important in fungal and TB meningitis, since India ink or acid-fast preparations are negative in >50%. Cultures for suspected fungal and TB meningitis require large volumes of CSF. In suspected partially-treated meningitis, the CSF should be cultured for at least 7 days.

EMERGENCY DEPARTMENT MANAGEMENT

The patient with headache, fever, and nuchal rigidity, with or without neurologic abnormalities, should be considered to have meningitis. A rapid examination should be done and laboratory studies sent, lumbar puncture done and antibiotics given. Antibiotics will not alter CSF within the first few hours. In early or atypical bacterial meningitis, a history and physical exam may suggest meningitis, confirmed by CSF examination. Because most patients are infected with pneumococcal or meningococcal organisms, empiric therapy includes crystalline penicillin G 50,000 U/kg every 4 hours. Alternatives include cefuroxime, moxalactam, cefotaxime, and ceftriaxone, all in a dose of 2 g IV. Penicillin-allergic individuals should receive chloramphenicol 25 mg/kg intravenously every 6 hours. Listeria monocytogenes meningitis is treated with ampicillin 50 mg/kg IV every 4 hours or chloramphenicol 25 mg/kg IV every 6 hours in the penicillin-allergic patient.

Staphylococcal meningitis is treated with nafcillin or oxacillin 2 to 3 g IV every 4 hours. Nosocomial meningitis may be treated with any of the cephalosporins mentioned above but may require the addition of an aminoglycoside. Admission to an ICU is appropriate. Patients with suspected TB or fungal meningitis require an infectious disease consultation but rarely require the institution of antimicrobial therapy in the ED. If viral meningitis is suspected but CSF demonstrates a predominant neutrophilia, a second lumbar puncture should be done in 8–24 hours, since >85% will show a significant decrease in the proportion of neutrophils. The decision to begin antibiotics before the second lumbar puncture is available must be made on the basis of the clinical picture, risk factors, and availability of staff to monitor the patient closely. Clear-cut cases of viral meningitis (except those caused by herpes simplex virus) do not require admission. Therapy consists of acetaminophen for headache and fever as well as supportive care and arrangements for appropriate follow-up.

CHEMOPROPHYLAXIS

Chemoprophylaxis after exposure to individuals with bacterial meningitis follws certain guidelines. Close contacts (e.g., families, roommates) of patients with meningococcal and *H. influenzae* meningitis have an increased risk (200- to 1000-fold) of contracting the disease and warrant chemoprophylaxis. Paramedics and hospital personnel with *close* contact (e.g., mouth-to-mouth resuscitation) also deserve chemoprophylaxis. Others, including schoolmates, do not require prophylaxis. Rifampin, 600 mg orally every 12 hours for a total of 4 doses, is the approved regimen for both *H. influenzae* and meningococcal meningitis. Individuals at risk for pneumococcal meningitis (e.g., postsplenectomy) should receive oral penicillin 500 mg every 6 hours for 7 days.

COMMON PITFALLS

- Do not rely on classic signs and symptoms alone for the diagnosis of meningitis; they may be absent in the elderly and the immunocompromised.
- There is occasional overlap of CSF findings in bacterial meningitis and aseptic meningitis.
- If a definitive diagnosis is not possible, err on the side of caution and institute treatment until the results of cultures are available.
- Delayed diagnosis and treatment directly relate to morbidity and mortality.
- If a mass lesion is seen on CT, blood cultures and cultures from sites of obvious infection should be obtained and antibiotics administered without delay. Antibiotics should not obscure the diagnosis of meningitis and there is no justification for withholding therapy since organisms remain detectable on Gram's stain of CSF in 60% of patients.

163   Localized and Disseminated Gonorrhea

Gonorrhea (GC) is a sexually transmitted disease caused by the small gram-negative diplococcus *Neisseria gonorrhoeae*. Complications include PID, epididymitis/orchitis, prostatitis, ophthalmitis, septic arthritis, endocarditis, meningitis, and perihepatitis. Chronic sequelae such as infertility, ectopic pregnancy, blindness, urethral strictures, and abdominal adhesions represent significant morbidity. Patients with GC fall into one of three categories: symptoms due to localized infection, symptoms attributable to disseminated disease, and asymptomatic contacts of partners known to be infected. In the ED, the diagnosis should be made, suitable specimens obtained for culture, appropriate antibiotics administered, and timely follow-up provided for.

CLINICAL PRESENTATION

The clinical manifestations of localized disease depend on the sex, site of the infection, and strain causing the infection. In heterosexual men, acute urethritis is the most common presentation. Primary GC in women is usually asymptomatic. Other local complications of GC include Bartholin's abscess and perihepatitis (Fitz-Hugh–Curtis syndrome). The pharynx is colonized in 3–7% of heterosexual men, 5–20% of women, 10–25% of homosexual men, and 39–96% of pregnant women. Oropharyngeal gonorrhea is usually asymptomatic but can present as an acute, exudative tonsillitis; a sore throat with minimal objective findings; or an acute, ulcerative gingivostomatitis. Anorectal involvement is common in both heterosexual women and homosexual men. Of women with GC, 26–63% may have positive rectal cultures, and in 4% the rectum may be the only site of infection. Positive rectal cultures for *N. gonorrhoeae* are found in 20–30% of homosexual men seen in VD clinics. Anorectal GC is often asymptomatic. When symptoms occur, they are usually mild, with pruritus ani, rectal discomfort, tenesmus, dyspareunia, hematochezia, and purulent or mucoid rectal discharge.

Disseminated gonococcal infection (DGI) may occur in 1–3% of patients with localized disease, but the majority of cases are seen in asymptomatic primary infection. About 80% occur in women, and about 2/3 occur within the first week following the onset of menses. Pregnant or puerperal women and homosexual men also are at risk for developing DGI. The most common presentations are the arthritis–dermatitis syndrome and acute gonococcal arthritis. Although relatively rare, endocarditis, meningitis, and myopericarditis also are manifestations of DGI.

The arthritis–dermatitis syndrome presents with fever, chills, polyarticular arthritis or arthralgias, a characteristic rash, and tenosynovitis of extensor tendons of the hands, wrists, or tendons about the ankles. The most frequently involved joints are the wrists, followed in frequency by the knees, hands, ankles, and elbows. Although painful, the joints are usually not red or warm, and the effusion, if present, is small and usually sterile. The characteristic rash begins as petechiae or painful red papules of the digits or distal extremities. These lesions either resolve spontaneously or evolve through vesicular and pustular stages to develop gray necrotic centers, often on hemorrhagic bases. It is generally accepted that they represent septic emboli during episodes of gonococcemia.

Gonococcal arthritis is characterized by an acute mono- or pauciarticular septic arthritis. The joint is red and warm and has an easily demonstrable effusion. The degree of systemic toxicity depends on the number and size of the joints involved. Although the occurrence of skin lesions may be elicited in the history, 25% have no evidence of antecedent gonococcemia.

DIFFERENTIAL DIAGNOSIS

Gonococcal proctitis should be suspected in homosexual men with rectal symptoms; however, no symptoms are specific for anorectal GC. Other causes of proctitis, including syphilis, herpes simplex, *Chlamydia, Entamoeba histolytica, Campylobacter,* anal fissure, anal fistula, and perianal abscess, should be sought.

The differential diagnosis of DGI depends on the clinical manifestations. With the classic arthritis–dermatitis syndrome, the major concern is with disseminated *Neisseria meningitidis.* Suggestive of meningococcemia are a larger number of skin lesions (>100) and leukocytosis. Acute rheumatic fever (ARF) and Reiter's syndrome (RS) should also be considered. The fever and migratory polyarthralgias of DGI may suggest ARF, but high temperature (>103°F) is unusual in DGI, and skin lesions, if present, are discriminatory. Features of DGI that distinguish it from RS are more acute onset, increased frequency of migratory polyarthralgias, upper limb predominance, female predominance, and the rarity of ocular involvement in DGI.

In men presenting with urethritis and arthritis, a Gram's stain of the urethral discharge may be helpful. The major differential in acute mono- or pauciarticular septic arthritis is between GC arthritis and other infectious arthritides. GC arthritis is the most frequent cause of septic arthritis in young, sexually active patients. It predominantly affects the wrists and small joints of previously healthy women in the 15-to-35-year age group. Other types of infectious arthritis are uncommon in this population. Diagnosis is based on culture and Gram's stain.

EMERGENCY DEPARTMENT EVALUATION AND MANAGEMENT

The diagnosis and treatment of men presenting with acute urethritis and women with possible PID are discussed elsewhere. Pharyngeal cultures for GC should probably be obtained in high-risk groups: homosexual men and prostitutes with pharyngitis, patients with sore throats and concurrent signs or symptoms of urogenital GC, pregnant women in whom gonorrhea is suspected, and patients with a history of exposure to GC and possible oropharyngeal involvement. Homosexual men with anorectal symptoms should have a careful examination for perianal erythema, ulcers, vesicles, fissures, tears, fistula, abscess, hemorrhoids, and other causes of symptoms. An anoscopic examination should be performed for mucosal lesions or exudate (which should be Gram-stained). The presence of other lesions does not rule out co-infection with GC, and all patients with a negative Gram's stain should have rectal cultures for GC.

Patients with signs or symptoms of DGI often have an asymptomatic primary infection. A careful examination for signs of complications should be done. Cultures of the pharynx, rectum, and urethra or cervix should be obtained before antibiotics. Blood cultures should be obtained, and any joint effusions should be aspirated and sent for cell count, Gram's stain, and culture. Pathologic cardiac murmurs or rubs suggest endocarditis or pericarditis, and if meningeal signs are present, a lumbar puncture is indicated. ECG (myocarditis or pericarditis) should be done if indicated. CDC guidelines are published regularly and these should be reviewed (Figure 163-1). *All* patients treated for GC should have blood samples drawn for syphilis serology. Patients with incubating syphilis will probably be cured by the regimens except spectinomycin alone. Patients with positive serologies should be treated as discussed elsewhere. Because of the high incidence of HIV in patients with sexually transmitted diseases, it is recommended that patients be offered testing for HIV and appropriate counseling.

DISPOSITION

Patients with uncomplicated GC may be managed as outpatients. All women and any patient with asymptomatic infection or an infection with PPNG should be referred for test-of-cure (TOC) cultures. Although hospitalization is recommended for patients with DGI, uncomplicated cases of arthritis–dermatitis syndrome may be successfully managed as outpatients. However, only reli-

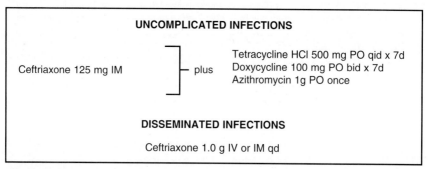

UNCOMPLICATED INFECTIONS

Ceftriaxone 125 mg IM]— plus   Tetracycline HCl 500 mg PO qid x 7d
Doxycycline 100 mg PO bid x 7d
Azithromycin 1g PO once

DISSEMINATED INFECTIONS

Ceftriaxone 1.0 g IV or IM qd

Figure 163-1. Treatment of gonococcal infection. (Adapted from Guide to Antimicrobial Therapy, 1994.)

able patients with a typical presentation and follow-up care should be considered for outpatient treatment. It is imperative that these patients understand that anything other than a prompt response to therapy (definite improvement within 24–48 hours and remission of symptoms within 72 hours of the initiation of therapy) necessitates an immediate return for possible hospitalization. Failure to respond rapidly to the recommended treatment suggests either an alternative diagnosis or, rarely, infection with an antibiotic-resistant strain of GC. Patients in whom the diagnosis is uncertain, who have purulent synovial effusions, in an area where PPNG accounts for >1% of the isolates, or who have psychosocial problems that may make compliance unlikely or follow-up difficult should probably not be considered candidates for outpatient therapy.

COMMON PITFALLS

- The most common error is failure to diagnose. A significant proportion of men with GC are asymptomatic, and the mild, nonspecific symptoms of primary GC in women requires suspicion; sexual history should be obtained from all patients with urogenital or rectal complaints, with a low threshold for cultures and antibiotics.

164   Syphilis

Syphilis is produced by the spirochete *Treponema pallidum,* an organism pathogenic only to humans. Syphilis is transmitted by sexual contact. The diverse manifestations of syphilis depend on the extent of spread of the spirochetes and the length of time between exposure and effective therapy.

CLINICAL PRESENTATION
PRIMARY SYPHILIS

After an incubation period of 3 weeks, the lesion of primary syphilis forms at the site of initial inoculation. In heterosexual males, this is usually a painless papule on the penis that soon erodes to form a smooth painless ulcer known as a chancre. Multiple chancres are seen in 30–50%. Within a week, painless unilateral or bilateral regional adenopathy is noted. The chancre heals without treatment in 3–6 weeks, but adenopathy may persist. Rectal and oral lesions may also be seen, particularly in homosexual men. Rectal chancres are often secondarily infected and may mimic a rectal abscess. Rectal syphilis may cause rectal bleeding and must be differentiated from other causes of proctitis in homosexual men. Oral chancres often appear as round indurated lesions. In women, painless lesions of the vulva, labia, clitoris, and cervix as well as mouth and rectum may be overlooked if syphilis is not suspected.

SECONDARY SYPHILIS

Secondary syphilis represents disseminated disease and occurs in virtually all cases of untreated primary infection. The lesions of secondary syphilis, noted 4–10 weeks after the primary lesions, affect the skin and mucous membranes. A macular pink rash that appears on the trunk and spares the face is often the first sign of disseminated disease. Several days later, a papular or papulosquamous eruption appears over the entire trunk and the extremities, including the palms and soles. Papulosquamous lesions are the classic cutaneous manifestations of secondary syphilis.

While skin and mucous membranes are most often affected, secondary syphilis is a disseminated infection and can affect any organ. Nonspecific symptoms such as fever, malaise, anorexia, weight loss, and arthralgias occur in 70% of patients. Syphilitic sore throat is seen, and generalized adenopathy, particularly the epitrochlear nodes, is common. At least 33% have subclinical central nervous system (CNS) disease as evidenced by abnormal cerebrospinal fluid protein and lymphocytosis. Syphilitic hepatitis is noted in 10%. The manifestations remit slowly even without treatment, but relapses occur in 20–25% of untreated cases, often 1 year following infection. Most often the oral cavity and anogenital region are involved, but condyloma lata are common.

LATENT SYPHILIS

In latent syphilis, specific treponemal serologic tests are positive but there are no signs of clinical illness. The absence of symptoms, however, does not mean the disease is not progressing; it is during "latency" that the major end-organ damage associated with syphilis occurs. In about 66% the latent period lasts for life with tertiary syphilis never appearing.

TERTIARY SYPHILIS

Tertiary syphilis is the result of longstanding untreated infection and is not clinically manifested until at least 10 years after infection. Neurosyphilis and cardiovascular syphilis are the two most important forms. Asymptomatic neurosyphilis (positive CSF VDRL or a mononuclear CSF pleocytosis with a positive blood serology) occurs in 33% of untreated patients. Symptomatic neurosyphilis falls into one of three major patterns. *Meningovascular syphilis* can present as chronic meningitis, stroke, seizures, or spinal cord syndromes. Prompt diagnosis is crucial because penicillin therapy can halt progression. In *general paresis,* nerve cells in the cerebral cortex are destroyed, causing progressive dementia often accompanied by dysphonia, weakness, gait disturbances, and hyperreflexia. *Tabes dorsalis* is the result of progressive demyelination of the posterior columns and dorsal nerve roots. Its manifestations are progressive ataxia, incontinence, and lancinating pains in the legs.

Cardiovascular syphilis becomes manifest after 20–40 years of untreated disease and causes symptoms related to the thoracic aorta. Late effects may include aortic valvular insufficiency and aneurysm of the ascending aorta. A characteristic chest x-ray finding is linear calcification of the ascending aorta.

Syphilis may present unique problems with concurrent HIV infection. Co-infection may be synergistic, resulting in more rapid progression of disease. Further, symptoms of neurosyphilis may be confused with CNS manifestations of HIV infection; moreover, serologic response may be altered in immunocompromised patients. There is evidence that standard treatment regimens may be inadequate in HIV-infected patients.

DIFFERENTIAL DIAGNOSIS

The reputation of syphilis as "the great imitator" is appropriate. The chancre of primary syphilis may be confused with chancroid, herpesvirus infection, lymphogranuloma venereum, or secondarily infected lesions. The painless nature of the ulcer, the absence of preceding vesicles, and the presence of a single ulcer are all clues that help to distinguish primary syphilis from other causes of the genital ulceroglandular syndrome.

Rectal diseases must be differentiated from gonococcal proctitis, anorectal herpes simplex, traumatic anal fissures, enteric pathogens of the "gay bowel syndrome," and noninfectious entities (e.g., neoplasms, inflammatory bowel disease). Pityriasis rosea, measles, tinea, sarcoid, granuloma annulare, lichen planus, and psoriasis may all be confused with the cutaneous manifestations of secondary syphilis, but findings of fever, malaise, generalized adenopathy, condyloma lata, or involvement of the palms and soles are more specific for syphilis. The diagnosis is seldom made on purely clinical grounds, but must always be suspected. Syphilis may be especially confusing in patients with HIV infection. Meningitis must be distinguished from the aseptic meningitis seen with HIV infection and from opportunistic CNS infection by *Toxoplasma, Cryptococcus, Coccidioides,* or TB. Neurosyphilis must be differentiated from the AIDS-dementia complex or other neurologic manifestations of HIV disease.

EMERGENCY DEPARTMENT EVALUATION

Any patient with compatible skin lesions or unusual systemic illnesses should be suspected of having syphilis, particularly homosexuals and those with recent sexually transmitted disease (especially gonorrhea) or a known exposure. Clues in the history include the time course of the illness, the presence of constitutional symptoms, previous episodes of syphilis, and any previous antibiotic therapy. The lesions of primary and secondary syphilis are highly infectious. Pay attention to any penile, rectal, or anal chancres; characteristic rashes, particularly involving the palms and soles; regional or generalized adenopathy; meningeal signs; and focal neurologic findings. The primary lesion may still be present while the patient is exhibiting signs of disseminated disease. Lesions should be scraped for dark-field microscopy, and blood should be drawn for serologic testing.

Diagnostic tests may be divided into three groups: direct examinations, nontreponemal tests, and treponemal tests. The *dark-field examination* may be performed on material aspirated from chancres, condylomata, and mucous patches. *Nontreponemal serologic tests* (VDRL, RPR, ART) use nonspecific reactions to screen for syphilis, to follow response to treatment, and to evaluate CNS disease. However, false-positive test results occur; transient false-positive reactions lasting <6 months are seen in viral illness (measles, hepatitis, infectious mononucleosis), *Mycoplasma* infection, malaria, or chlamydial infection. Chronic false-positive test results lasting >6 months are seen with aging, narcotic addition, autoimmune disease, and leprosy. Titers should begin to fall within several months of treatment. These tests should be nonreactive within 1 year following adequate treatment of primary syphilis, or 2 years after treating secondary syphilis. Longstanding disease may require 5 years for tests to revert to negative. Persistence of a reaction implies inadequate therapy, reinfection, or chronic "biological false-positive."

When a nontreponemal test yields a positive result, order a *treponemal serologic test* (FTA-ABS, MHA-TP, HATTS) to confirm the diagnosis, since these tests are very specific. Once positive, they remain positive for life.

EMERGENCY DEPARTMENT MANAGEMENT

The therapy for syphilis is penicillin. Treatment recommendations are summarized in Table 164-1. The Jarisch–Herxheimer reaction may occur several hours after the first dose of penicillin. This acute febrile reaction occurs in 30–50% of cases of primary syphilis, 70–90% with secondary syphilis, and 25–30% in late disease. The fever may be accompanied by hypotension. The reaction usually abates after 12 to 24 hours and should be treated with general supportive measures. Subsequent doses of antibiotics may produce milder reactions. Jarisch–Herxheimer reactions are not related to penicillin allergy and should not lead the clinician to discontinue antibiotic treatment.

DISPOSITION

Dermatology or infectious disease consultants may be helpful in recognizing or confirming the diagnosis in atypical or confusing cases. They may also assist in performing dark-field examinations or in interpreting inconsistent results of serologic tests. Patients suspected of having cardiovascular syphilis should be referred to cardiology or infectious disease consultants for evaluation and treatment.

TABLE 164-1. Current Recommendations for Treatment of Syphilis

Stage	Drug of Choice	Alternatives
Primary Secondary Latent, <1 year	Benzathine Penicillin G 2.4 million units IM, once	Tetracycline 500 mg QID x 15 days or Erythromycin 500 mg QID x 15 days
Latent, >1 year Cardiovascular	Benzathine Penicillin G 2.4 million units/week IM x 3 weeks	Tetracycline 500 mg QID x 30 days or Erythromycin 500 mg QID x 30 days
Neurosyphilis	Aqueous penicillin G 12–24 million units/day IV x 10 days followed by benzathine penicillin G 2.4 million units/week IM x 3 weeks	Tetracycline 500 mg QID x 30 days or Erythromycin 500 mg QID x 30 days

Patients with neurosyphilis or major CNS manifestation require admission for IV therapy. Uncomplicated cases may be referred to a local sexually transmitted disease clinic or public health clinic for follow-up and contact tracing.

COMMON PITFALLS

- Failure to consider the diagnosis of syphilis, especially in atypical presentations
- Failure to consider other sexually transmitted diseases in patients found to have syphilis and, conversely, failure to test for syphilis in patients with other sexually transmitted diseases
- Misinterpretation of serologic tests
- Failure to trace and treat contacts

165   Acquired Immunodeficiency Syndrome

Kaposi's sarcoma (KS) and *Pneumocystis carinii* pneumonia in homosexual men began to appear in 1981; these are now known as early manifestations of acquired immunodeficiency syndrome (AIDS). In the USA, cases are concentrated in large urban settings such as New York, Miami, and San Francisco.

EPIDEMIOLOGY

HIV infection results in a broad spectrum of clinical conditions ranging from an asymptomatic seropositive state to severe immunocompromise. AIDS itself is a specific diagnosis with a specific definition. Ninety percent have occurred in men, with 8% in women and 1.6% in children; >90% are in patients 20–49 years old. There is disproportionate infection among minority groups; 26% of adult and 53% of pediatric AIDS cases are among blacks; Hispanics represent

14% of adult and 23% of pediatric cases. Certain behaviors or risks are associated with an increased likelihood of acquiring HIV infection. These include homosexuality or bisexuality, IV drug abuse, prostitution, heterosexual exposure to a partner at risk, and receiving blood products before 1985.

The pattern of infection among high-risk individuals is changing; most new infections now occur among IV drug abusers. Seroprevalence among ED patients has been well documented; 6% of ED patients have evidence of HIV infection and in the majority the infection is unrecognized. Only a few modes of transmission have been proved: semen, vaginal secretions, blood or blood products, and transplacental transmission *in utero*. There have been no instances of casual transmission, although there has been one reported case of possible salivary transmission. HIV is a labile virus. It is easily neutralized by heat and common disinfecting agents such as 50% ethanol, 35% isopropyl alcohol, 0.3% hydrogen peroxide, Lysol, and a 1:10 solution of household bleach.

CLINICAL PRESENTATION AND EMERGENCY DEPARTMENT EVALUATION

The spectrum of disease caused by HIV ranges from an asymptomatic state to a wide variety of opportunistic infections, malignancies, and encephalopathy. Following exposure to the virus, seropositivity may develop in as little as 4 weeks or may be delayed for 6 months or even longer. There is no consistent pattern of disease progression. The average time from initial infection to clinical AIDS is estimated to be 9 years for homosexuals but may be different for other risk groups. The development of oral candidiasis is a poor prognostic sign, predictive of progression to AIDS; many of these patients can be expected to develop opportunistic infections within several months. Studies of large groups of homosexual men have shown that 15–20% develop AIDS and 5–10% develop AIDS-related complex (ARC) within 3 years of seroconversion. While not all cases progress to meet the definition of AIDS, the disease is considered to be uniformly and ultimately fatal for almost all. The average survival time following a diagnosis of AIDS is about 9 months.

Pneumocystis carinii pneumonia (PCP) is the most common opportunistic infection in AIDS, with over 80% of patients acquiring PCP at some point. It is the initial opportunistic infection in 60% of cases. The chest radiograph commonly shows a diffuse interstitial infiltrate but is not always abnormal at presentation. Bronchoscopy has been the mainstay of diagnosis with examination of sputum.

Toxoplasmosis is the most common cause of focal encephalitis in AIDS. Symptoms include headache, fever, focal neurologic deficits, altered mental status, and seizures. The diagnosis is usually made by a contrast-enhanced head computerized tomography (CT) scan showing one or more ring-enhancing lesions associated with edema. However, the CT may be falsely negative. Magnetic resonance imaging (MRI) is more sensitive and may be appropriate in certain cases. Unfortunately, clinical and radiologic features cannot distinguish CNS toxoplasmosis from a wide variety of other disorders (lymphoma, fungal infection, progressive multifocal leukoencephalopathy, cerebral tuberculosis, cytomegalovirus infection, Kaposi's sarcoma, and hemorrhage). Serologic tests are of no value because antibody to *Toxoplasma gondii* is prevalent in the general population. The presence of antibody to *T. gondii* in the CSF is helpful, however, although serology is often negative in documented cases. Often the diagnosis is established only with brain biopsy. Following treatment, improvement can be expected both clinically and on CT. Failure to improve suggests an alternative diagnosis, which may require a biopsy.

An atypical mycobacterium, *Mycobacterium avium-intracellulare* (MAI), causes disseminated disease in up to 50% of AIDS patients. It is usually associated with severe weight loss, diarrhea, and constitutional symptoms such as fever, malaise, and anorexia. It rarely causes significant pulmonary disease. The diagnosis is generally not difficult. Ziehl–Neelsen (acid-fast) stain of stool or other body fluids is frequently positive, and the organism also can be cultured from blood. Currently there is no effective therapy.

The incidence of *Mycobacterium tuberculosis* in HIV-infected patients is increasing, particularly in socioeconomically disadvantaged groups, including intravenous drug users. It may be the initial finding in HIV-infected patients. The typical pulmonary upper-lobe lesion is uncommon, and the radiographic findings may be indistinguishable from those due to a variety of other opportunistic infections. Extrapulmonary disease occurs in 75% of cases. Negative PPD tests are frequent. Attempts to diagnose tuberculosis by stain and culture of sputum may not be fruitful; bronchoscopy or biopsy of affected organs (e.g., lymph nodes, liver, brain) may be required.

Cytomegalovirus (CMV) is a frequent cause of opportunistic infection. Disseminated disease is common. It is usually associated with PCP in pulmonary infections. CMV is the most frequent cause of retinitis in HIV-infected patients. The gastrointestinal tract is involved frequently, and CMV should be considered when parasitic or other pathogens are not identified as the cause of diarrhea.

EMERGENCY DEPARTMENT MANAGEMENT

Opportunistic infections are rarely curable, and most of the infectious complications are not readily communicable (except for tuberculosis, herpes zoster infection, and possibly salmonellosis). Infections are rarely single, and thus a poor response to therapy may be due to a second or third unidentified cause. The type and frequency of opportunistic infections seen are directly related to the prevalence of asymptomatic infection in the local healthy population. Inquire about risk factors as part of the routine evaluation of all adult patients, especially in endemic areas. The infection rate may be surprisingly high. Many cases of early HIV infection may not be detected during ED evaluation because of low suspicion, particularly in areas where AIDS is not prevalent. Early presentations are listed in Table 165-1.

FEVER
Fever is a common complaint. When due to the HIV infection alone, it tends to occur in the afternoon or evening and is generally responsive to aspirin or acetaminophen. Evidence of an infectious or other cause of fever should be sought. Changes in the patient's usual fever pattern may indicate PCP, mycobacterial infection, cryptococcal meningitis or fungemia, toxoplasmosis, cytomegalovirus infection, disseminated herpes infection, or drug reaction. Patients with unexplained fever and AIDS should usually be admitted.

Laboratory evaluation includes blood cultures (aerobic, anaerobic, and fungal), blood tests for cryptococcal antigen and *Toxoplasma and Coccidioides* serologies, and chest radiography. Stool culture, stool examination for ova and parasites, urine culture for fungus and mycobacteria, and sputum smear and culture for fungus and mycobacteria may yield additional important

---

TABLE 165-1. Early and Initial Presentations of HIV-1 Infection

General	Gastrointestinal
Generalized lymphadenopathy	Persistent unexplained diarrhea
Unexplained fever	Oral thrush
Unexplained weight loss	**Dermatologic**
Fatigue	
Lassitude	**Herpes zoster**
Acute viral illness	**CNS**
Pulmonary	Seizure
Dyspnea	Altered mental status
Persistent cough	
Tuberculosis	

clues to diagnosis. If there is no contraindication, lumbar puncture should be performed if no other source of fever is identified or if there are neurologic signs or symptoms, particularly a change in mental status. A head CT may be done prior to the LP if indicated.

PULMONARY INVOLVEMENT

Pulmonary presentations account for frequent ED visits. The differential diagnosis includes viral, bacterial, mycobacterial, fungal, and protozoal pneumonias, as well as malignancies. Differentiation of these entities in the ED may be difficult, if not impossible. The physical examination is unlikely to establish a diagnosis. Patients with fever and productive cough often have a bacterial pneumonia, whereas a nonproductive cough is more likely to accompany PCP, CMV pneumonia, fungal infection, or neoplasm. Hemoptysis is most often associated with pneumococcal pneumonia and TB. Fulminant respiratory failure is most likely to be caused by PCP or CMV.

Patients with known HIV who present with pulmonary complaints generally require a CBC, electrolytes, ABG, serum lactate dehydrogenase, chest radiography, and sputum culture, as well as Gram's stain and special stains (Gomori, Giemsa, acid-fast). Obtaining blood cultures can avoid delays in antimicrobial therapy. Leukocytosis and focal infiltrates on chest radiography suggest bacterial pneumonia. A diffuse infiltrative process on CXR, especially in the absence of leukocytosis, is associated with PCP or CMV. PCP is suggested by an increased serum lactate dehydrogenase and hypoxia more severe than expected from radiographic findings. Hilar adenopathy with diffuse pulmonary infiltrates suggests cryptococcosis, histoplasmosis, mycobacterial infection, or neoplasm. Kaposi's sarcoma (KS) can present with cough, fever, and dyspnea, and the CXR may mimic that seen with PCP. PCP can be demonstrated by histologic techniques but cannot be cultured, and serology is unreliable.

Management includes O_2 and volume repletion, if indicated. Specific treatment can be instituted if the diagnosis is clear. If the symptoms are of new onset, or if there has been a change from previous status, the patient should be admitted. Decisions about patients with known pulmonary involvement are based on comparison to baseline status and the effectiveness of ongoing or previous treatment (i.e., treatment failure), as well as the individual's ability to obtain outpatient follow-up (see disposition considerations below).

Careful evaluation is warranted in patients with pulmonary symptoms who fall into high-risk groups but who do not carry a diagnosis of HIV infection. If ED tests (CXR, sputum examination, ABG) are not helpful, the patient should be referred (or admitted if warranted); voluntary HIV testing, counseling and follow-up, should be arranged. Patients admitted with pulmonary involvement in whom the diagnosis cannot be determined may require bronchoscopy. If the clinical suspicion of PCP is high, treatment should begin before diagnostic bronchoscopy.

NEUROLOGIC INVOLVEMENT

Central nervous system disease occurs in 30–40% of AIDS patients, and 10–20% initially present with CNS symptoms. Seizures and altered mental status are the most common neurologic manifestations, but headache, fever, and meningismus also are seen. Infection accounts for the vast majority of neurologic presentations and is usually accompanied by fever. AIDS dementia, a progressive process caused by HIV and commonly heralded by impairment of recent memory, occurs in >33%. Noninfectious causes of CNS dysfunction include lymphoma (primary and secondary) and KS. A specific diagnosis often can be established only with CT scan, CSF studies, and, in many cases (e.g., lymphoma), biopsy.

All patients with known HIV infection and those in high-risk groups who have a change in neurologic status or new neurologic symptoms or signs should have a lumbar puncture unless there is a clinical contraindication. Ideally a CT scan should be performed first if available. Besides routine CSF analysis, special studies may be required (e.g., viral and fungal cultures, India ink stain, cryptococcal antigen, and coccidiomycosis titre). Toxoplasmosis is the most common cause of focal encephalitis in HIV infection and should always be a major consideration.

Cryptococcosis may cause either focal cerebral lesions or diffuse meningoencephalitis. Presenting symptoms may be subtle (e.g., mild depression, headache, or dizziness without meningismus) but are often dramatic (e.g., cranial nerve palsies and seizures); there may also be extra-CNS involvement. The diagnosis depends on identifying organisms (by India ink preparation or fungal culture) or cryptococcal antigen in the CSF.

Tuberculous meningitis is suggested by characteristic CSF findings of low glucose, high protein, and lymphocytic pleocytosis, but similar findings may be noted with parameningeal abscess, *Listeria* meningitis, and the fungal meningitides (including that due to *Cryptococcus*). Diffuse or focal CNS involvement with *Nocardia, Cryptococcus, M. tuberculosis,* and other mycobacteria may be impossible to distinguish from cerebral toxoplasmosis by clinical and CT findings. Focal symptoms also may be due to progressive multifocal leukoencephalopathy or CNS lymphoma.

Bacterial meningitis in patients with AIDS is diagnosed by use of the same criteria applicable in other patients. Herpes simplex virus encephalitis may be suggested by a finding of enhanced cortical uptake on contrast-enhanced CT, but temporal lobe biopsy is usually required to establish the diagnosis. MAI and CMV also may be responsible for CNS disease. HIV itself can cause an acute meningoencephalitis, with an onset shortly before or at the time of seroconversion. CSF findings are nonspecific and CT is normal, but electroencephalogram (EEG) abnormalities become more severe as mental status deteriorates.

All AIDS patients with new or changed CNS symptoms or signs must be admitted to the hospital, even if the ED evaluation is unrevealing. CT scan and lumbar puncture should usually be performed although CSF culture and serologic results will not be available immediately. When the CT and all CSF studies are unrevealing, MRI has been helpful in identifying early CNS lesions.

OROPHARYNX

Oral candidiasis affects more than 80% of AIDS patients and typically involves the tongue and buccal mucosa. It can be distinguished from hairy leukoplakia by its characteristic whitish, lacy plaques that are easily scraped away from an erythematous base. Microscopic examination of the material on potassium hydroxide smear can confirm the diagnosis. Oral and esophageal involvement with *Candida* is considered predictive of a progressive course. Most oral lesions can be managed symptomatically on an outpatient basis. Painful oral and perioral ulcerations may be caused by herpes simplex virus (HSV) or MAI. HSV can be diagnosed by the identification of multinucleated giant cells in scrapings of the lesions; a diagnosis of MAI can be established if an acid-fast stain is positive. Both HSV and MAI also can be diagnosed by culture.

Oral KS may appear as nontender, well-circumscribed, slightly raised, violaceous lesions anywhere in the oropharynx. Definitive diagnosis requires biopsy.

GASTROINTESTINAL INVOLVEMENT

About one half of all AIDS patients have symptoms due to infection of the gastrointestinal tract at some point. The most common symptoms are abdominal pain, bleeding, and diarrhea.

ESOPHAGUS   Dysphagia or odynophagia are indicative of esophageal involvement. *Candida,* herpes simplex, and CMV infection may all cause painful esophagitis. Endoscopy, fungal stains, viral cultures, and occasionally biopsy may be required to establish the diagnosis. An air-contrast barium swallow can be obtained in the ED. An ulcerative pattern with plaques is characteristic of *Candida* esophagitis. Herpes esophagitis typically produces easily seen punched-out ulcerations without associated heaped-up plaques. Treatment is usually initiated with ketoconazole and/or acyclovir.

DIARRHEA   Diarrhea can vary in severity from a few loose stools per day to massive fluid loss with prostration, fever, chills, and weight loss. ED evaluation should be directed toward identifying those pathogens implicated in "gay bowel syndrome" (Table 165-2) and ruling out inflammatory bowel disease. *Cryptosporidium* and *Isospora* infection are associated with HIV infection, and both

TABLE 165-2. Pathogens Associated With Gay Bowel Syndrome

Shigella	*Chlamydia*	Herpes simplex
Neisseria gonorrhoeae	*Amoeba*	*Giardia*
Campylobacter		

organisms may produce prolonged watery diarrhea. Significant gastrointestinal bleeding has been associated with many pathogens, particularly CMV.

Salmonella infection appears to be a particular problem in patients with HIV, often producing recurrent bacteremia and other significant clinical disease. Occasionally, malignancy is the cause of significant symptoms; thus, KS and lymphoma are considerations. The ED evaluation of diarrhea *per se* is usually restricted to anoscopy (or sigmoidoscopy in some cases) and microscopic examination of the stool with methylene blue or Gram's, Wright's, or acid-fast stains, as well as stool specimens for cultures. When ordering stool cultures, it is important to specify which organisms are suspected, because not all are routinely cultured.

The diagnosis of infection with mycobacteria, *Cryptosporidium,* and *Isospora* is made by acid-fast stain. Because of intermittent shedding, repeated examination of the stool for trophozoites, cysts, and larvae is often necessary to diagnose infection with *Cryptosporidium* and *Isospora* as well as for amebiasis, giardiasis, and strongyloidiasis. If necessary, arrangements may be made for outpatient anoscopy, proctoscopy, or sigmoidoscopy (with or without biopsy) in patients who require further evaluation but do not require immediate admission.

LIVER   Several opportunistic organisms, including CMV, *M. avium-intracellulare, M. tuberculosis,* and *Histoplasma,* can produce a hepatitis-like picture. Most commonly, the patient presents with an elevation in the alkaline phosphatase disproportionate to that of other liver enzymes.

RECTUM   Proctocolitis is not uncommon and may be due to one or several organisms, among them *Campylobacter, Shigella, Salmonella, Giardia,* herpes simplex, *Entamoeba histolytica, Chlamydia,* and *Neisseria gonorrhoeae.* In patients with AIDS or with established risk factors for HIV infection, standard stool cultures, Thayer–Martin culture, and chlamydial culture or immunoassay should be ordered. In addition, stool should be examined microscopically for leukocytes, and a specimen should be sent for identification of ova and parasites. The diagnosis of anal gonorrhea can be confirmed on Gram's stain of stool by the presence of leukocytes and intracellular organisms. HSV can be diagnosed by viral culture or by the identification of multinucleated giant cells on scrapings of anal lesions.

CUTANEOUS INVOLVEMENT
KS has been involved in 25% of the known AIDS cases to date and is found predominantly among homosexual or bisexual males. The disease is usually widely disseminated with mucous membrane involvement, although most patients die from other complications unrelated to KS. Several common cutaneous manifestations of AIDS are likely to be seen in the ED. Varicella zoster eruptions involving several dermatomes are commonly seen; admission is usually warranted, and IV acyclovir (10 mg/kg three times daily) may hasten resolution of symptoms and prevent dissemination. Varicella immune globulin (VZIG) may be useful in patients with primary infection and visceral involvement.

Inguinal and perianal candidiasis have been noted commonly in AIDS patients, as have nail infections with *Candida* or *Trichophyton.* Other patients may present with multiple skin abscesses and impetigo usually due to staphylococci or streptococci. Treatment with oral antibiotics is often sufficient. Some patients develop a rash resembling seborrheic dermatitis, with erythematous, hyperkeratotic, scaling plaques involving the scalp, face (typically in a malar distribution), ears, chest, and genitalia. Treatment with topical steroids is effective in most patients. Other cutaneous manifestations of AIDS include alopecia and large painful venereal warts.

DIAGNOSING HIV-1 INFECTION

Diagnosing or testing for HIV in the ED is rarely if ever indicated. It is difficult to obtain informed consent, appropriate counseling (particularly the time involved) is all but impossible, confidentiality is difficult to maintain (at least for rapid "bedside" tests), and there may be low compliance with follow-up arranged from the ED. Testing to identify HIV-seropositive patients in the ED as a method to determine which patients require special infection control precautions may lull the treating providers into a sense of complacency. Testing may be appropriate for a few indications, such as when health care providers are exposed to patients' blood. On the other hand, emergency physicians should refer patients, particularly those with high-risk behaviors, for voluntary testing and counseling.

There are three approaches to establishing the diagnosis of HIV infection: isolation of the virus by culture, detection of viral-specific antigens, and detection of specific antibodies to HIV. Viral antibody is commonly detected by the enzyme-linked immunoassaytechnique (ELISA). ELISA tests are about 99% specific and about 95% sensitive. When the ELISA test indicates HIV antibodies, a second, more specific test such as the Western blot test is required before the diagnosis can be confirmed. Because HIV antibodies usually develop 6–12 weeks after initial exposure to the virus, it may be months before antibodies can be detected. Because of this "window" period between exposure to the virus and detectability of antibodies, negative test results cannot be relied on completely to identify infected patients.

TREATMENT

Treatment of AIDS and related illnesses consists of treatment or prevention of opportunistic infection or malignancy and attempts to eradicate or neutralize the virus. Opportunistic infection is more difficult to control than in other immunocompromised hosts, and many AIDS patients require long-term suppressive regimens (Table 165-3). The development of specific therapy active against HIV is still in its infancy. Initial treatment for *PCP* is with 20 mg/kg/day of trimethoprim (TMP) and 100 mg/kg/day of sulfamethoxazole (SMX), given either orally or IV for 2 to 3 weeks. A majority of patients (60%–80%) respond to therapy, although pneumocysts persist in the lungs of 66%. Three weeks of treatment is commonly recommended.

Those with radiologic or clinical disease progression after 4 to 5 days of TMP-SMX therapy, and those who fail to improve after TMP-SMX therapy, are considered treatment failures. Relapses are common; 65% of patients will have a reinfection within 18 months. Somewhat fewer reinfections respond to treatment. Adverse effects of TMP-SMX occur in up to 65% of AIDS patients and are 20 times more common than in the general population. They generally become apparent after 7 to 14 days of therapy. The most common adverse effects are nausea and vomiting, rash, fever, neutropenia, thrombocytopenia, hyponatremia, and hepatitis.

Treatment of *cryptococcal meningitis* usually begins with IV amphotericin B (0.4–0.6 mg/kg/day); flucytosine (75–100 mg/kg/day) may be added to this regimen. A response can be expected in about 60%. Some patients are able to be treated as outpatients with vascular access devices. The initial course of therapy lasts 6 weeks, and because of the high relapse rate (about 50%), chronic suppressive therapy is continued after successful treatment. The major adverse effect of treatment is bone marrow suppression.

CNS *toxoplasmosis* is treated for 3 to 6 months with oral sulfadiazine 100 mg/kg/day and pyrimethamine 25–50 mg/day, with folinic acid added to blunt hematologic toxicity. Short courses of high-dose steroids also are used. As with cryptococcal meningitis, chronic suppres-

TABLE 165-3. Guidelines for the Diagnosis, Treatment, and Prevention of HIV-Associated Infections

Infection	Therapy	Comments
P. carinii pneumonia	Oral TMP-SMX (15–20 mg TMP and 75–100 mg SMX/kg/day PO or IV) for 3 wk or pentamidine (4 mg/kg/day IV or IM) for 3 wk*	Primary prevention and post-treatment maintenance therapy are useful.
Central nervous system toxoplasmosis	Pyrimethamine (25–50 mg/day PO) plus sulfadiazine (100 mg/kg/day PO) for at least 3–6 mo	Maintenance therapy is required.
Cryptococcal meningitis	Amphotericin B (0.4–0.6 mg/kg/day—total dose at least 1.5–2 g)†	Maintenance therapy is required.
Disseminated M. avium-intracellulare	No effective therapy	
Tuberculosis	Isoniazid (5–10 mg/kg/day [usually 300 mg] PO), rifampin (9 mg/kg/day [usually 600 mg] PO), and either pyrazinamide (25 mg/kg/day PO) or streptomycin (0.75–1.0 mg/kg/day IM)‡	Isoniazid "prophylaxis" for all HIV- and PPD-positive persons not previously treated.
Disseminated cytomegalovirus	Ganciclovir (7.5–15 mg/kg/day)	Maintenance therapy is required.
Herpes simplex	Acyclovir (1000 mg/kg PO or 15 mg/kg/day IV for severe disease)	Maintenance therapy is required for severe recurrent disease.
Herpes zoster	Acyclovir (25–30 mg/kg/day IV)§	Strict isolation is necessary if patient is hospitalized
Salmonellosis	TMP-SMX (10 mg TMP and 50 mg SMX/kg/day IV or PO) or ampicillin (12 g/day IV)	Maintenance therapy is required.
Candidiasis	Clotrimazole (30–50 mg/day) or ketoconazole (200–400 mg/day)	Maintenance therapy is required. Amphotericin B is occasionally necessary for severe esophagitis.
Cryptosporidiosis	No effective therapy	

*Additional primary therapies include TMP and dapsone or inhaled pentamidine.
† Some would add flucytosine (100 to 150 mg per kilogram per day PO) for six weeks.
‡ This treatment is appropriate until sensitivities are known; then treat with at least two drugs (to which the pathogen is sensitive) for at least six months after cultures turn negative (9 months minimum).
§ Some have used 3 to 4 g per day PO in less severe cases.
From Glatt AE, Chirgwin K, Landesman S: Treatment of infections associated with human immunodeficiency virus. *N Engl J Med* 318:1439, 1988. Reproduced with permission.

sive treatment is usually indicated because of the high likelihood of relapse. Sulfadiazine and pyrimethamine frequently cause a rash and profound neutropenia (marrow suppression), requiring cessation of therapy in up to 45% of patients. Esophageal *candidiasis* is treated with ketoconazole 400 mg/day or with oral nystatin or clotrimazole troches. Relapses are common after cessation of treatment. Occasionally, IV amphotericin B must be employed. Disseminated candidiasis is managed with IV amphotericin B and flucytosine.

AIDS patients with *tuberculosis* usually receive standard triple therapy with isoniazid, rifampin, and ethambutol, which can be supplemented with pyrazinamide or streptomycin (Table 165-3). All HIV-infected patients with positive PPD should receive isoniazid prophylaxis. Infection with *M. avium-intracellulare* is difficult to treat. Most cultured organisms are resistant to isoniazid and rifampin, and all treatment regimens are generally ineffective, particularly for disseminated disease. There is no evidence that treatment of this infection improves the patient's outcome.

Herpes simplex infection in AIDS patients responds well to standard therapies, and toxic effects are infrequent. Oral acyclovir (e.g., 200 mg five times a day for 10 days) is effective for mucocutaneous infection and prevents recurrences. IV therapy (15–30 mg/kg/day) may be required in extensive disease. Multidermatomal herpes zoster responds well to IV acyclovir (5–10 mg/kg three times daily). Patients with these viral infections who require admission should be admitted to isolation beds. Suppressive therapy is effective.

CMV may be treated with DHPG (ganciclovir), notably CMV chorioretinitis and colitis. Its major adverse effects are neutropenia, thrombocytopenia, and azotemia. Because *Kaposi's sarcoma* in general is not associated with significant morbidity, therapy is indicated only for extensive or painful lesions, facial or lower extremity edema, disfigurement, or respiratory compromise. Chemotherapy (e.g., vincristine, vinblastine, or doxorubicin) or radiation therapy is used when treatment is necessary. In contrast, non-Hodgkin's lymphoma is often advanced by the time of diagnosis, and involvement of extranodal sites such as the CNS and bone marrow is common. Despite aggressive chemotherapy, outcome has been uniformly poor.

ANTIVIRAL AND IMMUNOMODULATOR THERAPY

Various agents are being investigated as immunomodulators: Azidothymidine (AZT) is the first antiviral agent to have demonstrated clinical benefit. AZT decreases the number and severity of opportunistic infections. AZT is associated with macrocytic anemia, headache, and leukopenia.

DISPOSITION

Disposition decisions for HIV-infected patients are based on clinical condition, outpatient resources, and the ability to arrange follow-up. Patients who are seropositive for HIV but not admitted should be referred for medical consultation and counseling. It is useful for each institution to arrange appropriate mechanisms for these referrals. Patients who have symptoms or signs suggestive of HIV infection (e.g., weight loss, generalized adenopathy, chronic diarrhea, oral thrush) but do not require admission also should receive similar referral. Indications for admission are shown in Table 165-4, and discharge considerations are shown in Table 165-5. When there is doubt about diagnostic or management options, consultation with specialists is appropriate: infectious disease specialist, neurologist, psychiatrist, AIDS specialist, and others.

Some contend that in advanced stages of AIDS, major resuscitative measures are not appropriate because of the uniformly poor prognosis. Many patients may agree as they approach the terminal stages of their disease. Decisions regarding the withholding of extraordinary resuscitation efforts are difficult to make in the ED, however. In general, when confronted with a patient with AIDS, it is best to take the same actions that would be taken with any other patient, unless specific information is available indicating that a contrary course should be followed.

TABLE 165-4. Indications for Admission

Patients with fever
  Unknown source
  CNS symptoms or findings
New-onset seizure or other CNS symptoms or
  findings
Suspected (but not yet diagnosed) PCP
Hypoxia worse than baseline
Intractable diarrhea
Herpes zoster infection
Marrow suppression
Extreme weakness
Inability to care for self or be cared for
Inability to obtain appropriate follow-up

TABLE 165-5. General Discharge Considerations From ED

Patient has stable medical condition with normal
  or baseline vital signs.
Appropriate follow-up and referral have been
  arranged.
Patient understands discharge instructions.
Patient or caretaker able to care for patient
Patient, partners, and family understand
  behaviors that lead to transmission and those
  which do not. If this is not the case, referral
  for counseling is indicated.

PREVENTION/PRECAUTIONS

Health care workers are often exposed to the blood and body secretions of AIDS patients or of other individuals who are at high risk of harboring the AIDS virus. Because there is no effective treatment for AIDS, the only available strategy is to take proper precautions in handling potentially infectious body fluids. The risk of acquiring HIV through occupational exposure appears to be low. Although the transmission of HIV has been documented after parenteral exposure and exposure of mucous membranes and inflamed skin, the risk of contracting AIDS is <0.5%. A substantial number of ED patients have unsuspected HIV infection and that HIV seroreactivity cannot be accurately predicted.

Because asymptomatic individuals who are HIV antibody-positive can transmit the disease, all contacts with patients' blood or body secretions must be considered potentially infectious by ED personnel. Although the risk of transmission of HIV to pregnant health care workers is no greater than that to nonpregnant employees, pregnant health care workers should probably avoid caring for AIDS patients. Furthermore, because of the potential for exposure to agents such as CMV and herpes simplex virus, pregnant women should avoid contact with AIDS patients. There is no evidence that HIV infection is transmissible to patients by ED personnel who are known to be HIV antibody-positive. Thus, routine screening of health care personnel for HIV infection is not justified.

166 Bacteremia and Septic Shock

Bacteremia is the presence of bacteria in the bloodstream. Its potentially explosive course and high mortality mandate antibiotics when suspected before cultures are known. Bacteremia is common following injury to mucosal surfaces (e.g., tooth brushing, urethral catheterization, sigmoidoscopy, angiography), but intact host defenses usually neutralize the bacteria and prevent infection. Septic shock is a state of circulatory insufficiency caused by bacterial products. Septic shock develops in <50% of cases of bacteremia; it occurs in about 40% of gram-negative bacteremia and about 20% of *Staphylococcus aureus* bacteremia. The organisms that most often produce bacteremia and septic shock: *Escherichia coli, Klebsiella* species, *Enterobacter* species, *Pseudomonas aeruginosa,* and *Proteus* species.

CLINICAL PRESENTATION

Bacteremia usually presents as an acute illness with symptoms of fever, chills, and prostration—the so-called "toxic" appearance. Not all patients have such a classic presentation, particularly those at the extremes of age or in debilitated states. Persistently low systemic vascular resistance is the major hemodynamic derangement in patients who die of septic shock. In advanced septic shock, depressed cardiac output and severe hypotension produce a vicious cycle of multiorgan failure usually unresponsive to volume and inotropic or vasoconstrictor therapy. ARDS is seen in 4–20% with bacteremia and 40–60% with septic shock.

DIFFERENTIAL DIAGNOSIS

Acute infections due to viruses, rickettsiae, mycobacteria, fungi, and parasites may present as acute "sepsis," but severe infection due to these organisms is less common than that due to bacteria, and most affected patients have underlying depressed immunity. Hyperthermia and heat stroke may mimic cardiopulmonary and neurologic manifestations of sepsis. Chills are, however, not expected with heat stroke. Shock from other causes should be considered. Septic shock should be suspected when hemodynamic measurements showing decreased vascular resistance and increased cardiac output are found. The prognosis of gram-negative bacteremia is primarily determined by the presence of underlying host disease.

EMERGENCY DEPARTMENT EVALUATION

Because sepsis may progress rapidly, the evaluation must be expeditious. Unexplained tachycardia or tachypnea may be early clues to infection. Oral temperatures do not accurately reflect core temperature; rectal temperature measurement is recommended with suspected hypothermia or fever. The examination should concentrate on potential sources for sepsis: the oral cavity, lungs, abdomen, urinary system, and skin are the most common locations. All indwelling catheters and lines should be suspected as possible sources. The laboratory and ancillary tests are potentially useful but the following yield the most information: chest radiograph; electrolytes, glucose, BUN, and creatinine; CBC including WBC and differential; urinalysis; blood cultures; and cultures of overt foci of infection. Initial antibiotic management is guided by the history and examination. Five factors are useful in predicting the likelihood of bacteremia or focal bacterial infection in adults with unexplained fever, the risk increasing with the number of factors present. High fever (>103°F) or a "toxic" appearance does not correlate with bacterial infection.

EMERGENCY DEPARTMENT MANAGEMENT

Stabilization may begin before assessment is complete. Adequate IV access, oxygen and cardiac monitoring should be done. All patients with sepsis require supplemental fluids with rate of infusion guided by the patient's volume and cardiovascular status. Because of vasodilatation and capillary leakage, large quantities of fluid may be required. Initial central venous pressure (CVP) or pulmonary artery occlusion pressure (PAOP) may provide confusing information about intravascular volume. Volume administration is best guided by observing the response of the CVP or PAOP to aliquots of fluid given over a short period of time. A rise of >5 cm H_2O or 5 torr after a volume infusion of several hundred milliliters indicates that the compliance of the vascular system is decreasing as further fluid is being given and the intravascular space is most likely "full." Colloids (albumin, hetastarch) have no proven benefit over crystalloids (normal saline or Ringer's lactate).

Further treatment has four components: (1) antibiotics, usually in combination; (2) removal or drainage of infected foci; (3) treatment of complications; and (4) pharmacologic interventions. Initial antibiotic treatment is empiric, based on an assessment of the patient's underlying host defenses, the potential sources for infection, and the most likely responsible organisms. Antibiotics must be "broad-spectrum," covering both gram-positive and gram-negative bacteria, since both classes produce an identical picture. Antistaphylococcal coverage is recommended in IV drug abuse or indwelling lines or devices. Coverage directed against anaerobes should be included for intra-abdominal or perineal infections. Antipseudomonal coverage is indicated with neutropenia or burns.

Because few antibiotics provide adequate coverage as single agents, combinations of drugs are usually recommended. For gram-negative coverage, most regimens include an aminoglycoside and a beta-lactam. The depressed cardiovascular system can be stimulated by inotropic and vasoconstrictive agents. Dopamine is the agent most commonly recommended: 5 10 µg/kg/min IV with the rate adjusted to blood pressure and other parameters. Norepinephrine can increase blood pressure, but has deleterious side effects on cardiac output and regional perfusion. If steroids are to be beneficial, and this is controversial, they should be given as soon as sepsis is recognized and given either as a single dose or for less than 24 hours. Most studies use methylprednisolone 30 mg/kg or its equivalent. Other agents perhaps of some benefit include naloxone, indomethacin, prostaglandin E_1, immune serum globulin, and antibodies.

DISPOSITION

The disposition of the patient with fever and no localizing signs of infection presents a dilemma. Young, otherwise healthy individuals with normal vital signs can generally be discharged with instructions for fever control and a warning to return if symptoms persist or worsen. A "toxic" appearance is of poor diagnostic value. Patients at risk for bacteremia should be admitted (IV drug abusers). Blood cultures for discharged adults are controversial.

COMMON PITFALLS

- Failure to consider bacterial infection as the cause of subtle or confusing symptoms and signs
- Fluid resuscitation may be restricted for fear of inducing pulmonary edema, but because of capillary leakage, large quantities of fluid may be required.
- Antibiotics may be delayed until cultures are collected, consultant is contacted, or the patient is admitted. All patients with suspected serious infections should receive antibiotics in the ED
- Patients with internal infection often require surgical drainage or excision. Because many have coexistent medical problems, surgery is often delayed to "get the patient into better shape." Experience teaches that such delays may not be in the patient's best interest.

167   Infections in the Compromised Host

Defects in our immunologic defense mechanisms result in increased susceptibility to infections with organisms of minimal risk for normal individuals and a tendency for infections to follow a fulminant and often fatal course. AIDS is the prototype of altered T-lymphocyte function and is manifested by infections with protozoans, fungi, viruses, and intracellular bacteria.

CLINICAL PRESENTATION

The presentation of infection can be diverse. The most challenging patients are those with immunodeficiency. Table 167-1 summarizes the primary diseases associated with immunodeficiency, their effect on the immune system, common sites of infection, common offending organisms, and

TABLE 167-1. Infections in the Compromised Host

Primary Disease Process	Immune Defects	Common Sites of Infection	Common Offending Microbes	Initial Antibiotic Regimens
Alcoholism	Phagocytosis Cell-mediated immunity Humoral factors	Lungs	S. pneumoniae S. aureus H. influenzae Mouth anaerobes M. tuberculosis Legionella	Timentin Cefazolin ± aminoglycoside 3rd-gen. cephalosporin plus erythromycin
		Skin/soft tissue	S. aureus S. pyogenes	Cefazolin
		Peritoneum	S. pneumoniae S. pyogenes S. aureus S. faecalis Enterobacteriaceae	Timentin Cefazolin or 3rd-gen. cephalosporin plus metronidazole
		Blood	S. aureus S. pneumoniae Enterobacteriaceae	Cefazolin plus aminoglycoside 3rd-gen. cephalosporin
Burns	External barrier Phagocytosis Humoral factors	Burn wound with secondary bacteremia	S. pyogenes S. aureus Enterobacteriaceae P. aeruginosa	Antipseudomonal penicillin plus aminoglycoside Cefazolin plus aminoglycoside Ceftazidime
Cystic Fibrosis	External barrier Phagocytosis	Lungs	P. aeruginosa	Antipseudomonal penicillin plus aminoglycoside

Diabetes Mellitus	External barrier	Skin/soft tissue	S. pyogenes
	Local environment		S. aureus
	Neuropathy		Enterobacteriaceae
	Hypoperfusion		Anaerobes
	Granulocyte function		Cefazolin plus metronidazole
			Timentin
		Urinary tract	Enterobacteriaceae
			Candida species
			3rd-gen. cephalosporin
			Cefazolin ± aminoglycoside
			TMP-SMX
			Ciprofloxacin
			Timentin
		Lungs	S. pneumoniae
			S. aureus
			K. pneumoniae
			Mouth anaerobes
			3rd-gen. cephalosporin
Intravenous Drug Abuse	External barrier	Skin/soft tissue	S. aureus
			S. pyogenes
			C. tetani
			Cefazolin
		Lungs	S. pneumoniae
			S. aureus
			Anaerobes
			M. tuberculosis
			Cefazolin
		Heart valves	S. aureus
			P. aeruginosa
			Candida species
			Oxacillin and gentamicin
		Joints	S. aureus
			S. pyogenes
			P. aeruginosa
			N. gonorrhoeae
			Cefuroxime ± gentamicin

(cont'd.)

TABLE 167-1. (Cont'd.)

Primary Disease Process	Immune Defects	Common Sites of Infection	Common Offending Microbes	Initial Antibiotic Regimens
Foreign Bodies				
Intravascular catheters	External barrier	Vessel Soft tissue Blood	S. epidermidis S. aureus Enterobacteriaceae P. aeruginosa Candida species	Vancomycin plus gentamicin Vancomycin plus aztreonam
Urinary catheter	External barrier	Urinary tract	S. faecalis Enterobacteriaceae P. aeruginosa Candida species	Aminoglycoside Ciprofloxacin
Nasal tube	External barrier Local environment	Sinuses	S. pneumoniae S. pyogenes H. influenzae	TMP-SMX Ampicillin
		Middle ear	S. pneumoniae B. catarrhalis H. influenzae	TMP-SMX Ampicillin
Vascular implants AV shunt Arterial graft Pacemaker	External barrier Local environment	Foreign body Blood	S. aureus S. epidermidis P. aeruginosa Enterobacteriaceae Candida species	Vancomycin plus aminoglycoside Vancomycin plus aztreonam
Prosthetic joint	Local environment	Foreign body	S. aureus S. epidermidis Enterobacteriaceae P. aeruginosa	Vancomycin plus aminoglycoside Vancomycin plus aztreonam

Condition	Host defense	Site	Organisms	Treatment
Ventriculoatrial and Ventriculoperitoneal shunts	Local environment	Meninges Foreign body	S. epidermidis S. aureus Enterobacteriaceae P. aeruginosa Diphtheroids	Vancomycin plus ceftazidime
Peritoneal dialysis catheters	External barrier	Peritoneum	S. aureus S. epidermidis Enterobacteriaceae P. aeruginosa Candida species	Cefazolin plus gentamicin Vancomycin plus gentamicin
Gastrectomy	Local environment	GI tract	Salmonellosis	Ampicillin TMP-SMX Ciprofloxacin
Malnutrition	Phagocytosis Cell-mediated immunity Humoral factors	Lungs	S. pneumoniae S. aureus K. pneumoniae H. influenzae Mouth anaerobes M. tuberculosis	Cefazolin ± aminoglycoside Timentin 3rd-gen. cephalosporin
Neoplastic Diseases and Their Treatment	Granulocytopenia Cell-mediated immunity Humoral factors	Blood	S. aureus S. epidermidis Enterobacteriaceae P. aeruginosa Candida species	Ticarcillin plus tobramycin Ceftazidime
		Lungs	S. aureus Enterobacteriaceae P. aeruginosa Aspergillus species P. carinii	Ticarcillin plus tobramycin Ceftazidime
		Urinary tract	Enterobacteriaceae P. aeruginosa Candida species	Ticarcillin plus tobramycin Ceftazidime

(cont'd.)

TABLE 167-1. (Cont'd.)

Primary Disease Process	Immune Defects	Common Sites of Infection	Common Offending Microbes	Initial Antibiotic Regimens
Neoplastic Diseases and Their Treatment *(cont'd.)*		Skin/soft tissue	S. aureus S. epidermidis Enterobacteriaceae P. aeruginosa Herpes simplex Varicella zoster	Vancomycin plus aztreonam or aminoglycoside Ticarcillin plus tobramycin
Organ Transplantation	Cell-mediated immunity Granulocyte function	Blood	S. aureus S. epidermidis Enterobacteriaceae P. aeruginosa L. monocytogenes Candida species	Ceftazidime plus ampicillin Ticarcillin plus tobramycin
		Lungs	S. aureus Enterobacteriaceae P. aeruginosa Nocardia species Mycobacteria Aspergillus species Pneumocystis carinii Cytomegalovirus Legionella	Ticarcillin plus tobramycin Ceftazidime TMP-SMX plus erythromycin
		Central nervous system	S. pneumoniae N. meningitidis Enterobacteriaceae P. aeruginosa L. monocytogenes C. neoformans	Ceftazidime plus ampicillin
		Urinary tract	Enterobacteriaceae P. aeruginosa Candida species	3rd-gen. cephalosporin Ciprofloxacin

Condition	Defect	Site	Organisms	Treatment
Rheumatic Diseases and Their Treatment (Especially Steroids)	Granulocyte function Cell-mediated immunity Inflammatory response External barrier	Skin/soft tissues	*S. pyogenes* *S. aureus*	Cefazolin
		Joints	*S. pyogenes* *S. aureus* *Enterobacteriaceae* *N. gonorrhoeae*	Cefuroxime 3rd-gen. cephalosporin
		Lungs	*S. pneumoniae* *S. aureus* *Enterobacteriaceae* *Mycobacteria* *Legionella*	Timentin plus erythromycin Cefazolin plus gentamicin plus erythromycin
		Urinary tract	*Enterobacteriaceae* *P. aeruginosa* *Candida species*	Ciprofloxacin TMP-SMX
Sickle Cell Disease	Spleen Humoral factors	Blood	*S. pneumoniae* *Enterobacteriaceae*	3rd-gen. cephalosporin
		Meninges	*S. pneumoniae* *H. influenzae* *N. meningitidis*	3rd-gen. cephalosporin
		Bone	*S. aureus* *Salmonella species* *Enterobacteriaceae*	Timentin Oxacillin plus ampicillin
		Lungs	*S. pneumoniae* *S. pyogenes* *M. pneumoniae* *H. influenzae* *Enterobacteriaceae*	Cefazolin ± erythromycin 3rd-gen. cephalosporin ± erythromycin Timentin ± erythromycin
Uremia	Granulocyte function Cell-mediated immunity Humoral factors	Urinary tract	*Enterobacteriaceae* *P. aeruginosa*	3rd-gen. cephalosporin TMP-SMX Ciprofloxacin Timentin
		Lungs	*S. pneumoniae* *S. aureus* *Enterobacteriaceae* *P. aeruginosa*	3rd-gen. cephalosporin
		Blood	*S. aureus* *S. epidermidis* *Enterobacteriaceae* *P. aeruginosa*	Vancomycin plus ceftazidime Timentin

567

suggested initial empiric antibiotic choices. Occult infections that may present with minimal localizing symptoms include otitis media, meningitis, sinusitis, osteomyelitis, skin and soft-tissue infections, cholecystitis, perinephric abscess, and peritonitis (particularly in the alcoholic with ascites or in the patient on corticosteroids), and diabetic ketoacidosis.

Patients who are suspected of being infected and who manifest signs of sepsis are particularly high-risk with about a 50% probability of having a positive blood culture and a mortality of 30%. Sepsis syndrome consists of: fever (>38.3°C) or hypothermia (<35.6°C), tachycardia (>90 beats/min), and tachypnea (>20 breaths/min or needing mechanical ventilation), plus inadequate organ perfusion manifested by one of the following—deterioration in mental status, hypoxemia (PaO$_2$ ratio <300), lactic acidosis, or oliguria (urine output <0.5 mL/kg/hr).

EMERGENCY DEPARTMENT EVALUATION AND MANAGEMENT

Studies include a CBC with differential (look for granulocytopenia); electrolytes, lactate level, ABG, and a coagulation profile (DIC); a urinalysis; and two sets of blood cultures as well as cultures of sputum, urine, abscess material, spinal fluid, joint fluid, or stool, as indicated. Radiographic studies should include a chest radiograph that shows the diaphragm, an abdominal flat plate, and any others as indicated. If there is significant concern about serious infection, an empiric regimen of broad-spectrum antibiotics should be started as soon as appropriate cultures have been obtained (Table 167-1). The immunocompromised patient with the sepsis syndrome or with septic shock (the sepsis syndrome plus a systolic blood pressure either <90 torr or >40 torr below the patient's usual systolic pressure) must be treated aggressively since sepsis can be lethal within hours in an immunocompromised individual. IV fluid resuscitation and other supportive measures should be started.

INFECTIONS IN GRANULOCYTOPENIC PATIENTS

An absolute granulocyte count <1000 cells/mm^3 places the patient at markedly increased risk for serious infection and for death. In general, the lower the number of neutrophils plus band forms, the worse the prognosis. A falling count is more ominous than a constant or rising one. The most common cause of granulocytopenia is cancer chemotherapy. Other etiologies include marrow replacement (usually by tumor), marrow fibrosis, radiation, toxic or allergic reactions to medications, cyclic neutropenia, sepsis, and congenital defects.

CLINICAL PRESENTATION

Infected granulocytopenic patients often present with only vague symptoms, a sense of lack of well-being, or fever. Fever even in the absence of localizing signs may represent serious or life-threatening infection and is considered an indication for evaluation and empiric antibiotics. Distinguishing between a fever from infection and a "tumor fever" is difficult. It is prudent to admit these patients.

EMERGENCY DEPARTMENT EVALUATION AND MANAGEMENT

A careful history and complete examination are mandatory. Attention should be directed toward: breaks in normal barriers (e.g., urinary catheters, indwelling vascular catheters, surgical sites, venipuncture sites, drains, and prosthetic devices). Other areas of concern include: pharynx, esophagus, lungs, perirectal/genital area, the urinary tract, and skin and soft-tissue sites. Most patients on cancer chemotherapy need a CBC with differential and platelet counts, for early recognition of granulocytopenia. Other tests include: electrolytes, creatinine, liver function tests, urinalysis, and chest radiograph. Blood, urine and sputum should be cultured as indicated. Any suspicious site should receive diagnostic attention.

Most granulocytopenic patients with possible infection require admission. Parenteral antibiotics should be started within 1 hour of recognition of the problem. Organisms commonly implicated are listed in Table 167-2. Antipseudomonal penicillin such as ticarcillin plus an amino-glycoside such as tobramycin are standard. If staphylococci are of concern (vascular catheter) vancomycin or a cephalosporin can be added. If an abdominal or pelvic infection is suspected, an anaerobe drug should be included (e.g., metronidazole or clindamycin).

INFECTIONS IN PATIENTS WITH IMPAIRED CELL-MEDIATED IMMUNITY

Although granulocytopenia is diagnosed with a CBC and differential, defects in cell mediated immu nity may be more difficult to recognize. A common cause is corticosteroid therapy and drugs used for autoimmune disease or transplanted organs. Other etiologies include malnutrition, uremia, sarcoidosis, lymphoma, and leprosy. Many cancer chemotherapy patients have a cell-mediated immune defect in addition to granulocytopenia. AIDS causes the most profound cellular defect.

CLINICAL PRESENTATION

The patient with altered cellular immunity may not demonstrate a normal inflammatory response to infection. Even apparently minor symptoms or signs should be evaluated thoroughly, with a low threshold for admission.

EMERGENCY DEPARTMENT EVALUATION AND MANAGEMENT

See principles outlined above for the granulocytopenic patient. Unfortunately, as seen in Table 167-3, the pathogens implicated with compromised cellular immunity are varied; most are intra-cellular organisms. Unlike the granulocytopenic in which empiric therapy is usually justified, sequential examination and close monitoring without empiric therapy are often appropriate if the source or its significance is unclear. Early aggressive attempts at pathogen identification (e.g., bronchoscopy, drainage procedures) are often justified because of the variety of pathogens and the need for specific therapy. If the need to treat is clear (threshold for initiating therapy should be low), the choice of antibiotics parallels that of the granulocytopenic patient. If diffuse pulmonary infiltrates are present, Bactrim should be considered for *Pneumocystis carinii*.

INFECTIONS IN ASPLENIC PATIENTS

The incidence of infection and death in individuals with either surgical or functional asplenia varies greatly depending on age and the condition resulting in asplenia. Infants and children are much more susceptible to overwhelming post-splenectomy syndrome (OPSI) than adults. Thalassemia major, malignancy with concurrent chemotherapy, radiotherapy, and immunosuppression have

---

TABLE 167-2. Organisms Commonly Associated With Infections in Granulocytopenic Patients

Gram-Positive Bacteria	**Yeasts**
Staphylococcus aureus	*Candida* species
Staphylococcus epidermidis	*Torulopsis glabrata*
	Cryptococcus neoformans
Gram-Negative Bacteria	**Filamentous Fungi**
Escherichia coli	*Aspergillus* species
Klebsiella pneumoniae	Agents of zygomycosis (mucormycosis)
Pseudomonas aeruginosa	
Anaerobic Bacteria	
Unusual	

TABLE 167-3. Organisms Commonly Associated With Infections in Patients With Impaired Cell-Mediated Immunity

Viruses	**Fungi**
Cytomegalovirus	*Cryptococcus neoformans*
Herpes simplex virus	*Candida* species
Varicella zoster virus	(mucocutaneous)
Epstein-Barr virus	*Aspergillus* species
Bacteria	**Parasites**
Listeria monocytogenes	*Pneumocystis carinii*
Salmonella species	*Toxoplasma gondii*
Nocardia species	*Strongyloides stercoralis*
Legionella species	*Cryptosporidium* species
Mycobacterium tuberculosis	
Atypical mycobacteria, especially	
M. avium-intracellulare	

the highest risk of OPSI. Adults who undergo splenectomy for trauma have no greater incidence of infection than the normal population, although they may have a higher mortality when they do become infected.

CLINICAL PRESENTATION

Septicemia, meningitis, and pneumonia account for most serious infections. The organisms in decreasing order of frequency are *Streptococcus pneumoniae, Neisseria meningitidis, Haemophilus influenzae,* other streptococci, and *Escherichia coli.* Many patients die within 12–24 hours of OPSI. High fever, shock, coma, and DIC may develop rapidly. Fever in an asplenic patient should be a cause for great concern, even without associated symptoms.

EMERGENCY DEPARTMENT EVALUATION AND MANAGEMENT

A rapid history and examination should be performed with emphasis on the respiratory and central nervous systems, since pneumonia and meningitis are the most likely sites of infection. IV access should be established and blood obtained for culture, CBC with differential, electrolytes, serum lactate, coagulation profile, urine culture and analysis, and other studies as indicated. A chest radiograph should be performed. A lumbar puncture should be done if there is suspicion of meningitis. Sick asplenic patients should be started on empiric parenteral antibiotics. The antibiotic choice should address the common pathogens and common sites of infection: ceftriaxone 2 g IV every 12 to 24 hours is an appropriate initial regimen.

DISPOSITION

All febrile granulocytopenic and asplenic patients should be admitted for observation and antibiotics. It is prudent to admit most patients with other types of immunologic compromise. However, if there is good evidence that the infection is of limited scope, immunosuppression is not severe, and the patient is reliable, outpatient management with oral antibiotics may be appropriate. Because the severity of illness in immunocompromised patients may be difficult to judge, admission for observation is often the safest decision. An ICU is appropriate for sepsis since these patients often need invasive hemodynamic monitoring, ventilatory support, and/or dialysis. Infectious disease consultation or critical care consultation may be appropriate depending upon the patient's complexity and severity of illness. If intensive care services are unavailable, prompt transfer to another facility must be arranged. Transfer requires a unit with ALS personnel. Patients who are discharged should be seen within 48 hours and should be instructed to return to the ED if they feel worse or develop high fever, dyspnea, vomiting, weakness, or confusion. It is wise to ask a family member or close friend to check in on the patient regularly. Single-dose antibiotic regimens are not appropriate for immunocompromised patients with urinary tract infections.

COMMON PITFALLS

- Failure to consider the diagnosis of infection in the absence of fever.
- Failure to obtain a white blood cell count and differential on all patients on cancer chemotherapy.
- Failure to consider admission for all questionable cases of infection in compromised hosts, even if it means only 24–48 hours of observation.
- Failure to institute empiric antibiotic therapy within several hours of presentation in the patient with a severely compromised immune system (e.g., granulocytopenia and asplenic patients) and suspected or documented infections.
- Delaying antibiotic therapy for complicated diagnostic tests or transfer in infected granulocytopenic or asplenic patients.

168   Hepatitis B and AIDS: Health Care Worker Exposure

See Figure 168-1 (p. 572).

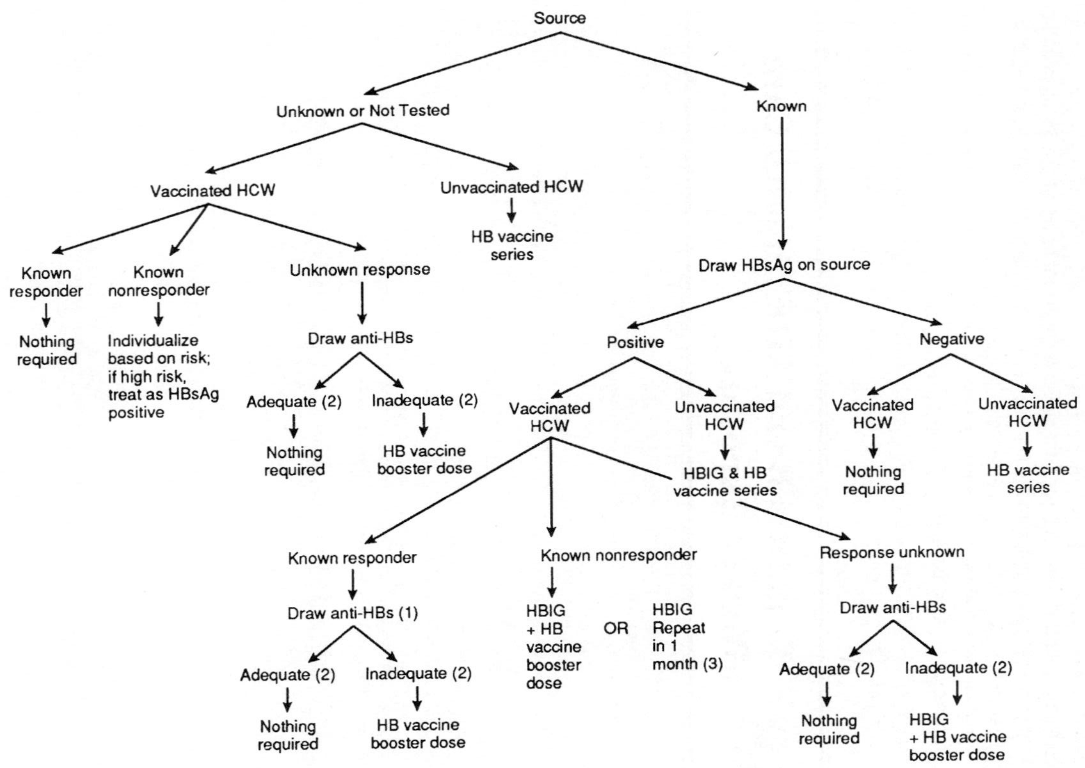

Figure 168-1. Hepatitis B postexposure algorithm. HCW, health care worker. **(1)** If not tested in previous 24 months. **(2)** Adequate antibody ≥10 SRU or positive by EIA. **(3)** Preferred for those who have failed to respond to at least 4 doses of vaccine. (Adapted from Centers for Disease Control: Protection against viral hepatitis: Recommendations of the Immunizations Practices Advisory Committee. MMWR 39 (RR-2); 19; 1990.)

PART VII

Neurologic Emergencies

169   Altered Mental Status and Coma

Coma is the most dramatic of the disorders of consciousness, but is the end point in a continuum of disease. Mental status is the most delicate and sensitive early indicator of advancing involvement of the nervous system. Evaluation of altered mental status always comes after the standard ABCs. Following initial stabilization, divide patients with severely altered mental status into two groups: diffuse metabolic/toxic causes of altered mental status, and focal disease that may require immediate surgical therapy. The differential diagnosis is exhaustive, but it is important to differentiate the two.

CLINICAL PRESENTATION

Patients with altered mental status may present in multiple ways. Patients may have altered mental status without actual depression of mentation. Acute confusional states exist in which the patient is alert and active but misinterprets external stimuli. Such findings are characteristic of toxic ingestions and metabolic encephalopathy, and occasionally accompany central nervous system infections.

DIFFERENTIAL DIAGNOSIS

There are a vast array of chemical agents and disease entities that can alter mental status. The neurologic examination and laboratory studies divide the causes of altered mental status into toxic/metabolic diseases and infratentorial lesions that affect the reticular activating formation (Tables 169-1 and 169-2).

EMERGENCY DEPARTMENT EVALUATION AND MANAGEMENT

ED evaluation requires a systematic approach. Support the patient with the basic ABCs, treat most obvious causes first, perform a detailed examination, produce the specific diagnosis, and begin specific therapy. Table 169-3 lists initial management steps that should be performed. Decisions on further examination must be made (Fig. 169-1). Normothermic patients who have not received neurologically active drugs and have no brain stem reflexes are considered to have unsalvageable brain tissue. Patients with evidence of focal herniation require immediate neurosurgical consultation; mannitol may be indicated. If CT scan results are normal, a lumbar puncture may be done. Bloody cerebrospinal fluid and a CT scan without a focal finding indicate subarachnoid hemorrhage.

TABLE 169-1. Toxic/Metabolic Disorders

Metabolic Disorders	Significant Differential Elements
Hyperglycemia/Hypoglycemia	Diabetics at high risk, both insulin-dependent and users of oral hypoglycemics; also more prone to infectious disease and renal failure. Hypoglycemia may be seen in patients with certain tumors, chronic alcoholics.
Hepatic failure	Most common in longstanding alcohol abusers and/or hepatitis. May lead to rapid rises in serum ammonia. May be associated with hypoglycemia due to decreased glycogen storage.
Uremia	Affects intracellular cerebral water content.
Oxygen deprivation	All aspects of cardiopulmonary system may be involved. Severe anemia, decreased cardiac output due to poor myocardial contractility, and arrhythmias. Cerebral hypoperfusion secondary to medications. Rapid increases in CO_2 despite adequate O_2 will alter mental status.
Endocrine disorders	Rapid changes in serum sodium affect osmolality and cerebral water content. Hypothyroidism: gradual alteration of mental status. Hyperthyroidism generally agitated and tremulous state; coma not seen until the patient is in extremely advanced disease.
Carcinoma	Remote effect of carcinoma and alteration of osmolality (i.e., syndrome of inappropriate ADH). Metabolic alkalosis with Cushing's syndrome. Hyper- and hypocalcemic states may alter consciousness, but progressive multifocal leukoencephalo-pathies seen with lymphomas may present with depression of consciousness.
Poisons and toxins	Alcohol still most widely used and commonly seen metabolic poison, relatively short duration. Barbiturate comas may be of several weeks' duration.
CNS infections	Meningitis (bacterial, viral, tuberculous, fungal, AIDS, encephalopathy); mechanism poorly understood.

DISPOSITION

Consultation with neurosurgery for an operable focal lesion is essential if the brain is to be saved. In patients in whom there is no surgically treatable disease, consultation with either neurology or internal medicine for ICU admission is indicated. All patients with significantly altered mental status require admission for continued evaluation and treatment.

COMMON PITFALLS

- A major mistake is to wait for laboratory results when physical examination findings clearly point to a focal process requiring immediate surgical intervention.
- Another common pitfall is failure to treat common causes first. Airway, cardiovascular support, and provision of adequate oxygen and glucose are critical.

TABLE 169-2. Structural Disease

Structural Problem	Significant Differential Elements
Subdural empyema	Recent otolaryngologic surgery, particularly involving sinuses. Meningitis not associated with focal neurologic findings, but findings become localized when empyema forms. *Streptococcus* most common offending organism.
Subdural hematoma	Suspect in trauma, elderly patients, alcoholics, and patients on anticoagulants. Even if not focal neurologic findings, consider subdural hematoma in these groups. Bilateral subdurals may compress structures diffusely, thus presenting much like a dementia or progressive encephalopathy. History of trauma, although helpful, is not necessary. In chronic subdural hematomas, symptoms can fluctuate mildly from day to day.
Epidural hematoma	Almost always related to major trauma; bleeding usually rapid in onset and related to involvement of the middle meningeal artery due to fractures in the basilar skull. Rapid downhill course generally seen.
Cerebral vascular accidents	Most thrombotic or embolic CVAs do not involve significant alteration of consciousness. Hemorrhagic CVAs commonly associated with unconsciousness. Bleeding associated with hypertension often doesn't disclose a discrete lesion. Controlled reduction of blood pressure may be important in patients becoming progressively more obtunded.
Intraventricular hemorrhage	Associated with poor prognosis and increased intracranial pressure. Clinically difficult to differentiate intraventricular hemorrhage from pontine bleeding without CT scanning.
Cerebral neoplasms	Neoplasms (primary or more commonly metastatic) are rare causes of coma. More common for patient to present with a seizure and postictal depression that leads to the diagnosis of tumor during radiologic evaluation. Slow-growing supraventricular tumors may produce mental status changes over time. Tumors in lateral and third ventricles may obstruct flow and cause acute pressure changes with rapidly deteriorating symptoms. In rare cases the tumor infiltrates reticular activating formation, causing irreversible coma.
Infratentorial compressive syndromes	Infratentorial compressive causes of coma are lesions that do not usually originate within the brain stem itself and by their proximity may compress the brain.
Basilar artery occlusion	Basilar artery represents principal blood supply to the brain stem through the vertebral-basilar system. Supplies blood to the reticular activating formation, necessary for consciousness. Posterior circulation transient ischemic episodes may present as drop attacks.

(cont'd.)

575

TABLE 169-2. *(cont'd.)*

Structural Problem	Significant Differential Elements
Traumatic posterior fossa hemorrhage	Severe trauma may lead to hemorrhage without the destruction of the brain stem proper. Decreased mental status due to external compression of the brain stem represents a surgically correctable cause of coma. Requires timely diagnosis.
Acute cerebellar hemorrhage	Bleeding into the cerebellum usually is a result of an arteriovenous malformation. Head pain with sudden vertigo and conjugate deviation of the eyes to the opposite side of the cerebellar lesion strongly suggest acute bleeding. Most treatable of the intraparenchymal hemorrhages.
Pontine hemorrhage	Devastating brain stem parenchymal lesion, difficult to initially separate from acute cerebellar hemorrhage or other forms of posterior fossa hemorrhage. Sudden decrease in consciousness, ataxia, irregular breathing, nonreactive pinpoint pupils, absent oculovestibular responses.
Brain stem tumors	Acute parenchymal lesions of brain stem (*i.e.*, angiomas, gliomas, ependymomas) causing brain stem compression or destruction of actual pathways. Other posterior fossa tumors, including meningiomas and acoustic neuromas, generally present with cranial nerve findings before alteration of mental status.

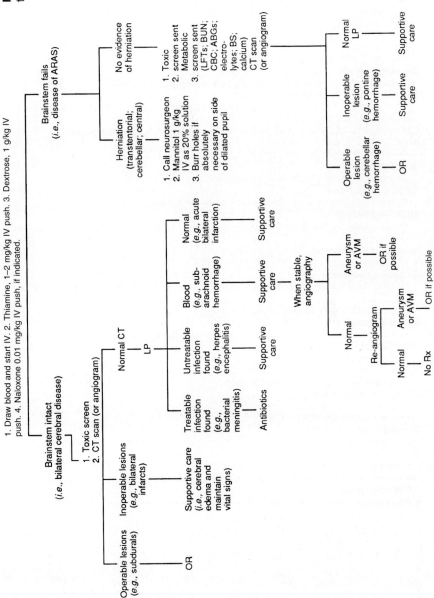

Figure 169-1. Diagnostic and treatment approach to coma.

1. Draw blood and start IV. 2. Thiamine, 1–2 mg/kg IV push. 3. Dextrose, 1 g/kg IV push. 4. Naloxone 0.01 mg/kg IV push, if indicated.

TABLE 169-3. Initial Evaluation and Management for Patients With Altered Mental Status

Initial management
  Airway established
  Breathing checked (including auscultation to rule out pneumothorax)
  Cardiac output assessed
  Cervical spine immobilized
  Obvious hemorrhage compressed
  IV line started
  Vital signs (full set)
  Thiamine 100 mg IV
  Glucose 50 ml 50% IV
  Naloxone 2 ampoules IV, repeated if no response
The stable patient
  Historical features obtained, including rate of onset, drugs, trauma, fever, prior episodes
General physical examination
  Signs of trauma; Battle's sign, hemotympanum, scalp hematomas and lacerations, subcutaneous
    emphysema of the chest, etc.
Obvious lesions of the abdomen, lesions of the pelvis, and long bone injuries
Skin
  Needle marks, cyanosis, pallor, rashes, dehydration
Breath odors
  Alcohol, acetone, fecal material, fetor hepaticus
Cardiac examination
  Rhythm, signs of decreased output, auscultation—endocarditis, valvular disease
Abdominal findings
  Organomegaly, ascites, bruits, flank ecchymoses (Grey Turner's sign), rectal and pelvic exam as
    time permits
Neurologic examination
  Observation
Respiratory pattern
  Normal, Cheyne-Stokes, hyperventilation, apneustic breathing, ataxic breathing, agonal breathing
Automatisms
  Yawning, coughing, hiccupping, vomiting
Mental status
  Responds to voice, responds to touch, responds to noxious stimuli
Cranial nerves
  Visual threat, inspection of fundi for papilledema and hemorrhages
Pupils
  Size, reactions (direct and consensual)
Extraocular movements
  Oculovestibular testing
  Oculocephalic testing (if appropriate)
Corneal reflex
Facial asymmetry
Motor system
  Posturing, ability of the limbs to move, stimuli
Decerebration, decortication, or true abduction by high-level centers
Pathologic reflexes

170   Headache

Headache is one of the most frequent ED complaints. It is not a disease but a symptom that may reflect the presence of disease. There are three primary headache types, classified by their pain-producing mechanism: (1) vascular headaches, including those resulting from cerebral artery dilatation; (2) muscle contraction headaches or "tension" headaches; and (3) traction and inflammatory headaches, which include those caused by infection of the bony and soft tissues of the head and mass lesions such as tumors, hematomas, and abscesses. About 10% of headaches seen in the ED are of the vascular type, often migraine or cluster headaches.

   Classic migraine may include a focal neurologic deficit or symptom that may occur before or, less commonly, during the headache. Common or simple migraine has no such neurologic deficit. Cluster headaches are characterized by several severe headaches per day over a period of weeks to months, after which there are no more headaches until the next "cluster" occurs, perhaps years later. Muscle contraction headaches are the most common, often associated with stress or emotional difficulties or, if chronic, with depression or anxiety. Traction and inflammatory headaches include those due to the most serious etiologies (e.g., subarachnoid hemorrhage due to a ruptured aneurysm or AVM, tumor or abscess, and inflammation from infection of the meninges). Stroke and hypertension may be included as may traumatic subdural or epidural hematoma.

   The comparative features of common types of headache are shown in Table 170-1.

EMERGENCY DEPARTMENT EVALUATION

The history is an especially important source of diagnostic information; inquire whether the headache is similar to others that the patient has had previously. The age when headaches first started should be ascertained. Vascular headaches rarely occur for the first time after the fourth decade of life. Headaches beginning later in life may have a psychogenic origin, but organic causes must be ruled out. On the other hand, in patients who have had the same type of headache for many years, an expanding lesion is rarely the cause. Precipitating factors, recent trauma, seizures, medication ingestion, or environmental exposures, may lead to more specific diagnostic testing. The location may also give clues: unilateral headaches are suggestive of migraine or inflammatory/traction headaches.

   Generalized pain is more often due to tension headache, although diseases that raise the intracranial pressure may also cause diffuse headache. Migraine headaches often switch sides, but they are typically unilateral. The timing of the pain's occurrence and its duration may also suggest the cause. Pain that awakens the patient from sleep and diminishes over time during the day may be due to hypertension. Muscle contraction headaches usually worsen as the day continues. Inflammatory headaches also usually get worse as the day progresses. Headache that is severe and of sudden onset suggests subarachnoid hemorrhage, even when there is no associated neurologic deficit or alteration of consciousness. The frequency should also be determined. Cluster headaches occur many times in a time period, with remissions for months or years, whereas muscle contraction headaches may occur daily during the week and be absent on the weekends, or vice versa.

   The quality and duration of the pain may be helpful clues. Headaches with an organic cause are usually acute in onset, persistent, and progressive. Migraine headaches may last

TABLE 170-1. Comparative Features of Common Types of Headache

Type	Frequency	Duration	Onset	Distribution	Pain Type
Migraine	Once weekly 1–2 per month	Variable, usually 12–18 hrs	Gradual, classic with prodrome	Unilateral, may become bilateral	Moderate to severe throbbing
Cluster	1–3 per day with long remissions	30–90 minutes	Sudden	Unilateral, often behind the eye	Continuous, severe
Muscular contraction	Variable, often continuous	Usually 8–12 hrs	Gradual, often related to stressful circumstances	"Bandlike," often radiates to neck	Dull, steady
Mass lesion	Variable on presentation	Variable on presentation	Variable on presentation	Often unilateral	Varied, often dull or throbbing
Temporal arteritis	Acute but may recur	Variable on presentation	Acute	Over affected artery	Sharp, burning

hours to days and are typically throbbing in character and severe. Cluster headaches are also usually throbbing and severely intense and rarely last more than 4 hours. A stabbing pain that lasts only seconds to minutes is often due to a neuralgia such as tic douloureux. Persistent, dull, aching pain is characteristic of tension headache but may also be due to an intracranial tumor. A neurologic prodrome (e.g., scotomata, flashing lights, strange odors, paresthesias, hypesthesias, vertigo, ataxia, diplopia, or hemiparesis) is typical of migraine.

Associated symptoms such as nausea and vomiting are also typical. Cluster headaches often present with unilateral lacrimation, facial flushing, and nasal discharge. A family history of migraine is common in migraine sufferers. Medications may predispose a patient to headache (e.g., nitroglycerin, oral contraceptives, niacin), and withdrawal of medications and substances may predispose to headache as well (e.g., ergot, caffeine, amphetamines, phenothiazines).

The physical examination begins with vital signs. A fever suggests an infectious process, and some inflammatory conditions (temporal arteritis may have low-grade fever). Severe hypertension may also cause headache. The head and neck should be examined for evidence of trauma and tenderness over the temporal arteries. The features of cluster headache, such as unilateral tearing or flushing, may be noted. Auscultation over the orbits, occiput, and temples may reveal the bruit of an arteriovenous malformation or aneurysm. Tonometry should be performed as indicated to assess intraocular pressure and rule out acute glaucoma. The fundi should be examined for the presence of venous pulsations and papilledema.

Hemorrhages or exudates suggest hypertension, diabetic retinopathy, or a bleeding disorder. Subhyaloid hemorrhage is pathognomonic of subarachnoid hemorrhage. The ENT exam may identify infection and other causes of referred pain. If focal deficits are found, CT scans or magnetic resonance imaging (MRI) studies should be obtained. A contrast CT scan may be indicated. Laboratory studies should be ordered, including an erythrocyte sedimentation rate (ESR) if temporal arteritis or another inflammatory etiology is suspected.

Emergency department management of headaches is outlined in Table 170-2.

DISPOSITION

If serious underlying disease is responsible, disposition includes prompt treatment. Patients with migraine should be referred to a neurologist, to a headache clinic, or to a family physician familiar with its management. The patient with intractable pain and vomiting associated with migraine requires admission and consultation with a neurologist. The use of narcotic analgesics should be restricted, if possible, to cases in which other treatments have failed.

COMMON PITFALLS

- Failing to obtain information about timing, location, and quality of the pain, precipitating events, and associated complaints.
- Failing to test gait and cerebellar function.
- Failing to document the history and physical examination. Documenting re-examination and symptomatic improvement is especially important.
- Making a diagnosis that is not supported by the clinical data. Patients with focal neurologic deficits should not be diagnosed as having psychogenic or muscle contraction headache.
- Not arranging adequate follow-up and failing to document instructions to the patient for follow-up or return to the ED.

TABLE 170-2. Signs, Symptoms, Predisposing Factors, and Treatment of Common Types of Headache

Type	Associated Symptoms	Signs	Predisposing Factors	Treatment
Migraine	Nausea with vomiting, aura in classic	Usually none but complicated, may have focal neurologic deficits	Tyramine, MSG, menstruation, other stress	Ergotamine tartrate 2 mg SL, P.O., or rectally, 0.25–0.50 mg IM or SC; chlorpromazine 25 mg IM or PO
Cluster	Usually none	Unilateral flushing, lacrimation	Alcohol	Ergotamine as above; lithium 300 mg tid for attacks longer than one year[7]
Muscular contraction	None	Muscle tension	Stress, Depression	Behavioral changes, sedatives, tricyclic antidepressants
Temporal arteritis	Visual loss	Blindness late, pain and redness over the artery	None known	Prednisone 80 mg PO Dexamethasone 8 mg IV

SC, subcutaneously; SL, sublingually; PO, orally; IV, intravenously; tid, 3 times a day.

171   Subarachnoid Hemorrhage

Hemorrhage into the subarachnoid space is a critical condition that may be missed initially, because the headache of a minor subarachnoid bleed may be dismissed as insignificant. Subarachnoid hemorrhage (SAH) is not rare; peak occurrence is seen in the fourth or fifth decade of life. An abrupt onset of headache, nausea and vomiting, light-headedness, lethargy, and nuchal rigidity is the classical picture, but the presentation may involve sudden severe headache, abrupt loss of consciousness, or sudden death.

The most common cause of subarachnoid hemorrhage is rupture of an intracranial aneurysm. Arteriovenous malformations are one seventh as common as intracranial aneurysms, and the majority present with subarachnoid hemorrhage or as symptoms of an intracranial mass before the fourth decade of life. Aneurysmal SAH has a high mortality. Death occurs as a result of cerebral edema, infarction, hydrocephalus, and rebleeding, as well as other secondary medical complications.

CLINICAL PRESENTATION

Clinical features depend on the severity of the hemorrhage. With catastrophic hemorrhage, there is persistent coma or sudden death. With major hemorrhage, severe headache, loss of consciousness, convulsion, vomiting, confusion, and ocular symptoms may be seen. It is with minor hemorrhage that difficulty in diagnosis occurs, because the presenting symptom may be headache alone. Always consider the possibility of SAH in patients presenting with headache.

DIFFERENTIAL DIAGNOSIS

The differential diagnosis is outlined in Table 171-1 and divided by the presenting complaint: headache, altered consciousness, persistent loss of consciousness, and acute focal neurologic deficit.

TABLE 171-1. Differential Diagnosis of Subarachnoid Hemorrhage

Headache	Persistent Loss of Consciousness
Migraine, cluster, or other vascular headache	Metabolic causes of coma
Acute hydrocephalus	Intracerebral hemorrhage
Muscle tension headache	Head injury
Meningitis/encephalitis	Encephalitis
Intracerebral hemorrhage	
Cerebral venous thrombosis/cavernous sinus thrombosis	**Acute Focal Neurologic Deficit**
Hemorrhagic infarction of the pituitary	Cerebral infarction
Cranial arteritis	Intracerebral hemorrhage
	Oculomotor palsy
Alteration or Loss of Consciousness	
Seizure	
Cerebral ischemia/stroke	
Myocardial infarction	

EMERGENCY DEPARTMENT EVALUATION

Goals are to (1) confirm the diagnosis, (2) identify the etiology, (3) localize the primary site of hemorrhage, and (4) detect complications. Noncontrast head CT is the most effective test and should not be deferred. High-density blood in the basal cisterns or elsewhere in the subarachnoid space is diagnostic of SAH. When a CT scan is interpreted as normal (or is unobtainable) and the clinical suspicion for SAH is high, lumbar puncture (LP) is indicated. If lateralizing signs and/or papilledema are present when a CT scan is not obtainable, LP should be deferred and immediate neurosurgical consultation obtained. In SAH, the lumbar puncture yields bloody cerebrospinal fluid (CSF), xanthochromia is frequently present and comparable numbers of red blood cells (RBCs) are present in the first and last tubes collected. Bloody CSF from a traumatic lumbar puncture has neither xanthochromia in the fresh specimen nor the same amount of blood (RBCs) in all tubes of CSF collected.

EMERGENCY DEPARTMENT MANAGEMENT

The patient should remain at strict bedrest, with the head of the bed elevated. Analgesia and sedation should be given; vital signs and neurologic assessment should be recorded frequently, and attention should be directed at lowering intracranial pressure and preventing seizures. If the blood pressure remains high despite general supportive measures, raised intracranial pressure may be present. Hypotensive therapy is generally not recommended in the preoperative management of patients with subarachnoid hemorrhage. If hypertension is severe, Nitroprusside may be indicated. In an unconscious patient, intubation and hyperventilation are indicated.

DISPOSITION

A neurosurgeon should be consulted immediately. Consultation is imperative if suspicion of SAH is high in a patient demonstrating signs of increased intracranial pressure and/or lateralizing signs, especially when a head CT scan is not obtainable. All patients with SAH should be admitted to the hospital. Any patient with a suspected SAH should not be discharged until diagnostic tests exclude SAH. If there is no angiographic capability or neurosurgeon available, expeditious transfer to a facility having the necessary resources is indicated.

COMMON PITFALLS

- Failure to diagnose SAH
- Deferring necessary tests (noncontrast CT scan of the head; lumbar puncture) when suspicion remains
- Lumbar puncture performed on patient with intracranial hematoma

172   Cerebrovascular Disease

Cerebrovascular diseases (CVD) are the most common neurologic disorders of adult life and the third most common cause of death in adulthood after heart disease and cancer. Occlusion or rupture of a cerebral vessel results in ischemic necrosis or hemorrhage, producing the signs and symptoms of stroke. The stroke syndrome is a focal neurological deficit of acute onset secondary to a localized alteration of cerebral blood flow. Its hallmark is its acute onset. The clinical presentation of stroke is extraordinarily variable, ranging from profound coma to subtle personality changes or minimal focal deficits. Three common stroke syndromes include thrombotic, embolic, and hemorrhagic. Subarachnoid hemorrhage is discussed elsewhere.

ANTERIOR CIRCULATION (INTERNAL CAROTID SYSTEM)

The internal carotid artery supplies the frontal, parietal, and anterior temporal lobes through the anterior and middle cerebral arteries. Lesions in the anterior circulation classically cause contralateral motor and sensory deficits, but there is great variation. Since the internal carotid artery supplies the retina and optic nerve, acute, painless, ipsilateral monocular blindness (amaurosis fugax) indicates a lesion of the anterior circulation. Anterior strokes do not cause cerebellar or cranial nerve deficits.

MIDDLE CEREBRAL ARTERY
Lesions of the middle cerebral artery typically cause contralateral hemiplegia and hemianesthesia (upper extremity typically more than lower) and homonymous hemianopia. Aphasia may result if the dominant hemisphere is affected. Signs of stroke in the nondominant hemisphere include apraxia, denial of deficits (anosognosia), and disorders of awareness of body and space (amorphosynthesis) such as right–left confusion. These deficits are occasionally mistakenly labeled dementia.

ANTERIOR CEREBRAL ARTERY
Lesions of the anterior cerebral artery classically present as contralateral sensorimotor deficits involving the lower extremity to a greater degree than the upper, with no involvement of the face. Frontal lobe stroke may present as personality or behavioral change, generalized psychomotor slowness, urinary incontinence, or gait apraxia.

POSTERIOR CIRCULATION (VERTEBRAL–BASILAR SYSTEM)

The vertebral-basilar system supplies the occipital lobes, cerebellum, thalamus, medial temporal lobes, auditory, and vestibular systems, and the brain stem, via the posterior cerebral arteries and the cerebellar arteries. Deficits tend to be bilateral and cranial nerve and cerebellar deficits are common. Patients with posterior circulation strokes may present with ophthalmoplegia, nystagmus, vertigo, nausea, vomiting, deafness, tinnitus, ataxia, and dysphagia. The "basilar artery syndrome" presents as quadriplegia and dense coma.

CAROTID BRUIT

A carotid bruit indicates significant vascular stenosis, usually from atherosclerosis; however, not all stenotic vessels generate a bruit. The significance, evaluation, and management of carotid bruits is controversial. Most patients have warning TIAs before they have a major stroke; as soon as a TIA occurs, admission and evaluation are indicated.

ATHEROTHROMBOTIC INFARCTION (ATI)

Hypertension, diabetes, and hyperlipidemia all predispose to and accelerate the development of atherosclerosis. Other risk factors are smoking and the combined use of oral contraceptives and cigarettes. Plaques occur at bifurcations and curves of the cerebral arteries. A stroke that evolves slowly (over several hours to days) in an intermittent fashion suggests a thrombotic process. It typically begins during sleep; the patient may awaken partially paralyzed. Occasionally it evolves over 1 to 2 weeks, and a subdural hematoma, tumor, or abscess must be considered. Patients may complain of a mild headache, but it is not severe and there are no meningeal signs. These patients are usually elderly and have a history of hypertension, diabetes mellitus, coronary artery disease, or peripheral vascular disease. ATI may also present with a seizure.

The course of ATI is unpredictable but usually progressive. If coma is present the prognosis is poor. Survival and recovery of neurologic function depends on protection of the airway, control of cerebral edema, prevention of respiratory and urinary tract infections, and maintenance of fluid and electrolyte balance. The only available medical treatment is anticoagulation. Its effectiveness in evolving stroke is controversial; it is not effective in completed stroke. Delays in improvement herald a worse prognosis.

TRANSIENT ISCHEMIC ATTACK (TIA)

A TIA is a focal, acute, reversible, ischemic, neurologic deficit lasting <24 hours. TIAs overlap with the embolic infarction; warning TIAs are present in 75% of patients with ATI. The majority of TIAs last <15 minutes. Medical therapy of TIAs includes anticoagulants (Coumadin) and antiplatelet agents such as aspirin and possibly dipyridamole (Persantin) and sulfinpyrazone (Anturane).

EMERGENCY DEPARTMENT EVALUATION AND MANAGEMENT

The diagnosis must be made and therapy instituted to restore circulation as soon as possible. Initially ATI is not detectable by CT scan. Within a few days the CT scan demonstrates areas of hypodense necrotic tissue and edema, and later cavitation. Nevertheless, the CT scan must be performed to determine if hemorrhage or mass effect is present, especially if surgery or anticoagulation is being contemplated. MRI and radionuclide scans show areas of ischemia within hours, but they are generally unavailable. Lumbar puncture is not helpful.

LACUNAR STROKES
Lacunar strokes are a subset of ATI in patients with atherosclerosis and hypertension. They are multiple, localized micro-infarcts of the deep gray matter, usually the pons or internal capsule, and do not affect higher functions or consciousness. Commonly, the infarcts are too small to cause symptoms and are discovered only at autopsy. Four syndromes should be identified: clumsy hand-dysarthria syndrome, unilateral leg paresis and ataxia, pure hemisensory loss, and pure hemiplegia. The mainstay of therapy is long-term control of hypertension.

EMBOLIC INFARCTION

Cerebral embolic infarction most frequently occurs from the atrial appendage during atrial fibrillation (AF) or from mural thrombi. Other causes of embolism are cardiac surgery or catheterization, prosthetic heart valves, valvular vegetations, and mitral valve prolapse. Although the majority of embolic infarctions are ischemic or "pale," approximately 30% become hemorrhagic. Embolic strokes are the most sudden in onset, often within seconds or minutes. They are rarely preceded by warning episodes. The course is highly variable. Long-term prognosis is determined by the severity and progression of the underlying heart disease. The head CT scan is usually normal. The mainstay of therapy is anticoagulation. In patients with minor deficits and a normal level of consciousness, immediate anticoagulation (after CT scan excludes hemorrhage) should be considered. Patients with larger infarcts should not receive anticoagulation immediately, since the risk of secondary hemorrhage is greater.

INTRACEREBRAL HEMORRHAGE (ICH)

The third most frequent stroke syndrome is primary hypertensive intracerebral hemorrhage. This occurs when a small artery ruptures into the brain, rendering an ischemic picture distally. In 50%, bleeding occurs in the putamen or internal capsule. Patients with hemorrhagic strokes tend to be younger than those with ischemic strokes and are likely to have a history of hypertension. The stroke begins abruptly without warning while the patient is active; onset during sleep is unusual.

The deficit progresses rapidly and steadily over minutes to hours and does not fluctuate. Patients who are conscious often complain of a headache and may have vomiting and nuchal rigidity. As the stroke progresses the level of consciousness may deteriorate.

Focal seizures occur in 10%; the mortality is 75% within 30 days, usually from temporal lobe herniation, intraventricular hemorrhage, or both. If the patient survives, some neurologic function may return slowly. The CT scan shows blood in the brain parenchyma and often in the ventricles. A LP is unnecessary. Initial treatment is supportive. Cerebral edema must be controlled. Blood pressure should be lowered gradually with sodium nitroprusside to 180–200 systolic and 120 mm Hg or less diastolic. Lowering the blood pressure too vigorously risks compromising cerebral perfusion and must be avoided.

CEREBELLAR STROKES

Cerebellar strokes are characterized by the rapid onset of occipital headache, vertigo, nausea, uncontrolled vomiting, nystagmus, hiccups, diplopia, facial numbness or weakness, dysphagia, dysarthria, and/or truncal ataxia. Patients are alert and have no hemispheric deficits. Cerebellar hemorrhage accounts for 10% of all ICH and is often associated with hypertension. Mortality for conscious patients is about 17%; comatose patients have a high mortality (80%). If cerebellar hemorrhage is suspected, a CT scan with special views to visualize the cerebellum should be obtained since patients may progress rapidly to coma and death. Lumbar puncture is contraindicated. Emergency neurosurgical consultation is indicated since evacuation of the hematoma prior to the development of coma can be lifesaving and is consistent with salvage of good neurologic function.

Subarachnoid hemorrhage is covered in the previous chapter.

EVALUATION AND MANAGEMENT OF THE STROKE PATIENT

The immediate goals are to confirm the diagnosis and eliminate other causes for a neurologic deficit. Fever and abnormal blood pressure should be noted. Look for head trauma and possible cervical spine injury. The eye grounds should be examined to detect hypertensive or diabetic retinopathy, the Roth spots of endocarditis, the preretinal hemorrhages of subarachnoid hemorrhage, or papilledema. The skin may reveal rashes, ecchymoses, or petechiae indicating infection or coagulopathy. The neck should be evaluated for abnormal position, tenderness, carotid pulsations, bruits, and nuchal rigidity. The heart should be auscultated for the presence of dysrhythmias or murmurs.

A complete neurologic examination should be performed. Intravenous access should be obtained, ECG monitoring begun, and supplemental oxygen given. If the patient has a depressed level of consciousness, naloxone (0.8–2.0 mg initially) and thiamine (100 mg IV or IM) should be administered. Serum glucose should always be assessed with a Dextrostick or Accucheck. Routine laboratory tests should be ordered. The CT scan is the diagnostic test of choice for suspected stroke. The CT scan provides immediate information about hemorrhage and mass effect. Anticoagulation or lumbar puncture should not be initiated until both hemorrhage and mass effect have been ruled out.

Another advantage of CT is that it may reveal a surgically treatable lesion (such as a subdural hematoma, tumor, or abscess) presenting as stroke. Ischemic strokes are not immediately visible on CT scan, but areas of hypodensity may be seen 2–3 days after the infarction has occurred. MRI scanning can provide detailed images of the CNS, but cannot accommodate a patient on respiratory support. Lumbar puncture is indicated if meningitis or subarachnoid hemorrhage are considered (after normal head CT). Clear CSF does not eliminate intracerebral hemorrhage, but simply indicates the absence of extension of hemorrhage into the ventricular system.

Intubation for airway protection should be considered in all patients with a depressed level of consciousness. Intubation is also indicated when hyperventilation is needed to control cerebral edema. Sedation before and after intubation is desirable to prevent further elevations in intracranial pressure due to the procedure. Clinical deterioration in a patient with acute stroke suggests cerebral edema. The degree of edema is directly related to the size of the infarction; in massive strokes cerebral edema may cause herniation and death. Signs of impending herniation include decreasing level of consciousness, ipsilateral nonreactive dilated pupil, hemodynamic and respiratory instability, and decorticate or decerebrate posturing. The most effective acute treatment for cerebral edema is hyperventilation to maintain the $PaCO_2$ in the 25–30 mmHg range. Mannitol may also be given. Direct intracranial pressure monitoring is the ideal method for guiding therapy.

Hypertension should be treated acutely only if the blood pressure is significantly elevated. Nitroprusside is the drug of choice. A reasonable target is a diastolic pressure of 110 mm Hg. Iatrogenic hypotension in the setting of a stroke can be disastrous. Anticoagulation with heparin may be initiated only after consultation with the neurologist or neurosurgeon. Prior to anticoagulation, a CT scan must be performed to rule out hemorrhage, and may need to be repeated in 24–48 hours. Coagulation studies, hematocrit, and type and crossmatch should be sent. Heparin is given as an IV bolus of 5000 units followed by a continuous IV infusion of 1000 units/h to maintain the PTT at 1.5 to 2 times normal. Heparin's effect can be reversed with protamine sulfate. If the patient deteriorates, heparin should be discontinued and a repeat CT scan ordered.

DISPOSITION

Any patient presenting with an acute or evolving stroke should be admitted to a monitored area until the clinical course is established. The critical or unstable patient requires ICU admission. Transfer to another hospital may be necessary to obtain CT scans, angiography, or neurosurgical consultation.

COMMON PITFALLS

- The "normal" CT scan: ischemic strokes are not visible acutely on CT scan. Even secondary hemorrhage may not be seen for several days. Thus, a normal CT should be considered a "baseline examination."
- Non-bloody CSF does not rule out intracerebral hemorrhage.
- About 20% of myocardial infarctions may be painless; the initial presentation of an AMI may be an embolic cerebral infarction from a mural thrombus, atrial dysrhythmia, or mitral valve prolapse. Therefore, an EKG is indicated.
- Post traumatic subacute or chronic subdural hematoma with mild headache, confusion, lethargy, and hemiparesis may be misdiagnosed as a stroke. A CT scan is indicated in every "stroke" patient to detect surgically treatable lesions.
- The cerebellar hemorrhage is a life-threatening and potentially treatable stroke. It may be misdiagnosed as alcohol or drug intoxication, labyrinthitis, or gastroenteritis. Finding no gross hemispheric deficits, the physician may neglect to test carefully the cranial nerves, cerebellar functions, and gait. The patient with a cerebellar infarct requires a CT scan to rule out expanding hemorrhagic lesions that may be operable.

173   Landry–Gullain–Barré Syndrome

See Tables 173-1 and 173-2.

TABLE 173-1. Differential Diagnosis of LGB—Other Acute Peripheral Neuropathies

Etiology	Characteristics and Examples
Infectious	
Mononucleosis	Typical signs and symptoms of mononucleosis.
Viral hepatitis	Onset follows jaundice by several days to weeks.
Diphtheria	Begins 5–8 weeks after the acute upper respiratory symptoms; bulbar weakness is common.
Toxic	
Thallium	Gastrointestinal symptoms, joint and back pain, hair loss that occurs 1–2 weeks after exposure, reflexes intact.
Arsenic	Gastrointestinal symptoms, confusion, seizures, coma.
Other	Triorthocresylphosphate, organophosphates, DDT, certain shellfish.
Metabolic	
Porphyria	Abdominal pain, psychosis, seizures.
Other	Polyarteritis nodosa, postdialysis fulminant uremic neuropathy, carcinomatous neuropathy, myelomatous neuropathy, nutritional neuropathy.

TABLE 173-2. Differential Diagnosis of LGB—Weakness Secondary to Other Diseases

Etiology	Characteristics and Examples
Infectious	
Poliomyelitis	Epidemic occurrence, fever, meningeal signs, asymmetric paralysis.
Botulism	Gastrointestinal symptoms, early cranial nerve findings, clustering of cases.
Tick paralysis	Rapidly resolves after tick is removed.
Myasthenia Gravis	Temporal variability of weakness, intact reflexes, improves with anticholinesterase drugs.
Acute Myelitis	Discrete sensory level, persistent bowel and bladder dysfunction.
Lumbar Disc	Sensorimotor symptoms in a specific nerve root(s) distribution.
Muscle Disease	
Polymyositis	Tender muscles, elevated creatine phosphokinase.
Other	Acute hypophosphatemia, periodic paralysis, hysteria, malingering.

174   Myasthenia Gravis

Myasthenia gravis, the most common disease of the neuromuscular junction, is an autoimmune disorder. The disease can occur at all ages but is most common in women in their mid-twenties. The peak incidence for men is in the sixth or seventh decade of life. Myasthenia gravis is of insidious onset, over weeks to months. The muscle weakness occurs transiently, at times precipitated by infection, stress, or pregnancy. The extraocular, facial, and bulbar muscles are most commonly affected, and some patients have involvement of the proximal limb, truncal, and respiratory muscles. The hallmark of myasthenia gravis is pathologic fatigue. Muscle weakness worsens with sustained activity and improves with rest; patients commonly report worsening of symptoms as the day progresses. A typical presentation is one of recurring episodes of diplopia and ptosis often noticed later in the day. There may also be weakness of eye closure, weakness of the muscles of facial expression, or difficulty chewing; transient dysarthria and dysphagia are common.

On physical examination, provocative maneuvers to demonstrate weakness after repetitive or sustained muscle activity assist in the diagnosis (e.g., ptosis or diplopia provoked by prolonged upward gaze, dysarthria or dysphonia with loud counting, inability to hold a tongue blade tightly in clenched teeth, or fatigue on holding the arms abducted or with repeated deep knee bends). The exam should also assess pupillary response, sensation, and deep tendon reflexes (normal in myasthenia gravis). Search for underlying or precipitating illness. The status and reserve of the respiratory system is important, especially the adequacy of resting tidal volume and the ability to manage secretions.

DIFFERENTIAL DIAGNOSIS

The differential diagnosis includes drug-induced myasthenia, Eaton–Lambert myasthenic syndrome, neurasthenia, botulism, inflammatory polyneuropathy (Guillain–Barré syndrome), periodic paralysis, and other causes of oculomotor palsy (diabetes, multiple sclerosis, aneurysm). However, myasthenia gravis (like periodic paralysis and multiple sclerosis) can easily be misdiagnosed as neurasthenia (psychoneurotic fatigue). Be extremely wary of making a diagnosis of a psychiatric or functional illness in a patient who complains of weakness, without carefully considering these possibilities.

EMERGENCY DEPARTMENT EVALUATION

A history of episodic weakness and fatigue involving extraocular, facial, and/or bulbar musculature suggests myasthenia gravis; it may be confirmed by noting improved strength in response to a short-acting anticholinesterase agent (edrophonium test) and by electrophysiologic testing. The edrophonium (or "Tensilon") test is performed by giving edrophonium chloride 2 mg IV push and observing for resolution of weakness in an affected muscle group. Usually, ptosis or extraocular motion is assessed and should improve within 30 seconds after giving the drug, with improvement lasting 5 minutes. If there is no response to the 2 mg dose, give 8 mg after 2 minutes, and again test muscle strength. Have atropine available to reverse possible bradycardic or hypotensive effects of the drug. A more definitive test is a repetitive nerve stimulation study. If myasthenia is suspected, further testing includes circulating anti-acetylcholine receptor antibodies. A chest x-ray or thoracic CT scan is may show a coexisting thymoma. Thyroid function tests and serologic testing for associated autoimmune diseases are often performed as well.

EMERGENCY DEPARTMENT MANAGEMENT

Anticholinesterase agents are the drugs of choice for symptomatic relief. Pyridostigmine at an initial dose of 60 mg t.i.d. is the agent most commonly chosen. A neurologist should initiate and monitor anticholinesterase therapy. A patient with known myasthenia gravis who presents with severe weakness may be suffering from either a rapid worsening of the disease ("myasthenic crisis") or a depolarizing neuromuscular block as a result of cholinergic overmedication ("cholinergic crisis"). The distinction between myasthenic crisis and cholinergic crisis may not be relevant clinically, since initial management does not involve the administration of cholinergic agents.

Management should focus on the patient's respiratory status and ability to handle secretions. ABG and bedside spirometry should be done and if there is any suggestion of respiratory compromise, endotracheal intubation should be done without delay. If intubation is not immediately required, the patient should be monitored in an ICU with frequent ABGs and spirometry. Respiratory infections are common precipitants of myasthenic crisis and must be diagnosed and treated aggressively. Electrolyte abnormalities may exacerbate the picture and should be identified. Prominent muscarinic side effects from cholinergic overmedication (bradycardia, abdominal cramping, bronchorrhea, etc.) may be treated with atropine 1 mg IV.

DISPOSITION

If weakness has worsened due to an underlying pneumonia or febrile illness, admit the patient for observation and treatment of the precipitating illness. If there is concern about the progression of severity of the disease, hospitalization is required. Acute medical and surgical problems in patients with myasthenia gravis should always be managed in consultation with a neurologist.

COMMON PITFALLS

- Failure to consider myasthenia in the patient with a history of episodic weakness; failure to consider other entities (e.g., periodic paralysis, myasthenia gravis, or multiple sclerosis).
- Failure to rule out electrolyte abnormalities in the patient with weakness.
- Failure to search for a precipitating illness in a patient with myopathy or myasthenia gravis with an exacerbation.
- Do not do an edrophonium test or other pharmacologic maneuvers in the myasthenic patient in crisis. ED treatment involves airway and ventilatory assessment and intervention, with a low threshold for endotracheal intubation. Drug decisions should be made in consultation with a neurologist.
- Prescribing medications that may exacerbate weakness in myasthenia gravis. Be aware of drugs that can impair neuromuscular function.

175   Grand Mal Seizures

Seizure activity is manifested in a variety of ways, from the generalized tonic–clonic and focal motor seizures to the subtle absence and psychomotor seizures. Most seizures are self-limited and are known as *simple seizures*. *Status epilepticus* is sustained or repeated seizures without an intervening return to normal consciousness. The etiology can be classified as intracranial, extracranial, or idiopathic.

CLINICAL PRESENTATION

Seizures can be dangerous. The precipitant of a seizure, such as intracranial hemorrhage, can be life-threatening; patients may sustain injury during seizure activity; finally, seizure activity itself may cause neuronal damage. The duration of seizures correlates with permanent neurologic sequelae. With status, the priorities are the airway and perfusion. Oxygen via bag–mask or endotracheal tube may be indicated. An IV line and a rapid bedside blood glucose should be done. If seizures do not cease, a benzodiazepine is the drug of choice, controlling seizures in 85–90% of patients. Most patients present after seizure activity has ceased. After stabilization, investigation is warranted to identify and treat etiologies.

Many have a documented seizure disorder. Determine if the present seizure fits the pattern of earlier seizures, and identify any new features or obvious precipitating cause. Common precipitants include low anticonvulsant drug levels, infection, and fatigue. An anticonvulsant drug level should be obtained in most cases. If new pathology is ruled out, adequate serum levels of anticonvulsant drugs are achieved, and appropriate follow-up care is arranged, most can be discharged. Patients with new onset seizures require an evaluation.

The history is the single most valuable diagnostic tool; the patient, the family, witnesses, prehospital personnel, and medical records are all potentially valuable sources of information. Elicit a description of the seizure activity and the circumstances of its onset, possible injury before or during the seizure, the past medical history, and information about medications (including possible ingestions and exposures). In the physical examination, seek evidence of injury as well as of concurrent illness. Although residual focal neurologic deficits may be due to Todd's paralysis, a structural intracranial lesion should also be considered.

Causes of seizure activity are shown in Table 175-1.

EMERGENCY DEPARTMENT EVALUATION

The evaluation includes identifying the etiology, but routine diagnostic testing is generally of low yield. Rectal temperature is advisable. Fever may reflect a CNS infection or sustained muscular

---

TABLE 175-1. Cause of Seizure Activity

INTRACRANIAL	EXTRACRANIAL
Structural	**Metabolic**
Neoplasm (primary and metastatic)	Electrolyte abnormality (hyponatremia, hypernatremia,
Hemorrhage	hypocalcemia, hypomagnesemia)
Intracerebral	Blood glucose derangements (hypoglycemia,
Subarachnoid	hyperglycemia, hyperosmolar states)
Arteriovenous malformation	Other organ system failure—respiratory (hypoxia,
	hypercapnia), uremia, liver failure, hypothyroidism
Degenerative	
Alzheimer's disease	**Toxic**
Multiple sclerosis	Drug ingestions
	Environmental exposures
Vascular Occlusion (New or Old)	Drug withdrawal
Cerebrovascular accident	
Transient ischemic attack	**MISCELLANEOUS**
Migraine headache	
Arteritis	**Eclampsia**
	IDIOPATHIC
Infection	
Meningitis	
Encephalitis	
Abscess	

contractions of the seizure. Blood studies are most useful in new-onset seizures and in those due to alcohol withdrawal. Glucose, electrolytes, BUN, CBC, creatinine, magnesium, and calcium levels are indicated. The CBC often shows signs of the demargination of mature white blood cells. ABG is indicated if hypoxia or hypercarbia are suspected. Blood gases drawn during or immediately after a seizure may reflect a mixed acid–base disorder, with both a respiratory acidosis and metabolic acidosis. Hypoxia is common and may not reflect steady-state or preseizure values. The serum creatine kinase may be elevated 24 to 48 hours after seizures.

Toxicology screens and drug levels should be considered if indicated. Blood alcohol levels may be helpful. Anticonvulsant drug levels are useful to guide drug therapy. Cultures should be done if there is evidence of infection. Lumbar puncture must be performed if meningitis is suspected. If a structural lesion is suspected, a head CT scan should precede the LP. If there is delay in the CT scan, give antibiotics empirically. A chest x-ray is indicated if underlying hypoxia, hypercarbia, pulmonary infection or sepsis are suspected, or if aspiration of vomitus or foreign bodies occurred during seizure activity. A chest x-ray with new-onset seizures may show pulmonary malignancy with cerebral metastases.

Emergency head CT in new-onset seizures is indicated if the following risk factors are present: head trauma, focal seizures, focal neurologic findings, multiple seizures, or malignancy. Be aware that 8–21% of patients with new-onset seizures and *no* risk factors have significant lesions demonstrable on CT. Obtain a CT scan on all patients with new-onset seizures.

EMERGENCY DEPARTMENT MANAGEMENT

Protect the airway and ensure adequate ventilation and circulation. Stabilize the neck if there is any possibility of cervical spine injury. Sequential examinations are necessary to document recovery from the postictal state. After giving IV glucose, anticonvulsants should be given when there is continuing seizure activity, when more than one seizure has occurred, or when a structural lesion is known to be present or is strongly suspected. Start antibiotics in suspected meningitis or sepsis. Antipyretics may be used to control fever. Lorazepam offers more prolonged anticonvulsant activity, and it may cause less respiratory depression and hypotension than diazepam when used in combination with other anticonvulsants. Lorazepam is given at a dose of 2 to 4 mg IV which may be repeated in 5 minutes if seizure activity continues.

Phenytoin is still the most commonly used medication for the treatment of generalized tonic–clonic seizures in adults. It is highly effective, and therapeutic levels can be achieved by the IV route. It does not produce respiratory depression or alteration of mental status. Phenytoin should be given no faster than 50 mg/min, with continuous monitoring. The loading dose is 18–20 mg/kg; oral maintenance therapy should begin 24 hours later. Oral phenytoin loading has been shown to be safe and effective, and may be an acceptable alternative to IV loading in stable patients with completed seizures. Phenobarbital is indicated if the patient is allergic to phenytoin, has a pre-existing cardiac conduction abnormality, or has continued seizures after therapeutic doses of phenytoin. The dose of phenobarbital is 7–10 mg/kg IV, no faster than 100 mg/min; this may be repeated in 30 minutes if necessary.

Status epilepticus, generalized seizure activity without an intervening period of consciousness, deserves special mention because if seizure activity persists for more than 1 hour, the potential for permanent neurologic sequelae or death rises. Patients who do not respond to benzodiazepines should be intubated to ensure airway control; give phenytoin and, if necessary, phenobarbital. Do a rapid evaluation seeking the cause of the seizures, and treat any identified precipitants. If seizure activity is not controlled within 40 minutes after the administration of diazepam, phenytoin, and phenobarbital, seek consultation from a neurologist and consider using general anesthesia, neuromuscular blockade, benzodiazepine infusion, or barbiturate coma. If possible, EEG monitoring is desirable if neuromuscular blockade and intubation are performed.

DISPOSITION

Admission depends more on the cause of the seizure and concomitant illness or injury than on the seizure itself. With new-onset seizures, if the evaluation is completed in the ED (LP, CT, etc), some authorities feel the patient may be discharged. All patients with status epilepticus require an ICU. Patients with known seizure disorder, a seizure similar to previous seizures, and a clear treatable precipitant (such as a low anticonvulsant level) may be discharged with reliable family or friends, with early follow-up arranged.

COMMON PITFALLS

- Failing to control the airway, leading to hypoxia
- Failing to recognize and treat status epilepticus
- Confusing an underlying disorder for the postictal state
- Failing to recognize an acute precipitant in a patient with a known seizure disorder
- Failing to recognize injuries
- Failing to consider seizure or postictal state as an etiology for acute confusion or a decreased level of consciousness
- Confusing true seizure and pseudoseizure

176 Neuroleptic Malignant Syndrome

Neuroleptic malignant syndrome (NMS) is a rare complication of neuroleptic drugs such as phenothiazines, butyrophenones, thiothixene, and rarely withdrawal of levodopa therapy. Symptoms include hyperthermia, hypertonicity, and altered mental status. Autonomic dysfunction may also occur and is manifested by sialorrhea, diaphoresis, hypertension, or hypotension. The incidence of NMS is about 1% of all patients receiving neuroleptic drugs.

CLINICAL PRESENTATION

NMS may develop at any time during therapy with neuroleptic drugs. Temperature ranges from 38.5°C to 42°C. All patients have abnormal mental status, ranging from mild confusion to profound coma. Blood pressure is usually elevated but may be labile. Late in the course hypotension develops. Diaphoresis is usually profuse and may be out of proportion to the fever. Sialorrhea may be present. Muscular rigidity, from mild cogwheel rigidity to opisthotonos, is invariably present. Neurologic features include dysarthria, mutism, dysphasia, abnormal deep tendon reflexes, and seizures. The white blood cell count is elevated. All patients have an elevated creatine phosphokinase (CPK) level, usually between 2,000 and 15,000 IU/L, and urine myoglobin may also be present. Transient elevations of BUN and sodium levels may occur secondary to the dehydration caused by diaphoresis. Lumbar puncture usually yields normal results. Computed tomography (CT) of the brain is normal but the EEG may show nonspecific abnormalities.

DIFFERENTIAL DIAGNOSIS

The differential diagnosis includes heat stroke, malignant hyperthermia, and sepsis. Patients on neuroleptic medications are at increased risk for heat stroke. Patients with heat stroke present with elevated temperature but with skin that is warm and dry. Malignant hyperthermia is a rare entity occurring during the induction of general anesthesia or after severe emotional stress or after trauma, particularly burns. Dantrolene sodium is used to treat both entities. In malignant hyperthermia the temperature falls rapidly during therapy as muscular rigidity is abolished. In NMS, however, dantrolene sodium abolishes muscular rigidity but does not lead to a decrease in temperature. Sepsis may present with altered mental status and hyperpyrexia, but rarely muscular rigidity or diaphoresis.

EMERGENCY DEPARTMENT MANAGEMENT

Treatment of NMS is directed at reversing manifestations while withdrawing the precipitating neuroleptic agent. Patients with Parkinson's disease who develop NMS from levodopa withdrawal must have the drug reinstituted. Treat hyperthermia with passive cooling using ice packs and hypothermia blankets, or active cooling using nasogastric and Foley catheter ice water lavage. In extreme cases (temperature $41°C$ with coma), consider iced peritoneal lavage. Treat muscular rigidity with IV dantrolene sodium. If the patient does not respond within 20-30 minutes, give a second dose IV. Abolishing rigidity prevents the release of myoglobin and potassium by preventing muscle damage. Pancuronium has been used to control muscular rigidity when dantrolene is contraindicated.

Treat hypotension and dehydration with appropriate fluids. If myoglobin is present in the urine, induce an alkaline diuresis with bicarbonate-containing fluids to prevent the precipitation of myoglobin in the renal tubules. Furosemide and mannitol may also be useful. Do an ABG early because some patients cannot ventilate adequately due to rigidity of the thoracic cage muscles. Such patients should be paralyzed, intubated and ventilated. Hyperkalemia is common acutely and should be treated aggressively. Neuroleptic malignant syndrome may be treated with bromocriptine or levodopa. Patients with NMS due to levodopa withdrawal respond well to bromocriptine or amantadine.

DISPOSITION

All patients with NMS should be admitted to a monitored care setting, usually an ICU.

COMMON PITFALLS

- Failure to recognize rhabdomyolysis. Order a CPK level and urinary myoglobin evaluations for all suspected NMS. Urine output should be carefully monitored.
- Failure to aggressively lower temperatures $>42°C$. Neurologic damage is proportionate to the duration of peak temperature.
- Failure to recognize hypoglycemia. Check the serum glucose early in the evaluation.

PART VIII

Hematologic and Oncologic Emergencies

177   Sickle Cell Anemia

Sickle cell disease is a hereditary disorder; homozygous Sickle cell genes (SS, Sickle cell disease) contain at least 90% hemoglobin S. The clinical severity is variable with some having a mild course with infrequent pain crises and a near-normal life span, while others are more severely affected. Infection remains the leading cause of death. Aggressive treatment of infection and current care has resulted in increased life expectancy into middle adulthood. Most SS patients develop painful crises before the age of 1 year; by age 5 years virtually all patients have experienced a crisis.

CLINICAL PRESENTATION AND DIFFERENTIAL DIAGNOSIS

The acute manifestations include hematologic crises and end-organ damage. Painful vaso-occlusive crisis is the most common presentation. Although an inciting event is not often discovered, many precipitants have been identified: infection, acidosis, dehydration, hypoxia, cold exposure, pregnancy, and physical stress. Sickle crisis may last 48 hours to several days. Bony pain is common during crises with back and proximal extremity pain. Search for other possible causes, such as trauma or infection. Repeated episodes of bony ischemia can lead to aseptic necrosis, often in the femoral head and carpal navicular areas. Osteomyelitis is another cause of bone pain. An association between Sickle cell anemia and *Salmonella* osteomyelitis has been described, but *Staphylococcus* remains the most common source of osteomyelitis.

    Abdominal pain, often with nausea and vomiting, is another common presentation. Local ischemia is thought to be the cause but a careful evaluation should assess for other medical and surgical causes: calcium bilirubinate gallstones (common), pancreatitis, appendicitis, renal colic, peptic ulcer disease and hepatitis (sicklers may have had blood transfusions and have a relatively high incidence of drug abuse. Jaundice may not indicate liver disease since it is occurs from chronic hemolysis). The pregnant Sickle cell patient with abdominal pain poses additional challenges: placental ischemia or active labor should be considered, since vaso-occlusive crises increase placental abruption and spontaneous abortion.

    Seizures or a strokelike syndrome with focal or generalized neurologic findings may be due to large vessel involvement. Acute retinal ischemia with visual loss may also occur. Chest pain, often pleuritic, is another common feature of crisis. Pleuritic chest pain may be from pulmonary infarction, but distinguishing it from an infection may be difficult since chronic interstitial changes are often seen. *Pneumococcus* is the most frequent cause of pneumonia. Always consider myocardial ischemia, especially when the pain is not pleuritic. Priapism may present in all age groups. It often responds to medical therapy including exchange transfusions, but surgical intervention is occasionally necessary. Rhabdomyolysis is a complication of vaso-occlusive crisis. Renal failure is seen due to multiple infarcts, often resulting in renal papillary necrosis. Fever during crisis is not uncommon, but when the temperature is >38°C infection should be ruled out. Due to autoinfarction of the spleen (with functional asplenia by age 5), Sickle cell patients are at risk for sepsis due to pneumococcus.

Less common crises include sequestration, hemolytic, aplastic, or megaloblastic crises. In sequestration crisis, acute anemia, hypotension, and even shock occur because of sequestration of RBCs in the spleen. This often follows a viral illness and usually occurs in younger children or in older patients with Sickle cell variants. Hemolytic crisis can occur during a fulminant vaso-occlusive episode. Severe anemia with increased reticulocytosis and jaundice is found; hypotension is not common. Marrow failure, caused by megaloblastic crisis (often due to folate deficiency) or aplastic crisis, presents with a rapidly falling hematocrit and an absence of a significant reticulocytosis.

EMERGENCY DEPARTMENT EVALUATION

Painful crisis is not the only type of crisis Sickle cell patients develop, and may mask serious pathology. The diagnosis of painful vaso-occlusive crises should be one of exclusion; a common error is to attribute all pain in Sickle cell patients to a vaso-occlusive crisis. The initial investigation should seek evidence of an acute infection or other precipitating event. Chest pain may be a manifestation of pulmonary embolism, pulmonary infarction, or myocardial infarction; abdominal pain may reflect a surgical emergency. By the third decade of life, many patients with SS disease have undergone cholecystectomy and appendectomy, either because of demonstrable pathology or because abdominal pain during vaso-occlusive crisis suggested an acute abdominal emergency.

The evaluation must include a history and a complete physical examination, focused on the most frequent, and most dangerous, manifestations. The upper respiratory tract, chest, abdomen, and genitalia must be examined. Especially ominous are any new neurologic signs or symptoms; if noted, a complete neurologic evaluation (including a head CT scan and lumbar puncture in many cases) is necessary. A CBC, reticulocyte and platelet counts are essential. Many patients have a baseline anemia, which may be moderately severe, and many have a persistent mild leukocytosis. An abnormally low reticulocyte count may indicate an aplastic crisis, whereas an extremely high count may be due to a hemolytic crisis. Many have a reticulocyte count of 8% to 12%. The ESR is usually low in SS disease and is generally not helpful unless quite elevated.

The urine should be screened for signs of infection or infarction, especially in patients with pelvic or back pain. Electrolytes, BUN, and creatinine are helpful. A chest x-ray, ECG, and/or blood cultures may be indicated. In unexplained abdominal pain an amylase, liver enzymes, abdominal x-rays, gallbladder ultrasound, or abdominal CT scan may be indicated. Neurologic complaints should be vigorously pursued, often with CT scanning. In previously undiagnosed cases, a sickle prep and hemoglobin electrophoresis must be obtained to confirm the diagnosis.

EMERGENCY DEPARTMENT MANAGEMENT

Treatment is usually supportive (rehydration and analgesia), since definitive treatment of crisis is still lacking. Some patients may be dehydrated; this is one of the few settings in which hypotonic fluid in a dehydrated patient is preferred. High-flow oxygen has never been demonstrated to affect the incidence, duration, or severity of crises. For significant infections, broad-spectrum antibiotics should be initiated pending culture results. Sickle cell patients should take folic acid supplements daily on a chronic basis.

Pain control is often a difficult issue; most adults are thought to require narcotics. Parenteral meperidine is commonly used but is a poor choice because of its short duration of action, its toxic metabolites, and its addiction potential. There is no ideal narcotic, but an agonist–antagonist (e.g., butorphanol) or a long-acting narcotic causing less euphoria (e.g., methadone) may be a more appropriate choice. Oral regimens may decrease the amount of narcotic used and the number of admissions required.

There is little place for transfusions in the ED. Anemia alone is usually not an indication for transfusion, since a chronic hematocrit of <20 is often well tolerated. The incidence of crises may increase if the hematocrit is elevated excessively. When transfusion is indicated (aplastic, sequestration, and hemolytic crises) exchange transfusion is generally preferable, since it helps prevent iron overload and is more efficacious than a simple transfusion. After a CVA, some neurologic symptoms may be reversed and the recurrence decreased in transfused patients. Priapism may also be relieved by exchange transfusion.

DISPOSITION

Patients with uncomplicated pain crises who are adequately hydrated and obtain pain relief can be discharged with close follow-up. A short course of oral analgesics can be prescribed. Patients should be discouraged from "shopping around"; the importance of obtaining all inpatient and outpatient care from the same institution should be emphasized.

Pain control is perhaps the most common indication for admission. Infection usually mandates admission. Fever without localizing signs or an unexplained elevation of the WBC count above baseline should mandate admission. Patients with sequestration, aplastic, or hemolytic crisis require admission, as do those with a significant decrease of hematocrit below baseline. A new neurologic sign or symptom, priapism, or an acute abdomen will also require admission.

Since continuity of care is important, the primary physician should be contacted during the ED visit. Consultation with internal medicine or hematology is advisable for routine admissions, and consultation with subspecialists is often necessary for medical or surgical problems or complications.

COMMON PITFALLS

- Do not assume that abdominal pain is due to a vaso-occlusive crisis without considering and properly ruling out surgical pathology.
- It is easy to overdiagnose pneumonia. Since an acute infiltrate may represent an infarct rather than infection, seek other signs of pneumonia. It is prudent to err on the side of caution and begin antibiotics.
- Some complications may be difficult to diagnose because of their similarity to "crisis" pain (e.g., osteomyelitis, aseptic necrosis of bone).
- Avoid pulmonary edema through excessive rehydration. Give IV fluids carefully and for standard indications.
- Transfusions are usually unnecessary. In the case of CVA, however, exchange transfusions are often not started soon enough.
- Provide adequate analgesia, while taking precautions to avoid analgesic abuse. Entering the patient into a well-regulated program can help control this problem.

178   Anemia

See Table 178-1.

TABLE 178-1. Differential Diagnosis of Anemia

ANEMIA SECONDARY TO BLOOD LOSS (ACUTE OR CHRONIC)

Intraperitoneal	Epistaxis
Retroperitoneal	Hemoptysis
Pelvic	External bleeding
Pleural	Drug-induced (coumadin, heparin)
Urinary tract	Trauma-induced
GI tract	
Gynecologic (vaginal bleeding, placenta previa, or abruption)	

ANEMIA SECONDARY TO DECREASED RBC PRODUCTION (INSIDIOUS ONSET, LOW RETICULOCYTE COUNT)

Hypochromic/microcytic
  Iron deficiency
  Thalassemia
  Sideroblastic (including lead)
  Chronic disease

Macrocytic
  Vitamin B_{12} deficiency
  Folic acid deficiency
  Liver disease
  Hypothyroidism

Normocytic
  Primary bone marrow disease (aplastic anemia, myeloid metaplasia, myelofibrosis, myelophthistic anemia)
  Secondary bone marrow disease (hypoendocrine, uremia, chronic inflammation, liver disease)
  Dilutional (anemia of pregnancy)

ANEMIA SECONDARY TO INCREASED RBC DESTRUCTION (ELEVATED RETICULOCYTE COUNT, HEMOLYSIS ON PERIPHERAL SMEAR)

Intrinsic
  Enzyme defect (G-6-P-D, pyruvate kinase)
  Membrane abnormality (spherocytosis, elliptocytosis, spur cell, paroxysmal nocturnal hemoglobinemia)
    Hemoglobin abnormality (hemoglobinopathy, thalassemia, unstable hemoglobin)

Extrinsic
  Immunologic (alloantibody, autoantibody)
  Mechanical (microangiopathic hemolytic anemia, prosthetic valve)
  Environmental (drugs, toxins, infections, hyperthermia, drowning)
  Abnormal sequestration (hypersplenism)

Modified from Hamilton GC: Anemia and white blood cell disorders. In Rosen et al (eds): Emergency Medicine: Concepts and Clinical Practice, 2nd ed, pp 1623–1640. St. Louis, CV Mosby, 1988

179 Transfusion Reactions and Complications

Transfusion reactions are any untoward effects of infusion of blood products. Transfusion of blood has significant morbidity and mortality in an estimated 0.5% of all transfusions.

CLINICAL PRESENTATION
HEMOLYTIC REACTIONS

Hemolytic transfusion reactions (HTRs) are the most serious adverse reaction, the most frequent cause for cessation of transfusion, and are seen in 1:300–4520 transfusions. Mortality averages about 40%. The most serious HTRs are caused by donor-recipient incompatibility between the major blood group (ABO). Less severe reactions can be caused by incompatibilities in the Rh_o, and other blood groups. The most common cause of HTR is clerical error. Signs and symptoms of acute HTR may begin after only a small amount of blood product has been infused. Most common are violent chills, high fever, and heat or pain at the infusion site; others include tachypnea, tachycardia, restlessness and anxiety; hemoglobinuria; oliguria or anuria; lumbar, flank, or joint pain; a sensation of chest restriction; vomiting or diarrhea; flushing; hypotension and shock; bleeding diathesis; and jaundice.

FEVER

A febrile reaction is the single most common adverse reaction to the administration of blood components, occurring in 0.6–3.0% of all transfusions. Simple febrile reactions are caused by anti-HLA, granulocyte-specific, and perhaps platelet-specific antibodies. Normally mild and inconsequential, febrile reactions are nonetheless important to recognize because fever may be the earliest sign of HTR or septic transfusion.

URTICARIA/ANAPHYLACTOID/ANAPHYLAXIS

Allergic reactions are the second most common type of complication of blood product infusion, reported in 0.3–1.0% of all blood-product infusions. Most allergic reactions occur in patients with a history of other allergies and are manifested by urticaria. These reactions often occur during or shortly after transfusion. Rarely, anaphylactoid or full-blown anaphylactic reactions may occur, with laryngeal and pulmonary edema, vasodilatation, and shock. Anti-IgA antibodies appear to play a role in the most severe reactions, and patients with IgA deficiencies are at greatest risk.

DELAYED REACTIONS

HEMOLYTIC   Delayed HTR is often manifested by unexplained post-transfusion anemia, appearing 7–10 days after a transfusion.

INFECTION   The most common delayed complication of transfusion is infection, and the most common post-transfusion infection is hepatitis. Although blood banks screen blood for hepatitis B surface antigen, non-A, non-B hepatitis is still a major risk, accounting for about 90% of post-transfusion hepatitis.

EMERGENCY DEPARTMENT EVALUATION

When an acute transfusion reaction is suspected, *stop the transfusion immediately* and contact the blood bank. Immediately check both at the bedside and in the blood bank to ensure that the patient has received the correct unit of blood product. Collect the blood bags from all transfusions the patient has had for analysis by the blood bank. Document vital signs, symptoms, and physical findings, and seek evidence for clotting or bleeding dysfunction, renal dysfunction, etc. Draw new blood samples (clot tube) for repeat ABO and Rh typing, direct antiglobulin testing, and visual comparison of the color of the serum with that of the serum of the pretransfusion sample retained in the blood bank. Additional tests can be run at the discretion of the blood bank and consulting pathologist.

If a delayed HTR is suspected, run a direct antiglobulin test. Evaluate for other causes of anemia.

EMERGENCY DEPARTMENT MANAGEMENT

Once the *transfusion has been stopped*, begin supportive care. In the case of HTR, IV saline and furosemide may help prevent acute renal failure. For febrile reactions, antipyretics and steroids are often useful. Allergic reactions can usually be treated with antihistamines alone; rarely are epinephrine, vasopressors, or steroids required.

DISPOSITION

The blood bank and consulting pathologist should both be involved in the evaluation of untoward reactions to infusions of blood products. They can advise the clinician of any special precautions necessary for continued or additional blood administration. An uncomplicated allergic or febrile reaction rarely requires admission, but pulmonary complications, sepsis, and acute HTR warrant admission, often to the ICU. Delayed HTR usually requires admission.

COMMON PITFALLS

- Overreacting to minor transfusion reactions such as allergic reactions is a common error. The transfusion can often be completed after a rapid clerical, clinical, and laboratory evaluation confirms that the reaction is minor. Do not continue the transfusion with blood units implicated in a febrile reaction or HTR.
- Failure to recognize the significance of signs and symptoms associated with acute HTR, particularly in the comatose patient. The presence of hemoglobinuria and hemoglobinemia should suggest the diagnosis.
- Remember that the patient with multiple sequential transfusions may be reacting to units previously transfused.

180   The Cancer Patient in the Emergency Department

Cancer patients deserve special attention because catastrophic oncologic emergencies often present with subtle complaints and findings (e.g., mild radicular low back pain with a positive "straight leg raising sign" can herald impending spinal cord compression; vague complaints of dyspnea may be due to a pericardial effusion). Minor aches may indicate the appearance of new metastases. A heightened suspicion is necesssary when treating a patient with a history of cancer: inquire about patterns of metastasis and previous complications, details about therapy (drugs, radiation, surgery). Early consultation with the patient's oncologist is useful, particularly with the foloowing questons: Is there hope for cure or palliation? Is the patient terminally ill? Is the patient/family aware of the gravity? How aggressive do they want treatment to be?

SHORTNESS OF BREATH

Upper airway obstruction is seen with far-advanced hypopharyngeal and laryngeal cancers. The patient with a malignant upper airway obstruction typically has a history of chronic, gradually increased dyspnea, worsened by exertion. The patient may also complain of hoarseness. Laryngoscopy and soft-tissue radiographs of the neck may be necessary. Treatment may involve surgery, radiation, or chemotherapy; steroids and, if there is significant obstruction, oxygen–helium mixtures may improve gas flow. Intubation may be necessary. Rapid obstruction is seen in fast-growing neck tumors, such as anaplastic thyroid cancers or Burkitt's lymphoma.

Partial upper airway obstruction from a laryngeal tumor may be exacerbated by infection, hemorrhage, or inspissated secretions and may present as a critical obstruction. Be prepared to establish a surgical airway, although there is usually time to use suction, administer nebulized racemic epinephrine, and attempt endotracheal intubation so that definitive intervention can be performed on a nonemergent basis. Tumors (usually lung, esophageal, or thyroid carcinomas) can impinge directly upon the trachea. Tracheal obstruction is often due to complications of treatment (such as tracheomalacia following prolonged intubation or edema secondary to radiation therapy). Be prepared to perform a cricothyroidotomy because endotracheal intubation is likely to be unsuccessful.

Bronchial obstructions are usually due to primary lung carcinoma and usually asymptomatic until there is >75% obstruction. The usual presentation is cough, hemoptysis, wheezing, or palpable rhonchi. A patient with breast cancer with "new-onset asthma" and a nonspecific chest radiograph may have widespread endobronchial metastases. Do not treat with bronchodilators without investigating this possibility.

Another cause of dyspnea (especially with lymphoma, lung, breast, or ovarian cancer) is pleural effusion. About 30% of patients with cancer develop malignant pleural effusions. In metastatic breast cancer, 48% will develop pleural effusions at some point. Malignant pleural effusion usually presents with dyspnea worse with exertion or supine position, and commonly with a dry cough. Chest examination reveals dullness to percussion, a pleural friction rub, and decreased breath sounds. Radiographs of the chest confirm the diagnosis. In new pleural effusions, thoracentesis is both diagnostic and therapeutic. Pleural fluid samples should be sent for cytology, culture, cell count, and protein and LDH determinations. Consult the oncologist.

Pericardial effusion presents with dyspnea and danger of cardiac tamponade. Pericardial effusions are not uncommon in advanced cancer (especially lung or breast); they can occur with lymphoma, leukemia, melanoma, sarcoma, or gastrointestinal tumors. Pericardial effusions with tamponade usually evolve into critical states over the course of a few hours. Nonconstricting pericardial effusion usually does not cause specific symptoms, but as compression worsens, patients develop dyspnea, chest pain relieved by leaning forward, cyanosis, or even dysphagia. Some with impending tamponade complain of hoarseness, epigastric discomfort, or hiccoughs.

On examination, the patient is anxious and diaphoretic, tachycardic with decreased systolic and pulse pressures. The lungs are clear; the neck veins are often engorged and the heart sounds may be muffled. An increased pulsus paradoxicus and Kussmaul's sign may be noted. With chronic pericardial constriction, peripheral edema, hepatojugular reflux, hepatomegaly, and eventually ascites may be seen. On chest radiograph, most have increased heart size, irregular heart borders, or a globular cardiac silhouette. The ECG shows sinus tachycardia and may show low-voltage QRS complexes or global ST elevation. Electrical alternans is pathognomonic of significant cardiac effusion, but can disappear as compression worsens. The diagnosis can be made by ECHO or cardiac catheterization. Vigorous IV fluids maintain filling pressure until surgery can be done. The indications for pericardiocentesis include shock, cyanosis, and decreased level of consciousness.

Superior vena caval obstruction can cause dyspnea; this syndrome is not rare, and is seen in 5–15% of lung cancer cases. Venous distention and facial swelling are seen, but most do not require emergent treatment. Indications for emergent therapy include decreased cardiac function, upper airway edema, or cerebral dysfunction secondary to brain edema. Always consider pulmonary embolism as a cause of dyspnea. Brain metastases do not preclude the use of anticoagulants.

Another cause of shortness of breath is pulmonary fibrosis, especially if bleomycin, high-dose cyclophosphamide, or radiation therapy to the chest have been given. A variety of pneumonias, sepsis, or metabolic acidosis may be seen in the immunocompromised host with cancer (especially leukemia and lymphoma) or because of immunosuppressive therapy with cytotoxic drugs, steroids, or radiation.

HEADACHE OR LETHARGY

A chief consideration is brain metastasis. The most common tumors that spread to the brain are lung, breast, genitourinary cancers and melanoma. There is an increasing incidence of brain metastasis; 10–30% of patients with metastatic breast cancer develop brain metastasis. Since >90% of brain metastases are located in the cerebrum, progressive lethargy, memory loss, aphasia, paresis, or sensory disturbance are seen. Cerebellar metastases account for 8% of metastases, and usually cause dysmetria or gait disturbance. Patients commonly complain of headache, typically worse on awakening and improved during the morning. Less than 25% with clinically significant brain metastasis have papilledema; about 15% present with new seizures. Brain metastasis is diagnosed by a head CT scan or MRI. Dexamethasone (4 to 10 mg IV) penetrates the CNS well. Steroids reduce headache and improve function in 60–75%. If increased intracranial pressure is suspected, 50 g mannitol IV and emergent consultation with the radiation therapist are indicated .

Carcinomatous meningitis can also present with headache or lethargy. It most commonly accompanies breast, lung, or genitourinary tumors, leukemia, and lymphoma, and is especially insidious because it can develop in the face of a systemic remission. Symptoms are usually subtle and tend to develop gradually; headache, nausea, photophobia, memory loss, and nonspecific mental status changes. Only 40% of patients have cranial nerve dysfunction, usually evidenced by diplopia, hearing loss, or facial numbness. With vague CNS symptoms in a patient with a predisposing cancer, suspect carcinomatous meningitis and do a lumbar puncture after the head CT. The CSF may be negative for malignant cells, since only 45% have the diagnosis made on the first tap; 30% have the diagnosis made on the second tap, 10% on the third tap. An opening pressure >160 mm, CSF leukocytosis, increased CSF protein, and decreased CSF glucose are suggestive of meningitis, although not specific for a malignant cause.

Metabolic disturbances are often the cause of lethargy or a change in mental status. Hypercalcemia is seen in breast, lung, renal, head and neck, esophageal, or thyroid cancers or multiple myeloma. Such patients usually respond well to saline infusion (diuretics may be used after the second liter of saline). Hyponatremia may cause lethargy; it is usually secondary to ectopic secretion of antidiuretic hormone in oat cell, prostate, adrenal, pancreatic, or esophageal tumors, brain metastases, or recent treatment with vincristine or cyclophosphamide. Hypoglycemia, seen in insulinoma, islet-cell tumors, sarcoma, hepatoma, and gastrointestinal or adrenal tumors, is easily diagnosed and treated if suspected.

MUSCULOSKELETAL PAIN

Musculoskeletal pain takes on a special importance in the cancer patient. The sudden onset of pain, especially in the upper arm or leg or pelvis, may mean pathologic fracture, especially in prostate, breast, or lung cancer or myeloma. These fractures often occur at previous radiation sites. The diagnosis is made by plain radiographs. Pathologic fractures or lytic lesions involving >25% of the cortex of a weight-bearing bone require immediate therapy from the orthopedic surgeon and radiation therapist. Fractures often require internal fixation, since poor results are obtained with casting or bracing. New onset back pain should suggest possible vertebral metastases, epidural metastases, and potential spinal cord compression. Patients with spinal cord compression face irreversible neurologic damage unless diagnosis and treatment are done rapidly. Most lesions causing spinal cord compression arise from metastasis to the vertebral bodies; 70% of are in the thoracic spine. Metastases from gastrointestinal cancers have a predilection for the lumbosacral spine.

Patients with malignant spinal cord compression typically have a history of 1–6 months of back pain, with features typical of radiculopathy. The earliest sign of cord compression is motor dysfunction, usually manifested by lower extremity weakness; about 50% have some loss of temperature or light touch sensation. Loss of pain sensation and bowel or bladder dysfunction are usually late signs. Patients with cauda equina syndrome exhibit "saddle anesthesia" with sensory disturbances in the urethral, vaginal, and perianal areas. Over 70% have positive spine radiographs, although lymphoma or retroperitoneal sarcomas are generally negative. In most, epidural metastases are detectable before the onset of cord injury.

Suspicion of epidural metastasis should result in immediate consultation with the neurologist or neurosurgeon. Steroids should be started. CT scanning with metrizamide injection or MRI scanning may be done. If positive, treatment options include radiation or laminectomy, usually emergently since compression and edema can progress rapidly to cause irreversible paraplegia or bowel or bladder dysfunction. Most cancer patients referred for rehabilitative treatment after malignant spinal cord compression lived for more than one year, so it is eminently worthwhile pursuing an aggressive plan.

Pain is seen in nearly all patients, but it almost always amenable to treatment. Mild to moderate pain is relieved by nonsteroidal anti-inflammatory drugs or acetaminophen; more severe pain requires narcotics. Give enough pain medication with adequate frequency: a patient who is still in obvious pain 1 hour after a dose of parenteral narcotic is *not* at high risk of ventilatory depression from an additional dose. No narcotic is more effective than morphine. Morphine allergy is rare (<1%); nausea and pruritus are more common but can be managed with antiemetics and antihistamines.

COMPLICATIONS OF CANCER TREATMENT

Most patients with cancer receive some sort of therapy, which can lead to complications requiring emergent treatment. The side effects of radiation therapy depend on the site of treatment and the dose administered. A common complaint with mediastinal radiation is severe dysphagia. This may be mild enough to treat with oral viscous lidocaine or it may be severe enough to cause significant dehydration and to require parenteral narcotics. Consult the radiation therapist or oncologist about complaints that relate to recent radiation treatment.

A special case is the patient with lymphedema who complains of swelling, pain, or redness in the involved extremity. Because of the high risk for infection secondary to impaired lymphatic drainage, cellulitis should be the diagnosis until proven otherwise. Venipuncture, IV lines, and even blood pressure measurement should be avoided in the affected extremity, and antibiotics for staphylococci and streptococci should be started immediately.

Cytotoxic chemotherapy has many side effects, some of which are life-threatening (Table

180-1). The most common and most serious side effect is delayed neutropenia. Many drugs used in cancer can also mask the signs of infection; this probably accounts in part for the fact that most cancer patients die of bacterial infection. Assume that any patient with a recent history of chemotherapy and even a minimal fever (>100.5°F) is neutropenic (and septic) until proven otherwise. Do not delay treatment: in the neutropenic patient with bacterial sepsis, death usually occurs within 48 hours of the onset of fever. Hospitalize patients with fever and an absolute granulocyte count of <1000/µL. Start antibiotics immediately after blood cultures. Since most lethal infections are caused by gram-negative bacilli, if there is no obvious source of infection, antibiotic treatment should include coverage for *E. coli, Enterobacter,* and *Pseudomonas* species. Initial treatment is a combination with overlapping gram-negative coverage, anti-pseudomonal penicillin and an aminoglycoside, or a third-generation cephalosporin. Severe nausea and vomiting are also seen, and may not be amenable to treatment with usual regimens. High-dose IV metoclopramide or parenteral benzodiazepines may be needed for severe nausea from chemotherapy.

TABLE 180-1. Chemotherapeutic Agents, Their Uses and Side Effects

Drug	Use	Common Side Effects
5-Azacytidine	Lymphoma, leukemia	Hypersensitivity reactions ranging from urticaria to anaphylaxis; nausea; acute pancreatitis; lethargy; coagulopathy
Azathioprine (Imuran)	Leukemia, various solid tumors Myeloma	Leukopenia and thrombocytopenia can occur 2 weeks after dose Anemia, thrombocytopenia, leukopenia; oral ulcers; pancreatitis, restrictive lung disease
Bacillus Calmette-Guerin (BCG)	Melanoma, leukemia, bladder cancer	Fevers, arthralgia, joint inflammation; lymphadenopathy can last up to 3 weeks
Bleomycin	Head and neck, penile, rectal, germ cell, and lung cancer, lymphoma	Delayed hyperpyrexic response in up to 50% of patients; rash, stomatitis, pneumonitis
Busulfan (Myleran)	Leukemia	Granulocytopenia, pancytopenia; hypogonadism
Carmustine (BCNU)	CNS tumors, lymphoma, myeloma	Leukopenia and thrombocytopenia can occur up to 5 weeks after treatment
Chlorambucil (Leukeran)	Leukemia, lymphoma, ovarian, breast cancer, choriocarcinoma	Neutropenia, thrombocytopenia
Cisplatin (Platinol)	Lymphoma, various solid tumors	Renal failure, which can be potentiated by gentamicin and cephalothin; hearing loss; peripheral neuropathy; neutropenia
Cyclophosphamide (Cytoxan)	Lymphoma, various solid tumors	Neutropenia, thrombocytopenia; hemorrhagic cystitis; SIADH, pneumonitis
Cytarabine (ARA-C, Cytosar)	Leukemia, lymphoma	Leukopenia, thrombocytopenia; various CNS side effects including ataxia, seizures, meningismus; GI hemorrhage, pseudo-obstruction
Dacarbazine (DTIC)	Melanoma	Myelosuppression; nausea; myalgias
Dactinomycin (Actinomycin-D)	Choriocarcinoma, Ewing's Wilms' tumor, melanoma	Neutropenia, mucositis
Doxorubicin (Adriamycin)	Various solid tumors, lymphoma	Neutropenia up to 2 weeks after dose; acute pericarditis/myocarditis; cardiomyopathy; tissue reactions in sites of previous radiation; stomatitis
Estrogens (DES, Premarin, Stilphosterol)	Prostate and breast cancer	Thromboembolic disease; nausea; uterine bleeding
Etoposide (VP-16)	Various solid tumors, leukemia, lymphoma	Neutropenia; nausea

Drug	Indication	Toxicity
Fluorouracil (5-FU)	Breast, GI tumors	Stomatitis, proctitis, diarrhea, esophagitis (these can all herald severe toxicity requiring hospitalization); leukopenia; thrombocytopenia; acute cerebellar dysfunction
Hydroxyurea (Hydrea)	Leukemia, prostate cancer	Neutropenia, thrombocytopenia, rash
Ifosfamide (Holoxan)	Testicular, breast, ovarian, lymphoma	Hematuria; hemorrhagic cystitis; uremia; moderate leukopenia
Lomustine (CCNU)	Brain tumors, Hodgkin's disease	Leukopenia and thrombocytopenia can occur 1 month after treatment; stomatitis; abnormal liver function tests
Mechlorethamine (nitrogen mustard)	Hodgkin's disease	Leukopenia; thrombocytopenia; vomiting
Melphalan (Alkeran)	Testicular, breast, ovarian, myeloma	Neutropenia; thrombocytopenia; stomatitis; dermatitis
Mercaptopurine (6-MP)	Leukemia, lymphoma	Hyperbilirubinemia; liver damage; mild neutropenia
Methotrexate (MTX)	Various solid tumors, lymphoma, leukemia	Pancytopenia; nausea and vomiting; stomatitis may predict severe GI toxicity and hepatotoxicity; renal failure; toxicity is enhanced by sulfonamide, aspirin, phenytoin
Mithramycin (Mithracin)	Brain, thyroid, gastric	Thrombocytopenia and coagulopathy; nausea and vomiting
Mitomycin-C (Mutamycin)	GI, esophageal, breast, bladder	Delayed bone marrow toxicity can occur up to 8 weeks after dosage; TTP-like syndrome
Mitotane	Adrenal carcinoma	Adrenal insufficiency requiring higher-than-usual replacement doses especially in cases of shock, trauma, or infection
Procarbazine (Matulane)	Lymphoma, melanoma, lung cancer	Severe drug interactions, which include disulfiramlike reaction with alcohol or sympathomimetics; hypertensive crises with antidepressants; profound sedation with narcotics, antihistamines, methyldopa, clonidine, phenothiazines; protracted myelosuppression up to 6 weeks after treatment
Progestins (Megace, Provera)	Breast, renal, endometrial cancer	Fluid retention; hypercalcemia
Streptozocin	Islet-cell tumors	Diabetes mellitus; renal failure
Tamoxifen (Nolvadex)	Breast cancer	Menopausal symptoms; vaginal bleeding; bone pain and hypercalcemia during initial treatment
Thioguanine (6-TG)	Leukemia	Neutropenia
Vinblastine (Velban)	Breast, choriocarcinoma, Hodgkin's, testicular, Kaposi's	Neutropenia; nausea
Vincristine	Breast, sarcoma, Hodgkin's leukemia	Peripheral and autonomic neuropathy; cranial nerve palsies; constipation may herald paralytic ileus; SIADH

PART IX

Allergy-Related and Immunologic Emergencies

181 Anaphylaxis

Anaphylaxis is an acute life-threatening condition; immediate recognition and treatment are critical. Its manifestations may range from minor nuisance symptoms such as rash or lip swelling to sudden death secondary to life-threatening upper airway obstruction or shock. Even the patient who presents with urticaria can subsequently develop hypotension, bronchospasm, or laryngeal edema, and should be treated with the same urgency as the patient with the full-blown anaphylactic syndrome. Anaphylactic symptoms result from massive release of chemical mediators from mast cells and basophils throughout the body. For anaphylaxis to occur, there must be previous sensitization to a foreign substance against which IgE is made by antibody-producing B lymphocytes. The term "anaphylactoid reaction" denotes a clinical syndrome identical to anaphylaxis but distinguished by the fact that mast cell mediator release results from an IgE-independent mechanism.

Penicillin is the most common cause of life-threatening anaphylaxis. About 1% of patients are sensitive to penicillin. Reactions most often involve urticaria alone, but an estimated 25:100,000 treated with penicillin will have severe anaphylaxis and one will die. The reaction rate to bee stings is about 0.4%, with 50 to 80 anaphylactic deaths per year. Iodinated contrast media (particularly in IVP) results in anaphylactoid reactions in 1–2%. Foods, food additives, and nonsteroidal anti-inflammatory agents are common causes of anaphylaxis, but the true incidences are unknown. Exercise, especially in combination with food or drug ingestion, can cause or aggravate anaphylaxis. Table 181-1 summarizes etiologic agents in anaphylaxis.

The more direct the route to the systemic circulation, the greater the likelihood and severity of reaction. The possible routes of exposure, in descending order of severity of potential reactions, are IV, IM, SQ, intradermal, oral, other mucous membranes, and skin. The onset of anaphylaxis usually occurs <30 minutes after exposure, but is often immediate. Antigens given orally may have a 2-hour delay. The more immediate the reaction, the more life-threatening it is. Symptoms may last only a few minutes even without therapy but on the average persist 3 to 4 hours; rarely, they may last for >24 hours. Steroids appear to be useful in preventing late exacerbation or delayed reaction.

CLINICAL PRESENTATION

Anaphylaxis is often heralded by premonitory symptoms (see Table 181-2). Pruritus of the palms and soles, tingling about the mouth and tongue, generalized warmth, tightness in the chest, or a lump in the throat are commonly described. Dizziness or syncope secondary to hypotension may

TABLE 181-1. Etiologic Agents in Anaphylaxis

Proteins

Insect venoms
Foods
Allergy extracts
Foreign serum and whole blood
Insulin
Streptokinase
Vaccines
Seminal fluid

Haptens

Penicillin and cephalosporins
Other antibiotics
Local anesthetics

Prostaglandin Inhibition

Aspirin (not sodium salicylate or Disalcid)
Nonsteroidal anti-inflammatory drugs (Zomax > ASA, indomethacin >
  tolmetin > ibuprofen naproxen, etc.)

Physical Factors

Exercise-induced anaphylaxis
Food or NSAID anaphylaxis unmasked by exercise
Cold-induced urticaria and anaphylaxis

Complement Activation/Mast Cell Degranulators (Anaphylactoid RXN)

IVP dye and other radiocontrast materials
Polysaccharides
Thiamine, vitamin K, morphine

Idiopathic Anaphylaxis

TABLE 181-2. Symptoms and Signs of Anaphylaxis

Reaction	Symptom	Sign
Urticaria	Itching	Raised wheals diffusely wandering, evanescent
Angioedema	Nonpruritic tingling	Swelling of lips, eyes, hands; no heat or erythema
Laryngeal edema	Hoarseness, dysphagia, lump in throat, airway obstruction, sudden death	Inspiratory stridor; intercostal and avicular retractions; cyanosis
Bronchospasm	Cough, dyspnea, chest tightness	Wheezing, high resp rate, retractions
Hypotension	Dizziness, syncope, confusion	Hypotension (mild to severe), tachycardia, oliguria
Rhinitis	Nasal congestion, itching and fluid	Mucosal edema
Conjunctivitis	Tearing, itching	Lid edema and injection
Gastroenteritis	Cramping, diarrhea, vomiting	Normal exam

also be manifestations in the absence of any other signs or symptoms of allergic reaction. Over 90% of patients have urticaria and/or angioedema. Urticaria is edema of the upper dermis, appearing as raised erythematous wheals in pruritic patches, whereas angioedema represents edema of the deep dermis and appears as puffy, nonpitting areas of skin or mucous membrane. Angioedema is generally painless and nonpruritic; patients note only tingling and swelling in the affected areas. It tends to be most prominent about the face and lips, and less so on the hands and arms.

Laryngeal edema resulting in upper airway obstruction is the principal cause of death from anaphylaxis. The onset can be dramatic, presenting as sudden death or "café coronary." Angioedema of the lips, uvula, tongue, and oropharynx are less likely to obstruct the airway, but must be treated aggressively because of the likelihood of concomitant edema of the larynx. Uvular edema in particular is a helpful marker for potential laryngeal involvement. Frequently, however, the patient complains of hoarseness and "a lump in the throat," and the examination of the oropharynx is completely normal. Indirect laryngoscopy may reveal supraglottic or laryngeal edema, but this examination should not delay the prompt administration of epinephrine.

Refractory hypotension is second only to laryngeal edema as a cause of death from anaphylaxis. A drop in blood pressure of 20–30 mm Hg is typical, but there is great variability. When sudden in onset, syncope or sudden death may occur. Although often overshadowed by other symptoms, abdominal cramping is common. Cardiac manifestations are thought to be secondary to hypotension, hypoxia, and overzealous epinephrine therapy, and not part of the allergic phenomenon.

DIFFERENTIAL DIAGNOSIS

The diagnosis of anaphylaxis is often obvious when antigen exposure is rapidly followed by urticaria, angioedema, bronchospasm, upper airway edema, and hypotension. Confusion may occur when a delay in symptoms obscures a cause-and-effect relationship or when the syndrome is only partially expressed. Anaphylaxis often presents as only one component of the syndrome. Serious confusion may arise when anaphylaxis presents as isolated hypotension; consider it in the differential of syncope and vascular collapse. Isolated angioedema of the skin and upper airway is a common presentation of anaphylaxis, but consider also hereditary angioedema. The latter is characterized by repeated episodes of angioedema of the skin, upper airway, and gut; these often date from adolescence and are provoked by minor trauma. Gastrointestinal involvement is usually prominent, often mimicking an acute abdomen. Other differentiating characteristics are that hereditary angioedema is never accompanied by urticaria and it does not respond to epinephrine.

Rapid onset of upper airway edema may also occur from viral or bacterial infections. Pain and fever rarely occur in acute allergic reactions, however, and erythema and exudate are not associated with allergic swelling. Rarely, patients may experience stridor and obstructive airway symptoms as part of an hysterical reaction; indirect laryngoscopy may be necessary. Scombroid fish poisoning may mimic anaphylaxis, with severe urticaria, nausea and vomiting, headache, and dysphagia. This syndrome occurs shortly after eating fish (tuna or mahi mahi) that has spoiled slightly so that the histidine is broken down to histamine. The "Chinese restaurant syndrome," a reaction to monosodium glutamate, may sometimes be confused with anaphylaxis, but the prominence of headache and burning chest discomfort distinguish it from an allergic reaction.

EMERGENCY DEPARTMENT EVALUATION AND MANAGEMENT

Immediate priorities include the upper airway and blood pressure monitoring. Angioedema of the lips, tongue, uvula, and soft palate, symptoms of hoarseness, stridor, dysphagia, or lump in the throat should suggest progressive airway compromise. Treat such patients immediately with epinephrine 0.3 cc (1/1000 dilution) subcutaneously. Cardiac monitor, oxygen by cannula, and an

IV line of normal saline should be done. If hypotension is profound and unresponsive to saline, or if airway obstruction is imminent (drooling and stridor), consider IV epinephrine. The most common error in this situation is giving *too* much epinephrine too fast, and precipitating cardiac arrhythmias. The preferred dose is 1.0 cc of 1/10,000 epinephrine diluted in 10 cc normal saline and given as a slow IV over 5–10 minutes.

If life-threatening symptoms persist, the IV dose may be repeated once or twice more, or epinephrine may be infused at 1–4 μg/minute. Be prepared to do a cricothyroidotomy if air exchange is further compromised. If symptoms are resolving, switch to epinephrine 0.3 cc subcutaneously at 20-minute intervals. Hypotension generally responds to saline infusion, with most adults requiring 1–2 L over the first hour. Epinephrine is an important part of therapy and can be given intramuscularly or subcutaneously if perfusion is adequate. Intravenous epinephrine should be considered a last resort. Most patients with anaphylaxis do not require such intensive therapy, with the majority responding to 2–3 doses of epinephrine subcutaneously at 15- to 20-minute intervals and a liter of saline IV. Even for the patient who presents with acute urticaria alone, epinephrine is suggested to stop progression to full-blown anaphylaxis. Bronchospasm in anaphylaxis is responsive to epinephrine, but occasionally inhaled beta agonists may be given.

Steroids are recommended in most patients with anaphylaxis. Although there is no immediate benefit, they might prevent the recurrence of symptoms several hours later. Dosage: hydrocortisone (Solu-Cortef) 250 to 500 mg, or methylprednisolone (Solu-Medrol) 50–125 mg IV push, repeated every 4 hours if symptoms persist. Give all patients with anaphylaxis an antihistamine such as diphenhydramine (Benadryl, 25–50 mg). The route of administration depends on the severity of the reaction. Antihistamines alone, however, are inadequate in the treatment of acute anaphylaxis, and should seldom be relied upon as the sole treatment.

It is critical to stop further exposure to antigen: place a tourniquet above an injection site, remove the bee stinger, wash off any offending chemicals, stop the IV line, etc. Throughout therapy, assess the vital signs frequently, check for edema of the uvula or oropharynx, observe for laryngeal edema or bronchospasm, stridor, retractions, or wheezing. These checks should be made at 1- or 2-minute intervals at first, with the intervals lengthened as the patient stabilizes.

When treating patients over 50 or those with a cardiac history, give steroids and antihistamines routinely, but generally in the lower dose range. Saline loading for hypotension should be done cautiously, while monitoring closely for volume overload. Do *not* withhold epinephrine if potential upper airway obstruction exists or in hypotension unresponsive to volume loading. A test dose of epinephrine 0.15 cc (1/1000) subcutaneously or intramuscularly can generally be given safely. If no chest pain or cardiac arrhythmias develop, give another test dose or a full dose. Avoid IV epinephrine in this group unless death appears imminent without its use.

Another special situation arises when anaphylaxis occurs in a patient who is taking a beta-adrenergic blocking agent, in which case epinephrine therapy may have a net alpha-adrenergic effect only, thereby limiting its efficacy. In this situation, glucagon 1 to 2 mg IV over 5 minutes appears to be of great benefit. Terbutaline 0.25 mg subcutaneously or an isoproterenol drip may also be considered. Table 181-3 summarizes treatment guidelines for anaphylaxis.

DISPOSITION

If there is complete and rapid resolution of all symptoms with initial therapy, observe the patient in the ED without further treatment. If there is no recurrence of symptoms in the next 3 hours, the patient may safely be discharged and should continue on a 2- to 3-day course of prednisone (40 mg per day) and diphenhydramine (25 mg every 4 hours as needed). Discharge instructions should caution the patient to avoid the suspected inciting cause, such as medications, foods, chemicals, or even exercise. Instruct the patient to return immediately if hoarseness, dysphagia, wheezing, dyspnea, dizziness, or worsening rash and swelling develop. Recommend follow-up with an allergist, particularly if no obvious etiology has been identified. Admit patients with a life-

TABLE 181-3. Treatment of Anaphylaxis

1. Remove antigen, delay absorption.
2. Maintain an adequate airway.
3. Epinephrine:
   0.3 cc SC (0.01 cc/kg in a child) 1/1000;
      repeat at 10- to 20-minute intervals.
      May give IM if severe episode.
   If in shock or incipient airway obstruction, give 1/100,000 dilution IV, 1–2 cc/min to a total of 10 cc (0.1 mg).
   If persistent shock, may start a drip: 1 mg in 250 cc D_5W, 1–4 µg/min.
   If patient is >50 or has a cardiac history, and life-threatening symptoms exist, give a test dose of 0.1–0.15 cc SC or IM (1/1000). If shock resistant to other measures or imminent airway closure, consider a drip as above.
4. Volume expansion with saline or lactated ringer's
   Shock:
      Adult: 1 L over 15 min, then reassess.
      Child: 20 cc/kg bolus
5. Methylprednisolone:
   50–125 mg IV push (1 mg/kg in a child), may repeat every 4 hours if persistent symptoms (hydrocortisone 250–500 mg as alternative). If discharging home, prednisone 40 mg/day, for 2 to 3 days.
6. Diphenhydramine:
   25–50 mg IV push, then every 2 to 4 hours as needed. If being discharged, 25 mg q 6hr prn for 3 days.
7. If resistant hypotension:
   MAST suit, dopamine infusion.
8. If beta-blocker-accentuated anaphylaxis:
   Terbutaline 0.25 mg SC, isoproterenol drip, glucagon 1–2 mg IV push
      over 4 to 5 minutes.

threatening manifestation, such as shock or upper airway obstruction, even if it has resolved with acute therapy; those who have a slow or incomplete response to therapy or worsening of symptoms during ED treatment; and any elderly, debilitated, or cardiac patient with the full syndrome.

COMMON PITFALLS

- Giving dangerously large doses of epinephrine IV (cardiac epinephrine should be further diluted as described above).
- Don't withhold epinephrine therapy in the elderly or cardiac patient with imminent airway obstruction or refractory shock.
- Failure to recognize possible recrudescence of symptoms 4-8 hours after resolution of symptoms.
- Failure to identify common causes of anaphylaxis [anti-inflammatory drugs (ibuprofen, aspirin), foods (shellfish, nuts), antibiotics, anti-hypertensive drugs (beta-blockers, ACE inhibitors), and exercise].
- Failure to treat upper airway symptoms, such as hoarseness and dysphagia, with appropriate aggressiveness. These patients should be observed in the ED after resolution or should be admitted if symptoms persist or recur.
- Not recognizing uvular and pharyngeal angioedema as warning signs of laryngeal involvement.
- Overdiagnosing the "Chinese restaurant syndrome" (MSG), when in fact the reaction was anaphylaxis.

182   Angioedema

Angioedema is characterized by areas of cutaneous and visceral swelling, with a predilection for the face, oral areas, distal extremities, and genitalia; it may also involve the larynx, gastrointestinal tract, and central nervous system. The swelling is deep rather than superficial. Unlike urticaria, the cutaneous lesions are not usually pruritic. There are two main forms of angioedema: acquired and hereditary. The *acquired* form is more common, often occurring in association with urticaria and is usually the result of a reaction to certain stimuli. *Hereditary* angioedema (HAE) is manifested by recurrent attacks of angioedema not associated with urticaria. Compromise of the airway occurs in 66% of patients and is the cause of death in 25%.

CLINICAL PRESENTATION

The presentation depends on the affected sites or systems. Most commonly, localized cutaneous swelling may occur with urticaria after appropriate stimulus exposure. The patient often complains of pruritus due to urticaria and tightness or burning in the angioedematous areas. Involvement of the gastrointestinal tract, seen more commonly in HAE, can cause abdominal pain, nausea, vomiting, and diarrhea. The most serious is upper airway obstruction with dysphagia, a "tightness" in the throat, dyspnea, cough, hoarseness, and stridor. In acquired angioedema, airway involvement is rare but can progress rapidly. In HAE, airway edema can progress over several hours, with increasing hoarseness and difficulty swallowing prior to complete airway obstruction.

DIFFERENTIAL DIAGNOSIS

Consider other entities that can cause swelling, including cellulitis and erysipelas, CHF, lymphedema, renal disease, and venous obstruction.

EMERGENCY DEPARTMENT EVALUATION

Most important is a meticulous history and examination to identify inciting agents, to assess the severity of illness, and to consider HAE or other underlying disorders. The airway status is vital; avoid underestimating the extent of airway involvement and potential for obstruction. Laboratory studies are seldom useful, except to eliminate other causes of edema.

EMERGENCY DEPARTMENT MANAGEMENT

The mainstays of drug treatment of acute acquired angioedema are epinephrine and H_1 antihistamines such as diphenhydramine, hydroxyzine, and cyproheptadine. In chronic angioedema, corticosteroids have been used in conjunction with H_2 antagonists with varying success. If the patient presents with uncomplicated cutaneous swelling, treatment consists of oral or intramuscular diphenhydramine (25–50 mg) or hydroxyzine (25–50 mg). With gastrointestinal involvement, give additional symptomatic and supportive therapy as indicated. For upper respiratory involvement, the most important aspect is maintenance of a patent airway. These patients should receive subcutaneous epinephrine (0.3 cc of 1:1000), followed by a parenteral H_1 antihistamine. There is no added benefit of IV epinephrine. Monitoring of airway status is important; when indicated, perform intubation or cricothyrotomy.

Acute attacks of HAE do not benefit from epinephrine, antihistamines, and corticosteroids. Androgen derivatives, such as danazol, and antifibrinolytic agents, such as epsilon-amino-caproic acid and tranexamic acid, have been shown to decrease the frequency of attacks, but do not arrest acute episodes. Significant improvement has been seen with infusion of C1 INH concentrates. For simple cutaneous episodes, no therapy is required; gastrointestinal attacks require only symptomatic and supportive care. With impending airway obstruction, maintenance of airway patency is of prime consideration, while infusion of C1 INH concentrate, where available, may be beneficial.

DISPOSITION

Consider consultation with anesthesia or surgery if airway control is problematic. In previously diagnosed HAE, discuss the management with the physician who follows the patient. In both acute and hereditary forms of angioedema, patients with simple cutaneous swellings can usually be discharged with follow-up in 1 to 2 days. Admit patients with airway problems or worsening symptoms despite therapy. An ICU is mandatory for airway compromise or severe neurologic symptoms.

COMMON PITFALLS

- The most grievous error made is inadequate airway control and subsequent airway obstruction.
- Another common pitfall is misdiagnosis of gastrointestinal and neurologic involvement. Careful attention to associated cutaneous lesions or to a history of previous episodes should alert the physician to the diagnosis of angioedema.
- Another error in HAE is to rely on epinephrine and antihistamines, which are **not** beneficial in the hereditary form of angioedema.

183 Monoarticular Arthritis

The evaluation of monoarticular arthritis involves a history, and physical and synovial fluid analysis. This identifies specific groups: hemorrhagic, infectious (septic), crystal-induced, and inflammatory arthritides.

ETIOLOGY, PATHOPHYSIOLOGY, AND CLINICAL PRESENTATION

Hemorrhagic arthritis (hemarthrosis) may occur from trauma or secondary to coagulopathy. Coagulopathy may be congenital (hemophilia) or a reaction to the drugs that interfere with normal clotting mechanisms, such as coumadin. Traumatic hemorrhagic effusion most often is due to intra-articular or osteochondral fracture, or from cartilaginous or ligamentous injury.

Etiologies of infectious arthritis vary. The condition may result from traumatic penetration with direct seeding of the joint capsule, from a contiguous focus of osteomyelitis, or from arthrocentesis and arthrotomy. More commonly, infectious arthritis occurs because of hematogenous dissemination from a remote focus of infection. Bacterial infection is of concern because it has the greatest potential to cause rapid joint destruction. While viral, mycobacterial, and fungal infections do cause septic arthritis, they are more likely to present as a polyarticular (viral) or chronic (fungal and mycobacterial) process.

After age 2, gram-positive cocci predominate. *Neisseria gonorrhoeae* predominates from adolescence until about age 40. In adults, about 75% of nongonococcal septic arthritis is caused by gram-positive cocci, particularly *S. aureus* and the pneumococci. With *S. aureus* arthritis, the focus of primary infection may be cellulitis, cutaneous abscess, or endocarditis; all may be from IV drug abuse. With pneumococcal arthritis, pulmonary or pericranial infections (i.e., sinusitis, otitis media) are considerations. Also consider *Pseudomonas aeruginosa* and *E. coli* in IV drug abusers, immunosuppressive drugs, and urinary tract obstruction, infection, or recent instrumentation. In most cases of nongonococcal septic arthritis, one or more contributing factors can be identified, including prior arthritis in the involved joint, an extra-articular infection, a debilitating disease, and immunosuppressive therapy.

The common crystal-induced arthropathies, gout and pseudogout, result from the deposition within the joint of monosodium urate and calcium pyrophosphate dihydrate crystals, respectively. The etiology and pathophysiology of other inflammatory monoarticular arthropathies are less clear. Many of these systemic disorders (e.g., rheumatoid arthritis, systemic lupus erythematosus) are believed to have an autoimmune etiology with formation of immune complexes within the synovial fluid.

DIFFERENTIAL DIAGNOSIS AND EMERGENCY DEPARTMENT EVALUATION

See Table 183-1. The signs and symptoms of monoarticular arthritis (i.e., pain, fever, joint swelling, limitation of motion) are similar regardless of etiology.

SYNOVIAL FLUID ANALYSIS

See Table 183-2. Synovial fluid analysis by arthrocentesis is the most important diagnostic step in acute monoarticular arthritis.

EMERGENCY DEPARTMENT MANAGEMENT AND DISPOSITION

Arthrocentesis not only is critical for diagnosis, but is therapeutic if the joint can be decompressed. In hemophiliac patients with hemarthrosis, replacement therapy with factor VIII in hemophilia A and plasma prothrombin complex (factors II, VII, IX, and X) in hemophilia B should be administered. In patients with hemarthrosis due to anticoagulants, the anticoagulant should be stopped temporarily. In acute gouty arthritis, do not reduce the serum uric acid level acutely, since this may precipitate another acute attack by mobilizing uric acid crystals. Additional treatment and disposition guidelines are outlined in Table 183-3.

COMMON PITFALLS

- Negative Gram's stain of synovial fluid does not rule out infectious arthritis.
- Consider infectious arthritis in all patients with a history of previous crystal-induced or inflammatory arthropathy who present with acute monoarticular arthritis.
- Do not reduce the serum uric acid level in gouty arthritis acutely during an exacerbation. A sudden decrease in the uric acid level may mobilize uric acid crystals and initiate another acute attack.
- Acute gout may mimic cellulitis.

TABLE 183-1. Differential Diagnosis of Monoarticular Arthritis

Type of Arthritis	History	Physical Examination	Laboratory Analysis (Excluding Synovial Fluid Analysis)	Radiologic Analysis
Hemorrhagic	Trauma, coagulopathy		Clotting studies	Fracture
Infectious	Penetrating joint injury, arthrocentesis/arthrotomy, osteomyelitis	Penetration site	Gram's stain and culture focus	Traumatic (foreign body, "air arthrogram")
	Underlying infection	Gonococcal: petechial-pustular rash with necrotic center; tenosynovitis of wrist/ankles	Gonococcal: culture urethra, cervix, pharynx, rectum	Acute infection: normal; chronic: joint erosion
	Intravenous drug abuse Prior arthritis	"Track marks"		
Crystal-induced	Hyperuricemia Drugs: diuretics;, alcohol (gout)	Gout: may mimic cellulitis; tophi in joint margin, tendons, helix of ear	Gout: uric acid (can be normal)	Gout: soft-tissue swelling (acute); "punched-out" lesion (chronic)
	Metabolic/endocrine disorders (pseudogout)	Pseudogout: clinical signs of underlying metabolic/endocrine disorder	Pseudogout: per underlying disorder	Pseudogout: chondrocalcinosis
Inflammatory	Extra-articular manifestations (see text)	Psoriatic: nail pitting, psoriasis; distal interphalangeal joint	See text	Chronic: juxta-articular osteopenia; joint space narrowing
		Reiter's: urethritis (nongonococcal), conjunctivitis, iritis, keratodermia blenorrhagica, circinate balanitis, Achilles tendinitis		Psoriatic: "sausage-shaped" digit

TABLE 183-2. Synovial Fluid Analysis in Monoarticular Arthritis

Type of Arthritis	Appearance	Viscosity	Cell Count	Crystals	Gram's Stain	Glucose (mg/dL)
Hemorrhagic	Bloody	Varies	Preponderance of erythrocytes	Negative	Negative	<10
Infectious	Opaque, turbid	Low	Often >50,000 WBC/μL	Negative	Positive in 75%, but negative Gram's stain does not rule out diagnosis	>40
Crystal-induced	Opaque	Low	2,000–50,000 WBC/μL	Gout: monosodium urate Pseudogout: calcium pyrophosphate dihydrate	Negative	<30
Inflammatory	Opaque	Low	2,000–50,000 WBC/μL	Negative	Negative	<30

*The synovial fluid glucose should be compared to plasma glucose. The values presented are the difference between plasma and synovial fluid glucose levels.

TABLE 183-3. Treatment of Monoarticular Arthritis

Type of Arthritis	Treatment	Admission Criteria	Disposition/Referral
Hemorrhagic	Soft compression dressing, splint, ice, elevation/no weight bearing, analgesia Coagulopathy: see text	Surgery for fracture	Orthopedics: intra-articular fracture Hematology: coagulopathies
Infectious	Gram-positive: Methicillin, nafcillin, oxacillin 125 mg/kg/day IV or 3rd-generation cephalosporin Gram-negative bacillus: Gentamicin 3–5 mg/kg/day IV plus carbenicillin 400–500 mg/kg/day IV H. influenzae: Ampicillin 200 mg/kg/day IV plus chloramphenicol 50–75 mg/kg/day IV N. gonorrhoeae: Penicillin G 10 million units/day IV	Until organism is isolated Surgery for joint disruption/foreign body removal; surgical drainage except in gonococcal infection	Orthopedics: trauma-related Rheumatology for inpatient treatment
Crystal-induced	Indomethacin 50 mg q8h until pain tolerable, then 25 mg q8h Colchicine: most effective if given within 24 hrs of onset. Drug of choice if patient cannot take indomethacin (heart failure, coagulopathy, ulcer disease). 0.6 mg P.O. qlh until symptoms subside or nausea/diarrhea occurs; or single 2-mg IV dose	Only if required for pain control	Rheumatologist/general medicine
Inflammatory	Indomethacin 25 mg q6–8 h for Reiter's, rheumatoid, and psoriatic arthritis Aspirin 12–15 tablets/day for rheumatoid arthritis	Only if required for pain control	Rheumatologist for follow-up care

184   Polyarticular Arthritis

Many polyarthritic syndromes have a gradual onset and sometimes defy precise diagnosis despite months of workup (Table 184-1). There is significant overlap between symptoms of systemic lupus erythematous (SLE), RA, and other collagen-vascular diseases, and laboratory test results are often equivocal. A definitive diagnosis will not usually be made in the ED (Table 184-2).

EMERGENCY DEPARTMENT EVALUATION

Sudden onset of joint pain (developing over several hours, rather than days) strongly suggests gout (almost always monoarticular) or infection. The most important joint disorder to diagnose early is infectious arthritis. The pattern of joint involvement is important. Symmetric involvement argues for RA or SLE. Asymmetric joint involvement is seen in the seronegative arthritides (e.g., Reiter's syndrome); migratory involvement (leaving one joint before involving another) is typical of acute rheumatic fever (ARF). A family history of arthritis supports a diagnosis of RA or one of the seronegative spondylarthropathies. Thiazides are known to increase the serum uric acid level and may precipitate gout. Hydralazine, procainamide, isoniazid, and phenytoin can induce a lupus-like reaction.

TABLE 184-1. Polyarthritic Syndromes

Rheumatoid arthritis: symmetric, additive involvement initially of small joints, morning stiffness, + rheumatoid factor 75%.

Systemic lupus erythematosus: multiple organ system involvement, symmetric evanescent involvement of any joint, serologic autoreactivity (anti-DNA, etc).

Osteoarthritis: lower extremities, DIP (Heberden's nodes), lack of inflammatory signs.

Ankylosing spondylitis: insidious involvement of spine (occasionally hips and shoulders), uveitis in 25%, HLA-B27 + 90%.

Colitic arthritis: large joints; parallels course of ulcerative colitis or regional enteritis.

Psoriatic arthritis: DIP, symmetric or asymmetric, skin disease begins first, 80% have pitting of nails.

TABLE 184-2. Acute Polyarticular Arthritis: Clinical Features

Acute rheumatic fever: Migratory polyarthritis, carditis, erythema marginatum, subcutaneous nodules, chorea.

Gonococcal arthritis: Early tenosynovitis and diffuse arthralgias, common wrist involvement, characteristic rash.

Lyme disease: Brief, recurrent, involving knees, preceded by characteristic rash (erythema chronicum migrans), cardiac and neurologic involvement.

Reiter's syndrome: Asymmetric involvement of lower extremities, urethritis, conjunctivitis, skin lesions.

Viral arthritis: Symmetric involvement of fingers, wrist, and knees.

Serum sickness: Migratory involvement of large and small joints, associated rash.

Inflammation in the periarticular soft tissues (tendons, bursae) can cause swelling and limitation of motion, and mimic joint disease. Arthritis usually limits both active and passive motion equally, whereas acute tendonitis or bursitis usually limits active motion significantly more than passive. Synovitis is always indicative of joint inflammation but usually results from chronic disease and does not necessarily indicate active disease. The most specific physical finding to indicate acute joint inflammation is an effusion. A diagnosis of polyarthritis demands objective evidence of inflammation in at least two joints.

Examine all the joints, not only those currently symptomatic, patterns of involvement and chronicity. All of the most important acute polyarthritides are associated with a characteristic rash. Subcutaneous nodules are seen in 35% of patients with RA (2%–3% of those with ARF). Psoriatic arthritis usually has characteristic pitting of the nails and the typical rash. A general examination may note such important findings as a pleural effusion in SLE or RA, or hepatomegaly (with or without jaundice) with the arthritis of hepatitis. Do a pelvic examination on all sexually active women with unexplained arthritis to rule out *N. gonorrhoeae*.

For both the undiagnosed and the patient with known disease, the single most important laboratory test is examination of the joint fluid; it is the only way to diagnose acute infection. Tests such as antinuclear antibody or rheumatoid factor are seldom available in the ED. These studies should be ordered, however, in appropriate patients for subsequent care. The erythrocyte sedimentation rate (ESR) is of little help. It is, however, useful for chronic conditions such as RA. Significant arthritis can occur in the presence of a normal ESR. Radiographs are of little help with nontraumatic joint pain. Radiographic inflammatory changes (symmetric erosions of the wrist and metacarpophalangeal joints in RA) occur late in the disease, and a normal radiograph does not rule out arthritis. The main utility is to exclude complications in chronic arthritis.

RHEUMATOID ARTHRITIS (RA)   The most commonly encountered chronic polyarthritis is RA, a syndrome characterized by symmetric polyarthritis, constitutional symptoms, and in some cases extra-articular organ system involvement. The diagnosis is based on the clinical course over a period of months to years. Rheumatoid factor, although not a specific marker, is in the serum of 75–80% of patients.

ACUTE RHEUMATIC FEVER (ARF)   There are recent reports of dramatic increases in ARF. The diagnosis requires fulfillment of the modified Jones criteria (Table 184-3). The arthritis is typically migratory and most often affects the large joints of the lower extremities, but rarely the hips. *Carditis,* seen in 40–50%, is the most serious finding. The diagnosis requires one of the following: new organic heart murmur (usually mitral regurgitation), cardiomegaly, pericarditis, or congestive heart failure. A recent report found ECHO evidence of mitral regurgitation in many patients with no clinical sign of carditis. The diagnosis requires laboratory confirmation of recent streptococcal pharyngitis. An elevated antistreptolysin O (ASO) titer is seen in the majority of patients.

GONOCOCCAL ARTHRITIS (GA)   Gonococcal arthritis is by far the most common bacterial arthritis in young people; it is discussed in detail elsewhere.

TABLE 184-3. Modified Jones Criteria for Diagnosis of Rheumatic Fever

Major Criteria	Minor Criteria
Carditis	History of ARF
Polyarthritis	Fever
Chorea	Arthralgia
Erythema marginatum	Elevated sed rate
Subcutaneous nodules	Prolonged PR interval

The diagnosis of ARF requires two major criteria or one major and two minor PLUS evidence of recent streptococcal infection (positive culture or increased ASO).

LYME DISEASE (LD)   Lyme disease is caused by the spirochete *Borrelia burgdorferi,* which is transmitted by the deer tick *Ixodes;* 60% of patients develop erythema chronicum migrans. It starts as a single red macule that expands to form a large annular lesion with a red outer border and central clearing and induration. Several days after the initial lesion, 50% develop multiple secondary lesions, which are similar in appearance but not as large. Two weeks to 2 years after the initial skin lesion, 60% develop acute arthritis, mainly in the knees, which is transient and intermittent. About 10% develop cardiac abnormalities, most often AV block. Some patients require temporary pacemakers. Eleven percent of patients develop significant neurologic abnormalities, including meningitis, encephalitis, and cranial neuropathies.

REITER'S SYNDROME   Reiter's syndrome, a common cause of arthritis in young men, consists of nongonococcal urethritis, asymmetric polyarthritis, and conjunctivitis. The arthritis is usually acute and involves the large joints of the lower extremities, particularly the knees and ankles. Achilles tendonitis ("lover's heel") is also common. This entity is discussed elsewhere.

EMERGENCY DEPARTMENT MANAGEMENT

Treatment for all the polyarthritides is nonsteroidal anti-inflammatory drugs (NSAID), to control both pain and inflammation. If one NSAID fails to control symptoms, another agent in a different class may work quite well. Except under unusual circumstances, do not initiate therapy with agents other than the NSAIDs without consultation with the patient's physician. Disorders that require specific treatment are discussed below.

Patients with *acute rheumatic fever* should be hospitalized and monitored for carditis and arrhythmias; the most common is first-degree AV block. High-dose salicylates are used for arthritis; steroids are reserved for significant carditis. Penicillin is recommended to eradicate remaining streptococci; thereafter, the patient should be kept on penicillin prophylaxis indefinitely.

Treatment of *gonococcal arthritis* with high doses of penicillin is usually effective. While most patients should be admitted, a compliant patient without involvement of a weight-bearing joint can be followed as an outpatient.

Treatment of *Lyme disease* during the erythema chronicum migrans stage is with tetracycline. During the late stages of arthritis, high doses of penicillin have been advocated. Most authorities treat *Reiter's syndrome* with a course of tetracycline.

COMMON PITFALLS

- Failure to analyze synovial fluid in a patient with undiagnosed arthritis
- Failure to recognize an acute septic joint in a patient with underlying polyarthritis
- Failure to recognize rheumatic fever and initiate appropriate therapy
- Failure to recognize symptoms due to therapy rather than to the underlying disease
- Failure to appreciate extra-articular manifestations of chronic polyarthritis

PART X

Dermatologic Emergencies

185 Varicella

Varicella (chicken pox) is not uncommon in adults. It presents with a polymorphic rash, predominantly on the trunk, consisting of vesicles, umbilicated pustules, and hemorrhagic crusts, which heal to leave atrophic scars. A key diagnostic feature is the simultaneous presence of lesions in all stages of development. It is often accompanied by a prodrome of fever, malaise, myalgia, and coryza, and there may be a clear history of exposure 10–14 days prior to the rash. Pruritus may be severe. The patient is contagious until all the lesions have crusted over, generally 5–6 days after the first appearance of the eruption. A Tzank smear and viral culture may aid in making the diagnosis. Pneumonia and encephalitis are uncommon but potentially life-threatening complications. Treatment is symptomatic, with oral antihistamines and tepid compresses.

186 Life-Threatening Dermatoses

Cutaneous lesions are often the first sign of serious systemic disease. Common life-threatening dermatoses are listed in Table 186-1. They can be grouped into diffuse red rashes, vesiculobullous eruptions, localized or discrete lesions, and purpuric or hemorrhagic lesions.

Generalized exfoliative erythroderma (formerly called exfoliative dermatitis) is a diffuse widespread dermatitis that covers most of the body surface. This condition not only causes pruritus and pain, but may also be complicated by fluid, electrolyte, and protein loss; invasion of bacteria and opportunistic organisms through the skin; hypothermia; and high-output CHF from vasodilatation. The causes of exfoliative erythroderma include previously existing skin diseases (e.g., psoriasis, atopic eczema, contact dermatitis) (50%); drug eruptions (10%); lymphoproliferative disorders (e.g., Hodgkin's disease, leukemia, Sezary syndrome) (15%); and idiopathic (25–40%). Mortality is <5%. Angioedema and disseminated herpetic infection are discussed elsewhere.

DIFFUSE RED RASHES

Toxic epidermal necrolysis (TEN) is a disease of adults in which the skin sloughs in large sheets. Although similar in appearance to scalded skin syndrome, it is quite different. It may actually represent the most severe form of erythema multiforme, and begins, like erythema multiforme, with

TABLE 186-1. Life-Threatening Dermatoses

Diffuse Red Rashes	Vesiculobullous Diseases
Urticaria with anaphylaxis	Pemphigus
Toxic shock syndrome	Pemphigoid
Kawasaki disease	Stevens-Johnson syndrome
Toxic epidermal necrolysis	Toxic epidermal necrolysis
Staphylococcal scalded skin	Disseminated zoster
syndrome	Disseminated herpes simplex
Generalized exfoliative erythroderma	
Pustular psoriasis	
Cutaneous T-cell lymphomas	
Systemic lupus erythematosus	
Localized or Discrete Lesions	**Purpuric or Hemorrhagic**
Erysipelas and cellulitis	Meningococcemia
Gonococcemia	Gonococcemia
Ecthyma gangrenosum	Disseminated intravascular coagulation
Brown recluse spider bite	Palpable purpura
Behcet's syndrome	Brown recluse spider bite
Malignant melanoma	Rocky Mountain spotted fever
Kaposi's sarcoma and AIDS	Miscellaneous hematologic disorders

With permission from Krusinski PA, Flowers FP: Life-threatening dermatoses. In Flowers FP, Krusinski PA: Dermatology in Ambulatory and Emergency Medicine. A Clinical Guide with Algorithms. Chicago, Year Book Medical Pub. 1984.

constitutional symptoms of fever, malaise, and myalgia. The skin is initially diffusely painful, hot, and red. Within 24 hours, blisters and large areas of denuded skin develop; erosive, sloughing lesions of the oral mucosa are common. Nikolsky's sign is positive.

TEN almost always occurs in adults and is precipitated by drugs such as sulfas, phenylbutazone, phenytoin, or penicillin, or by graft-versus-host reactions (e.g., after bone marrow transplantation) or blood product transfusions. Erosive oral lesions are common. TEN desquamates the entire thickness of the epidermis, accounting for TEN's high mortality rate (>50%). Diagnosis is made by presentation and biopsy. Treatment is removal of the precipitating agent, if possible, and as in burn patients, fluid and electrolyte therapy and prevention of infection.

Toxic shock syndrome is an acute febrile illness associated with localized infection by strains of *S. aureus* that produce an exotoxin (TSST-1). Early macular skin rash, hypotension, abnormalities in multiple organ systems, and acral desquamation occur 1–2 weeks after the onset of illness; 85–90% are reported in menstruating women. The remaining cases are associated with localized infection in men, children, and nonmenstruating women. Strict criteria for the diagnosis are fever, hypotension or orthostasis, an erythematous macular rash, involvement of at least three organ systems (Table 186-2), and the presence of an *S. aureus* infection. Hypotension may appear early; most patients will present to the hospital with orthostasis.

The differential diagnosis includes Rocky Mountain spotted fever, scarlet fever, sepsis, Kawasaki disease (rare in those >8 years old), leptospirosis, Colorado tick fever and other viral infections. Supportive treatment for dehydration and hypotension includes fluid replacement and pressors. The adult respiratory distress syndrome (ARDS) is common in serious cases. A penicillinase-resistant penicillin or a first-generation cephalosporin is considered mandatory if the diagnosis cannot be excluded; vancomycin or clindamycin are alternatives. All patients suspected of having TSS require admission for vigorous supportive treatment.

TABLE 186-2. Revised Case Definition of Toxic Shock Syndrome

Fever: temperature ≥ 38.9°C (102°F)
Rash: diffuse macular erythroderma
Desquamation 1 to 2 weeks after onset of illness, particularly of palms and soles
Hypotension: systolic blood pressure ≤ 90 mm Hg for adults or below fifth percentile by age for
   children below 16 years of age, orthostatic drop in diastolic blood pressure ≥ 15 mm Hg from
   lying to sitting, orthostatic syncope, or orthostatic dizziness
Multisystem involvement—three or more of the following:
   GI: vomiting or diarrhea at onset of illness
   Muscular: severe myalgia or creatine phosphokinase level at least twice the upper limit of normal
      for laboratory
   Mucous membrane: vaginal, oropharyngeal, or conjunctival hyperemia
   Renal: blood urea nitrogen or creatinine at least twice the upper limit of normal for laboratory or
      urinary sediment with pyuria (≥ 5 leukocytes per high-power field) in the absence of urinary tract
      infection
   Hepatic: total bilirubin, SGOT*, SGPT† at least twice the upper limit of normal for laboratory
   Hematologic: platelets ≥ 100 000/µL
   CNS: disorientation or alterations in consciousness without focal neurologic signs when fever and
      hypotension are absent
   Negative results on the following tests, if obtained:
   Blood, throat, or cerebrospinal fluid cultures (blood culture may be positive for *Staphylococcus
      aureus*)
   Rise in titer to Rocky Mountain spotted fever, leptospirosis, or rubeola

---

   *SGOT denotes serum aspartate transaminase.
   †SGPT denotes serum alanine transaminase.
   Reproduced with permission from Reingold AL et al: Toxic shock surveillance in the United States
1980–1981. Ann Intern Med 96 (pt 2): 875—880, 1982.

VESICOBULLOUS DISEASES

Bullous erythema multiforme forms part of the spectrum of acute immunologic reactions known
as erythema multiforme. The classic lesion is the target lesion, a central gray wheal or bulla surrounded by concentric rings of erythema and normal skin. Many types of lesions may be present
simultaneously–macules, papules, urticaria (though nonpruritic), and bullae. The extremities are
involved more than the trunk; the palms and soles are often affected. The rash appears abruptly
and may be accompanied by fever, malaise, and pruritus.

   Further along the spectrum is *Stevens–Johnson syndrome* (bullous erythema multiforme
accompanied by constitutional symptoms and involving at least two mucous membranes). A prodrome of fever, malaise, and myalgia is followed by the explosive appearance of blisters on mucous
membranes and skin. Symmetric blistering begins on the dorsa of the hands and feet and on extensor surfaces. Erosive lesions begin on oral mucosa, lips, and bulbar conjunctiva and can extend to
the pharynx, larynx, esophagus, and genital mucosa. Ocular lesions can result in corneal ulceration,
panophthalmitis, and even blindness. Stevens–Johnson syndrome may progress to an illness clinically indistinguishable from TEN, with large confluent bullae and sloughing of epidermis in sheets. It
carries a mortality rate of 40–50%. Milder cases can be treated with oral antihistamines and topical
corticosteroids; more severe cases require systemic corticosteroids and hospital admission.

LOCALIZED OR DISCRETE LESIONS

Patients with gram-negative sepsis may manifest the skin lesions termed *ecthyma gangrenosum*.
Because the lesions are manifestations of life-threatening illness, the diagnosis must be made
early; this is a true dermatologic emergency. These patients are critically ill and usually immunocompromised (e.g., with leukemia or lymphoma).

Disseminated gonococcal infection (DGI) usually occurs in individuals with asymptomatic infection of the pharynx, rectum, or genitalia. This infection is discussed elsewhere.

Erysipelas is a superficial cellulitis that progresses rapidly and involves the associated lymphatic channels. Group A streptococcus, group C and D streptococci and *Staphylococcus aureus* have been isolated. The infection is most common in infants and children and in the elderly. The source of the infection in most cases is probably an inapparent wound. Erysipelas may range from a self-limited process with spontaneous resolution, to a rapidly progressive and severe infection leading to bacteremia. The involved skin is erythematous, warm, and tender to palpation, and has an advancing margin that is slightly elevated. Fever is common. The diagnosis is usually clinical since local aspiration is rarely positive. Penicillin is effective if erysipelas is due to streptococci, but either a first-generation cephalosporin or a penicillinase-resistant penicillin should also be used to cover *Staphylococcus*. Admission is based on the clinical status. Some affected individuals may be treated as outpatients with close follow-up, and admitted if there is no response or worsening after 1–2 days of oral antibiotics.

Cellulitis, an acute spreading inflammation of the skin and subcutaneous tissue, appears as a warm, tender, erythematous area with indistinct margins. Its differentiation from erysipelas is based on the appearance of the advancing edge of the infection: in cellulitis, it is not raised. In practice, the management of erysipelas and cellulitis is similar. Erysipelas is more likely to require prompt antibiotics since it may progress so rapidly.

PURPURIC OR HEMORRHAGIC LESIONS

Neisseria meningitidis colonizes the nasal mucosa in humans (5–15%), but may, depending on the host's immunologic status, invade the bloodstream and cause disease. Most cases occur in children and adolescents, although any age group may be affected. The mortality of *meningococcemia* is higher than that of meningitis. The early skin lesions in both forms of the disease are a result of vascular damage. Early recognition of the skin lesions may result in a better outcome. Meningococcemia usually follows an upper respiratory infection with flu-like symptoms of headache, myalgias, nausea, and vomiting. The severity can range from an indolent, slowly evolving infection to a fulminating illness causing prostration within a few hours after the onset of symptoms.

The classic skin lesions may be petechial, raised with pale gray vesicular centers, macular, or maculopapular. All are a few millimeters in size, on any part of the body early on and may progress to a hemorrhagic rash. Meningitis presents with the usual symptoms of meningeal irritation—neck soreness, photophobia, headache—while meningococcemia does not present with meningeal signs. Gram's stain and culture of skin lesions are positive in only 50%. Diagnosis often rests on clinical findings and is confirmed by positive cultures of blood and/or cerebrospinal fluid.

Consider meningococcemia in any patient with fever, malaise, and a petechial or maculopapular rash, and include it in the differential diagnosis of other bacteremias (e.g., *H. influenzae, S. pneumoniae, S. aureus*), subacute bacterial endocarditis, gonococcemia, vasculitis, enteroviral exanthems, and Rocky Mountain spotted fever. Penicillin G (2 million units every 2 hours), ampicillin (2 g every 4 hours), chloramphenicol (4–6 g/day), or ceftriaxone are all effective. Supportive care is necessary for those with complications such as shock, disseminated intravascular coagulation (DIC), ARDS, or metabolic acidosis. Prophylaxis is recommended for close school and household contacts. Rifampin 600 mg is given orally twice daily for 2 days (doses of 10 mg/kg for children, and 5 mg/kg for infants less than 1 month old).

Rocky Mountain spotted fever (RMSF) is an acute infectious disease caused by *Rickettsia rickettsii* and transmitted by the bites of several species of ticks (*Dermacentor andersoni* in the western United States, *Dermacentor variabilis* in the eastern United States, and *Amblyomma americanum* in some southwestern areas). It is not limited to the Rocky Mountain area. The highest incidences are in the south-Atlantic region and west–south central states. The disease causes fever, rash, myalgia, and headache. It ranges in severity from a mild self-limited illness to a severe life-threatening disease. The skin rash appears between the second and sixth days of illness, on the wrists, ankles, and forearms as a macular erythematous rash and extending to the palms, soles, and torso. The lesions become maculopapular in a few days in most cases and become petechial shortly thereafter (2 to 4 days after the start of the rash). The diagnosis is clinical based on fever, headache, rash, and other associated symptoms and signs. Only 70% give a history of tick exposure; serologic testing can confirm the diagnosis. See chapter 219.

COMMON PITFALLS

- Toxic epidermal necrolysis (TEN) can be confused with scalded skin syndrome. TEN requires the removal of any possible precipitating agent, most commonly a drug; prognosis is markedly different.
- The rash of TSS may be indistinct. Consider the diagnosis with fever and volume depletion, even without tampon use.
- Bullous pemphigoid can be confused with pemphigus vulgaris. Early consultation with a dermatologist may be necessary to avoid misdiagnosis and inappropriate treatment.
- In a febrile, seriously ill patient, suspect that a skin lesion is a manifestation of sepsis.
- Rapid diagnosis and treatment are crucial in ecthyma gangrenosum. The underlying septic process can be fatal if not treated promptly.
- The diagnosis of gonococcemia is often overlooked in tendonitis without injury.
- The early rash of meningococcemia may be macular or maculopapular as well as petechial.
- In Rocky Mountain spotted fever, the rash is absent in a significant proportion of patients. Increased suspicion is necessary for a viral-like illness in the late spring or early summer.

PART XI

Psychiatric Emergencies

<table>
<tr><td>

187

</td><td>

Disturbed Behavior: Functional and Organic Illnesses

</td></tr>
</table>

Undiagnosed medical illness in psychiatric patients is a major concern with 5–30% of psychiatric patients having undiagnosed medical illness that causes or exacerbates their psychiatric symptoms. Focussing on aberrant and often violent behavior may preclude consideration of medical illness as an underlying etiology.

CLINICAL PRESENTATION

Most organic mental syndromes present as delirium, a reversible disturbance secondary to an extracerebral insult such as infection or metabolic disturbance. Delirium is characterized by impairment of memory, thinking, perception, and attention. It has an acute onset and develops over a few hours to a few days. Patients at highest risk are elderly, children, postcardiotomy patients, burn patients, patients with pre-existing brain damage, and patients suffering drug addiction. While the neurologic and physical exams are important, the mental status examination is essential.

Delirium is characterized by clouding of consciousness, which can range from loss of awareness of self or surroundings to stupor or coma. Generally, patients with clouded consciousness are apathetic or stuporous. Clouding of consciousness is frequently misinterpreted as malingering, hysteria, or negativism. Attention span is severely impaired in delirium and patients are easily distracted. Thought processes are disjointed and incoherent. Failure to appreciate impairment of attention can lead to a misdiagnosis of "loose associations or flight of ideas". Delirious patients cannot register events. Recent and remote memory are impaired. Patients frequently misidentify familiar persons or familiarize the unfamiliar (for instance, claim to have known a stranger for years). They are often disoriented to place and time, but very rarely disoriented to person.

All have perceptual disturbances, including delusions, hallucinations, and illusions, often woven into a vague, paranoid delusional system. Illusions in which actual stimuli are misinterpreted (e.g., a dropped stethoscope is misinterpreted as a gunshot) are also common. Visual hallucinations are frequent and more common than auditory hallucinations; tactile hallucinations are the least common.

A central feature of delirium is fluctuation of symptoms. A cooperative, alert, pleasant patient may be confused, paranoid, agitated, and uncooperative several hours later. Lucid intervals alternating with periods of confusion is usually diagnostic of delirium. The time course of is also important: delirium is almost always marked by an acute onset, usually over hours or days. An acute change in mental status or behavior should **always** suggest an underlying medical event. Several features of delirium are so common and so characteristic that they indicate delirium until proven otherwise: *clouding of consciousness, age >40 with no psychiatric history, disorientation, abnormal vital signs, visual hallucinations, and illusions.*

DIFFERENTIAL DIAGNOSIS

The differential diagnosis of delirium is so extensive that there may be a tendency to avoid searching for an etiology. For example, an elderly delirious patient may have pulmonary insufficiency, cardiac failure, pre-existing brain damage, and may be taking multiple medications. Each is a possible contributor to delirium and must be pursued and evaluated independently. It is useful to think of the differential diagnosis in two categories: emergent and urgent. Emergent conditions that are life-threatening and require immediate intervention include:

Meningitis and encephalitis
Hypoglycemia
Hypertensive encephalopathy
Diminished cerebral oxygenation
Anticholinergic delirium
Intracranial hemorrhage (spontaneous or traumatic)
Wernicke's encephalopathy.

Most other causes may be urgent enough to require ED treatment (Table 187-1).

EMERGENCY DEPARTMENT EVALUATION

Studies helpful in ruling out life-threatening illnesses include a CBC, glucose, electrolytes, BUN, chest radiograph, ECG, and ABG. Patients with acute change of behavior and clouded consciousness not explained by these labs require head CT followed by a lumbar puncture.

TABLE 187-1. Treatable Causes of Organic Mental Disease

Cardiac
Arrhythmias
Congestive heart failure
Myocardial infarction

Pulmonary
Chronic obstructive pulmonary disease
Pulmonary emboli

Hepatic
Cirrhosis
Hepatitis
Wilson's disease

Renal
Worsening of mild nephritis by urinary tract
    infection
Dehydration with elevation of (BUN) > 50 mg/dL

Vascular
Subdural hematoma
Cerebrovascular accident

Infection

Endocrine Disease
Thyroid disease
Cushing's disease
Diabetes
Addison's disease
Hypoglycemia

Electrolyte Imbalance
Hyponatremia
Hypernatremia
Hypercalcemia

Vitamin Deficiencies
Thiamine
Niacin
Riboflavin
Folate
Ascorbic acid
Vitamin A
Vitamin B_{12}

Drug-Induced
Alcohol
Tranquilizers
Over-the-counter preparations
Any drug used to treat medical illness (e.g.,
    Dilantin, aminophylline, digitalis, steroids)

Exogenous Toxins
Carbon monoxide
Bromide
Mercury
Lead

Tumors

Normal Pressure Hydrocephalus

Depression

EMERGENCY DEPARTMENT MANAGEMENT

Agitation is often part of delirium and can impede evaluation. Pharmacologic intervention is necessary. Rapid tranquilization can be helpful. Haloperidol is effective in quieting delirious patients with well established safety. Antipsychotic medications may be given intramuscularly or orally. The most common side effects are dystonic reaction and akathisia. These are effectively treated with diphenhydramine (50 mg IM) or benztropine mesylate (2 mg IM). Psychological support is important.

DISPOSITION

Treatment is based on the underlying cause. Admit the patient if no specific etiology can be identified but the patient's inappropriate behavior interferes with required medical care; if a specific etiology or several etiologies have been identified and the patient's inappropriate behavior interferes with his or her medical care; or if the patient's medical condition is such that the he or she is at risk for increased morbidity or mortality.

COMMON PITFALLS

- Despite the importance of rapid recognition, evaluation and treatment, delirious patients with bizarre and agitated behavior are often inappropriately referred to a psychiatrist.
- Psychiatric patients cause discomfort for many because of bizarre disruptive behavior; as a result, they are not approached with the same sense of urgency or seriousness as are patients with nonpsychiatric disease. Too often, decisions are based on a previous diagnosis.
- Disordered Perceptions: A common misunderstanding is that delusions, hallucinations, and disorganized thoughts are diagnostic of functional psychiatric illness. On the contrary, these are nonspecific and occur in both functional and organic illnesses as well as personality disorders.
- Violence creates anxiety with a tendency to refer violent patients prematurely to a psychiatrist. Yet, like disordered perceptions, violence is etiologically nonspecific. Violence in psychiatric settings often results from underlying organic illness. The evaluation of the violent patient must always include a search for organic disease.
- Self-Induced Illness: The least tolerated patients are those who are believed to create their own disease, such as alcoholics, drug abusers, and suicidal patients.
- Ageism: Clinicians often fail to take complaints of elderly patients seriously, often attributing symptoms to old age. This attitude is particularly unfortunate when the patient is demented, since 30–40% of all dementias are treatable or reversible. For many, dementia implies a chronic, progressive, irreversible deterioration of higher intellectual functions. However, dementia is not etiologically specific and does not imply irreversibility. Premature labelling tends to preclude the proper evaluation necessary to determine the etiology of dementia.

188   Depression and Suicide

Depression is the most common psychological disturbance with a prevalence of 10–20% in the general population. Suicide is the 6th most common cause of death in the US, with 30,000 deaths/year. Recent trends show suicide to be the second most common cause of death in the college-age population and the most common cause of death in young black women.

CLINICAL PRESENTATION

Depressed patients may present with suicidal ideation or after a frank suicide attempt, but more often they come to the ED with vague, ill-defined somatic symptoms, pains in a wide variety of anatomic sites, or nervous symptoms such as increased tension and feelings of anxiety. The coexistence of psychiatric and medical disorders is the rule rather than the exception. Drug overdose accounts for 70–90% of all suicide attempts. Major and minor tranquilizers and antidepressants have replaced barbiturates and other sedatives as the major agents. Less common but important presentations include apparently unintentional overdoses, self-induced gunshot wounds, wrist cutting, falls from heights, and MVAs of unclear etiology. Evaluate injured patients for potential suicide whenever the mechanisms of injury are unclear and the possibility of self-induced harm exists.

DIFFERENTIAL DIAGNOSIS

Symptoms of depression include a diminished sense of self-esteem and general physical and mental well-being; loss of interest in, or enjoyment of, pleasurable activities; loss of energy; poor appetite; sleep disturbances including insomnia or hypersomnia; decreased attention span and concentration ability; decreased effectiveness or productivity at school, work, or home; episodes of tearfulness or crying; irritability or excessive anger; a pessimistic attitude toward the future; and recurrent thoughts of death or suicide.

A number of psychiatric and medical disorders may present with symptoms of depression. About 80% of persons suffering bereavement have one or more symptoms of depression for a year or more following the death of a loved one. Persons suffering from an adjustment disorder may develop similar symptoms within 3 months of the onset of psychosocial stresses (e.g., economic loss, physical illness, or trouble with interpersonal relations). The diagnosis of organic affective syndrome is made when symptoms of depression are found to accompany organic neurologic disease such as organic brain syndrome, stroke, tumor, or trauma. Symptoms of depression may be exacerbated or even caused by medications: antihypertensive drugs (beta blockers, clonidine, methyldopa, reserpine), antidepressants, antihistamines, neuroleptic agents, sedative–hypnotic drugs, cimetidine, and alcohol are common offenders.

When these diagnostic possibilities have been eliminated in a patient with symptoms of depression, entertain a final diagnosis of dysthymic disorder (depressive neurosis or minor depression) or major affective syndrome (major depression). The difference is one of degree, and best left to a psychiatrist.

EMERGENCY DEPARTMENT EVALUATION AND MANAGEMENT

Patients considered markedly depressed or potential suicide risks should be relieved of medications or weapons and placed in a quiet area. Physicians and nursing staff who observe, evaluate, and care for them should exhibit an accepting, supportive attitude. Physicians, particularly house staff, often have negative and sometimes hostile attitudes toward patients who have made a suicide attempt. Outward expression of this attitude by an authority figure reinforces the patient's diminished self-worth and increases the likelihood of another suicide attempt. Chemical restraints inhibit psychiatric evaluation and should be avoided if possible. Mechanical restraints should be used if they are necessary to protect the patient or health-care providers.

After medical management of overdose, injury, or associated medical problems, assess the degree of depression and potential for suicide. A significant proportion of suicide victims (14%–87%) have seen a physician during the few weeks to months before committing suicide. Unfortunately, most physicians are poor at recognizing and assessing suicidal potential. Patients likely to engage in self-destructive behavior may show high-risk characteristics (SAD PERSONS) (Table 188-1). The standard for determining the need for hospitalization of a potentially suicidal

TABLE 188-1. SAD PERSONS Score

	Description	Points
S = Sex	Male	1
A = Age	<19 or >45 years	1
D = Depression or hopelessness	Admits to depression or decreased concentration, appetite, sleep, libido	2
P = Previous attempts or psychiatric care	Previous attempt, or previous inpatient or outpatient psychiatric care	1
E = Excessive alcohol or drug use	Stigmata of chronic addiction or recent frequent use	1
R = Rational thinking loss	Organic brain syndrome or psychosis	2
S = Separated, divorced, or widowed	Recent or on anniversary	1
O = Organized or serious attempt	Well-thought-out plan or life-threatening presentation	2
N = No social supports	No close family, friends, job, or active religious affiliation	1
S = Stated future intent	Determined to repeat attempt, or ambivalent	2
		SCORE

Score	Risk
<6	Low
6–8	Intermediate
>8	High

patient is a trained and experienced psychiatrist's objective impression following formal evaluation. In an unintoxicated patient whose history can be corroborated by friends or family, the
numerical SAD PERSONS score appears to correlate closely with the clinical decision made by a
psychiatrist after an in-depth evaluation.

Patients with a low SAD PERSONS score may be suitable for outpatient psychiatric follow-
up. About 50% with intermediate scores may require hospitalization, and almost all with high
scores hospitalized. When psychiatric consultation is not immediately available, the SAD PER-
SONS score serves as a useful baseline for the assessment of the potentially suicidal patient and
can facilitate communication between with psychiatric colleagues. It is both medically and legally
necessary for the emergency physician to assess the degree of depression or suicidality and to
document that assessment. Use of the SAD PERSONS score can facilitate this process. A low
SAD PERSONS score should not preclude psychiatric consultation if a true risk for suicide exists
or when a patient asks to see a psychiatrist.

DISPOSITION

A potentially suicidal patient generally requires admission to a psychiatric unit. Do not consider
discharge unless the following conditions are met:

1. The patient has been evaluated and is deemed a low suicide risk. In general, nonpsychotic
   younger patients whose attempts involved low risk, high likelihood of rescue, and high manipulative intent can be discharged safely.
2. Psychiatric consultation has been obtained (at least by telephone) and hospitalization has been
   judged unnecessary or inadvisable.
3. Short-term outpatient follow-up can be arranged.
4. The patient agrees to return immediately if further self-destructive urges arise.
5. A positive, supportive environment of family or friends is available.

Do not transfer a potentially suicidal patient to another medical facility or to a psychiatrist's
office unless the patient is accompanied by paramedical personnel or family members who have
agreed to observe the patient closely. Since about 12% of those who attempt suicide will eventually kill themselves, 2% within the year following their first attempt, all patients who have made
a suicide attempt, who express suicidal ideation, or who exhibit marked signs of depression
require in-depth psychiatric evaluation. The reliability in scheduling and keeping follow-up appoint-
ments is notoriously poor. When ED staff demonstrate a supportive attitude and when the patient
is given a scheduled outpatient follow-up appointment at the time of discharge (ideally within 2–3
days), compliance with follow-up improves markedly.

COMMON PITFALLS

- "Accidental" trauma may be a manifestation of self-destructive behavior. When the mechanism is questionable or inconsistent with the injuries, an evaluation of the patient's mental
  state and motives is warranted.
- Corroborate with family or friends the information obtained from a potentially suicidal patient.
  Patients who vehemently deny suicidality, give abrupt answers to questions, and appear
  anxious to leave may be committed to finishing the act they began.

189   The Agitated, Acutely Psychotic, or Violent Patient

A patient who is aggressive or assaultive can present a danger to himself and bystanders. The care of most psychiatric patients has shifted from chronic care in state hospitals to acute care in community hospitals. Trends in reimbursement have led to a further shift from inpatient to out-patient care. ED visits for psychiatric care have tripled in the past 20 years.

Agitation, acute psychosis, violent acting out, functional psychosis, organic psychosis, toxic states, and personality disorders may each manifest differently. Always suspect an organic cause; behavior management and physical control of patients is also important. Control must often be achieved before diagnosis can begin. The acutely psychotic patient may harm himself or others out of confusion or in an effort to avoid some imagined or projected threat. Among life-threatening organic conditions that may present with behavioral agitation are subdural hematoma, intracerebral hemorrhage, meningitis, hypertensive crisis, hypoglycemia, and drug intoxications, especially atropine and tricyclic antidepressants.

CLINICAL PRESENTATION AND DIFFERENTIAL DIAGNOSIS

Patients are likely to be male (60%), white (75%), single, and slightly younger than the average ED patient and are described as angry, belligerent, or negative. In about 1/3, functional psychosis is eventually diagnosed; the remainder suffer from toxic psychosis, organic psychosis, or personality disorders. These patients present with agitation, abnormal behavior, violence, or a history of violence.

The differential diagnosis centers on determining organic versus functional. The patient with an organic condition tends to be more confused and disoriented, and exhibits more bizarre behavior. If violent, the violence is less directed and occurs when he is frightened or personal space is violated. The onset of confused or bizarre behavior >age 40 should be considered to be due to organic causes until proven otherwise. The patient with altered mental status in the presence of any other medical illness should be considered to be experiencing a complication of that illness (or its treatment) until proven otherwise. Drugs, or drug withdrawal, are responsible in most cases. Anticholinergic drugs, steroids, and sedative or alcohol intoxication or withdrawal are the most common causes of delirium; cocaine, phencyclidine, and other street drugs are also common. Hypoglycemia must always be considered. Fever suggests meningitis or encephalitis. Hypertensive encephalopathy, intracranial hemorrhage, subdural hematoma and thyrotoxicosis are treatable conditions that should not be overlooked.

EMERGENCY DEPARTMENT EVALUATION

The history is often obtained from others. Ask about the onset of abnormal behavior, psychiatric history, and history of violent behavior or assault. Questions must be asked frankly and without using euphemisms: for instance, "Have you ever used a car, a weapon, or your fists to hurt any-one?" When asking about medications, be specific: ask about "pain pills," "nerve pills," "sleeping pills". If the patient is confused, his wallet, purse, or pockets should be searched for medications, identification, and physician appointment cards. The patient's speech, if loud or profane, may indi-cate impending loss of control. Motor activity, such as restlessness or pacing, especially if it is escalating, is another clue. Signs of drug or alcohol intoxication call for caution, since an intoxi-cated patient is unpredictable.

EMERGENCY DEPARTMENT MANAGEMENT

When dealing with acutely agitated, psychotic, and violent patients, management and behavior control can be more pressing than diagnostic considerations. Behavioral management can be achieved by verbal, chemical, or physical means.

VERBAL RESTRAINTS

It is important to define acceptable and unacceptable behavior, and the consequences of unacceptable behavior. When limits are set, they must be applied in a nonhostile, nonpunitive manner. Recognize the need to reduce environmental stimuli. It is usually easy to determine whether family or friends exert a calming or adverse effect; it is helpful to isolate patients from them when necessary. Staff members should not allow themselves to be isolated with a potentially assaultive patient. Do not turn your back on a patient, and never place a patient between you and the door. Avoid provoking the patient to more violence, and avoid invading the patient's personal space. Using force and punishment to deal with violent and assaultive behavior often causes the situation to escalate. Remember that the patient's aggressive behavior is a defensive stance against overwhelming feelings of helplessness and fragility. Intervention is aimed at helping the patient control these impulses.

CHEMICAL RESTRAINTS

A typical dose of haloperidol is 5 to 10 mg every 30 minutes, up to a total of eight doses. Equivalent doses of other agents are chlorpromazine (Thorazine) 100 mg, trifluoperazine (Stelazine) 10 mg, and thiothixene (Navane) 10 mg. Prophylactic administration of antiparkinson drugs is unnecessary. When extrapyramidal side effects develop, they are usually easily managed with anticholinergic drugs (e.g., benztropine 2 mg IM). Adding lorazepam (Ativan) 1 mg IM to each dose of neuroleptic will increase sedation and accelerate control of symptoms. These drugs are especially useful in treating atropine psychosis, phencyclidine psychosis, or sedative withdrawal (Table 189-1).

SECLUSION AND PHYSICAL RESTRAINTS

If four-point leather restraints are to be used, the patient is placed on a stretcher and first the legs, then the arms, are secured to the stretcher one at a time. The physician should document the indications for restraint, the planned time course of restraint, and the planned frequency of monitoring.

DISPOSITION

Agitated or violent patients who require restraints or medication should in almost all instances be evaluated by a psychiatric consultant. Even after behavioral control is achieved, longer-term treatment is necessary, and more complete medical assessment is often needed as well. Intoxicated patients may develop repeated episodes of agitation, since acute pharmacologic measures may not outlast the intoxicant. Psychiatric hospitalization can be either voluntary or involuntary. The ideal disposition is to a voluntary unit in a general hospital. Civil statutes governing involuntary hospitalization vary from state to state, but most statutes require a determination of the potential for harming self or others, or being unable to care for himself. In some states the patient's ability to understand the need for treatment is an issue.

COMMON PITFALLS

- Most errors in management of agitated behavior occur when treatment is unduly delayed.
- Recognize the need to protect the patient from harming himself or others.

TABLE 189-1. Neurologic Side Effects of Antipsychotic Agents

Reaction	Overall Incidence	Predisposing Factors	Usual Onset	Clinical Manifestations	Treatment
Acute dystonia	2–10%; higher with potent agents	Young, male, higher starting doses	24–48 hours, may occur after a single dose	Bizarre muscle spasms involving tongue, face, eyes, neck, back; difficulty in speech and swallowing	Antiparkinson agents are diagnostic and curative.
Akathisia	21–50%	Female, middle-aged	1–8 weeks, rarely presents early	Motor restlessness, agitation, inability to stand or sit still	Reduce dose or change drug; antiparkinson agents, benzodiazepines, or propranolol may help.
Parkinsonism	15%	Elderly, female	Variable, usually 1–10 weeks	Tremor, rigidity, bradykinesia, shuffling gait, masked facies	Reduce dose; antiparkinson agents.
Tardive dyskinesia	0.5–56%	Elderly, female, higher doses, long duration of treatment	Usually after years of therapy	Oral-facial dyskinesia, choreoathetoid movements; usually worsens on withdrawal of antipsychotic	None effective; prevention is crucial.
Neuroleptic malignant syndrome	Rare	Unknown	Variable	Fever, catatonia, tachycardia, altered consciousness, diaphoresis; autonomic instability, rhabdomyolysis; fatal in 20%	Stop antipsychotic immediately; dantrolene or bromocriptine may be helpful.

- The use of chemical and physical restraints can be life-saving. Failing to treat a psychotic patient who "refuses" to give consent is a serious ethical and legal error.
- Recognize the potential for violence. Do not try to negotiate with a patient whose aggressiveness is escalating, when the time for verbal management has long passed.
- Serious errors in the initial evaluation include failure to obtain/use history, vital signs not taken, patients may not be searched, and important clues may be overlooked.
- Always consider organic causes for strange or agitated behavior.

PART XII

Special Topics

190 Medical Complications of Alcohol Abuse

Alcoholism is the dependence upon alcohol and the development of tolerance and withdrawal symptoms. At least 50% of MVA fatalities, 67% of drownings, 70–80% of fire-related deaths, and 67% of murders involve alcohol. Many organic problems caused by alcoholism are the result of the way ethanol is oxidized to carbon dioxide and water.

CLINICAL PRESENTATION

Phsycians should suspect alcohol-related illness in adolescents, patients involved in violent activity or trauma (especially single motor vehicle accidents), caretakers accused of child abuse, suicidal individuals, and those with other neuropsychiatric disturbances. The alcoholic patient is a diagnostic challenge; the homeless or indigent alcoholic may be easy to identify, but the affluent middle-class alcohol abuser can be difficult to diagnose (see Table 190-1). Always consider the many other causes of altered mental status (hypoglycemia, sepsis, drug or other toxins, carbon monoxide poisoning, Wernicke–Korsakoff syndrome, tumor, meningitis, epidural or subdural hematoma, subarachnoid hemorrhage, and dementia). Adulterating liquor with less expensive and potentially lethal substitutes such as isopropanol, methanol, or ethylene glycol should also be considered.

EMERGENCY DEPARTMENT EVALUATION AND MANAGEMENT

Table 190-2 summarizes important aspects of the evaluation. Like all patients with altered mental status, the alcoholic should receive a dex-stick and/or 50–100 mL of 50% dextrose solution, 100 mg of thiamine, and high-flow O_2, as well as naloxone 0.4 to 2 mg if opiates are suspected. Institute appropriate cervical spine immobilization for suspected head, neck, or other major trauma, since inebriated patients have altered pain perception and may be unable to protect the cervical spine. The vital signs, rectal temperature, should be noted. ECG monitoring and a 12-lead ECG may be useful to evaluate for ischemia and signs of electrolyte imbalances such as hypomagnesemia, hypokalemia, and hypocalcemia, which are commonly noted in the alcoholic.

The examination should proceed with a fully disrobed patient, so that trauma is not overlooked. The patient who is not fully alert needs to be serially re-examined; frequently, trauma or progressive illness is not noted on initial examination. Intravenous rehydration should include electrolytes, vitamins, and glucose, since many alcoholics have inadequate glycogen stores and become hypoglycemic with stress. Consider aspiration pneumonia if the patient is obtunded; a chest radiograph should not be based solely on the presence of fever. If the patient is admitted, withdrawal is likely to occur during hospitalization.

TABLE 190-1. Clinical Presentation of Alcohol Abuse

CNS
Inebriation
Seizures
Dementia
Coma
Wernicke-Korsakoff's psychosis
Polyneuropathy

CV
Autonomic dysfunction
Alcoholic congestive myopathy
"Holiday heart"

GI
Alcoholic hepatitis
Alcoholic cirrhosis
Peptic ulcer disease
GI bleeding
Pancreatitis
Pancreatic pseudocyst
Varices and hemorrhoids
Ascites
Malabsorption and malnutrition
Cancers of the GI tract

GU
Uric acid nephropathy
Acute tubular necrosis secondary to
   rhabdomyolysis
Hepatorenal syndrome

Hematologic
Myelosuppression
Coagulopathies
Microcytic anemia
Megaloblastic anemia
Thrombocytopenia

Infectious
Pneumonia
Meningitis
Endocarditis
Cellulitis
Bacteremia
Spontaneous bacterial peritonitis

Metabolic
Ketoacidosis
Electrolyte abnormalities
Vitamin deficiencies

Musculoskeletal
Myopathies
Gout
Rhabdomyolysis

Pulmonary
Sleep apnea
Chronic respiratory insufficiency

The metabolism of ethanol will influence the care. Since ethanol is metabolized via zero-order kinetics, the blood alcohol level can be expected to fall by 15 to 45 mg/dL per hour. The physician can approximate when the patient should theoretically be functional and therefore capable of safe discharge. Knowing the blood alcohol level can be advantageous in observing an intoxicated patient; if the patient does not show appropriate improvement within a reasonable amount of time, then further studies are indicated. This approach helps to avoid the pitfall of failing to diagnose occult trauma, or medical problems such as meningitis and sepsis, in the intoxicated individual.

ALCOHOL WITHDRAWAL

Alcohol withdrawal presents with a spectrum of symptoms ranging from mild abstinence syndrome manifested by minimal tremulousness to the full-blown syndrome of delirium tremens with severe autonomic derangements. The sedative–hypnotics are most efficacious for treating withdrawal: phenobarbital, chlordiazepoxide, diazepam, oxazepam, and lorazepam. Since chlordiazepoxide and diazepam are erratically absorbed when administered intramuscularly, they should not be given via this route. Phenobarbital may be most useful for severe withdrawal, since its anticonvulsant activity lasts much longer than that of the benzodiazepines. In severe withdrawal, the patient may develop delirium tremens with hallucinations, confusion, and insomnia, as well as manifestations of adrenergic excess including agitation, tachycardia, hypertension, tachypnea, tremor, diaphoresis, hyperthermia, and altered mental status.

Large amounts of IV medications may be required; patients in severe withdrawal should be in the ICU and all medications given IV and titrated to normalize the vital signs. Avoid discharging

TABLE 190-2. Laboratory and Radiologic Evaluation

Laboratory	Radiologic
CBC	Chest Radiograph
Cell counts for evaluation of marrow function	Pneumonitis
Indices for folate, iron, pyridoxine, B_{12}	Aspiration
deficiencies	Tuberculosis
Electrolytes/BUN/creat/glucose	Pneumothorax
Anion gap	Fractured ribs/
Hypoglycemia or hyperglycemia	trauma
Renal function	Cardiac size
Electrolyte imbalance	Abdominal radiograph
Calcium/magnesium/phosphorus	Pancreatic
Hypocalcemia	calcifications
Hypomagnesemia	Free air
Hypophosphatemia	Ileus
Hyperphosphatemia	Limb radiograph
Coagulation profile	Fractures
Hepatic insufficiency reflected in elevated PT	Dislocations
and PTT and abnormal liver function	Osteomyelitis
tests	Foreign bodies
Arterial blood gas with co-oximeter	CT Scan
Hypoxemia	Extra-axial
Acid-base disturbances	hemorrhage
Carbon monoxide exposure	Intracerebral
Therapeutic drug monitoring	hemorrhage
Anticonvulsant levels	Intracerebral
ECG	contusion
Arrhythmia	Intra-abdominal
Evidence of electrolyte abnormalities	trauma
Ischemia	
Osborn waves (hypothermia)	
Urinalysis	
Crystalluria	
Myoglobinuria	
Hemoglobinuria	

alcoholics on sedating drugs, since if alcohol is again abused the additive effect of these depressants may contribute to a more severe problem. In addition, sedative–hypnotic drugs have a potential for abuse in their own right. Neuroleptic agents such as the phenothiazines and butyrophenones offer no advantage over the benzodiazepines and phenobarbital and can have potentially serious adverse effects (reduced seizure threshold, promote hyperthermia, dystonic reactions).

Beta blockers and clonidine are effective in treating some of the peripheral signs of adrenergic excess, but they do not prevent central effects such as hallucinosis, agitation, hyperthermia, and seizures. By masking the peripheral signs of withdrawal without modifying the dangerous central effects, they make it difficult to titrate treatment.

WITHDRAWAL SEIZURES

Many studies document the ineffectiveness of phenytoin in treating pure withdrawal seizures. Withdrawal seizures are usually single, grand mal and not sustained. Focal seizures suggest a different etiology. Status epilepticus should not be ascribed to withdrawal. Alcoholics presenting with a first seizure require evaluation before being discharged with a diagnosis of alcohol withdrawal seizures. This should include head CT, lumbar puncture, toxicologic testing, a blood carboxyhemoglobin level, and EEG, as well as others deemed necessary by a neurologic consultant. These patients may benefit from initiation of anticonvulsant treatment after consultation with a neurologist.

HEAD INJURIES

Significant injuries in intoxicated patients are frequently overlooked because of the inebriated state. This is particularly true for head injuries. These patients are distracted, do not have a normal response to pain, and may not express discomfort. They may be abusive, violent, or dirty, and it is easy to attribute their altered mental status to alcohol. The diagnosis of intracranial bleeding may be delayed. Other sources of confusion are carbon monoxide poisoning or hypothermia. When an inebriated-appearing patient presents, a blood alcohol level is useful in determining the need for further diagnostic evaluation for suspected head injury, metabolic derangement, or central nervous system (CNS) infection. A level inconsistent with the level of consciousness suggests that intracranial pathology may be present; a patient with a moderate to high blood alcohol level who does not steadily improve over a reasonably short period of observation is one who is at significant risk. Even if the patient improves, focal neurologic findings, abnormal respiratory patterns, or subtler signs of CNS dysfunction should trigger further evaluation. **An elevated blood alcohol level should never be an excuse for an incomplete evaluation.**

MEDICOLEGAL ISSUES

Since alcoholic patients can be uncooperative, belligerent, or violent, the physician must be familiar with the medicolegal issues involved in their treatment. With the violent patient, the need to protect staff may conflict with the need to evaluate fully a dangerous, agitated patient for serious medical problems. The risk of instituting appropriate and cautious restraint, whether physical or chemical, is much lower than the risk of ignoring potential medical problems or of allowing the patient to leave the ED prematurely and possibly cause injury to himself or others. Measuring the blood alcohol level is useful: if it is low, it should focus attention on other causes of abnormal behavior; if high, it aids in judging the patient's mental competence and ability to care for himself.

The inebriated patient who wants to leave against medical advice, either before or after evaluation and treatment, should be considered analogous to the patient who wants to leave against medical advice but has an altered mental status for other reasons. It is the ED's responsibility to protect patients who are incompetent to make decisions. Blood alcohol levels help document that the patient is under the influence of alcohol and may not be competent. Psychiatric consultation is also often helpful. When in doubt, err on the side of safety and restrain the patient rather than allowing a patient to leave and risk injury or other mishaps. Ideally, the inebriated patient should not be discharged until he is sober and able to think clearly, and until provision has been made for social assistance and appropriate medical follow-up.

COMMON PITFALLS

- Failure to consider that altered mental status may not be due to intoxication
- Failure to fully evaluate an agitated, combative patient
- Failure to restrain an obviously intoxicated but ill or injured patient who is attempting to leave against medical advice
- Failure to check a rectal temperature
- Failure to fully disrobe the patient
- Failure to administer 50% dextrose and thiamine
- Failure to clear the cervical spine in the intoxicated patient with evidence of trauma
- Failure to acknowledge that an adolescent intoxication may be a serious suicide attempt

- Failure to reevaluate the patient frequently
- Failure to check an alcohol level in trauma patients
- Failure to treat withdrawal adequately
- Failure to evaluate for occult infection
- Failure to involve social services
- Failure to evaluate for carbon monoxide poisoning in the obtunded alcoholic.

191 Use of Sonography in Emergency Medicine

CHOLELITHIASIS/CHOLECYSTITIS

Sonography (US) has changed the diagnostic approach to biliary tract disease; the diagnosis of gallbladder calculi can be accomplished with an accuracy of 90%–95%. However, gallstones in the patient with right upper quadrant pain is not the equivalent of a diagnosis of acute cholecystitis. Since only about one third with clinical features of acute cholecystitis will, in fact, prove to have an acutely inflamed gallbladder, it is important to separate those with asymptomatic calculi from the patients with acute cholecystitis and cholelithiasis. The normal gallbladder wall measures <3 mm, but wall thickening is a non-specific sign of acute cholecystitis and may be seen in a variety of conditions, including non-fasting patients, hepatitis, hypoalbumenemia, ascites, and cirrhosis. Pericholecystic fluid collections are highly specific for acute cholecystitis, although false positives can result from a perforated peptic ulcer or loculated ascites. US is the imaging procedure of choice for acute calculous cholecystitis. The sensitivity of US for the detection of acalculous cholecystitis is only 67%, and cholescintigraphy is often employed. Cholescintigraphy with ^{99m}Tc-IDA derivatives has a sensitivity and specificity of 95% in acute cholecystitis, but can take 2–24 hours to complete, whereas US can be accomplished with minimal delay. The choice between these modalities should be largely dependent on the time and local expertise available.

ABDOMINAL AORTIC ANEURYSM

US detects abdominal aortic aneurysms with almost 100% sensitivity. US can not only detect the aneurysm, but also can reliably measure the AP diameter. An AP diameter exceeding 30 mm is considered diagnostic of an aneurysm. The imaging of types I and II thoracic aortic dissections is beyond the capability of US.

TESTICULAR TORSION

The acutely painful or swollen scrotum requires immediate diagnosis and treatment. Scintigraphy relies on the physiologic parameter of a change in blood flow to diagnose acute scrotal conditions, and has a reported sensitivity of 95% and specificity approaching 100% in detecting acute torsion and differentiating it from epididymitis. Sonography depicts the anatomic contents of the scrotum, and can accurately demonstrate a broad range of abnormalities of the scrotum and its contents. The scan is best performed with high-resolution, real-time equipment, causes no discomfort, and is a relatively quick and easy procedure. US has been more useful in the chronic or missed torsion 1 to 10 days after the onset of symptoms. The combination of scintigraphy and

US has been shown to change the diagnosis and improve the clinical management when compared to scintigraphy alone. Doppler US has been utilized in the diagnosis of torsion, but its interpretation is more difficult. In blunt trauma, US is useful in assessing for testicular rupture.

OTHER APPLICATIONS

Doppler sonography in the diagnosis of flow disorders in both the arterial and deep venous system are available. The diagnosis of thrombosis of the deep veins of the calf is possible through either conventional, Doppler, or color flow Doppler mapping. Superficial radiolucent foreign bodies can frequently be demonstrated at US, and superficial clot or infection can be seen using the newer high resolution linear array systems. Sonography is particularly useful in the pediatric population in the diagnosis of hypertrophic pyloric stenosis as well as intracranial hemorrhage in the neonatal intensive care unit setting.

OBSTETRICS AND GYNECOLOGIC DISORDERS

Sonography has a vital role in the detection of ectopic pregnancy. It also can distinguish the variety of disorders that may be associated with first trimester bleeding. In the latter stages of pregnancy, placenta previa or abruption can be identified accurately. In the patient with pelvic pain, sonography can detect findings associated with adnexal torsion.

ECTOPIC PREGNANCY AND OTHER FIRST TRIMESTER DISORDERS   Sonography has a pivotal role in the evaluation of the patient with suspected ectopic pregnancy. First, by identification of a gestational sac within the uterus as early as 4 to 5 weeks' menstrual age, sonography can exclude the possibility of an ectopic pregnancy. Transvaginal sonography is particularly helpful in identifying the normal gestational sac associated with a normal intrauterine pregnancy as well as the adnexal mass and other findings associated with ectopic pregnancy. Transvaginal sonography can usually delineate the presence of adnexal mass in ectopic pregnancy.

Sonography can diagnose molar pregnancy as early as 10 to 12 weeks.

PLACENTA PREVIA   Transabdominal sonography and transvaginal sonography can establish placenta previa.

ADNEXAL TORSION   Adnexal torsion typically occurs when there is mass or significant enlargement of the ovary. In the early stages of adnexal torsion, the ovary enlarges and appears edematous. With torsion of a few days' duration, there typically is a collection of fluid within the cul-de-sac. Adnexal torsion occurs when there is a hemorrhagic mass within the ovary.

SECTION VI

PEDIATRICS

PART I

Pediatric Resuscitation

192   Newborn Resuscitation

Most newborns require no resuscitation. Of the few who need intervention, the majority require only oxygen, stimulation, and warming. Most of the remaining infants will respond to bag–valve–mask ventilation. Only very few infants will require chest compressions and endotracheal intubation, and an even smaller number will require vascular access and administration of drugs for successful resuscitation.

The most important parameter to monitor in a resuscitation is the heart rate. Because the newborn has a relatively fixed stroke volume, bradycardia results in poor cardiac output. Airway intervention and, if unsuccessful, pharmacologic intervention is initiated to raise the heart rate. Pulselessness mandates cardiopulmonary resuscitation (CPR) in the older child, but in a newborn the relative bradycardia of 60 with pulses present requires CPR. In the ED, the heart rate should be monitored manually by palpating the brachial artery or the proximal end of the umbilical cord. Rarely is there time or accessible equipment to monitor the heart rate with ECG equipment. For the same reason, blood pressure measurements are difficult to obtain and unnecessary as a guide to ED resuscitation.

Heart rate and respiratory status should serve as the guides to successive steps of resuscitation.

RESUSCITATION

As soon as the infant is born, the umbilical cord should be clamped and cut and the baby placed on the resuscitation table under the radiant warmer. A rapid assessment of color, respiratory effort, and heart rate should be made immediately. The pulse can be easily palpated at the base of the umbilical cord or the brachial artery. Drying the baby provides gentle stimulation to breathe and reduces heat loss by evaporation. For the healthy neonate who is moving actively and has a vigorous cry, suctioning of secretions in the nares and mouth with a bulb syringe is sufficient.

The distressed neonate should be placed supine in a slight Trendelenburg position with the head in midline. If the infant remains cyanotic, or the rate and depth of respirations do not increase with drying and stimulation, oxygen should be given and the pulse monitored. If assisted ventilation is required, positive-pressure ventilation should be given with a bag and mask at 40 per minute. Such ventilation should provide adequate and equal chest expansion and bilateral breath sounds. If adequate chest expansion cannot be achieved, the infant's head should be repositioned and ventilation attempted again. It is important to ensure a good seal between the mask and the infant's face. Bag and mask ventilation may produce gastric distention, which can compromise diaphragmatic excursion. Stomach decompression with a nasogastric tube may be necessary.

645

If the infant resumes effective spontaneous respirations following assisted ventilation and if the heart rate remains above 100 beats per minute, positive-pressure ventilation may be discontinued. It may be necessary to provide gentle tactile stimulation to ensure continued spontaneous respirations. If the infant's heart rate is 60 to 100 bpm and rising after 15 to 30 seconds of assisted ventilation, positive-pressure ventilation should continue (Table 192-1). Chest compressions will not be necessary unless the heart rate falls, but they should be started if the heart rate remains less than 60 bpm, or when it is less than 80 bpm and does not rise despite adequate ventilation with 100% oxygen for 30 seconds. The sternum should be compressed 120 times per minute to a depth of 1/2 inch to 3/4 inch. Compressions should be accompanied by positive-pressure ventilation at a rate of 40 to 60 breaths per minute. (For an older child, a ratio of five chest compressions per ventilation is maintained, but this is not advocated for neonatal CPR.) Compressions and ventilations may be performed simultaneously and need not be synchronized.

Endotracheal intubation will be necessary whenever bag–mask ventilation is ineffective, when tracheal suction is necessary, or when prolonged positive-pressure ventilation is required. Following intubation, proper tube placement should be ensured using physical examination and chest radiograph. Chest expansion should be equal and adequate bilaterally when hand ventilation is provided.

Pharmacologic support is necessary if the infant's heart rate remains less than 80 bpm following ventilation with 100% oxygen (Table 192-2). Sodium bicarbonate should be given only during prolonged resuscitation to correct documented metabolic acidosis. Epinephrine is indicated for asystole, or for a heart rate <80 bpm despite adequate ventilation with 100% oxygen. A dose of 0.1–0.3 mL/kg of 1:10,000 solution should be given intravenously or through the endotracheal tube. If the endotracheal tube is used, epinephrine should be diluted with 1 or 2 mL of normal saline (Table 192-3). The drug may be given every 5 minutes during resuscitation.

POSTRESUSCITATION

Assume that until proven otherwise any infant who has been resuscitated prior to ED arrival has an airway complication. It is very easy for a tube to become dislodged or plugged and for pneumothoraces to be produced by overzealous ventilation. Always check

---

TABLE 192-1. Indications for Assisted Positive-Pressure Ventilation

1. Apnea unresponsive to drying, stimulation and suctioning.
2. Heart rate < 100/min.
3. Persistent central cyanois with 100% O_2.

Indications for Intubation

1. When bag-mask ventilation is ineffective.
2. When tracheal suctioning is necessary (e.g., meconium aspiration)
3. When prolonged positive-pressure ventilation is anticipated.

Indications for Chest Compression

1. Heart rate < 60/min.
2. Heart rate < 80/min and not rising despite provision of adequate ventilation with 100% O_2 for 30 seconds or more. (These values are guidelines and in the emergency department setting clinical judgment should be exercised).

Indication for Medications

1. Heart rate < 80/min following adequate ventilation with 100% O_2.

TABLE 192-2. Resuscitation Drug/Equipment Card

Indication for Medications:

HR 80, *after* adequate CPR and ventilation with 100% O_2

Resuscitation Drug Doses

DRUG	CONCENTRATION	DOSE
Epinephrine	1:10,000 (0.1 mg/mL)	0.01 mg/kg
Sodium bicarbonate	1 mEq/mL	2 mEq/kg

Formula for Bicarbonate Calculation

mEq Na HCO_3 = 0.3 x weight (kg) x base deficit (mEq/L)

CPR

Compression rate	120/min
Ventilation rate	40–60/min
Depth	1/2–3/4 inch

---

these immediately when the infant arrives in the ED. Transfer the neonate, once stabilized, to the nursery as soon as possible. Obtain the following laboratory data on all postresuscitation infants who will remain in the ED for any period of time: Hemoglobin and hematocrit, Arterial blood gas, Dextrostix. Obtain a chest radiograph to assess tube placement and the possibility of pneumothorax.

SPECIAL CONCERNS AND TECHNIQUES

POSITIONING, SUCTIONING, STIMULATION   Due to the suddenness of the resuscitation, it is often impossible to set up adequate wall suction. Manual suction with a bulb syringe or DeLee suction trap is preferred and the complications of excessive wall suction pressures can be avoided.

TEMPERATURE REGULATION   It is critical to maintain adequate temperature. The alert, active infant should be dried promptly and wrapped in a warm blanket. In depressed or immature infants who may have asphyxiated or have reduced energy stores, an overhead radiant warmer helps maintain body temperature while allowing access to the infant during resuscitation.

BAG–VALVE–MASK VENTILATION   Tidal volumes in small and premature newborn infants are small compared to older children and adults. Many iatrogenic problems, such as pneumothorax, are caused by overzealous bagging of infants. Begin bag–valve ventilation with very small volumes and rapidly increase the tidal volume, through small increments, until adequate tidal volume (as measured by a chest rise) is achieved. A tight seal during bag–valve–mask ventilation is imperative.

INTUBATION FOR MECONIUM ASPIRATION   Meconium aspiration is the other indication for intubation. The DeLee suction catheter or manual suction through the endotracheal tube are preferred. Particulate or thick meconium should always be removed, but thin meconium need not be suctioned directly from the trachea.

VASCULAR ACCESS   When vascular access is needed, employ the umbilical vein using sterile technique.

PNEUMOTHORAX   A pneumothorax is not uncommon but can be difficult to diagnose. The pneumothorax can be released by inserting a needle or catheter into the fifth intercostal space in the mid-axillary line.

TABLE 192-3. Drug Dosages and Equipment Sizes

Size	Epinephrine		Sodium Bicarbonate*		ET Tube/Suction Catheter	Laryngoscope Blade
	Dose	Vol	Dose	Vol		
Small (1.0–2.0 kg)	0.01–0.02 mg	0.1–0.2 mL	2.0–4.0 mEq	2.0–4.0 mL	2.5/5F	0
Medium (2.0–3.0 kg)	0.02–0.3 mg	0.2–0.3 mL	4.0–6.0 mEq	4.0–6.0 mL	3.0/8F	0–1
Large (3.0–4.0 kg)	0.03–0.04 mg	0.3–0.4 mL	6.0–8.0 mEq	6.0–8.0 mL	3.5/8F	0–1

*Dilute 1:1 with sterile H_2O

193   Resuscitation in Children

Childhood cardiopulmonary arrest is most often the final result of respiratory failure or arrest. The outcome of isolated respiratory failure is much better than combined cardiac and pulmonary failure. **The primary focus in childhood cardiorespiratory arrest is the respiratory system.** Children rarely experience primary ventricular fibrillation. Children also manifest differences consisting of size-dependent variables.

EMERGENCY DEPARTMENT MANAGEMENT
AIRWAY

The cornerstone of any pediatric resuscitative attempt is adequate, timely airway management. Positioning the infant requires careful attention to the tendency of the prominent occiput, which can cause neck flexion and airway occlusion. Mild extension of the head to achieve the "sniffing" position will provide airway patency. Overextension may cause airway obstruction by compressing the pliant trachea. The large tongue–mandible complex may still occlude the airway, even with proper head–neck position. When hypotonia occurs, the mandible will no longer be maintained in a stable open position by the child, so the tongue will fall against the posterior pharyngeal wall into a stable closed position. Chin lift or jaw thrust will open the airway. Nasopharyngeal tubes for conscious children or oropharyngeal airways in unconscious patients may be helpful once the airway has been opened manually. When the airway cannot be maintained or other indications exist, an oral endotracheal tube may need to be inserted. If intubation is indicated, preparations for this procedure should be started while the child is being properly positioned and oxygenated. A bag-valve-mask device can provide ventilation until intubation preparations are complete. In general, a straight blade is preferable in children <5 years of age; the curved blade should be used for older children. Endotracheal tubes without cuffs should be used in children <7 or 8 years of age since the cricoid ring is small enough to produce an air seal.

The appropriately sized endotracheal tube can be found by using a table of approximate sizes. These tables require an accurate age or weight estimation for access to appropriately sized equipment. Two additional tubes should be available, one-half size smaller and one-half size larger. The child's small finger can serve as an approximation of his or her tracheal diameter. Length has been shown to be the most accurate predictor of correct endotracheal tube size. The Broselow Tape (a length-based tape) provides accurate equipment selection as well as resuscitation drug doses with single length measurement. Endotracheal tubes are easily dislodged from the trachea, so be wary of tube movement and carefully secure the tube in position. Holding the tube and the corner of the mouth together until the tube is taped or otherwise held in position usually maintains this security. An endotracheal vapor cloud may be seen and apparent breath sounds may be heard even with esophageal intubation, especially in small infants. The *sine qua non* of proper endotracheal tube placement is a patient whose vital signs improve, whose chest rises, and whose tissue perfusion improves. If the patient does not improve or if doubt exists, tube position must be checked by direct visualization using a laryngoscope.

BREATHING

Proper bag–valve–mask use demands a good mask—face seal with an appropriately sized mask and the use of a bag that allows the provider to supply the necessary tidal volume. The mask must fit over the nose and mouth without compressing the eyes (which may lead to vagal-induced brady-cardia) and without extending beyond the chin. A self-inflating bag is used most commonly. Overventilation may lead to unilateral or bilateral pneumothoraces; underventilation will lead to carbon dioxide retention and respiratory acidosis. Whether using a mask or endotracheal tube, the clinician should provide a tidal volume that causes the chest to rise. A pop-off valve, if present, allows for a preset maximum inspiratory pressure. Additional tidal volume can be delivered at higher pressures by holding a finger on the valve while delivering the breath with the self-expanding bag. Ideally, an in-line manometer should be used to monitor peak inspiratory pressure. Resting tidal volume in children and adults is 5 to 7 mL/kg, while ventilatory supported tidal volume may be 10 to 15 mL/kg. Rather than calculating a value, pay attention to lung and chest-wall compliance while bagging, and vary the volume according to chest rise. Resuscitation bags with 500-mL capacity should be used for infants and small children. Adolescents require 750-mL bags.

CIRCULATION

Adequacy of circulation is a clinical determination. The primary indication for assisting circulation with chest compressions is pulselessness. In newborns, chest compressions are also indicated when the heart rate remains <60 bpm despite effective airway intervention.

Compression rate varies with age because cardiac output in neonates and infants depends principally on rate: in the newborn, 100–120 per minute, older children and adults, 80 to 100 per minute. Compression depth should be sufficient to produce a brachial and femoral pulse.

Vascular access in the infant or small child can be obtained in the dorsal hand veins, superficial veins on the dorsum of the foot, antecubital veins of the forearm, superficial scalp veins, the external jugular veins, and the femoral vein in the inguinal canal. Once the airway is patent and maintained, any one or more of these sites may be used. Both the external jugular vein and the femoral vein may provide passage to the central venous circulation through guide wire and long-line insertion. These procedures should not be first-line attempts; rather, short, reasonably large-bore cannulas should be placed first. When the patient is stable, these lines can be replaced under more controlled conditions.

An alternate site is the bone marrow. Intraosseous cannulation can be accomplished using either the distal femur or the proximal tibia. All the drugs of resuscitation, as well as needed fluids for volume resuscitation, may be given intraosseously.

For drug administration, either the endotracheal or the bone marrow route is valid, although appropriate doses, dilutions, and intervals have not been identified for pediatric use. The dose for endotracheal epinephrine is 0.1 mg/kg of the 1:1000 concentration. All other drugs given via the ET should have their doses increased. Epinephrine, with both alpha and beta receptor action, is a potent medication to help reverse cardiac collapse. The cardiac beta action may improve output when heart rate is slow. Epinephrine is often used in neonates and young infants to accelerate heart rate. Epinephrine is indicated for the treatment of symptomatic bradycardia associated with poor systemic perfusion or pulseless arrest. Epinephrine remains the first line drug for resuscitation. For bradycardia, the following is advised: all IV/IO doses: 0.01 mg/kg (1:10,000); all ET doses: 0.1 mg/kg (1:1,000). For pulseless arrest, first IV/IO dose: 0.01 mg/kg (1:10,000); all ET doses: 0.1 mg/kg (1:1,000); second and subsequent IV/IO/ET doses: 0.1 mg/kg (1:1,000); IV/IO doses as high as 0.2 mg/kg may be effective; administer every 3–5 minutes during arrest.

Atropine is the standard parasympatholytic drug used in cardiorespiratory arrest. Atropine increases heart rate; dose is 0.01 to 0.02 mg/kg, with a minimum of 0.1 mg in even the smallest infant. It may be given every 5 minutes to a maximum of 1.0 mg in the child <1 year and 2 mg in the older child. The maximum individual dose in any child is 1 mg. Atropine may also be given endotracheally or via the bone marrow.

Glucose: in infants and small children, glucose is readily exhausted during stress. Accucheck should be done on all critically ill children. If needed, glucose can be given intravenously or intraosseously in a dose of 2 to 4 mL/kg of 25% dextrose in water. Because dextrose concentrations over 12.5% may cause loss of integrity of small peripheral veins, it should be given in as large a vein as possible.

Sodium bicarbonate is the principal agent used to ameliorate metabolic acidosis. During CPR, sodium bicarbonate should be given intravenously or through the bone marrow only after the airway is patent and maintained, hyperventilation is ongoing, and cardiac compressions are being performed with suitable forward blood flow.

The dose of sodium bicarbonate is 1 mEq/kg of the 8.4% solution. In the neonate, the dose is the same but the solution should be 4.2%. Ideally, bicarbonate should be given according to the child's acid–base status, but if arterial blood gas measurements are unavailable the first dose can be given after the first dose of epinephrine and repeated in 10-minute intervals at a dose of 0.5 mEq/kg.

Electrical dysfunction of cardiac muscle in childhood is most often secondary to respiratory failure. Also, the arrhythmias noted differ from those of the adult cardiac arrest victim: they are more recalcitrant to therapy since they tend to occur in circumstances of respiratory acidosis and hypoxia. The most common rhythm disturbance is sinus bradycardia. It will respond to adequate ventilation and oxygenation, if given early enough, and rarely requires medication. Sinus tachycardia is also seen and may be the earliest sign of impending cardiopulmonary arrest. If cardiac dysfunction includes the rhythms associated with cardiovascular collapse (asystole, electrical mechanical dissociation, ventricular fibrillation, and rarely ventricular tachycardia without pulses) the patient should be treated just as the adult. (See the management algorithms shown in Figures 193-1 and 193-2.)

Electrical conversion of cardiac rhythms associated with collapse in the pediatric patient should follow the guidelines accepted for adult patients; only the dose of electrical energy changes. Suggested energy levels for paroxysmal atrial tachycardia (PAT) are 0.25 J/kg to 1 J/kg, while delivered energy for ventricular fibrillation or pulseless ventricular tachycardia starts at 2 J/kg. Use appropriate-sized paddles and place them in appropriate position. The recommended paddle size for small children is 4.5 cm in diameter and up to 8 cm in diameter in larger children and adolescents. If only large paddles are available, place them in the anterior-posterior position. Regardless of position, ensure that proper conducting medium is used with full paddle contact on the chest wall.

Summary: Assess the child for hypothermia or hyperthermia, hypoglycemia or hyperglycemia, and alterations in oxygen, potassium, calcium, sodium, and magnesium. Correct acid–base alterations rapidly. Treat mechanical causes, such as hypovolemia due to dehydration, cardiac tamponade, tension pneumothorax, endotracheal tube obstruction or misplacement, and assorted other causes for the collapsed state.

Bradycardia Decision Tree
Pediatric Advanced Life Support

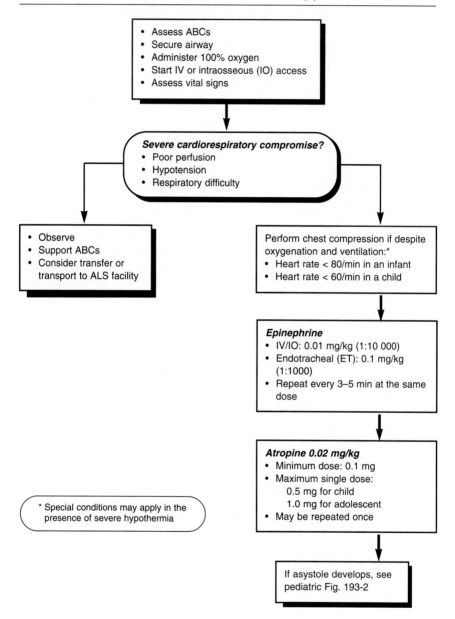

- Assess ABCs
- Secure airway
- Administer 100% oxygen
- Start IV or intraosseous (IO) access
- Assess vital signs

Severe cardiorespiratory compromise?
- Poor perfusion
- Hypotension
- Respiratory difficulty

- Observe
- Support ABCs
- Consider transfer or transport to ALS facility

Perform chest compression if despite oxygenation and ventilation:*
- Heart rate < 80/min in an infant
- Heart rate < 60/min in a child

Epinephrine
- IV/IO: 0.01 mg/kg (1:10 000)
- Endotracheal (ET): 0.1 mg/kg (1:1000)
- Repeat every 3–5 min at the same dose

Atropine 0.02 mg/kg
- Minimum dose: 0.1 mg
- Maximum single dose:
  0.5 mg for child
  1.0 mg for adolescent
- May be repeated once

* Special conditions may apply in the presence of severe hypothermia

If asystole develops, see pediatric Fig. 193-2

Figure 193-1. *(Figures 193-1 and 193-2:* Standards and guidelines for cardiopulmonary resuscitation and emergency care. JAMA 1992 June; 268:2171–2302. Copyright 1992, American Medical Association. Reprinted with permission.)

Asystole and Pulseless Arrest Decision Tree
Pediatric Advanced Life Support

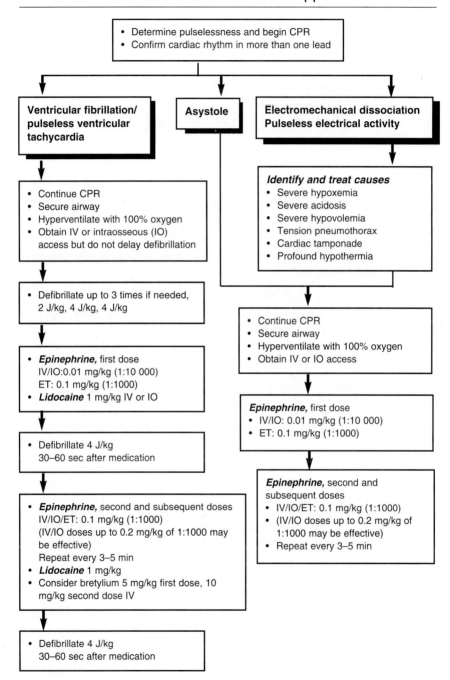

- Determine pulselessness and begin CPR
- Confirm cardiac rhythm in more than one lead

**Ventricular fibrillation/
pulseless ventricular
tachycardia**

Asystole

**Electromechanical dissociation
Pulseless electrical activity**

- Continue CPR
- Secure airway
- Hyperventilate with 100% oxygen
- Obtain IV or intraosseous (IO)
  access but do not delay defibrillation

Identify and treat causes
- Severe hypoxemia
- Severe acidosis
- Severe hypovolemia
- Tension pneumothorax
- Cardiac tamponade
- Profound hypothermia

- Defibrillate up to 3 times if needed,
  2 J/kg, 4 J/kg, 4 J/kg

- Continue CPR
- Secure airway
- Hyperventilate with 100% oxygen
- Obtain IV or IO access

- ***Epinephrine,*** first dose
  IV/IO:0.01 mg/kg (1:10 000)
  ET: 0.1 mg/kg (1:1000)
- ***Lidocaine*** 1 mg/kg IV or IO

Epinephrine, first dose
- IV/IO: 0.01 mg/kg (1:10 000)
- ET: 0.1 mg/kg (1:1000)

- Defibrillate 4 J/kg
  30–60 sec after medication

Epinephrine, second and
subsequent doses
- IV/IO/ET: 0.1 mg/kg (1:1000)
- (IV/IO doses up to 0.2 mg/kg of
  1:1000 may be effective)
- Repeat every 3–5 min

- ***Epinephrine,*** second and subsequent doses
  IV/IO/ET: 0.1 mg/kg (1:1000)
  (IV/IO doses up to 0.2 mg/kg of 1:1000 may
  be effective)
  Repeat every 3–5 min
- ***Lidocaine*** 1 mg/kg
- Consider bretylium 5 mg/kg first dose, 10
  mg/kg second dose IV

- Defibrillate 4 J/kg
  30–60 sec after medication

Fig. 193–2.

PART II

Presenting Signs and Symptoms in the Pediatric Patient

194 Pediatric Anaphylaxis

CLINICAL PRESENTATION

Most fatalities result from respiratory failure secondary to inadequate control of the airway or insufficient alveolar gas exchange. Respiratory failure may result from upper airway obstruction due to mucosal edema, bronchospasm of small airways, and hypersecretion of mucus. Consequently, patients may be tachypneic with grunting and may have intercostal and subcostal retractions. They may have nasal flaring and may be using accessory muscles of respiration. However, if the episode has progressed long enough, compensations may have already failed; the child then is close to cardiopulmonary arrest. Children may be restless, anxious, and unconsolable. Pain at the site of injection of insect venom or medication may cause the child to cry, but incipient anaphylaxis will cause systemic findings out of proportion to the pain. Sweating, sneezing, coughing, rhinorrhea, and urinary and fecal incontinence may also occur. Cardiac rhythm disturbances may occur; tachycardia is the most common.

Because small children rarely have vasovagal reactions, bradycardia should signify impending cardiac collapse. Tachypnea, tachycardia with weak central and/or peripheral pulses, stridor, wheezing, rales, vomiting, and diarrhea in a child who was well minutes before requires the clinician to act immediately. Many reactions occur within seconds to minutes after exposure. Most occur within 30 minutes, but some may not occur for 2 to 8 hours. Resolution of signs and symptoms usually begins promptly with therapy; the attack may completely resolve within minutes. Some children will slowly improve over 12 to 36 hours, even with continued therapy. Bronchospasm may take several days to resolve fully.

EMERGENCY DEPARTMENT MANAGEMENT

Prevention: a complete history regarding an allergic reaction is imperative before prescribing any potentially anaphylaxis-generating drug or procedure. In patients with severe systemic anaphylaxis (i.e., major features), obtain vascular access and provide immediate therapy. Stabilize the airway and rapidly identify and treat laryngeal spasm or edema, shock, and cardiac dysfunction. Anaphylaxis can be classified in terms of any minor, major, and late features (Table 194-1). When only minor features are present and there is no progression to any major signs, the child may

TABLE 194-1. Manifestations of Anaphylaxis

	Target Organ	Dysfunction
Minor	Eye	Pruritus, tearing, conjunctival edema
	Nose	Rhinitis, congestion, sneezing
	Skin	Sweating, urticaria, rash, flush, angioedema
	Gastrointestinal	Nausea, vomiting, abdominal pain, diarrhea, increased gastric secretion
	Neurologic	Dizziness, syncope, lethargy, fear of impending doom, metallic taste, headache
Major	Respiratory	Common: Laryngeal edema, bronchospasm Uncommon: Hemoptysis, pulmonary edema
	Cardiac	Common: Shock, tachycardia, arrhythmia, capillary leak Uncommon: Congestive heart failure, disseminated intravascular coagulation
	Neurologic	Common: Prolonged unconsciousness, seizures Late: Headache
	Gastrointestinal	Common: Hematemesis, melena, bloody diarrhea

require only subcutaneous epinephrine. Intravenous fluids with or without H_1 and H_2 histamine receptor blocking agents may also be used (Tables 194-2 and 194-3).

If histamine blocking agents are used, they may be given by mouth or intravenously. Diphenhydramine (5 mg/kg/day divided q 6–8 hours) can be given as outpatient therapy for a minor reaction. An observation period of at least 24 hours is appropriate, since late sequelae may manifest 8 to 24 hours following the initial reaction. For intravenous antihistamine therapy, diphenhydramine can be given at 1 mg/kg/dose and H_2 histamine receptors can be blocked with ranitidine at 1 mg/kg initially. If intravenous antihistamines are used, the child should be admitted, preferably to the ICU. In addition to volume resuscitation and oxygen, epinephrine is the drug of choice if a major feature of the anaphylactic reaction occurs.

Any child given epinephrine should be admitted to an intensive-care setting for observation. Epinephrine can be given subcutaneously, intramuscularly, intravenously, in intraosseous bolus or infusion, as well as via the endotracheal route. The usual subcutaneous or intramuscular dose of epinephrine is 0.01 mg/kg of 1:1000 concentration. The subcutaneous or intramuscular route should be used for patients with minor reactions. The subcutaneous or intramuscular route can also be used before placement of intravenous or intraosseous vascular access. Intravenous or intraosseous epinephrine is the mainstay of therapy when laryngeal spasm/edema and/or shock are present. If the patient requires endotracheal intubation, epinephrine can be given endotracheally. The intravenous, intraosseous, or endotracheal dose of epinephrine is 0.01 mg/kg of the 1:10,000 solution. Epinephrine may need to be continued as an infusion, along with continued fluid resuscitation (0.1 µg/kg/min) titrated up to 1 to 1.5 µg/kg/min. Epinephrine infusions should be given through central venous access. For intravenous or intraosseous infusion, epinephrine can be mixed as follows: $0.6 \times$ wt (in kg) to make 100 mL of solution; run at 1 mL/hr provides 0.1 µg/kg/min infusion rate.

TABLE 194-2. Signs and Symptoms of Anaphylactic Shock

Time	Symptoms	Signs	Therapy
0–2 min	Nasal congestion, dyspnea Syncope, fainting	Mucosal edema, laryngeal stridor, vocal cord edema, hypotension	Epinephrine SQ, epinephrine SQ, IM, IV, oxygen, airway control Fluid resuscitation, epinephrine IM, epinephrine IV, oxygen, airway control, Trendelenburg position, tourniquet, site infiltration with epinephrine
	Cardiac arrest	Asystole, electromechanical dysfunction, ventricular fibrillation, no pulses, no respirations	Pediatric Advanced Life Support procedures, CPR
2–5 min	Cough, wheeze, chest discomfort Pruritis, hives Nonpruritic swelling (face, hands, feet); ocular itching, tearing	Cough, wheeze, rales, tachypnea, respiratory distress Urticarial lesions Asystemic edema Conjunctival inflammation	Epinephrine SQ,, inhaled beta-agonists, oxygen Epinephrine SQ,, H_1 and H_2 histamine blockers PO, IV Epinephrine SQ,, H_1 and H_2 histamine blockers PO, IV Epinephrine SQ,, H_1 and H_2 histamine blockers PO, IV
2–5 min to >5 min*	Nausea, vomiting, abdominal pain, diarrhea		Epinephrine SQ,, H_1 and H_2 histamine blockers PO, IV

*If bronchospasm, laryngeal edema, and hypotension persist for >5 min, in addition to IV fluids, pressors, and beta-agonists consider hydrocortisone 1.5–5 mg/kg initially followed by 1–2 mg/kg IV q 4–6 hr for 24–36 hr.

TABLE 194-3. Drugs Used in Treatment of Anaphylaxis

Time	Drug	Dose	Frequency	Route*
0–2 min	Epinephrine	0.01 mg/kg of 1:1000	q 15–20 min	SQ, IM
	Oxygen	100%	Continuous	As tolerated
	(Consider venous and lymphatic obstructing tourniquet proximal to injection site. Consider infiltration of epinephrine with half of above dose at antigen site.)			
2–5 min	Diphenhydramine	1 mg/kg	q 4–6 hr	IV
	Ranitidine	1 mg/kg	q 6 hr	IV
	(If shock is present or persistent, consider infusions of dopamine 5–20 μg/kg/min, L-norepinephrine 1–3 μg/kg/min, epinephrine 0.1–1.0 μg/kg/min. If bronchospasms present or persistent, consider inhaled beta-agonists: Albuterol 2.5 mg/dose, terbutaline 1–2 mg/dose.)			
Beyond 5 min	Hydrocortisone	1.5–5 mg/kg	q 6 hr	IV
	(Continue IV infusions and inhaled beta-agonists if reaction persists. Transfer to pediatric intensive care unit for continued inpatient care. Consider epinephrine bolus IV at 0.01 mg/kg of 1:10,000 dilution if hypotension/shock is unresponsive to prior measures.)			

*All drugs listed for IV infusion or bolus can also be given intraosseously.

Special circumstances (such as bronchospasm not responsive to epinephrine, severe progressive edema, pulmonary edema, disseminated intravascular coagulopathy, or persistent hypotension) require additional therapy beyond fluids, epinephrine, and oxygen. Bronchospasm can be treated with inhaled or intravenous adrenergic agonists and corticosteroids. Shock unresponsive to volume loading and epinephrine infusion may respond to dopamine or L-norepinephrine. Trendelenburg position and medical antishock trousers may also be required. Drugs such as epinephrine, L-norepinephrine, or dopamine must be used with appropriate monitoring.

Children on beta antagonists will respond differently to the usual therapeutic maneuvers; use great care in treating these children. Glucagon may be beneficial in these patients.

Corticosteroids are of benefit for prolonged attacks. Hydrocortisone can be given at 1.5 mg/kg to 5.0 mg/kg initially and continued for 24 to 48 hours at 5-hour intervals. Methylprednisone has also been used at an initial dose of 1 mg/kg up to 30 mg/kg.

DISPOSITION

Anaphylaxis can be, and usually is, rapidly progressive; with proper therapy, it can be rapidly reversed and the child can be stabilized. Occasionally it is slow in onset, and the reaction then is also slow to reverse, even with proper treatment. Most children can be discharged with proper instruction and prescriptions for H_1-blocking antihistamines; they should be observed long enough to assure that no further immediate therapy is needed. Remember that late reactions may occur 8 to 24 hours after the initial inciting stimulus. Document instructions to parents on the record; indicate the need for follow-up evaluation with the child's pediatrician.

The child who has had a severe life-threatening anaphylactic reaction, regardless of how easily controlled or how rapidly reversed, should be admitted to a pediatric ICU. This child is at increased risk of exacerbation of the reaction. The child who responds slowly to therapy should also be transferred to an ICU. This child may require large volumes of fluid (30–80 mL/kg or more), continuous infusions of catecholamines, airway control, and ventilator management. If poor response continues, pulmonary artery catheterization has been advocated. Although subcutaneous epinephrine before intravenous or intraosseous administration may reverse laryngeal edema if circulation is adequate, do not rely on it in cardiovascular collapse.

195   Fever of Acute Onset in Children

Fever accounts for 25% of pediatric ED visits. Age and the presence or absence of an identifiable source of infection are important.

CLINICAL PRESENTATION

A rectal or oral temperature of 38°C defines fever. Axillary temperatures are unreliable and should not be used. Although the height of the temperature bears some relationship to the severity of illness, the relationship is too weak to greatly affect clinical decision-making to any great extent. This is particularly true if a patient has received antipyretics within 4 hours before the ED visit, because the degree of fever *response* to antipyretic therapy bears no relationship to severity of illness. Therefore, the fact that the fever is lower after antipyretics should not decrease the extent of the work-up. Table 195-1 lists key presenting signs and symptoms.

TABLE 195-1. Key Historic and Physical Findings Relevant to the Evaluation of the Acutely Febrile Infant or Child*

History

Behavior	Intermittently playful, irritable when moved (sign of meningitis), fluid intake
Respiratory symptoms	Cough, difficulty breathing
GI symptoms	Vomiting, diarrhea (with blood or mucus)
Renal symptoms	Abdominal pain, dysuria, frequency, urgency
Other	Pain (limp, sore throat, earache, abdominal pain), rash, urine output, chronic illness, exposures

Physical Examination

General appearance	Activity, eye contact, muscle tone, color, consolability, vocalization, hydration
Respiratory	Grunting, respiratory rate, rales, bronchial breath sounds (often the only auscultatory finding in infants with pneumonia), retracting
HEENT	Fontanelle, adenopathy, meningismus, pharyngitis, otitis (bulging, decreased mobility—redness only is not sufficient to diagnose otitis)
CV	Peripheral perfusion, murmur, heart rate
Abdomen	Tenderness or organomegaly, CVA tenderness
Skin	Rash (diffuse erythema, petechiae, erythema of the mucous membranes and palms [Kawasaki's disease])
Musculoskeletal	Bone/joint tenderness, swelling or erythema

*Of necessity, the emergency department evaluation of the febrile child is a *focused* evaluation. Therefore, the clinician is not necessarily expected to pursue every aspect of the above work-up. If, for example, there is clear upper respiratory symptomatology, it would not be time-effective to pursue signs and symptoms of urinary tract infection.

DIFFERENTIAL DIAGNOSIS

The challenge is to recognize the subtle signs of meningitis, pneumonia, and sepsis/bacteremia.

EMERGENCY DEPARTMENT MANAGEMENT AND DISPOSITION

See Table 195-2.

0 TO 28 DAYS   Ampicillin (200 mg/kg/day) and gentamicin (7.5 mg/kg/day, or 5 mg/kg/day if less than 1 week post-term age) are generally used if the lumbar puncture is negative. If positive, the same antibiotics or ampicillin and a cephalosporin such as cefotaxime (150 mg/kg/day) may be used.

1 TO 3 MONTHS   It is unrealistic to perform a lumbar puncture and admit and treat all of these infants. The recommendations in Table 195-2 represent a compromise. The suspicion of bacteremia is grounds for intravenous or intramuscular antibiotic therapy because of the potential for rapid deterioration. Ruling out meningitis in this age group prior to antibiotic therapy is imperative.

3 TO 36 MONTHS   Careful assessment of general appearance is the key to ruling out meningitis. Benign general appearance does not rule out other significant infections, such as urinary tract infection, pneumonia, and bacteremia. Three to 5% of infants with temperatures >39.5°C will be bacteremic with *Pneumococcus, Haemophilus influenzae,* or *Meningococcus.* Blood culture is recommended for children with temperatures >39.5°C and no source of infection. An alternative approach would be very close follow-up. Expectant antibiotic therapy for occult bacteremia is controversial. Antibiotic choices would be intramuscular ceftriaxone 50 mg/kg or oral amoxicillin 50 mg/kg/day divided into three doses. (Cefaclor in the same dose might be used in areas where the incidence of beta-lactamase-positive *H. influenzae* is high.)

TABLE 195-2. Evaluating the Acutely Febrile Child*,†

Age‡	Fever Without a Source§	Fever With a Source¶
<28 days	**A** Admit, septic work-up‖ IV or IM antibiotics	**B** Same as A. If the infant is near 28 days and has a URI or OM and the initial septic work-up is negative, may consider admission for observation (URI) and oral antibiotics (OM).
1–3 months	**C** UA and UC, stool culture, CBC, ESR** ILP and BC if T ≥ 39°C or WBC > 15,000 or ESR > 30 or irritability, lethargy, grunting, or age near 1 month and +U/A; CXR for cough, tachypnea, lethargy, grunting, toxicity, irritability, T ≥ 39°C, WBC > 15,000 or ESR > 30. Admission and antibiotic therapy dependent on 1. General appearance,†† change during observation 2. Results of LP, CXR, U/A, CBC, ESR 3. Exposures (e.g., NICU, household, day care) 4. If a BC is performed, IV or IM antibiotic therapy should be strongly considered.	**D** Same as C; if diarrhea, perform stool smear and, if positive, admit.
3–36 months	**E** BC if T >39.5°C,‡‡, CBC (see below), UA and UC (esp. in female or uncircumcised male). Additional work-up (LP, CXR) and therapy dependent upon 1. General appearance and change in general appearance with time and antipyretics 2. Specific physical findings (meningismus, tense fontanelle, cough, tachypnea, retracting, rash, etc.) 3. WBC count may be used to guide expectant IM antibiotic therapy for occult bacteremia, particularly if BC results require more than 24 hours or follow-up is uncertain.	**F** Entire work-up dependent on 1. General appearance 2. Specific physical findings/source of infection.¶¶
>36 months	UA and UC for female,§§ otherwise as in F above	As in F above

*Too many variables exist in the evaluation of a child with fever to be incorporated into a single outline. Therefore, this table is offered as one approach to the infant or child with fever in an emergency (ED) setting.

†This table applies to patients without identified chronic illness and assumes no antipyretic therapy in the 4 hr before ED arrival. Sickle-cell status of all febrile black children <6 yr of age must be determined.

‡Age is defined as post-term age. Also, these age groups should not be interpreted rigidly. For example, an 11-wk-old infant might best be evaluated according to categories E or F and 13-wk-old infant according to categories C or D. Body weight, exposures, and past medical history would be factors to consider when determining which category is most applicable to a given infant or child.

§This includes infants with URI when age is > 1 month. (In one study, 79% of infants with pneumococcal bacteremia had URI symptomatology.)

¶This includes otitis media, gastroenteritis, exudative pharyngitis, and, for infants <28 days of age, URI.

‖Blood culture, urinalysis, urine culture, lumbar puncture, chest x-ray, CBC, stool culture.

**Acute phase reactants are most useful in this age group. However, because of false-negatives they should be used only to alter evaluation in the direction of being more aggressive than planned before knowing their results.

††General appearance includes activity, alertness, color, strength of cry, consolability, irritability, eye contact, social responsiveness, and respiratory effort.

‡‡Choice of 39.5°C is arbitrary and is only meant to highlight the concept that, in this age, the height of the fever has some relevance to the extent of evaluation performed.

§§If not toxic in appearance, discharge to return in 12 hr with urine may be considered.

¶¶In this age group, exudative pharyngitis, gastroenteritis, and illness associated with a fine maculopapular rash (viral exanthem) are not often complicated by bacteremia unless there is a toxic general appearance. Therefore, a blood culture will, generally, not be indicated even when the temperature is >39.5°C. If pneumonia is present, a blood culture is indicated. The incidence of bacteremia with otitis media is somewhat lower than when no source is identified but is still significant. The decision to perform a blood culture in this situation is controversial. Individualization based on the age, general appearance, exposures, and height of fever, is recommended.

661

OVER 36 MONTHS   History and physical examination should entirely guide work-up and disposition. The only exception would be a urinalysis and urine culture on girls without an obvious source of infection.

DISPOSITION

Fever control with acetaminophen (15 mg/kg every 4 hours), cool clear liquids, and light dressing are advised. Sponging may be used, but is of questionable value. If fever persists, an infant <3 months old should be seen in 12–24 hours.

COMMON PITFALLS

- Failure to understand the importance of infant age in the evaluation
- Over-reliance on the white blood cell count or sedimentation rate
- Failure to evaluate and document general appearance
- Failure to consider noninfectious processes in the differential

196   Vomiting in Children

See Table 196-1.

197   Diarrhea in Children

See Table 197-1.

198   Seizures in Children

Seizures in childhood are not uncommon. Four to six percent of children will experience a seizure at some time (including febrile seizures). *Status epilepticus* describes a state of prolonged or repetitive epileptic seizures in which the patient does not regain consciousness for 30 minutes or longer. Status epilepticus is a medical emergency. Most cases of life-threatening status and resultant neurologic sequelae can be prevented by early recognition and treatment.

TABLE 196-1. Life-Threatening Causes of Vomiting

Newborn (Birth to 2 Wk)

A. Anatomic anomalies—esophageal stenosis/atresia, intestinal obstructions, especially malrotation and volvulus, Hirschsprung's disease
B. Other GI causes
    1.Necrotizing enterocolitis
    2.Peritonitis
C. Neurologic—kernicterus, mass lesions, hydrocephalus
D. Renal—obstructive anomalies, uremia
E. Infectious—sepsis, meningitis
F. Metabolism—inborn errors, especially congenital adrenal hyperplasia

Older Infant (2 Wk to 12 Months)

A. Gastroesophageal reflux, severe
B. Esophageal disorders
C. Rumination
D. Intestinal obstruction, especially pyloric stenosis, intussusception, incarcerated hernia
E. Other GI causes, especially gastroenteritis (with dehydration)
F. Neurologic—mass lesions, hydrocephalus
G. Renal—obstruction, uremia
H. Infectious—sepsis, meningitis, pertussis
I. Metabolic—inborn errors
J. Drugs—aspirin, theophylline, digoxin

Older Child (Over 12 Months)

A. GI obstruction, especially intussusception
B. Other GI causes, especially appendicitis, peptic ulcer disease
C. Neurologic—mass lesions
D. Renal—uremia
E. Infectious—meningitis
F. Metabolic—diabetic ketoacidosis, Reye's syndrome, adrenal insufficiency
G. Toxins, drugs—aspirin, ipecac, theophylline, digoxin, iron, lead

Reproduced from: Henritig FM: Vomiting. In Fleisher G, Ludwig S (eds): Textbook of Pediatric Emergency Medicine, pp 331—339. Baltimore, Williams & Wilkins, 1988.

TABLE 197-1. Emergency Department Management of Acute Diarrhea With Mild Dehydration

Estimate degree of dehydration and daily maintenance fluid requirements. If dehydration is 5% or less and otherwise uncomplicated, the child is a candidate for emergency department oral rehydration.

Maintenance requirements are 100 mL/kg for first 10 kg plus 50 mL/kg for each additional kg, and 11–20 kg plus 20 mL/kg for each kg over 20 kg.

Deficit requirements for 5% dehydration are 50 mL/kg.

An oral rehydration solution such as Pedialyte RS or Rehydralyte should provide maintenance and deficit fluids over the following 24 hr. In the ED give estimated deficit over 3–4 hours with frequent reassessment during the ED stay. Total fluid should be given over the next 20 hr.

If they are stable and retaining fluids, the child may be discharged from the ED after deficit fluid is replaced, with phone contact 3–4 hr later.

Beyond 24 hr, a maintenance oral hydration solution such as Pedialyte, Lytren, or Resol should be used to ensure that maintenance plus ongoing fluid losses are met.

Infants should be offered breast milk or half-strength formula in gradually increasing amounts. Older infants and children should be offered rice cereal, rice, potatoes, toast, crackers, bananas, or noodles.

DIFFERENTIAL DIAGNOSIS

Several conditions may mimic seizures: syncope, breath-holding spells, cardiac arrhythmias, and pseudoseizures.

Syncope is the most common cause of loss of consciouneess (other than seizure) in the school-age child. The most common distinguishing feature is that syncope has a precipitating event. Common among teen-agers is orthostatic syncope, strong emotional stimulus (the sight of an accident, loss of a loved one, fear of hospitalization and/or surgery), mechanical influence and illness (e.g., prolonged bed rest). Other characteristics of syncope are the short duration of loss of consciousness, absent motor activity, and lack of incontinence of urine or feces.

Breath-holding spells involve brief loss of consciousness; the usual precipitating event is frustration. Breath-holding spells are usually found in young infants between the ages of 6–18 months and follow a period of vigorous crying that is usually provoked by frustration. The breath-holding spells are benign.

Cardiac arrhythmias should be considered, as well as positive family history for sudden death in children, congenital heart disease, and prolonged QT interval. Pediatric ECG and sometimes 24-hour Holter monitor and stress test are needed to make the diagnosis.

A pseudoseizure is a feigned seizure in which the patient fully produces stereotypical behavior that mimics a true seizure, with abrupt onset and other bizarre clinical features such as complaints of paralysis, paresthesias, blindness, or diplopia. No abnormal activity is detected by EEG before, during, or after the event.

ETIOLOGY

Two groups exist: in the first, 53% have no apparent cause but half of these have coexisting fever; in the second group, 21% had chronic encephalopathy (brain malformation, cerebral palsy, anoxic or birth injury) or seizure disorder. In these patients, the two most common antecedents included rapid discontinuation of anticonvulsive medication and hyperpyrexia secondary to a non-central nervous system infection. The remaining 26% had an acute insult to the central nervous system (12% infection, 3% trauma) or a metabolic/toxic disorder (11% electrolyte disorder, hypocalcemia, hypoglycemia or exogenous toxin).

EMERGENCY DEPARTMENT EVALUATION

Key history: past neurologic and medical disorders, recent head injury, central nervous system infection, and ingestion of drugs or toxic substances. In children with seizures on anticonvulsants, the most common cause of seizures is a sudden reduction in dosage or total discontinuation of anticonvulsant medication. Do a rapid examination for signs of trauma, meningeal irritation, and raised intracranial pressure. Laboratory tests may be helpful: serum glucose and accucheck, CBC, sodium, potassium, calcium, phosphorus, magnesium, and BUN, anticonvulsant levels, a toxic screen, and blood lead levels may be indicated. Blood cultures should be obtained if sepsis is suspected. Liver function tests are occasionally helpful. Urinalysis and toxic screen may be indicated.

A lumbar puncture should be done in all children with a first seizure, in all children <18 months of age with a febrile seizure, and in older children with a seizure in whom central nervous system infection is suspected. Latex agglutination or counterimmunoeletrophoresis (CIE) should be done on the CSF and urine. Examination of the cerebrospinal fluid should include measurements of opening pressure, glucose and protein, cell count and morphology, and a Gram's stain.

Evidence of chronically raised intracranial pressure may be evident (in the younger child, look for separation of the cranial sutures). A computed tomography (CT) scan will identify intracranial bleeding, brain edema, tumors, and structural abnormalities of the brain. It also will give indirect information of the possibility of raised intracranial pressure. Focal seizures suggest the possibility of a mass lesion and increased intracranial pressure. With focal seizures and fever, antibiotics are begun and a CT scan is done prior to the LP.

EMERGENCY DEPARTMENT MANAGEMENT

Position the patient to avoid aspiration or suffocation. Establishing an airway is the first priority. Use suctioning for excessive secretions, and give oxygen. Bag–valve–mask ventilation or intubation and bag ventilation may be necessary. Start an intravenous infusion with 5% dextrose in normal saline. Give a bolus of 1 to 2 mL/kg of body weight of 25% dextrose if immediate Dextrostix is not available.

PHARMACOTHERAPY

There is no single drug of choice. The benzodiazepines, diazepam (Valium), and lorazepam (Ativan), are widely used in status epilepticus.

Diazepam (0.2–0.3 mg/kg IV) rapidly penetrates the blood–brain barrier and has an onset of action within 1 to 3 minutes. It may be repeated every 5 to 10 minutes. Large doses can produce respiratory depression, hypotension, and cardiac arrest. If diazepam and phenobarbital are used, be prepared for respiratory depression and possibly intubation. Lorazepam (0.05–0.1 mg/kg IV) has a rapid onset of action (within 1–3 minutes), longer duration of anticonvulsant effect (about 2 hours), and less respiratory depression.

Phenobarbital is given intravenously at a loading dose of 10 to 30 mg/kg, with a maximum infusion of 100 mg/min. Phenobarbital has an onset of action of 10 to 20 minutes. The major side effects are hypotension if infused too rapidly, sedation and respiratory depression. Long-term effects on cognitive function have led to decreased use for older children and adults.

Phenytoin is given intravenously at a loading dose of 10 to 20 mg/kg. Onset of action is 20 to 25 minutes, with a duration of action of 24 hours. The rate of infusion should not exceed 50 mg/min. Phenytoin causes little respiratory depression and its onset of action is 20 to 25 minutes. The maintenance dose for phenytoin is 5 mg/kg/day. Paraldehyde is used rarely and the intravenous preparation is no longer available. Rectal paraldehyde, 0.3 mL/kg mixed with an equal amount of mineral oil, may be used, with a maximum dose of 6 mL. The major side effect is bronchospasm.

ROUTES OF DRUG ADMINISTRATION

Alternate routes include intraosseous, rectal, endotracheal, and intramuscular routes. The intraosseous route is an effective alternate means of rapid administration of anticonvulsants and fluids. Rectal administration of diazepam and paraldehyde is effective. Undiluted preparation of diazepam per rectum requires higher doses than intravenous administration (0.5 to 0.75 mg/kg). Endotracheal administration of diazepam is effective. Intramuscular route has no place in the treatment of status epilepticus since drugs such as phenobarbital require up to 45 to 60 minutes to achieve adequate levels, and other drugs such as diazepam, phenytoin, and paraldehyde may cause sterile abscesses.

FEBRILE SEIZURES

A febrile seizure occurrs between the ages of 3 months and 5 years. A simple febrile seizure usually lasts less than 10 minutes. It is generalized and associated with a fever usually >102°F. The seizure occurs within 24 hours of the onset of the fever. The postictal examination reveals no focal findings. EEG examination is normal. Febrile seizures may recur in approximately 30–40%, but intelligence and learning are not affected. Lumbar puncture is recommended when meningitis is suspected, or for children <18 months old, and for all first cases of febrile seizures. Prophylaxis is not recommended because of potential side effects (behavioral changes, sleep pattern disturbances, and interference with cognitive functioning).

199   Abdominal Pain in Children

Infants and preverbal toddlers localize pain poorly. Abdominal pain may manifest as nonspecific signs of tachycardia, tachypnea and shallow or grunting respirations, and irritability. Abdominal distention, vomiting, flexed thighs, and refusal of the bottle or breast may be more specific and should be considered to represent a primary abdominal process until proven otherwise. In older toddlers, the location of pain to the abdomen becomes more obvious. If a young child can lateralize point tenderness, it is more likely to be due to a process of surgical concern. Signs such as rebound tenderness are less reliable. Likewise, in both infants and toddlers bowel sounds are less helpful and may be present even in advanced peritonitis. In school-age children typical signs, such as rebound tenderness and the obturator sign, become more reliable. In the mentally retarded child, signs can be difficult to interpret and the child's affect may be inappropriate.

In infants, the most common causes of abdominal pain are: colic, intussusception, and the malrotation–volvulus complex. In toddlers and preschool children, acute gastroenteritis, urinary tract infection, pain referred from other processes (e.g., pneumonia), and constipation are the most common causes. In the school-age child, the most common causes include idiopathic recurrent abdominal pain, appendicitis, acute gastroenteritis, constipation, and urinary tract infections. In the teenager, appendicitis, peptic ulcer disease, mittelschmerz, benign ovarian cysts, pelvic inflammatory disease, and ectopic pregnancy are common.

Many disorders can cause pain at any age: trauma, hepatitis, sickle-cell disease, discitis, strangulated hernia, testicular torsion, ovarian torsion, primary peritonitis, DKA, esophagitis, mesenteric adenitis, systemic diseases (e.g., streptococcal pharyngitis), and lactose or other food intolerance. Unique childhood entities occasionally have abdominal pain as a major feature (e.g., Henoch–Schönlein purpura). Children with nephrotic syndrome, ascites, immunodeficiency, and the postsplenectomy state are prone to primary peritonitis.

CLINICAL PRESENTATION

Colic: prolonged, continuous crying with a vague impression that the baby is experiencing abdominal pain. The child may have mild distention, may pull the knees up against the abdomen, and may be inconsolable, although rocking, swinging, or a car ride often seem to help. The pain pattern is often predictable, coming on suddenly in the late afternoon or early evening. Feeding irregularities such as excessive air swallowing and gulping, poor burping, or bottle-propping by the caregivers may be discovered. The physical examination is generally unremarkable.

In contrast to the colicky baby, an infant with pain brought on by surgical disorders usually has signs of intestinal obstruction with vomiting and distention. Babies with bilious vomiting have bowel obstruction until proven otherwise.

Surgical causes:

Malrotation complicated by midgut volvulus is a surgical emergency of infancy with acute-onset pain followed soon by distention and vomiting, often bile-stained.

Intussusception: dramatic, acute onset in a thriving baby (5–10% have experienced a similar attack that abated spontaneously.) Vomiting follows, pain seems to come in waves. Currant-jelly stools occur later. Mental status changes may exist.

Appendicitis in the infant presents as peritonitis in 50%. Crying and irritability, with fever, distention, vomiting, shallow and grunting respirations, and, at times, shock, are seen. In older children, the earlier presentation reduces the rate of perforation. *Yersinia* infections may mimic appendicitis.

Abdominal pain with fever and peritoneal irritation in the child with nephrotic syndrome, ascites, or immunodeficiency suggests primary peritonitis.

Acute bacterial gastroenteritis presents with fever, abdominal pain, bloody diarrhea, and occasionally striking neurologic signs including seizures or meningismus.

Chronic functional constipation or Hirschsprung's disease may present with crampy, recurrent abdominal pain. In the infant, Hirschsprung's disease may be complicated by toxic megacolon and present as an acute abdomen with signs of peritonitis and obstruction.

Chronic recurrent abdominal pain is the most common somatic complaint of school-age children and is usually psychophysiologic. Periumbilical or epigastric pain lasts <3 hours and does not awaken the child from sleep.

Recurrent abdominal pain associated with fever, diarrhea, and growth or sexual maturational arrest suggests inflammatory bowel disease.

The postpubertal girl with lower abdominal pain may have an ectopic pregnancy or a corpus luteal cyst.

DIFFERENTIAL DIAGNOSIS

Obstruction: incarcerated hernia, intussusception, malrotation, Hirschsprung's disease, and adhesions from previous surgery.

Peritonitis: appendicitis, ruptured viscus from trauma, foreign body, or as a complication of bowel obstruction.

Nonabdominal conditions: pyelonephritis or sickle-cell disease.

EMERGENCY DEPARTMENT MANAGEMENT

Laboratory investigations may include complete blood count, electrolytes, blood urea nitrogen, glucose, liver enzymes, bilirubin, amylase, blood cultures, and urinalysis with culture. A urine specimen is crucial and may require bladder tap or catheterization. Radiographic studies are obtained primarily to rule out an intestinal obstruction or perforation or an occult lower lobe pneumonia. Computed tomography is appropriate in trauma. If there are signs of hemodynamic instability, promptly obtain vascular access. If there are signs of intestinal obstruction, establish nasogastric decompression with a small sump tube. Prompt pediatric surgical or general surgical and pediatric consultation are in order whenever obstruction, peritonitis, bleeding, or testicular torsion is suspected. Midgut volvulus is an emergency requiring rapid detorsion of the mesenteric vessels.

DISPOSITION

THE ROLE OF THE CONSULTANT   Volvulus, intra-abdominal bleeding, or torsion warrant immediate surgical consultation. If there are signs of septic shock, cardiovascular collapse, or respiratory compromise, pediatric critical care consultation is indicated.

INDICATIONS FOR ADMISSION   All children with intestinal obstruction, intra-abdominal trauma or bleeding, peritonitis, or cardiorespiratory instability should be admitted promptly to an ICU. A legitimate reason to admit is parental exhaustion or inability to cope with the child's illness.

TRANSFER CONSIDERATIONS   Surgical emergencies in infants require a surgeon with specific expertise and may require transfer to another facility. Transfer may be precluded, however, in the extreme conditions of volvulus, bleeding, or torsion.

COMMON PITFALLS

- Intussusception is common and easily missed.
- Commonly missed pathology arises from the urinary tract. It should always be considered in pediatric abdominal pain of obscure cause.

200   Limp in Children

DIFFERENTIAL DIAGNOSIS

There are a wide variety of medical problems that share a presenting complaint of limp. See Table 200-1.

MAJOR EMERGENCY ENTITIES

An early presumptive diagnosis for the cause of gait disturbance must be established for a limited number of conditions. Failure to consider these disease states may lead to deformity, functional disability, or death.

DIAGNOSTIC APPROACH

Distinguish children who require immediate hospitalization and treatment from those who may be observed. Febrile patients with nuchal rigidity; limitation of joint motion; lower limb direct metaphyseal pain; compression tenderness over a spinal process; or back pain enhanced with Valsalva movement, heel strike, or straight leg raising should be considered to have one of the diseases that require prompt treatment. Those who have a gait disturbance with altered consciousness, cranial nerve weakness, subjective or objective sensory disturbance, ataxia, alteration of sphincter tone, urinary retention, or altered deep tendon reflexes require prompt establishment of the definitive diagnosis.

TABLE 200-1. Principle Causes for Altered Childhood Locomotion

Overt and occult trauma
Cellulitis
Osteomyelitis
Pyarthyrosis
Sickle cell, vasooclusive crisis
Drug intoxication
Transient synovitis
Legg-Perthes disease
Appendicitis
Juvenile rheumatoid arthritis

Modified and reproduced with permission from Singer J: The cause of gait disturbance in 425 pediatric patients. In Ludwig S, Fleisher G (eds): Pediatric Emergency Care, Vol 1, p 7. Baltimore, Williams & Wilkins, 1985.

A complete blood count may facilitate the diagnosis of systemic infection, hemoglobinopathy, or blood dyscrasia. The sedimentation rate (ESR): 70% with an ESR of >30 mm/hr have arthralgia or arthritis of infectious or inflammatory origin. An ESR of >40 mm/hr have bacterial infections.

Radiographs have proven diagnostic efficacy. Plain radiographs may aid in the diagnosis of periostitides, osteochondroses, benign and malignant tumors, mechanical disturbances, metabolic derangements, and infectious diseases. Films that appear negative should never hinder therapeutic strategies. Several conditions may be associated with normal radiographs: tibial fracture in the toddler, septic hip in the child over 1 year of age, osteomyelitis of the long bone or pelvis, sacroiliac joint infection, or intervertebral disk infection. Radionuclide scans provide important positive and negative information. A positive technetium scan reflects any condition that results in increased bone formation or blood flow. A negative technetium scan should be followed by a gallium scan. A positive gallium scan supports a provisional diagnosis of infection, and negative technetium and gallium scans refute it. Computerized tomography is useful for tumors and inflammatory and infectious problems of the musculoskeletal system. Magnetic resonance imaging is superior to both plain film and computerized tomography for soft tissue detail.

201   Dehydration in Children

For clinical assessment of dehydration, see Table 201-1.

EMERGENCY DEPARTMENT MANAGEMENT

If the patient is in shock, fluid boluses of 20 mL/kg of an isotonic solution should be given until clinical improvement is noted. If the child is not in shock but is dehydrated, the 20 mL/kg fluid bolus may be given over a period of .5–1 hour. Subsequent maintenance and deficit therapy is less urgent and usually addressed by the physician.

DISPOSITION

Most children with dehydration requiring intravenous fluids will also require hospital admission.

TABLE 201-1. Clinical Assessment of Hydration Status

	Mild (5%–8%)	Moderate (8%–12%)	Severe (12%–15%)
Mucus membranes	+	+	++
Skin turgor	±	+	++
Anterior fontanelle	±	+	++
Sunken eyeballs	±	+	++
Depressed mental status	−	±	++
Increased pulse	−	±	++
Hypotension	−	−	++

−, not present; ±, variable; + present; ++, extreme

202   Pediatric Intoxications

Age-dependent pharmacokinetic variations, the unpredictability and variability in handling of toxins, and differences in sensitivity to the effects of toxic exposures dictate a modified approach to the management of the poisoned child. Transit time through the gastrointestinal tract is shorter and more variable in the infant, approaching adult values after about 2 to 3 years of age. This may affect the time course of an overdose. *History is the most important indicator of poisoning.* Most accidental ingestions in children involve only a single substance. The accidental ingestion of a bad-tasting household product often results in only one swallow (5 mL) in the child, whereas the suicidal adolescent may ingest much larger quantities. Medications mistaken for candy by children, or those intentionally flavored for pediatric use, are often ingested in multiple quantities. The following information allows assessment of whether the victim is in danger:

1. Source of the exposure
2. Severity of the symptomatology
3. The nature of the toxin
4. Other medications or products available in the environment
5. Time of exposure
6. Approximate amount involved
7. Actions taken before emergency department presentation
8. Reliability of the informant
9. Assessment of intent (accidental, suicide attempt)

Accidental ingestions, whether toxic or nontoxic, may warrant investigation into the home situation if:

1. The ingestion occurs in a child over age 5 years. This usually signals a cry for help.
2. More than one episode of "accidental" ingestion occurs. This may signal inadequate parental concern, inadequate poison prevention education, or possibly neglect.
3. The "accidental" ingestion occurs in a child under 1 year of age. Infants this young often do not possess the physical or mental capabilities required to self-administer a toxin.

STABILIZATION

Evaluate the airway and cardiac function. Patients with severe central nervous system or respiratory depression should be intubated with an endotracheal tube (cuffed in a patient over age 9 years to protect against aspiration). The comatose patient should receive:

1. Oxygen
2. 0.5 g/kg glucose as 10% to 25% dextrose in water (do accucheck and a blood specimen for glucose)
3. Naloxone 0.1 mg/kg up to 2 mg in a child every 3 to 5 minutes for two doses. If suspicion of opiate intoxication exists, dosing should proceed up to a total of 10 mg. If adequate response is obtained with bolus dosing, consider using a naloxone infusion (two thirds of the initial reversal dose per hour).
4. Assessment (if warranted and guided by toxidrome recognition) of arterial blood gases, BUN, creatinine, liver function tests, blood ammonia and electrolytes, blood culture, osmolality, toxicology screen.

5. Identify the toxin. Most ingestions in young children involve nontoxic products or those that cause only minor toxicity. A common error is to treat all ingestions aggressively, even when such treatment is unnecessary.

OCULAR AND DERMAL EXPOSURES

Ocular exposures warrant immediate attention by irrigation with copious amounts of water or saline. Dermal exposure requires removal of clothes followed by complete soap-and-water washing of the child (including the hair, fingernails, and navel) to limit further percutaneous absorption.

CAUSTIC OR CORROSIVE EXPOSURES

Dilution with milk or water is warranted. Contraindications to such therapy include the patient's inability to swallow and signs of upper airway obstruction, esophageal perforation, or shock. Giving more than 15 mL/kg in a child (up to a maximum of 250 mL) may result in undesireable vomiting and enhanced gastrointestinal absorption of certain toxins. Specific neutralization techniques with caustic or corrosive ingestions have been abandoned.

GASTROINTESTINAL DECONTAMINATION

Most cases present to the ED within 1 to 3 hours after the ingestion. The substance has either been substantially absorbed (in the case of liquids) or has already passed through the pylorus on its way through the small bowel. Gastrointestinal evacuation after the toxin has left the stomach is useless and delays the administration of activated charcoal. Ipecac should be reserved for those instances where gastrointestinal evacuation (if indicated) is to be performed at home or in those cases where the ingestion occurred only minutes before presentation to the ED.

Contraindications to ipecac:

1. Relative contraindications
    a. The ingestion of a high-viscosity petroleum distillate, and other certain hydrocarbons in small quantities
    b. The ingestion of an agent likely to produce rapid depression of consciousness or convulsions
    c. A child under 6 months of age
    d. The ingestion of a foreign body
2. Absolute contraindications
    a. The ingestion of a caustic or corrosive product
    b. A comatose or seizing patient
    c. The presence of hemetemesis
    d. Lack of or depression of upper airway protective reflexes

Some clinicians have advised that ipecac is safe to administer at home in children 6 months or older. The appropriate dose of ipecac should be based on the child's age: less than 1 year of age, 10 mL; 1 to 5 years old, 15 to 30 mL; 5 years old to adult, 30 mL. This dose of ipecac may be repeated only once if the child does not vomit within 15 to 20 minutes. Patients who present less than 30 to 60 minutes after ingestion with apparent signs of toxicity, or those who arrive asymptomatic but have ingested a highly toxic compound, will benefit from rapid gut evacuation followed by charcoal administration. If ipecac is used, the delay in onset of emesis will allow continued absorption of the toxin, and the duration of vomiting incurred by the use of ipecac will again delay the administration of activated charcoal. Gastric lavage should be performed, followed immediately by activated charcoal. If a patient presents more than 1 hour after ingestion, charcoal administration alone is necessary, unless delayed gastric emptying or concretions are suspected.

TABLE 202-1. Pediatric Dosages of Selected Antidotes

Antidote	Indications	Pediatric Dose
N-Acetylcysteine	Acetaminophen toxicity	Loading: 140 mg/kg Maintenance: 70 mg/kg q 4 hr for 17 doses orally as a 5% solution
Atropine	Organophosphates/carbamates and other severe cholinergic poisonings	0.05 mg/kg (2 mg max) every 2–5 min until cessation of symptoms (e.g., pulmonary secretions)
Cyanide Kit	Cyanide poisoning	See below

Hemoglobin	Sodium Nitrite 3% (initial dose: max 10 ml)	Sodium Thiosulfate (initial dose: 12.5 g max)
8 g	0.22 mL/kg (6.6 mg/kg)	1.10 mL/kg
10 g	0.27 mL/kg (8.7 mg/kg)	1.35 mL/kg
12 g*	0.33 mL/kg (10 mg/kg)	1.65 mL/kg
14 g	0.39 mL/kg (11.6 mg/kg)	1.95 mL/kg

*If hemoglobin unknown, use this dose.

Antidote	Indications	Pediatric Dose
Deferoxamine	Iron intoxication	Therapeutic dose: 90 mg/kg IM or IV to a max of 1 g, every 4–12 hours; not to exceed 6 g in 24 hr. IV slow infusion up to 15 mg/kg/hr Diagnostic trial: 20 mg/kg IM (up to 1 g)
Diazepam	Seizures resulting from intoxication	0.1–0.3 mg/kg up to 10 mg IV slowly over 2 min
Dimercaprol (BAL)	Intoxications from lead, arsenic, gold, mercury, copper, nickel, antimony	IM use only: 3–5 mg/kg initially, followed by 2.5 mg/kg q 4 hr for 2 days, then q 6–12 hr. Note: dosage and duration vary with specific intoxicant and severity; see recommendations for each poisoning
Diphenhydramine	Dystonic reactions from phenothiazine and related compounds	1–2 mg/kg IM or IV over 2 min
Ethanol	Methanol, ethylene glycol	Loading: 7.6–10 mL/kg of a 10% solution in D_5W over 30 min IV; or 0.8–1.0 ml/kg 95% ETOH diluted to a 20–30% solution for oral administration Maintenance: 1.4 mL/kg/hr of a 10% ETOH solution IV (0.15 mL/kg/hr PO 95%); add 91 ml/hr if patient on dialysis

(cont'd.)

TABLE 202-1 (Cont'd.)

Antidote	Indications	Pediatric Dose
Glucagon	Beta blocker intoxication	50–150 µg/kg IV over 1 min followed by infusion of 1–5 mg/hr tapered over 5–12 hr. *Note:* do not use supplied diluent (contains phenol)
Methylene Blue	Methemoglobinemia	0.1–0.2 mL/kg of a 1% solution (1–2 mg/kg) IV over 5 min
Naloxone	Opioid toxicity	0.1 mg/kg IV if no response to initial dose Note: many clinicians use normal adult doses in children; maintenance infusion is 2/3 the initial reversal dose used, per hr
Physostigmine	Severe anticholinergic poisoning	0.5 mg IV over 2 min repeated to a max dose of 2 mg if required *Note:* reserved for severe, life-threatening toxicity when conventional therapy has failed
Pralidoxime (2-PAM)	Organophosphate poisoning	25–50 mg/kg IV over 2 min or IM; repeat every 8–12 hr if needed; if severe can be infused at <0.5 g/hr

From Schauben JL, Mofenson HC, Caraccio TR: Problems in the management of intoxications. In Luten RC (ed): Problems in Pediatric Emergency Medicine, pp 245–277. New York, Churchill Livingstone, 1988

Contraindications to gastric lavage:

1. Caustic or corrosive ingestions without previous assessment of esophageal damage
2. Uncontrolled seizures
3. Absence of protective upper airway reflexes without previous insertion of an endotracheal tube
4. Significant arrhythmias
5. Certain petroleum distillates or hydrocarbons

The best results are obtained with gastric lavage when the largest-bore tube that can be reasonably and safely inserted is used. A 36 French orogastric hose can be safely passed in children. Aspiration of gastric contents should precede instillation of any lavage fluid.

If the child is to be intubated before lavage, do not use a cuffed endotracheal tube in a child less than 9 years. Children should be lavaged with 0.45% saline. The use of an alternative fluid composition in children may lead to hypernatremia, hypocalcemia, or other severe electrolyte imbalances. Aliquots of 15 mL/kg lavage fluid should be used in children. If these volumes are exceeded, the stomach contents may be forced through the pylorus into the intestine or vomiting may result. The lavage should be continued until a consistently clear fluid return is achieved. Give activated charcoal after the lavage is completed.

Ingestants that cause gastric concretions, such as ferrous sulfate, meprobamate, glutethimide, salicylates, and large amounts of dry tablets may require prolonged, forceful lavage to dissolve, break up, or otherwise remove the bolus of material. This may be an indication for the use of multiple-dose activated charcoal or possibly whole gut lavage. Endoscopic or surgical removal may be required. Clues to the presence of concretions include failure to respond to appropriate treatment, continued deterioration despite therapy, or measured blood concentrations that do not decrease with adequate gastrointestinal decontamination.

For asymptomatic patients presenting after more than 1 hour post ingestion, or for patients who present before 1 hour with an ingestion of low toxic potential, give activated charcoal without prior gut evacuation.

Charcoal should not be given with ingestions involving a caustic or corrosive product because it will not effectively adsorb these compounds, may cause vomiting, and will most probably hinder any endoscopic attempts to evaluate the esophageal or gastric mucosa. Remember that activated charcoal cannot adsorb all known toxins. It has limited usefulness with boric acid, caustics, corrosives, cyanide, ethylene glycol, iron, iodides, lithium, as well as other elemental metal ingestions. Certain pesticides and other poorly water-soluble compounds also may not be effectively captured by the charcoal complex. The alcohols may be adsorbed to a limited extent by charcoal, but this has little clinical significance since absorption of the alcohols is so rapid.

The dose of standard-grade activated charcoal is usually 1 to 2 g/kg/dose in children, given as a slurry in at least 100 mL of water or sorbitol solution, either orally or through a gastric tube. The suspension should be sipped through one or two straws, alternating with sips of a clear fluid such as water. If attempts to get the child to drink within 15 to 20 minutes have failed, a nasogastric tube should be placed and the charcoal slurry administered through it. Multiple doses of activated charcoal, given every 2 to 6 hours, is gaining widespread acceptance. Multiple-dose therapy appears useful in cases of long-acting or sustained-release agents, preparations resulting in concretions, and in agents undergoing enterohepatic or enterogastric recirculation. Do not indiscriminantly administer multiple-dose charcoal without evaluating the risks, the clinical symptomatology, and its reported usefulness for a particular compound. Do not give charcoal to a patient who has absent bowel sounds or any evidence of an ileus. The use and relative efficacy of multiple-dose charcoal in the pediatric literature is limited to case reports. For multiple dosing in children, give 1 g/kg of standard-grade activated charcoal (or superactivated charcoal) every 2 to 4 hours with water.

The utility of whole gut lavage in children is still undefined.

Cathartics are used to shorten the transit time of the toxin or toxin/charcoal mixture through the gastrointestinal tract and prevent the formation of "charcoal briquets" in the gastrointestinal tract. Despite the almost universal use of cathartics in the management of poisonings, there has been no scientific or clinical proof to support their efficacy. Fleet's Phosphosoda, a favorite with adults, should not be used in children due to the risk of severe electrolyte complications. Sorbitol improves the palatability of charcoal and is a better cathartic than magnesium or sodium salts. The use of sorbitol in children is not without concern, because it may induce significant diarrhea and electrolyte imbalances. For this reason, do not use prepared charcoal/sorbitol mixtures. Sorbitol is not recommended for children under 1 year of age and should be used with caution in those under 3 years of age. Sorbitol can be given in doses of 1 to 1.5 g/kg of no greater than a 35% solution, once every 12 hours.

ANTIDOTAL THERAPY

See Table 202-1 above.

OBSERVATION GUIDELINES

ED observation for 6 to 8 hours is usually long enough to unmask most of the delayed-onset toxic reactions. Consider children under 1 year of age to be at a higher risk for toxicity. Because they often do not show the classic adult symptomatology, use caution with early discharge.

Indications for admission: patient with toxic signs and symptoms, exposure to an agent known to be highly toxic, a dose or exposure to a toxin sufficient to anticipate the development of toxicity, or a history of an intentional ingestion. Assess the adequacy of the home environment before discharge. Evaluate older children with suicidal ideation before their release.

COMMON PITFALLS

* Inappropriate application of adult poisoning management to children, without regard for the differences between the adult and pediatric protocols

203   Altered Mental Status in Children

Assess the degree of alteration with the modified Glasgow Coma Scale for children.

DIFFERENTIAL DIAGNOSIS

Table 203-1 contains key diagnostic considerations. Table 203-2 lists substances associated with altered mental status.

EMERGENCY DEPARTMENT MANAGEMENT

Focus on rapid diagnosis and treatment.

DISPOSITION

Disposition depends on diagnosis and degree of alteration of level of consciousness. Any persistent alteration or profound alteration in the level of consciousness requires admission. If intubation is required, the ICU must be experienced in dealing with children. Until admission, the child with an altered level of consciousness requires both continuous electronic monitoring and continuous nursing monitoring. In particular, the child with an altered level of consciousness should *not* be sent to the radiology department without *both* forms of monitoring.

TABLE 203-1. Key Diagnostic Considerations

A — Alcohol
E — Encephalitis/meningitis
I — Insulin
O — Overdose
U — Uremia/metabolic encephalopathy
T — Trauma, tumor
I — Intracranial hemorrhage
P — Psychiatric
S — Seizure
O — Other

TABLE 203-2. Substances Associated With AMS*

Alcohols—osmolar gap
Antihistamines
Barbiturates
Carbon monoxide—carboxyhemoglobin
Narcotics—miosis, response to a Narcan trial dose
Salicylates—hyperpnea, overcompensated metabolic acidosis
Phenothiazines
Tricyclic antidepressants—atropinic signs, widened QRS complex
Atropinics
Anticonvulsants
Organophosphates insecticides—increased respiratory secretions, miosis
PCP
Heavy metals (Pb)—basophilic stippling, lead lines, paint chips on KUB, elevated
CSF protein

*Substances for which emergency treatment beyond the general support of vital functions may be indicated are in boldface.

COMMON PITFALLS

- Failing to consider certain unusual diagnoses that present with AMS: infectious encephalopathy without CSF pleocytosis, selected poisonings, selected metabolic encephalopathies, cerebral infarction with a negative CT scan, hysterical coma, seizures without tonic-clonic activity and intussusception
- Failing to prioritize the evaluation of the child with AMS in a fashion that considers *both* the relative emergent nature of various diagnoses *and* the potential for iatrogenic complications: Lumbar puncture causing cerebral herniation; intubation or uncontrolled fluid therapy resulting in an exacerbation of increased intracranial pressure; positioning for a CT scan resulting in exacerbation of an unstable cervical spine injury

204 Shock and Vascular Access in Children

Therapy involves vascular access for administration of volume expanders, vasoactive infusions, or both. Early intervention is necessary for survival, since cellular ischemia leads to irreversible damage. Death from shock can occur immediately in the form of a cardiac arrest unresponsive to resuscitation even if the arrest is witnessed, or in a delayed fashion as the result of multiple organ system failure.

CLINICAL PRESENTATION

The diagnosis of shock is made by an examination that focuses on the adequacy of perfusion since hypotension is a late and often premorbid sign of pediatric shock. One should assess the central nervous system, skin, muscle tone, pulses, heart rate, blood pressure, and urinary output. The fluctuating mental status in shock reflects impairment of cortical perfusion. Initially, the patient is awake and recognizes his or her parents, but progressively the patient becomes lethargic, combative during procedures, unable to recognize the parents, unarousable, and finally unresponsive to painful procedures such as venipuncture or lumbar puncture.

The skin loses perfusion early in shock to preserve blood flow to more vital organs. Capillary refill of blanched areas on distal extremities should be <2 seconds. Coolness of distal extremities is a sign of poor perfusion due to low cardiac output or increased systemic vascular resistance, or both.

Poor muscle tone also reflects shunting of blood to more vital organs. Palpation of peripheral pulses provides a qualitative assessment of heart rate, stroke volume, blood pressure, and systemic vascular resistance. Absence of peripheral pulses from low stroke volume occurs while the patient is still normotensive. As cardiac output continues to fall, hypotension develops before loss of central pulses and arrest.

In the newborn, the normal heart rate ranges from 120 to 160 beats per minute. Sinus tachycardia from 180 to 210 is not uncommon from a variety of benign causes in the first years of life (fever, agitation, etc.), but also can be an important early sign of hypovolemic shock.

The normal newborn systolic blood pressure is 60 mm Hg. After 6 months of age, normal values (50th percentile) can be estimated by the formula:

$$\text{Systolic blood pressure} = 90 + (2 \times \text{age in years}).$$

Substituting the number 70 for 90 in the above equation gives the systolic values for the fifth percentile.

Finally, urine output reflects glomerular filtration rate, which reflects renal blood flow. When shock is suspected, early catheterization of the bladder is indicated.

DIFFERENTIAL DIAGNOSIS

The most common causes of pediatric shock are hypovolemia, sepsis, cardiogenic, neurogenic, and anaphylactic.

EMERGENCY DEPARTMENT EVALUATION

The history most often determines the cause of shock. Cardiopulmonary assessment can be performed by inspection and palpation of pulses. Airway, breathing, and circulation are examined to determine adequacy of oxygenation, ventilation, and perfusion. Exact determination of vital signs is a secondary priority.

EMERGENCY DEPARTMENT MANAGEMENT

Once the diagnosis is made, immediate management includes oxygen, monitoring of heart rate and rhythm, transcutaneous pulse oximetry if available, and vascular access. Before the last goal is accomplished, venous return can be enhanced by the Trendelenburg position. Volume expansion or vasoactive infusions are given in accordance with the underlying cause.

VOLUME EXPANSION

Shock resulting from absolute or relative hypovolemia is treated by volume expansion with a fluid that will remain in the intravascular space. These fluids are classified as crystalloids (lactated Ringer's, normal saline, 3% saline), colloids (plasmanate, albumen, all other blood products), and synthetic colloids (hetastarch, dextran). The immediate goal is to restore perfusion as rapidly as possible so that volume expansion is initiated with readily available fluids. Replacement of red cell mass and clotting factors is an important secondary concern, but is dependent on blood bank response time.

In pediatric shock, volume expansion is performed in multiple aliquots of 10 to 20 mL/kg of body weight administered over 2- to-10-minute intervals until the desired effect on perfusion is obtained. Initial cardiovascular response includes a lowering of heart rate and a resolution of hypotension. The end point of volume expansion, however, needs to be determined by improvement in organ perfusion and function, not cardiovascular stability. Clinically, the patient should become alert and active, with improved skin perfusion, muscle tone, peripheral pulses, and urinary output. These parameters are continuously reassessed after each therapeutic maneuver. In severe hypovolemia, 60 to 100 mL/kg of fluid or more may be necessary.

VASOACTIVE INFUSIONS

Lack of unusual fluid losses by history, pre-existing heart disease, hepatomegaly, rales, cardiomegaly, and failure of perfusion to improve with volume expansion suggests either a primary cardiogenic shock or a strong cardiogenic component to another form of shock. Given appropriate volume expansion, vasoactive infusions can further improve cardiac output. Dopamine, at dosages of less than 5 µg/kg/minute, exerts dopaminergic effects include increasing contractility without changing heart rate, and improving renal and mesenteric blood flow. At 5 to 20 µg/kg/minute, its beta effects include increase in heart rate and contractility. At higher dosages, its alpha effect may improve blood pressure at the expense of perfusion by increasing systemic vascular resistance.

Dobutamine in the range of 2 to 10 µg/kg/minute increases contractility without increasing heart rate or myocardial oxygen consumption. It does not improve renal or mesenteric blood flow. Its beta-2 effects limit its usefulness when profound hypotension is a problem.

To improve cardiac output, infants respond to stress primarily by increasing heart rate as opposed to increasing contractility. This fact, combined with the absence of ischemic heart disease, leads many pediatric centers to prefer epinephrine or isoproterenol infusions. The initial dosage for both is 0.05 to 0.1 µg/kg/minute, with upward titration until the desired effect is achieved.

DISPOSITION

To prevent cardiac arrest, shock must be treated swiftly and steps taken to correct the underlying cause. Additional therapies are diverse (antibiotics for septic shock, hemostasis for traumatic injury, surgical correction or palliation of congenital heart lesions, etc.). Hence, choice of the consultant depends upon the underlying condition. All cases need admission for monitoring and ongoing management.

The admitting hospital must be fully staffed and equipped for the intensive-care needs of the pediatric patient. Transfer and selection of transport personnel should be made with the referral institution.

COMMON PITFALLS

- The most common pitfall is *difficulty in early diagnosis* due to normal blood pressure and fluctuating level of consciousness. Both mislead because at times the infant or child may appear normal
- *Failure to rapidly administer the appropriate amount of volume.*

PART III

Specific Pediatric Diseases

205 Meningitis and Encephalitis in Children

Bacterial meningitis and viral disease presenting as meningitis, encephalitis, or meningoencephalitis are the most commonly encountered forms of CNS infection in children.

Bacterial meningitis occurring in the neonatal period is usually due to the group B streptococcus, gram-negative enteric bacilli such as *Escherichia coli*, or *Listeria monocytogenes*. Over the age of 3 months, *Haemophilus influenzae* type b, *Neisseria meningitidis*, and *Streptococcus pneumoniae* are the major pathogens. The enteroviruses (ECHO, coxsackie) are the most common viral pathogens infecting the CNS, followed by the arboviruses (La Crosse strain of the California encephalitis virus, St. Louis encephalitis), and *Herpes simplex* virus (HSV).

CLINICAL PRESENTATION

Fever, lethargy, and irritability suggest possible meningitis. Inflammation of the meninges is generally associated with headache, back pain, nuchal rigidity, nausea, vomiting, irritability, and changes in sensorium. Clinical findings such as seizures, a bulging fontanelle, focal neurologic signs (hemiparesis, quadriparesis, cranial nerve palsies, visual field defects), and ataxia also suggest meningitis, but no one sign is pathognomonic. Symptoms and signs of meningitis are variable and depend in part on the patient's age, the duration of the illness, and the host's response to the infection. This is especially true when dealing with neonates and young infants, where the clinical findings may be quite subtle and include disinterest in feeding, increased sleep, respiratory distress, jaundice, and diarrhea. As a result of the bacteremia that often precedes meningitis, other focal infection (cellulitis, pneumonia, septic arthritis, myocarditis, and pericarditis) may be present. Cutaneous petechiae and purpura are most commonly associated with meningococcal infection but can be seen with other bacterial pathogens. Alteration in consciousness is apparent in all children with encephalitis. This may be manifested by only lethargy or delirium, but in severe cases the lethargy may progress to a stuporous state or frank coma.

EMERGENCY DEPARTMENT EVALUATION
HISTORY

With neonates, question the mother about infections during pregnancy and at delivery, antibiotic usage during pregnancy, previous babies with neonatal infections, and parental history of or exposure to HSV. No matter what the child's age, seek an exposure history to sick individuals (tuberculosis, another individual with infection due to *H. influenzae* type b or *N. meningitidis*).

PHYSICAL EXAMINATION

A quick appraisal determines how to progress: a bulging anterior fontanelle in an infant in the seated position is an indication of increased intracranial pressure. Papilledema should raise concern for a brain abscess, subdural empyema, or venous sinus occlusion. A complete neurologic examination is required. In children, this includes head circumference. Seek meningeal irritation and examine for nuchal rigidity. In young infants, this can be facilitated by placing the infant supine with the shoulders at the edge of the examining table or bed and the head supported by the examiner's hand. Involuntary rigidity will persist in this position when an attempt is made to flex the neck.

LABORATORY EVALUATION

The lumbar puncture (LP) should include an opening pressure, cellular analysis, glucose (including simultaneous serum glucose) and protein determination, Gram's stain smear, and appropriate cultures (typically bacterial and viral). In only four situations is it reasonable to delay a lumbar puncture:

1. Clinically significant cardiopulmonary instability
2. Signs of significantly increased intracranial pressure (retinal changes, altered pupillary responses, increase in blood pressure with bradycardia, cranial nerve palsies, hemiparesis, posturing, etc.)
3. Focal seizures
4. Infection of the skin, soft tissue, or epidural areas that the needle will traverse to obtain the CSF.

In the case of significantly increased intracranial pressure, obtain a contrast-enhanced, cranial CT scan first. Typical bacterial meningitis has polymorphonuclear leukocyte (PMN) pleocytosis in excess of 500/µl, with hypoglycorrhachia (less than 50% of the simultaneous serum glucose in infants/children and 75% in neonates) and an elevated protein. Viral CNS infections are associated with a lymphocyte pleocytosis of less than 500/µl, with relatively normal glucose and protein concentrations initially. However, the first CSF examination in a child with enterovirus meningitis may have a predominance of PMNs, and the cell count may be in excess of 1000/µl.

Antibiotic pretreatment of a child with bacterial meningitis usually does not markedly affect the CSF chemical parameters or Gram's stain characteristics, but it may result in sterile CSF in those with pneumococcal or meningococcal disease. The rapid antigen diagnostic tests, including countercurrent immunoelectrophoresis, latex particle agglutination, and enzyme-linked immunosorbent assay, may be helpful in establishing the etiology. Interpreting a traumatic tap is difficult; parameters, such as the CSF glucose concentration, Gram's stain, and antigen detection studies, may help determine the presence of infection.

Obtain blood cultures in all patients, especially in those not having an LP, since culture of blood reveals the bacterial pathogen in more than 80% of previously untreated cases of meningitis. Also obtain cultures of other associated foci of infection (joint fluid, sputum, skin lesions, etc.). Additional laboratory evaluation should include a CBC with differential and platelet count, coagulation studies if thrombocytopenia is present, serum calcium, serum electrolytes and urine sodium concentration, urine analysis, and liver function studies when nonbacterial disease is suspected.

EMERGENCY DEPARTMENT MANAGEMENT

Supportive care and stabilization are critical. Treatment of septic shock, control of intracranial hypertension, control of seizures, and appropriate therapy of hyponatremia resulting from inappropriate antidiuretic hormone secretion are problems the physician handle. In all patients with suspected intracranial hypertension, elevate the head 30 degrees. Mannitol (1 g/kg infused over 10 minutes) may be used. Hyperventilation is an effective means of decreasing the intracranial pressure—$PaCO_2$ should be 25–30 mm Hg. Patients requiring hyperventilation and mannitol should have a ventricular catheter or subarachnoid bolt.

Dexamethasone at 0.15 mg/kg every 6 hours for 4 days results in less hearing loss in infants and children with *H. influenzae* type b meningitis treated with cefuroxime. The timing of the first dexamethasone dose is critical and in order to be beneficial it should precede antibiotic administration by 5–10 minutes. Early seizure activity occurs in 20–30% with bacterial meningitis. It is commonly the result of cerebritis and less commonly associated with cerebral edema, cortical venous thrombosis, or metabolic derangements (hypoglycemia, hyponatremia, hypocalcemia). Effective anticonvulsants include diazepam or lorazepam acutely, and phenobarbital or phenytoin as maintenance. Seizures associated with hyponatremia will require correction of the hyponatremic state by slow infusion of hypertonic sodium chloride and possibly Lasix in the stable patient. The dose of hypertonic saline is determined by: mL of 3% NaCl = (120 − present Na+) (weight in kg) (0.6)/0.513.

Treating the underlying disease is the best way to reverse DIC. If the patient is actively bleeding from peripheral sites or from the gastrointestinal or urinary tracts, platelet transfusions to counts above 50,000/µl, vitamin K to correct a prolonged prothrombin time (PT), and fresh frozen plasma to correct a prolonged activated partial thromboplastin time (APTT) may be required. In the setting of DIC and thrombotic manifestations, consider heparin therapy (loading dose of 50–75 units/kg followed by 10 units/kg/hr as a continuous infusion). If the patient is not dehydrated and vitals are stable, fluid administration of a 0.2 or 0.3 normal saline solution at 1000 mL/m2/24 hours should be instituted with close monitoring of the serum sodium, urine specific gravity and sodium concentration, and urine output.

ANTIMICROBIAL THERAPY

Table 205-1 lists the drugs and doses suggested for the initial therapy of suspected bacterial meningitis. If the LP is to be delayed, antimicrobial therapy should be instituted. If HSV encephalitis is strongly suspected, institute acyclovir therapy at 10 mg/kg every 8 hours.

DISPOSITION

All patients with potential bacterial meningitis or HSV encephalitis require immediate hospitalization with intensive monitoring. Those CNS infections of probable enteroviral or arboviral origin may require hospitalization for diagnostic purposes or for supportive care. In some patients, the results of the initial CSF examination do not distinguish between a bacterial or viral process. If the patient has been pretreated with antibiotics, is <1 year of age, or is clinically unstable, institute antimicrobial therapy. Otherwise, carefully observe the patient and repeat the LP in 8 hours to

TABLE 205-1. Antimicrobial Therapy for Bacterial Meningitis

Age	Drug	Dosage
Newborn–30 days	Ampicillin	100 mg/kg q 12 h 0–6 days 100 mg/kg q 8 h 7–30 days
	and Gentamicin	2.5 mg/kg q 12 h 0–6 days 2.5 mg/kg q 8 h > 7 days
30 days–3 months	Ampicillin and a 3rd-generation cephalosporin Ceftriaxone loading dose 75–100 mg/kg, then 50 mg/kg q 12 h Cefotaxime 50 mg/kg q 6 h	75 mg/kg q 6 h
>3 months	Ceftriaxone or cefotaxime or Ampicillin and chloramphenicol 18.75–25 mg/kg q 6 h	

help differentiate the infectious process (with aseptic meningitis due to an enterovirus, a lymphocyte predominance typically develops).

It is advisable to manage infants and children with meningitis in a hospital that has specialized equipment and staff with expertise in caring for infants and children who are critically ill. Infants and children with septic shock, significant intracranial hypertension, or difficult-to-control seizures should be transported to a referral center. This is best accomplished by contacting the regional referral center directly; personnel there will suggest appropriate management options and assist in making the necessary transportation arrangements. If an LP had been performed, send an aliquot of the CSF with the patient, along with documentation of the management that the patient has received.

COMMON PITFALLS

- Failure to consider bacterial meningitis and perform an LP in a febrile, lethargic, irritable infant without the classical signs of meningitis
- Failure to perform an LP in a neonate with suspected sepsis (about 15% of neonates with bacterial meningitis have a negative blood culture)
- Failure to consider meningitis and perform an LP in an infant with another obvious focus of infection such as arthritis, pneumonia, or facial cellulitis
- Failure to consider HSV encephalitis in a neonate just because skin lesions are absent, and failure to question the mother as to the presence of vaginal blisters or burning/pruritic lesions during the pregnancy in a neonate with meningoencephalitis
- Failure to do a Gram's stain of the CSF just because it looks clear or has no cells present
- Failure to consider the possibility of a CNS infection in a child who apparently has had a simple febrile seizure. Unless the physician is confident that the child is alert and well and has no suggestion of signs of meningitis, LP should be considered.
- Failure to recognize the signs of warm shock and to take appropriate action to reverse it
- Failure to recognize the signs of increased intracranial pressure and to institute therapy to reduce it and prevent herniation
- Failure to recognize the seriousness of the situation and to call for assistance
- Failure to obtain a blood culture before instituting antibiotic therapy, especially in the patient who has not had an LP
- Because bacterial meningitis is a rapidly progressive disease process, children at the first visit may have a positive blood culture only, with a negative CSF culture, and may return 8 to 72 hours later with culture-proven meningitis. Carefully evaluate for the presence of meningitis in febrile infants without a focus, and document this in the hospital record to provide quality care and also for protection in case litigation attempts to prove that meningitis was missed.

206   Otitis Media in Children

OTITIS MEDIA
CLINICAL PRESENTATION

The usual presentation is seen in a child who has had several days of symptoms of an upper respiratory tract infection and suddenly develops ear pain, fever, decreased hearing, or ear drainage. In infancy, irritability, crying and difficulty sleeping can be the presenting symptoms.

Some children have minimal symptoms or none at all and OM is diagnosed during a routine physical exam. Tugging at the ears may be a sign for OM, but this is often misleading because children may tug or pull at their ears for other reasons.

Thus, the diagnosis of OM is based on the appearance and the mobility of the tympanic
membrane rather than on the symptomatology. The tympanic membrane is red or yellow, dull,
bulging, and has decreased or absent mobility when examined with a pneumatic otoscope.
Bulging is best interpreted by the absence of the normal bony landmarks, which in an early case
may be limited to the pars flaccida. Some of the difficulties in diagnosing OM include the presence of wax in the ear canal, which obscures the visualization of the tympanic membrane, and a
crying or febrile child in which a hyperemic tympanic membrane could be falsely interpreted as
early OM. Bullous myringitis is a form of acute OM in which bullae form between the outer and
middle layers of the tympanic membrane. These children usually present very acutely with severe
otalgia. Purulent otorrhea constitutes a reliable sign for an OM with perforation. Hearing loss may
be a presenting sign of OM, but this will not be the complaint in the young child and it can also
easily be missed by parents.

The diagnosis of OM in the newborn and very young infant is even more difficult because
their tympanic membranes may be naturally gray and dull in appearance. In these babies, the
diminished or absent mobility may be the only physical findings for OM. If tympanocentesis is performed, a purulent middle-ear aspirate is usually obtained. Although not an emergency department (ED) procedure, tympanometry usually reveals an effusion pattern.

The microbiology of OM from middle-ear aspirates demonstrates that the most common
pathogens are *Streptococcus pneumoniae, Haemophilus influenzae, Branhamella catarrhalis, S.
pyogenes* Group A, and *Staphylococcus aureus. Mycoplasma pneumoniae* and viruses have been
isolated from the middle ear in less than 5% of the cases. The microbiology of acute otitis media in
the newborn (the first 6 weeks of life) is different from that in later life. *S. aureus* and gram-negative
enteric organisms should be considered in addition to the other organisms that cause otitis media
in the older child. *Chlamydia trachomatis* also may cause acute OM in the first few months of life.

DIFFERENTIAL DIAGNOSIS

Earache could be caused by pain referred from sore throat, toothache, external otitis, parotitis,
foreign body in the ear canal, or impacted ear cerumen. Injected blood vessels at the periphery
of the tympanic membrane and along the malleus can be seen with fever or crying.

COMPLICATIONS

Acute OM may resolve without treatment, but spontaneous rupture of the tympanic membrane
and otorrhea may occur. Complications such as ossicle necrosis, retraction pockets,
cholesteatoma, mastoiditis, meningitis, and cerebral thrombophlebitis are rare. The introduction
of antimicrobial therapy has produced a decline in the frequency of these complications.

EMERGENCY DEPARTMENT MANAGEMENT

Most children who present with symptomatology of OM or fever can be easily diagnosed by examining the tympanic membranes and pneumatoscopy. Clean the ear canals if obscured by cerumen, remembering that irrigation of the ear canal could cause a temporary injection of the blood
vessels in the tympanic membrane.

Tympanocentesis is not a routine ED procedure but consultation with an ENT specialist
and diagnostic aspiration of the middle ear may be necessary in some circumstances. Indications
for tympanocentesis or myringotomy include the following: OM in patients who appear seriously
ill, unsatisfactory response to antimicrobials for 72 hours, OM in patients already receiving an
appropriate antimicrobial agent, OM with suppurative complications, and OM in the very young

infant or in the immunodeficient individual. The decision to perform tympanocentesis must be individualized. Send the fluid obtained to the laboratory for Gram's stain and bacterial cultures.

SYSTEMIC ANTIBIOTICS

Antimicrobial therapy is directed against the major pathogens: *S. pneumoniae, H. influenzae, B. catarrhalis*, and *Streptococcus* Group A. In the United States, the incidence of beta-lactamase-producing *H. influenzae* varies but can be as high as 20% to 25% (for *B. catarrhalis*, up to 70%).

In spite of this, most physicians choose amoxicillin as the drug of choice. Amoxicillin is inexpensive and has only few side effects (diarrhea, rash). In those regions where ampicillin-resistant organisms cause a significant percentage of OM and frequent therapeutic failures, alternative agents should be used. In the very ill-appearing and febrile child (particularly the young infant or the child already on amoxicillin), rather than risk therapeutic failure, use an alternative drug. For the beta-lactamase-producing *H. influenzae* and *B. catarrhalis*, alternatives include Cefaclor, trimethoprim-sulfisoxazole, erythromycin-sulfa and amoxicillin-clavulinic acid. All sulfonamides carry the risk of Stevens–Johnson syndrome. Cefaclor is associated with rashes, diarrhea, and rarely a serum sickness-like reaction. Amoxicillin-clavulinic acid is associated with the same side effects as amoxicillin, plus a higher incidence of gastrointestinal symptoms. In suspension, Cefaclor and amoxicillin are more palatable. Amoxicillin and trimethoprim-sulfamethoxazole are the least expensive.

Most physicians choose amoxicillin as the first-line drug and reserve the others for the young infant or the ill-appearing child, or in the case of treatment failure. For dosages, see Table 206-1. The length of therapy is 10 days. In newborn infants, Cefaclor or amoxicillin-clavulinic acid may have advantage of activity against coliforms and *S. aureus*.

In the child who clinically responds well to therapy, a re-examination must be performed by the child's physician in 2 to 3 weeks, looking for resolutions of acute signs of OM. At this checkup, about half of the children still have evidence of serous effusion of the middle ear.

ANTIBIOTIC EAR DROPS

In the child with considerable purulent drainage from the ear, occasionally ear drops can be prescribed. Gentle cleansing with normal saline solution or diluted sterile vinegar may be followed then by antibiotic-corticosteroid ear drop suspension for a few days. Symptomatic relief should occur within 48 to 72 hours after the initiation of therapy. The patient and the parents should be

---

TABLE 206-1. Antimicrobial Therapy of Otitis Media

Amoxicillin
40 mg/kg/d PO q 8 h

Erythromycin-Sulfa Combination
40 mg/kg/d of erythromycin component PO q 6 h

Cefaclor
40 mg/kg/d PO q 8 h

Trimethoprim-Sulfamethoxazole
6–8 mg/kg/d of the TMP component PO q 12 h

Amoxicillin-Clavulinic Acid
40 mg/moxicillin component/kg/d PO q 8 h

Adapted from Nelson JD: Pocketbook of Pediatric Antimicrobial Therapy, 7th ed. Philadelphia, BC Decker, 1986

advised to seek medical attention if symptomatology continues beyond that time. If at this point the child still has very red and bulging tympanic membranes, a change to a broader-spectrum antimicrobial (a beta-lactamase-resistant one) should be considered.

Also, careful evaluation as to possible complications of the acute OM or to a coexisting condition (meningitis, brain abscess, or mastoiditis) should be done. In addition, the emergency physician needs to advise the parents to seek prompt medical attention if, during the course of treatment, symptoms of lethargy, irritability, vomiting, or relapse of the fever develop.

ANALGESICS AND ANTIPYRETICS

The child with severe earache may need acetaminophen or even codeine during the first 2 or 3 days of treatment. The use of an oral decongestant is ineffective in the treatment of OM; it should be prescribed only for the relief of symptoms of a concomitant upper respiratory tract infection.

DISPOSITION

The vast majority of children with acute OM can be discharged with subsequent follow-up by their physician in about 2 weeks. Most infants in the first 6 weeks of life, and those older children who appear toxic and severely ill, must be evaluated for a coexisting, more serious infection, such as sepsis or meningitis. Some of these children will require hospital admission. Children who have mastoiditis complicating OM need ENT consultation and hospital admission.

COMMON PITFALLS

- Otitis media is often overdiagnosed by making the diagnosis of early OM in a febrile or crying child who has only hyperemic (injected) tympanic membranes on otoscopic exam.
- Another common pitfall is the failure to consider other diagnoses and neglecting to consider a more serious and even life-threatening disease such as meningitis, sepsis, or pneumonia coexisting with acute OM.

207 Management of Diabetic Ketoacidosis in Children

CLINICAL PRESENTATION

Children with DKA have a readily recognizable clinical picture, particularly if the patient is known to have diabetes. Presenting features include nausea, vomiting, abdominal pain, hyperpnea, fruity breath odor, dehydration, and lethargy or coma. Polyuria, polydypsia, and polyphagia, the three classic symptoms of diabetes, are also usually present. Children with new-onset IDDM who present with DKA may be inappropriately diagnosed as having viral gastroenteritis or a urinary tract infection. This is particularly true in very young children in whom the possibility of diabetes may not be considered.

EMERGENCY DEPARTMENT EVALUATION

The initial evaluation of a child who presents with the clinical picture described above should be directed at the following areas:

1. Establishing the diagnosis of DKA
2. Assessing the degree of dehydration and electrolyte imbalance
3. Searching for the precipitating event for the DKA.

The first step in establishing the diagnosis of DKA in children is to test the urine for the presence of glucose and ketones. Their presence confirms the diagnosis of IDDM in a child with the appropriate clinical picture. The presence of a partially compensated metabolic acidosis on venous or capillary blood gas measurement confirms the diagnosis of DKA. The plasma glucose level is usually but not always above 300 mg/dL.

The physical examination can be used initially to assess the degree of dehydration as well as to search for underlying infectious or inflammatory processes that may have precipitated the DKA. Remember that since the extracellular fluid of children with DKA is hyperosmolar, the percentage of dehydration is usually greater than that estimated by the usual physical signs (i.e., dry mucous membranes, sunken eyes, decreased skin turgor, cool extremities, etc.). In general, assume at least 10% dehydration.

Serum electrolyte levels in DKA may be misleading. First, the sodium level is often decreased because of renal compensation for hyperosmolarity generated by high plasma glucose levels. Second, the serum potassium level is usually normal or slightly elevated despite the fact that the patient's total body potassium stores are depleted. This happens because intracellular potassium ions are exchanged for extracellular hydrogen ions in the presence of acidosis. Low-normal potassium levels in DKA indicate extreme total body potassium depletion. The serum calcium concentration is usually normal but the phosphate level is often low.

EMERGENCY DEPARTMENT MANAGEMENT

Fluid replacement and correction of dehydration should begin as soon as possible after the child with DKA arrives in the emergency department (ED). Normal saline, 20 mL/kg, is usually given as fluid bolus during the first hour of therapy. Avoid fluid boluses of more than 20 mL/kg unless needed to maintain normal blood pressure because of the risk of cerebral edema. Ringer's lactate solution is less commonly used, to avoid the theoretical potential of hyperchloremic acidosis.

After the first hour, the fluids are usually adjusted to replace the remainder of the patient's fluid deficit over the next 24 hours. If the patient is extremely hyperosmolar, slower correction may be desirable. Maintenance fluids are calculated in the usual manner (100 mL/kg for the first 10 kg, 50 mL/kg for the second 10 kg, and 20 mL/kg for every kilogram after that). Daily maintenance sodium is 2 to 3 mEq/kg. Maintenance potassium is 1 to 2 mEq/kg/day. The potassium deficit is about 6 mEq/kg and the sodium deficit is about 10 mEq/kg. This can usually be done with a solution of 0.45% NaCl plus KCl 40 mEq/L. The use of KPO_4 instead of KCl has been proposed because of the deficiency of 2–3 diphosphoglycerate but has been shown to be of no clinical benefit in children with DKA. Its use should be limited to those patients with extremely low serum phosphate concentrations (less than 1 mg/dL). Dextrose is added when the plasma glucose level falls below 300 mg/dL to maintain the glucose level between 200 and 300 mg/dL.

The use of bicarbonate is also highly controversial in the treatment of DKA. Its use has both theoretical advantages and disadvantages. The potential advantages of the use of bicarbonate are more rapid correction of the acidosis and improvement of the cardiovascular status. The major potential disadvantage to the use of bicarbonate is the possibility of the generation of paradoxical cerebrospinal fluid acidosis due to increased formation of carbonic acid and CO_2. The clinical studies that have been done show no advantage or disadvantage to the use of bicarbonate. If bicarbonate is used, give it as a slow infusion over several hours, not as a bolus. The use of a bicarbonate bolus adds to the patient's extreme hyperosmolarity.

A low-dose insulin infusion of 0.1 units/kg/hour has become the accepted standard for the treatment of the insulin deficiency present with DKA. This method of treatment allows for slower, more even correction of hyperglycemia and less hypoglycemia than do other forms of insulin administration. The insulin concentration for the infusion should be at least 0.5 units/mL to avoid problems with insulin binding to the intravenous infusion equipment. Begin the insulin infusion after the first hour of hydration to allow time for the initial laboratory results to return.

Plasma glucose levels should be monitored hourly. Serum electrolyte concentrations and venous blood gases should be monitored every 2 hours and calcium and phosphorous concentrations every 8 hours. The rate of glucose fall averages 75 mg/dL/hour.

DISPOSITION

During recovery, closely watch children in moderate to severe DKA for signs of cerebral edema, the leading cause of death due to DKA in children. Bradycardia, hypertension, sluggish pupillary reflexes, or mental status changes may be the first sign of brain herniation. The cause of this devastating complication is unknown, but overhydration and hyponatremia have been implicated. In addition, cardiac monitoring is needed because rapid changes in the serum potassium concentrations can lead to cardiac arrhythmias. Children in moderate to severe DKA should be treated in a facility with a pediatric intensive or intermediate care unit. Also, children with new-onset diabetes, especially those under 6 years of age, need to be transferred to a facility where age-appropriate diabetes education can be given.

Patients who can retain adequate amounts of oral intake without vomiting and who are not significantly acidotic (pH above 7.25) or dehydrated may be discharged home from the ED if appropriate follow-up care can be arranged. This includes frequent telephone contact with an individual knowledgeable in diabetes over the first 24 hours after leaving the ED.

COMMON PITFALLS

- Failure to administer insulin adequately is the most common cause of persistent DKA. This is often due to errors in insulin dilution or infusion. If a patient fails to respond to insulin treatment, discard the old insulin and examine the infusion system closely. In addition, hypoglycemia should be prevented by adding dextrose to the fluid replacement, not by slowing or stopping the insulin infusion.
- Failure to treat an underlying infectious or inflammatory process adequately is a second cause of persistent DKA in children. Thoroughly re-examine patients who fail to respond to treatment, looking for underlying infections. In particular, intra-abdominal disorders such as pancreatitis or appendicitis may be missed because of the abdominal pain associated with DKA.
- Failure to rehydrate the patient adequately is another problem that leads to poor treatment response. This usually results from failure to monitor the patient's fluid input and output adequately.
- Overhydration and too-rapid correction of the hyperosmolarity may lead to cerebral edema and brain stem herniation.
- Hypokalemia may result from inadequate potassium replacement during the correction of the acidosis, which leads to a shift of potassium into the cells.

208   Bleeding Disorders in Children

Bleeding disorders in childhood are most commonly related to deficiencies of plasma clotting factors (the hemophilias) or qualitative or quantitative platelet defects. This chapter will describe three of the most common childhood bleeding disorders: the hemophilias, von Willebrand's disease, and immune thrombocytopenic purpura.

HEMOPHILIA

Hemophilia is a deficiency of a soluble clotting factor, most commonly factor VIII or factor IX. Factor VIII deficiency is also known as "classical hemophilia" or hemophilia A; factor IX disease is also called Christmas disease or hemophilia B. Both are inherited as X-linked recessive conditions. The incidence of factor VIII deficiency is approximately one in 10,000 males, with factor IX only one fourth as common. Deficiencies of other less-common soluble clotting factors will not be discussed.

Diagnosis of these two conditions is suggested in the laboratory by a prolonged partial thromboplastin time (PTT) and normal prothrombin time (PT), with specific factor assays then performed. Clinically severe disease, with spontaneous hemorrhage into muscles or joints, is associated with factor assays of less than 1% activity (normal 50%–150% activity). Moderate disease, with increased bleeding with minor trauma, is seen with factor activity of 1% to 5%. Mild disease, with only occasional clinically significant hemorrhage, is seen with activity in the 6% to 25% range.

The usual treatment of significant hemorrhage in a hemophiliac involves the use of factor concentrate. Lyophilized powder concentrates of factors VIII and IX are available in various dose amounts. Use only heat-treated products to essentially eliminate the risk of HIV transmission; the risk of hepatitis B and non-A, non-B hepatitis remains. Once a bottle is entered, the entire contents should be given, not just a portion. Factor VIII at a dose of 1 unit/kg will increase activity by 2%; factor IX at 1 unit/kg will increase activity by 1%. Alternatively, cryoprecipitate at 0.2 units/kg or fresh-frozen plasma at 10 mL/kg may be used for minor hemorrhages. Intravenous desmopressin (DDAVP) may be used in mild to moderate hemophilia.

Trauma to the hemophiliac patient presents special problems. Intracranial hemorrhage may be severe, and factor replacement to the 80% to 100% activity level is indicated. Hematoma formation or hemorrhage in the neck may obstruct the airway, and aggressive management may be necessary. In addition to possible intubation, factor replacement to the 80% to 100% level should be undertaken. Extremity trauma with hemorrhage compromising the neurovascular bundles again requires aggressive immediate therapy. Hematologic consultation should be obtained in such instances. In general, patients can be prepared for surgery with bolus factor replacement. More bloody procedures require levels approaching 100% activity, while procedures with better hemostatic control can be done at levels closer to 50% activity.

The most common problems seen are secondary to muscle or joint bleeds. The joint may be warm, red, and swollen, with decreased range of motion; alternatively, the patient may sense a bleed, with no signs clinically present. Joint bleeds should be treated as early as possible, optimally when sensed by the patient and before clinical signs of hemorrhage appear. Replacement to the 40% activity level is usually sufficient, with follow-up for possible further therapy arranged.

Oral bleeding may occur due to trauma, loss of a tooth, or biting the tongue. Factor replacement to the 30% to 40% level (to form an initial clot) should be followed by oral epsilon aminocaproic acid (Amicar) at a dose of 100 mg/kg every 6 hours for 7 days. Amicar helps block the clot-dissolving effects of plasminogen in the saliva.

Factor deficiencies (e.g., XI, V, etc.) for which no commercially available concentrate exists can generally be treated with fresh frozen plasma 10 mL/kg; the frequency of dosing is determined by the half-life of the specific factor. Cryoprecipitate is a good source of fibrinogen.

VON WILLEBRAND'S DISEASE

Von Willebrand's (vW) disease is an autosomal dominant condition associated with a prolonged bleeding time secondary to decreased platelet adhesion to vascular endothelium, which normally is potentiated by the vW factor. Patients with this disorder either have decreased amounts of vW factor (Type I) or, less commonly, functionally abnormal moieties (Type II). In either case, a defect in the platelet phase of coagulation is noted.

Patients classically have prolonged bleeding after cuts, and gum or tooth bleeding and epistaxis are not uncommon. Muscular or joint bleeds are seen in the unusual homozygous form of this disease. If vW disease is suspected, hematologic evaluation including PT, PTT, factor VIII level, bleeding time, ristocetin co-factor, and factor VIII—related antigen studies are needed. The diagnosis may be difficult, and test results may vary over time.

Two basic therapeutic approaches may be used with the bleeding vW patients:

1. The vW factor is present in cryoprecipitate. The usual dose is 0.2 units/kg (minimum 2 units). This infusion has all the potential risks of any transfused blood product.
2. Intravenous DDAVP (Stimate) (dose, 0.3 µg/kg) will within 20 to 30 minutes increase the release of endogenous vW factor. This will temporarily increase plasma levels to a degree sufficient for all but major trauma. It can only be used for patients with Type I disease, however, because Type II vW patients cannot produce functional vW factor, and in some cases thromboses have been reported. Patients treated with DDAVP should also receive Amicar 100 mg/kg P.O. every 6 hours for 7 days, to prevent activation of plasminogen, which is also released by DDAVP.

Again, patients with oral bleeding should receive Amicar 100 mg/kg P.O. every 6 hours for 7 days to stabilize the clot formed by inhibiting lysis by plasminogen in the saliva.

IMMUNE THROMBOCYTOPENIC PURPURA

Immune (or idiopathic) thrombocytopenic purpura (ITP) in children is an acquired hemorrhagic disorder that results from excessive destruction of circulating platelets. Most childhood cases (85%) are acute, lasting less than 9 months; the remainder become chronic. The basic pathophysiology is that platelets are bound with IgG and are rapidly destroyed in the spleen. Although marrow platelet production is increased, the extremely rapid platelet clearance leads to profound thrombocytopenia and possible hemorrhage.

CLINICAL PRESENTATION

The classic clinical presentation is that of an otherwise healthy child with a recent viral syndrome, noted to have the onset of petechiae and ecchymoses. Apart from the bleeding diathesis, the history and physical examination are normal. In particular, history of significant fever, weight loss, bone pain, and anorexia are absent. The physical examination discloses no significant adenopathy or hepatosplenomegaly. Bruising can range from rare, scattered petechiae to diffuse ecchymoses and oral mucosal hemorrhage. Occasionally gastrointestinal, renal, or intracranial hemorrhage may occur. Muscle or joint hemorrhages, such as in hemophilias, are extremely rare.

Laboratory studies should include a complete blood count with manual differential, platelet count, reticulocyte count, and careful morphologic review. Most children with ITP have profoundly low platelet counts, usually less than 20,000/mm. Giant (young) platelets are often observed on the peripheral smear. Evidence of abnormality of any other cell line (RBC or WBC) without obvious explanation necessitates a full hematologic evaluation. Remember that half the children with acute lymphoblastic leukemia have normal or low WBC counts at diagnosis.

The optimal evaluation of a child with apparent ITP is controversial. Anything in the history, physical examination, or laboratory studies inconsistent with ITP necessitates a full evaluation, including a bone-marrow aspiration. Many hematologists will perform marrows on essentially all such patients to confirm the diagnosis and allay parental (and physician) fears of a misdiagnosis.

DIFFERENTIAL DIAGNOSIS

The differential diagnoses in these children include several major disease categories: a platelet defect, humoral defect, child abuse, aplastic anemia, leukemia or metastatic tumor. Bacterial sepsis, disseminated intravascular coagulation, or both are usually clinically apparent. Marked splenomegaly requires specific evaluation.

TREATMENT

Treatment of ITP is again controversial. Aspirin should be avoided, as should activities that may induce trauma, such as tree climbing or bicycle riding. In general, children with platelet counts above 10,000/mm and only mild to moderate bleeding require no specific therapy. Prednisone can frequently elevate the platelet count but has no effect on preventing chronic disease. Steroids should be avoided unless there is no question as to the diagnosis, as some patients with acute lymphoblastic leukemia can be placed in a temporary remission with prednisone alone. A typical course of prednisone is 4 mg/kg/day in two or three divided doses for 4 days, followed by 2 mg/kg/day to complete a 14-day course. Intravenous immunoglobulin (IVIG) can rapidly increase platelet counts, but because of its cost it is appropriate in only very limited instances.

Spontaneous intracranial hemorrhage is very unusual in ITP, with an incident of far less than 1%. In such cases, or in cases of ITP and major trauma, therapeutic interventions could include platelet transfusion (with little effect, due to the prompt destruction of transfused platelets), IVIG 1 g/kg, and emergency splenectomy.

COMMON PITFALLS

- Failure to recognize that platelet defects cause oral and cutaneous hemorrhage, while soluble clotting factor defects cause deep (muscle and/or joint) bleeds
- Failure to recognize that hemorrhage into joints and/or muscle in hemophiliacs are to be treated early, when they are sensed by the patient and before they are clinically apparent
- Failure to recognize that vW disease may be difficult to diagnose, and may be treated with either cryoprecipitate (often) or with intravenous DDAVP
- Failure to recognize that epsilon aminocaproic acid (Amicar) is of great benefit in oral bleeding in hemophiliacs
- Failure to recognize that children with ITP are well aside from their bleeding abnormality, and have no significant adenopathy or organomegaly.

209   Sickling Syndromes in Children

Sickle-cell anemia is an autosomal recessive hemoglobinopathy characterized by hemolytic anemia, recurrent vaso-occlusion, and end-organ dysfunction. The heterozygous state (AS), sickle-cell trait, is found in 8% to 10% of American blacks. The homozygous state (SS), sickle-cell anemia, occurs in one in 400 to 600 black newborns. The disease is seen less commonly in the Hispanic, southern European, and Middle Eastern populations.

Hemoglobin electrophoresis permits the accurate diagnosis of sickle-cell anemia, sickle-cell trait, hemoglobin SC disease, and other sickle variants as early as in the newborn period.

The sickle-cell prep (or Sickledex) is inaccurate before 4 to 6 months of age. In the older infant or child, the average child with sickle-cell anemia has a hemoglobin of 8 gm%, hematocrit of 24%, reticulocyte count of 10%, with an elevated platelet count and white blood cell count of 13,000 to 17,000.

Unexplained anemia in a black child should raise the issue of a hemoglobinopathy. The presence of any sickle forms on a peripheral smear is presumptive evidence of sickle-cell anemia. Children with sickle-cell trait have normal hematologic values.

Evaluation in the emergency department is dictated by the presentation or "crisis" of the present illness. Clinical symptoms may begin as early as 3 to 4 months of age, when significant amounts of hemoglobin S become present. Referral for ongoing treatment and parent education, preferably through a sickle-cell center, is vitally important.

DACTYLITIS (HAND-FOOT SYNDROME)

The hand-foot syndrome is the most common presentation of the child between 6 and 24 months of age with sickle-cell anemia. Painful swelling of the hands and/or feet results from symmetric infarction of the metacarpals and metatarsals. Low-grade fever (below 101.5°F) is common, and no significant changes in hematologic values are noted. Radiographs initially show only soft-tissue swelling, but osteolytic and periosteal changes are seen 2 to 3 weeks after the onset of symptoms. The presentation is often classic but must be differentiated from osteomyelitis (either unifocal or multifocal) and trauma. Therapy consists of hydration at one-and-a-half to two times maintenance (and/or intravenous fluids) and analgesia. Pain and swelling commonly require 2 to 5 days to resolve. Recurrence is not rare, but the syndrome generally ends by age 2 as the vascular supply to these bones collateralizes.

INFECTION

Bacterial infection is the most common cause of serious morbidity and mortality in children with sickle-cell anemia. The primary pathogens are the encapsulated organisms *Streptococcus pneumoniae* and *Hemophilus influenzae*, but *Salmonella* osteomyelitis and severe *Mycoplasma pneumoniae* infections are also seen. The primary cause is functional asplenia secondary to auto-infarction, which may occur as early as 5 months of age but is routine by age 5 years. Defects in complement and opsonization also have been noted in sickle-cell patients.

Consider the following statistics when evaluating any child with sickle-cell anemia and fever:

1. Bacterial meningitis and septicemia are more than 600 times more common in sicklers than normal children.
2. Bacterial pneumonia is 100 times more common in sicklers.
3. Pneumococcal sepsis in sicklers carries a 14% mortality, often within hours of presentation, even when recognized and treated.
4. Pneumococcal disease is most common before age 6, and particularly common in the first 2 to 3 years of life.

Prophylactic daily penicillin should be started at age 3 to 4 months and continued at least until age 5 years at a dose of 125 mg P.O. twice daily. A dose of 250 mg P.O. twice daily is given from age 3 to 5 years. Additionally, HiB and Pneumovax should be administered routinely. Educating the family is critical.

Despite optimal treatment, children with sickle-cell anemia may present with fever and potential bacterial infections. Initial evaluation should include:

1. A careful history of the present illness. Bacteremia is somewhat more likely to be of only several hours' duration and associated with a fever of above 103°F.
2. A careful review of the child's medical history, including penicillin prophylaxis and possible missed doses.
3. A careful physical examination. Focal sites of infection can coexist with bacteremia.
4. For fever of above 101.5°F, a complete blood count with differential, reticulocyte count, and a blood culture are probably minimal requirements. Marked leukocytosis (above the baseline 13,000–17,000) or left shift should be noted. Urine bacterial antigen screen, lumbar puncture, and chest radiographs may be indicated. Erythrocyte sedimentation rate (ESR) and C-reactive protein (CRP) are unreliable.

In general, the child less than 3 years of age with a fever above 101.5°F and no focal source of infection requires appropriate bacterial cultures and intravenous antibiotics. Children with lower fever, benign focal infection (e.g., otitis media), or older children can often be cultured, observed for several hours, and discharged home on oral antibiotics with good follow-up. Antibiotic choice should depend on local patterns of bacterial sensitivity, but coverage of both *H. influenzae* and *S. pneumoniae* is necessary in the young child. Children older than 8 or 9 years can often be managed with penicillin alone.

VASO-OCCLUSIVE EPISODES

The hallmark of sickle-cell anemia is the "painful crisis" caused by artery occlusion by irreversibly sickled cells. Vaso-occlusion may be precipitated by dehydration, hypoxia, acidosis, or infection, but often occurs without ready explanation. Symptoms vary according to the location of vascular obstruction, but pain secondary to tissue hypoxemia is common. Pain episodes commonly involve the extremities or abdomen, but head pain (calvarial) and chest wall (rib, sternal) pain are common in older children. Low-grade fever is often noted.

Therapy consists of aggressive hydration (twice maintenance) and analgesics. For mild pain, aspirin or acetaminophen may be adequate. For moderate pain, intravenous or intramuscular morphine sulfate or meperidine may be appropriate, followed by hydration and transfer to oral agents such as Tylenol with codeine. Severe pain requires intravenous morphine sulfate, fluids, and hospitalization. Avoid giving multiple doses of meperidine because of its short duration of action and because of the seizure-threshold-lowering effects of the metabolic byproduct nor-meperidine.

CEREBROVASCULAR ACCIDENT

About 7% of sickle-cell patients will sustain a central nervous system event, often a stroke. In the younger child, the event is usually thrombotic; in the adolescent or adult, it may be hemorrhagic. These events are unpredictable. They routinely involve major cerebral arteries and can be devastating. In the emergency department, any untoward neurologic event in a sickle-cell patient is a cerebrovascular accident (CVA) until proven otherwise.

Initial evaluation should include taking a careful history for precipitating events, doing a formal neurologic examination, placing an intravenous line, and obtaining baseline laboratory values.

CT scanning without contrast is needed routinely. Neurology and hematology consultations should be obtained. Arteriography is usually not needed and can precipitate further sickling in the untransfused patient.

Acute therapy usually includes intravenous hydration and exchange transfusion to decrease the percentage of hemoglobin S to below 30%. Prompt recognition and treatment in an intensive-care setting usually results in a gratifying outcome.

Long-term treatment necessitates hypertransfusion for several years to reduce the 66% chance of recurrent CVA in these patients.

ACUTE SPLENIC SEQUESTRATION

Splenic sequestration is a life-threatening condition seen in young children before the onset of auto-infarction of the spleen. Over a period of hours, a significant portion of the circulating blood volume is sequestered in the spleen because of vaso-occlusion in the splenic vein. Thus, the patient develops hypovolemia, pallor, massive splenomegaly, and occasionally shock and death. Families should be educated in splenic palpation. Evaluation will demonstrate splenomegaly (often massive), anemia, and reticulocytosis.

Treatment is aimed at sustaining blood volume until the condition spontaneously reverses, releasing the sequestered blood. Careful monitoring and frequently a transfusion of 10 mL/kg of packed red blood cells may be required. Overtransfusion should be avoided, as the condition will reverse.

APLASTIC CRISIS

Aplastic crisis refers to acute anemia that may be superimposed on sickle-cell patients by episodes of marrow hypoplasia. The severely decreased red cell survival in these patients necessitates a marked reticulocytosis (above 10%) to maintain their baseline hemoglobin levels. Episodes of erythroid hypoplasia, manifested by progressive anemia with reticulocytopenia (below 1%), occur both sporadically and epidemically in association with the human parvovirus. Packed red blood cell transfusion may be necessary until erythroid production returns, usually within a few weeks. Patients with aplastic crisis require close monitoring, because their hemoglobin may fall to 4 gm% or lower within a few days.

ACUTE CHEST SYNDROME

Episodes of cough, chest pain, fever, and pulmonary infiltrates are common. In older children the cause is usually infection, and in older children and adolescents, infarction. A syndrome of progressive infection and infarction may develop, with diffuse lung involvement. Consider *M. pneumoniae,* which can produce severe and unusual patterns of infection in these patients. Focus treatment on appropriate antibiotic coverage. Oxygen supplementation, transfusion, or both may be indicated.

PRIAPISM

Priapism refers to painful, involuntary penile erection. Sickling within the penile cavernous sinuses is most common in adolescents and young adults. Any episode lasting more than 3 hours is unlikely to resolve spontaneously and requires intravenous hydration and narcotic analgesia. Hematologic consultation regarding transfusion or exchange transfusion should be considered. Episodes persisting for more than 24 hours require surgical intervention. Physiologic sexual impotence commonly occurs from chronic scarring of the erectile tissue.

COMMON PITFALLS

- Failure to recognize that any sickled cell on peripheral smear is presumptive evidence of sickle-cell anemia
- Failure to appreciate the immune status of the sickle-cell patient. The febrile sickle-cell child requires careful evaluation, and often hospitalization and intravenous antibiotics.
- Failure to recognize that sickle-cell anemia can be diagnosed in the newborn; symptoms may begin by age 3 to 4 months

- Failure to recognize that the sickle prep is inaccurate before 4 to 6 months of age
- Failure to remember that the evaluation of any untoward neurologic event in a sickle-cell patient should include consideration of a CVA
- Failure to consider aplastic crises and acute splenic sequestration in the acutely anemic sickle-cell patient.

210   Asthma in Children

Asthma is a chronic illness characterized by increased reactivity of pulmonary airways to various stimuli; resultant episodes of increased work of breathing are due to inflammation, increased secretions, or narrowing of the airways due to bronchospasm. These episodes vary in severity and duration, and improve either spontaneously or after pharmacologic intervention.

CLINICAL PRESENTATION

The hallmark of asthma is respiratory distress (increased work of breathing). A clinical spectrum of respiratory distress exists in acute asthma. Some patients will present in frank respiratory failure, requiring immediate respiratory assistance to preclude cardiovascular failure. Most patients will present with mild to moderate symptoms, however, and the ED physician will have time to evaluate the history and perform a physical exam before beginning therapy. Most children will have tachypnea and a prolonged expiratory phase of respiration. Chest auscultation will usually reveal diffuse expiratory wheezes. Inspiratory wheezes, intracostal retractions, supraclavicular retractions, nasal flaring, and use of accessory muscles to assist breathing all develop progressively as work of breathing increases. As a child tires, wheezing may diminish because of decreased air exchange. Agitation, confusion, and, in the older child, complaint of headache are clinical signs often associated with hypoxia; lethargy is associated with hypercapnea or fatigue. Cyanosis in an asthmatic usually indicates hypoxia sufficient to produce at least 5 g/dL of reduced (ferrous) hemoglobin—an ominous clinical sign.

Acute respiratory failure is a clinical diagnosis.

DIFFERENTIAL DIAGNOSIS

Pulmonary diseases can be divided into three broad categories: upper airway disease, lower airway disease (asthma is classified as a lower airway disease even though some degree of large airway pathology may also be involved), and alveolar disease. The initial step in differential diagnosis is to exclude upper airway and alveolar disease.

1. Inspiratory stridor is the hallmark of upper respiratory disease. Inspiration is prolonged and usually accompanied by suprasternal/supraclavicular retractions. Because the pathology is above the carina, intracostal retractions are less prominent or absent. Examples of commonly acquired upper airway diseases are croup, epiglottitis, and aspiration of a foreign body (which lodges above the glottis).
2. Rales are the hallmark of alveolar disease. Examples of commonly acquired alveolar diseases are pneumonia and pulmonary edema.

Having located the pathology in the lower airways, the next step is to determine whether distress is from asthma or some other cause of lower airway disease. What makes this difficult is the fact that some degree of bronchospasm is present in many lower airway diseases other than asthma. Thus, treating for asthma may produce improvement despite the fact that the primary pathology is not asthma.

A common cause of tachypnea and wheezing in the infant is bronchiolitis. Relationships exist between asthma and bronchiolitis, but because the discussion is lengthy, this subject is assigned a separate chapter in this text (Chapter 211). Fever may be present in bronchiolitis, and can be useful in differentiating it from "pure" asthma, in which fever is absent.

Pulmonary congestion from left heart failure or a large left-to-right shunt will present with tachypnea and wheezing. Cardiac examination may reveal cardiac murmur, lateral displacement of point of maximum impulse (PMI), hepatomegaly, distended neck veins, or edema.

Aspiration of a foreign body may produce tachypnea and wheezing. Onset is sudden. Careful observation of respiratory pattern may reveal chest asymmetry; auscultation may reveal localized wheezes. Left and right decubitus radiographs or fluoroscopy often demonstrate air trapping indicative of a foreign body.

Look at the patient's fingers for clubbing. If present, a disease other than asthma must exist because "pure" asthma rarely, if ever, produces clubbing.

Cystic fibrosis (CF) will present with recurrent episodes of respiratory distress (often pneumonia) accompanied by wheezing. Clubbing of the fingers is associated with cystic fibrosis. Often the patient shows signs of poor nutrition, indicative of malabsorption associated with cystic fibrosis. Rectal prolapse occurs in a minority of patients with CF. Nevertheless, this history should be sought because its presence argues strongly in favor of a presumptive diagnosis of CF, and referral for a sweat chloride test should be arranged.

EMERGENCY DEPARTMENT TREATMENT

Examination should include assessment of the general status of the child and evaluation of the work of breathing. Palpation of neck and chest may reveal subcutaneous emphysema, indicating pneumomediastinum. Low-grade fever may mean pneumonia but often reflects merely a viral illness that precipitated the respiratory distress. Lab tests in acute asthma are primarily useful to confirm clinical impressions and should be deferred in the absence of specific indications. If pneumonia, pneumothorax, or pneumomediastinum is suspected, an A–P and lateral chest radiograph should be ordered. Arterial blood gases are painful and often increase respiratory distress in the anxious patient; pulse oximetry can determine oxygen saturation painlessly and is usually a preferable alternative. Older children will often cooperate in assessment of peak pulmonary flow or FEV_1 before and after treatment, especially if encouraged by a parent. Most asthmatic children will benefit from supplemental oxygen. Hyperhydration does not produce liquefaction of pulmonary secretions and SIADH may result from overhydration. Thus, intravenous therapy should be reserved for patients with specific indications, and should not be automatic.

PHARMACOLOGIC THERAPY AEROSOLS

Acute asthma is optimally treated with a pharmacologic agent with rapid onset of action and high efficacy. For decades, subcutaneous injection of epinephrine has been effective initial ED treatment. Recently, beta-agonist aerosols have been shown to be equally effective; they have fewer cardiovascular side effects and do not require painful injections. Therefore, beta-agonist aerosols are preferred for initial treatment of acute asthma. Albuterol is a popular choice for aerosol therapy. Dosage is 50 to 100 µg/kg (0.01–0.02 mL/kg of 0.5% solution) to a maximum dose of 2.5 mg (0.5 mL of 0.5% solution). Dilute the albuterol in 2 to 3 mL of sterile normal saline. Metaproterenol may be used at a dosage of 0.5 mg/kg (0.1 mL/kg of 5% solution) to a maximum dose of 15 mg (0.3 mL of 5% solution). Dilute in 2 to 3 mL of sterile normal saline. Ipratropium bromide, a quaternary ammonium derivative of atropine, is an anticholinergic agent with few side effects when given by aerosol. Pharmacologically, cholinergic blockade differs from the action of beta agonists, and ipratropium has been shown to be a useful alternative to beta agonists in treatment of adults. Studies to date in children indicate that it is likely to be useful when given alone or in combination with albuterol. Inhaled beta agonists produce more rapid and more potent bronchodilatation than intravenous theophylline.

CORTICOSTEROIDS

Corticosteroids are useful in treating acute asthma, even though clinical improvement lags behind intravenous infusion by several hours. Glucocorticoids are often given when beta agonists fail to produce satisfactory clinical improvement, but debate exists over the dosage, timing, and even the choice of glucocorticoid. An initial bolus of 6 to 7 mg/kg of hydrocortisone or 1 to 2 mg/kg of methylprednisolone are commonly used dosages. Subsequent glucocorticoids may be given orally or intravenously. Steroids may be prescribed for patients who are discharged from the ED. We have used prednisone (1–2 mg/kg/24 hr, maximum dose 40 mg/24 hr) two or three times daily for 5 days with good clinical results.

DISPOSITION

Considerable variation in response to treatment exists not only between patients, but also between attacks suffered by the same patient. It is unwise to expect improvement in symptoms because a patient appears to be having an attack analogous to a previous attack that improved readily. Even if the patient is well known, always observe and record response to therapy. Decisions regarding disposition usually can be made reliably after the second or third aerosol treatment. Disposition for patients at the mild and severe ends of the clinical spectrum of asthma is usually straightforward.

Patients who improve after treatment in the ED can be discharged home. Oral medications are usually prescribed for acute asthma; inhaler medications are usually reserved for use after the acute episode has resolved. Oral metaproterenol has proven to be as effective as theophylline over a 4-week period. Oral medications frequently prescribed: metaproterenol, albuterol, and prednisone. Accepted pediatric dosages for these medications are listed in Table 210-1. The discharged patient (and family) should be instructed to return to the ED if the respiratory condition unexpectedly worsens or becomes uncertain. Accordingly, the wise physician will inquire about the family situation and make alternative plans (including admission) if the patient does not have the ability to return promptly should his or her condition worsen.

Patients who improve with initial therapy but remain too ill to be discharged may be treated further and observed in the ED to determine whether admission will be necessary. We usually place the patient in a monitored bed, start an intravenous line, glucocorticoids, and search for any underlying condition that may be exacerbating the attack. Since corticosteroids may require several hours to produce observable clinical effects, we usually wait 4 to 8 hours before admitting. Obtaining chest radiographs routinely at admission seldom provides useful information. If chest radiographs are clinically indicated, always obtain a lateral view in addition to an anteroposterior (or posteroanterior view).

Sometimes, however, a patient will progress to respiratory failure despite prompt and appropriate therapy. Treatment of the patient with respiratory failure may include any of the previously discussed therapies for acute asthma, plus tracheal intubation and mechanically assisted ventilation. Continuous beta-agonist aerosol is often useful for the intubated patient. Alternatively, a continuous isoproterenol infusion may be given at an initial rate of 0.1 µg/kg/min, with incremental increases in rate as clinically indicated. Heart rate above 200 bpm is generally accepted as a contraindication to increasing the rate of isoproterenol infusion. Isoproterenol drip infusion: patient's weight in kg $\times$ 0.6 equals mg isoproterenol added to 100 mL normal saline. At this concentration, 1 mL/hr delivers 0.1 µg/kg/min.

TABLE 210-1. Accepted Pediatric Dosages

Theophylline

<1 y/o = 0.2 x (age in weeks) + 5 = mg/kg/day
1–9 y/o = 22 mg/kg/day q 8–12 hr
9–12 y/o = 20 mg/kg/day q 8–12 hr
12–16 y/o = 18 mg/kg/day q 8–12 hr
>16 y/o = 13 mg/kg/day q 8–12 hr

Metaproterenol

<6 y/o = 1.3–2.6 mg/kg/day TID or QID
6–9 y/o = 10 mg/dose TID or QID
>9 y/o = 20 mg/dose TID or QID

Albuterol

2–5 y/o = 0.1 mg/kg/dose q 8 hr (max 12 mg/day)
6–11 y/o = 2 mg/kg/dose PO TID (max 24 mg/day)
>11 y/o = 2–4 mg/kg/dose PO TID or QID

Prednisone

0.5–1.0 mg/kg/24 hr (max 40 mg/24 hr)

From Cole CH (ed): The Harriet Lane Handbook, 11th ed. Chicago Year Book Medical Pub, 1987. Reprinted with permission.

COMMON PITFALLS

- Remember that the usual ED environment is often a totally new experience for many children and can be frightening.
- Try to avoid painful procedures that may worsen respiratory distress.
- Respiratory failure is a clinical diagnosis. Assessment of the "work of breathing" is more essential than relying on laboratory tests.

---

211   Bronchiolitis in Children

Bronchiolitis is an acute infectious disease that presents with respiratory symptoms. The patient usually has a history of rhinitis, cough, dyspnea, and poor feeding. Another family member often has had a recent, usually mild, respiratory infection. Fever is variably present. Physical examination commonly reveals tachypnea, a prolonged expiratory phase of respiration, wheezing, rales, and inspiratory retractions. Cyanosis is uncommon. Bronchiolitis can occur at any age, but is most commonly a disease of infancy. There is an incidence of 11.4% in the first year of life, 6% in the second year of life, and further decreases in incidence thereafter. The principal etiologic agents in the preschool child were respiratory syncytial virus (RSV) and parainfluenza virus; the principal agent in the school-aged child was Mycoplasma pneumoniae.

Epidemics of bronchiolitis occur often, usually in the winter and spring. RSV has been shown to be the primary pathogen during these epidemics, a fact with therapeutic implications.

EMERGENCY DEPARTMENT EVALUATION

Respiratory difficulty is a salient finding on physical examination. The chest is often hyperexpanded due to air trapping and hyperresonant to percussion. The liver and spleen are often displaced into the abdomen from diaphragmatic flattening, but are not truly enlarged. Coryza, conjunctivitis, or otitis media may be present. Hypoxia is common; place patients on a cardiac monitor and assess oxygen saturation via a pulse oximeter. Increased work of breathing often interferes with ingestion of fluids, producing mild or moderate dehydration. A normal white blood cell count is common. Chest radiographs, if ordered, should always include a lateral view. Hyperinflation, characterized on the lateral view by flattening of the diaphragms, and on the anterior view by increased radiolucency with small heart size, is a common finding. Areas of opacity may be present: these most often represent atelectasis, but pneumonia usually cannot be excluded as a cause.

EMERGENCY DEPARTMENT MANAGEMENT

Assess not only the degree of respiratory distress, as indicated by the work of breathing, but also the infant's ability to ingest liquids and avoid dehydration. Because hypoxia is common and may be clinically inapparent, offering humidified supplemental oxygen should be routine if the patient tolerates.

Chest radiographs often reveal areas of opacity consistent with atelectasis or pneumonia. We find it difficult to withhold antibiotic therapy in a febrile, tachypneic infant with rales and an abnormal radiograph, even though atelectasis usually turns out, in retrospect, to be the correct diagnosis. Avoiding routine radiographs and ordering chest films only if clinically indicated will minimize the occurrence of this clinical dilemma. There is no significant benefit from routine antibiotic usage in patients with bronchiolitis. Bronchodilators in bronchiolitis is controversial.

All patients are given humidified oxygen. Bronchodilator therapy is continued based on the results of an initial treatment given the patient. We begin intravenous rehydration if clinically indicated, but avoid routine intravenous therapy in these patients.

Ribavirin has been reported to be effective specific therapy for bronchiolitis caused by RSV. The American Academy of Pediatrics recommends that hospitals have the ability to perform rapid diagnostic testing for RSV to confirm the diagnosis before using ribavirin to treat certain categories of hospitalized infants (infants at high risk for severe or complicated RSV infection, infants with severe lower respiratory tract RSV disease, and infants <6 weeks of age or with certain underlying conditions). Therapy is via a nebulized aerosol given over several days; ribavirin should not be given without first arranging for inpatient care of the patient.

Patients with respiratory failure should be intubated and have mechanically assisted ventilation. If sedation is necessary, chloral hydrate (20–50 mg/kg/dose; maximum dose 1000 mg) via nasogastric tube, or morphine sulfate (0.1 mg/kg/dose IV) have been reported as effective alternatives to paralyzing the patient.

DISPOSITION

Most patients with bronchiolitis do not require admission to the hospital. Age, however, is important: most fatalities occur in patients <6 months of age. Admission rates are highest during the first year of life, with most of these occurring in the first months of life. Young infants are at risk for apnea. Pre-existing pulmonary disease, congenital heart disease, immunodeficiency, and immunosuppression are associated with more severe illness, especially when the etiologic agent is RSV. Admit patients in the high-risk categories, and other patients based on clinical assessment of respiratory and fluid status. Patients discharged home should be instructed to return for re-evaluation if the condition worsens. A follow-up visit within 24 hours should be arranged for all but the mildest cases.

COMMON PITFALLS

- Don't mistake congenital heart disease, cystic fibrosis, or foreign body aspiration for bronchiolitis.
- Corticosteroids and prophylactic antibiotics have not been shown to benefit patients with bronchiolitis.
- Allow the older child to assume his own position of comfort.
- Do not place infants on the stretcher unless the head of the stretcher is elevated; even better is in the arms of a parent. Avoid placing infants with respiratory distress in an infant seat.
- Hypoxia is common and may be clinically inapparent. Give humidified oxygen, unless specifically contraindicated.
- If giving supplemental oxygen to a child produces fear and agitation, a parent may be able to persuade the child to accept therapy. If the child cannot be comforted, it is probably better not to insist on therapy that increases oxygen consumption and work of breathing. Remove the oxygen; watch the child closely.
- Ordering radiographs or starting an intravenous line should be based on clinical indications and should not be routine.
- Premature and very young infants are at risk for apnea and should be admitted to the hospital even if they look relatively well in the ED.
- Patients with underlying medical conditions such as congenital heart disease, pulmonary disease, immunodeficiency, or immunosuppression are at risk for complications or a more severe illness. This is especially true for bronchiolitis caused by RSV.
- The decision to discharge a patient should include the ability to take oral fluids as well as work of breathing.
- If a patient is discharged home, it is prudent to arrange for a repeat examination within 24 hours.

212   Ingested Foreign Bodies

Infants enjoy using their mouths to help them assess new objects. They continue this into the toddler years, when they are mobile and therefore have greater opportunities to find small objects.

CLINICAL PRESENTATION

When children present with a history of foreign body ingestion, a choking or gagging episode has usually been witnessed by an adult or has been reported to the parent by an older child. Many of these children are asymptomatic on presentation. The greater diagnostic challenge is the symptomatic child who presents without a positive history. Diagnosis in this case requires awareness of the range of presenting symptoms. In one review of 125 children with foreign body ingestions, the most frequent complaints were gagging/vomiting, choking, neck and throat pain, foreign body sensation, and dyspnea. In a review of esophageal foreign bodies, the most common presenting symptoms of the 343 children were refusal to take feeds, salivation, pain and discomfort on swallowing, and vomiting.

In addition to the more common presentations, children with esophageal foreign bodies may present with symptoms referable to the respiratory tract (i.e., stridor, persistent cough, wheezing, and chronic pneumonia).

DIFFERENTIAL DIAGNOSIS

When there is a positive history for ingestion, localizing the foreign body within the gastrointestinal tract is important even if the child is asymptomatic. One study showed that 17% of asymptomatic children with a history of coin ingestion were found to have coins in the esophagus. Delay in removal of esophageal foreign bodies may result in obstruction, because an inflammatory reaction and edema develop with the resultant possibility of aspiration; perforation or erosion through the esophagus; or formation of a tracheoesophageal fistula.

Esophageal foreign bodies may present very much like airway foreign bodies. Again, it is important to remember that stridor, cough, or wheezing may represent an esophageal foreign body.

EMERGENCY DEPARTMENT EVALUATION

When there is a clinical suspicion of ingested foreign body, radiographic evaluation should include a lateral soft-tissue view of the neck in addition to an anteroposterior view, as well as films of the chest and abdomen. Foreign bodies are often missed when only an anteroposterior view is ordered. Lateral views are also necessary to demonstrate multiple coins in rouleau. Nonradiopaque items can usually be demonstrated with barium.

EMERGENCY DEPARTMENT MANAGEMENT

Most foreign bodies pass through the digestive tract without problems. Objects lodged in the esophagus require immediate removal because of the reasons listed above. Once objects have been demonstrated to have passed beyond the esophagus, however, they rarely represent a hazard to the patient: 95% pass without incident. A brief observation period (12–24 hours) has been recommended by some for asymptomatic patients with coins in the esophagus. It is important to know that the object has been eliminated. Sometimes objects enter a Meckel's diverticulum or the appendix. A repeat radiograph should be done in 1 week if examination of the stool has not detected the foreign body. Sharp objects pose an increased risk for perforation if detained at one site.

Elongated objects sometimes cannot traverse the C loop of the duodenum or the area of the ligament of Treitz. For such objects, closer follow-up is needed to monitor development of signs of potential obstruction or peritonitis. Endoscopic removal is indicated for objects retained in the stomach or rectum. Operative removal is indicated if the object remains at the same site in the duodenum or small intestine longer than 7 days or if symptoms develop. Enemas are usually successful at dislodging retained colonic foreign bodies. The amount of time it takes for a foreign body to pass through the entire gastrointestinal tract varies widely. but 85% usually pass within 72 hours, 99.9% within 7 days.

Removal of esophageal foreign bodies traditionally has been done using a rigid endoscope. The flexible scope may be an alternative for select patients. when done by those skilled in its use with children. Removal of blunt objects using a Foley catheter under fluoroscopy avoids general anesthesia necessary for rigid endoscopy but should be used only with recent ingestions of blunt, nonorganic radiopaque objects in a cooperative patient with a normal esophagus. Disc batteries lodged in the esophagus pose a high risk for serious injury to the patient although a benign course occurs with batteries that passed beyond the esophagus. The success rate for endoscopic removal from the stomach is low (33%). An attempt is recommended for batteries 23 mm in diameter retained in the stomach for >48 hours, because delayed transit occurs with batteries of this size. Ipecac is not recommended.

DISPOSITION

Children with esophageal foreign bodies should be referred immediately to a person skilled in the removal of foreign bodies in children. Children with foreign bodies beyond the gastroesophageal junction may be observed as outpatients, with instructions to the parents to screen the stools. If the object is not passed in 4 to 7 days, obtain radiographic studies. Earlier (4 days) studies and closer clinical follow-up is recommended for disc batteries and for sharp and elongated objects; 48 hour follow-up radiographs are recommended for disc batteries lodged in the stomach that are >23 mm in diameter.

COMMON PITFALLS

- Failure to recognize an esophageal foreign body in a child with *respiratory* symptoms
- Failure to obtain lateral radiographic views, which may result in failure to visualize opaque foreign bodies

213   Pediatric Pneumonias

Pneumonias are disease processes marked by inflammation of the lungs. They may be acute or chronic, caused by viruses, bacteria, fungi, and physical or chemical agents. This chapter will be limited to acute pneumonias with an infectious cause; inflammatory lung processes such as asthma and those caused by physical and chemical agents are treated elsewhere in this text. In children, particularly those of preschool age, acute respiratory infections commonly affect conducting airways and lung parenchyma simultaneously. The term "acute lower respiratory tract infections" (LRTI) circumvents the need to separate diseased lung components and is widely used. In this chapter, pneumonias will be defined as those LRTI with auscultatory (inspiratory rales, suppression of breath sounds) or radiographic (abnormal densities) findings of parenchymal involvement.

For practical purposes, LRTI will be divided into two categories: bacterial and nonbacterial infections. A clinical and epidemiologic approach to a specific etiologic diagnosis is of utmost importance to guide the initial empiric therapy and laboratory investigations. Nonbacterial pneumonias are those caused by viral agents, *Mycoplasma pneumoniae* and Chlamydiae. They are the most common respiratory infections affecting children. Some are treatable. Bacterial pneumonias, including Mycobacteria, although less common still occur frequently. They are amenable to specific curative therapy.

Certain agents have clear preferences for certain age groups. In the first 3 months of life, *Chlamydia trachomatis* is reportedly the most commonly recovered agent (not true during respiratory syncytial virus outbreaks); presumably it reflects intrapartum acquisition of the organism. Respiratory syncytial virus (RSV) is a common pathogen in this group of young infants during cold weather, potentially causing severe disease. The parainfluenza, especially Type 3, and influenza viruses also have seasonal peaks. Other viruses are recognized less frequently. Croup, tracheobronchitis, and bronchiolitis are three syndromes of acute LRTI typically caused by viral agents.

Bacteria are the major cause of pneumonia in the neonate. A sick newborn infant with findings of rales, radiographic lung densities, or both should be hospitalized because of possible sepsis.

Beyond the newborn period, it has been estimated that bacteria are responsible for one tenth to one third of all acute pneumonias. In infants, toddlers, and preschool-age children, RSV, parainfluenza, and influenza viruses, in decreasing frequency, are the leading causes of pneumonia. Adenoviruses and measles (in the absence of measles immunization) virus are not uncommon. The bacterial agents reported for this age group infants are *Pneumococcus, Hemophilus influenzae* type B, *Staphylococcus aureus,* and Group A *Streptococcus. Pneumococcus* is responsible for 50%, *H. influenzae* type B for 32%, *S. aureus* 16%, and Group A *Streptococcus* 2%. Half of *S. aureus* pneumonias occur before age 3 months, whereas the medians for *Hemophilus* and *Pneumococcus* were 9 and 15 months, respectively.

In school-age children (6–16 years of age), *Mycoplasma pneumoniae* is the leading cause of pneumonia. Viruses continue to play an important epidemiologic role. Influenza and parainfluenza viruses are frequent offenders. Adenoviruses and Epstein–Barr virus are not uncommon. Bacteria other than Mycoplasma are not a common cause of pneumonia in older children. When they do occur, the lobar infiltrate caused by the pneumococcus seems to lead the list.

CLINICAL PRESENTATION

Acute lower respiratory tract infections in children can be divided into four clinical syndromes. Certain agents have a predilection for a given syndrome, but no syndrome is specific for a selected agent.

1. Laryngeal symptoms predominate in *croup:* hoarseness, barky cough, and stridor. It is predominantly caused by parainfluenza viruses, especially type 1. Its peak incidence is in the fall.
2. *Tracheobronchitis* is characterized by cough and rhonchi without laryngeal obstruction or wheezing. It is predominantly caused by Influenza viruses, but is also common with most other agents, including Mycoplasma. Peak incidences are in spring and winter.
3. *Bronchiolitis* is the diagnosis when expiratory wheezing with or without tachypnea, air trapping, and substernal retractions predominate. RSV is the agent most frequently associated with this syndrome. Peak incidence is in winter and spring.
4. *Pneumonia* is characterized by the presence of rales and pulmonary consolidation. Such abnormal lung density can be diffuse parenchymal with peribronchial cuffing as seen commonly in nonbacterial infections, including Mycoplasma, or they can be localized to a given segment, lobe (lobar) or contiguous lobes (bronchopneumonia). The latter patterns are typically seen with bacterial processes. Often these syndromes overlap.

In infants and young children, 1 or 2 days of rhinitis, poor appetite, low-grade fever, and irritability are usually the prodrome. Gradually the child becomes more irritable and more congested, coughing and vomiting occur, and fever may rise higher. Diarrhea is often seen. Apnea may occur in younger infants. The older child and adolescent will usually complain of malaise, myalgia, or sore throat. On physical exam there may be intercostal, subcostal, and suprasternal retractions as well as tachypnea, tachycardia, and nasal flaring. Grunting is not uncommon. Cyanosis may be present and can be continuous or associated with apneic or coughing spells.

The chest exam may range from unrevealing to floridly abnormal. The chest may be hyperresonant, suggestive of air trapping, or may have areas of dullness, suggestive of lobar consolidation or pleural effusion. Vocal fremitus may be normal, increased (lung consolidation), or decreased (pleural effusion). On auscultation, localized or diffuse rales may be present. Breath sounds may be diminished to absent over consolidated segments or may have a bronchial quality. Wheezing is common in children with a bronchiolitis component or in those with underlying increased airway reactivity. Conjunctivitis, otitis media, pharyngitis, mouth ulcers, and skin rashes are often found concomitant with the lung infection.

Clinical characteristics that may alert the physician to a bacterial process are high fever (above 39°C), abrupt onset or sudden deterioration during a "common cold," and toxicity.

Pleuritic chest pain is common in bacterial processes. The chest radiograph in bacterial pneumonias usually shows a lobar or subsegmental distribution. Pleural fluid can be present in large effusions.

Mycoplasma pneumoniae infections usually present with fever below 38°C, headache, sore throat, and myalgias. The presenting respiratory symptom is usually a gradually worsening paroxysmal cough that sometimes is productive. There is often a family history of similar illness weeks apart in different individuals. Occasionally there is conjunctivitis, myringitis, rash, or enanthem. The chest radiograph may show a diffuse or lobar infiltrate. This agent is the most commonly identified pathogen in school-age and adolescent patients with pneumonia.

DIFFERENTIAL DIAGNOSIS

The four distinct LRTI syndromes characterized in the previous section will commonly overlap during nonbacterial infections. Bacterial lung infections will cause a more distinct pneumonia with few if any airway symptoms. Noninfectious lung problems may present with signs and symptoms that may be confused with an LRTI. Conditions to keep in mind include the following.

> *Foreign body aspiration.* Foreign body aspiration will present with symptoms of either large or small airway obstruction depending on the site of lodging. Small foreign bodies lodged in secondary or tertiary bronchii can cause long-term chronic symptoms of cough and focal parenchymal densities due to volume loss and secondary infection. The initial episode of aspiration is not always elicited during the interview with the parents. They may not have actually witnessed it, or the initial episode may have had only short-lasting symptoms and may have been disregarded. A recurrent focal lung infiltrate should raise this suspicion, and subspecialty consultation should be sought. Foreign bodies lodged in the large airways are life-threatening emergencies that can be diagnosed with the history (sudden choking followed by respiratory distress), auscultatory findings of either stridor or wheezing, and radiographic findings. This diagnosis or suspicion should prompt immediate hospitalization and consultation with the appropriate service for retrieval of the foreign body.
>
> *"Aspiration pneumonia"/chemical pneumonitis.*
>
> *Reactive airways disease (asthma).* Reactive airways disease, especially chronic cough-variant asthma, is often confused with acute pneumonia during episodes of exacerbation. Often these children are labeled as having "recurrent" or "chronic" pneumonia and are given courses of antibiotics almost continuously. They are often suspected of having some form of immunodeficiency and undergo investigations. Children with "chronic" or "recurrent" pneumonia should be referred to the pediatric pulmonologist.
>
> *Pulmonary contusion.*
>
> *Pulmonary infarction.*
>
> *Acute or chronic pulmonary edema.* Acute pulmonary edema can present as acute respiratory distress with wheezing and rales and an abnormal chest radiograph. An enlarged heart will usually be seen when the edema is cardiogenic in origin from either congenital or acquired heart disease. Noncardiogenic lung edema occurs in children associated with other processes (i.e., nephrosis and seizures). They should be relatively easy to differentiate. Infants with congenital left-to-right shunts that sometimes are difficult to diagnose in the early postnatal period may present in "unexpected" overt congestive heart failure in their second or third month of life. The chest radiograph may be deceiving: hyperinflation is common and it can make the lung hyperemia and cardiomegaly less striking in appearance.
>
> *Lung involvement of other chronic diseases: sickle-cell anemia, uremia.* Chronic lung diseases will often have chronic symptoms and should pose little difficulty to differentiate. Remember that children with chronic lung disease are at increased risk for more frequent and

severe LRTI. Early hospitalization is strongly advised for some of these children when lung infections occur.

EMERGENCY DEPARTMENT EVALUATION

The diagnosis of LRTI can be made on the basis of history and physical examination. Pre-existing respiratory disorders or other chronic illnesses should always be sought. Laboratory studies contribute little in mild and low-risk cases. The amount of laboratory studies should vary in direct proportion to the severity of the illness and the risk level (pre-existing conditions) of the patient. A chest radiograph may be all that is needed in the ED to confirm the diagnosis and guide the therapy and disposition of the patient.

Once pneumonia is diagnosed on clinical grounds, the next step is to search for the causative agent. The immediate concern is to differentiate between bacterial, nonbacterial, and Mycoplasma infections. This differentiation may be difficult. Bacterial pneumonias are sometimes preceded by a "viral syndrome." Most viral respiratory infections do not lead to bacterial superinfections. Some clinical features can help differentiate between bacterial and nonbacterial infections, albeit not flawlessly. Diffuse wheezing strongly suggests a nonbacterial cause. Sudden onset and high fever are more common in bacterial processes, as is a toxic appearance. Pleuritic chest pain is more common with bacterial infections, as are large pleural effusions.

The rational use of laboratory resources is of great importance. Specific tests that may give indirect or direct evidence of the presence of a given organism are most helpful in moderate and severe cases requiring hospitalization. Bacterial infections tend to cause higher white blood cell counts, with a relatively greater number of neutrophils. However, the difference is too small in less than moderate cases and not always helpful. A bone marrow suppressive response can occur during viral infections and overwhelming bacterial sepsis.

Assessing the child's general condition is as important as the diagnostic evaluation to judge expected outcome and decide disposition and management.

EMERGENCY DEPARTMENT MANAGEMENT

Astuteness is required for managing children with pneumonia since the specific etiologic diagnosis will rarely be available for the initial therapeutic decisions. Differentiation between viral and bacterial processes can only be approximated with the information that will be commonly available in the initial few hours of presentation. Furthermore, documenting a viral infection by a rapid diagnostic assay (i.e., viral antigens in nasopharyngeal secretions) does not negate a concomitant bacterial infection. After diagnosing pneumonia in a child, several important decisions arise: Should the child be hospitalized or should specialty consultation be sought? Is there any potential benefit in administering or withholding antibiotics? Both socioeconomic and medical issues will play a role in these decisions.

GENERAL MEASURES

Support measures and symptomatic therapy are independent of the cause of the infection. Neonates and young infants with pneumonia should be hospitalized. Two important areas need careful consideration: *hydration* and *oxygenation*. Net oral intake may be diminished either because the child refuses fluids, or there is frequent vomiting. Emesis in this clinical setting may be related to coughing paroxysms or to actual involvement of the gastrointestinal tract in the infectious process. Thus, it is important to ascertain the child's ability for oral intake. This judgment can be made by history: How much has the child had to drink over the preceding few hours? How much emesis has occurred and is it associated with coughing? How well hydrated does he or she appear now? Can he or she drink clear fluids in the ED? What is the respiratory rate? Are there severe coughing paroxysms? A toxic-appearing child (lethargic/encephalopathic) is not a candidate for ambulatory management.

Oxygenation is difficult and often impossible to assess on clinical grounds alone. The child with minimal respiratory symptoms who is not anemic and has a pink appearance clearly does not need to have objective measurements of oxygen in blood. The child in moderate to severe distress with a doubtful color (pale, grayish, or blue) and perhaps anemic should have an objective arterial blood oxygen, CO_2, and pH measurement. In less severe cases, a transcutaneous oximetry reading of hemoglobin saturation is acceptable.

The child with pneumonia who is well hydrated, well oxygenated, and likely to maintain good oral intake is a good candidate for ambulatory management. The home environment should be appropriate for the surveillance such a child will need. Two particular symptoms are traditionally treated with more or less aggressiveness: fever and cough.

Fever should be treated with antipyretics (acetaminophen preferably) in children with a convulsive disorder. In the absence of such a condition, its treatment is optional. To the best of our knowledge, dangerous hyperthermia does not occur in the well-hydrated child as a result of acute infectious processes. It is important to recognize environmental factors that may obstruct the natural paths for body heat losses. Advise the parents to avoid overclothing and to keep the patient away from room heating elements; encourage lukewarm water baths.

Three types of cough can be clinically differentiated: a loose productive type and a dry type that may or may not have a strong laryngeal component (hoarse, barking, metallic, or brassy are terms used to describe the laryngeal component). In any of these categories, the cough may be hacking or paroxysmal (the latter often culminating in emesis). It often has a protective role in enhancing mobilization of secretions, but at times certain receptors may be stimulated in the absence of secretions.

A loose productive cough is desirable. The use of narcotic antitussives is generally *not* indicated. This type of cough may be helped by chest physiotherapy. The bouts of coughing will be more severe during the sessions, but in between sessions less coughing should be seen. Dry, persistent nonlaryngeal cough during acute infectious respiratory processes appears to be related to bronchial smooth muscle spasms. Clinical improvement is often achieved by the use of bronchodilators (inhaled or oral B_2 adrenergic agents).

Treat a dry cough, whether hacking or paroxysmal, with B_2 adrenergic agents. For children <6 years old, albuterol 0.1 mg/kg/dose (maximum 2 mg to start) q 6 to 8 hours should be tried. In older children and adolescents, the maximum dose may be increased to 4 mg q 6 hours if adequate response is not obtained with the lower dose. A preferred option for this older group of patients is the use of inhaled albuterol (by metered-dose inhaler) 2 puffs q 4 to 8 hours. The concomitant use of oral and inhaled routes may not have additive benefits while tachycardia and striated muscle tremor, the two most common side effects, may be more intense. Other B_2 adrenergic agents may be equally effective, but different dosing schedules may be needed. Terbutaline seems to be interchangeable with albuterol using slightly higher dosages and frequency of administration. Other adrenergic agents are much less desirable.

The dry laryngeal cough can be a more challenging, or frustrating, symptom to manage. In young children (infants and preschool age) this cough may be associated with stridor. The presence of stridor at rest is an indication for hospitalization. In older children, it is often associated with hoarseness. The most important aspect in managing this cough is to give the large airway and larynx a rest. The young uncooperative child must be kept comfortable, consoled, undisturbed, entertained, reassured, etc.; in other words, avoid agitation. The next aspect of therapy is the use of cool mist. Narcotic antitussives do not have clear indications for use in pediatric cough. Other antitussive agents are not recommended. Adequate hydration, *not* overhydration, is the best expectorant we can recommend.

DRUGS—ANTIBIOTICS

Penicillin, amoxicillin, cefaclor, and erythromycin are effective against pneumococci. Erythromycin and tetracycline are effective against *M. pneumoniae*. Amoxicillin and cefaclor are effective against more than 50% of the recovered *H. influenzae* type B. Most pediatric LRTIs have a viral cause. The routine use of antimicrobials is not indicated. Empiric antimicrobial coverage may be appropriate in children with certain chronic lung diseases (other than asthma) during LRTI, but in otherwise healthy children, routine use of antibiotics during LRTI is unnecessary.

In view of our modest diagnostic capabilities (the best attempts at etiologic diagnosis still have only a 50% yield), children with pneumonia in whom a bacterial or mycoplasmal cause is suspected are candidates for empiric antibiotic coverage. Findings that may exclude a child less than 5 years old from the use of antibiotics are low-grade fever, nontoxicity (level of activity and playfulness), WBC count below 15,000 with less than 50% neutrophils (if a CBC is obtained), wheezing, and negative antigenuria for pneumococcus and *H. influenzae* if available. Close observation by a reliable caretaker should provide reassurance as good as the "empiric" use of antimicrobials. Reevaluation in 24 hours is desirable.

In the absence of a specific bacterial diagnosis, when bacterial pneumonia is suspected the empirically chosen antibiotic should be effective against the most likely agents epidemiologically for the child's age. Neonates and young infants should be hospitalized.

Bacterial pneumonias in children between 1 month and 5 years of age are most commonly caused by either pneumococcus or *Hemophilus*. Moderate and severely ill children should be hospitalized. For the mildly ill child, ampicillin 150 mg/kg/day divided q 6 hours for 10 days suffices. Alternatives are amoxicillin 40 mg/kg/day divided q 8 hours, or the combination of amoxicillin/clavulanic acid or cefaclor 40 mg/kg/day divided q 8 hours.

In children older than 5 years, *M. pneumoniae* is the leading cause of pneumonia and should be treated with erythromycin 40 mg/kg/day (2 g/day maximum) divided q 6 hours for 7 to 10 days. Tetracycline may be used in children older than 8 years. When bacterial pneumonia is suspected in those older children, Pneumococcus is by far the most common agent. The antibiotic of choice is penicillin. For less severe cases, penicillin V orally, 50–100 mg/kg/day divided q 6 hours for 10 days is adequate. Very ill children should be hospitalized for intravenous penicillin G. Erythromycin is a good alternative for penicillin-sensitive children. It is effective against *M. pneumoniae* and pneumococcus. These organisms are the two most common treatable causes of pneumonia in school-age children, adolescents, and young adults.

DISPOSITION

Pneumonias are part of the spectrum of LRTI in children. A nonbacterial cause is most common in preschool-age children. Symptomatic therapy and observation is all that is needed in most instances. Antibiotics are not routinely needed and should be used only when a bacterial or Mycoplasma cause is documented or strongly suspected.

The mildly ill, well hydrated, and active child with a reliable caretaker will be best served by painless but thorough clinical evaluation followed by supportive/symptomatic treatment and close observation at home. The child's condition should be reviewed within 24 hours to confirm the benign outcome expected from the initial evaluation.

The moderate to severely ill child and those in whom prediction of outcome is difficult (i.e., young infants, underlying chronic lung disease) should be hospitalized and/or referred for specialty care.

COMMON PITFALLS

- A common pitfall is antibiotic overuse in the undiagnosed asthmatic child. Cough-variant asthma and cases with a strong hypersecretory component frequently fall under this misdiagnosis.

- The prophylactic use of antibiotics in children of good baseline health during nonbacterial LRTI has no proven benefit and does not represent good medical care. In certain chronic lung diseases, however, there may be good reasons for such prophylaxis.
- Radiographic hyperinflation of the chest is a common sign of congestive heart failure in infants with congenital cardiovascular abnormalities.

214 Croup

Croup is a term used to describe an infraglottic inflammatory process. The two most common forms are spasmodic and viral (laryngotracheobronchitis). The latter is usually due to parainfluenza type 1 and 3, respiratory syncytial virus, parainfluenza type 2, or rhinovirus. Its peak incidence is during late fall with a smaller peak in late spring. It occurs year round. The true incidence is unknown but approximated at 50 per 1,000 children. Croup can occur in all age groups but is mostly seen during the second year of life. There is a 2:1 male to female ratio with a recurrence rate of 5%. Stridor is audible when 75% to 90% of the airway is blocked. The supraglottic structures are normal.

CLINICAL PRESENTATION

Inspiratory stridor, a barking cough, and hoarse voice with mild to moderate respiratory distress are the common presenting symptoms of laryngotracheobronchitis (LTB) (Table 214-1). One to two days of upper respiratory infection with a low grade fever is the usual prodrome. The symptoms peak for 2 to 3 days, with improvement and resolution noted by 5 to 7 days. Respiratory distress worsens when the patient cries or becomes agitated. A standardized clinical scoring sys-

TABLE 214-1. Comparison Between Epiglottitis and LTB

Characteristic	LTB	Supraglottitis
Age	6 months–3 yr	2–6 yr
Onset	Gradual	Rapid
Etiology	Viral	Bacterial
Swelling site	Subglottic	Supraglottic
Symptoms		
Cough-voice	Hoarse cough	No cough
		Muffled voice
Posture	Any position	Sitting
Mouth	Closed; nasal flaring	Open-chin forward, drooling
Fever	Absent to high	High
Appearance	Often not acutely ill	Anxious, acutely ill
Radiograph	Narrow subglottic area	Swollen epiglottis and supraglottic structures
Palpation larynx	Nontender	Tender
Recurrence	May recur	Rarely recurs
Seasonal incidence	Winter	None

From Backofen JE, Rogers MC: Upper airway disease. In Rogers MC: Textbook of Pediatric Intensive Care, vol 1 pp 171–197. Baltimore, Williams & Wilkins, 1987.

tem to assess pulmonary function is helpful. This enables the physician to assess the degree and progression of respiratory insufficiency and to decide when to intubate. In spasmodic croup, a family history of allergy, asthma, and recurrent episodes of croup is elicited. The same barking, croupy cough, stridor, and respiratory distress are observed, but the patient usually gets better by time of arrival at the emergency department. Spasmodic croup is usually responsive to cool, humidified air.

DIFFERENTIAL DIAGNOSIS

Epiglottitis is classically differentiated by its more acute and fulminant presentation (Table 214-2). Bacterial tracheitis is suspected when there is no response to the standard management for croup, or when the patient's symptoms worsen. Aspirated or swallowed foreign bodies along with retropharyngeal abscess, peritonsilar abscess, and severe bronchospasms must be considered. For recurrent or persistent stridor or a clinical presentation of LTB during an atypical time of the year, the following also should be considered: congenital airway anomalies, acquired tracheal stenoses secondary to previous intubations, congenital heart disease with associated vascular anomalies, tracheal hemangiomas, recurrent angioneurotic edema.

EMERGENCY DEPARTMENT EVALUATION

The child in respiratory distress should not be separated from parental comfort unless impending respiratory arrest is suspected. Minimal manipulation and stimulation is necessary so as not to increase the child's work of breathing and worsen the respiratory distress. Oxygen can be delivered in a manner tolerable to the child. Physical examination should be done and the clinical scoring system applied. Sequential clinical scoring is done at least every 30 minutes and after each patient manipulation or treatment. In the majority of patients, a clinical diagnosis is adequate. (If the child is stable, an inspiratory lateral neck x-ray and chest x-ray may be obtained, but only if there is a question as to the diagnosis of croup versus epiglottitis. The steeple sign (a gradual narrowing at the subglottic area) is observed on all views. This sign also may be seen as a normal variant, but may not be present in spasmodic croup due to its rapid resolution. All supraglottic structures should appear normal.

EMERGENCY DEPARTMENT MANAGEMENT

All patients with a clinical score of 4 or greater should receive oxygen and nebulized racemic adrenaline (0.5 mL of a 2.25% solution diluted in 4 mL of saline or water, repeated as necessary). There should be an immediate clinical improvement due to the reduction of the edema and vasoconstriction of the inflamed subglottic mucosa through the stimulation of the alpha-adrenergic receptors. Parents should be encouraged to deliver the nebulized treatment in a nonthreatening manner. Endotracheal intubation must be decided on quickly for all patients with a clinical score of 7 or greater and no immediate improvement with the nebulized treatment. Patients should be intubated with an endotracheal tube 0.5 to 1.0 mm in diameter less than that predicted for their age or weight.

All patients who receive a nebulized treatment with or without an initial clinical score of 4 or greater should be admitted in the hospital because of possible rebound effect. The rebound effect, which produces an equal or greater clinical score than pretreatment, usually occurs within 2 to 4 hours after treatment. Continuous EKG monitoring is recommended during treatment with nebulized sympathomimetics. The treatment should be stopped when the heart rate exceeds 200 beats per minute or if arrhythmias occur. Humidified oxygen must be given by a method best tolerated by the patient, usually by croup tent. It may be necessary for the parent to be inside the tent as well in order to maintain comfort.

TABLE 214-2. Differential Diagnosis of Croup Syndrome

Illness	Mimics Epiglottitis	Mimics Viral Croup	Diagnostic Aids
Severe pharyngitis	+	–	"Febrile dysphagia"
Infectious mononucleosis	+	–	"Febrile dysphagia"
Peritonsillar abscess	+	–	"Febrile dysphagia"
Retropharyngeal abscess	+	–	"Febrile dysphagia"
Caustic (e.g., lye) ingestion	+	–	History suggestive; patient usually afebrile
Pharyngeal neoplasm	+	–	Chronic; gradual onset
Hypopharyngeal foreign body	+	+	History suggestive; patient usually afebrile
Angioneurotic edema	+	+	History suggestive; patient usually afebrile
Trauma to neck	+	+	History suggestive; patient usually afebrile
Tetany	+	+	Seizures; hypocalcemia
Diphtheria	+	+	Membranous pharyngitis
Tracheo-(laryngo-) malacia	–	+	Chronic; nonprogressive
Laryngeal or tracheal foreign body	–	+	History suggestive; patient usually afebrile
Spasmodic croup	–	+	Patient afebrile
Measles	–	+	Rash; clinical course
Bacterial tracheitis	–	+	Prolonged and severe croup
Vascular ring	–	+	Chronic; nonprogressive
Mediastinal tumor	–	+	Chronic; gradual onset
Laryngeal tuberculosis	–	+	Gradual onset; PPD–
Chemical (e.g., smoke) inhalation	–	+	History suggestive
Congenital or acquired (postintubation) tracheal stenosis	–	+	Recurrent or prolonged croup

From Dickerman JD, Lucey JF: Smith's The Critically Ill Child: Diagnosis and Medical Management, pp 1–17. Philadelphia, WB Saunders, 1972.

Antibiotics are unnecessary. Intravenous steroids are controversial but can be given if the clinical presentation is serious (Decadron 0.1 mg/kg IV every 6 hours). Supportive treatment includes intravenous fluids, antipyretics, mild sedation, and chloral hydrate (20–50 mg/kg/dose every 4 hours PR/PO).

DISPOSITION

Patients with minimal to no response to nebulized adrenergic treatment must be admitted. Intubated patients must be transferred to a pediatric ICU. Instructions to parents whose children are sent home include: monitor the child's work of breathing (increases in respiratory rate, retractions, and agitation), humidifier at bedside, and minimal stimulation.

COMMON PITFALLS

- Separation of child from parents.
- Under-estimation of the child's respiratory failure.
- Use of too large an endotracheal tube.
- Delay in establishment of artificial airway.
- Failure of skilled personnel to accompany the child during transport
- Not having adequate airway equipment available.

215   Acute Pharyngitis in the Pediatric Patient

A sore throat often brings the pediatric patient to medical attention. Most of these children will have acute pharyngitis. Many infectious agents cause acute inflammation of the tonsils and pharynx, including Epstein–Barr virus, adenovirus, parainfluenza, Group A and other beta-hemolytic streptococci, and *Mycoplasma pneumoniae*. Although nonbacterial agents are the most common causes, especially in children under 2 years of age and in adolescents, the most important agent for diagnostic, treatment, and public health considerations remains Group A beta-hemolytic streptococci (GABHS). If inadequately treated, infection with GABHS can lead to suppurative complications including peritonsillar and retropharyngeal abscesses, mastoiditis, and cervical adenitis as well as the nonsuppurative complication of acute rheumatic fever.

CLINICAL PRESENTATION

Most children will present with subjective complaints of sore throat, rhinitis, cough, headache, abdominal pain, or vomiting. The parent may report that younger children will not drink. On physical examination these children may have fever, pharyngeal inflammation with or without tonsillar exudate, and tender cervical adenopathy. Children with GABHS infection may have a fine, diffusely papular erythroderma ("sandpaper rash") or palatal petechiae. Numerous studies have demonstrated that clinicians can differentiate GABHS from nonbacterial pharyngitis with only 50% to 75% accuracy. Although GABHS-infected patients often have more pharyngeal inflammation and tender lymphadenopathy, these findings are not reliably predictive.

DIFFERENTIAL DIAGNOSIS

These clinical entities must be excluded: peritonsillar and retropharyngeal abscesses. Peritonsillar cellulitis is characterized by marked pharyngeal erythema, leukocytosis, and fever. This may progress to abscess formation either in a tonsil or in the parapharyngeal space. Patients with abscesses will present with fever, trismus, a muffled ("hot potato") voice, and swelling of the affected tonsil with deviation of the uvula. Sore throat may not be a primary complaint. Retropharyngeal abscesses are commonly seen in young children who may develop lymphadenitis of retropharyngeal nodes during the course of acute pharyngitis. This should be considered in a toxic-appearing child with dysphagia, drooling, airway obstruction, and neck stiffness.

Neisseria gonorrhoeae/Gonococcal pharyngitis should be considered in both the sexually active adolescent and the younger child in whom sexual abuse is suspected.

EMERGENCY DEPARTMENT EVALUATION AND TREATMENT

The goal is to diagnose GABHS infection. This is most commonly done by obtaining a throat culture from the posterior pharynx and tonsillar pillars. Within 48 hours, GABHS can be identified. In the ED, where patient follow-up is a problem, the use of rapid antigen detection kits for GABHS providea highly specific identification of the GABHS antigen but lacks sensitivity (75%–85%). If used without throat culture back-up, the rapid detection kits may miss as many as 25% of cases. Other blood studies such as sedimentation rate, C-reactive protein, or white blood cell count are not helpful.

It is important to assess for airway patency and hydration status. If GABHS is the responsible organism, penicillin is indicated. Current recommendations suggest either benzathine penicillin G 600,000 units intramuscularly in children less than 60 lbs, and 1.2 million units in larger children or oral penicillin V, 200,000–400,000 units (125–250 mg) three or four times daily for 10 days. In penicillin-allergic patients, erythromycin ethylsuccinate 40 to 50 mg/kg/day in three or four divided doses for 10 days is recommended.

Empiric treatment is indicated if the child has a past history of acute rheumatic fever, has a family member with acute rheumatic fever, or presents with pharyngitis during a community epidemic of acute rheumatic fever or acute glomerulonephritis. In most cases, it is best to wait for the culture results.

DISPOSITION

Most children with pharyngitis can be evaluated and managed as outpatients. Those in whom abscess or cellulitis is suspected should be seen by an otolaryngologist to determine the need for surgical intervention. These patients should be admitted for intravenous antibiotics and surgical treatment. Admission should be considered if intravenous hydration is necessary or if there is evidence of airway obstruction. In the case of airway compromise, a nasopharyngeal airway may be necessary to ensure airway patency. These patients should be evaluated by the otolaryngologist and admitted to monitored beds.

COMMON PITFALLS

- Overtreatment of nonbacterial pharyngitis with antibiotics
- Underdiagnosis of GABHS infection if rapid antigen detection kits are used without throat culture confirmation of negative results or if an inadequate culture is obtained
- Overlooking the presence of an abscess (peritonsillar, retropharyngeal)
- Inadequate patient follow-up for treatment of positive cultures.

216   Pediatric Epiglottitis

Epiglottitis is an acute inflammatory disease that involves the supraglottic structures and progresses to bacteremia. It is usually caused by *Hemophilus influenzae* Type b, although *Staphylococcus aureus,* beta-hemolytic, catarrhalis, and pneumococcus have been isolated. It occurs mainly in preschool children (2–6 years old) but it can present in almost any age group, including adults. It does not recur after the first infection. The onset is usually rapid with a fulminant course that leads to respiratory arrest from either complete airway obstruction or fatigue from a partial obstruction.

CLINICAL PRESENTATION

The typical presentation is an abrupt onset of sore throat, high-grade fever, and one or more of the four D's: dysphagia, dysphonia, drooling, and distress. One series reported normal or near-normal temperature in 40% of patients, and drooling as a late sign. An inspiratory stridor may be audible but there is usually no cough. The stridor has a low-pitched, gurgling sound when the child is at rest and becomes high-pitched if the child is agitated. Secretions, laryngospasm, and fatigue can further compromise breathing. Classically, patients assume a tripod sitting position with their mandible extended forward. Palpation of the larynx reveals tenderness. Patients may appear very apprehensive and often toxic due to sepsis.

DIFFERENTIAL DIAGNOSIS

Epiglottitis must be differentiated from laryngotracheobronchitis and bacterial tracheitis. An inspiratory soft-tissue lateral neck radiograph may be helpful. Radiographic signs of epiglottitis include the thumb sign, the swelling of the aryepiglottic folds, the blunting of the vallecula, and the obliteration of the pyriform sinuses. A widening of the soft tissue between the air column and cervical vertebrae points to retropharyngeal abscess or cellulitis. If membranes are noted in the oropharynx, diphtheria and infectious mononucleosis must be considered. If the patient is afebrile and has a history of choking, the possibility of aspiration of a foreign object must be investigated.

EMERGENCY DEPARTMENT EVALUATION

The child with suspected epiglottitis should be held and comforted by the parents unless respiratory arrest is imminent. The physical examination by inspection and observation can be done from a comfortable distance from the patient. Oxygen can be given by the parents in a gentle, nonthreatening manner. Venipuncture for blood samples or intravenous lines should be deferred to avoid distressing the patient. When epiglottitis is highly suspected, the patient needs to be brought to the operating room to secure an artificial airway immediately. Further evaluation of the airway during anesthesia by direct visualization can then be done. A physician experienced in airway management must accompany the child during transport to the operating room. If the physician is in doubt of the diagnosis and the patient is stable, an inspiratory soft-tissue lateral film can be obtained.

EMERGENCY DEPARTMENT MANAGEMENT

An epiglottitis protocol that can be rapidly activated must be established in each institution (Table 216-1). Once the diagnosis of epiglottitis is made, the personnel must be notified. The patient must be taken to the operating room immediately, where inhalation anesthesia is given in a sitting position. The hypopharynx is then visualized and rapid oral intubation is performed. Intubation is preferred

TABLE 216-1. Protocol for Epiglottitis and Upper Airway Obstruction

1. All children referred to seen in the hospital emergency department with acute upper airway obstruction under emergency conditions will be evaluated in the ED immediately upon arrival by the ED attending and referring physician (who must accompany the child) or a senior pediatrician.

2. Children with suspected epiglottitis or bacterial tracheitis should be accompanied to the ED by the referring physician in an ambulance with a parent.

3. Upon arrival in the ED, experienced personnel should make a rapid clinical assessment of the patient as to the severity and emergent nature of the obstruction. A history should be taken to rule out other forms of upper airway obstruction if time allows.

4. The child should be left in the parent's lap, sitting up, and should not be disturbed, examined, or have any procedure done and placed in a trauma-code room equipped for pediatric intubation/tracheostomy/codes.

5. The following "team" should be assembled *immediately* in the ED: anesthesiologist, surgeon skilled in pediatric tracheostomy; senior pediatrician, and respiratory therapist.

6. If the patient progresses from respiratory failure to arrest before reaching the OR, the following sequence of procedures is followed to re-establish adequate oxygenation and ventilation: 1) bag-valve-mask ventilation using $F_1O_21.00$ and the two-hand technique to secure the mask; 2) rapid oral intubation; 3) needle cricothyrotomy.

7. If the judgment of the team is that the child has epiglottitis, severe viral croup, or bacterial tracheitis but is stable, then the patient should be transported by the team with a code cart to the OR in the parent's lap in a wheelchair. Direct visualization and evaluation for intubation should then take place in the OR under controlled conditions.

8. If the judgment of the team is that the patient has viral croup and is stable, the team should accompany the child to x-ray where a lateral neck and chest (PA or AP) x-rays must be taken to rule out epiglottitis or radiopaque foreign body.

9. Administer low concentration (30%) oxygen on arrival by mask if tolerated by the child.

10. Examine child, draw blood, or start an intravenous line only when the patient is stable and the above have been done.

11. If the diagnosis is viral croup and racemic epinephrine is given via nebulizer, the child *must* be admitted to the hospital.

12. Criteria for intubation
    a. Epiglottitis—*all*
    b. Bacterial tracheitis—*all*
    c. Severe viral croup
    d. Clinical evidence of progressive, severe obstruction, respiratory failure
    e. CO_2 retention
    f. Hypoxemia with supplemental O_2
    g. Acidosis
    h. Fatigue

Hen J Jr: Current management of upper airway obstruction. Pediatr Ann 15(4):274, 1986.

instead of tracheostomy. After suctioning of secretions through the endotracheal tube, a more secure nasopharyngeal airway is then established. Hypopharyngeal cultures (positive in 20%–39% of patients), complete blood count, and serum counter immunoelectrophoresis (CIE) are then obtained.

Intravenous access is performed either before or after induction of anesthesia. Intravenous cefuroxime (200 mg/kg/day given at 8-hour intervals) or chloramphenicol (100 mg/kg given at 6-hour intervals) is administered in the OR. Steroids have no role in the management of epiglottitis. Bronchospasm secondary to secretions can be treated with beta-2 agonist nebulization (i.e., albuterol, metered doses of 2.5 mL and 5 mL, or terbutaline 0.1–0.5 mg diluted in 2 mL normal saline) and suctioning. Racemic epinephrine is unnecessary. The well-sedated patient can then be transferred to a pediatric ICU. Should the patient extubate during transport, proper bag–valve–mask ventilation is usually effective. A secure artificial airway still must be re-established.

For patients who present in impending or complete respiratory arrest, the airway must be addressed immediately. Bag–valve–mask ventilation with 100% oxygen should be started. Higher positive pressures are sometimes necessary, requiring a two-handed technique to obtain an adequate chest rise. If these measures are not successful within 15 to 30 seconds, a rapid oral intubation should be tried first and then an emergency tracheostomy must be done. Insertion of a 14- or 16-gauge angiocatheter through the thyrocricoid membrane and attaching a 3.5-mm endotracheal tube can give a temporary, open airway for bag ventilation or direct attachment to pressurized continuous flow oxygen. Ketamine (1–4 mg/kg/dose IM) can be given for sedation without depressing the respiratory effort during establishment of an artificial airway.

Associated early complications of both the disease and the artificial airway placement include pulmonary edema, tension pneumothorax, subcutaneous emphysema, pneumomediastinum, bleeding, endotracheal tube plugging, accidental extubation, and bronchospasm.

DISPOSITION

The majority of patients with a diagnosis of epiglottitis with or without respiratory distress must be intubated by a qualified team of physicians. All such patients must have continued care in an ICU. Intrahospital and interhospital transport of the well-sedated patient must be accompanied by personnel with intubation skills and proper airway equipment.

COMMON PITFALLS

- Separating the child from the parents
- Increased agitation and respiratory distress secondary to obtaining vital signs, laboratory studies, etc.
- Obtaining radiographic studies when the diagnosis by history and presentation already suggests epiglottitis
- Failing to have the patient accompanied by a physician skilled in artificial airway placement

217   Acute Rheumatic Fever

Acute rheumatic fever (ARF) is an inflammatory disease involving mainly the joints and heart; less frequently, the central nervous system, skin, and subcutaneous tissues are affected. Rheumatic fever occurs in all ages except infancy. The incidence peaks at 5 to 15 years, coincident with the ages when Group A streptococcal pharyngitis is most prevalent. Environmental factors of overcrowding and poor access to medical care have been suggested to play a role because the attack rate is highest in developing countries. The incidence of rheumatic fever in the United States has steadily declined over the last 40 years. Recently, however, several areas of the country have reported a resurgence in the attack rate for rheumatic fever in their pediatric populations.

ARF is a sequela of group A beta-hemolytic streptococcal infection of the upper respiratory tract. The mechanisms whereby the Group A *Streptococcus* brings about the manifestations of ARF are poorly understood. An autoimmune mechanism has been suggested.

CLINICAL PRESENTATION

The presentation of ARF varies widely, depending on the areas of involvement and the severity of the attack. The onset is usually acute when arthritis is the presenting symptom and more gradual when carditis or chorea is the presenting feature. Joint symptoms are the most common presenting complaint, occurring in about 75% of patients. Symptoms range from mild arthralgia to frank arthritis. The pain is often disproportionately severe in its intensity when compared with the objective findings of joint involvement. The arthritis is usually migratory and the knees, ankles, elbow, and wrists are the joints most commonly affected. Joint symptoms subside in 3 to 4 weeks with no permanent deformity.

Carditis presents as a new significant murmur in 40% to 50% of initial attacks, with the highest incidence in young children. Carditis is recognized to be less frequent and less severe than in the past. Chorea occurs in 10% to 15% of children with acute rheumatic fever. It is characterized by involuntary purposeless movements, most often of the face and upper extremities. Skin nodules occur in 5% to 10% of patients and are round, hard, freely movable nodules, usually over bony prominences. Erythema marginatum is the rash of acute rheumatic fever but occurs in fewer than 5% of patients. The lesions are evanescent, slightly raised, red, nonpruritic macules that extend outward to form wavy lines or rings with sharp margins. Fever is usually present at the onset of an acute attack and ranges from 38.3°C to 40°C.

DIFFERENTIAL DIAGNOSIS

Because arthritis is the most common presenting symptom, the differential is usually that for arthritis. Several forms of juvenile rheumatoid arthritis (JRA) can mimic rheumatic fever early in the course of the illness. Systemic JRA can present with fever, rash, polyarticular arthritis, and heart, liver, spleen, and lymphatic involvement. These patients also may have an elevated erythrocyte sedimentation rate (ESR). The antinuclear antibody (ANA) is rarely positive and the rheumatoid factor is negative. In pauciarticular JRA, fewer than five joints are affected and the arthritis is of the lower extremities. The ANA is positive and the ESR is elevated in 50% of the cases. Polyarticular JRA may have either an acute or insidious onset with symmetrical involvement of more than four joints of both the upper and lower extremities. Numerous infections may have an associated arthritis. These include infectious mononucleosis, hepatitis, and influenza. Suppurative bacterial arthritis is usually monoarticular and is confirmed by examination and culture of the joint fluid.

Leukemia presenting with arthritis is diagnosed by the findings on complete blood count (CBC). Sickle-cell anemia also may be confirmed by CBC or a known history of the disease. Children who present with hip pain must be evaluated for Legg–Perthes disease, slipped capital femoral epiphysis, and toxic synovitis. These entities are generally distinguished on the basis of age at presentation and the results of hip radiographs. Hemophiliacs usually have a known history and single joint involvement. Patients who have multiple joint manifestations and cardiac involvement with Kawasaki disease might be thought to have ARF at initial presentation. Collagen

TABLE 217-1. Revised Jones Criteria for the Diagnosis of Acute Rheumatic Fever

Major Criteria	Minor Criteria
Carditis	Previous ARF
Polyarthritis	Arthralgia
Chorea	Fever
Subcutaneous nodules	Laboratory acute phase reactants (*i.e.*, ESR or CRP)
Erythema marginatum	Prolonged P–R interval on ECG

The diagnosis may be made when two major criteria or one major and two minor criteria are present.

From Brewer EJ: Pitfalls of the diagnosis of juvenile rheumatoid arthritis. Pediatr Clin North Am 33:1015, 1986.

vascular diseases such as systemic lupus erythematosus, dermatomyositis, or scleroderma are distinguished by other manifestations of the illness. Henoch–Schönlein purpura or anaphylactoid purpura is recognized by the characteristic rash, as is psoriasis. Inflammatory bowel disease may present with only arthritis initially, but other Jones criteria will be lacking.

EMERGENCY DEPARTMENT MANAGEMENT AND DISPOSITION

Management includes an assessment for evidence of a preceding streptococcal infection and an evaluation of the patient for the revised Jones criteria. Laboratory tests for evidence of a recent streptococcal infection include an ASO titer, anti-DNase B, and anti-DPNase. The revised Jones criteria are divided into major and minor criteria (Table 217-1). The diagnosis may be made when two of the major criteria or one major and two minor criteria are present. A chest radiograph is indicated if cardiomegaly or pericardial effusion is a consideration. All patients with ARF should be hospitalized and placed on bed rest. Treatment with anti-inflammatory drugs should be initiated.

COMMON PITFALLS

- Failure to thoroughly examine the child's joints
- Failure to place significance on the child's complaints of joint pain
- Failure to consider the diagnosis in the patient with vague complaints of joint pain
- Failure to give special attention to differentiating between a new or changing murmur that may be indicative of carditis from one noted previously

218   Urinary Tract Infections

Urinary tract infections (UTI) pose particular problems in diagnosis and management. Infants present with varied symptomatology not always related to the urinary tract. Also, the significance of the infection and necessary workup will vary depending on age and sex. The male:female ratio of 2.5:1 during the first month of life reverses to 1:20 in childhood. Most infections in early infancy involve the renal parenchyma. In this age group symptoms are nonspecific.

CLINICAL PRESENTATION

The clinical presentation of patients with UTI varies with age. In infancy, common presenting symptoms include fever, sepsis, failure to thrive, irritability, and those related to the gastrointestinal tract such as poor feeding, diarrhea, vomiting, and jaundice. Of particular importance is the increased incidence of sepsis in the young infant with UTI (31% of neonates with UTIs are bacteremic). With increasing age, the incidence declines to 21% of infants between 1 and 2 months of age, 14% between 2 and 3 months of age, and 6% of those between 3 and 8 months old. Preschool children may present with traditional symptoms of suprapubic pain, urgency, dysuria, and frequency. At this age, they still have symptoms not localized to the urinary tract, such as fever (febrile seizure), generalized abdominal pain, and diarrhea. Enuresis in a previously continent child also is an indicator of possible infection. In the school-age child with a UTI, symptoms referable to the urinary tract are usually present. Fever is often present, and although it suggests upper tract disease, alone it is not a good marker since fever may be seen with cystitis. Also, fever may be absent in a patient with significant renal scarring.

DIFFERENTIAL DIAGNOSIS

Although the infant will present with nonspecific symptoms, careful questioning may uncover additional symptoms that would direct attention to the urinary tract. Symptoms such as dribbling, poor stream, frequency, and malodorous urine may be present, although not the presenting complaint. When the preschool-age and older child present with urgency, dysuria, or frequency, the differential should include chemical urethritis, pinworms, vaginitis, and possible child abuse.

EMERGENCY DEPARTMENT EVALUATION

Voided specimens are often obtained from infants and incontinent children by placing a bag over the previously cleaned perineum. Contamination rates are so high with voided specimens in infants that they are useful only if no growth appears on culture. Growth of even 100,000 colony-forming units (cfu)/mL of such specimens is unreliable as a test for true infection. Presence of bacteria on microscopic examination is most likely to be from contamination. If a UTI is suspected in an incontinent patient, a urine specimen should be obtained by catheter or suprapubic aspiration. This is especially true for those patients to whom antibiotics are to be given for suspected sepsis or other source of infection. Bacteria may be introduced into a specimen when obtained with a catheter.

So, microscopic examination may be helpful only if the specimen is negative or if bacteria are present in large numbers (>100/high-power field of sediment). With growth of 100,000 cfu/mL from such a specimen, there is a 95% likelihood of infection; with 10,000 cfu/mL, there is a 50% likelihood of infection. Any bacteria seen on examination per high-power field or growth on culture from a specimen obtained by suprapubic aspiration probably represents infection. In the continent patient, contamination rates are still high enough to preclude an accurate diagnosis. However, if two voided specimens show 100,000 cfu/mL of the same organism, the diagnostic accuracy increases from 80% (achieved with one voided specimen) to 95%. Therefore, two voided specimens should be obtained before beginning antibiotic therapy. The indications for obtaining a urine culture are listed in Table 218-1.

There is no agreement on what constitutes significant pyuria on spun specimens. Presence of pyuria is nonspecific, since children with other febrile illnesses, dehydration, appendicitis, or other inflammatory processes also may have this finding. Nitrite striips are useful screens. Radiographic assessment of the urinary tract for detection of renal scarring, obstructive lesions, and vesicoureteral reflux is accomplished using ultrasound or intravenous pyelography (IVP) for evaluation of the upper tract and a voiding cystourethrogram (VCUG) for evaluation of the lower tract. All males of any age and infants of both sexes should have an ultrasound (or

TABLE 218-1. Indications for Obtaining Urine Specimens for Analysis and Culture

Age

<12 months	Febrile	Absolute	All febrile infants <2 months
		Consider	Febrile infant females and uncircumcised males 3–12 months (usually based on level of temperature elevation, ≥104°F, and toxicity)
	Afebrile	Absolute	Failure to thrive
		Consider	Infants with vomiting, diarrhea, poor feeding, irritability if presentation is atypical or protracted
>12 months	Febrile	Absolute	Enuresis in previously continent child, UTI symptomatology
		Consider	Protracted or atypical diarrhea, abdominal pain

IVP) as soon as possible to detect any obstructive process or renal disease. VCUG for evaluation of reflux may be delayed until after the infection has cleared, as infection predisposes to reflux. In the past, radiographic evaluation of girls >1 year of age was reserved for those with pyelonephritis and those with recurrent lower tract infections. Most experts now recommend radiographic evaluation for all symptomatic girls under 3 years of age with their first UTI. One study found fever to be indicative of a treatable urologic problem in 42% of girls less than 5 years of age with UTIs.

EMERGENCY DEPARTMENT MANAGEMENT

For patients with equivocal clinical and laboratory findings, treatment may be postponed until culture results are available. Treatment is indicated if there is any growth from a specimen obtained by suprapubic aspiration. Growth of >100,000 cfu/mL of a single organism from a catheter specimen or two voided specimens represents infection and should be treated. With less growth on such specimens, treatment also may be indicated, depending on the degree of clinical suspicion. For patients who are febrile or otherwise symptomatic, treatment before availability of culture results may be indicated. Findings highly suggestive of infection and of the need to initiate treatment include:

1. Presence of any bacteria on the UA (spun or unspun) collected by suprapubic aspiration
2. Presence of bacteria on Gram's stain of unspun urine obtained by catheterization or midstream clean-catch specimen in the older child
3. Presence of >100 bacteria per high-power field via catheterization or midstream catch in older child

Antiobiotic therapy: Infants <3 months of age should receive parenteral antibiotics; aminoglycoside, gentamicin or amikacin, and ampicillin will provide broad-spectrum coverage. High doses should be used for possible bacteremia: gentamicin 7.5 mg/kg/day divided q 8 hrs, amikacin 15 to 30 mg/kg/day divided q 8 hrs, ampicillin 100 mg/kg/day divided q 6 hrs. Keep in mind the ototoxicity and nephrotoxicity of aminoglycosides. For the older child with suspected pyelonephritis, options for parenteral antibiotic therapy include gentamicin (6 mg/kg/day divided q 8 hrs IV or IM) and trimethoprim–sulfamethoxazole (6 mg TMP, 30 mg SMX/kg/day divided q 12 hrs IV). Change to an appropriate oral drug may be made after clinical response.

Outpatient treatment with proven efficacy includes sulfonamides (sulfisoxazoles), aminopenicillins (amoxicillin/ampicillin), trimethoprim–sulfamethoxazole, nitrofurantoin, and cephalosporins (cefaclor, cefadroxil). Culture and sensitivity should be obtained before antibiotics and follow-up cultures obtained within 48 hours. Recommendations on the duration of therapy vary. Because short-course and single-dose therapies have been successful with adult women, proven regimens may be acceptable for uncomplicated cystitis in adolescent females. Before adolescence, 7 to 10 days of one of the antibiotics listed above is recommended, since studies of short-course therapy in children have yielded conflicting results. In addition, the difficulty with accurately identifying all cases of upper tract disease in children make short-course therapy less acceptable. There is no added benefit from continuing therapy beyond 10 days, although a prolonged course may be chosen for prophylaxis.

DISPOSITION

Hospital admission is indicated for all infants less than 3 months old with UTI because of the frequent accompanying bacteremia. Clinical judgment may be used for those infants who do not appear ill and who are >3 months old. All infants need evaluation by ultrasound or IVP for possible obstruction and renal involvement within 24 hours. For those patients who are treated as outpatients, it is essential to establish follow-up for radiographic evaluation of the urinary tract, if indicated, and repeat cultures, both for adequacy of therapy and screening for asymptomatic recurrence.

COMMON PITFALLS

- Failure to obtain appropriate specimens before antibiotics in the septic infant may lead to delay in diagnosis of obstructive lesions of the urinary tract.
- Mild respiratory and gastrointestinal symptoms do not preclude UTI as the source of fever in the young child.
- Failure to arrange adequate follow-up for radiographic studies and repeat cultures may result in failure to find treatable causes of renal disease.

219   Life-Threatening Rashes of Childhood

Many potentially life-threatening diseases in children present with rash. In the newborn, herpes simplex, varicella zoster, enterovirus, and virtually any bacterial infection may be seen. In infants and older children, Rocky Mountain spotted fever, meningococcemia, *Haemophilus influenzae,* staphylococcal scalded skin syndrome, Stevens–Johnson syndrome, Kawasaki syndrome, leukemia, and ITP may all present with skin manifestations. In adolescents (and less often in younger children), toxic shock syndrome is a potentially fatal illness.

ROCKY MOUNTAIN SPOTTED FEVER

Rocky Mountain Spotted Fever (RMSV) is a widespread small-vessel vasculitis caused by *Rickettsia rickettsia*. It is transmitted to humans primarily by tick vectors. There is a marked seasonal character: 95% of cases occur between April 1 and September 30, time of maximal tick activity. Two thirds of cases occur in children <15 years old, with the highest incidence in the 5-to-9 age group. Prevalence is widely variable, with the south Atlantic and western south-central regions of the United States considered endemic. Early recognition is important because in classic cases, virtually all patients treated appropriately before day 6 of illness will survive, compared with a 25% mortality for untreated patients.

CLINICAL PRESENTATION

Fever, headache, rash, and myalgias are the classic early manifestations of RMSF. Children (under 15 years) will fit this typical pattern more consistently than adults. A history of tick bite is present in 70% to 93% of children. This is followed by a 2-to-14-day incubation period (usually 4 to 8 days). Onset is typically although not invariably abrupt, with headache and fever of 40° to 40.6°C. Myalgias and muscle tenderness, particularly of the calves and thighs, are also characteristic. The rash of RMSF begins on the second or third day of illness, although onset occasionally may be delayed up to a week. Failure of a rash to develop (Rocky Mountain spotless fever) is less common in children than in adults. A rash never develops in up to 5% of pediatric cases. Typically the lesions are small erythematous macules and maculopapules that later become petechial. They first appear peripherally on the wrists and ankles, subsequently spreading centrally to the trunk. Involvement of the palms and soles is characteristic and helpful diagnostically when present. Firm nonpitting edema, initially in the periorbital region, is a common diagnostic clue. This finding is common in other vasculitides, however, and is not unique to RMSF.

Cardiac, pulmonary, and gastrointestinal involvement may occur. Central nervous system involvement is common late in the disease and is the primary cause of death. Ophthalmologic findings of conjunctivitis, photophobia, and petechiae of the bulbar conjunctiva are also common.

DIFFERENTIAL DIAGNOSIS

Measles, meningococcemia, enteroviral infections, and occasionally Kawasaki disease are the major concerns in the differential diagnosis. The classic measles rash begins on the head and neck and spreads peripherally. The respiratory prodrome of measles, presence of Koplik's spots, and winter-spring seasonality all help to distinguish it from RMSF. Meningococcemia is usually a more fulminant disease than RMSF. The rash begins earlier, typically within 24 hours of the appearance of fever, is petechial at onset, and lacks a characteristic pattern. The meningococcal organism can frequently be detected by Gram's stain of cerebrospinal fluid and skin lesions, as well as by counterimmunoelectrophoresis or latex agglutination of CSF or urine. If differentiation is impossible, treatment of both diseases should be instituted.

Enteroviruses are the most difficult infections to differentiate from early RMSF. They produce febrile exanthems with maculopapular rashes that usually start centrally, but may be petechial and involve the palms and soles. Aseptic meningitis is common with enteroviral infections and further confuses the picture. The diagnosis of RMSF is supported by myalgias, edema, hyponatremia, thrombocytopenia, a history of tick exposure, and a characteristic progression of disease. Unfortunately, none of these findings are reliable, and thus some patients with enteroviral illness will require treatment for presumptive RMSF. Early in its course, Kawasaki disease, with its fever, conjunctivitis, and rash, may be mistaken for RMSF. Although children with Kawasaki disease tend to be younger (80% under 4 years) than patients with RMSF, considerable overlap exists. The characteristic clinical course of Kawasaki disease ultimately distinguishes it from RMSF.

EMERGENCY DEPARTMENT EVALUATION

In the ED, RMSF is a clinical diagnosis based on signs, symptoms, and epidemiology. None of the serologic tests available are reliably positive in the first week of illness when therapy is most beneficial. Evaluation of a child with suspected RMSF should include a complete blood count with differential, a platelet count, and serum electrolytes. The white count is normal or low in the first week, often with an increased number of band forms. Thrombocytopenia and hyponatremia are common early in the course of RMSF. Serologic tests for RMSF are available at most state health departments and acute titers should be drawn. Further evaluation depends on the clinical status of the patient. Consideration should be given to ECG, chest radiograph, liver function studies, and lumbar puncture, as involvement of the heart, liver, and central nervous system are all common in more advanced disease.

EMERGENCY DEPARTMENT MANAGEMENT

ED management consists of cardiovascular stabilization and appropriate antibiotic therapy. Myocardial dysfunction is common, presenting with congestive heart failure, pulmonary edema, and arrhythmias. Severity of left ventricular dysfunction appears to reflect the clinical severity of the illness. Caution with volume resuscitation is imperative. Inotropic agents may be necessary. Antibiotic therapy for stable patients older than 9 years without significant vomiting includes oral tetracycline or doxycycline. The dose of tetracycline is 30 to 40 mg/kg/day divided q 6 hr with a maximum of 2 g/day. Doxycycline requires a loading dose of 4.4 mg/kg/day divided q 12 hr for the first day of therapy; thereafter, a maintenance dose of 2.2 mg/kg/day divided q 12 hr is appropriate. The maximum daily dose of doxycycline is 300 mg/day.

The unstable, more severely ill patient should initially be treated with parenteral antibiotics: Chloramphenicol and the tetracyclines are equally efficacious. The dose of intravenous doxycycline is identical to the oral dosage. The dose of intravenous tetracycline is 20 to 30 mg/kg/day divided q 12 hr. The dose of chloramphenicol is 50 to 100 mg/kg/day intravenously or by mouth divided q 6 hr to a maximum of 3 g/day. In RMSF patients <8 or 9 years old, controversy exists as to the appropriate therapy. Chloramphenicol avoids the tooth enamel hypoplasia and discoloration associated with the use of tetracycline in young children. However, chloramphenicol is associated with a rare but potentially fatal bone marrow aplasia. Concern for this possible complication has led others to recommend doxycycline even in young patients, provided they have no previous exposure to the tetracyclines. Doxycycline is preferred over tetracycline because it is less bound to calcium than tetracycline and, therefore, potentially less likely to discolor or damage tooth enamel. Patients should be treated until they are afebrile for 3 to 5 days. Chloramphenicol has the advantage of covering for meningococcemia as well as RMSF. If differentiation is in doubt, penicillin can be added to tetracycline therapy to achieve the same results.

DISPOSITION

Indications for admission include evidence of significant cardiovascular, pulmonary, or central nervous system involvement. Patients who vomit to the extent that oral therapy is impossible also require admission. More common is a mildly ill child with an uncertain diagnosis. Therapy is often indicated based on epidemiologic and clinical signs, despite the fact that many, if not most, of these patients will ultimately be found not to have RMSF. If close follow-up and good compliance can be ensured, outpatient therapy is an appropriate alternative to admission. Response to early therapy is prompt and predictable.

COMMON PITFALLS

- Failure to consider RMSF
- Failure to give therapy in the absence of rash (absent in up to 5%)
- Failure to obtain informed consent before therapy (both chloramphenicol and tetracycline may have significant risks and documented informed consent is warranted.)

MENINGOCOCCEMIA

Meningococcemia is an emergency. The disease spectrum ranges from transient bacteremia to fulminant septic shock and death within hours. Peak incidence occurs in the late winter and early spring; 90% of cases are in infants <age 2.

CLINICAL PRESENTATION

Onset is usually abrupt with high fever, petechiae, lethargy, and headache. The rash may initially be petechial, urticarial, or maculopapular. Maculopapular lesions are often tender. Lesions are sparse and generalized in distribution. Purpura and ecchymosis indicate fulminating disease with a high incidence of shock and disseminated intravascular coagulation. Other signs and symptoms include evidence of an upper respiratory tract infection, myalgias, and joint pains. Meningitis occurs in 50% with meningococcemia.

DIFFERENTIAL DIAGNOSIS

Sepsis and/or meningitis due to *Haemophilus influenza* and occasionally to *S. pneumoniae* can present with a picture identical to meningococcemia. In one series, 20% with fever and petechiae had an invasive, potentially life-threatening disease. Half of these were due to *N. meningitides*.

Severe RMSF may initially be difficult to distinguish from meningococcemia, and therapy for both diseases is often begun in the ED.

EMERGENCY DEPARTMENT EVALUATION

A rapid septic workup is required for suspected meningococcemia: chest radiograph, complete blood count with differential and platelet count, PT, PTT, erythrocyte sedimentation rate, electrolytes including glucose and calcium, blood culture, and urine for culture and urinalysis. A lumbar puncture should be performed in all stable patients. Counterimmunoelectrophoresis or latex agglutination to detect meningococcal antigen in urine, spinal fluid, or serum may be helpful in cases when diagnosis is in doubt. Cardiovascular monitoring and close observation for signs of shock are necessary as these patients can deteriorate rapidly. Deterioration shortly after antibiotic administration, possibly secondary to endotoxin release, has been noted.

EMERGENCY DEPARTMENT MANAGEMENT

Although most patients will do well, some will rapidly develop shock, coma, and disseminated intravascular coagulation. Factors associated with a poor prognosis: onset of petechiae within 24 hours of admission, the presence of purpura or ecchymosis, shock (systolic blood pressure <70 mmHg), coma, disseminated intravascular coagulation, thrombocytopenia (platelet count <150,000/µl), metabolic acidosis (pH <7.30 or serum bicarbonate <15 mEq/l), and the absence of meningitis. Since hypotension is a late manifestation of shock in children, repeated evaluation of mental status, skin perfusion, urine output, pulse pressure, and pulse quality are important.

Evidence of inadequate tissue perfusion should initially be treated with volume expansion. Myocardial dysfunction is common and inotropic agents may be required. Intravenous penicillin

G, 250,000 units/kg/day divided q 4 hr should be given. Chloramphenicol is an acceptable alternative in the penicillin-allergic patient or when other organisms such as *H. influenzae* or *R. rickettsiae* have not been ruled out. Antibiotic prophylaxis is recommended for household, day-care center, and nursery-school contacts. Persons who have had contact with the patient's oral secretions (including kissing, sharing food and beverages, mouth-to-mouth resuscitation, intubation, or suctioning) should receive prophylaxis. *N. meningitides* and *H. influenzae* are the two most common causes for sepsis associated with a petechial rash in children. Rifampin 10 mg/kg q 12 hr for 8 doses (adults 600 mg q 12 hr for 8 doses) is effective for both organisms.

DISPOSITION

All patients with meningococcemia should be admitted to a facility able to handle children in septic shock, ideally under the care of a pediatric intensivist.

If transfer is planned, the potential for rapid deterioration during transport should be anticipated. Dopamine should be mixed in advance and infusion rates established. Intubation before transport should be strongly considered in all unstable patients. Two intravenous lines are desirable if possible.

COMMON PITFALLS

1. Failure to diagnose shock in infants and children is common. Once recognized, inadequate resuscitation is also common. Children can require massive amounts of volume and potent inotropic agents. True septic shock necessitates a Swan–Ganz catheter.
2. Failure to provide prophylaxis to contacts

220   Acute Childhood Exanthems and Classic Childhood Diseases

ACUTE CHILDHOOD EXANTHEMS

Most patients with childhood exanthems have a benign, nonspecific, self-limited viral illness rather than a classic disease such as measles. The physician should focus on identifying diseases that require specific therapy (e.g., scarlet fever) or have public-health implications, and should exclude life-threatening illnesses with rash. The history should focus on initial location, spread, duration, and any changes noted in the appearance of the rash. Prodromal symptoms such as fever and other complaints including sore throat, cough, vomiting, headache, and neck pain should be characterized. A history of recent exposure to a highly contagious disease such as varicella or measles is often helpful. Recent medication use may suggest a drug eruption. In addition, if either the patient or a household contact is a neonate, pregnant, or immunocompromised, the management of an otherwise benign illness may be altered.

Physical examination should focus on assessing the general severity of illness (e.g., irritability, state of hydration) and thoroughly characterizing skin and mucous membrane lesions (Figure 220-1). Search carefully for complications such as otitis media, pneumonia, and encephalitis.

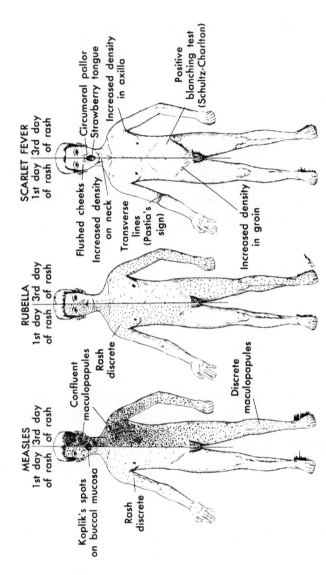

Figure 220-1. Differences in appearance and progression of rashes in measles, rubella, and scarlet fever (Krugman S et al: Infectious Diseases of Children, 8th ed. St. Louis, CV Mosby, 1985. Reproduced with permission.)

DISEASES WITH MACULOPAPULAR ERUPTIONS

Most common, nonspecific viral eruptions have maculopapular lesions, often resembling the classic childhood diseases. Differentiating features of illnesses with characteristic maculopapular eruptions are shown in Table 220-1.

EPIDEMIOLOGY AND CLINICAL PRESENTATION OF SPECIFIC DISEASES

MEASLES   Measles (rubeola) is caused by a paramyxovirus. The incidence of measles greatly declined after widespread vaccination began, but outbreaks still occur in preschool children, schools, and college campuses. Vaccine failures account for about 38% of cases. The diagnosis of measles has important public-health implications, since prevention of spread requires prompt recognition of a local outbreak. Measles has a characteristic 3-to-4-day prodrome, beginning with fever, chills, and malaise, followed a day later by cough, coryza, and conjunctivitis. An enanthem known as Koplik's spots precedes the rash and consists of small red patches capped by bluish-white specks, seen first on the buccal mucosa opposite the molars with subsequent spread and coalescence within the mouth (resembling sprinkles of salt).

Koplik's spots are pathognomonic of measles; unfortunately, they resolve by the second or third day of rash and are often absent when the patient is seen. The exanthem consists of purplish-red maculopapules that begin at the hairline and spread downward, tending to be confluent on the face and neck. The child with full-blown measles appears miserable with high fever, conjunctivitis, marked cough, and rhinorrhea. The severity of symptoms peaks on the second day of the rash, with subsequent rapid recovery. Otitis media and pneumonia are common complications of measles. Rare but potentially fatal complications include acute encephalitis (0.1–0.4% of cases), and severe, obstructive laryngotracheitis. Measles is highly contagious, with infectivity from about 2 days before onset of illness to 4 days after the rash appears.

RUBELLA   Rubella (German measles) is a mild disease caused by a rubivirus. Its major significance is its ability to cause severe illness and birth defects in prenatally infected infants. Since vaccination began, the incidence of rubella has decreased, but 10% to 20% of adults remain susceptible. Rash is usually the first symptom of rubella, beginning with discrete pink-red maculopapules on the face that rapidly spread downward. A nonspecific enanthem of small reddish dots on the soft palate (Forchheimer spots) may be seen. The rash often coalesces on the trunk and usually fades within 3 days. Generalized lymphadenopathy, particularly postauricular and suboccipital, is typical. Adolescents and adults tend to have a febrile prodrome and commonly develop arthralgias or arthritis. First-trimester prenatal infection may cause severe anomalies and illness in the fetus.

ROSEOLA INFANTUM   Roseola infantum (exanthem subitum) is common in young children. Human herpes virus 6 (HHV-6) has recently been implicated as the causative agent in most cases of roseola. Roseola has a characteristic history of abrupt onset of high fever for 3 to 4 days, followed by sudden defervescence coinciding with the onset of rash. The skin lesions are small, discrete, rose-pink macules or maculopapules that appear first on the trunk before spreading to the rest of the body. The rash resolves within 1 to 2 days. When seen during the febrile phase, the child may be mildly irritable but usually appears remarkably well. A febrile seizure may be the first symptom; physical findings may include mild pharyngitis and cervical adenopathy. Serious complications such as encephalitis are rare.

ERYTHEMA INFECTIOSUM   Erythema infectiosum ("fifth disease") is caused by human parvovirus B19, which also causes aplastic crises in patients with chronic hemolytic anemia. It typically affects school-age children in epidemics. Most patients are asymptomatic, although mild fever may occur. The skin findings appear in three stages: the first is characterized by a bright-red, raised macular rash on the cheeks that spares the nasal bridge and mouth, giving the child a distinctive "slapped-cheek" appearance. The second stage begins about a day later with a variable rash on the extremities and trunk (noted first on extensor surfaces), which appears "lace-like" as confluent areas clear.

TABLE 220-1. Differentiating Features of Selected Diseases With Maculopapular Eruptions

Disease	Ages Most Affected	Typical Seasons	Type/Distribution of Skin and Oral Lesions	Common Associated Symptoms/Signs	Complications
Measles	Children, young adults	Winter, spring	Skin—purple-red maculopapules spreading from the hairline downward, confluent on face and neck Oral mucosa—Koplik's spots	Prodrome of high fever, coryza, cough, conjunctivitis	Common: otitis media, pneumonia Rare: encephalitis, severe laryngotracheitis
Rubella	Children, young adults	Winter, spring	Skin—discrete, pink-red maculopapules spreading from face downward Soft palate—Forchheimer's spots	Children—lymphadenopathy, minimal fever Adolescent/adult—febrile prodrome, joint pains	Common: arthritis in older patients Very rare: encephalitis, purpura Prenatal exposure: congenital rubella syndrome
Roseola infantum	6 months to 3 yr	Spring, fall, summer	Discrete, small rose-pink macules spreading from trunk to rest of body	High fever for 3–4 days before rash, mild pharyngitis, otitis, and adenopathy	Common: febrile seizures Very rare: encephalitis
Erythema infectiosum	2 to 12 yr	Late winter, spring	1st stage—"slapped-cheek" malar rash 2nd stage—trunk/extremity rash, fading in lacelike pattern 3rd stage—recurrence of rash with stimuli	Asymptomatic or mild fever	Rare: arthritis (esp. adults), hemolytic anemia, encephalitis, fetal loss
Scarlet fever	3 to 12 yr	Winter, spring	Skin—face flushed with circumoral pallor, trunk/extremities with "sandpapery," blanching pinpoint red rash most prominent in creases, Pastia's lines Mucosa—pharyngitis/tonsillitis, palatal petechiae, strawberry tongue	Fever, sore throat, vomiting, abdominal pain, tender anterior cervical nodes	Early: otitis media, peritonsillitis, cervical adenitis Late: rheumatic fever, glomerulonephritis

During the third stage, lasting weeks to months, the rash may reappear with various stimuli such as bathing, temperature extremes, or local irritation. Occasional complications include arthralgias and arthritis (more common in adults), hemolytic anemia, and, rarely, encephalitis. Prenatal infection may cause fetal death.

SCARLET FEVER   Scarlet fever (scarlatina) is a rash seen in association with Group A beta-hemolytic streptococcal infections caused by strains producing an erythrogenic toxin. The importance of appropriate antibiotics for this infection has been underscored by a recent increase in cases of acute rheumatic fever. Scarlet fever is most common in school-age children in the winter and spring and is more prevalent in temperate or colder climates. The clinical symptoms are those of streptococcal pharyngitis. Rash appears within 1 to 2 days, beginning on the trunk and spreading rapidly. The skin is red, blanches, and has fine "sandpapery" punctate bumps. The face is flushed and has circumoral pallor. The rash is prominent in skin folds, and Pastia's lines (areas of hyperpigmentation and petechiae) may be seen in joint creases such as the antecubital fossae. Desquamation after resolution of symptoms is very characteristic. The complications of scarlet fever are those of streptococcal pharyngitis. The diagnosis of scarlet fever is confirmed by throat culture (or rapid strep test). Leukocytosis is usually present. Serology (anti-streptolysin-O titer, etc.) may be helpful in evaluating post-streptococcal illnesses or desquamation.

OTHER AGENTS   Many other agents ause nonspecific maculopapular eruptions. *Infectious mononucleosis* is accompanied by an exanthem in about 10% to 15% of cases; the rash is usually maculopapular but may be urticarial, vesicular, hemorrhagic, or erythema multiforme. The appearance of a rash in 80% to 90% of patients with mononucleosis who are given ampicillin is well known. *Mycoplasma pneumoniae* infections have a wide variety of associated rashes, including maculopapular and vesicular types. *Enteroviruses* are a common cause of nonspecific febrile exanthems and more distinctive vesicular lesions (see below). *Adenovirus* infections may have a rash, particularly in association with conjunctivitis and pharyngitis.

DIFFERENTIAL DIAGNOSIS

Important conditions associated with maculopapular skin lesions include drug eruptions, rheumatic diseases, and Kawasaki disease. Toxic shock syndrome and staphylococcal scalded skin syndrome may resemble scarlet fever. Other life-threatening infections such as meningococcemia and Rocky Mountain spotted fever occasionally present with a benign-appearing rash.

EMERGENCY DEPARTMENT EVALUATION

The child's overall degree of illness is the most important assessment, as laboratory tests are rarely helpful or indicated in the child who is only mildly ill. A throat culture should be obtained if the child has a sore throat or suspected scarlet fever. Acute and convalescent antibody titers are important for confirming suspected cases of measles and rubella. White blood cell counts and blood cultures are helpful in evaluating the ill-appearing child who is suspected of having complications or a more serious disease. Further workup should be aimed at confirming clinically suspected complications such as pneumonia or encephalitis.

EMERGENCY DEPARTMENT MANAGEMENT

A child with an uncomplicated, presumably viral illness should be treated symptomatically with acetaminophen and oral fluids. Antibiotics should be reserved for secondary bacterial infection. Scarlet fever requires treatment with penicillin or an alternative. Avoid ampicillin and amoxicillin in patients who appear to have infectious mononucleosis. Isolate the child with suspected measles or rubella within the ED and report the case to the appropriate local health authority. Attempts at prevention or amelioration of measles may be indicated for susceptible household contacts, particularly infants younger than 1 year or immunocompromised persons. Preventive therapy includes measles vaccination within 72 hours of exposure (contraindicated in the immunocompromised) or intramuscular immune globulin given within 6 days of exposure.

DISPOSITION

Consultation with a pediatrician or infectious disease specialist should be obtained if the child appears to have a serious complication, is a neonate or immunosuppressed, or if a potentially serious disease is under consideration. Indications for admission: dehydration, pneumonia with respiratory distress, encephalitis, and toxicity.

Patients discharged should have follow-up scheduled. Phone contact is sufficient if the illness improves, but the child should be seen by a physician if symptoms worsen or change.

COMMON PITFALLS

- Children with benign, nonspecific febrile exanthems do not need lengthy diagnostic evaluation; however, occasionally signs of serious illness are missed because of the unimpressive nature of a rash. Early scarlet fever is often overlooked.
- Misdiagnosis of rubella in a pregnant women could have serious medical and legal consequences.

DISEASES WITH VESICULAR OR PUSTULAR LESIONS

Viral vesicular rashes and enanthems are frequently distinctive, allowing a presumptive diagnosis in most cases.

VARICELLA (CHICKEN POX)

Chicken pox is a common and contagious childhood disease caused by the varicella zoster virus. Ninety percent of cases occur in children 1 to 14 years old, but adolescents and adults tend to have a severe course with more frequent complications. Chicken pox is common in late fall, winter, and spring.

Varicella in healthy children presents with mild systemic symptoms, fever, and rash after an incubation period of 10 to 21 days. The skin lesions appear in crops, beginning as macules with rapid progression to papules, then vesicles that umbilicate and crust. The early vesicle is small and surrounded by erythema, resembling "a dewdrop on a rose petal." Early lesions are often present on the face and scalp. Lesions of all stages are characteristically present within a single area of the body, with concentration on the trunk and proximal extremities. Shallow ulcers often occur in the mouth but may also be seen on other mucous membranes. The extent of skin lesions varies but in general correlates with the height of fever and severity of symptoms. Pruritis is a common complaint, and scarring may result if the lesions are traumatized by severe scratching or if secondary infection occurs. The patient is contagious from 1 day before onset of the rash until all the lesions are crusted over.

Serious complications are unusual in childhood varicella. Secondary bacterial skin infections, manifested by impetigo, cellulitis, or local abscess, are seen most commonly in young children. Neurologic problems, ranging from acute cerebellar ataxia (incidence: 1 per 4000 cases in children under 15) to more serious manifestations such as encephalitis and Reye's syndrome, are the most common serious complications in childhood. Varicella pneumonia is rare in children but often seen in older patients. Severity ranges from subclinical to fatal; chest radiographs typically demonstrate nodular infiltrates. Unusual complications include liver disease, eye involvement (conjunctivitis or uveitis), coagulopathy, arthritis, orchitis, nephritis, and invasive bacterial infection (e.g., sepsis, osteomyelitis seeded from infected skin). Patients with altered cell-mediated immunity, such as leukemic children on chemotherapy, are susceptible to disseminated varicella, with hemorrhagic lesions, pneumonitis, and encephalitis. Newborns exposed to perinatal maternal varicella are at risk for severe illness.

EMERGENCY DEPARTMENT EVALUATION AND MANAGEMENT

Assess hydration and ability to take oral fluids. Laboratory evaluation is indicated for suspected complications or in high-risk patients in whom definitive diagnosis is necessary. Suspected sexual acquisition of herpes simplex in a prepubertal child warrants virus isolation and typing. Symptomatic therapy includes acetaminophen (avoid aspirin in varicella because of its association with Reye's syndrome) and fluids. Topical measures such as cool baths, calamine lotion, and colloidal oatmeal baths (Aveeno) may be helpful for the pruritus associated with chicken pox; oral antihistamines (e.g., diphenhydramine 5 mg/kg/day in four divided doses) may be added for severe itching. Topical antihistamines are not recommended because of the risk of sensitization and excessive systemic absorption.

Refusal to drink with viral stomatitis (especially herpetic) may be problematic. Cold substances such as Popsicles, ice cream, and nonirritating fluids are often tolerated best. Topical anesthetics (e.g., viscous lidocaine) are seldom helpful and should be used sparingly to avoid toxicity. Intravenous hydration may be required. Antibiotics should be given only for secondary bacterial infections. There is limited experience using oral acyclovir for otherwise healthy children with varicella-zoster or herpes simplex infections. Oral acyclovir (20 mg/kg/dose qid for 5 days, maximum dose 800 mg) given to children over 2 years old within 24 hours of the onset of chicken pox lesions has been shown to decrease the duration of fever and severity of skin lesions; however, it is controversial whether the modest benefits seen justify universal use. Patients with varicella should be isolated in the ED. Passive immunization with varicella zoster immune globulin (VZIG) may be indicated within 48 to 96 hours of exposure of a susceptible, high-risk patient.

DISPOSITION

Neonates or immunocompromised patients with suspected varicella zoster or herpes simplex infection should be seen in the ED by the appropriate specialist (infectious disease, oncology, neonatology, pediatrics, etc.). If sexual abuse is suspected in a child with genital herpes, obtain consultation with the appropriate person or team (e.g., child abuse social worker or pediatrician).

Hospitalization is indicated for significant complications or when a more serious disease is under consideration. Most neonates and immunocompromised patients with varicella zoster or herpes simplex infections will require hospitalization for observation and antiviral therapy (e.g., IV acyclovir). Children with uncomplicated varicella are discharged on symptomatic therapy, with outpatient follow-up as needed if further symptoms develop or if the child does not improve within a few days.

CLASSIC CHILDHOOD DISEASES WITHOUT RASH
MUMPS

Mumps infection commonly presents with parotid gland swelling, but other glands in the body as well as the nervous system are often affected. The mumps vaccine was not used routinely until the late 1970s, and significant numbers of children and adults remain susceptible to mumps.

CLINICAL PRESENTATION

Classic mumps parotitis presents with fever and progressive, painful parotid gland swelling. Although 75% of patients have bilateral involvement, often the second side is affected several days after initial symptoms appear. The submaxillary or sublingual salivary glands may be involved with or without parotid swelling. Inflammation of the opening of the parotid (Stensen's) or submaxillary (Wharton's) duct is often detectable. Occasionally, presternal edema may be seen and is presumed to be due to lymphatic obstruction. Fever generally resolves within a week, and parotid swelling subsides by 7 to 10 days. When other organs are affected, the patient may have preceding, concurrent, or later parotid involvement; some have no parotitis.

The most common complication is meningoencephalitis; about 65% have spinal fluid pleocytosis, and 10% are symptomatic. About 30% of postpubertal males develop epididymo-orchitis (usually unilateral); symptoms include fever, chills, vomiting, lower abdominal pain, and painful testicular swelling. Subsequent testicular atrophy is common, although infertility is unusual. Postpubertal females may similarly develop oophoritis with lower abdominal pain. Other rare manifestations of mumps infection include pancreatitis, thyroiditis, mastitis, dacryoadenitis, bartholinitis, myocarditis, arthritis, hematologic abnormalities, and nephritis. Sudden hearing loss may present with nausea, tinnitus, and ataxia. Patients are contagious up to 6 days before parotid swelling and until the swelling has resolved.

EMERGENCY DEPARTMENT EVALUATION AND MANAGEMENT

In unclear cases, a serum amylase (elevated in about two thirds of cases of parotitis) may be helpful. White blood cell counts may be normal or elevated. Obtain further tests if complications (e.g., encephalitis) are suspected or if a more serious diagnosis is being considered. Although not useful in the ED, definitive diagnosis may be obtained by virus isolation or titers. Therapy is supportive (analgesia, rest) in uncomplicated mumps. Mumps is a reportable disease in almost all states.

DISPOSITION

Consultation should be obtained if the physician is considering other diagnoses requiring definitive therapy. Patients with severe symptoms (e.g., pancreatitis, severe orchitis/oophoritis, encephalitis) may need hospitalization. Patients with uncomplicated mumps are discharged on symptomatic therapy, with outpatient follow-up as necessary.

COMMON PITFALLS

The physician may have difficulty recognizing mumps since it is no longer common. Accordingly, some patients receive unnecessary diagnostic evaluation or antibiotic therapy.

CHILDHOOD IMMUNIZATIONS

Table 220-2 is a synthesis of recent recommendations regarding childhood immunizations. Immunization practices are changing rapidly. Areas where new developments are likely include combination vaccines to decrease the number of simultaneous injections, and new *Haemophilus influenzae type B*, acellular pertussis, and varicella vaccines. Serious complications from currently used vaccines are rare; minor febrile and local reactions are common. Informed consent should be obtained before administering vaccines. Detailed written information about risks and benefits, such as pamphlets provided by the CDC is required before giving DPT, MMR, or polio vaccines. When a vaccine is administered, the date, manufacturer, lot number, site, and the person administering the vaccine should be recorded. Serious events related to vaccine administration, such as anaphylaxis, encephalopathy, shock-like state, hypotonic-hyporesponsive collapse, residual seizures, and paralytic polio must be reported to the U.S. Department of Health and Human Services Vaccine Adverse Event Reporting System (VAERS, phone 1-800-822-7967).

Table 220-2. Recommended Schedule for Immunization of Healthy Infants and Children*

Recommended Age†	Immunization‡	Comments
Birth	HBV§	
1–2 mo	HBV§	
2 mo	DTP, Hib, OPV	DTP and OPV can be initiated as early as 4 wk after birth in areas of high endemicity or during outbreaks.
4 mo	DTP, Hib, OPV	2-mo interval (minimum of 6 wk) recommended for OPV.
6 mo	DTP, (Hib‖)	
6–18 mo	HBV§, OPV	
12–15 mo	Hib, MMR	MMR should be given at 12 mo of age in high-risk areas. If indicated, tuberculin testing may be done at the same visit.
15–18 mo	DTaP or DTP	The 4th dose of diphtheria-tetanus-pertussis vaccine should be given 6 to 12 mo after the 3rd dose of DTP and may be given as early as 12 mo of age, provided that the interval between doses 3 and 4 is at least 6 mo and DTP is given. DTaP is not currently licensed for use in children younger than 15 mo.
4–6 y	DTaP or DTP, OPV	DTaP or DTP and OPV should be given at or before school entry. DTP or DTaP should not be given at or after the 7th birthday.
11–12 y	MMR	MMR should be given at entry to middle school or junior high school unless 2 doses were given after the 1st birthday.
14–16 y	Td	Repeat every 10 y throughout life.

*Table is not completely consistent with all package inserts. For products used, also consult manufacturer's package insert for instructions on storage, handling, dosage, and administration. Biologics prepared by different manufacturers may vary, and package inserts of the same manufacturer may change from time to time. Therefore, the physician should be aware of the contents of the current package insert.

†These recommended ages should not be construed as absolute. For example, 2 mo can be 6 to 10 wk. However, MMR usually should not be given to children younger than 12 mo. If measles vaccination is indicated, monovalent measles vaccine is recommended, and MMR should be given subsequently, at 12–15 mo.

‡Vaccine abbreviations: HBV = Hepatitis B virus vaccine; DTP = diphtheria and tetanus toxoids and pertussis vaccine; DTaP = diphtheria and tetanus toxoids and acellular pertussis vaccine; Hib = Haemophilus influenzae type b conjugate vaccine; OPV = oral poliovirus vaccine (containing attenuated poliovirus types 1, 2, and 3); MMR = live measles, mumps, and rubella viruses vaccine; Td = adult tetanus toxoid (full dose) and diphtheria toxoid (reduced dose), for children ≥. 7 y and adults.

§An acceptable alternative to minimize the number of visits for immunizing infants of HBsAg-negative mothers is to administer dose 1 at 0–2 mo, dose 2 at 4 mo, and dose 3 at 6–18 mo.

‖(Hib: dose 3 of Hib is not indicated if the product for doses 1 and 2 was PedvaxHIB [PRP-OMP], available from Merck & Co, West Point, PA).

221   Child Abuse

An awareness of child abuse and neglect is of particular importance in the ED. Any visit by a child may provide a chance to protect him or her from further harm. The visit may also provide a rare window into a family that may desperately need intervention and supportive services. Child abuse affects about 2 million children yearly in the USA and results in the death of 2000 to 5000 children. Since many of these children receive only episodic medical care or care at a time of medical crisis, the ED or acute clinic plays a special role in identifying and reporting child abuse and neglect. Although the physician is legally required to report suspected child abuse and is protected from liability for making a report in all states, a more important responsibility of the physician is to protect the child from further harm and therefore to cause an investigation to be done by the appropriate agency.

Physical abuse occurs in all cultural, ethnic, socioeconomic, and racial groups. There are some geographic and regional differences in the prevalence of given types of abuse, but not in overall incidence. The incidence of abuse in a socioeconomic subgroup is most closely related to the presence of significant stresses in that population (i.e., joblessness, homelessness, drug and alcohol abuse). The parent with caretaking responsibilities is more likely to abuse a child. Abusive parents usually are not psychotic and generally are responding to their children in a pattern similar to that experienced in their own childhoods. They fairly consistently have unrealistic expectations of their children and limited knowledge of developmental norms, and cannot cope with the child's failure to meet expectations. Triggering behaviors in the child such as excessive crying or colic are often seen.

CLINICAL PRESENTATION

The history from an abused child or an abusive parent remains the most important evaluative tool for the physician. The veracity of a child's history must be assumed until there is good reason to assume otherwise. If children do lie, they usually do so to hide the abuse rather than to bring it to light. The history from an abusive parent usually reflects a significant delay in seeking medical attention; if a primary physician exists, parents have usually not sought his or her advice. There is almost always a history disparate from the severity or type of injury. If repeated questioners are used to elicit the history, there is usually considerable variation in detail. Injury may be attributed to a sibling or to someone not present to verify the occurrences. Parents often simply cannot give any explanation for the injuries sustained. A brief interview of witnesses to trauma can often quickly obviate a need for investigation of a case.

The initial physical assessment may show findings that are strong indicators that further evaluation for abuse is necessary. These include:

1. Bruises in unusual locations or where an accidental cause is implausible due to the age or developmental status of the child (i.e., a nonambulatory infant with multiple bruises)
2. Bruises that have a characteristic pattern suggesting an object used to inflict the injury (i.e., hand print, belt mark, etc.)
3. Second-degree burns without bullae that show a characteristic pattern (i.e., the sole plate of an iron)
4. Second-degree burns with bullae, no evidence of splash marks, and an unusually sharp line of demarcation (i.e., glove or stocking burns of an extremity)
5. Burns limited to the perineum

6. Swelling of any body part out of proportion to the severity of described injury (may indicate an underlying fracture)
7. Unexplained or implausibly explained sudden changes in neurologic status
8. Retinal hemorrhages
9. Failure to thrive without a history suggestive of chronic or debilitating disease.

The finding most commonly present in abused children is bruises, but bruises are also the most commonly found accidental injury in children. Accidental bruises are located in areas most frequently exposed to injury in play or other normal childhood activities. the elbows, knees, and skin over the anterior tibia. The occasional bruise in less usual locations is of little concern and generally occurs over a bony prominence. The only commonly occurring lesion that may be mistaken for a bruise is the Mongolian spot. Mongolian spots are most common in darker-skinned infants and are characteristically shiny, blue-black, and limited to the back. Bruises that occur in clusters and in unusual locations such as the abdomen, back, or buttocks and that show unusual severity or varying stages of resolution are rarely accidental and should cause concern.

Resolution of bruises takes place in a predictable sequence. The bruise less than 48 hours old is swollen, tender, and red-purple. As the bruise begins to resolve, the tenderness, swelling, and redness disappear and the bruise becomes blue or dark purple. This takes place by the second day and remains for 5 to 7 days after injury. The bruise then heals through a green-brown-yellow color sequence and disappears after about 2 to 4 weeks. Much more specific sequencing can be accomplished by experience in observing many bruises. Photographs and a descriptive documentation of these findings may become critically important to those pursuing the investigation of abuse; this must be anticipated in the record.

LABORATORY EVALUATION

Laboratory evaluation should include bleeding and clotting studies when bruises are present and when there is any suggestion of easy bruisability: prothrombin time, partial thromboplastin time, and platelet count. A photographic record of any finding is always better than a written or schematic description alone. Radiographic studies are indicated where evidence of trauma is noted and in children where abuse is identified by some other means. These studies should include the chest, skull, and long bones in addition to the area of suspected injury. Films should be reviewed for fractures as well as evidence of osteopenia, increased trabeculation, and presence of excessive numbers of Wormian bones in the skull. These findings, along with an appropriate family history, might suggest the presence of osteogenesis imperfecta.

If fractures are seen, they should be related to the history of the type of injury. For example, spiral fractures occur in response to a torsional force, and chip fractures of the metaphysis occur with traction of the extremity. Metaphyseal chip fractures, in our experience, are rarely accidental. It is often necessary to estimate the age of fractures in comparison to the history. Fractures of differing ages without good evidence of multiple accidental trauma are virtually diagnostic of physical abuse. Healing of a fracture takes place in a predictable sequence. Periosteal new bone is formed as early as 4 to 10 days after the fracture and soft callus formation may be seen as early as 10 to 14 days. Hard callus formation may occur as early as 14 days and remodeling may begin by 3 months after the acute fracture.

A CT scan of the head is indicated in children with retinal hemorrhages or evidence of acute neurologic deterioration. The presence of intracranial hemorrhage with or without skull fracture and in the absence of a history of major trauma is diagnostic of child abuse until proven otherwise. Magnetic resonance imaging will be a useful tool in identifying small areas of bleeding and in determining areas of bleeding that have occurred at different times. The use of bone scans is usually not indicated except under special circumstances where abuse is clearly a possibility and where fractures may be suspected that are not yet visible on routine films.

With abdominal trauma, one might expect to see evidence of acute anemia associated with intra-abdominal bleeding or an elevated amylase with trauma to the pancreas. Hematuria is not uncommon with paddling or spanking where one or more blows have strayed cephalad.

ASSOCIATED SYNDROMES
SHAKEN BABY SYNDROME

Shaken babies rarely present with a history of shaking. The most common presentation is respiratory difficulty or unexplained seizures. The basic insult is the presence of intracranial bleeding, which may be characterized as subdural, epidural, interhemispheric or intraparenchymal, and symptoms are usually a result of increased intracranial pressure. Retinal hemorrhages are the single most common physical finding, and outside the newborn period provide presumptive evidence of intracranial bleeding due to trauma. While retinal hemorrhages may be seen with other head trauma, they should be considered the hallmark of the shaken baby syndrome until another plausible explanation is found. The hemorrhages are usually superficial and diffuse compared with the deeper flame-type hemorrhages seen in hypertension.

The diagnosis is made by a careful history after documentation of intracranial bleeding by CT scan or MRI. The mechanism of injury was once thought to be totally due to rotational and shear forces created by the to-and-fro motion of the head in shaking, but later studies strongly suggest that similar lesions can be caused by significant increased venous pressure transmitted from squeezing of the chest as part of shaking, or in any type of injury where significant increases in intra-abdominal or intrathoracic pressure are sustained.

Other skeletal injuries can be seen with shaking. The child is commonly held by the thorax or the extremities with enough force to cause fractures at those sites. The combination of intracranial bleeding and metaphyseal chip fractures of the distal tibias is indicative of the child's being held by the feet and cracked like a whip. The clinical outcome is dismal: about 65% will die or suffer significant neurologic sequelae as a result. Milder forms of this syndrome undoubtedly exist, with milder neurologic sequelae, but are yet to be carefully documented.

FAILURE TO THRIVE

Failure to thrive is often categorized as organic and nonorganic, although there are often some elements of both types in most individual cases. The child presents with a weight more than two standard deviations below the mean expected for age, and there may be associated growth failure as well. In most cases of organic failure to thrive, a strong suggestion of the underlying cause will be evident from the history and/or physical examination. Suggestions of a nonorganic cause may be evident by observing the interactions between the mother and child: they often show little interaction, and no nurturing behavior is evident on the mother's part. The child often shows little eye contact and generally is withdrawn from the environment. Most commonly, nonorganic failure to thrive requires a period of observation in a hospital setting for accurate diagnosis.

EMERGENCY DEPARTMENT MANAGEMENT

After a decision to report has been made, the next dilemma is to decide whether to tell the parents about the report. Under most circumstances it is better to calmly inform the parents that a report is being made because state law requires it and that you have no choice in the matter. It is better not to inform the parents when you believe they are likely to flee with the child and further endanger his or her health and welfare. Meticulous attention to the chart is essential in all abuse cases. The examiner is often called on to recall the encounter with the patient and parents and careful documentation is essential. The use of direct quotes from the child is helpful in avoiding questions of hearsay information. The use of detailed body charts to delineate injuries and findings, including careful measurements, is important; even better is the inclusion of photographs as part of the medical record.

The most common pitfall is the physician's failure to seriously consider this cause in the differential diagnosis of trauma to children. The presence of documented findings of trauma with an implausible history should provide more than adequate impetus for further evaluation and then careful documentation.

222 Congenital Heart Disease and Supraventricular Tachycardia

The incidence of congenital heart disease is 8 per 1000 births. The lesions are classified anatomically as shunts, obstructions, transpositions, and complex lesions. They are classified physiologically as cyanotic or noncyanotic, depending on the presence and severity of a right-to-left shunt. Definitive diagnosis and treatment of congenital heart disease is a complex topic. We will address eight syndromes based on clinical presentation (Table 222-1).

CLINICAL PRESENTATION AND DIFFERENTIAL DIAGNOSIS
CYANOSIS

Failure of the arterial pO_2 to rise above about 60 torr when the infant is placed on 100% oxygen is indicative of a cyanotic lesion. Most of these lesions are discovered before the infant leaves the nurs-

TABLE 222-1. Clinical Presentation of Congenital Heart Disease and SVT

Cyanosis	TGA, TOF, TA, TAt, TAVR
Congestive heart failure	PDA, HPVL, Coart, VSD, SVT
Failure to thrive	See above two categories
Murmur in an asymptomatic patient	Shunts: VSD, PDA, ASD
	Obstructions
	Valvular incompetence
Abnormal pulses	
Bounding	PDA, AI, AVM
Decreased	Coart., HPLV
Hypertension	Coart.
Syncope	
Cyanotic	TOF
Acyanotic	Critical AS
Tachycardia	
Sinus	Shock, benign causes
Supraventricular	Idiopathic, WPM

AI = aortic insufficiency; AS = aortic stenosis; ASD = atrial septal defect; AVM = arterial venous malformation; ECG = electrocardiogram; HPLV = hypoplastic left ventricle; PDA = patent ductus arteriosus; SVT = supraventricular tachycardia; TA = truncus arteriosus; TAt = tricuspid atresia; TAVR = total anomalous venous return; TGA = transportation of the great arteries; TOF = tetralogy of fallot; VSD = ventricular septal defect; WPW = Wolff-Parkinson-White.

ery, so that the parents are aware of the diagnosis during any subsequent visits to an ED. Tetralogy of Fallot, however, is a common cyanotic lesion that may escape detection in the nursery. Diagnosis can be delayed because the severity of the right-to-left shunt and, therefore, the degree of cyanosis, depend on the extent of pulmonary stenosis. If the stenosis is mild, the infant may be acyanotic or cyanotic only when crying or feeding. Other findings include a holosystolic ventricular septic defect (VSD) murmur in the third intercostal space at the left sternal border, a boot-shaped heart with decreased pulmonary vascular markings on chest radiography, and right ventricular hypertrophy with right axis deviation on electrocardiogram. The classic signs of clubbing and a history of exercise intolerance relieved by squatting are seldom seen due to early surgical repair. Hypercyanotic spells or syncope with cyanosis are still seen before total surgical repair.

CONGESTIVE HEART FAILURE

In infants, tachypnea and hepatomegaly are the first signs of left-sided and right-sided failure, respectively. The tachypnea is usually quiet or effortless because of lack of airway obstruction. Sweating during feeding and stopping to breathe after an ounce of formula are symptoms of dyspnea on exertion. Cardiomegaly is evident on chest radiography. Rales and peripheral edema are late signs of congestive heart failure in children. In premature infants who require mechanical ventilation, patent ductus arteriosus is a common cause of heart failure. In full-term infants, hypoplastic left ventricle is the most common cause of congestive heart failure in the first week of life, and coarctation of the aorta is the most frequent cause in the second week. Both of these conditions can present with the infant in the extremes of cardiogenic shock. The difference in strength of pulses and blood pressure between the upper and lower extremities makes bedside diagnosis of the latter possible. In hypoplastic left ventricle, pulses are uniformly diminished and the diagnosis usually is confirmed by echocardiogram. Large ventricular septal defects also can present in the first 2 months of life with progressive congestive heart failure. The failure slowly worsens and becomes more obvious as pulmonary vascular resistance falls from high fetal values to normal, causing the shunt from left to right to increase.

FAILURE TO THRIVE

Congenital heart disease can present as growth failure, particularly if the infant has cyanosis, congestive heart failure, or other associated anomalies. These last three factors help determine the differential diagnosis.

MURMUR IN AN ASYMPTOMATIC PATIENT

Auscultation for heart murmurs should be part of the routine physical examination for all pediatric patients. Pathologic murmurs are caused by turbulent flow produced by shunts, obstructions, or incompetent valves. Murmurs that should arouse suspicion for further workup are those that are holosystolic, diastolic, or grade 3 or louder, and those associated with any of the other clinical syndromes listed in this section.

ABNORMAL PULSES

The two most common cardiac causes of diminished pulses have been mentioned above. Vascular causes of bounding pulses include patent ductus arteriosus, palliative shunts from the systemic to pulmonary circulation, aortic insufficiency, and arterial-venous malformations or fistulas. Nonvascular causes include fever, sepsis, anemia, and hyperthyroidism.

HYPERTENSION

Coarctations of the aorta that are not severe enough to produce congestive heart failure in the second week of life when the ductus arteriosus closes can present at any time in life as hypertension.

SYNCOPE

Loss of consciousness from cardiac causes in the pediatric age group is rare but can be caused by dynamic obstruction to pulmonary outflow in tetralogy of Fallot resulting in an increased right-to-left shunt, or to critical aortic stenosis. Hypercyanosis aids in the diagnosis of the former, and signs of left ventricular hypertrophy on electrocardiogram are evident in the latter. These episodes can be fatal and require prompt medical and surgical intervention.

TACHYCARDIA

In the first few years of life, sinus tachycardia with rates as high as 180 to 200 beats per minute is not uncommon. Although the cause is usually benign (fever, stress, mild infection, etc.), shock and congestive heart failure should be considered and excluded by physical examination. Supraventricular tachycardia occurs in both infants and adolescents and is usually not associated with structural congenital heart disease. It is readily recognized by the rapid heart rate (220–360 beats per minute, as opposed to rates of 150–200 seen in adults). In infants, there is usually a history of sudden onset of poor feeding within the last 24 to 48 hours, accompanied by tachypnea, pallor, and lethargy. In adolescents, palpitations and chest pain can be prominent symptoms. Physical examination reveals thready pulses with a heart rate that is too rapid to be accurately counted. Clinically, the low cardiac output is secondary to inadequate diastolic filling time and can vary from a picture of congestive heart failure to cardiogenic shock.

EMERGENCY DEPARTMENT EVALUATION, MANAGEMENT, AND DISPOSITION

FEVER IN A CHILD WITH A KNOWN HEART LESION

Primary concerns include subacute bacterial endocarditis and of decompensation into acute congestive heart failure due to the stress of fever. Clinical signs of failure and a change in heart size on the chest radiograph are important observations in the latter situation. Admission for observation is often advisable. In endocarditis, blood cultures drawn before starting antibiotics can be invaluable. If the patient is alert and smiling, routine infections can be treated on an outpatient basis. If the patient has prominent lethargy or other signs of systemic compromise, consider admission for observation.

CYANOSIS

In infants with a known cyanotic lesion, recent onset of growth failure and progressive polycythemia are subacute signs that the child has reached a point of decompensation due to the lesion. Reevaluation by a pediatric cardiologist is prudent.

CONGESTIVE HEART FAILURE

Place the infant in an upright position and keep him or her comfortable. Give an increased FiO_2 in a way acceptable to the infant. Diuresis with 1 mg/kg of furosemide intramuscularly or intravenously can be given promptly. The decision to digitalize is usually made in conjunction with a pediatric cardiologist. The total digitalizing dosage ranges from 0.03 to 0.06 mg/kg (30–60 µg/kg). Half this dosage is given initially, preferably intravenously.

MURMUR IN AN ASYMPTOMATIC PATIENT

Initial evaluation of these patients includes a chest radiograph and electrocardiogram. Key radiographic signs include abnormalities in heart size and shape, and diminished or increased pulmonary vascular markings. Axis deviation, ventricular hypertrophy, and atrial enlargement are important findings on electrocardiogram. Referral to a pediatric cardiologist can be made on an elective outpatient basis.

SYNCOPE

In patients with uncorrected tetralogy of Fallot, initial management of hypercyanotic spells consists of placement in a knee-chest position and administration of 0.1 mg/kg of intravenous morphine and as high an FiO_2 as possible. Keep the patient in a position of comfort and minimize any stress from administering oxygen and performing venipuncture. The morphine can be repeated if necessary before transfer to the pediatric cardiology service.

Intravenous propanolol also relieves the subpulmonic, infundibular spasm that causes these episodes. Administration of propanolol should be done in conjunction with the cardiovascular surgeon.

Children with acyanotic syncope due to critical aortic stenosis should be kept at strict bed rest, using sedation if necessary. Referral for evaluation and possible emergency repair should be immediate.

SUPRAVENTRICULAR TACHYCARDIA

Electrocardiogram will confirm the diagnosis by showing narrow, regular QRS complexes and absent or abnormal P waves. In the stable patient, multiple methods of management are available, excluding the use of verapamil in infants (see below). Digoxin is still the preferred form of chronic therapy by many pediatric cardiologists, and half of the digitalizing dosage of 0.03 to 0.06 mg/kg can be given intravenously in the ED. It usually takes 4 to 6 hours for digoxin to convert the rhythm. Adenosine has now emerged as a safe, effective medication for rapid conversion of SVT to a sinus rhythm. Adenosine is metabolized rapidly. Therefore, it must be given rapidly, but it also has a wide range of safety in dosage. Starting with 0.1 mg/kg, adenosine is given as a rapid bolus, followed by an equally rapid bolus of 2–10 cc of normal saline, to help deliver the adenosine bolus to the myocardium. To facilitate this quick delivery, both the adenosine and the saline syringes can be inserted into the IV hub in advance preparation for the push. Oftentimes, there are a few seconds of asystole before the reappearance of a normal sinus rhythm. If necessary, repeat the bolus at 0.2 mg/kg, then 0.4 mg/kg, to a maximum of 12 mg. Vagal maneuvers, particularly ice water submersion, are more likely to be effective after digitalization. Cardioversion with 0.25 to 1 watt-second/kg is indicated when profound cardiogenic shock with impending arrest is present.

COMMON PITFALLS

- *Unrecognized cyanosis.* Cyanosis represents the presence of 5 g% or more of unoxygenated hemoglobin. It may be difficult to detect in milder degrees in infants with undiagnosed lesions or in those with dark skin. The workup should include a hematocrit, an arterial blood gas, a chest radiograph, and electrocardiogram. Consultation with a pediatrician or pediatric cardiologist can then be performed to determine the optimal time of referral.
- *Pneumonia vs. congestive heart failure.* Congestive heart failure can be misdiagnosed as pneumonia, since the latter is more common. At times, pneumonia may be the precipitating factor that causes an undiagnosed lesion to decompensate into failure. Cardiomegaly, hepatomegaly, chronicity of symptoms, and failure to thrive point to congestive heart failure.
- *Supraventricular tachycardia.* Due to sudden deaths from cardiac decompensation, the use of verapamil is now contraindicated for treatment of supraventricular tachycardia in infants.

223   Intussusception

Intussusception, an invagination of a proximal portion of the intestine into a distal adjacent part, is a common cause of intestinal obstruction in children <2 years old, with >60% of cases in the first year of life. Early diagnosis is essential: the duration of intussusception before treatment bears a close relationship to its morbidity and mortality.

CLINICAL PRESENTATION

The cardinal symptoms of intussusception are abdominal pain, vomiting, and rectal bleeding. In a typical case, there is a sudden onset of severe abdominal pain that may last several minutes. After an asymptomatic interval, repeated paroxysms will cause the child to cry out again. The child may be impossible to console or may seem comfortable only in a knee-chest position in the arms of an attendant. Vomiting may occur either with the initial painful episode or soon after. Concurrent with vomiting, the child usually has one or more bowel movements, which vary from thin liquid to formed stools. Within 12 to 24 hours, mucus, blood, or both may be passed per rectum, creating currant-jelly stools. Whereas abdominal pain and vomiting are found in 60% to 80% of patients, rectal bleeding is a less constant feature. The classic triad is found in <30% of patients. Apathy or listlessness may occasionally be the dominant concern of the parent.

The appearance of the child may be variable. Most children will be alert, well nourished, and hydrated. Those with advanced disease complicated by either fluid or electrolyte imbalance or blood loss may appear less responsive. Not uncommonly, a child with a very brief history of enteric manifestations may be obtunded at presentation. Other findings are limited to the abdominal examination. A sausage-shaped, sometimes ill-defined, and variably tender mass is present in 25–89% of patients. Abdominal guarding and distention are infrequent. On rare occasions, the advancing mass prolapses through the anus. Otherwise, the rectal examination reveals only bloody mucus on the finger as it is withdrawn.

DIFFERENTIAL DIAGNOSIS

Intussusception is readily diagnosed in a small percentage of children with the constellation of abdominal pain, vomiting, rectal bleeding, and abdominal mass. When the picture is less complete, other diagnoses entertained include intestinal obstruction, pseudomembranous or infectious enterocolitis, acute gastroenteritis, Hirschsprung's disease, appendicitis, Meckel's diverticula, and anaphylactoid purpura. Metabolic derangement, endocrinopathy, intoxication, occult cranial trauma, sepsis, and meningitis may be considered in those patients with intussusception with altered mental status.

EMERGENCY DEPARTMENT MANAGEMENT

Nontoxic hydrated children with a provisional diagnosis of intussusception should be placed NPO. Those who appear dehydrated should be given polyionic intravenous fluids pending serum electrolytes. A nasogastric tube should be inserted. Plain abdominal films in two views should be obtained. Those patients with evidence of complete bowel obstruction, perforated viscus, peritonitis, or generalized sepsis should not be subjected to attempts at hydrostatic reduction. All remaining patients with a tentative diagnosis of intussusception should have either an air insufflation reduction or a barium enema performed. The former has gained acceptance as the initial method for evaluation and treatment of intussusception overseas. Those patients who cannot be successfully reduced by either means will require operative intervention.

DISPOSITION

Air insufflation or barium enema reductions should never be done except with the consent of, and in the presence of, the surgeon who must accept the responsibility of operating if the reduction is unsuccessful. All patients with intussusception, even if successfully reduced with hydrostatic barium, should be admitted for a 24-hour observation period.

COMMON PITFALLS

- Failure to recognize the typical history
- Failure to perform a rectal examination
- Reluctance to accept the diagnosis in a well-appearing child with a prolonged history
- Failure to consider the disease in older children.
- A less than classic picture may lead to misdiagnosis (absence of pain, lack of a mass, or the presence of bright-red rectal bleeding or altered mental status)

---

224   Appendicitis in Children

Obstruction of the appendiceal lumen is the primary cause of appendicitis, most commonly due to a fecalith (calcified fecal material).

CLINICAL PRESENTATION

About 33% of appendices occupy locations other than the most common intraperitoneal location. Thus 30% of children with appendicitis will have localized pain in a region other than the right lower quadrant (retrocecal location may cause back or flank pain, while a pelvic appendix may cause suprapubic pain or a retroileal location may cause testicular pain). Although the classic triad of pain, vomiting, and fever may not always be present, the initial periumbilical pain shifting to another variable location several hours later is almost always present. It is important to note that the pain precedes the nausea, vomiting, and fever.

Anorexia is usually not present in children. Diarrhea is even less common, and if present is a small volume of mucoid feces. If the disease is allowed to progress without surgical intervention, appendiceal rupture will occur. The diagnosis of perforation is not difficult to make. The child is ill, toxic, dehydrated, and prostrated. In the younger child in particular, the incompletely developed greater omentum is incapable of walling off the inflammatory process. Therefore the abdominal pain is more diffuse and may decrease in intensity just after perforation, becoming much more severe as peritonitis develops.

The physical examination includes noting a hesitation to climb onto the examination table, and inability to stretch the right leg. The child usually prefers to lie still in the supine position with the thighs drawn up, particularly the right, since any motion increases pain. Vital signs are usually normal. Bowel sounds are usually normal. With progression of disease, advanced inflammation, perforation, or both results in ileus and a quiet abdomen. Abdominal palpation should start on the side opposite the pain. Muscular resistance to palpation of the abdomen parallels the severity of the inflammatory process. Early in the disease process, resistance, if present, consists of voluntary guarding. With the progression of peritoneal irritation, muscle spasm increases and becomes involuntary.

The most important physical finding is point tenderness at McBurney's point. Specific physical signs usually associated with acute appendicitis are Rovsing's sign, Psoas sign, and Obturator sign. A positive psoas or obturator sign suggest retrocecal or retrocolic inflammation. Nonspecific signs of peritoneal inflammation include cough tenderness and rebound tenderness. The diagnostic value of the rectal examination in children is limited. Rectal tenderness is present in 50% of children with or without appendicitis. A rectal examination must always be performed in the adolescent female to rule out uterine or tubo-ovarian disease.

DIFFERENTIAL DIAGNOSIS

The differential diagnosis in children depends on three major factors: the anatomic location of the inflamed appendix, the stage of the process (simple or ruptured), and the age and sex of the patient. The five main groups of differential diagnoses are:

1. Intestinal diseases: mesenteric adenitis, viral and bacterial enteritis, Meckel's diverticulitis, intussusception, enteric duplication
2. Uterine or tubo-ovarian pathology: gonadal torsion, acute epididymitis, pelvic inflammatory disease, tubal pregnancy, endometriosis, mittelschmerz
3. Urinary tract infection: acute pyelonephritis, cystitis
4. Respiratory and systemic diseases: basal pneumonia, Henoch–Schönlein purpura, sickle-cell crisis, primary bacterial peritonitis
5. Trauma: child abuse, accident.

Some of the distinguishing features of the major differential diseases are discussed below.

ACUTE MESENTERIC LYMPHADENITIS   Mesenteric adenitis is most often confused with acute appendicitis in children. Careful history almost invariably reveals the presence of upper respiratory symptoms. Laboratory studies are of limited value in differentiation, although a relative lymphocytosis may suggest mesenteric adenitis or a generalized viral syndrome. The abdominal pain is usually more diffuse and less severe, and generalized lymphadenopathy may be noted on physical examination. These patients may be observed for a few hours, but if any doubt persists, surgery is the only safe treatment.

PELVIC INFLAMMATORY DISEASE   Pain is most often bilateral and lower in location. History of vaginal discharge can be elicited. Physical examination reveals Chandelier's sign (pain with motion of the cervix).

ACUTE GASTROENTERITIS   Acute gastroenteritis usually can be differentiated from appendicitis without difficulty. These patients have profuse watery diarrhea, nausea, and vomiting, all of which usually precede the onset of pain. The pain is intermittent and crampy in nature, and localizing signs are absent. The abdomen is relaxed between cramps.

MECKEL'S DIVERTICULITIS   Preoperative differentiation is unnecessary, since the signs and symptoms of this disease are similar to acute appendicitis and surgical treatment is indicated for both.

INTUSSUSCEPTION   Differentiating between intussusception and acute appendicitis is extremely important and relatively straightforward. Age is an important factor. Appendicitis is very rare in children under 2 years of age, whereas nearly all intussusceptions occur in children under the age of 2 years.

HENOCH–SCHÖNLEIN PURPURA   This disease usually occurs a few weeks after a streptococcal infection. Abdominal pain may be a prominent symptom but joint pains, purpura, and nephritis also can be present, and the development of these symptoms can be delayed.

MITTELSCHMERZ   The pain is usually diffuse in nature. History-taking is important because these patients are at the midpoint of their menstrual cycle.

GONADAL TORSION   A number of nonspecific symptoms may exist, including anorexia, nausea, and vomiting. The correct diagnosis can be made by including the genitalia in the physical examination, which will usually reveal the subtle findings of asymmetry in gonadal size and position.

URINARY TRACT INFECTION   Bacteria in freshly catheterized urine specimens may be present in about 17% of children with acute appendicitis if the appendix lies near the ureter or bladder. The UA is normal in >80% of children with acute appendicitis.

EMERGENCY DEPARTMENT EVALUATION

The most important steps are the history and physical examination, including the external genitalia in males and an internal pelvic exam in adolescent females. Laboratory studies and other tests may assist in differentiating appendicitis from other entities: complete blood count with differential and urinalysis. Moderate leukocytosis (10,000–18,000/µl) accompanied by polymorphonuclear predominance is the rule; however, the total white count is usually not elevated in the early phase of appendicitis. A left shift in the differential precedes leukocytosis in most children.

Abdominal radiographs are not particularly helpful in making the diagnosis of appendicitis. A chest film may be required to rule out right lower lobe pneumonia. Ultrasonography is useful to differentiate appendicitis from tubo-ovarian disease and appendiceal phlegmon from appendiceal abscess.

Symptoms suggestive of perforation are:

1. Duration of symptoms >36 hours
2. Temperature >102°F
3. White count >15,000/µL
4. Physical findings of peritonitis.

The most common erroneous preoperative diagnoses, in descending order of frequency, are acute mesenteric lymphadenitis, no organic pathologic condition, acute pelvic inflammatory disease, twisted ovarian cyst, mittelschmerz, and acute gastroenteritis. These account for >75% of all misdiagnoses. History and physical examination should result in a correct diagnosis in 80% of cases. Perforated appendicitis has a mortality rate of 5% and a morbidity rate up to 46% in some series, compared with a mortality rate of 0.1% in nonperforated appendicitis.

EMERGENCY DEPARTMENT MANAGEMENT

Appendicitis is a surgical emergency. Children with significant abdominal pain should be evaluated by a surgeon. The initial management of simple and perforated appendicitis is the same. Once the diagnosis has been made, the child must receive intravenous fluids and kept NPO. Start dextrose 5% in 1.5 normal saline and 20 mEq/L of KCl at 1.5 maintenance initially. Give lactated Ringer's solution boluses at 10 mL/kg to maintain urine output at 1 to 2 mL/kg/hour. If the patient has eaten or vomited within 6 hours of the operation, consider inserting a nasogastric tube to empty the stomach. In a child who has been vomiting, obtain serum electrolytes. If the patient's temperature is above 101.5°F, give an acetaminophen suppository to lower the temperature.

Routine antibiotics with acute nonperforating appendicitis remain controversial. Absolute indications for antibiotic therapy are systemic signs, suspected perforation, and the presence of underlying conditions that predispose to complications of bacteremia (i.e., infants under 6 months of age, children with congenital or acquired cardiac anomalies, diabetes mellitus). The most common intravenous antibiotics are ampicillin (100 mg/kg/24 hours ÷ 4), gentamicin (5 mg/kg/24 hours ÷ 3), and clindamycin (40 mg/kg/24 hours ÷ 4). This ensures coverage of aminoglycoside-resistant enterococci, gram-negative bacilli, and anaerobes, respectively.

DISPOSITION

Children with appendicitis should be admitted to the hospital for surgical exploration. If doubt persists as to the correct diagnosis and the surgeon opts not to operate immediately, the child should be admitted for serial physical examinations.

COMMON PITFALLS

- Time is of essence in the diagnosis of acute appendicitis in children. Rapid progression of disease in this age group demands early suspicion, diagnosis, and operation if the complication of perforation is to be avoided. Late diagnosis results in a significantly higher morbidity and mortality.
- The physician must be thorough in obtaining the history and performing the physical examination.

---

225   Sexual Abuse in Children

Until a few years ago, sexual abuse in children was considered uncommon. It is now clear that sexual abuse or sexual molestation will affect at least one in four female and one in seven male children at some time before age 18. The short-term and long-term physical and psychological effects of this problem depend on many factors, including the severity of the abuse, the length of time of involvement, the relationship of the abuser to the child, and the sensitivity of intervening professionals and family members after the problem has come to light. The ED response to sexual abuse must address the child's medical needs as well as the need for accurate collection of evidence, but must be equally considerate of every aspect of the child's psychological needs.

CLINICAL PRESENTATION

Sexual abuse cases may present with a medical emergency, usually with vaginal bleeding or clinical suggestions of acute abdominal trauma or peritoneal irritation. In these cases, all matters of evidence collection, forensic evaluation, and reporting are secondary to the need for immediate intervention to stabilize the child's medical condition. Resuscitative measures take precedence.

The more typical case of child sexual abuse will present in one of two ways. First, the child may present with a chief complaint of sexual abuse by or because of a caretaker's suspicion of sexual abuse. Second, the child may present with a seemingly unrelated chief complaint, and the examiner suspects sexual abuse because of other findings in the examination.

The approach to these cases may be somewhat different, but each case mandates the involvement of a team of professionals to elicit a complete history, to recommend and carry out necessary intervention, and to ensure the child's immediate safety as well as access to treatment for the child and family. This requires the involvement of the local child protection agency, law enforcement, and ideally a multidisciplinary child protection team in the community. In all cases when there is a suspicion of sexual abuse, a physician must report that suspicion to child protective services or to a local law-enforcement agency. Local and state laws determine the physician's detailed responsibility for reporting.

HISTORY

In cases where the presenting complaint is sexual abuse or sexual molestation, record in the chart the history and source of the history. Where possible, the history should be from the child.

PHYSICAL ASSESSMENT

The examination of the genitalia should always be done in the context of a complete standard physical examination. This approach is necessary to ensure that other significant problems are documented. Abnormal findings should never be reported in the presence of the child. Long after the minor trauma of the examination itself has faded, the child will remember assurance by a medical figure that he or she is not at fault. With adequate preparation and patience, examination under anesthesia or with sedation is rarely necessary.

Examining the genitalia of a prepubertal child is a process of description and observation. Preferable positions from the viewpoint of the examiner are the knee-chest or the frog-leg position. In the frog-leg position, direct inspection and moderate downward and outward traction of the labia majora will give adequate visualization of all structures germane to the examination. In the knee-chest position, structures can usually be visualized directly without traction on the labia.

There are significant differences in appearance of normal anatomical structures in different positions as well as in differing degrees of relaxation in the same child. For this reason, only findings that clearly indicate scarring or consistent loss of reflex response should be considered definitive. Invasion with a speculum or finger is seldom necessary or helpful. Culture or specimen collection should be carried out with the smallest swab available. Inspection of the labia and introitus should include attention to evidence of old or new lacerations, chafing, or irritation.

Hymenal configuration should be noted and may be described as annular, crescentic, cribriform, septate, or imperforate. Congenital absence of the hymen does not occur. Thickness of the membrane should be described, with any scarring located and recorded in relation to the hour hand of a clock. Hymenal lateral and anterior-posterior opening diameter should be carefully measured and recorded. In the past, lateral hymenal diameter was believed to be of extreme import in diagnosing sexual abuse or molestation, but currently it seems to be of less importance than evidence of chronic scarring or acute injury. If the vaginal canal can be visualized, a description of general appearance, ruggal folds, and any scars is important.

Abnormalities indicative of sexual abuse in the prepubertal child include:

Lacerations of the hymen (acute or healed)
Thickening and rolling of the hymeneal margin
Perineal scars
Absence of the hymen
Scarring of the hymen with associated vaginal scarring
Anal scarring
Loss of the anal wink reflex or reflex anal relaxation with stimulation
Gaping hymeneal orifice

In cases of documented sexual abuse, definite physical findings are present in only about 50% to 60% of cases. Findings should be recorded on a standard anatomical chart for future reference. Color photography is recommended but is not always readily available in the ED. Remember that overt sexual activity may not leave physical scars, and a negative examination does not rule out sexual abuse. You may conclude that the examination is consistent with but not diagnostic of sexual abuse, or you may conclude that the physical examination neither confirms nor denies a history of sexual abuse. It is likely you will be asked to support your conclusions at a later date.

LABORATORY EVALUATION

If forensic evidence is needed, an evidence collection packet must be available from local law-enforcement sources, and the physician must be knowledgeable about the use of the kit before the examination is done. Useful forensic evidence is almost never found beyond 72 hours after an assault. Assessment for sexually transmitted diseases is always necessary, but the extent of the search is a matter of clinical judgment. Cultures for *Neisseria gonorrhoeae* should be sought from all prepubertal patients from the vagina, rectum, and throat. Cultures for the presence of *Chlamydia trachomatis* are useful. Wet mounts should be done with anogenital discharges and dark-field examinations are done on genital ulcers when present. Viral cultures from vesicular lesions for herpes simplex and routine bacteriologic cultures should be done in all patients with a demonstrable discharge.

EMERGENCY DEPARTMENT MANAGEMENT

Treatment should be designed to alleviate any urgent or life-threatening medical needs. Subsequent treatment is usually limited to the treatment of sexually transmitted diseases if present. Presumptive treatment is not advisable, and treatment should only be undertaken with definitive culture or clinical evidence that a disease is present.

COMMON PITFALLS

- The examining physician is often confused when a child recants a history of sexual abuse. This phenomenon is common in the child sexual abuse syndrome and often results from fear, parental coaching, the observed response of authority figures to the report, or the realization that intervention may result in jail or family separation. The physical examination may be even more important in these cases if abnormal findings are present to help corroborate the original allegation.
- A common pitfall is the physician's failure to record all data; meticulous attention to detail in the examination and in the recording of the examination are essential.

226   Sudden Infant Death Syndrome

Sudden infant death syndrome (SIDS) is the sudden and unexpected death of an apparently healthy infant in whom a complete autopsy fails to reveal an adequate cause of death. SIDS is responsible for about 7,000 deaths a year in the United States, making it the most common cause of death in infants between 1 week and 1 year of age.

EPIDEMIOLOGY

Virtually all SIDS deaths appear to have occurred during sleep, with the vast majority of infants found dead during usual sleeping hours. There have been rare reports of infants being seen awake shortly before being found dead, but these account for a very small proportion of SIDS deaths. The age distribution of SIDS is striking and unlike any other known pediatric disorder. SIDS is extremely rare in infants under the age of 2 weeks. More than 50% of deaths occur during the second and third months of life. SIDS is rare after the age of 6 months. SIDS is more common among blacks and lower socioeconomic classes. About 65% of SIDS victims have evidence of a mild viral infection at autopsy.

THE EMERGENCY DEPARTMENT AND SIDS

SIDS is both sudden and unexpected; the family's grief reaction cannot begin until the patient's death. Initial reactions consist primarily of shock, denial, anger, and guilt. The grief process can go on for years and can have profound effects on the lives of the family members. Warm, sympathetic, and understanding ED personnel can greatly reduce the psychological morbidity of the grief reactions. Informing the parents that the cause of SIDS is unknown and that it cannot be predicted or prevented can greatly ameliorate their feelings of guilt.

Written information for the parents is available from many local health departments and from the National SIDS Foundation in Chicago. Hospital social workers, nurses, and chaplains can help the family notify friends, relatives, and clergy and help the family deal with their grief process. Some families will wish to hold the baby and say good-bye. They should be allowed to do so in the presence of a caring, sympathetic individual. Others may not wish to see the baby and should not be coerced into doing so.

Autopsies of potential SIDS victims are now required in most states. In about 15% of suspected SIDS cases, an identifiable cause of death will be found. The parents should be informed of the result of the necropsy as soon as possible. Finally, continued family support should be arranged. Visiting nurses, parents' groups, public health nurses, and mental health resources are useful to carry on family support as long as necessary.

COMMON PITFALLS

- Failure to perform a postmortem examination and laboratory studies in the ED. Examining the infant's body may reveal signs of trauma or other causes of death. Postmortem blood and spinal fluid cultures also may be informative.
- Failure to arrange for an autopsy. Autopsy results may have implications for genetic counseling of parents as well as ruling out other causes of sudden, unexpected infant death.
- Failure to arrange for immediate and continuing family support after a SIDS death.

PART IV

Pediatric Trauma

227 Approach to the Pediatric Multiple Trauma Patient

The major causes of pediatric trauma include motor vehicle accidents, auto–pedestrian collisions, burns and smoke inhalation, falls, poisonings, and child abuse. Data from the National Pediatric Trauma Registry indicate that about 90% of childhood injuries are due to blunt trauma. The remaining 10% of pediatric injuries tend to occur in urban settings or are due to farm-related accidents or hunting injuries.

THE PRIMARY AND SECONDARY SURVEYS

The Primary Survey is an initial assessment of the patient's airway, oxygenation, ventilation, circulation, perfusion, and overall level of consciousness (Table 227-1). The patient is fully undressed for a detailed Secondary Survey, a directed evaluation of each body area. The Secondary Survey assesses the type and severity of injury, as well as the body system's potential contribution to physiologic instability. The examination should not delay evaluation or treatment of life-threatening injuries.

AIRWAY

The highest priority is providing a patent airway with adequate ventilation and oxygenation. However, significant differences in the pediatric airway require an approach different from that for an adult (Figure 227-1). While cervical spine injuries are less common in children, it is important to protect the cervical spine since 2/3 of all children with spinal cord injuries have no radiographic abnormalities apparent on initial radiographs or follow-up tomograms. Most of these children have symptoms

---

TABLE 227-1. Primary Survey Approach to the Pediatric Trauma Patient

A—Airway (with cervical spine immobilization)
B—Breathing
C—Circulation
D—Disability
    Diagnosis and Treatment of Shock
E—Expose
    Environment

Adapted from American College of Surgeons Committee on Trauma: Textbook of Advanced Trauma Life Support. Chicago, American College of Surgeons, 1985.

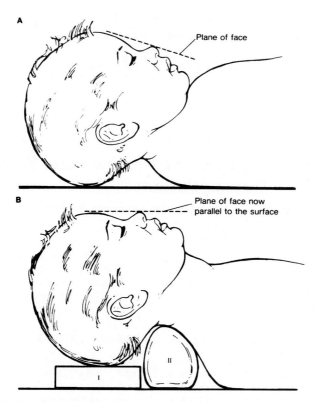

Figure 227-1. (A) Airrway at high risk for occlusion. Flexion of the neck on the thorax is caused by a prominent occiput **(B)** Sniffing position, which gives maximum possibility for a patent airway. Note the mild extension of the head. Flexion is now corrected by elevation of the head (I) and/or posterior neck support (II).

of transient paresthesias or numbness that occur at the time of the impact injury. Because of the devastating consequences of missing a cervical spine injury, any patient with an injury to the chest or above should be considered to have a cervical spine injury until proven otherwise.

In-line cervical immobilization is effective in children, although it often requires a two-res-cuer approach in the struggling child. It is often possible to use both a rigid cervical collar and sandbags and tape to immobilize a child's cervical spine without compromising the airway. Concurrently with stabilizing the cervical spine, the airway should be evaluated and positioned. The most frequent and obvious error is failure to position the airway properly. Because the larynx is both more anterior and more cephalad in a child, position the child in the "sniffing position" (neck slightly flexed on the spinal axis and the head slightly extended on the neck).

Once the airway has been positioned, a rapid assessment should be made for airway patency and adequacy of ventilation. If airway obstruction exists, manual clearing or suction with a rigid tonsillar suction should be provided, after which the airway should be repositioned. In addi-tion, the respiratory effort should be at the appropriate rate and should provide adequate bilat-eral chest wall rise. Cyanosis should also be noted. Supplemental oxygen should be provided. A second common error is failure to recognize problems with ventilation. Because children have small tidal volumes, the chest wall rise that is usually present may be subtle.

BAG-AND-MASK VENTILATION

Most children can be initially ventilated in an adequate fashion via bag-and-mask ventilation.

NASOGASTRIC TUBE PLACEMENT

Whenever assisted ventilation is provided, a nasogastric tube should be placed. Aerophagia and gastric distention are common and may result in distention of the left hemidiaphragm, compromising ventilation. The best means to assess appropriate positioning of the nasogastric tube is to place 15 cc of normal saline through the tube and ensure that a like quantity can be aspirated easily.

ENDOTRACHEAL INTUBATION

There are three general indications for ET intubation:

1. Inability to adequately ventilate the child by bag-and-mask methods
2. The need for prolonged control of the airway, including prevention of aspiration
3. The need for controlled hyperventilation in serious head injury.

When any of these indications are present, continue adequate bag-and-mask ventilation with 100% oxygen until appropriate preparations can be made for ET intubation. To select the appropriate-sized ET tube, recall that the narrowest portion of the pediatric airway is at the level of the cricoid cartilage. In children, the airway narrows below the level of the vocal chords at the area of the cricoid cartilage. A tube that passes through the vocal chords may encounter resistance at the level of the cricoid cartilage and cause later necrosis and resultant subglottic stenosis. Chose a tube about the size of the cricoid cartilage. There are two anatomic means of doing this. The distal portion of the fifth finger at the level of the distal phalanx, and the size of the child's naris both closely approximate the size of the diameter of the cricoid cartilage. A formula that approximates ET tube sizing:

$$\text{Tube size in mm} = \frac{\text{Age in years} + 16}{4}$$

Length has been shown to be the most accurate predictor of the correct size endotracheal tube for a child. The Broselow Tape can be used to select pediatric equipment using a single length measurement.

Other preparations necessary before ET intubation include adequate preoxygenation of the patient via bag-and-mask ventilation with 100% oxygen. A straight laryngoscope blade is more helpful in children. Airway positioning is critical during ET intubation. Place the child in the sniffing position and use Sellick's maneuver to prevent vomiting and aspiration. Never interrupt assisted ventilation for more than 30 seconds for any reason. If the tube cannot be easily placed within that time, continue bag-and-mask ventilation for an additional 60 to 90 seconds, after which an additional attempt at ET intubation can occur. The presence of bilateral, symmetrical chest wall rise and improvement in the child's overall color and condition should confirm placement of the tube. Obtain a chest radiograph to ensure proper position.

Additional means of securing the pediatric airway include needle cricothyroidotomy and rapid sequence intubation. Needle cricothyroidotomy should be used only in rare circumstances in children. It is largely a means to avoid surgical cricothyroidotomy, which is difficult in the child.

In those circumstances in which an airway is needed immediately because of massive facial or laryngeal trauma in the child, needle cricothyroidotomy is an alternate technique. A 14-16G catheter is placed in the midline through the cricoid cartilage and is advanced distally.

RAPID SEQUENCE INTUBATION

Rapid sequence intubation is an effective technique of securing the airway when intubation is needed. Whenever possible, place a nasogastric tube before intubation to allow suctioning of fluid, secretions, and particulate matter from the stomach. *Always* perform Sellick's maneuver to ensure that vomiting and aspiration do not occur. Maintain this maneuver until it is certain that the tube is placed within the trachea. Maintain in-line cervical stabilization and adequate airway positioning during the entire rapid sequence intubation procedure.

The technique uses an anticholinergic drug (atropine 0.02 mg/kg) to decrease secretions, as well as a short-acting barbiturate (thiopental 2–4 mg/kg) and a neuromuscular blocking agent (either succinylcholine or pancuronium bromide) to provide anesthesia and muscular relaxation. Other drugs to produce paralysis include vercuronium, which produces a duration of action between that of succinylcholine and pancuronium bromide, but with fewer cardiovascular side effects. Succinylcholine is an extremely short-acting neuromuscular blocking agent with an onset of action at 1 minute and a peak at 1.5 to 2 minutes, with a duration of action of 8 minutes. It is generally given in a dose of 1.5 mg/kg to effect complete paralysis. In cases in which *immediate* intubation is required, succinylcholine or the newer agents, such as vercuron, can be given without thiopental.

CIRCULATION

The major goals are to assess to overall circulatory status, including pulse and perfusion, while obtaining reliable venous access and controlling any internal or external hemorrhage. Circulatory assessment should include palpating the pulse for quality (strong, normal, thready) rate and regularity. While tachycardia is a normal response to hypovolemia, the tachycardic response to blood loss is much more profound in children than in adults. The earliest sign of hypovolemia in children is tachycardia.

VENOUS ACCESS

Rapid venous access is among the most challenging problems. Options include percutaneous peripheral venous cannulation, intraosseous infusion, peripheral venous cutdown, and percutaneous central venous access. Select the route that is the most rapid.

INTRAOSSEOUS INFUSION
In children up to age 5 years, intraosseous infusion is the second-best access to the peripheral circulation.

PERCUTANEOUS CENTRAL VENOUS ACCESS
When percutaneous venous cannulation and/or intraosseous infusion are unsuccessful, the physician should use whatever technique is most likely to be successful. Depending upon training and expertise, that may be either central venous cannulation or peripheral venous cutdown. When central venous access lines are obtained, the most common sites are the subclavian vein and the internal jugular vein. The internal jugular vein is often used but is less likely to be successful in a resuscitative situation in which airway manipulation is being used and access to the internal jugular vein is more difficult. The subclavian vein is difficult to cannulate in children, particularly those in shock or in need of resuscitative measures.

PERCUTANEOUS VENOUS CUTDOWN
Percutaneous venous cutdown can be used at either the saphenous vein in the ankle or the brachial or cephalic veins in the antecubital space. Percutaneous peripheral cutdown should take no longer than percutaneous central venous access and is far safer, with a much lower incidence of complications.

HEAD INJURY

Head injuries are present in nearly 80% of all severely injured multiple trauma patients. The best way to assess central nervous system injury is the patient's level of consciousness. The ATLS course recommends the "AVPU": mnemonic:

A: Alert
V: Responsive to verbal stimuli
P: Responsive to painful stimuli
U: Unresponsive

In general, a patient who responds only to painful stimuli or does not respond at all should be assumed to have a major head injury until a GCS score can be assessed. Check for the size and reactivity of the pupils and the presence of any posturing or lateralizing findings. Do a more detailed mini-neurologic examination in the Secondary Survey.

SHOCK

The earliest finding in pediatric patients in shock is tachycardia. Table 227-2 lists the maximal pulse values by age. Rapidly establish a rapid vascular access line and give at least 20 cc/kg of lactated Ringer's.

SECONDARY SURVEY

Remember that infants and small children, up until the age of about 2 years, may require warming lights and/or blankets to maintain their temperature at a normal level. The major threats to life in the *early* evaluation come from the cardiorespiratory system. While head injury is the most common cause of death, airway and shock are the earliest threats to life (Table 227-3).

TABLE 227-2. Maximum Pulse Rates and Respiratory Rates by Age

	Infants	Preschool	School Age
Maximum Pulses Rate	≤140	≤120	≤100
Maximum Respiratory Rate	≤30	≤20	≤15

Mayer TA: Initial evaluation and management of the injured child. In Mayer TA (ed): Emergency Management of Pediatric Trauma. Philadelphia, WB Saunders, 1985.

TABLE 227-3. Checklist for Sudden Deterioration

Airway

Adequate airway position?
Adequate tidal volume?
Adequate rate?
Pneumothorax?
Tension pneumothorax?

Endotracheal Tube

Dislodged?
Plugged?
Right mainstem bronchus?

IV Access

Functional?
Adequate size?
Medications infusing?

Unrecognized Bleeding

Pelvis
Chest
Abdomen
Thighs
Retroperitoneum

Unrecognized Injuries

CERVICAL SPINE

There is a higher risk for cervical spine injury in children injured from motor vehicle accidents over 45 m.p.h., motor vehicle accidents in which the occupant is unrestrained, auto–pedestrian collisions, falls greater than 10 feet in height, and direct trauma to the posterior neck. Up to two thirds of children with spinal cord injuries have no radiographic abnormality. So, whenever either focal muscular splinting or neurologic findings are present or if the history strongly suggests a cervical spine injury, the neck should remain immobilized.

CHEST

Because the chest wall in children has less muscle and fat, forces applied to the external thorax can be transmitted to the underlying pulmonary parenchyma. The presence of retractions is significant and indicates significant respiratory difficulty. Obtain a chest film to evaluate underlying pulmonary contusion or hemopneumothorax.

ABDOMEN

The child's abdomen should be examined for evidence of splinting, contusions, abrasions, ecchymosis, or distention. Examine both the front and back of the abdomen. *The most helpful portion of the abdominal examination is palpation.* In conscious patients, ask where they hurt and begin the examination as far away from that site as possible. Repeated examinations commonly reveal significant findings that would have been missed with a single examination.

A rectal examination should be done gently and with a well-lubricated gloved finger. Most children can be talked through this examination quite easily, and the entire pelvic rim can be palpated for signs of injury.

PELVIS

After the abdominal examination, inspect the bony pelvis and the perineum. Palpate the entire bony pelvis for instability or tenderness. Ask the patient to gently flex and abduct the hip, since this may detect subtle pelvic fractures. Assess for urethral meatal blood and evidence of scrotal hematoma or swelling.

MUSCULOSKELETAL EVALUATION

Palpate carefully over the entire bony skeleton for tenderness or swelling. Visually examine all bony areas for deformity, abrasion, contusion, or hematoma. Splint obvious deformity; obtain appropriate radiographs. Document the pulse and neurologic status of the extremities.

NEUROLOGIC EXAMINATION

Do a mini-neurologic examination. The most critical aspect in the head-injured patient is the overall level of consciousness. The Glasgow Coma Scale (Table 227-4) assesses patients with regard to eye opening, verbal stimuli, and motor responses. In children in the preverbal age group (<2–3 years old), the score is modified by giving any child who cries a full verbal score; this reflects the fact that comatose children do not cry.

LABORATORY STUDIES AND RADIOLOGIC EVALUATION

Possible or documented evidence of shock, altered level of consciousness, or evidence of either single- or multisystem injury are indications for a complete set of radiographic trauma series and laboratory studies (blood count, electrolytes, glucose, blood urea nitrogen, amylase, urinalysis, type and screen or crossmatch, prothrombin time, partial thromboplastin time, and platelet count). In patients with respiratory compromise or on whom artificial ventilation is being performed, obtain an arterial blood gas analysis. Examine the nasogastric and rectal contents for occult blood. In older children, alcohol or other intoxicants may contribute so obtain appropriate toxicologic studies. The need for additional laboratory studies should be guided by the patient's physical findings and clinical course.

TABLE 227-4. Glasgow Coma Scale

Eye Opening	Never	1
	To pain	2
	To speech	3
	Spontaneously	4
Best Verbal Response*	None	1
	Garbled	2
	Inappropriate	3
	Confused	4
	Oriented	5
Best Motor Response	None	1
	Extension	2
	Abnormal flexion	3
	Withdrawal	4
	Localizes pain	5
	Obeys commands	6

*Children 2 years of age or younger who cry are given a verbal score of 5.

Radiography: the cervical spine may need radiographic evaluation, although its limitations have been pointed out. Chest radiograph should be done next, followed by pelvis films. Computed tomography (CT) scanning of the head, and abdomen should be guided by the findings and clinical course.

DISPOSITION

CONSULTATION   *Immediate surgical consultation is required for any pediatric multiple trauma victim with either single- or multisystem injury, or in whom there has been an altered level of consciousness or documented shock.* Because 80% of children have head injuries in association with multiple trauma, neurosurgical consultation may be indicated.

INDICATIONS FOR TRANSFER   The decision to transfer a pediatric multiple trauma patient depends largely on the patient's stability and on the availability of a pediatric trauma center. In some cases, severe intra-abdominal bleeding may require immediate operative intervention to obtain appropriate hemostasis. However, these cases represent a small minority of pediatric trauma cases.

INDICATIONS FOR ADMISSION   A child with a GCS score of 8 and major cardiovascular instability needs to be admitted. Determining the criteria for admission for the "gray area" patients is much more difficult. In general, any pediatric patient who has lost consciousness or in whom a single- or multisystem injury has required the placement of an intravenous line should be observed in the hospital for at least 24 hours. This is to ensure that continued and complete observation of the patient results in a clear delineation of the extent and severity of injuries.

OUTCOME FROM PEDIATRIC MULTIPLE TRAUMA

The single most important determinant of outcome in pediatric multiple trauma patients is the presence or absence of severe head injury. Patients with severe head injuries have a poorer outcome than those without such injuries. However, the outcome from head injury in pediatric patients is much better than in adults. Even in patients with GCS scores of 3 or 4, a good recovery can be expected in 30%. All pediatric multiple trauma patients should be resuscitated aggressively. The overall mortality from severe pediatric trauma (in which two or more body systems are injured to a severe degree) is still only 10% to 15%.

Component	+2	+1	−1
Size	>20 kg	10–20 kg	<10 kg
Airway	Normal	Maintainable	Unmaintainable
CNS	Awake	Obtunded	Coma
Systolic BP	>90 mm Hg	90–50 mm Hg	<50 mm Hg
Open Wound	None	Minor	Major
Skeletal	None	Closed Fx	Open/Mult Fx's

Figure 227-2. Pediatric trauma score.

PEDIATRIC TRAUMA SCORING

Tepas and Ramenofsky developed the Pediatric Trauma Score (PTS) in an attempt to recognize the unique needs of the pediatric trauma victim (Figure 227-2). PTS has a high validity as a predictor of injury severity.

228 Hemorrhagic Shock in Children

During the immediate phase of care of the pediatric trauma victim, shock is nearly always due to hypovolemia, usually caused by external or internal hemorrhage. In the vast majority of pediatric trauma victims presenting in shock, the shock is caused by hemorrhagic factors (Table 228-1). An exception would be patients suffering from major burns, in which plasma is the major volume constituent lost.

EMERGENCY DEPARTMENT EVALUATION

Because the child's response to the early catecholamine output is more profound than in adults, recognizing shock in children (Table 228-2) requires a complete understanding of this difference. Until the child loses about 15% of total blood volume, the only signs of shock will be local swelling and bleeding and an increased heart rate. For this reason, *tachycardia out of proportion to that seen in adults is often the only finding early in the course of hemorrhagic shock in the pediatric patient.* However, children's pulse rates vary widely according to age. Remember that the pulse should be <140 in infants, <120 in preschool children, and <100 in school-age children (Table 228-3). *Assume that any child with a heart rate above these levels is in shock.*

The best general estimate for general circulating blood volume in children is 85 mL/kg. Children's blood pressure also varies according to age. Below is a simple formula for a *minimal* systolic blood pressure:

$$\text{Blood pressure} = 80 + (\text{age in years} \times 2)$$

The diastolic blood pressure in a child should be about two thirds of the systolic blood pressure. When the child has lost about 15% of total blood volume, the sole sign of shock may

TABLE 228-1. Classification and Causes of Shock

Class	Clinical Causes
Hypovolemic	Hemorrhage
	Burns
	Peritonitis
	Vomiting
	Heat loss
Cardiogenic	Myocardial infarction
	Cardiomyopathy
	Myocardial contusion
	Arrhythmias
	Valvular disease
	Heart failure
Obstruction	Tension pneumothorax
	Cardiac tamponade
	Flail chest
	Pulmonary embolus
	Hemopneumothorax
	Hypotension
Distributive	Spinal cord injury
	Anaphylaxis
	Septicemia
	Drugs
	Anesthesia

Mayer TA: Management of hypovolemic shock. In Mayer TA: Emergency Management of Pediatric Trauma, Philadelphia, WB Saunders, 1985

TABLE 228-2. Clinical Signs of Acute Hemorrhagic Shock

% Blood Loss	Clinical Signs
≤15	Slightly increased heart rate
	Local swelling, bleeding
15—25	Increased heart rate
	Increased diastolic blood pressure
	Prolonged capillary refill
25—50	Above findings plus:
	Hypotension
	Confusion
	Acidosis
	Decreased urine output
>50	Refractory hypotension
	Refractory acidosis

TABLE 228-3. Maximal Baseline Pulse and Respiratory Rate

	Infants	Preschool	School-Age
Maximum pulse rates	≤140	≤120	≤100
Maximum respiratory rates	30	20	15

be a slight increase in pulse rate. When 15% to 25% of blood volume has been lost, additional factors come into play. Adrenergic stimulation is maximal, venous beds are fully contracted, and peripheral resistance is elevated, resulting in increased diastolic blood pressure (or decreased pulse pressure). In addition, prolonged capillary refill time and further increases in heart rate may be seen. While up to 25% of the child's total blood volume may have been lost, shock can be detected only by looking at the heart rate, the diastolic blood pressure, and the capillary refill time. *Not until blood loss reaches 25% to 30% of total blood volume are hypotension, confusion, decreased urine output, and acidosis seen.*

If blood loss continues or progresses, decreased urine output, altered mental status, and the development of systemic acidosis occur.

EMERGENCY DEPARTMENT TREATMENT

There are three primary goals of shock therapy: to restore effective circulatory volume, to maximize oxygen delivery, and to decrease ongoing blood loss.

RESTORING EFFECTIVE CIRCULATORY VOLUME

Insert an intravenous line in pediatric patients with signs of trauma, a heart rate above 140 in infants, 120 in preschool children, or 100 in school-age children.

In any child with tachycardia or decreased pulse pressure, place an intravenous line and rapidly infuse 20 cc/kg over 5 to 10 minutes. The patient's weight can be estimated (Table 228-4) or length can be measured using the Broselow Tape to determine fluid boluses. The initial fluid bolus therapy may be lactated Ringer's or lactated Ringer's with glucose. Normal saline can also be used, but large fluid infusions with 0.9% sodium chloride can result in hyperchloremic acidosis. Children who present with hypotension in addition to tachycardia and a decreased pulse pressure have lost at least 25% to 30% of their total circulating blood volume and are in extreme danger of decompensating rapidly. Under such circumstances, immediately infuse an initial fluid bolus of 40 cc/kg. *The single most important determinant of the adequacy of ongoing fluid resuscitation is the child's response to the fluid infusion.* Following infusion of the fluid bolus, reassess the shock parameters to determine if the patient is improving, staying the same, or deteriorating.

The second aspect of restoring effective circulatory volume is transfusion. Infuse packed red blood cells if the patient fails to respond to a total of 40 cc/kg of crystalloid infusion. Based

---

TABLE 228-4. Estimating Pediatric Weight by Patient's Age

Age (years)	Weight (kg)
<1	Age in months/2 + 4
1–2	(Age in yr x 2) + 10
>2	(Age in yr x 2) + 15

TABLE 228-5. Total Fluid Infusion in Pediatric Shock

% Blood Loss	Replacement
<25	3 mg LR per mg blood loss
25–50	1/2 Volume = 3 cc LR per cc blood loss
	1/2 Volume = 1 cc PRBC per cc blood loss
>50	Type specific or O⁻ or O⁺
	Amount titrated to ongoing urine output

LR = Lactated Ringer's solution; PRBC = Packed red blood cells.

on the extent of physical findings (Table 228-5), rapidly infuse 5 to 10 cc/kg of packed red blood cells, through a blood warmer if possible. Rapidly infusing cold blood into a child can cause major problems with hypothermia, which may make the child resistant to the usual resuscitative measures.

If the child's cardiovascular parameters respond to the initial fluid bolus of 20 cc/kg, monitor the child closely. If the cardiovascular parameters remain stable, the total fluid infusion should be according to the principles in Table 228-5. If the child has lost less than 25% of total blood volume, the total amount of blood lost should be replaced with 3 cc of lactated Ringer's for each estimated cc of blood lost. Observe closely all patients who require transfusion since major hemorrhage has occurred.

MAXIMIZING OXYGEN DELIVERY

The second goal of shock therapy is to maximize oxygen delivery. By far the most important aspect in doing so is to ensure an adequate airway. All multiple trauma patients should receive 100% humidified and warmed oxygen.

DECREASING BLOOD LOSS

Put pressure on any external bleeding points. Patients who continue to hemorrhage either externally or internally may need surgery.

DISPOSITION

THE ROLE OF THE CONSULTANT   The immediate resuscitation of the pediatric trauma victim with hemorrhagic shock is the emergency physician's responsibility. A pediatric surgeon or a general surgeon skilled in the care of the pediatric trauma patient should be consulted for final disposition. Patients who receive intravenous lines and fluid bolus therapy and those whose shock parameters do not immediately return to normal should be observed for at least 24 hours to rule out bleeding.

In most cases in which fluid therapy is required, radiologic imaging is indicated. Pediatric neurosurgery, pediatric intensive care, and other surgical subspecialties may be necessary depending on the type and extent of the patient's injuries.

INDICATIONS FOR ADMISSION   Admit any patient who manifests signs or symptoms of hemorrhagic shock. Exceptions are patients who present with relatively minor trauma and tachycardia who respond immediately to initial fluid bolus therapy and are not found to have any significant injuries; observe these patients in the ED for several hours prior to discharge.

TRANSFER CONSIDERATIONS   Children who are transferred to a regional pediatric trauma center should have an intravenous line, an adequate airway, Foley catheter, and a nasogastric tube.

COMMON PITFALLS

- The most common pitfall is failure to recognize subtle signs and symptoms of early hemorrhagic shock
- The second major pitfall is failure to recognize that tachycardia is the earliest and most consistent sign of shock in the pediatric patient.
- The third pitfall is the tendency to attribute such tachycardia to factors such as anxiety or pain rather than to shock. Because tachycardia's role in the early development of shock often goes unrecognized, many physicians fail to place an intravenous line and give an appropriate fluid bolus.
- There is a tendency to underinfuse with intravenous fluids (give at least 20 cc/kg over 5–10 minutes) of lactated Ringers.

229   Pediatric Head Trauma

Pediatric head trauma is the most frequent cause of hospitalization in the United States, accounting for 200,000 admissions annually. Trauma in general is the leading cause of death in children over 1 year of age, and 80% of these deaths are associated with significant central nervous system (CNS) injury. Most head injuries in children occur from falls. In children less than 3 years old, these occur indoors; in older children, the typical causes of injury are traffic accidents, as either a pedestrian or a bicyclist.

The presence of skull fractures means that significant force has been applied to the cranium. Seventy-five percent of skull fractures are *linear fractures. Basilar skull fractures* involve the frontal, ethmoid, sphenoid, temporal, and/or occipital bones. Signs of basilar skull fracture include "raccoon eyes," Battle's sign, cerebrospinal fluid (CSF) otorrhea or rhinorrhea, and hematotympanum. *Compound fractures,* those with laceration of the scalp, carry a risk of complicating infection of the CNS. *Depressed skull fractures* are seen when force is applied over a small surface area. A depressed fracture greater than a few millimeters needs surgical elevation. *Diastatic fractures* are unique to children and are seen in the first 4 years of life. These fractures represent separation of the sutures.

Traumatic intracranial hemorrhage includes subdural, epidural, and subarachnoid hemorrhages. *Subdural hemorrhages* occur 5–10x as often as epidural bleeds. Signs and symptoms are secondary to increased intracranial pressure. In infants these hemorrhages may present with seizures. Although rare in children, the mortality rate of 10% to 20% associated with *epidural hematomas* makes early recognition essential. The usual presentation is one of rapid and focal neurologic deterioration. The classic triad is of concussion with an intervening lucent phase followed by deterioration. These bleeds usually represent a tear in the middle meningeal artery. In the child, hemorrhages from the meningeal and diploic veins are also seen. *Subarachnoid hemorrhages* are a common computed tomography (CT) finding in severe pediatric head trauma.

Penetrating head injuries are less common in children. Puncture wounds are seen with lawn darts, other missile-type projectiles, and dog-bite wounds in young children. These injuries are often associated with lacerations of the brain.

Contusions and lacerations of the cerebral cortex are often adjacent to sites of significant focal impact or at locations that predispose the brain to accelerative forces. Coup injuries represent contusions directly beneath the site of impact, while contra-coup injury occurs against the skull surface opposite the site of impact. The signs are often focal and are associated with local swelling on a computed tomography scan. These injuries are not necessarily the cause of unconsciousness.

Concussions are a functional injury. Mild concussions are associated with brief impairment of consciousness. Associated symptoms include anorexia, vomiting, pallor, or abnormal behavior lasting up to several hours. Severe concussions may present with signs ranging from lethargy to coma. All grades have an associated amnesia either retrograde, permanent retrograde, or temporary post-traumatic antegrade. Alternative presentation in infants and younger children includes lethargy, irritability, and vomiting not associated with loss of consciousness. These symptoms usually subside within 48 hours.

Cerebral edema and increased intracranial pressure account for significant morbidity in the pediatric patient. Cerebral edema and increased intracranial pressure as a result of severe head injury occur in 80% of pediatric cases, as opposed to 40% to 50% of the cases in adults.

EMERGENCY DEPARTMENT EVALUATION

The history is often obtained from an adult caretaker who may or may not have been present at the time of injury. Elicit and document details of the accident, including the height of any falls and the type of surface struck. Include a history of loss of consciousness, memory loss, disorientation, and visual disturbance. A brief seizure at the time of impact may be part of the history but may have no diagnostic or prognostic significance, in contrast to seizures that occur after injury. Vomiting is another useful symptom, especially when it is protracted and/or occurs more than 6 hours after injury.

Do not limit the physical examination to the head; significant physical findings may be found elsewhere. Quickly evaluate the level of consciousness using the mnemonic "AVPU" (**A**lert, responds to **V**oice, responds to **P**ainful stimuli, **U**nconscious). The Glasgow Coma Score, a fast, objective, and reproducible scoring system, evaluates the best eye opening, verbal, and motor response of the patient (Table 229-1) and has been modified for the preverbal child (Table 229-2). Check ocular signs, including pupil size and response and extraocular movement, and do an early fundoscopic examination looking for retinal hemorrhages and papilledema. Examine the head for signs of trauma including scalp lacerations and abrasions, hematomas, hematotympanum, Battle's sign, raccoon eyes, and CSF leaks from the ears or nose. A complete neurologic examination should be part of the secondary survey. This should also include looking for signs of injury at other sites.

In general, obtain radiographs if a fracture is strongly considered based on high-yield criteria and if demonstration of the fracture would be helpful in management (Table 229-3). Computed tomography is an effective tool for evaluating cranial trauma. It can delineate facial, orbital, and sinus injuries, as well as linear and depressed skull fractures, epidural, subdural, and intracerebral hematomas. In general, the following criteria are useful for determining which children should have a CT scan:

TABLE 229-1. Glasglow Coma Scale

Eye Opening

Spontaneous	4
To voice	3
To pain	2
None	1

Verbal Response

Oriented	5
Confused	4
Inappropriate words	3
Incomprehensible words	2
None	1

Motor Response

Obeys command	6
Localizes pain	5
Withdrawal	4
Abnormal flexion	3
Extensor response	2
None	1
	E + V + M = 3 to 15

Raimondi AJ, Hirschauer J; Head Injury in the infant and toddler. *Child's Brain.* 11:12, 1984

TABLE 229-2. Glasgow Coma Scale Modified for the Preverbal Child

Eye Opening

Spontaneous	4
To voice	3
To pain	2
None	1

Verbal Response

Coos, babbles	5
Irritable cries	4
Cries to pain	3
Moans to pain	2
None	1

Motor Response

Spontaneous movements	6
Withdraws to touch	5
Withdraws to pain	4
Abnormal flexion	3
Extensor response	2
None	1
	E + V + M = 3 to 15

Raimondi AJ, Hirshauer J: Head injury in the infant and toddler. *Child's Brain,* 11:12, 1984

TABLE 229-3. Risk Groups for Intracranial Injury

Low-Risk Group

Asymptomatic
Headache
Dizziness
Scalp laceration
Scalp contusion or abrasion
Absence of other group criteria

Moderate-Risk Group

Age less than 2 years (except minimal injury)
Suspected physical abuse
History of change of consciousness at the time of injury or subsequently
History of progressive headache
Unreliable or inadequate history of injury
Post-traumatic seizure
Vomiting
Post-traumatic amnesia
Multiple trauma
Serious facial injury
Signs of basilar skull fracture
Possible skull penetration or depression fracture

High-Risk Group

Depressed level of consciousness not due to drugs
Focal neurologic signs
Penetrating skull injury or palpable depressed fracture

Masters SJ, McClean PM, Ancarese JS, et al: Skull x-ray examinations after head trauma. N Engl J Med 316:84, 1987

1. Children <1 year old who have a full fontanelle, split sutures on plain skull films, prolonged unconsciousness, or bradycardia
2. Children >1 year who are conscious at presentation but develop progressive disturbance of consciousness or focal neurologic deficit, or who have a depressed skull fracture
2. Children >1 year who are unconscious at presentation or who have a history of unconsciousness.

EMERGENCY DEPARTMENT MANAGEMENT
MAJOR HEAD TRAUMA

Patients with major head trauma are at the highest risk for intracranial injury. They may have findings of depressed level of consciousness, focal neurologic signs, decreasing level of consciousness, and/or penetrating injury or palpable depressed skull fracture. Airway and cervical spine control are critical. Assist with bag–valve–mask ventilation in an attempt to keep the PaO_2 above 100 mm Hg. Cricoid pressure is useful to avoid regurgitation and aspiration. A secure airway must be maintained. Consider endotracheal intubation in children with a Glasgow Coma Score <8; rapid sequence intubation is the method of choice. With an assistant providing cricoid pressure and oxygenation, give atropine sulfate 0.02 mg/kg intravenously to reduce secretions and for vagolytic effect, then diazepam 0.05 to 0.1 mg/kg or thiopental 2 to 4 mg/kg if the patient is normotensive as an amnestic. Confirmation that the patient can be ventilated manually is followed by the administration of succinylcholine 1 to 2 mg/kg or pancuronium 0.1 mg/kg for muscle relaxation.

Maintain circulation within normal physiologic limits. Shock may be explained by large scalp lacerations in older children or epidural hemorrhage in infants, but more commonly the source of blood loss is elsewhere. Treat shock with crystalloid boluses (Ringer's lactate) of 20 mL/kg to a limit of 40 to 60 mL/kg, at which time vasopressors may be used. Once normal blood pressure is established, give fluids at one half to two thirds maintenance.

The goal of treatment of increased intracranial pressure is to prevent displacement (herniation) of the brain. Elevating the patient's head to 20 degrees promotes venous drainage. Controlled hyperventilation reduces cerebral blood flow by reducing arteriolar diameter. Maintain $PaCO_2$ in the 25–30 mm Hg range. Use diuretic therapy in an attempt to shift water from the brain into the vascular compartment, but use these agents cautiously in the hypovolemic patient. Intravenous mannitol at 0.25 g/kg is generally recommended. Intracranial pressure increases initially after mannitol administration as a result of an increase in cerebral blood flow secondary to expansion of the vascular volume and increased cardiac output. Intravenous furosemide (Lasix) 0.5 to 1 mg/kg is useful in cases of diffuse cerebral edema.

Patients in the high-risk group require emergency CT as soon as they are stable enough to tolerate the procedure. Obtain neurosurgical consultation as soon as possible.

MINOR HEAD TRAUMA

The major concern is missing the child with intracranial hematoma. At low risk for intracranial injury are those children with few or no complaints or physical findings. No high-risk or moderate-risk criteria are met. Possible findings include headache, dizziness, scalp hematoma, scalp laceration, and/or scalp contusion or abrasion. These patients are best managed with observation alone. They should be discharged home with a reliable, responsible adult and with a head injury information sheet.

Children at moderate risk have a history of change of consciousness at or after the time of injury or a history of progressive headache. An unreliable or inadequate history of injury, as well as suspected child abuse, places a patient in the moderate-risk group. Patients in the moderate-risk group may have symptoms or physical findings of post-traumatic seizures, vomiting, post-traumatic amnesia, multiple trauma, serious facial injury, signs of basilar skull fracture, possible skull penetration, or depressed skull fracture. Any patient under 2 years, except in trivial circumstances (i.e., a fall from the patient's height), is included in this group. Managing these moderate-risk children includes extended close observation and in most centers, head CT.

DISPOSITION

Seek neurosurgical consultation for high-risk patients and consider it for moderate-risk patients. Seek pediatric consultation for patients requiring admission and in those in whom abuse is suspected. Hospitalization provides an environment for early recognition and treatment of developing complications. There are no simple admission criteria, except for patients in the high-risk group. Signs of moderate risk that indicate need for possible hospitalization for observation include failure of prompt return of normal function, loss of consciousness greater than 2 minutes, abnormal neurologic examination, amnesia, and early post-traumatic seizures.

A patient with major head trauma should be stabilized and transported to a facility with a pediatric ICU. The patient should be transported with an ECG monitor, and personnel should be able to monitor the blood pressure with a cuff or Doppler. Neurologic status must be assessed en route. The patient's head should be maintained at 30 degrees and the patient should be hyperventilated. In transport, an intravenous infusion of dextrose 5% in one-half normal saline should be given at one half to two thirds maintenance.

| COMMON PITFALLS |

- The open fontanelle and sutures in the younger child, along with the larger subarachnoid space and cisterns, offer a greater extracellular space, and a better tolerance of expanding mass lesions
- Poor history, incomplete examination, and failure to recognize signs of retinal hemorrhage and increased intracranial pressure in an infant can lead to a delay in diagnosis and treatment.
- Suspected child abuse, especially "shaken baby" syndrome, must be considered.
- When there are no obvious signs of trauma, consider other causes of altered mental status such as CNS infections, metabolic disorders such as hypoglycemia, and toxins.

230   Evaluation of the Pediatric Cervical Spine

A significant percentage of pediatric spinal cord injuries occur without radiographically identifiable fractures and dislocations.

NORMAL VARIANTS AND CONGENITAL ANOMALIES

Due to the laxity of the ligaments in the pediatric cervical spine as compared to the adult spine, absent lordosis is a frequent finding on the lateral radiograph. The finding of anterior wedging in not one but several adjacent vertebrae sugggests that this is a developmental finding and not a compression fracture. The extreme laxity of ligaments in children <8 years old can create a pseudosubluxation of adjacent vertebrae. This finding is most pronounced at the level of C2 to C3. This pseudosubluxation is seen in 46% of children less than 8 years old. In normal children <8 years old, 20% will demonstrate a predental space of 3 mm or more, and distances up to 5 mm may be seen in nonpathologic instances. However, one should consider distances greater than 3.5 mm abnormal until proven otherwise. Widening of the prevertebral soft tissue due to hemorrhage and edema is an important adult radiographic finding. In children, suggested norms have included soft-tissue space less than 7 mm anterior to C2 or less than three quarters of the adjacent vertebral body's width. However, the younger the child is, the more unreliable are these norms, as dramatic increases in soft-tissue density occur during expiration or when the neck is held in mild flexion.

CLINICAL PRESENTATION

Radiographically apparent cervical spine injury is extremely rare in children. About 2% of all cervical spine fractures and dislocations occur in children less than 16 years old, and only about 1.2% of all pediatric cervical spine radiographs reveal an abnormality. The incidence of cervical spine fractures and dislocations increases with age. Radiographically apparent cervical spine injury is virtually nonexistent in children less than 16 months old, excluding birth trauma.

The etiology of cervical spine fractures and dislocations is broad: motor vehicle accidents account for about 35% to 45%, diving injuries and falls, about 30% to 35%, and sports injuries, about 20% to 25%. Pediatric cervical spine injuries can be divided into those of the upper cervical spine (C1 to C2) and those of the lower cervical spine (C3 to C7). Types of injuries most commonly seen in the upper cervical spine are fracture or synchondral separation of the odontoid with atlanto-axial dislocation, and the hangman's fracture of the neural arches of C2. Types of abnormalities most frequently encountered in the lower cervical spine are anterior subluxation/dislocation, compression fractures, teardrop fractures, and spinous process fractures.

Children older than 12 years have a distribution of injuries resembling that of adults, with a preponderance of low cervical lesions. Children aged 8 to 12 years are in a transition state between high cervical lesions and low cervical lesions. Children under 8 years old have a high preponderance of upper cervical spine fractures and dislocations; this is thought to be due to the fact that children under 8 years of age have heavy heads, lax ligaments and nearly horizontal facet joints. These result in high torques and shear forces being applied to the C1 to C2 regions.

The incidence of pediatric spinal cord injuries has been reported to range from less than 1% to 9.4% of all spinal cord injuries. The reported incidence of spinal cord deficits resulting from cervical spine fractures and dislocations is approximately 30%. Of those with a spinal deficit, approximately 12% are quadriplegic. The incidence of neurologic deficit with cervical spine fractures and dislocations increases with age, with 20% of children less than 8 years and about 40% of children age 8 to 16 years having a neurologic deficit.

The reported incidence of spinal cord injury without radiographic abnormality (SCIWORA) ranges from 4% to 67% of all pediatric spinal injuries. SCIWORA is thought to result from disruption of the microvascular blood supply from hyperextension with inward bulging of the interlaminar ligaments, reversible disc prolapse, flexion compression of the cord, longitudinal distraction of the cord, and vertebral artery spasm.

EMERGENCY DEPARTMENT MANAGEMENT

The neck of a child with potential cervical spine injury should be immobilized. Pre-hospital cervical spine immobilization is best accomplished with a rigid plastic cervical collar and a backboard combined with tape, sandbags, or a head immobilization device. However, in the case of an alert child vigorously resisting attempts at immobilization, these attempts could potentially worsen an injury.

Oral intubation is preferred in younger children and is best performed using manual in-line traction to maintain cervical immobilization. Fortunately, young children require little, if any, extension to visualize the glottis. Nasotracheal intubation should only be attempted in older children with spontaneous respirations.

The presence of any one of the following should suggest obtaining radiographs of the cervical spine: history of direct neck trauma, neck pain, neck tenderness, limitation of mobility, abnormality in flexion, strength, or sensation, or decreased mental status. Standard lateral radiographs detect 95% of injuries and 100% when combined with the AP view (Figure 230-1).

Due to the potential for SCIWORA, question all children with potential spinal injury about transient paresthesias at the time of the injury. If such paresthesias were present, assume that these children have a spinal injury until a neurosurgical consultation establishes otherwise. The diagnosis of SCIWORA should be a diagnosis of exclusion and should not be made until occult bony, ligamentous, or disc injuries have been ruled out by fluoroscopic guided flexion and extension radiographs, computed tomography (CT) scanning, and myelography.

COMMON PITFALLS

- Synchondroses and secondary ossification centers may be confused as fractures
- Remember that absent lordosis, anterior wedging of cervical bodies, pseudosubluxation of C2 on C3, increased prevertebral soft-tissue density, and widening of the predental space can be normal variants.

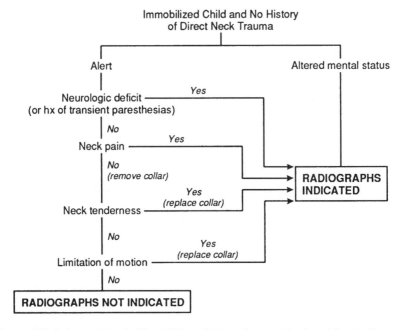

Figure 230-1. Protocol for deciding which pediatric patients arriving immobilized in the emergency department need radiographs. (Modified with permission from Wales LR, Knopp RK, Morishima MS: Recommendations for evaluation of the acutely injured cervical spine: A clinical radiologic algorithm. Ann Emerg Med 9:422, 1980)

- A normal radiograph does not rule out cervical spinal cord injury in children, as spinal cord injuries occur without radiographically detectable injuries. All children with suspected neck injury should be questioned specifically for transient paresthesias at the time of the injury, as about half of all patients with delayed onset of SCIWORA have this finding.

231 Abdominal Trauma in Children

Motor vehicles are the major mechanism of pediatric blunt abdominal trauma. The child, either as passenger or pedestrian, suffers sudden changes in acceleration and deceleration, and solid and hollow abdominal viscera must bear these forces with the risk for significant injury. Additional causes of abdominal trauma are sports-related injuries, falls from heights, self-inflicted wounds, and child abuse. Although child abuse accounts for a small number of pediatric abdominal injuries, it must be considered.

EMERGENCY DEPARTMENT EVALUATION
PRIMARY SURVEY

Examine the injured child immediately upon arrival for the presence of catastrophic intra-abdominal exsanguination. A rapid primary survey will identify life-threatening circumstances that may affect the airway, breathing, and circulation. The child's cervical spine is stabilized throughout the primary survey. Children with exsanguinating intra-abdominal hemorrhage require a rapid sequence of events:

Airway and ventilation secured, usually by endotracheal intubation
Two large-bore intravenous catheters via upper extremity veins, and Ringer's lactate infusion
Transfusion of type O, Rh-negative whole blood
Plans for urgent laparotomy initiated

The surgeon must evaluate these children immediately, since prompt operation is necessary for survival in massive intra-abdominal hemorrhage. Fortunately, most children with abdominal trauma do not have exsanguinating injuries. An orderly approach to fluid resuscitation and monitoring of vital signs becomes essential to the diagnosis of intra-abdominal injury. Hypotension signifies at least 20–25% loss of intravascular volume. Administer a 20 mL/kg bolus of Ringer's lactate solution over 10 minutes. Following the bolus infusion, give the Ringer's lactate solution at maintenance rate and determine the child's vital signs (pulse, blood pressure, and capillary refill time). If hemodynamic stability is obtained without clinical deterioration, assume the child's blood volume has been restored and that the patient lost less than 25% of circulating blood volume.

If the initial bolus results in no response or rapid deterioration of vital signs, give a second bolus of 20 mL/kg Ringer's lactate over 10 minutes. If hemodynamic instability persists or recurs, rapidly infuse whole blood (20 mL/kg) or packed red blood cells (10 mL/kg). Assume that children who require two bolus infusions of Ringer's lactate followed by urgent blood transfusion have lost between 25–50% of circulating blood volume from hemorrhage from the following areas: chest, abdomen, pelvis or femur. Prompt surgical intervention is usually required in the management.

Complete exposure of the injured child is necessary to check for occult trauma. Check for tire marks, contusions, seat belt impressions, or other visible signs of compressive injury across the chest or abdomen that may indicate underlying organ damage. Children with penetrating trauma require examination for entrance and exit wounds anteriorly, posteriorly, and on the perineum.

SECONDARY SURVEY

The secondary survey of the abdomen includes an orderly physical examination and identification of presumed injuries. The secondary survey should document the presence of intra-abdominal injury. Palpation of the abdomen should begin away from the area of subjective pain. Ascertain the presence of localized versus diffuse tenderness with peritoneal irritation. Most important, repeated examination by the same physician is necessary to detect changes in abdominal findings. A careful rectal examination includes observation of the perineum for bruises or hematomas, assessment of intact rectal and perirectal anatomy, quality of anal sphincter tone, and presence of blood. Examination of the perineum is necessary in impalement injuries and in girls suspected as victims of rape. Significant perineal trauma generally requires examination under anesthesia.

Appropriate tubes for decompression of the stomach and bladder should be inserted in children with abdominal trauma. A nasogastric tube relieves distention, reduces the risks of respiratory embarrassment and aspiration, and allows for an accurate examination. In a child with massive maxillofacial injuries or cribriform plate and basal skull fractures, do not insert a nasogastric tube; instead, pass an orogastric tube. Insert an indwelling bladder catheter if no blood is evident at the urethral meatus, rectal examination is normal, and pelvic fractures are not obvious.

Suspicion of urethral disruption warrants a retrograde urethrogram prior to bladder catheterization. In males less than 2 years of age, inserting the Foley catheter requires careful technique to avoid urethral trauma.

LABORATORY AND RADIOGRAPHIC STUDIES

Studies include a hemoglobin and hematocrit and type and cross match. Less urgent tests include white blood cell and platelet counts, serum amylase, and urinalysis. An elevated amylase level is not uncommon in major injury, but a serial rise would suggest possible pancreatic or small intestinal injury.

Initial radiologic studies include a lateral cervical spine, chest film, flat plate of the abdomen and pelvis. If the patient's clinical status allows, obtain upright films of the chest and abdomen to detect pneumoperitoneum. Gross hematuria warrants an intravenous pyelogram or abdominal CT.

SURGICAL CONSULTATION

A pediatric or general surgeon should evaluate children with major trauma. Those patients who mandate urgent surgical consultation include:

Life-threatening hemorrhage
Gunshot wound to chest or abdomen
Stab wound
Pneumoperitoneum
Pelvic fracture
Evisceration
Abdominal tenderness
Mental obtundation
Multiple injuries

To expedite surgical consultation, the emergency physician should be familiar with the criteria for urgent operative management. Children with exsanguinating hemorrhage require immediate laparotomy. Urgent laparotomy is necessary for children with gunshot wounds and some stab wounds. Pneumoperitoneum indicates hollow viscus perforation and requires operative intervention. Evisceration may result in laparotomy. The child with increasing localized or diffuse abdominal tenderness and peritoneal irritation may have intraperitoneal spillage of intestinal contents, requiring urgent laparotomy. Children with significant central nervous system or spinal injury and an altered level of consciousness, as well as children with multisystem trauma, require prompt abdominal examination by a surgeon.

DIAGNOSTIC PERITONEAL LAVAGE

Diagnostic peritoneal lavage (DPL) is used in diagnosing intra-abdominal bleeding. In children with blunt abdominal trauma, DPL is used infrequently and for relatively specific indications: a child with altered level of consciousness and hemodynamic instability or questionable abdominal findings, or in a child who requires general anesthesia for operative treatment of an associated injury. DPL should be performed by the surgeon responsible for the child's care and decision making. DPL is contraindicated with a history of multiple abdominal operations or an obvious indication for laparotomy.

Aspiration of gross blood, bile, or food particles is indicative of intra-abdominal injury. If aspiration is initially clear, Ringer's lactate (10 mL/kg) is instilled into the peritoneal cavity, retrieved by gravity drainage, and sent for laboratory analysis. Positive results include more than 100,000 red blood cells or more than 500 white blood cells per cubic millimeter, amylase twice the serum level, or the presence of bile or bacteria. Once DPL has been performed, the quality and reliability of the abdominal examination are altered.

SPECIFIC INJURIES
SPLEEN

The spleen is the most commonly injured abdominal organ in children. Typical mechanisms of injury to the spleen are motor vehicle accidents, kicks to the left side, and bicycle and sledding accidents. Suspect a spleen injury in a child whose trauma is mainly left-sided, such as fractures of the ribs on the left and a left femur fracture. A contusion to the left upper quadrant or flank may be present. The child may complain of left shoulder pain (Kehr's sign), indicative of diaphragmatic irritation. In most instances of pediatric splenic trauma, the child is minimally hypotensive and quickly responsive to intravenous restoration of blood volume. Serial determination of a falling hemoglobin and hematocrit, especially if normal on admission, indicates ongoing bleeding. Abdominal and chest radiographic findings that should arouse suspicion of splenic injury include:

Fractured ribs
Elevated left hemidiaphragm
Enlarged splenic shadow
Medial displacement of the splenic shadow

Surgical consultation is mandated for any child suspected of splenic trauma. Since most non-exsanguinating splenic injuries in children are managed by nonoperative observation, ideally, centers capable of such an expectant approach with immediate surgical expertise should care for these patients.

LIVER

Life-threatening hemorrhage from liver injury is the leading cause of mortality in children with abdominal trauma. Massive abdominal distention with profound cardiovascular shock at the accident scene or upon arrival usually indicates a severe liver laceration with disruption of the hepatic veins or retrohepatic inferior vena cava. These children have a poor chance of survival, even with immediate surgical intervention. Non-exsanguinating liver lacerations may present with right upper quadrant pain, minimal abdominal tenderness, and signs of controlled blood loss. As with splenic injury, certain liver injuries in children are managed nonoperatively. Immediate surgical consultation and a pediatric trauma facility are necessary for all children with suspected liver injury.

KIDNEY

Gross hematuria or microscopic hematuria associated with hypotension suggest renal injury. A rapid infusion intravenous pyelogram (IVP) should be performed in a child with gross hematuria. Failure to visualize a kidney by IVP should be followed by abdominal CT or ultrasound to rule out congenital unilateral renal agenesis. Most pediatric renal injuries are contusions that donnot require operative treatment. If the kidney cannot be visualized by IVP, immediate surgical consultation or transfer to a pediatric trauma facility is warranted. Successful salvage of a major vascular injury to the kidney requires revascularization, generally within 6 hours of injury.

GASTROINTESTINAL INJURIES

Blunt trauma to a hollow viscus results from compressive forces between the intestine and the spine and the anterior abdominal wall. Seat belts, bicycle handlebars, and kicks to the abdomen may cause serious intestinal injury. The hallmark of an isolated intestinal injury in children is increasing abdominal distention with worsening abdominal tenderness. Serial examination of the abdomen is essential to the diagnosis of intestinal injury. Pneumoperitoneum, absent on an initial abdominal radiograph, may be present on a later one. A rising white blood cell count and serum amylase may accompany small-bowel injuries.

PELVIC FRACTURES

Pelvic fractures can result in significant blood loss and retroperitoneal hemorrhage. Diagnostic features of pelvic fractures include ecchymoses below the anterior iliac crest and asymmetry of the bony structure. Compression of the pelvic bones elicits pain, and examination of the perineum may show scrotal or labial hematomas. Suspicion of a pelvic fracture warrants a plain film of the pelvis and if positive for fracture, evaluation for urethral disruption prior to bladder catheterization. It is extremely uncommon for the female urethra to be injured, even with severe pelvic fractures.

BLADDER/URETHRA

Consider injuries to the bladder and urethra in children with pelvic fractures. Urethral disruption may occur in straddle injuries or penetrating perineal trauma. Blood at the urethral meatus is an absolute indication for a retrograde urethrogram. Once the urethra is demonstrated to be intact, a Foley catheter can be inserted and a retrograde cystogram can be performed. Extravasation of bladder contrast material identifies either an extraperitoneal or intraperitoneal injury; surgical consultation is required for appropriate management of either injury.

DIAPHRAGM

Suspect injuries to the diaphragm in penetrating trauma to the lower chest and upper abdomen and in blunt trauma from a fall or crush injury. This injury is often diagnosed late. Clues to early detection include gas-filled loops of bowel within the chest, an obscure diaphragm or a persistent abnormality of the lower lung fields on repeated chest radiographs. Any child suspected of a diaphragmatic injury warrants surgical consultation.

DISPOSITION

ADMISSION   Indications for admission or transfer to an appropriate pediatric trauma facility of a child with abdominal injury include:

Documented or suspected abdominal injury
Presence of associated injuries
Child involved in an automobile accident in which other passengers were killed or seriously
    injured
History of significant trauma despite no apparent injury
Injury suspicious for child abuse or self-infliction
Abdominal pain
No reliable caretaker

Infants, regardless of clinical status, should be routinely admitted for overnight observation. Children who have sustained minor trauma, are several hours postinjury without abdominal pain or tenderness, and have normal laboratory tests and radiographs and reliable caretakers may be discharged. Give clear instructions, verbally and in written form, to the parents or caretakers regarding warning signs of abdominal injury (i.e., fever, vomiting, abdominal distention).

COMMON PITFALLS

- Failure to recognize major intra-abdominal exsanguinating hemorrhage
- Failure to decompress the stomach
- Failure to administer appropriate intravenous fluids
- Failure to monitor serial vital signs
- Failure to suspect abdominal injury
- Failure to recognize clinical deterioration

- Failure to obtain surgical consultation for suspected abdominal injury
- Failure to suspect child abuse
- Failure to identify associated injuries
- Inappropriate performance of diagnostic peritoneal lavage

232   Burns in Children

Burns represent a significant cause of morbidity and mortality in children, accounting for 1200 deaths in children under 15 years old in the United States. The most common mechanism of burn injury in children under 3 years of age is scalding, typically by accidental spillage of hot liquid. The usual toddler scald burn results from pulling a pot of boiling water or coffee off a stove or table onto the head, chest, and arms. Flame burns are generally more severe in extent and depth of injury and can be associated with inhalation injury. Less frequent causes of thermal trauma in children include contact burns, chemical injury, and high-voltage electrical burns. The possibility of child abuse must be considered in all pediatric burns, especially in children under 3 years of age. Scald burns, specifically tap water immersion, account for most cases of inflicted thermal trauma. Any of the following should raise the suspicion of intentional injury:

A well-demarcated burn of the perineum or buttocks
A circumferential extremity burn
Contact burn depicting the outline of an object
Coexistent soft-tissue trauma
Delay in seeking medical attention
History of injury incompatible with the burn or the child's developmental stage
Prior history of accidents
Unstable family situation

MAJOR BURNS
ASSESSMENT

The severity of a thermal injury is determined by the etiology, extent and depth of injury, age of the patient, and associated inhalation injury. Certain causative agents, such as grease, chemicals, and electricity, have the potential to cause a deeper, more severe injury. Depth of burn trauma refers to the level of destruction of the epidermal and dermal skin layers. Infants and young children have a much thinner dermal layer than adults, with a greater propensity for deep burns.

A first-degree burn extends to the epidermis only and is characterized by erythema and pain. The protective functions of the skin remain intact and healing is uneventful. Overexposure to sunlight and brief scalding account for most first-degree burns in children.

Second-degree or partial thickness burns involve the entire epidermis with extension to a variable depth of dermis. A superficial second-degree burn, characterized by erythema, blisters, and pain, damages a minimal amount of dermis and heals without significant scarring in 10 to 14 days. A deep second-degree burn extends farther into the dermis and is covered by tough, usually erythematous blistered skin. Pressure over the skin causes blanching that is relieved with release of pressure. A deep second-degree burn may be anesthetic for the first few days of injury, so that absence of pain is not a reliable sign for differentiation from a third-degree injury. The deep second-degree burn heals by epithelial regeneration from sweat glands and hair follicles within 3 or 4 weeks if infection can be prevented.

Third-degree or full thickness burns involve destruction of epidermis and dermis down to the underlying subcutaneous tissue. The injured area becomes tough, leathery, white, and insensate. This injury will not heal spontaneously and, unless very small in size, requires skin grafting. Differentiating between a deep second-degree and third-degree burn in infants and children may be difficult or impossible in the ED.

The *extent of burn injury* is described in terms of total body surface area involvement. An accurate assessment is essential for calculating fluid requirements and determining severity of injury. Children have relatively larger heads and smaller lower extremities than adults, making the "rule of nines" inaccurate for patients under 10 years of age. A modification of the Lund and Browder chart considers these unique anatomical factors in children (Fig. 232-1). Calculating the extent of the injury requires complete examination of the undressed patient and should be performed only after initial stabilization.

INITIAL STABILIZATION

The immediate resuscitation of a burn patient should be carried out as with any other trauma victim. Determining the patency and adequacy of the child's airway is the most important aspect of initial treatment. Assume that any patient whose burn occurred within an enclosed space has an inhalation injury.

AIRWAY CONSIDERATIONS

Carbon monoxide poisoning is the most immediate cause of fire mortality. Smoke inhalation may produce a wide spectrum of injury to the upper and lower respiratory tracts. Oxygen therapy should continue throughout the initial assessment. Physical findings associated with inhalation injury include facial burns, singed nasal hairs, carbonaceous sputum, altered level of consciousness, stridor, hoarseness, wheezing, and rales. An extrapolated carboxyhemoglobin blood level above 10% indicates carbon monoxide poisoning, but symptoms, not the absolute level, should be used to guide therapy. Chest radiography is not reliable in the early phase of inhalation injury.

Indications for endotracheal intubation in the burned infant or child include upper airway obstruction, inhalation injury, respiratory depression, facial and/or neck burns, posterior pharyngeal edema, and nasolabial full thickness burns. Circumferential burns of the chest or abdomen may lead to respiratory compromise, requiring intubation. The choice of nasotracheal or orotracheal intubation depends on the patient's clinical condition and physician's technical skill. Of paramount importance is secure taping of the endotracheal tube, since reintubation of a patient with edema of the neck or posterior pharynx may be very difficult.

FLUID RESUSCITATION

Children with burns of >20% total body surface area require intravenous fluid resuscitation. Patients with lesser burns who have facial and mouth burns or suspected inhalation injury should also be treated with intravenous fluids. The child's weight must be known to calculate the fluid requirements. Place a large-bore intravenous catheter under sterile conditions in an unburned area; two intravenous catheters will be required in patients with burns of greater than 50% total body surface area. If an intravenous catheter cannot be placed percutaneously, perform a saphenous vein cutdown at the ankle using sterile technique.

The Parkland formula is used to calculate the intravenous fluids for the first 24 hours: Ringer's lactate at 4 mL/kg/% burn. Half the day's requirement is given in the first 8 hours. For example, a child weighing 20 kg with a 40% burn should receive 3200 mL Ringer's lactate in the first 24 hours, of which 1600 mL is given in the first 8 hours.

CHILDREN'S HOSPITAL
COLUMBUS, OHIO

Date_____19____

BURN SHEET

Name_____ Age_____ Number_____

Burn Record. Ages—Birth-7½   Date of Observation_____

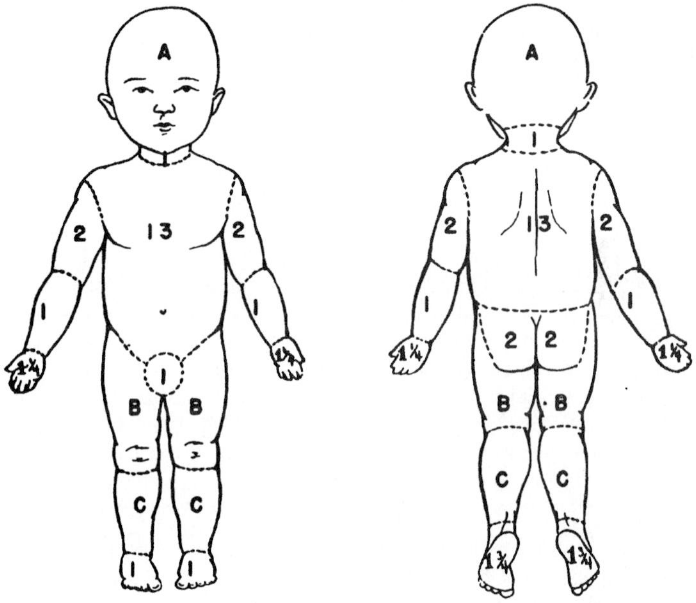

RELATIVE PERCENTAGES OF AREAS AFFECTED BY GROWTH

Area	Age 0	1	5
A = ½ of Head	9½	8½	6½
B = ½ of One Thigh	2¾	3¼	4
C = ½ of One Leg	2½	2½	2¾

% BURN BY AREAS

Probable 3rd˚ Burn	{ Head_____ Neck_____ Body_____ Up. Arm_____ Forearm_____ Hands_____			
	{ Genitals_____ Buttocks_____ Thighs_____ Legs_____ Feet_____			
Total Burn	{ Head_____ Neck_____ Body_____ Up. Arm_____ Forearm_____ Hands_____			
	{ Genitals_____ Buttocks_____ Thighs_____ Legs_____ Feet_____			

Sum of All Areas_____ Probably 3rd˚ _____ Total Burn_____

Figure 232-1. Modified Lund and Browder chart for estimation of body surface area burn involvement in infants and children.

A Foley catheter is necessary for accurate monitoring of urinary output and response to fluid administration. Maintain an hourly urinary output of at least 1.5 mL/kg. Additional parameters that are useful for assessing response to intravenous fluids are pulse, blood pressure, and peripheral circulation. The Parkland formula offers only a guideline to intravenous fluid replacement; adjustment of fluid needs must be regularly re-evaluated according to the child's clinical condition.

Initial laboratory tests should include complete blood count, electrolytes, type and cross-match, urinalysis, and arterial blood gas analysis. Obtain a carboxyhemoglobin level in patients with suspected inhalation injury. Screen the urine for free hemoglobin or myoglobin.

Gastric distention and ileus often develop in children with burns greater than 25% of body surface area. A nasogastric tube of appropriate size should be inserted, attached to suction, and checked at frequent intervals.

ESCHAROTOMY

Circumferential full thickness burns of the chest and upper abdomen may lead to constriction of the chest wall, restriction of breathing and chest expansion, and respiratory embarrassment. Extremity circumferential burns may cause vascular compromise of the fingers and toes. These conditions may warrant an escharotomy, an incision through the burn eschar to the underlying subcutaneous fat. Immediate surgical consultation is indicated. Indications for chest wall escharotomy are impending respiratory failure and inability to ventilate a patient with a circumferential chest and upper abdominal burn. The escharotomy should be placed bilaterally on the chest along the anterior axillary line. Extension of the incisions along the costal margins and horizontally across the sternum may be necessary if improvement does not occur with the axillary escharotomies.

Indications for extremity escharotomy are cyanosis of the distal unburned skin, impaired capillary filling, and progressive neurologic change. Serial Doppler flow measurements are useful in deciding if an escharotomy is needed. On the extremity, the incision should be placed along either the medial or lateral aspect, including involved joints and avoiding superficial blood vessels and nerves. Response is assessed by improved capillary refill, neurologic status, and Doppler flow.

CARE OF THE BURN WOUND

Cleanse the burn wound with warm sterile saline, and remove loose soot and tissue. Gently remove tar and asphalt; do not peel them off since damage to skin and hair can result. Useful agents for tar removal include mineral oil, petroleum ointment, neosporin ointment, and Medisol. Leave intact blisters unopened. For patients who require transfer to a regional burn unit, cover the burns with saline-soaked gauze and wrap them with an occlusive dressing. For patients who are to be admitted, apply 1% silver sulfadiazine (Silvadene) cream to second- and third-degree burns of the trunk and extremities, and cover the wounds with an occlusive dressing. Neosporin spray or ointment may be used on the face.

INFECTION CONTROL

Give tetanus toxoid (0.5 mL intramuscularly) to any child who has not had a booster in the last 5 years or whose last immunization date is unknown. If the child has had no immunizations, give 250 units of intramuscular tetanus human immune globulin and the first of a series of active immunizations with tetanus toxoid.

Systemic prophylactic antibiotic administration is controversial in children: some burn centers routinely give a 3-to-5-day course of penicillin, while others prefer no antibiotic prophylaxis. Give systemic antibiotics only after consulting with the physician who will be ultimately caring for the patient.

PAIN CONTROL

Once the child's airway and respiratory parameters are secure and vital signs are stabilized, adequate pain control should be undertaken by giving morphine sulfate (0.1 mg/kg) intravenously. Do not give intramuscular analgesics, because they have an unpredictable absorption in patients with major injury.

DISPOSITION

Admit patients with any of the following:

Greater than 10% body surface area involvement with second-degree burns
Greater than 2% body surface area involvement with third-degree burns
Inhalation injury
Electrical injury
Burns of hands, feet, face, perineum, and genitalia
Wringer injury
Suspicion of child abuse or neglect
Inadequate social support.

Transfer to a regional burn center patients with partial thickness burns greater than 20% body surface area, inhalation injury with burns, electrical burns, and presence of associated injuries. Pay meticulous attention to stabilizing the patient prior to transport. The patient's airway must be secured; if there is any question about the child's respiratory status, intubation should be performed prior to transport. Appropriate intravenous fluid resuscitation should be in progress. All patients should be transferred on a cardiac monitor. The nasogastric tube should be placed on portable suction or the end left open for free drainage of gastric contents. The nasogastric tube should be frequently aspirated during transport to minimize the risk of aspiration. The Foley catheter should be taped in place and the urine output recorded during transfer. The patient should be covered by sterile sheets. The referring physician should telephone the receiving physician. A written transfer record should accompany the patient and should include history, vital signs, physical examination, intravenous fluid record, urine output, laboratory results, radiographs, and parental consent. An accurate flow chart that includes hourly intravenous fluids and urine output inclusive of the transport period should be readily available for the receiving physician. Follow-up communication should include the patient's condition on arrival and ultimate outcome.

COMMON PITFALLS

- Delayed recognition of inadequate oxygenation and ventilation
- Delayed intubation
- Inadequate estimation of depth and extent of burn
- Failure to decompress gastric distention
- Underestimated severity of electrical injury
- Failure to recognize suspected child abuse
- Failure to identify associated injuries

SPECIFIC BURNS
ELECTRICAL BURNS

Electrical burns may present with small, unimpressive external wounds that obscure extensive deep-tissue destruction. The electrical current passes along neurovascular bundles, causing thrombosis of blood vessels and damage to adjacent muscle and bone. Myocardial injury from the electrical current can result in infarction and arrhythmias. An injury peculiar to children is the burn to the lip and commissure of the mouth caused by chewing an electrical cord.

Evaluation of the patient should include color, perfusion, and pulses of the extremities. An ECG and cardiac isoenzymes should be obtained.

Patients with extensive muscle damage may develop myoglobinuria and may require intravenous fluids to maintain a vigorous diuresis. All patients with electrical injuries should remain on a cardiac monitor. Children with electrical lip burns should be admitted and observed for delayed hemorrhage of the labial artery and oral splinting.

WRINGER INJURY

Although wringer washers are no longer manufactured, children may present with soft-tissue crush injuries from inserting an arm between the rollers of the wringer apparatus. The skin is often abraded and a severe soft-tissue contusion with hematoma and edema may result. Treat the skin as a second-degree burn, elevate the extremity, and observe carefully for the development of a compartment syndrome.

CHEMICAL BURNS

Household cleaners often cause chemical burns in children. Suspect ingestion in any young child with a chemical burn. Copiously irrigate the burn with water or normal saline for 20 minutes after removing the child's clothing. Then assess the extent and depth of the burn and treat it with appropriate topical agents.

MINOR BURNS

Use the same principles as for major burns to determine the severity of a minor thermal injury. Outpatient management is suitable for patients with partial thickness burns of no more than 10% body surface area and full thickness burns of no more than 2%. Deep burns of the face, hands, or feet, and all genital or perineal burns should not be treated on an outpatient basis. Do not discharge the child if the injury is suspicious for abuse or neglect or if the caretakers are unreliable. Thoroughly and gently wash the wound and irrigate it with water or normal saline. Dirty wounds should be debrided only after the child has been sedated with an appropriate pain medication; it is advisable to apply cool, clean towels and wait about 30 minutes after administration of the pain medication. Suggested medications include intravenous morphine (0.1 mg/kg), intravenous meperidine (0.5 mg/kg) or intramuscular meperidine (0.5–1 mg/kg). Leave intact blisters undisturbed, but debride ruptured blisters. Apply Silvadene cream over the wound, cover it with nonstick porous gauze, and wrap the wound in a bulky occlusive dressing of Kerlex. Minor burns of the face and neck may be treated by an open method, washing the wound three or four times daily and applying Neosporin ointment or spray.

It is our policy to administer prophylactic oral penicillin for 5 days to children receiving outpatient burn care. Tetanus prophylaxis should be given following the same principles outlined for major burns. The patient should be given prescriptions for Tylenol with codeine for pain control and Benadryl for pruritus.

Carefully instruct the child's caretakers in dressing care and give them prescriptions for necessary supplies and topical medications. Dressings should be changed twice daily. It is the emergency department's responsibility to arrange close follow-up care. The burn should be reexamined within 48 hours, either in the emergency department or by the child's pediatrician or family physician.

COMMON PITFALLS

- Failure to recognize full thickness injury
- Failure to explain dressing care to caretakers
- Failure to provide adequate pain control
- Failure to arrange appropriate follow-up
- Failure to provide necessary supplies for wound care

233   Fractures in Children

The most important consideration of fracture care in children is the diagnosis. A good history from the parent, the child, or both can guide the physician toward the injured area, but the most important aspect is a good physical examination. After the physician has an idea of the injured area, an appropriate radiographic evaluation should be performed.

RADIOLOGIC EVALUATION

Radiology is crucial to the evaluation of fractures in children, but fractures in children are not always easy to visualize radiographically. Obtain as many views as necessary to rule out a fracture; ultimately, the diagnostic proof of a fracture is the radiograph showing the fracture. Try to visualize the suspected fracture in at least two views 90 degrees to each other. Obtain an anterior–posterior and lateral projection. Because some fractures are not apparent on standard anterior–posterior and lateral radiographs, an oblique radiograph may be necessary. Oblique radiographs are essential in all ankle injuries. Another important tool in radiologic examination of the extremities is a comparison view of the other extremity. A comparison view is sometimes necessary to avoid confusion, multiple re-examinations, and inappropriate treatment. Because of the elastic capacity of the child's bone and soft tissue, the injured part often springs back into its anatomical position and is not always visible on radiologic examination. In these instances, a clinical decision is sometimes made to treat a given injury as a fracture at the initial presentation.

Soft-tissue lines can also help the physician diagnose fractures. The shadows of fatty tissue may serve as a contrast density, outlining the margins of other soft tissues. Thus, injuries to soft tissues are often comminuted into fractures. This should be assessed as accurately as possible as part of the evaluation.

Ligamentous injuries are rare in the child. More commonly, an injury of the growth plate is seen, a weak area of the ligamentous attachment. Stress films should be taken when there is a question of growth plate injuries in both varus and valgus modes. Such stress films should be done by the physician.

If there is every clinical indication of a fracture but the radiograph does not show one, further films may be necessary.

CLASSIFICATION OF FRACTURES

Once the fracture has been diagnosed, it should be classified.

DIAPHYSEAL FRACTURES

Diaphyseal fractures involve the central shaft between the metaphyses.

METAPHYSEAL FRACTURES

Metaphyseal fractures involve the area between the diaphysis and the epiphysis. Fractures in this area are often seen because there is more cancellous bone than cortical bone, thus creating compression (torus-type) fractures. The subcapital and supracondylar fractures are found at both the level of the condyles and epicondyles in the femur and humerus respectively. Fractures in this area usually heal without problems, but in supracondylar fractures of the humerus, adequate alignment and rotation should be achieved to prevent long-term deformity.

GROWTH PLATE INJURIES

The growth plate usually repairs well, but occasionally these injuries have the potential to cause angular deformity. If part of the plate is injured or a bony bridge has formed, progressive shortening of the limb and angular deformity of the limb may occur. The Salter–Harris classification is an accurate method of describing growth plate injuries in children (see Table 233-1). Special attention should be given to Salter–Harris types III and IV because of their intra-articular component. If displaced >1 mm, the injury should be reduced anatomically in the operating room.

TREATMENT

Some fractures can be treated by casting or splinting and referred to the orthopedic surgeon, while others must be treated on an emergency basis. The objective is to completely restore func-

TABLE 233-1. Salter-Harris Classification of Epiphyseal Injuries

Description	Diagram
Type I: Fracture extends through the epiphyseal plate, resulting in displacement of the epiphysis.	
Type II: As above; additionally, a triangular segment of metaphysis is fractured.	
Type III: The fracture line runs from the joint surface through the epiphyseal plate and the epiphysis.	
Type IV: Fracture line occurs as in Type III but also passes through the adjacent metaphysis.	
Type V: Crush injury of the epiphysis; may be difficult to determine on radiograph.	

tion while causing the least amount of risk, pain, and inconvenience to the child and the least amount of anxiety to the parents and physician. A common mistake is to see a child with a displaced fracture in the emergency department, to splint the fracture, then refer the child to the orthopedic surgeon. Children's bones react more quickly to a fracture than do adult's bones: within a few days, the bony fragments are joined by callus and reduction is impossible.

CLOSED TREATMENT

A splint should be used only as a temporary method of immobilization. The splint should be placed after a fracture has been satisfactorily reduced or to transfer a patient prior to reduction. Before applying the splint, the extremities should be well padded and the padding should be free from gaps and folds. Remember that the splint should include the joint above and the joint below the fracture. There are many types of commercial splints, but a well-molded plaster of paris splint is usually sufficient.

OPEN TREATMENT

Open reduction is indicated only when a closed reduction fails. Open reduction is indicated mainly in fractures of both bones of the forearm, tibial spine fractures, and radial neck fractures. Open reduction with internal fixation should be the initial method of treatment of fractures in which remodeling would not help, including displaced intra-articular fractures and Salter–Harris types III and IV.

COMPLICATIONS

Complications can occur at any stage of treatment. Complications may occur when an incorrect diagnosis is made, especially in growth plate injuries. Remember that a displaced intra-articular fracture can give the child deformities secondary to growth plate malalignment producing angular deformity and growth discrepancies. Early and correct diagnosis is a must. Complications may also arise from inadequate early treatment. Intra-articular fractures become fixed and deformed if not reduced within a week postinjury. Within a few days, a fracture that was initially reducible becomes fixed in deformity, requiring surgery to make it acceptable. As a general principle, fractures should always be reduced as early as possible to prevent deformity and to prevent soft-tissue swelling.

SPECIAL PROBLEM FRACTURES
FRACTURES ABOUT THE SHOULDER

Fractures of the clavicles are benign, but if they occur in the outer third, they are equivalent to acromion clavicular separation and may benefit from closed percutaneous K-wire fixation. Midshaft fractures of the clavicle can be treated with a figure-of-eight splint. Proximal diaphyseal separation of the humerus with less than 40 degrees of angulation can be treated with a sling, but angulation of more than 40 degrees requires closed reduction and percutaneous K-wire fixation.

FRACTURES OF THE ELBOW

Fractures of the elbow in children are the most difficult to diagnose. Errors in diagnosis can complicate treatment, producing deformity.

SUPRACONDYLAR FRACTURES   These are fractures of the distal humeral metaphysis just above the epicondyles. They are classified as types I, II, and III, depending on the angulations and deformity. They usually occur from forced hyperextension or flexion. Posterior and medial displacement of the distal fracture fragment with respect to the proximal humerus is the most common finding. Accurate reduction is essential. Closed reduction, overhead traction, and closed reduction with percutaneous pinning are treatment choices that depend on the degree of displacement, the severity of associated soft-tissue swelling, and the physician's experience.

FRACTURES OF THE LATERAL CONDYLE   The lateral condyle of the distal humerus articulates with the radial head and forms the lateral half of the elbow joint. Fractures of the lateral condyle might be a Salter–Harris type III or IV. Lateral condyle fractures are intra-articular fractures, requiring anatomical reductions.

FRACTURES OF THE MEDIAL CONDYLE   The medial condyle articulates with the proximal ulna and forms the medial half of the elbow joint. Isolated medial condyle fractures are uncommon. As with other articular fractures, anatomic reduction is necessary. Open reduction and internal fixation with K-wire is usually the treatment of choice.

FRACTURES OF THE MEDIAL EPICONDYLE   The medial epicondyle is a secondary ossification center of the medial aspect of the distal humerus. There is controversy over the best method of treatment, but in most instances surgeons operate to reduce the duration of disability.

FRACTURES OF THE RADIAL NECK AND OLECRANON   These fractures are rare in children. Fractures of the radial neck, when nondisplaced, are treated in a cast. When there is more than 20 degrees of angulation, reduction is required, preferably closed if possible. Fractures of the olecranon are usually intra-articular. A displacement of more than 2 mm or a gap greater than 2 mm is best managed with open reduction and internal fixation. K-wires are usually the treatment of choice.

FRACTURES OF THE WRIST

Fractures of the distal radius and ulnar metaphysis are common in children. They often result from minor trauma. Salter–Harris types I and II are common epiphyseal injuries of the distal radius and ulna. In most cases, closed reduction is usually successful. A lower arm splint is appropriate to prevent neurovascular compromise from closed reduction and swelling. This is used for 3 to 4 weeks, then the splint or short arm cast is applied for another 3 to 4 weeks.

FRACTURES OF THE KNEE

Fractures of the distal femur and proximal tibia are common in children and are more frequent than ligamentous injury. In children, a ligamentous disruption should be the last diagnosis considered. Meniscal injuries are also rare. Like any other intra-articular fractures, Salter–Harris types III or IV of the distal femur proximal tibia should be treated by anatomical reduction. Because these fractures are intra-articular fractures, when they are displaced open reduction is necessary.

METAPHYSEAL FRACTURES OF THE PROXIMAL TIBIA

In spite of, or perhaps because of, their innocuous appearance, proximal metaphyseal fractures have been described as among the worst fractures in children. Metaphyseal fractures of the tibia lead to valgus deformity of the extremity.

FRACTURES OF THE ANKLE JOINT

Fractures around the ankle joint usually result from a combination of twisting and bending forces. Careful radiologic evaluation of the patient with a suspected ankle injury is essential: anterior–posterior, lateral, and oblique views are a must. An intra-articular fracture must be treated by open reduction and internal fixation.

234   Minor Trauma in Children

PUNCTURE WOUNDS

EMERGENCY DEPARTMENT EVALUATION

Puncture wounds can be caused by sharp or blunt objects and teeth. They appear minor in nature but can hide a serious injury below the surface. They may become infected and are tetanus-prone wounds. Tetanus prophylaxis is especially important since these wounds favor anaerobic organism colonization. If the child is inadequately immunized, unimmunized, or allergic to tetanus toxoid, give human immune globulin (Table 234-1).

EMERGENCY DEPARTMENT MANAGEMENT

Evaluation of the wound includes checking neurovascular status and cleansing and debriding surface contamination. Radiographs are indicated in some cases to check for retained foreign bodies or air in joint spaces. Most metallic, nonsharp foreign bodies do not result in infection and are left in the soft tissues if they are not in joint spaces and if no vascular injury is suspected. Wood or vegetative materials must be removed. Some wounds, such as puncture wounds through rubber-soled shoes, should be anesthetized, incised, and irrigated. Antibiotic use is controversial for most puncture wounds. However, puncture wounds to the feet with signs of infection should be covered for staphylococcus and streptococcus organisms. Suspect Pseudomonas infection if signs of infection are present 1 week after injury or if osteomyelitis is present. Refer the patient to an orthopedic surgeon. Animal bites carry the risk of rabies. See Table 108-1 for Guidlines on Rabies Prophylaxis.

TABLE 234-1. Tetanus Prophylaxis—CDC Guidelines*

History of Tetanus Immunization (Dose)	Clean Minor Wounds		All Other Wounds	
	Td†	TIG‡	Td†	TIG‡
Uncertain	Yes	No	Yes	Yes
0–1	Yes	No	Yes	Yes
2	Yes	No	Yes	No§
≥3	No‖	No	No¶	No

*Refer to text on specific vaccines or toxoids for contraindications, precautions, dosages, side effects and adverse reactions, and special considerations. Important details are in the text and ACIP recommendation (MMWR 30:392, 1981).

†The combined preparation Td, containing both tetanus and diphtheria toxoids, is preferred to tetanus toxoid alone.

‡Tetanus immune globulin.

§Yes, if wound more than 24 hours old.

‖Yes, if more than 10 years since last dose.

¶Yes, if more than 5 years since last dose (more frequent boosters are not needed and can accentuate side effects.)

Adult Immunization Supplement MMWR 33(15):15.

For the routine puncture wound, the foot should be soaked 3 to 4 times a day to keep the wound edges open. Puncture wounds to the foot also benefit from nonweight bearing for 1 to 4 days. Consider broad-spectrum antibiotics for dirty wounds after debridement and high-pressure irrigation.

Pain from a puncture wound should resolve in 2 to 3 days; if not, orthopedic consultation for possible infection should be considered. If you suspect violation of a joint space, plantar fascia, nerve, tendon, or vascular injury, consult an orthopedic surgeon. Hand injury with significant flexor tendon injury or neurovascular injury should be referred to a hand surgeon.

In order to properly cleanse, explore and repair the injury, consider what form of anesthesia is needed (Table 234-2).

COMMON PITFALLS—PUNCTURE WOUNDS

- Failure to obtain radiographs for retained foreign bodies, evaluation of joint space violation and associated injuries, and inadequate tetanus prophylaxis.
- Other errors include incomplete wound cleansing, irrigation, debridement, improper use of antibiotics, and lack of follow-up.

DENTAL EMERGENCIES

Injuries to the teeth are common in children. The most common dental emergencies include soft-tissue lacerations, tooth fractures and avulsions, tooth displacement, alveolar fractures, and maxillary or mandibular fractures.

EMERGENCY DEPARTMENT MANAGEMENT

The goals of management are the preservation of the teeth and dental arch, proper occlusion, and normal development of the mandible and maxilla.

PRIMARY TEETH

Displacement is the most common injury to primary dentition, more so with maxillary incisors than any other teeth. Displacement can cause disruption of the neurovascular supply with pulp necrosis and abscess formation or may damage unerupted permanent teeth. Concussion is a mild nondisruptive blunt injury with no tooth motion and pain only to percussion. Subluxation, with lateral or back-and-forth movement, has pain with tooth movement and requires splinting and dental follow-up. In intrusion, the tooth is pushed inward into the alveolar socket, requiring radiographic and dental evaluation. In extrusion, the tooth is lower than surrounding teeth and may be torn from its apical neurovascular bundle; it requires dental evaluation and splinting. Minimally displaced teeth may be repositioned and splinted, if necessary, unless the tooth is near exfoliation or pathologically involved.

Primary simple dental fractures involving enamel only may appear shiny or dull, have no apparent symptoms, and can be referred to the dentist to have the rough edges smoothed. If the child complains of sensitivity to cold air or fluids, the fracture extends into the dentin or pulp. If the surface is dull with reddish marking, the fracture extends into the pulp and the dentist should apply a temporary zinc oxide or calcium hydroxide cap within 45 minutes of injury to avoid further injury to the pulp. The child will need a permanent cap and evaluation on a periodic basis for pulpal necrosis. A root fracture extends into the gingival groove and the alveolar socket. The dentist will need to evaluate the tooth promptly and will usually extract the fragments to avoid pulpal necrosis and injury to the permanent root bud.

Avulsion injuries occur more frequently as root resorption occurs. Avulsed primary teeth have short, small roots and should not be replaced. Direct pressure should stop bleeding, but

TABLE 234-2. Local Anesthetics

Name	Procaine	Lidocaine	Tetracaine[*]	Bupivacaine[*]	Mepivacaine
Concentration for infiltration[†]	1%	0.5–1%	1%	0.2%	1%
Onset of action[‡]	5–15 min	5–10 min	10–20 min	10–20 min	5–10 min
Duration of action[‡]	45–60 min	30–60 min	1.5/2–3 hr	2–4 hr	1–3 hr
Dosage	7 mg/kg	5 mg/kg	1.5 mg/kg	2 mg/kg	7 mg/kg
Group	Ester	Amide	PABA	Amide	Amide

[*]Not recommended for children under 12 years of age
[†]Recommended concentration for children
[‡]Onset and duration varies from source to source
Schafermeyer RW: Problems in pediatric minor trauma care. In Luten R: Problems in Pediatric Emergency Medicine. New York, Churchill Livingstone, 1988

occasionally a 4-0 chromic suture will be needed to help stop the bleeding. Identify the whole tooth or all of the fragments. Occasionally, dental radiographs will be needed to identify intruded pieces or to identify fragments in the lacerated lip or gingival spaces. A chest–abdomen scout film may be needed to rule out an aspirated or ingested tooth.

PERMANENT TEETH

The maxillary incisors are the most commonly injured permanent teeth, especially in boys ages 8 to 12 years. Crown fractures are the most common injury. Sports are the leading cause of these injuries, and it is important to tell parents and coaches to insist that children use protective appliances. Malocclusion can predispose a child to dental injuries, and early orthodontic treatment may reduce the likelihood of injury. Displacement of permanent teeth is common. Digitally reduce the tooth and stop bleeding with direct pressure. Dental wax can be used as a temporary splint until the dentist can see the child. Dentists will use a direct bonding acrylic resin for splints that will stay in place from 1 to 8 weeks. The vast majority of patients will require root canal therapy and constant evaluation for pulp necrosis. All intruded teeth will need root canal therapy to prevent ankylosis and inflammatory root resorption.

Fractures may involve enamel, dentin, and pulp. Enamel injuries require radiographs to evaluate the tooth for an occult root fracture and periodic evaluation by the dentist for pulp vitality. The rough surface can be smoothed. When enamel and dentin are involved, there is a dull, off-white surface and temperature sensitivity. The exposed dentin should be protected, as mentioned earlier, followed by prompt referral for evaluation of pulp vitality, dental radiographs, and tooth restoration.

Coronal fractures that involve the pulp must receive immediate dental evaluation and therapy because pulp exposure for more than 45 minutes will increase the possibility of pulp necrosis. Root formation is not completed until 2 to 4 years after eruption. Although root canal therapy can be performed, the long-term prognosis of that tooth is diminished.

Root fractures within the alveolar socket are treated with a dental splint and need frequent checks for pulp vitality. Fractures of the root that communicate with the oral cavity will not heal. The coronal segment is extracted and, if the root is long enough, root extrusion may be achieved orthodontically and dental restoration completed.

Avulsion of permanent teeth are true emergencies, as the success of reimplantation is inversely proportional to the time the tooth is out of its socket. Ideally, all teeth should be reimplanted immediately. If the tooth is dirty, rinse it gently with water to remove debris and to avoid injuring the periodontal membrane remnants. If there is a clot in the socket, remove it with gentle irrigation. Reposition the tooth; a dental wax splint can be used until the dentist arrives. If you cannot replant the tooth, or if a parent calls who cannot replant the tooth, place the tooth between the child's gum and cheek if he is old enough so that he will not swallow or choke on it, or have the parent place it in his own buccal pouch. The tooth can be placed in a glass of milk or physiologic saline while seeking immediate dental care.

If the tooth is reimplanted within 30 minutes, there is good prognosis for long-term retention. Reimplantation can be achieved much later, but extensive root resorption and ankylosis will occur. All avulsed permanent teeth will need a pulpectomy within a week to avoid inflammatory root resorption and abscess formation.

Always check occlusion and ask the child if his teeth feel okay and bite normally, and check for any temporomandibular joint tenderness or pain to palpation and movement of the jaw. This may help identify subtle mandibular fractures or mild disruption of a tooth's alignment that will require radiographs and dental evaluation in the near future. Clues of mandibular injury include pain, crepitus, gingival tears, or sublingual ecchymosis. Most mandibular fractures will require referral to a specialist and hospitalization.

DISPOSITION

Most dental injuries should receive dental consultation. Some injuries requiring immediate attention are airway compromise, mandibular fractures, intrusion/extrusion of primary and permanent teeth, fractures into the dentin/pulp, root fractures, and avulsion of permanent teeth. Admission may be required for excessive hemorrhage, potential for swelling that may compromise the airway, and maxillofacial or mandibular fractures.

COMMON PITFALLS—DENTAL EMERGENCIES

- Check tetanus immunization status for all but the most minor of dental injuries.
- Account for all teeth; radiographs may be necessary to evaluate for aspiration of the tooth. Occasionally a tooth or fragment is embedded in soft tissues or deep in the lacerated tissues and will lead to infection and poor healing.
- If pulp is exposed or a permanent tooth avulsed, time is of the essence and the patient must be evaluated, treated, and consulted promptly.
- Preservation of the growing dental arch and proper growth of the maxilla and mandible are important. Look beyond the tooth injury and evaluate the mandible, maxilla, occlusion, and temporomandibular joints.
- Use of penicillin for intraoral lacerations is controversial and, if used, should be used for 1 or 2 days after the injury.

Appendix

Figure A1

Universal Algorithm for Adult Emergency Cardiac Care (ECC)

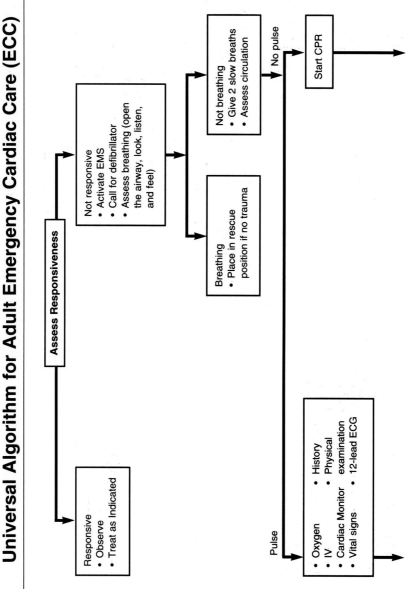

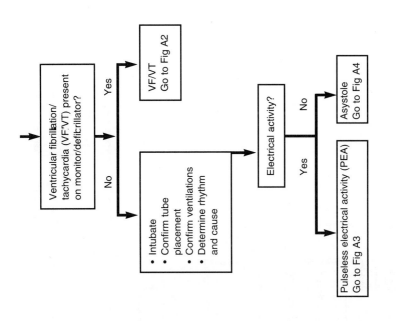

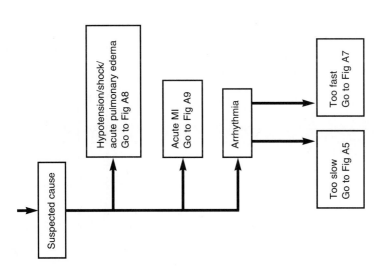

787

Figure A2

Ventricular Fibrillation/
Pulseless Ventricular Tachycardia Algorithm (VF/VT)

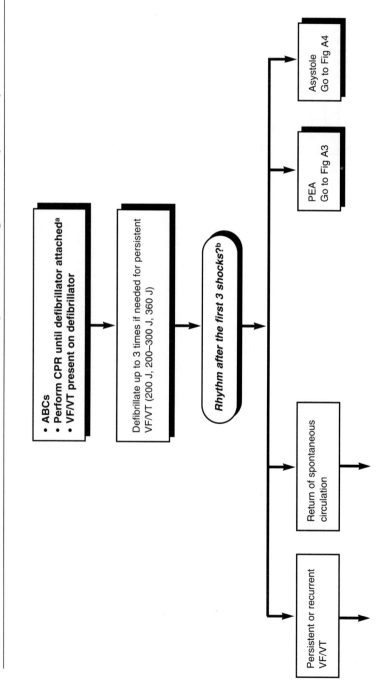

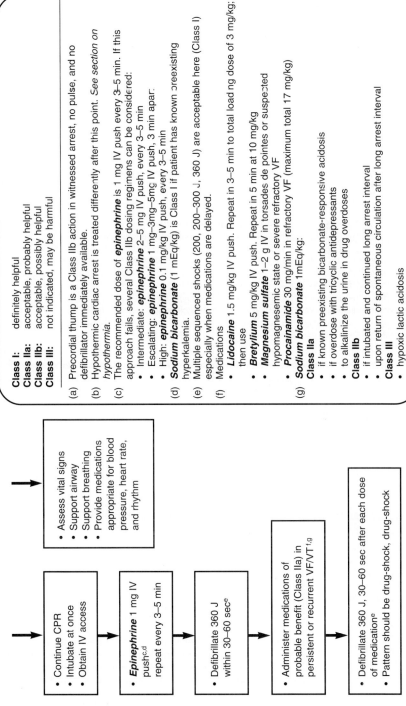

- Assess vital signs
- Support airway
- Support breathing
- Provide medications appropriate for blood pressure, heart rate, and rhythm

- Continue CPR
- Intubate at once
- Obtain IV access

- *Epinephrine* 1 mg IV push[c,d] repeat every 3–5 min

- Defibrillate 360 J within 30–60 sec[e]

- Administer medications of probable benefit (Class IIa) in persistent or recurrent VF/VT[f,g]

- Defibrillate 360 J, 30–60 sec after each dose of medication[e]
- Pattern should be drug-shock, drug-shock

Class I: definitely helpful
Class IIa: acceptable, probably helpful
Class IIb: acceptable, possibly helpful
Class III: not indicated, may be harmful

(a) Precordial thump is a Class IIb action in witnessed arrest, no pulse, and no defibrillator immediately available. *See section on hypothermia.*

(b) Hypothermic cardiac arrest is treated differently after this point. *See section on hypothermia.*

(c) The recommended dose of *epinephrine* is 1 mg IV push every 3–5 min. If this approach fails, several Class IIb dosing regimens can be considered:
- Intermediate: *epinephrine* 2–5 mg IV push, every 3–5 min
- Escalating: *epinephrine* 1 mg–3mg–5mg IV push, 3 min apart.
- High: *epinephrine* 0.1 mg/kg IV push, every 3–5 min

(d) *Sodium bicarbonate* (1 mEq/kg) is Class I if patient has known preexisting hyperkalemia.

(e) Multiple sequenced shocks (200, 200–300 J, 360 J) are acceptable here (Class I) especially when medications are delayed.

(f) Medications
- *Lidocaine* 1.5 mg/kg IV push. Repeat in 3–5 min to total load ing dose of 3 mg/kg; then use
- *Bretylium* 5 mg/kg IV push. Repeat in 5 min at 10 mg/kg
- *Magnesium sulfate* 1–2 g IV in torsades de pointes or suspected hypomagnesemic state or severe refractory VF
- *Procainamide* 30 mg/min in refractory VF (maximum total 17 mg/kg)
- *Sodium bicarbonate* 1mEq/kg:
  Class IIa
  - if known preexisting bicarbonate-responsive acidosis
  - if overdose with tricyclic antidepressants
  - to alkalinize the urine in drug overdoses
  Class IIb
  - if intubated and continued long arrest interval
  - upon return of spontaneous circulation after long arrest interval
  Class III
  - hypoxic lactic acidosis

Pulseless Electrical Activity (PEA) Algorithm
(Electromechanical Dissociation [EMD])

Includes:
- Electromechanical dissociation (EMD)
- Pseudo-EMD
- Idioventricular rhythms
- Ventricular escape rhythms
- Bradyasystolic rhythms
- Postdefibrillation idioventricular rhythms

- Continue CPR
- Intubate at once
- Obtain IV access
- Assess blood flow using Doppler ultrasound

Consider possible causes
(parenthesis = possible therapies and treatments)

- Hypovolemia (volume infusion)
- Hypoxia (ventilation)
- Cardiac tamponade (pericardiocentesis)
- Tension pneumothorax (needle decompression)
- Hypothermia (see hypothermia algorithm)
- Massive pulmonary embolism (surgery, **thrombolytics**)
- Drug overdoses such as tricyclics, digitalis, beta-blockers, calcium channel blockers
- Hyperkalemia[a]
- Acidosis[b]
- Massive acute myocardial infarction (go to Fig. A9)

- **Epinephrine** 1 mg IV push [a,c] repeat every 3–5 min

- If absolute bradycardia (<60 beats/min) or relative bradycardia, give **atropine** 1 mg IV
- Repeat every 3–5 min to a total of 0.04 mg/kg[d]

Class I:	definitely helpful
Class IIa:	acceptable, probably helpful
Class IIb:	acceptable, possibly helpful
Class III:	not indicated, may be harmful

(a) **Sodium bicarbonate** 1mEq/kg is Class I if patient has known preexisting hyperkalemia

(b) **Sodium bicarbonate** (1mEq/kg):
Class IIa
- if known preexisting bicarbonate-responsive acidosis
- if overdose with tricyclic antidepressants
- to alkalinize the urine in drug overdoses
Class IIb
- if intubated and long arrest interval
- upon return of spontaneous circulation after long arrest interval
Class III
- hypoxic lactic acidosis

(c) The recommended dose of **epinephrine** is 1 mg IV push every 3–5 min. If this approach fails, several Class IIb dosing regimens can be considered:
- Intermediate: **epinephrine** 2–5 mg IV push, every 3–5 min
- Escalating: **epinephrine** 1 mg–3 mg–5mg IV push 3 min apart
- High: **epinephrine** 0.1 mg/kg IV push, every 3–5 min

(d) Shorter **atropine** dosing intervals are possibly helpful in cardiac arrest (Class IIb).

Figure A4

Asystole Treatment Algorithm

- **Continue CPR**
- **Intubate at once**
- **Obtain IV access**
- **Confirm asystole in more than one lead**

Class I: definitely helpful
Class IIa: acceptable, probably helpful
Class IIb: acceptable, possibly helpful
Class III: not indicated, may be harmful

(a) TCP is a Class IIb intervention. Lack of success may be due to delays in pacing. To be effective TCP must be performed early, simultaneously with drugs. Evidence does not support routine use of TCP for asystole.

Consider possible causes
- Hypoxia
- Hyperkalemia
- Hypokalemia
- Preexisting acidosis
- Drug overdose
- Hypothermia

(b) The recommended dose of *epinephrine* is 1 mg IV push every 3–5 min. If this approach fails, several Class IIb dosing regimens can be considered:
- Intermediate: *epinephrine* 2–5 mg IV push, every 3–5 min
- Escalating: *epinephrine* 1 mg–3mg–5mg IV push, 3 min apart
- High: *epinephrine* 0.1 mg/kg IV push, every 3–5 min

Consider immediate transcutaneous pacing (TCP)[a]

(c) *Sodium bicarbonate* 1 mEq/kg is Class I if patient has known preexisting hyperkalemia.

(d) Shorter *atropine* dosing intervals are Class IIb in asystolic arrest.

(e) *Sodium bicarbonate* 1mEq/kg:
Class IIa
- if known preexisting bicarbonate-responsive acidosis
- if overdose with tricyclic antidepressants
- to alkalinize the urine in drug overdoses

- *Epinephrine* 1 mg IV push[b,c] repeat every 3–5 min

Class IIb
- if intubated and continued long arrest interval
- upon return of spontaneous circulation after long arrest interval
Class III
- hypoxic lactic acidosis

- *Atropine* 1 mg IV repeat every 3–5 min up to a total of 0.04 mg/kg[d,e]

(f) If patient remains in asystole or other agonal rhythms after successful intubation and initial medication and no reversible causes are identified, consider termination of resuscitative efforts by a physician. Consider interval since arrest.

Consider termination of efforts[f]

Figure A5

Bradycardia Algorithm
(Patient is not in cardiac arrest)

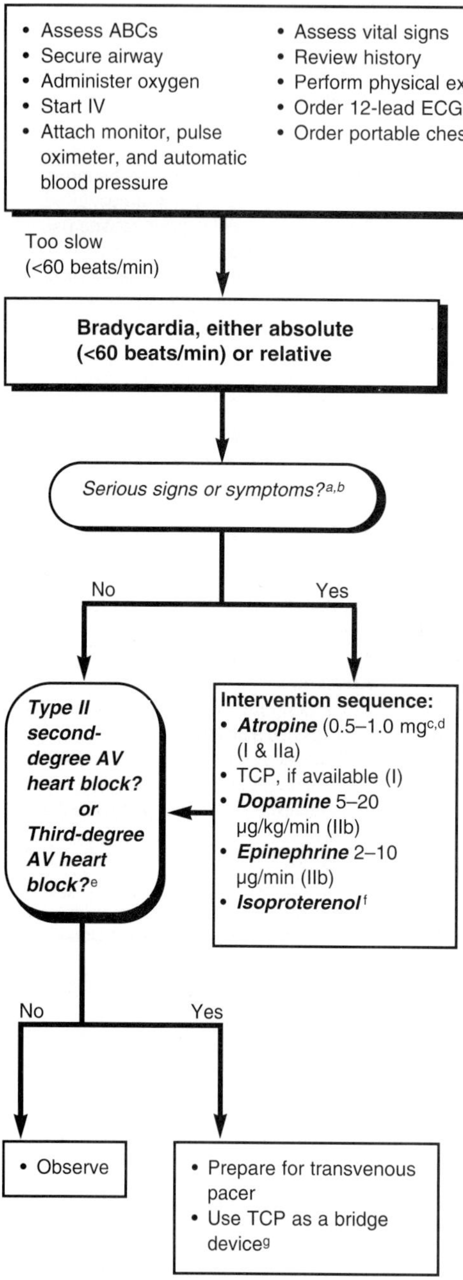

- Assess ABCs
- Secure airway
- Administer oxygen
- Start IV
- Attach monitor, pulse oximeter, and automatic blood pressure

- Assess vital signs
- Review history
- Perform physical examination
- Order 12-lead ECG
- Order portable chest roentgenogram

Too slow
(<60 beats/min)

Bradycardia, either absolute (<60 beats/min) or relative

Serious signs or symptoms?[a,b]

No →

Type II second-degree AV heart block? *or* **Third-degree AV heart block?**[e]

Yes →

Intervention sequence:
- *Atropine* (0.5–1.0 mg[c,d] (I & IIa)
- TCP, if available (I)
- *Dopamine* 5–20 µg/kg/min (IIb)
- *Epinephrine* 2–10 µg/min (IIb)
- *Isoproterenol*[f]

No →
- Observe

Yes →
- Prepare for transvenous pacer
- Use TCP as a bridge device[g]

(a) Serious signs or symptoms must be related to the slow rate. Clinical manifestations include:
  - symptoms (chest pain, shortness of breath, decreased level of consciousness)
  - signs (low BP, shock, pulmonary congestion, CHF, acute MI).

(b) Do not delay TCP while awaiting IV access or for *atropine* to take effect if patient is symptomatic.

(c) Denervated transplanted hearts will not respond to *atropine*. Go at once to pacing, *catecholamine* infusion or both.

(d) *Atropine* should be given in repeat doses in 3–5 min up to total of 0.04 mg/kg. Consider shorter dosing intervals in severe clinical conditions. It has been suggested that *atropine* should be used with caution in atrioventricular (AV) block at the His-Purkinje level (type II AV block and new third-degree block with wide QRS complexes) (Class IIb).

(e) Never treat third-degree heart block plus ventricular escape beats with *lidocaine*.

(f) *Isoproterenol* should be used, if at all, with extreme caution. At low doses it is Class IIb (possibly helpful); at higher doses it is Class III (harmful).

(g) Verify patient tolerance and mechanical capture. Use analgesia and sedation as needed.

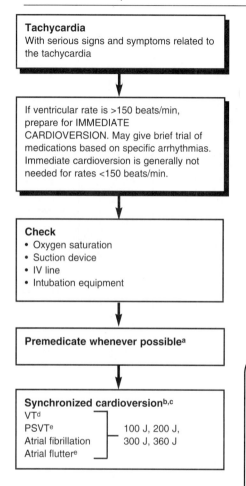

Figure A6

Electrical Cardioversion Algorithm
(Patient is not in cardiac arrest)

Tachycardia
With serious signs and symptoms related to the tachycardia

↓

If ventricular rate is >150 beats/min, prepare for IMMEDIATE CARDIOVERSION. May give brief trial of medications based on specific arrhythmias. Immediate cardioversion is generally not needed for rates <150 beats/min.

↓

Check
- Oxygen saturation
- Suction device
- IV line
- Intubation equipment

↓

Premedicate whenever possible[a]

↓

Synchronized cardioversion[b,c]
VT[d]
PSVT[e]
Atrial fibrillation
Atrial flutter[e]

100 J, 200 J, 300 J, 360 J

(a) Effective regimens have included a sedative (eg, *diazepam*, *midazolam*, *barbiturates*, *etomidate*, *ketamine*, *methohexital*) with or without an analgesic agent (eg, *fentanyl*, *morphine*, *meperidine*). Many experts recommend anesthesia if service is readily available.
(b) Note possible need to resynchronize after each cardioversion.
(c) If delays in synchronization occur and clinical conditions are critical, go to immediate unsynchronized shocks.
(d) Treat polymorphic VT (irregular form and rate) like VF: 200 J, 200–300 J, 360 J.
(e) PSVT and atrial flutter often respond to lower energy levels (start with 50 J)

Figure A7

Tachycardia Algorithm

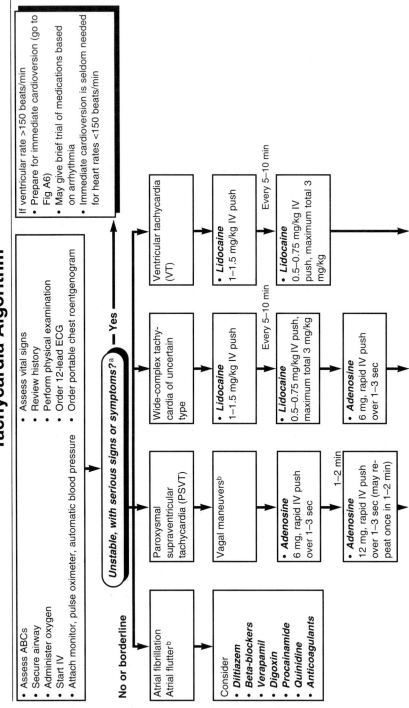

- Assess ABCs
- Secure airway
- Administer oxygen
- Start IV
- Attach monitor, pulse oximeter, automatic blood pressure

- Assess vital signs
- Review history
- Perform physical examination
- Order 12-lead ECG
- Order portable chest roentgenogram

Unstable, with serious signs or symptoms?[a] — **Yes**

If ventricular rate >150 beats/min
- Prepare for immediate cardioversion (go to Fig A6)
- May give brief trial of medications based on arrhythmia
- Immediate cardioversion is seldom needed for heart rates <150 beats/min

No or borderline

Atrial fibrillation
Atrial flutter[b]

Consider
- *Diltiazem*
- *Beta-blockers*
- *Verapamil*
- *Digoxin*
- *Procainamide*
- *Quinidine*
- *Anticoagulants*

Paroxysmal supraventricular tachycardia (PSVT)

Vagal maneuvers[b]

- *Adenosine*
  6 mg, rapid IV push over 1–3 sec

1–2 min

- *Adenosine*
  12 mg, rapid IV push over 1–3 sec (may repeat once in 1–2 min)

Wide-complex tachy-cardia of uncertain type

- *Lidocaine*
  1–1.5 mg/kg IV push

Every 5–10 min

- *Lidocaine*
  0.5–0.75 mg/kg IV push, maximum total 3 mg/kg

- *Adenosine*
  6 mg, rapid IV push over 1–3 sec

Ventricular tachycardia (VT)

- *Lidocaine*
  1–1.5 mg/kg IV push

Every 5–10 min

- *Lidocaine*
  0.5–0.75 mg/kg IV push, maximum total 3 mg/kg

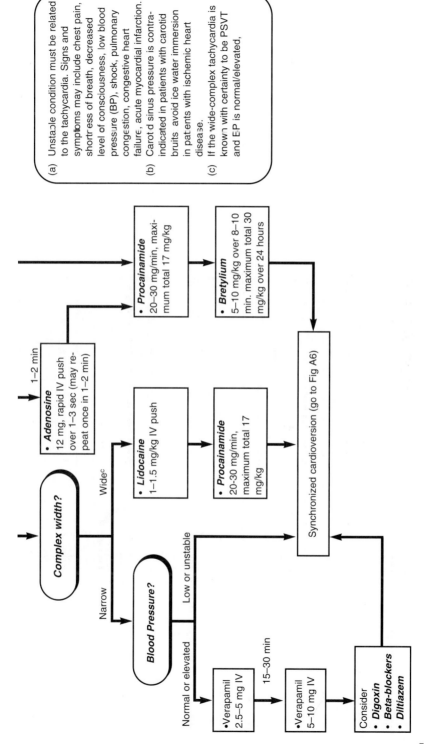

(a) Unstable condition must be related to the tachycardia. Signs and symptoms may include chest pain, shortness of breath, decreased level of consciousness, low blood pressure (BP), shock, pulmonary congestion, congestive heart failure, acute myocardial infarction.

(b) Carotid sinus pressure is contra-indicated in patients with carotid bruits; avoid ice water immersion in patients with ischemic heart disease.

(c) If the wide-complex tachycardia is known with certainty to be PSVT and EP is normal/elevated,

Complex width?

Wide^c

Blood Pressure?

Narrow

Low or unstable

Normal or elevated

• *Adenosine*
12 mg, rapid IV push over 1–3 sec (may re-peat once in 1–2 min)

1–2 min

• Lidocaine
1–1.5 mg/kg IV push

• *Procainamide*
20–30 mg/min, maximum total 17 mg/kg

• *Procainamide*
20–30 mg/min, maxi-mum total 17 mg/kg

• *Bretylium*
5–10 mg/kg over 8–10 min. maximum total 30 mg/kg over 24 hours

Synchronized cardioversion (go to Fig A6)

•Verapamil
2.5–5 mg IV

15–30 min

•Verapamil
5–10 mg IV

Consider
• *Digoxin*
• *Beta-blockers*
• *Diltiazem*

795

Figure A8

Hypotension/Shock/Acute Pulmonary Edema Algorithm

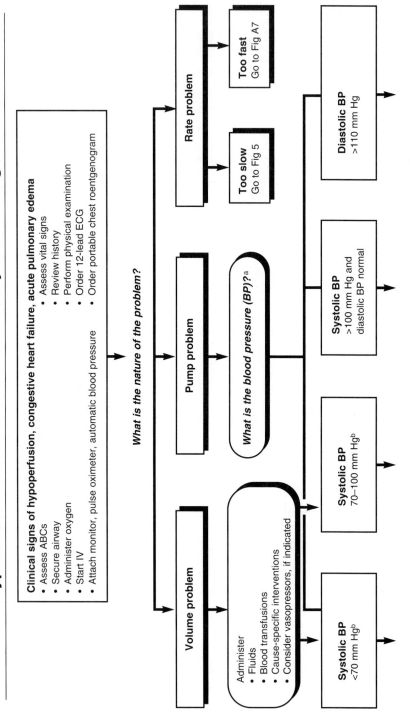

Clinical signs of hypoperfusion, congestive heart failure, acute pulmonary edema
- Assess ABCs
- Secure airway
- Administer oxygen
- Start IV
- Attach monitor, pulse oximeter, automatic blood pressure
- Assess vital signs
- Review history
- Perform physical examination
- Order 12-lead ECG
- Order portable chest roentgenogram

What is the nature of the problem?

Volume problem

Pump problem

Rate problem

Administer
- Fluids
- Blood transfusions
- Cause-specific interventions
- Consider vasopressors, if indicated

What is the blood pressure (BP)?[a]

Too slow
Go to Fig 5

Too fast
Go to Fig A7

Systolic BP
<70 mm Hg[b]

Systolic BP
70–100 mm Hg[b]

Systolic BP
>100 mm Hg and
diastolic BP normal

Diastolic BP
>110 mm Hg

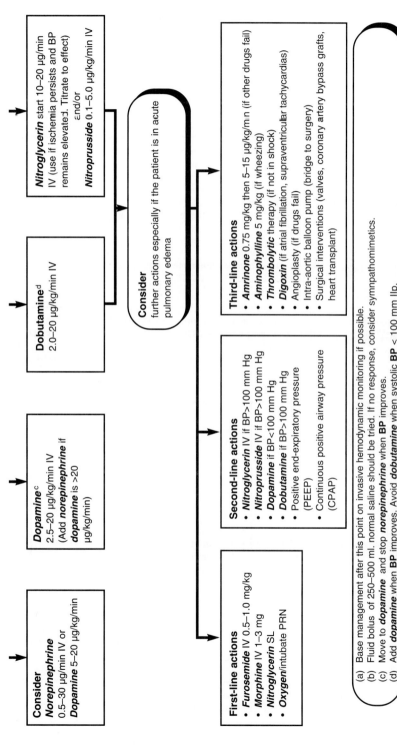

Consider
Norepinephrine
0.5–30 µg/min IV or
Dopamine 5–20 µg/kg/min

Dopamine[c]
2.5–20 µg/kg/min IV
(Add *norepinephrine* if
dopamine is >20
µg/kg/min)

Dobutamine[d]
2.0–20 µg/kg/min IV

Nitroglycerin start 10–20 µg/min
IV (use if ischemia persists and BP
remains elevated. Titrate to effect)
and/or
Nitroprusside 0.1–5.0 µg/kg/min IV

Consider
further actions especially if the patient is in acute
pulmonary edema

First-line actions
• *Furosemide* IV 0.5–1.0 mg/kg
• *Morphine* IV 1–3 mg
• *Nitroglycerin* SL
• *Oxygen*/intubate PRN

Second-line actions
• *Nitroglycerin* IV if BP>100 mm Hg
• *Nitroprusside* IV if BP>100 mm Hg
• *Dopamine* if BP<100 mm Hg
• *Dobutamine* if BP>100 mm Hg
• Positive end-expiratory pressure
  (PEEP)
• Continuous positive airway pressure
  (CPAP)

Third-line actions
• *Amrinone* 0.75 mg/kg then 5–15 µg/kg/min (if other drugs fail)
• *Aminophylline* 5 mg/kg (if wheezing)
• *Thrombolytic* therapy (if not in shock)
• *Digoxin* (if atrial fibrillation, supraventricular tachycardias)
• Angioplasty (if drugs fail)
• Intra-aortic balloon pump (bridge to surgery)
• Surgical interventions (valves, coronary artery bypass grafts,
  heart transplant)

(a) Base management after this point on invasive hemodynamic monitoring if possible.
(b) Fluid bolus of 250–500 ml. normal saline should be tried. If no response, consider sympathomimetics.
(c) Move to *dopamine* and stop *norepinephrine* when **BP** improves.
(d) Add *dobutamine* when **BP** improves. Avoid *dobutamine* when systolic **BP** < 100 mm IIp.

797

Acute Myocardial Infarction Algorithm
Recommendations for early management of patients
with chest pain and possible AMI§

COMMUNITY

Community emphasis on "Call First, Call Fast, Call 911"

EMS SYSTEM

EMS system approach that should address
- Oxygen–IV–cardiac monitor-vital signs
- *Nitroglycerin*
- Pain relief with narcotics
- Notification of emergency department
- Rapid transport to emergency department
- Prehospital screening for *thrombolytic* therapy*
- 12-lead ECG, computer analysis, transmission to emergency department*
- Initiation of *thrombolytic* therapy*

EMERGENCY DEPARTMENT

"Door-to-drug" team protocol approach
- Rapid triage of patients with chest pain
- Clinical decision maker established (emergency physician, cardiologist, or other)

Time interval in emergency department

Assessment
Immediate:
- Vital signs with automatic BP
- Oxygen saturation
- Start IV
- 12-lead ECG (MD review)
- Brief, targeted history and physical
- Decide on eligibility for *thrombolytic* therapy
Soon:
- Chest X-ray
- Blood studies (electrolytes, enzymes, coagulation studies)

§For information on the National Heart Attack Alert program, contact the National Institutes of Health Information Center, P.O. Box 30105, Bethesda, MD 20824-0105
*Optional guidelines

Treatments to consider if there is evidence of coronary thrombosis plus no reasons for exclusion:
(some but not all may be appropriate)
- *Oxygen* at 4L/min
- *Nitroglycerin* SL, paste or spray (if systolic blood pressure > 90 mm IIg)
- *Morphine* IV
- *Aspirin* PO
- *Thrombolytic* agents
- *Nitroglycerin* IV (limit systolic BP drop to 10% if normotensive: 30% drop if hypertensive; never drop below 90 mm Hg systolic)
- *Beta-blockers* IV
- *Heparin* IV
- Routine *lidocaine* administration is **NOT** recommended for all patients with AMI
- *Magnesium sulfate* IV
- Percutaneous transluminal coronary angioplasty

30–60 min to *thrombolytic* therapy

Index

Numbers followed by an *f* indicate a figure; *t* following a page number indicates tabular material.